Breast Disease

Adam I. Riker
Editor

Breast Disease

Comprehensive Management

Springer

Editor
Adam I. Riker, MD, FACS
Advocate Center for Breast Health
Advocate Cancer Institute
Advocate Christ Medical Center
Oak Lawn
Illinois
USA

ISBN 978-1-4939-1144-8 ISBN 978-1-4939-1145-5 (eBook)
DOI 10.1007/978-1-4939-1145-5
Springer New York Heidelberg Dordrecht London

Library of Congress Control Number: 2014952366

Printed on acid-free paper

Springer is part of Springer Science+Business Media (www.springer.com)

Contents

Contributors

Akram Abdoue, MD Department of Anesthesia, Advocate Christ Medical Center, University of Illinois College of Medicine at Chicago, Oak Lawn, IL, USA

Summer V. Allen, MD Department of Family Medicine, Mayo Clinic, Rochester, MN, USA

Ricardo H. Alvarez, MD, MSc The Morgan Welch Inflammatory Breast Cancer Research and Clinic Department of Breast Medical Oncology, The University of Texas MD Anderson Cancer Center, Houston, TX, USA

Peter D. Beitsch, MD, FACS Dallas Breast Center, Dallas, TX, USA

Richard Betzold, MD Department of Surgery, University of Arkansas for Medical Sciences, Little Rock, AR, USA

Christie Brenzek, BA, MBA Suburban Plastic Surgery, Oak Lawn, IL, USA

John Chipko, MD Department of General Surgery, Tampa General Hospital, Tampa, FL, USA

Charles E. Cox, MD Department of Surgery, USF Breast Health Program, Morsani College of Medicine, University of South Florida, Tampa, FL, USA

Massimo Cristofanilli, MD Breast Cancer Center, Jefferson Medical College, Thomas Jefferson University-Kimmel Cancer Center, Philadelphia, PA, USA

Paul Crossan, MD Department of Radiation Oncology, Advocate Christ Hospital Medical Center, Oak Lawn, IL, USA

Mary B. Daly, MD, PhD Department of Clinical Genetics, Fox Chase Cancer Center, Philadelphia, PA, USA

Shaheenah Dawood, MRCP, MPH Department of Medical Oncology, Department of Health and Medical Services, Dubai Hospital, Dubai, United Arab Emirates

J. Michael Dixon, OBE, MD, FRCS. FRCEd FRCP The Edinburgh Breast Unit, Western General Hospital, Edinburgh, Scotland, UK

Charles Dupin, MD Division of Plastic Surgery, Department of Surgery, Louisiana State University Health Sciences Center, New Orleans, LA, USA

Çağatay H. Erşahin, MD, PhD Department of Pathology, Silver Cross Hospital, New Lenox, IL, USA

Adela Fernandez, MD Department of General Surgery, Tampa General Hospital, Tampa, FL, USA

Julia A. Files, MD Division of Women's Health Internal Medicine, Mayo Clinic Arizona, Scottsdale, AZ, USA

Richard E. Fine, MD, FACS Division of Oncology, Department of Surgery, University of Tennessee Health Science Center, College of Medicine, Memphis, TN, USA

Education and Research, West Clinic Comprehensive Breast Center, Germantown, TN, USA

Andrea Forman, MS, CGC Department of Clinical Genetics, Fox Chase Cancer Center, Philadelphia, PA, USA

Shom Goel, MBBS, FRACP Division of Women's Cancers, Dana-Farber Cancer Institute, Boston, MA, USA

Donald A. Goer, PhD Intraop Medical Corporation, Sunnyvale, CA, USA

William J. Gradishar, MD Medicine – Division of Hematology/Oncology, Maggie Daley Center for Women's Cancer Care, Robert H. Lurie Comprehensive Cancer Center, Northwestern University Feinberg School of Medicine, Chicago, IL, USA

Richard J. Gray, MD Department of Surgery, Mayo Clinic Arizona, Phoenix, AZ, USA

Rebecca Grutsch, MD Department of Anesthesiology and Critical Care Medicine, The Johns Hopkins Hospital, Johns Hopkins University School of Medicine, Baltimore, MD, USA

Rasheed Hammadeh, MD Department of Pathology, Advocate Christ Hospital and Medical Center, Oak Lawn, IL, USA

Hannah W. Hazard, MD, FACS Department of Surgery, Health Sciences Center – South, West Virginia University School of Medicine, Morgantown, WV, USA

Hugo St.Hilaire, MD, DDS Division of Plastic Surgery, Department of Surgery, Louisiana State University Health Sciences Center, New Orleans, LA, USA

M'liss Hogan, MD Division of Plastic Surgery, Department of Surgery, Louisiana State University Health Sciences Center, New Orleans, LA, USA

Roohi Ismail-Khan, MD, MS Division of Breast Oncology & Experimental Therapeutics, H. Lee Moffitt Cancer Center & Research Institute, Tampa, FL, USA

Philip Israel, MD Department of Surgery, The Breast Center, Marietta, GA, USA

James W. Jakub, MD Department of Surgery, Mayo Clinic, Rochester, MN, USA

Haiqiao Jiao, MD Department of Surgery, Louisiana State University Health Sciences Center, New Orleans, LA, USA

Michelle Jung, BS Department of Surgery (USF), University of South Florida (Morsani), Tampa, FL, USA

Virginia G. Kaklamani, MD Department of Medicine Hematology/ Oncology, Northwestern University, Chicago, IL, USA

Ramasamy Kalimuthu, MD, FACS Department of Plastic, Hand, and Reconstructive Surgery, Advocate Christ Medical Center, University of Illinois Chicago, Oak Lawn, IL, USA

Sarah Keck, MD Santa Rosa Medical Group, University of California San Francisco, Santa Rosa, CA, USA

Nazanin Khakpour, MD, FACS Department of Women's Oncology, H. Lee Moffitt Cancer Center & Research Institute, Tampa, FL, USA

Maria A. Kimovec, MD Department of Anesthesia, Advocate Christ Medical Center, University of Illinois College of Medicine at Chicago, Oak Lawn, IL, USA

Barbara L. Krueger, MD, FACS Breast Cancer Program, Advocate Cancer Institute, Advocate Christ Medical Center, Oak Lawn, IL, USA

Peggy Kupres, BSN, MA Advocate Christ Medical Center, Cancer Institute, Oak Lawn, IL, USA

Yanxia Li, MD, PhD Department of Pathology, Loyola University Medical Center, Maywood, IL, USA

Elgene Lim, MBBS, FRACP, PhD Division of Women's Cancers, Dana-Farber Cancer Institute, Boston, MA, USA

Jared Linebarger, MD Department of General Surgery, Gundersen Health System, La Crosse, WI, USA

Norma J Vinger Center for Breast Care (NJVCBC), La Crosse, WI, USA

E. Jane Macaskill, MBChB, MD, FRCSEd Department of Breast Surgery, Ninewells Hospital, Dundee, Scotland, UK

Melanie Majure, MD Department of Medicine, University of California San Francisco, San Francisco, CA, USA

James Mayo, MD Division of Plastic Surgery, Department of Surgery, Louisiana State University Health Sciences Center, New Orleans, LA, USA

Susan Minton, DO Division of Breast Oncology & Experimental Therapeutics, H. Lee Moffitt Cancer Center & Research Institute, Tampa, FL, USA

Tracy-Ann Moo, MD Department of Breast Surgery, Memorial Sloan Kettering Cancer Center, Evelyn H Lauder Breast Center, New York, NY, USA

Pamela N. Munster, MD Division of Hematology and Oncology, Department of Medicine, Helen Diller Family Cancer Center, University of California, San Francisco, San Francisco, CA, USA

Atilla Ömeroğlu, MD Department of Pathology, McGill University, Montreal, QC, Canada

Department of PathologyDuff Medical Building, Montreal, QC, Canada

Gülbeyaz Ömeroğlu, MD Department of Pathology, McGill University, Montreal, QC, Canada

Department of PathologyDuff Medical Building, Montreal, QC, Canada

Barbara A. Pockaj, MD Department of Surgery, Mayo Clinic Arizona, Phoenix, AZ, USA

Pamela R. Portschy, MD Department of Surgical Oncology, University of Minnesota, Minneapolis, MN, USA

Vanessa Prowler, MD Department of Surgery, Tampa General Hospital, Tampa, FL, USA

Sandhya Pruthi, MD General Internal Medicine, Mayo Clinic, Rochester, MN, USA

Adam I. Riker, MD, FACS Advocate Center for Breast Health, Advocate Cancer Institute, Advocate Christ Medical Center, Oak Lawn, IL, USA

Monica Rizzo, MD, FACS Division of Surgical Oncology, Department of Surgery, Emory University School of Medicine, Winship Cancer Institute, Atlanta, GA, USA

Hope S. Rugo, MD Department of Medicine, University of California San Francisco Helen Diller Family Comprehensive Cancer Center, San Francisco, CA, USA

Ali Sadeghi, MD Division of Plastic Surgery, Department of Surgery, Louisiana State University Health Sciences Center, New Orleans, LA, USA

Christopher Sanders, MD Division of Plastic Surgery, Department of Surgery, Louisiana State University Health Sciences Center, New Orleans, LA, USA

Miraj G. Shah-Khan, MD Division of Surgical Oncology, Medical College of Wisconsin, Milwaukee, WI, USA

Steven C. Shivers, PhD Department of Surgery, USF Breast Health Program, Morsani College of Medicine, University of South Florida, Tampa, FL, USA

Paulomi Shroff, MD Department of Surgery, The Breast Center, Marietta, GA, USA

Melvin J. Silverstein, MD Gross Family Foundation Endowed Chair in Oncoplastic Surgery, Hoag Breast Program, Hoag Memorial Hospital Presbyterian, Newport Beach, CA, USA

Clinical Professor of Surgery, Keck School of Medicine, University of Southern California, Los Angeles, CA, USA

Rache Simmons, MD, FACD Department of Surgery, New York Presbyterian Hospital, New York, NY, USA

Patrice A. Stephens, MSN, APN, AOCN-BC Advocate Christ Medical Center, Cancer Institute, Oak Lawn, IL, USA

Evan Tummel, MD Department of Surgery, Tampa General Hospital, Tampa, FL, USA

Todd M. Tuttle, MD Department of Surgical Oncology, University of Minnesota, Minneapolis, MN, USA

Michelle Vice, BS Department of General Surgery, Morsani College of Medicine, Tampa, FL, USA

Jami Walloch, MD Department of Pathology, Advocate Cancer Institute, Advocate Christ Medical Center, Oak Lawn, IL, USA

J. Ben Wilkinson, MD Department of Radiation Oncology, Willis-Knighton Health System, LSU Feist-Weiller Cancer Center, Shreveport, LA, USA

Eric P. Winer, MD Division of Women's Cancers, Dana-Farber Cancer Institute, Boston, MA, USA

M. Whitten Wise, MD Division of Plastic Surgery, Department of Surgery, Louisiana State University Health Sciences Center, New Orleans, LA, USA

S. Sarah Yegiyants, MD, MS Division of Plastic, Reconstructive, and Cosmetic Surgery, Department of Surgery, Division of Plastic, Reconstructive, and Cosmetic Surgery, Department of Surgery, University of Illinois, Chicago, Chicago, IL, USA

Jon Zellmer Department of Medical Education, Gundersen Lutheran Medical Foundation, La Crosse, WI, USA

Wei Wei Zhang, MD Department of General Surgery, University of South Florida, Tampa, FL, USA

Anatomy of the Breast, Axilla, and Chest Wall

1

Ramasamy Kalimuthu, S. Sarah Yegiyants, and Christie Brenzek

Introduction

The breast is an organ that has captured the imagination of mankind since the beginning of our existence. It serves the dual function of an end organ, influenced by the endocrine system, with the ability to produce milk in mammals, sustaining the offspring, and functioning as a secondary sex organ in humans. The breast is evaluated and treated by a multitude of specialists, for both aesthetic and disease processes. In this chapter, we will focus on the anatomy of the breast with respect to the treatment of breast disease. The breast aesthetics, while an important aspect of the breast evaluation, is beyond the scope of discussion in this chapter.

R. Kalimuthu, MD, FACS (✉)
Department of Plastic, Hand, and Reconstructive Surgery, Advocate Christ Medical Center, University of Illinois Chicago, 5346 West 95th Street, Oak Lawn, IL 60453, USA
e-mail: kali@suburbanplastic.com

S.S. Yegiyants, MD, MS
Division of Plastic, Reconstructive, and Cosmetic Surgery, Department of Surgery, University of Illinois, Chicago, 820 South Wood Street, 515 CSN, Chicago, IL 60612, USA
e-mail: syegiyants@yahoo.com

C. Brenzek, BA, MBA
Suburban Plastic Surgery, 5346 West 95th Street, Oak Lawn, IL 60453, USA
e-mail: christie@suburbanplastic.com

Evolution and Comparative Anatomy of the Breast

To fully appreciate the anatomy and physiology of the human breast, one must delve into the evolution and comparative anatomy of the organ. The mammary glands, closely tied to reproduction, are unique features of mammals and their evolutionary development. The Anamniota, the "lower vertebrates," are a group comprising the fish and the amphibians. Their eggs lack an amnion, which serves to transport oxygen and expel carbon dioxide, causing the anamniotes to lay eggs in water which helps in the diffusion of waste products. In contrast, the amniotes are a group of "higher vertebrates" whose eggs possess an amnion, allowing for an adaptation to lay eggs on land.

Amniotes, like reptiles, lay eggs away from water and maintain egg moisture by secretion from sweat glands [1–3]. The amniotic egg represents a critical divergence within the vertebrates, which allowed for terrestrial reproduction. The monotremes, like the platypus and echidna, are mammals that lay eggs instead of giving birth. Monotremes have mammary gland, which they have derived from an ancestral apocrine-like gland that lactates through mammary hair follicle openings. This provides moisture and other nutrients which permeate to hatch the eggs. This association is retained by monotreme mammary glands and is evident as vestigial mammary hair during development of marsupials.

The nipple has evolved from the vestigial hair opening seen in marsupials. There is evidence

A.I. Riker (ed.), *Breast Disease: Comprehensive Management*,
DOI 10.1007/978-1-4939-1145-5_1, © Springer Science+Business Media New York 2015

that lactose, secreted by apocrine-like glands, also continues to secrete complex nutrient-rich milk in marsupials. This, in turn, causes the decline in egg size development of the underdeveloped fetus in marsupials. Marsupials have more developed nipples present in the pouch, such as a kangaroo. To feed the incompletely developed offspring born without an immune system [4] and lacking fur to maintain warmth, they stay attached to the nipples in the pouch for the remainder of their development.

The mammary gland development is closely related with the evolution of the cloaca and the placenta. Monotremes with a single cloaca, performs the reproductive, intestinal, and urinary excretion, thus, laying an egg. Conversely, marsupials have a choriovitelline placenta, in which the embryo is nourished from an egg yolk sac, also capturing nutrition from the uterus, which later matures in the pelvic pouch.

Progression of evolution led to the development of the eutherians, the fully developed placental mammals, which have the ability to maintain a warm, internal temperature. This ability led to the development of bigger fetuses, which are secondary to the development of the placenta. Initially, the placenta was attached via the choriovitelline, which lacked the hormones to fully support the development of the fetus. In contrast, the more evolved chorioallantoic placenta has the ability to secrete choriogonadotropin to maintain the fetus to full development.

The eutherians also have well-developed genital organs, urinary tracts, and anal opening. The mammary gland formation from skin apocrine glands coincides with the development of the cloaca and the placenta in the eutherians. A further evidence shows that it has led to the development of the pre-maxilla, palate, and limb posture and development of the corpus callosum.

The mammary gland is a modified epidermal appendix of an apocrine gland, which arises from a dense cluster of the mammo-pilo-sebaceous unit. The development led to other evolutionary changes in higher mammals to nourish their offspring. This has allowed placental structures to accept lactation which is truncated in the mammary gland of eutherians.

Vitellogenin is a glycoprotein molecule, with an egg yolk precursor present in oviparous female species of most invertebrates, amphibian fish, reptiles, birds, and monotremes like the platypus and echidna [1]. This glycoprotein declines in placentation and lactation in placental mammals and is replaced by the progressive casein. Casein has similar properties, a phosphoprotein that is a main nutrition source for offspring. This progression shows the placentation in oviparous to placentation and lactation in placental animals.

Embryology

The skin consists of two main layers, the dermis and epidermis. The epidermis is derived from ectoderm and consists of epidermal cells, melanocytes, Merkel cells derived from neuroendocrine cells and Langerhans cells from the bone marrow. Melanocytes produce melanin to protect the skin from sun damage. The Merkel cell is a nerve ending for pressure-sensitive end organs, and Langerhans cells are responsible, in part, for antigen presentation. The dermis is derived from mesoderm and contains supporting structures like blood vessels, nerve endings, and a collagen layer. The single layer of ectoderm with its underlying mesoderm begins to proliferate to form multilayers and specialized epidermal structures like hair and hair follicles, nails, and teeth and gives rise to sebaceous, eccrine, apocrine, and mammary glands during the fourth week of intrauterine life [5].

The sebaceous, eccrine, and mammary glands are epidermal glands that develop as downgrowths or diverticula of the epidermis to the dermis. The mammary gland is a modified apocrine gland. During the fourth week of gestation, a paired epidermal thickening develops called mammary ridges that are a part of the milk duct line that extends from the axilla to the medial thigh (Fig. 1.1). This mammary ridge or milk line

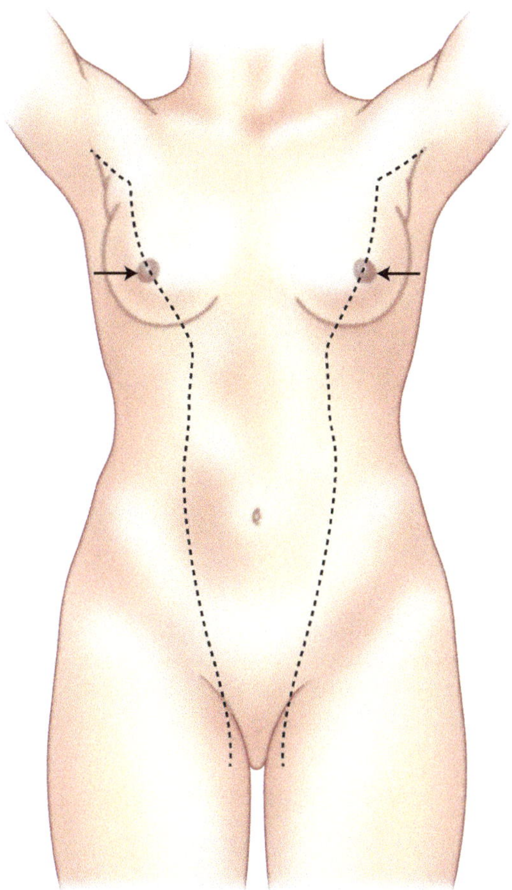

Fig. 1.1 Milk line from the axilla to the groin

becomes curvilinear due to the differential epidermal growth around the umbilical cord and lateral folding during development. In humans, the mammary ridges disappear, except at the fourth intercostal space on the mid-axillary thorax. There are two pairs of mammary glands that develop in human beings. These numbers and locations vary in different species corresponding to the number of offspring.

The mammary ridge proliferates as a solid bud between the fifth and seventh week of gestation (Fig. 1.2). The mammary bud grows downward into the dermis and starts branching to the secondary bud around the twelfth week. This downward growth and branching is due to inductive influence of the extracellular matrix of the primary mesoderm on the mammary bud. This epithelial and mesenchymal signaling is through paracrine and juxtacrine mechanisms. The mesoderm and underlying adipose tissue around the bud produce growth factors and hormones, which interact with receptors on the mammary bud ectodermal cells to proliferate and grow downward. These hormones and growth factors derive from lipids from adipose tissue. These buds elongate to form lactiferous ducts at about the twentieth week.

The canalization of the mammary bud that is transformed into lactiferous ducts is influenced by placental hormones that are circulating through the fetal circulation. The placental hormones consist of progesterone, growth hormone, insulin-like growth hormone, estrogen, prolactin, adrenoglucocorticoid, and triiodothyronine. There are about 15–20 lobes of glandular tissue formed with lactiferous ducts. The mammary gland is surrounded by mesenchyme, which forms connective tissue, fat, and vasculature and intersects mammary nerves.

By the end of prenatal life, the mammary ectoderm, with modified apocrine glands, branches into 15–20 solid buds that then canalize and form the lactiferous ducts and lobes of the lung alveoli. The mammary gland proliferates and the ducts elongate; further divisions occur to form the mammary glands and ductal system. Initially, the lactiferous ducts open into a small mammary epithelial pit, which is transformed into the nipple by proliferation of the underlying mesenchyme. Mesodermal proliferation also gives rise to the circular and longitudinal smooth muscle fibers of the nipple-areola complex. A failure of mesenchymal proliferation causes the ducts to open into a shallow pit resulting in an inverted nipple. At birth, the male and female anatomies appear alike due to maternal circulating prolactin in the mother. While the male breast remains the same, the female breast undergoes further transformation at the time of puberty, pregnancy, and lactation due to hormonal influence.

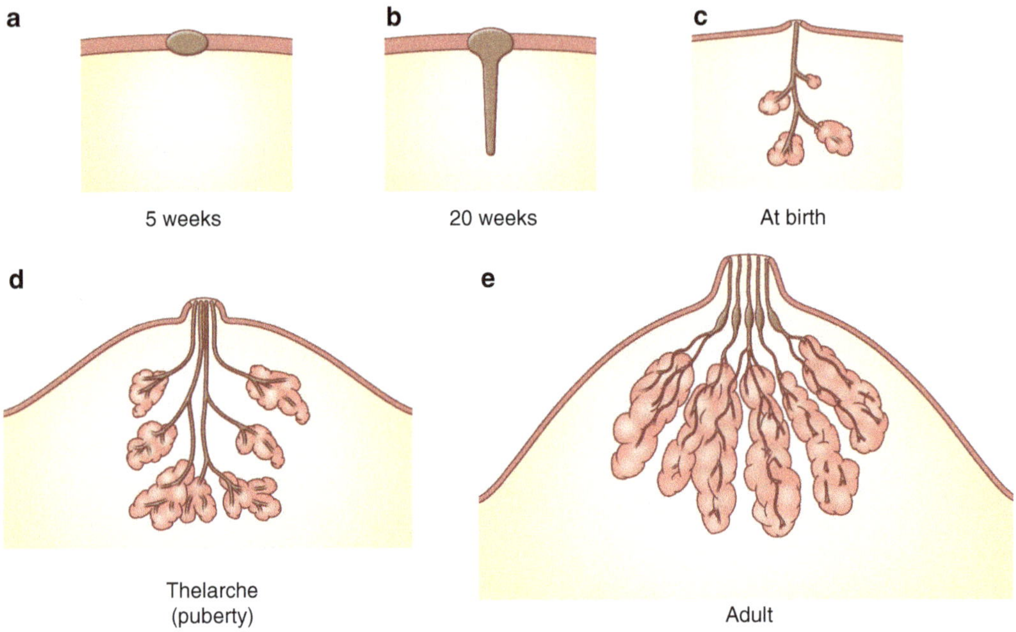

Fig. 1.2 Development of breast. (**a**) Mammary ridge. (**b**) Elongation of the mammary bud and canalization of the lactiferous duct in 20 weeks. (**c**) Rudimentary mammary glands. (**d**) Further development to form the adult ductal system in the mammary gland during puberty. Connective tissue and deposition of fat. (**e**) Functional gland with secretary alveoli

Areola

During the neonatal period, the nipple is a small pit at the center of the thickened areola. The areola contains sweat glands and sebaceous gland with its Montgomery tubercle. The nipples become elevated and protrude, with the areola developing increased pigmentation. Prolactin secretion in the pituitary gland is stimulated by falling estrogen levels in the neonatal period and may result in the acini to develop and produce witch milk, milk secreted from the breasts of newborns [6].

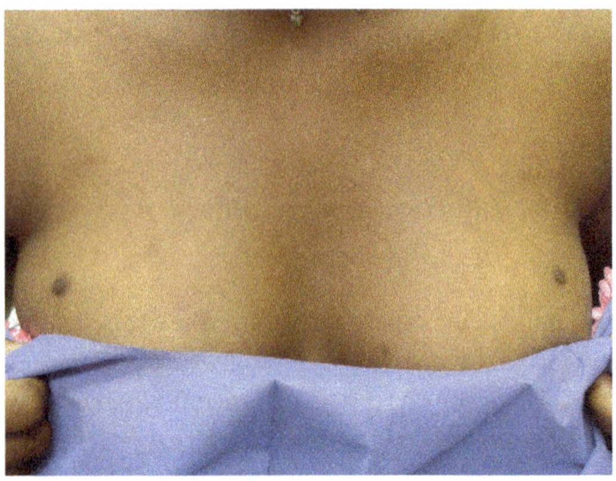

Fig. 1.3 Accessory nipple. Accessory nipple seen on the superior aspect of both breasts

Congenital and Acquired Deformity of the Breast

Occasionally, fragments of the mammary ridge may persist, giving rise to accessory nipples (polythelia) or developing into a complete breast, also known as polymastia, along the mammary line (Fig. 1.3) [7–11]. The most common location of an accessory nipple is within the inframammary fold, while accessory breasts are most commonly found in the axilla (Figs. 1.4 and 1.5).

There is a wide variation of congenital and acquired deformities (Table 1.1). For example, the congenital deformities are hyperplasia, hypoplasia, and a combination of these. The hyperplastic breasts are unilateral or bilateral with hyperplasia, polythelia, polymastia, hematoma, and giant fibroadenoma occurring in the female and gynecomastia in the male (Fig. 1.6). The hypoplasia of the breast may occur in one or both breasts. Hypoplasia can be seen in tuberous breasts due to a fibrous cord and the absence of superficial fascia under the areola causing hypertrophy and a herniated areola (Figs. 1.7 and 1.8). There are various abnormalities of the hypoplastic breast and athelia of the breast, which can occasionally be seen in Poland syndrome (Fig. 1.9).

The acquired deformity is due to iatrogenic injury caused by thoracotomy or biopsy of the breast for a tumor, and post-radiation deformity is due to radiation for a hemangioma or tumor. Such injuries may be the result of thermal burns

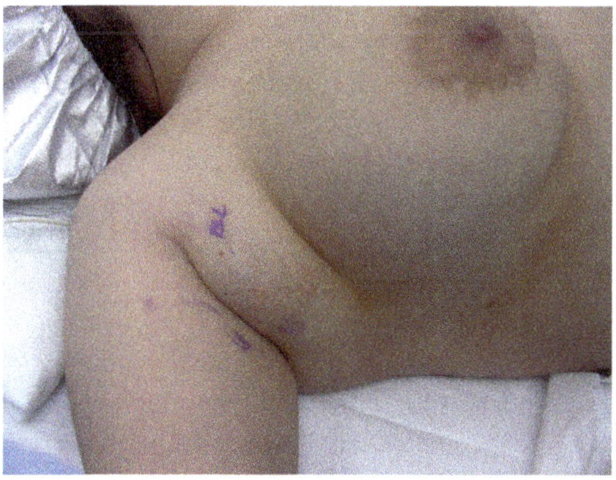

Fig. 1.4 Axillary breast. Patient has axillary breast in the axilla of the right breast

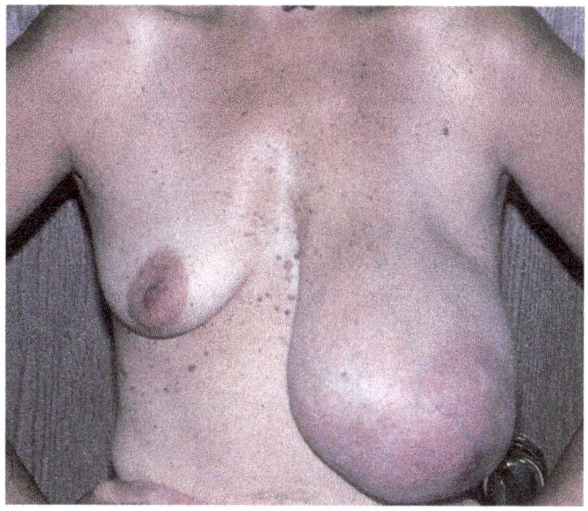

Fig. 1.6 Hematoma of the breast. This patient presents with a hematoma of the left breast and hypoplasia of the right breast. It is slow in growth, 5 years

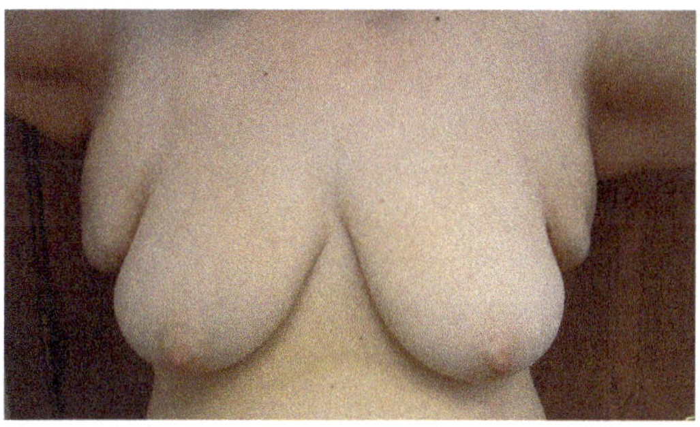

Fig. 1.5 Axillary breast. The patient has bilateral axillary breasts

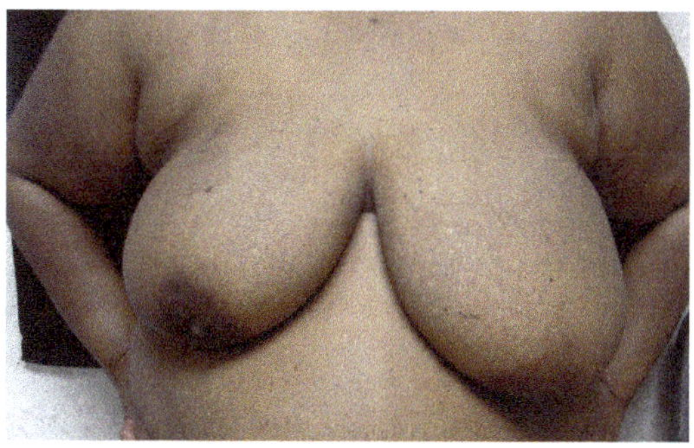

Fig. 1.7 Asymmetry breast. This patient has hypertrophy breast with asymmetry

Table 1.1 Congenital and acquired deformity of the breast

Congenital		Acquired	
Hyperplastic breast	Hypoplasia of the breast	Iatrogenic	Trauma
Hypertrophy	Hypoplasia	Thoracotomy	Thermal burn
Unilateral and bilateral	Unilateral and bilateral	Breast biopsy	Penetrating injury to the breast
Polythelia	Athelia	Lumpectomy	Breast ironing
Polymastia	Poland syndrome	Radiation	
Male gynecomastia	Tuberous breast		
Giant fibroadenoma	Inverted nipple		

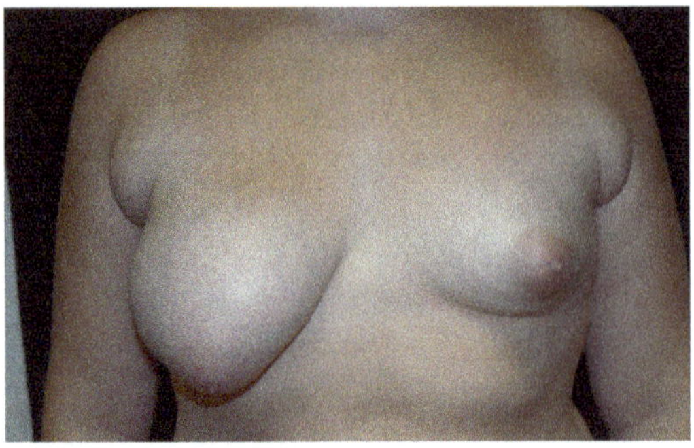

Fig. 1.8 Asymmetrical breast. This patient has hypertrophy of the breast with asymmetry

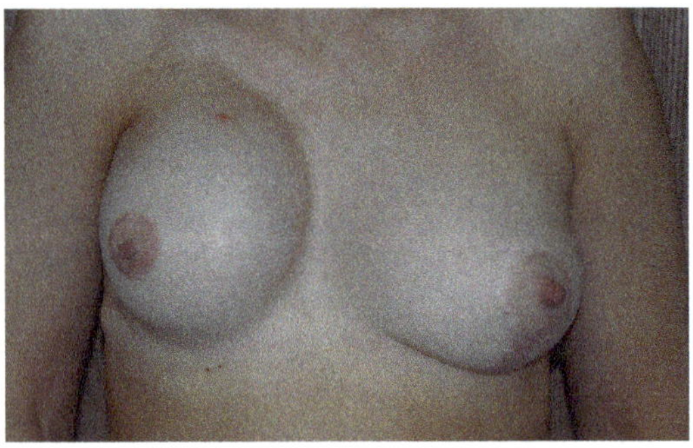

Fig. 1.9 Poland syndrome. Patient has hypoplasia of the right breast, absence of pectoral muscle, and a small areola. The patient has nipple tattooing of the right breast. The patient has mastopexy with implant on the left side

in childhood that may cause scars, contracture, and deformity. Other examples describe an alarming number of worldwide reports that have identified vicious practices of "breast ironing" [12] in teens in order to suppress the growth of breasts and prevent teen pregnancy in Central and West Africa.

Development and Physiology of the Breast Parenchyma

During puberty, enlargement of the mammary glands is primarily due to ovarian estrogen. The lactiferous ducts branch to form a solid spherical mass of glandular cells that are potentially still able to develop into alveoli. At the end of puberty, there is dense fibrous stroma that separates the scattered ducts lined with epithelium and fat in the mammary gland. Increasing serum estradiol concentrations promote fat deposition and the formation of new ducts by branching and elongation.

During pregnancy, the lactiferous ducts branch and secretory alveoli appear due to the influence of placental progesterone, estrogen, prolactin, and lactogen. The adipose tissue increases under the influence of a robust blood flow.

The abrupt withdrawal of progesterone upon delivery leaves the breast under the influence of prolactin. In the presence of growth hormone, insulin, and cortisol, prolactin converts the epithelial cells to secretory cells, resulting in the production of milk by alveolar cells. Oxytocin is then released from the posterior pituitary gland in response to nipple-areola stimulation, causing the ductal myoepithelial cells to contract and eject milk. After parturition, there is reduction of estrogen and progesterone levels that stimulates prolactin secretion from the anterior hypophysis. This promotes the apocrine gland to secrete milk with fat droplets. Placental lactogen and sex hormones maintain the mammary epithelium in a pre-secretory phase by antagonizing the effects of prolactin and thyroid hormone [6]. During the post-lactational period, the prolactin level decreases with an inhibitory effect of non-expelled milk that results in a return to a nonfunctional state. During the pre- and postmenopausal period, the gland becomes senescent, with resulting involution of the mammary gland and deposition of connective tissue and fat [5].

Adult Breast

Overview

The breasts are located on the anterior chest wall and are composed of the skin envelope which contains the nipple-areola complex with adnexal structures and mammary parenchyma containing glandular tissue and adipose and fibrous connective tissue which support the gland (Fig. 1.10). The adult female breast rests within the superficial and deep fascia held in position with

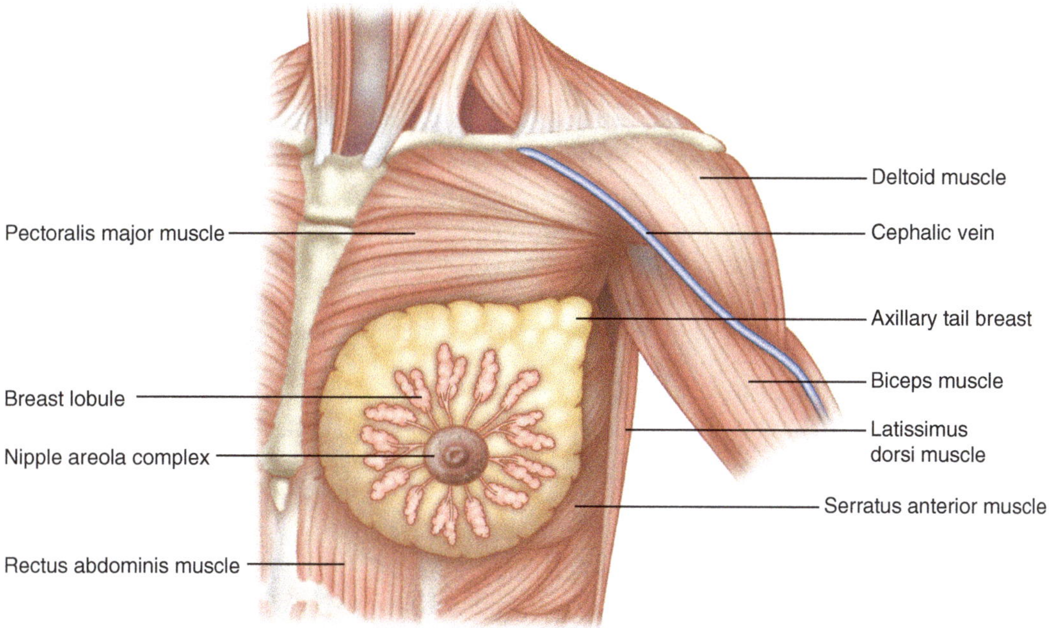

Fig. 1.10 Anterior view: breast shows mammary glands, lobules situated over the pectoralis major muscle, axillary tail projecting into the axilla

suspensory ligaments on the anterior upper thoracic wall. The breast extends from the second rib to the inframammary fold located at the level of the sixth or seventh rib [13–15]. Medial extension of the breast is to the sternum, and the lateral border extends to the mid-axillary line terminating as the axillary tail of Spence. The posterior surface of the gland rests upon the fascia of the pectoralis major and serratus anterior muscle. The inferior aspect rests on the external oblique muscle and upper portion of the rectus sheath with inframammary support.

The size and shape of the breast vary with individual race and age. The breast can develop into a variety of shapes, including hemispherical, conical, pendulous, tuberous, piriform, thin, or flattened. Due to the development of the human infant jaw relative to primates, the conical shape of the breast is primarily due to fat accumulation during lactation period aids. This aids with breastfeeding without suffocation of the baby and further helps to feed without retraction of the pre-maxilla.

Skin Envelope and Nipple-Areola Complex

The skin of the breast surrounds the underlying parenchyma, with the nipple-areola complex located at the apex of the breast. The quality of the skin varies from patient to patient. During youth, the skin has greater elasticity and provides firm support to the underlying parenchyma. With age, weight gain, and pregnancy, the skin loses its elasticity, becoming thinner and often developing stria (tears and separations in the thinned dermis) with diminished support of the underlying parenchyma. Thinning of the central breast skin and absence of elastic support of the parenchyma can lead to a constricted breast associated with tubular or tuberous breasts.

The nipple stays within the center of the areolar skin which is of ectodermal origin. It contains sebaceous glands that when enlarged form Montgomery tubercles. The areola also has sweat glands that secrete lipoid material that helps lubricate and protect this structure. The areolar size ranges from about 28 to 50 mm in diameter for the typical breast. Enlarging during pregnancy, the areola is under hormonal influence that results in hyperpigmentation of the nipple and areola. The areolar pigmentation depends upon two polymers, eumelanin and pheomelanin, which cause brown and red pigments to be secreted. The extent of pigmentation varies with skin tone. The areola and nipple have no hair and are devoid of fat underneath the areolar skin. The areola is composed of sweat and sebaceous glands located within the periphery and the accessory glands of Montgomery, which produce small elevations on the surface of the areola.

The areola secretes both lubricants and pheromones to facilitate breastfeeding, with the latter facilitating the baby to nurse. It has been suggested that the differing color of the nipple-areola complex is for a higher visibility for the infant. The nipple contains openings for the lactiferous ducts and smooth muscle that aid in lactation and breastfeeding. The areola also contains tissues that cause erection of the nipple-areola complex during lactation.

The nipple stays at the level of the fourth intercostal space in the nulliparous woman or young adult. The nipple contains multiple sensory nerve endings, Meissner's corpuscles, Ruffini's corpuscles, Krause's corpuscles, and autonomic nervous system. The sensory innervation of the nipple plays a great functional significance during lactation. The nipple contains openings for the lactiferous ducts and circular nonstriated smooth muscle that aid in lactation and breastfeeding. The longitudinal muscle may retract the nipple and circular muscles that, in turn, causes erection of the nipple.

Parenchyma of the Breast

The parenchyma of the breast is composed of the glandular tissue supported by fibrous tissue that holds the gland and interlobular adipose tissue that is also enriched with blood vessels and nerves. The breast parenchyma is pale yellow in color, with the lobulated tissue supported by connective tissue. It is usually composed of 15–20 lobes, with each lobe comprised of the same number of tubuloalveolar lobules connected by a single lactiferous duct. They are arranged in a radial pattern and orientation from the areola. These lobules drain to the lobes through the lactiferous duct and sinuses just underneath the areola. The sinuses are reservoirs that are connected to the narrow papilla that transmit milk to the orifices in the nipple. The lactiferous ducts, lined with stratified squamous epithelium, transition into lactiferous sinuses lined with cuboidal and myoepithelial cells located beneath the areola.

Each of the lobules contains hundreds of secretory acini. The ducts have columnar epithelia and lined by the basal lamina and myoepithelium at the periphery of the ducts. It is from within these ducts that invasive ductal carcinoma arises. Larger ducts have two or three layers of epithelium, becoming keratinizing stratified squamous epithelium at the opening. The morphology of the secreting gland varies greatly with age and hormonal influence. The inactive breast undergoes mild cyclical changes associated with the menstrual cycle. Conversely, significant cellular hypertrophy of the breast occurs throughout pregnancy. The breast also contains varying amounts of fat, which contributes to the contour, shape, and softness of the breast. Fat deposition is influenced by genetic and hormonal factors. For example, postmenopausal women have more fat in their breasts, often making it easier to evaluate the tissue with mammography [16]. Lacking the alveoli, the male breast tissue is structurally different than the female breast. The male breast ducts are solid with little adipose tissue and no extension of the ducts beyond the areola. The nipple papilla and areola are small.

Gynecomastia

The early stages of breast development are independent of the sex steroid hormones, causing similarity of the breasts in both genders. During this time, the male mammary glands become responsive to the hormonal environment, with the presence of testosterone leading to the normal involution of the male mammary gland. However, in testicular feminization syndrome, where there are higher circulating levels of testosterone and a lack of testosterone receptors, the individual develops a female phenotype, including the typical female breast development.

Fascia and Ligaments

Scarpa's fascia extends onto the chest and splits into an anterior and posterior lamella that encompasses the breast (Fig. 1.11). The anterior lamella forms inframammary fold and encloses the breast [13, 14, 17, 18]. The anterior lamella serves as the dissection plane when performing a mastectomy. The posterior lamella [19] separates the breast from the underlying pectoralis major muscle and is the plane of dissection for sub-glandular breast augmentation. There is a retromammary space between the breast parenchyma and posterior lamella on the pectoralis major muscle. This is called the loose areolar membranous layer and allows the overlying breast tissue to move upon the pectoral fascia. Occasionally, we see invasion of the fascia and muscle with invasive breast cancer, with the capacity to also invade the suspensory ligaments and retromammary space. The latter is often associated with visible skin retraction and lymphatic tumor cell invasion of the skin, referred to as peau d'orange, for its typical thickened appearance of the skin similar to that of an orange peel.

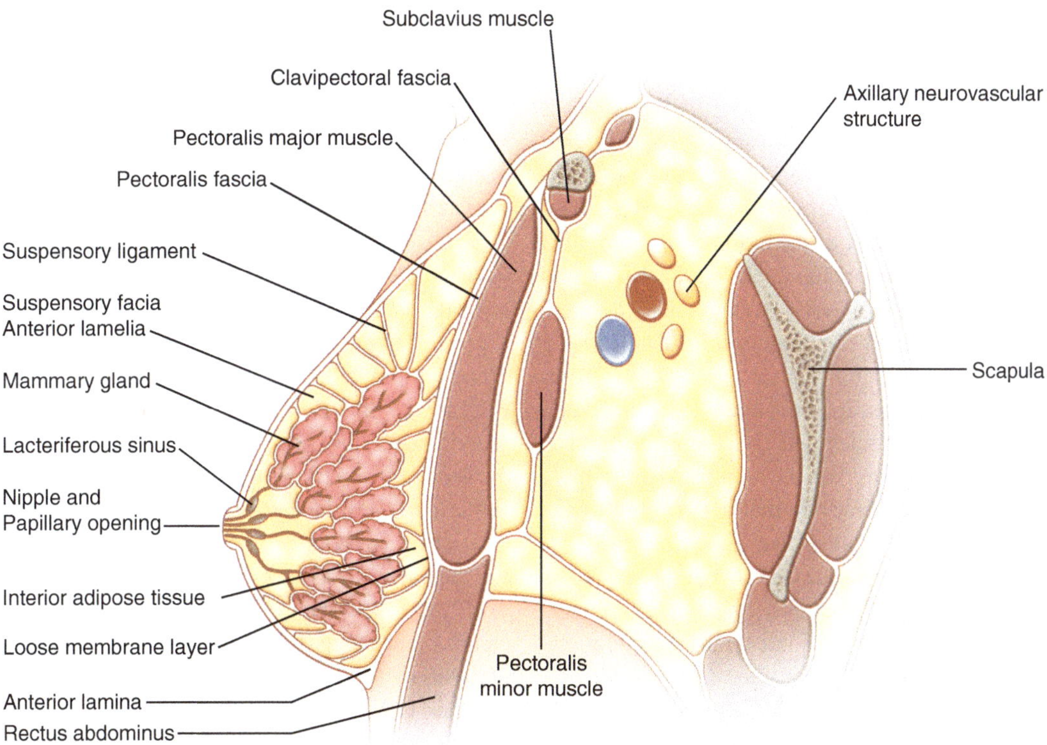

Fig. 1.11 Lateral view of breast. The rectus fascia, Scarpa's fascia, splits into the anterior and posterior laminae. The posterior lamina called pectoral fascia spreads across the pectoralis major muscle and to the clavicle. The anterior lamina (fascia) envelops the breast. The suspensory ligaments anchor the anterior lamina and mammary gland to the pectoral fascia. The clavipectoral fascia attached to the clavicle splits around subclavius muscle and to the pectoralis minor and reaches the axilla through which the axillary vessels and nerves travel to the axilla

There are multiple interdigitating connective tissue fibers within the breast and between the lamellae called Cooper's ligaments, which contribute to the shape of the breast and support it. In addition, there is a horizontal fascial septum originating from the lower, lateral border of the pectoral fascia at the level of the fifth rib that splits the breast into a superior two-thirds and inferior one-third. This septum was first described by Wuringer and colleagues and is associated with a well-formed neurovascular supply that courses within this fascia and provides support for the nipple-areola complex. The axillary tail of the breast has additional support via the suspensory ligament of the axilla. Retaining ligaments of the lateral chest wall suspend the lateral portion of the breast parenchyma and are often divided during a mastectomy [20].

Anatomy of the Axilla

The axilla is a distinct, pyramidal-shaped compartment located between the thoracic wall and the upper extremity and has four boundaries and one apex. The apex of the axilla extends into the posterior triangle of the neck via the cervicoaxillary canal. The anterior wall includes the pectoralis major and minor muscles as well as the clavipectoral fascia. The posterior wall is composed of the subscapularis, teres major, and latissimus dorsi muscles and overlying fascia. The medial wall is based on the serratus anterior muscle and the first four ribs that are covered by the intercostal muscles and fascia that is continuous with Scarp's fascia. The lateral wall is bounded by the intertubercular sulcus of the medial humerus with the insertion of the latissimus dorsi, coracobrachialis, and biceps muscle. The base is composed of the axillary fascia that extends from the pectoralis major to the latissimus dorsi muscle and encloses the axillary contents.

The pectoral fascia invests the pectoralis major muscle, while the clavipectoral fascia extends from the clavicle to the axillary fascia within the floor of the axilla and encloses the pectoralis minor muscle. The part of the clavipectoral fascia attaches to the clavicle, enclosing the subclavius muscle to the first rib and referred to as Halsted's ligament. It then unites to form one layer that covers the axillary neurovascular bundle. This fascia again divides to enclose the pectoralis minor muscle. This part of the fascia covers the axillary neurovascular bundle and axillary lymph nodes.

The fascia units below the pectoralis minor form the axillary fascia and terminate within the axilla as the suspensory ligaments of the axilla or Gerdy's ligament (coracoaxillary fascia). This fascia is pierced by the cephalic vein, lateral pectoral nerve, and vascular branches from the thoracoacromial trunk. The suspensory ligament is pierced by the axillary tail of the breast (tail of Spence). The upper part of the clavipectoral fascia and Halsted's ligament extends from the clavicle to the first rib, covering the thoracic inlet as an axillary sheath. The thickened fascia from the first rib to coracoid is called the costocoracoid ligament. A tubular sheath emerges from the thoracic inlet in order to cover the axillary neurovascular bundle, referred to as the axillary sheath. The axillary contents are composed of fibroadipose tissue that is pierced by the axillary tail, lymphatic system, and second lateral intercostal sensory nerves that innervate the upper inner aspect of the arm. The axilla also contains the great vessels and nerves that supply the upper extremity. These nerves and vessels are enclosed within the axillary sheath.

There are several nerves in the axilla that need to be identified during a formal axillary dissection. The long thoracic nerve, which is located on the medial wall of the axilla, arises from the C5 to C7 and enters the axilla via the cervicoaxillary canal. It lies along the lateral aspect of the serratus anterior muscle that it innervates. Injury to this nerve will result in the "winged scapula." The thoracodorsal nerve originates from the posterior cord (C6 to C8) of the brachial plexus, accompanied by the subscapular artery and innervates the latissimus dorsi muscle. The intercostobrachial nerve is a purely sensory nerve that provides sensation to the skin of the axilla and the upper medial aspect of the arm.

Vascular Anatomy of the Breast

The breast receives blood supply from the perforating branches of the internal mammary artery medially, the lateral branches of the posterior intercostal arteries, and the lateral thoracic and pectoral branches of the thoracoacromial artery superiorly [21–25]. There is a mesentery as described by Wuringer that connects the lateral thoracic artery and chain of lateral intercostal vessels from the lateral border of pectoralis major to the medial anterior perforating intercostal vessels arising from the internal mammary artery.

These form the mesentery arc at the base of breast (Figs. 1.12 and 1.13) and traverse through the gland to the superficial vascular system (Fig. 1.14) [26–28]. The blood supply to the skin is primarily from the subdermal plexus with communications to the underlying perforators from the external mammary artery, anterolateral and anteromedial intercostal artery, and internal mammary artery. There is an abundant and substantial collateralization of arterial flow within the breast.

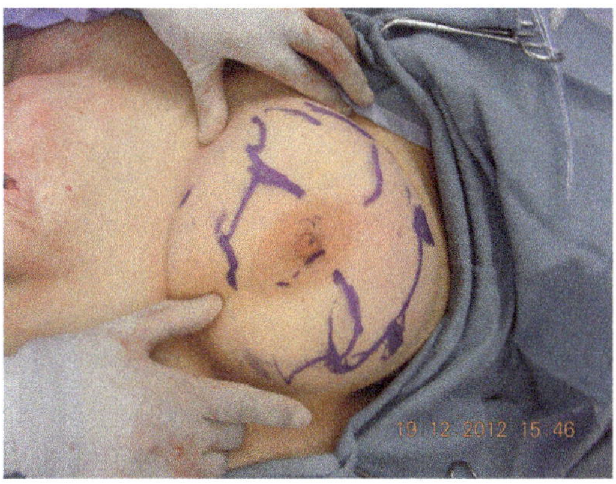

Fig. 1.12 Venous outflow. The subdermal plexus of the vein travels in a radial direction from the nipple-areola complex

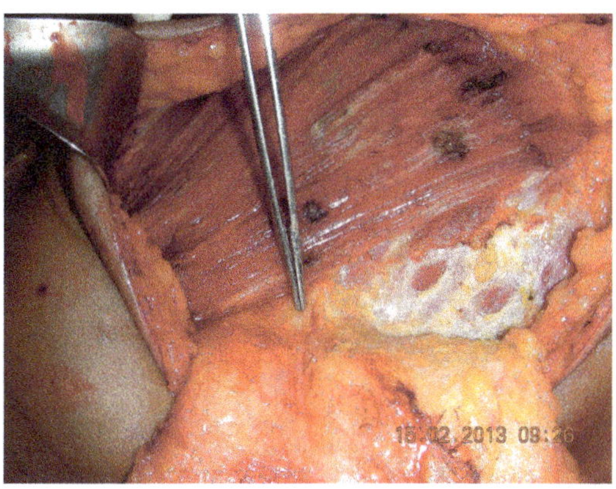

Fig. 1.13 Vascular mesentery. This dissection shows lateral thoracic vessel arches, lateral to the pectoral muscle and form arc to supply blood flow to the breast

The venous drainage of the breast closely follows the arterial blood supply and is directed towards the axilla. The superficial veins have extensive collateralization that may be visible just underneath the skin. The major venous drainage of the breast occurs through (A) perforating branches of the internal mammary artery, (B) tributaries of the axillary vein, and (C) perforating branches of the posterior intercostal veins. The posterior intercostal veins are in continuity with the vertebral plexus of veins, the Batson's plexus that extends from the base of the skull to the sacrum. This pathway may provide a direct and efficient route of hematogenous spread of breast cancer to the skull, vertebrae, pelvic bones, and central nervous system [29]. The blood supply to the nipple-areola complex is contributed from both the parenchyma beneath and the rich subdermal plexus surrounding the complex [20, 23, 30–32].

Lymphatic Drainage of the Breast

The lymphatics of the breast are located within the parenchyma itself, with individual lymphatic drainage to each of the lobules and ducts (Fig. 1.15). The main route of drainage of the breast, greater than 75 %, is through the axillary lymph node groups. The remainder of lymphatic drainage is through the parasternal nodes and likely the internal thoracic lymph nodes, which are a group of smaller lymph nodes located about a centimeter lateral to the sternal border. These nodes are located within the intercostal spaces along the internal mammary vessels. The skin of the breast drains via the superficial lymphatic vessels into the axillary lymph nodes.

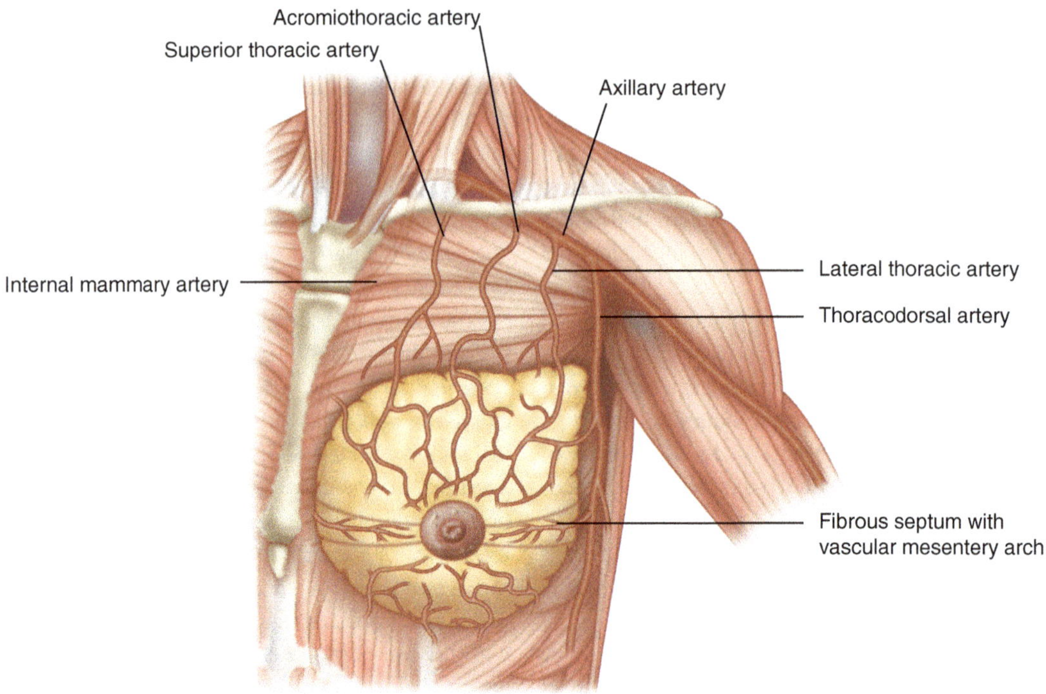

Fig. 1.14 Arterial vessels to the breast fibrous septum forming central pedicle to supply major part of the breast and nipple-areola complex described by Dr. E. Wuringer

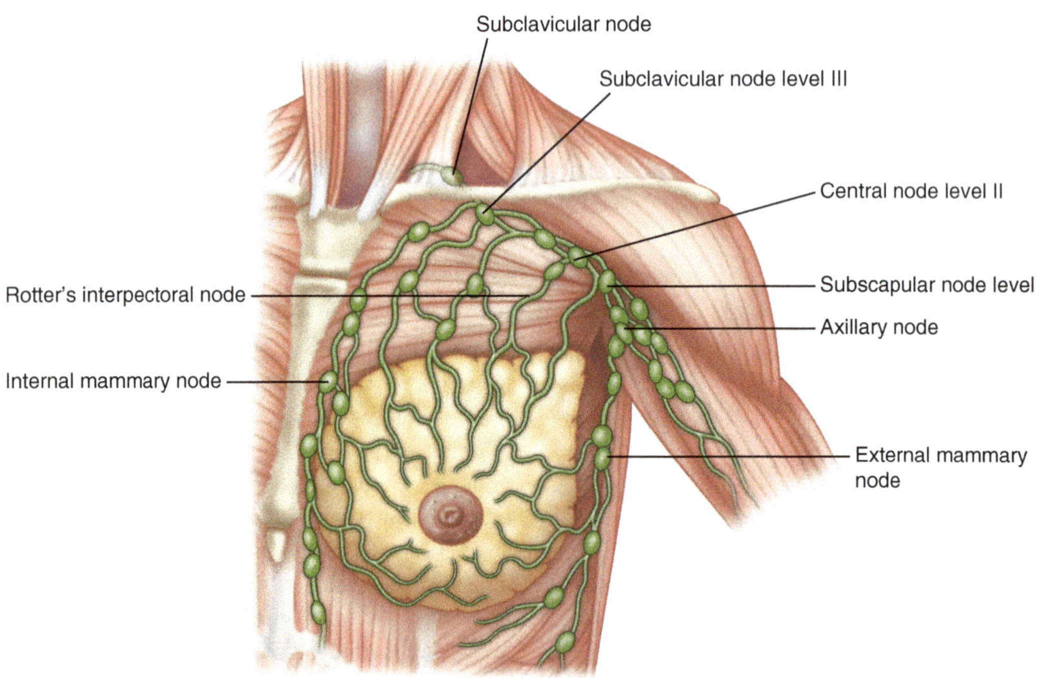

Fig. 1.15 Lymphatic drainage of the breast

There are six commonly described groups at three anatomic levels [29, 33–37]:

1. The *axillary vein group* consists of four to six lymph nodes located posterior to the axillary vein and receives drainage from the deltopectoral lymph nodes and upper extremity.
2. The *external mammary group* is composed of four to six lymph nodes, located along the lower border of the pectoralis minor muscle, in close proximity to the lateral thoracic vessels. These nodes receive the majority of lymph drainage from the breast.
3. The *scapular group* is composed of six to seven lymph nodes located at the posterior wall of the axilla, in proximity to the lateral border of the scapula. These nodes receive drainage from lower aspects of the neck and the posterior skin and subcutaneous tissues of the trunk.
4. The *central group* is composed of three to four lymph nodes located posterior to the pectoralis minor muscle. These nodes receive drainage from the preceding nodal basins (axillary, external mammary, and scapular) and afferent lymphatic from the breast.
5. The *subclavicular group* is the apical group composed of 6–12 lymph nodes located superior to the pectoralis minor, extending into the apex of axilla. These nodes receive drainage from all other nodal groups. The lymphatic drainage of the group is into the subclavian trunk which empties into the internal jugular vein or the subclavian vein. On the left side, the subclavian trunk may terminate into the thoracic duct.
6. *Rotter's group* is composed of one to three lymph nodes located between the pectoralis major and minor muscles. Lymphatic drainage from these nodes is to the central and subclavicular systems.

The axillary lymph node groups are divided according to their lateral and medial relationship to the pectoralis minor muscle into levels I–III. Level I nodes are located inferior to the lower border of the pectoralis minor and are composed of external mammary, axillary vein, and scapular lymph node groups. Level II nodes are located posterior to the pectoralis minor and include the central lymph node group. Level III nodes are located superomedial to the pectoralis minor and are composed of the subclavicular group.

Innervation of the Breast

The sensory innervation of the breast is supplied primarily by the lateral and anterior cutaneous branches of the second through the sixth intercostal nerves (Fig. 1.16). The sensation of the breast skin is segmental and is derived from the dermatomes of breast development. The third through the sixth branches, known as the lateral mammary branches, supply the majority of the skin covering the breast. The medial parts of the breast skin are innervated by the sensory anterior intercostal nerve, although the supraclavicular nerve supply below the clavicle does not contribute any sensory innervation to the skin covering the breast [38–43]. The intercostobrachial nerve originates from the lateral branch of the second intercostal nerve and courses through the fascia of the floor of the axilla to join the medial cutaneous nerve of the arm. This nerve is often divided during an axillary lymph node dissection resulting in the loss or decrease in sensation to the upper inner aspect of the arm. The innervation of the nipple-areola complex and the central breast is primarily from the T3–T5 branches of the anterolateral and anteromedial intercostal nerves. The nipple is innervated by the third, fourth, and fifth lateral intercostal nerves [44–49].

Muscles Supporting the Breast

The breast is situated on top of the pectoralis fascia and anterolateral chest wall musculature. The upper central and medial portions of the breast lie over the pectoralis major muscle, with the lower portions of the breast covering the anterolateral serratus anterior muscle and the upper external oblique muscle, and fascia over the upper origins of the rectus abdominis muscle inferomedially.

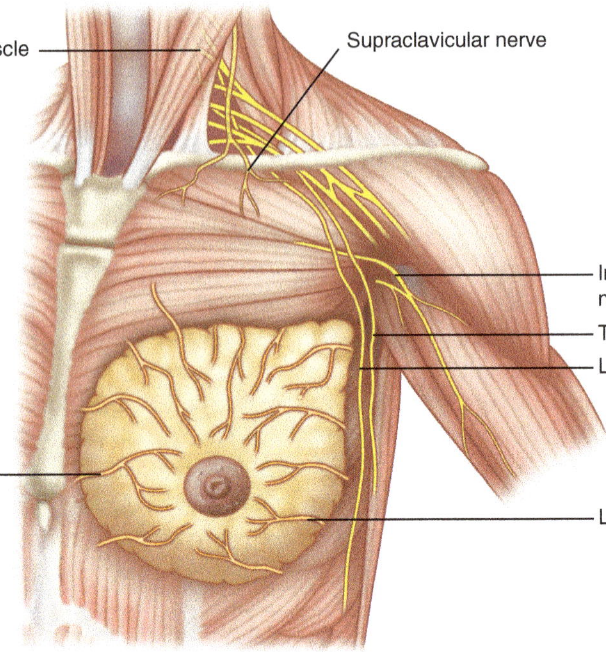

Fig. 1.16 Nerves of axilla. Thoracodorsal nerve (posterior cord) supplies the latissimus dorsi muscle. Long thoracic nerve (C5, C6, C7 root) innervates the serratus muscle. Second intercostal brachial nerve travels axilla to medial border arm. The supraclavicular nerve arises from C3 and C4 and innervates the infraclavicular part of the chest wall. The breast is innervated by the thoracic medial 1–6 and lateral 2–7 intercostal nerves. The nipple is innervated by lateral and anterior cutaneous branches of the 3rd, 4th, and 5th intercostal nerves and equally medial and. Lateral branch of thoracic 4th intercostal nerve provides the major innervation

Pectoralis Major Muscle

The pectoralis major is a thick, triangular-shaped muscle that covers most of the upper thoracic area, with two muscular heads, the clavicular and sternal heads that are separated by a cleft (Fig. 1.17). The clavicular head of the pectoralis major originates from the medial half of the clavicle. The sternal head of the pectoralis major takes origin from lateral anterior part of sternum to the first through seventh ribs and costal cartilage. It also traverses the sternal end of the sixth and seventh ribs and aponeurosis of the external oblique muscle. The muscle is composed of a flat tendon that inserts into the lateral lip of the intertubercular sulcus of the articular capsule and into the deltoid tubercle of the humerus. It has two laminae, the anterior lamina from the clavicle and sternum manubrium and the posterior deep lamina derived from the sternum and ribs. The anterior lamina inserts lower than the posterior lamina. The insertion of the pectoralis major muscle is anterior to the coracobrachialis muscle and is also covered by the anterior portion of the deltoid.

The thoracoacromial artery, internal mammary artery perforators, and anterolateral cutaneous branches of the intercostal vessels contribute to the blood supply. The pectoralis major adducts and internally rotates the humerus, and these two heads of the muscle function differently while swinging the arm. The clavicular head is innervated by C5–C6, while the sternal head is innervated by C7–T1. This is the only muscle in the body that is innervated by all of the branches from the brachial plexus. This muscle forms the major component of the anterior axillary fold. The deep fascia of the pectoralis major is continuous with the axillary fascia and the investing fascia of the latissimus dorsi muscle.

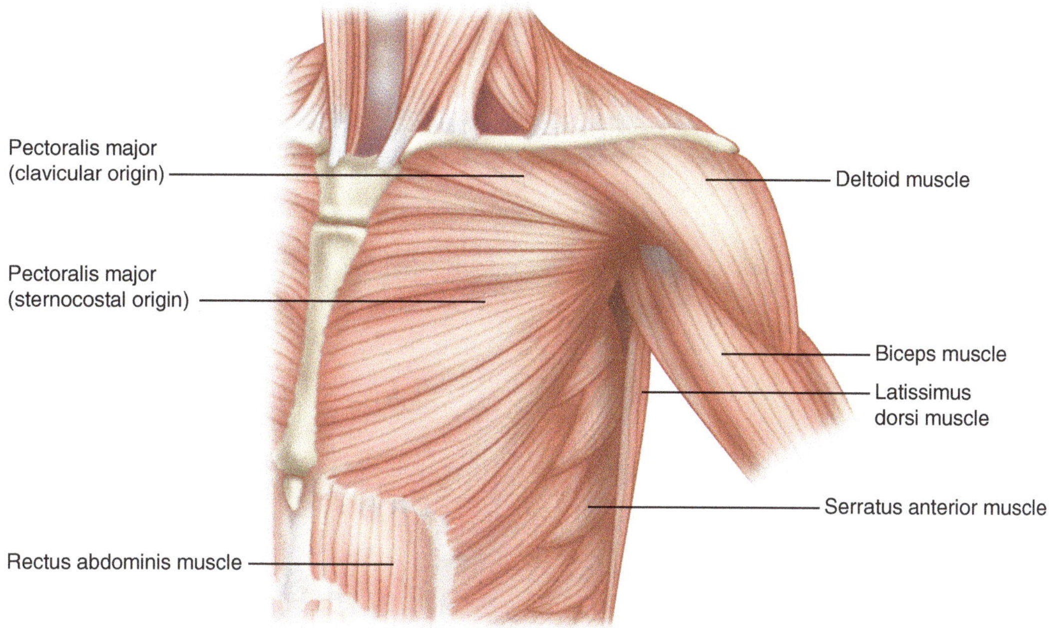

Fig. 1.17 Pectoralis major with relationship to the rectus abdominis serratus muscle and latissimus dorsi muscle

The sternal and clavicular portions are distinct embryologically and separated by a fascial component. The functional deficit caused by removal and denervation of the pectoralis major muscle is not significant.

Pectoralis Minor Muscle

This muscle is covered by the pectoralis major muscle. The pectoralis minor originates from the third to fifth ribs and inserts onto the medial border of the upper surface of the coracoid process. This attachment may cross the coracoid process and attach as the coracoacromial and coracohumeral ligament (Fig. 1.18). The blood supply is via the thoracoacromial artery and the lateral thoracic artery, and it is innervated by the medial pectoral nerve via the C6–C8 nerve roots. The pectoralis minor is a triangular muscle that protracts the scapula. It covers part of the axilla and is an important landmark for performing a complete axillary lymph node dissection.

Serratus Anterior Muscle

This muscle is a large muscle that lies upon the lateral wall of the thorax and originates from the first eight ribs laterally. This muscle inserts onto the ventral surface of the medial border of the scapula. It is a segmental muscle and is attached to medial border of scapula at various levels from the superior scapula angle to the triangle area along the inferior border of scapula. Its blood supply is via the segmental intercostal perforators and external serratus branch arising from the thoracodorsal artery. It is innervated by the long thoracic nerve via the C5–C7 nerve roots and acts to stabilize the scapula. It also draws the medial scapula onto the thoracic wall, preventing the winging of the scapula, when injured. It also assists with abduction of the arm.

Rectus Abdominis Musculature

The rectus abdominis muscle originates from the pubic crest and the symphysis pubis. It inserts

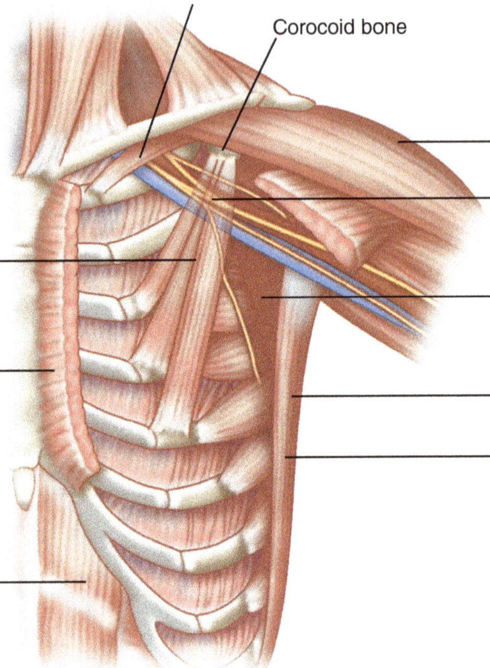

Fig. 1.18 Pectoralis minor originates from the third, fourth, and fifth rib and is inserted into the medial and upper border of coracoid process. It is a landmark for division of axillary vessels as the vessels pass under the muscle. The pectoralis major muscle is reflected

onto the fifth through seventh costal cartilages. Three major sources supply vascular flow to the muscle: the deep inferior epigastric artery, superior epigastric artery, and segmental intercostal arteries (seventh through the twelfth). It is innervated by seventh through twelfth intercostal nerves and acts to flex the vertebral column. Preservation of the epigastric vessels may help with the reconstruction of the breast utilizing the deep inferior epigastric perforating (DIEP) vessels.

Latissimus Dorsi Muscle

The latissimus dorsi muscle forms the lateral boundary of the axilla as it passes around the teres major muscle to be inserted in the intertubercular sulcus located in front of the teres major and behind the pectoralis major muscle (Fig. 1.19). The latissimus dorsi is a very large muscle that takes its origin from the thoracolumbar fascia, spines of lower six thoracic vertebrae and from the outer lip of the iliac crest lateral to the erector spinae and third and fourth lower ribs interdigitating with the external oblique muscle. The muscle fibers have a horizontal direction to them, oblique in the middle and vertical along the anterior aspect. The two triangles, lumbar and auscultation triangle, are associated with the latissimus muscle. The lumbar triangle is surrounded by the external oblique anteriorly, iliac crest inferiorly and lower fibers of the latissimus dorsi muscle posteriorly. The floor is covered by the internal oblique muscle. Weakness within the muscular floor of this triangle may result in a lumbar hernia. The triangle of auscultation is formed by the medial border of the scapula, trapezius muscle and latissimus dorsi muscle. This is the thinnest part of chest wall where one is able to auscultate the lungs with a stethoscope.

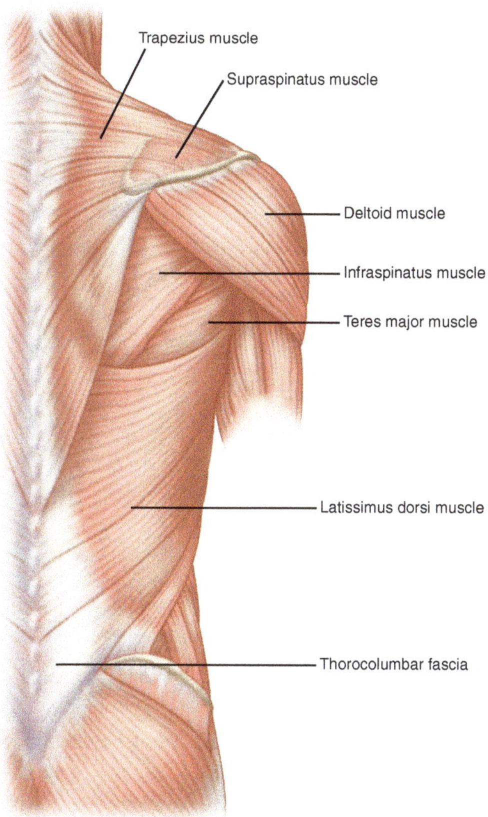

Fig. 1.19 Latissimus dorsi muscle takes origin from thoracolumbar fascia lumbar spine inserts in the bicipital grove in anterior to teres major. This muscle travels posterior to anterior and winds around the teres major muscle

The vascular supply is mainly from the subscapular artery that supplies the subscapularis muscle through the circumflex scapular artery. It is a branch to the serratus anterior muscle and terminates with the latissimus dorsi muscle. Additional blood flow is provided by the perforating lower intercostal and lumbar arteries. This vascularity provides a rich vascular supply to a variety of myocutaneous flaps that are utilized for reconstruction. The innervation is through the thoracodorsal nerve from the posterior cord, C6–C8.

External Oblique

The external oblique muscle originates from the lower eight ribs and inserts onto the linea semilunaris of the rectus sheath. Its vascular supply is via seventh through twelfth segmental intercostal arteries and it is innervated by the seventh through twelfth segmental intercostal nerves. It acts to laterally flex and rotate the trunk.

Anomalous Muscles

There are several possible anomalous muscles that may be present. Limb muscles generally arise in situ from the somatopleuric layer of lateral plate of the mesoderm around the developing bones. Some primordial muscles of different layers fuse to form a single muscle. Grim et al. reported this in 1972, observing that while the primordial stage disappears in some muscles, others may persist to the formation of muscle slips [50, 51]. The most common anomalies that are seen include the presence of an accessory "slip" and an abnormal origin or insertion of the pectoralis major muscle (Poland syndrome) (Fig. 1.20) [15, 52–54]. A second set of anomalies is associated with abnormal muscles, which may include the rectus, sternalis, and abnormal insertion of the latissimus dorsi muscle, known as Langer's muscle (Fig. 1.21) [55–58].

The sternalis muscle is a well-known, documented normal anatomic variant seen in humans [59–62].

It can be unilateral or bilateral, and usually lies within the anterior chest wall superficial and medial to the sternal origins of the pectoralis muscle. The sternalis usually courses longitudinally adjacent to the sternum and does not cross the midline. Several variations regarding the superior and inferior insertion have been noted. The superior insertions can include the tendon of the sternocleidomastoid muscle, sternum, clavicle, pectoralis major, platysma, and the upper ribs and costal cartilages. The inferior insertions can include the third to eighth costal cartilages, the fourth to eighth ribs, the anterior rectus sheath, the pectoralis major fascia, and the subcutaneous adipose tissue overlying these muscles (Figs. 1.22, 1.23, and 1.24). The presence of the sternalis muscle is not associated with any known symptomatic findings. However, its presence may

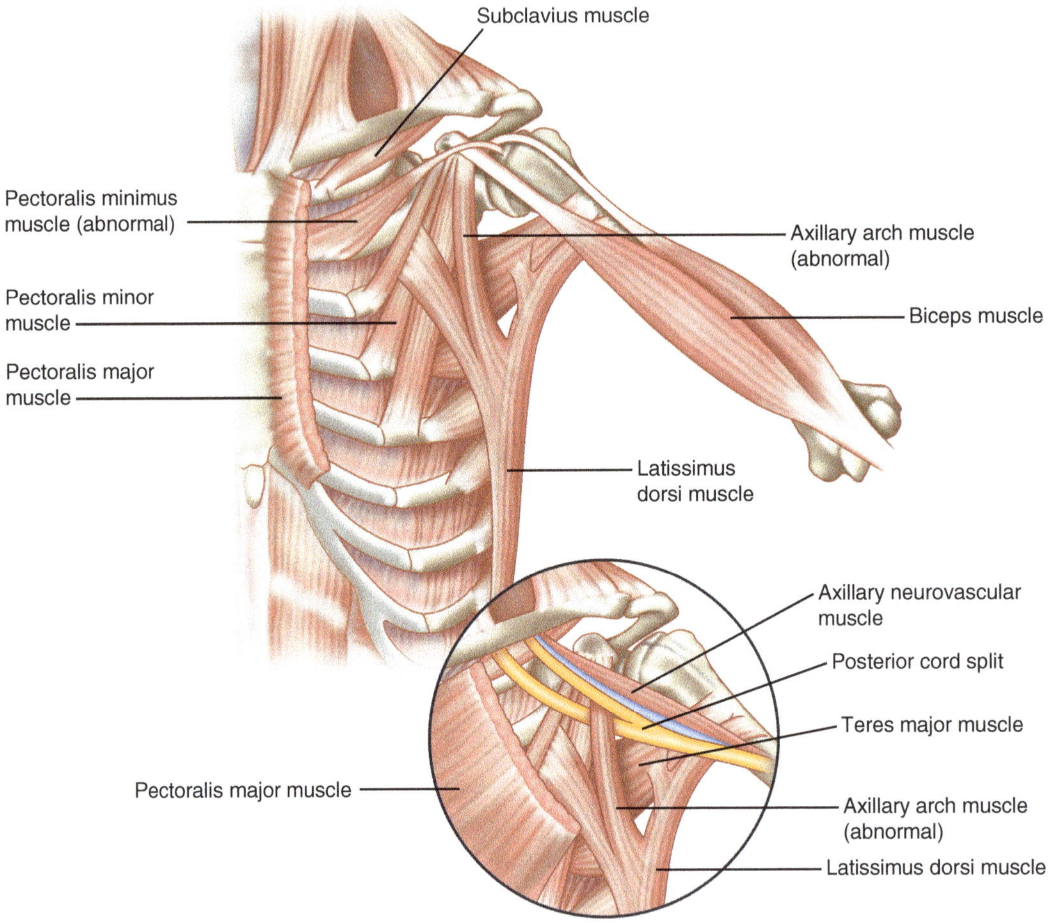

Fig. 1.20 Latissimus dorsi sends anomalous slips to form the axillary arch muscle and teres major, infraspinatus, and pectoralis minor causing difficult-to-do axillary dissection and nerve compression. Abnormal pectoralis minimus muscle is seen in deep chest wall dissection

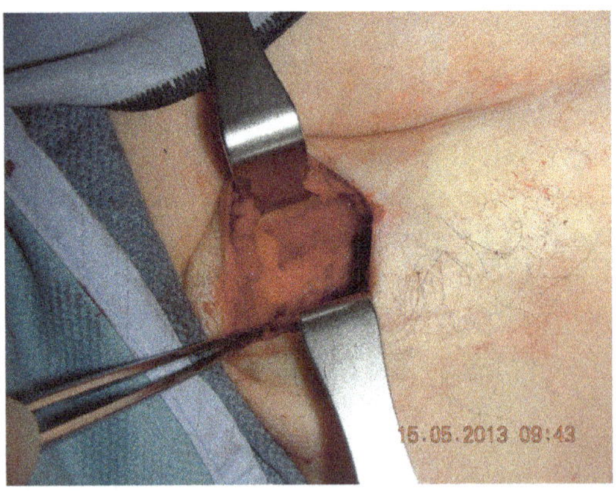

Fig. 1.21 Langer's arch muscle. This patient has Langer's muscle presents in the axilla, anomalous muscle takes a slip from Latissimus muscle and inserts into the pectoral muscles causing compression of nerves at the axilla. This may cause difficult axillary dissection

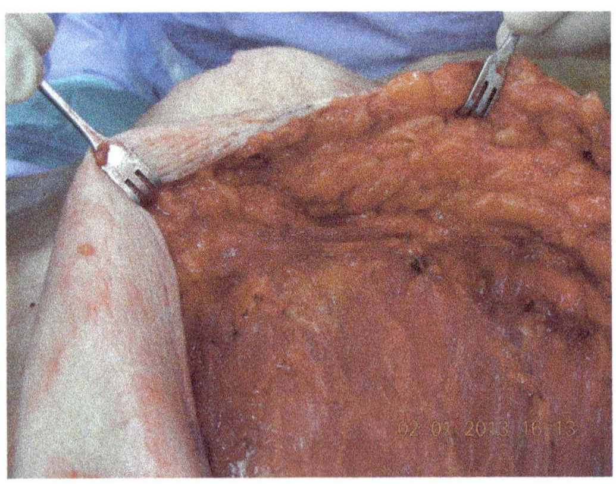

Fig. 1.22 Rectus sternalis. This muscle is analogous to the rectus abdominis. This muscle is present over sternal bone and takes origin on the sternal bone. Insertion varies and is multiple

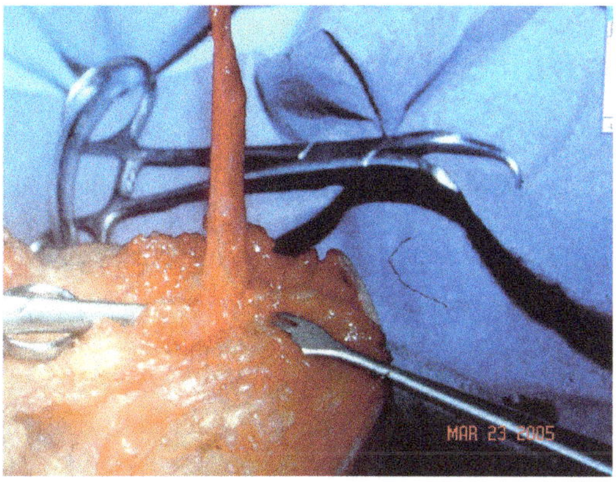

Fig. 1.23 Sternomastalis. The sternomastalis is a part of the rectus sternalis inserts of the breast; it can be seen in X-ray. It deforms the breast appearance

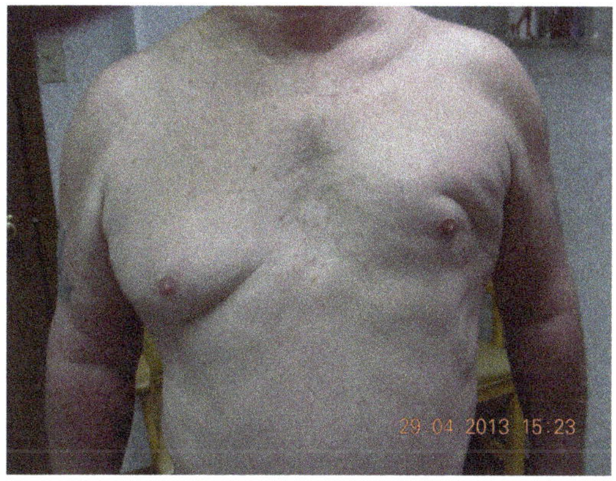

Fig. 1.25 Poland syndrome. This male patient shows Poland syndrome, hypoplasia of the pectoral and serratus muscle

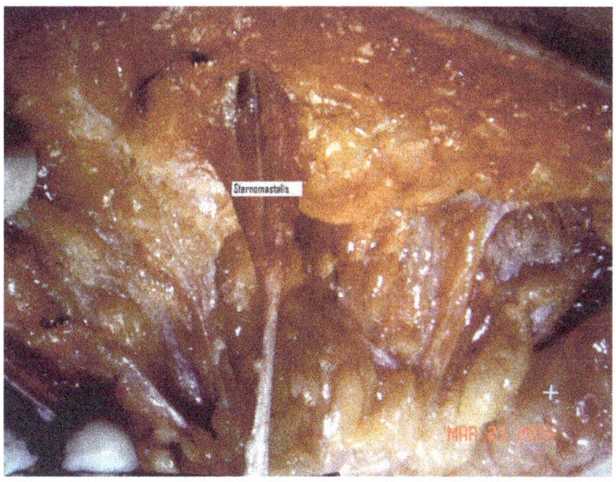

Fig. 1.24 Sternomastalis. This picture is showing the origin of the sternomastalis, an analogue muscle that corresponds to the rectus abdominis. This is a superficial muscle under the fascia. It is sometimes seen in the breast, X-rays, and surgery. Insertion varies

be interpreted as an abnormal breast mass when first observed by mammography. Sternomastalis is a variant of the sternalis muscle, with attachments to Cooper's ligaments of the breast or to the substance of the breast tissue.

Langer's axillary arch muscle is an anomalous muscular slip of latissimus dorsi muscle, first described by Ramsay in 1795, and subsequently confirmed in cadaver dissections to be present in 7–13 % of humans [51]. The muscle arch extends from the proximal border of the latissimus dorsi muscle as it arches across anteriorly to the axillary vessels at the level of posterior border of axillary fold. It then inserts onto the undersurface the pectoralis major tendon and the tendon of coracobrachialis muscle and fascia of the long head of the biceps muscle.

Another variation is described by Pillay [51], with the muscle originating from the latissimus dorsi and teres major muscle. It passes upwards through the posterior cord of the brachial plexus and can be seen under the axillary neurovascular bundle. It then splits in two slips and inserts into the coracoid process and the lesser tubercle of humerus. The latissimus dorsi muscle connects to the triceps tendon, called dorsoepitrochlearis brachii. These muscles may be seen as a mass within the axilla, leading to difficulty in performing an axillary dissection, especially along the lower part of the axilla. Additionally, this anomalous muscle may produce lymphedema and neurovascular impingement.

There are several anomalies involving the pectoralis muscle [63–69]. Complete absence of the muscle is usually associated with congenital syndromes. Poland [53] described a condition associated with the absence of a unilateral pectoralis major and cutaneous syndactyly of the ipsilateral hand (Fig. 1.25) [53, 70]. It may also be associated with microtia. Other variations include a normal pectoralis major muscle, but with breast malformation secondary to anterior thoracic hypoplasia and associated vascular impairment in utero. There are varying degrees of hypoplasia described by Paraskevas et al., including bilateral hypoplasia of the clavicular head associated with associated vascular anomalies of the external jugular vein in an atypical Poland syndrome.

Other anomalies involving the pectoralis include a cleft between origin of pectoralis muscle from the clavicle, sternum and cephalic vein as it traverses over the clavicular origin of the pectoralis muscle. There are also variations of the insertion of the pectoralis muscles. These are named according to the various slips of insertion and include the chondrohumeralis, axillopectoral, and chondroepitrochlearis. The chondrohumeralis takes origin from the pectoralis major muscle and inserts superficial to the axillary neurovascular bundle and the biceps. This is a remnant of the axillopectoral muscle. The chondroepitrochlearis is a rare anomaly where the muscle takes origin from the inferior border of the pectoralis muscle and inserts onto the epitrochlear bone. It runs parallel to the biceps.

There are various slips of the pectoralis major muscle, which may not be fused and, as such, leads to the formation of a single muscle with various names, such as the pectoralis quartus, pectoralis intermediate, and, pectoralis minimum. The pectoralis quartus arises from the costochondral junction of the sixth rib and passes laterally under the border of pectoralis major and inserts onto the intertubercular groove of humerus. The pectoralis intermediate takes origin from third and fourth ribs and passes as a fleshy slip and inserts onto the short head of the biceps. The pectoralis minimum arises from the second costal cartilage and passes between the pectoralis major and minor muscle, inserting into the superior surface of the coracoid process. The oblique pectoralis anterior muscle, described by Huber et al., originates from the sternum medially and courses inferiorly, inserting onto the sixth and seventh ribs and anterior rectus aponeurosis. The anomalous pectoralis major muscle with an accessory head of pectoralis arises from the serratus anterior muscle and inserts onto the intertubercular groove of the humerus. Anomalies involving the rectus muscle include the rectus thoracis bifurcalis, which takes origin from external oblique aponeurosis and splits into a Y shape at the sternal angle and inserting into the sternocleidomastoid bilaterally called the rectus thoracis [71, 72].

Principles to the Surgical Approach of the Breast

In the surgical approach to the breast, one has to carefully plan the incisions incorporating both the need for future reconstructive procedures and breast aesthetics. In patients undergoing excisional biopsy for high-risk tumors, the incisions should be placed along future mastectomy incisions whenever possible. When the tumor is close to the areola, a periareolar incision should be utilized. Lumpectomy incisions should be placed along Langer's lines in order to minimize the visual scar. Every attempt should be made to avoid scar placement above the bra line. The surgeon should be familiar with the vascular supply of the breast, especially in the setting of a lumpectomy pocket closure to prevent parenchymal necrosis, hematoma, and infection. It is important to preserve the anterior intercostal perforator artery, especially the second intercostal perforator. The knowledge of anomalous muscles must be considered during surgical dissection. Additionally, too much traction during glandular dissection may result in damage to the skin flaps and leading to wound healing complications. A well-planned and executed incision will achieve a nice aesthetic result and maintain maximum vascularity to the skin flaps in order to allow for future breast reconstruction. The papillary ducts are directed radially and any incision around the nipple should be made in a similar fashion [20]. The mammary ducts are present within 1 mm from the areolar surface, also present within the dermis of the areola. It is difficult to remove all of the ducts during nipple coring or a nipple-sparing mastectomy.

References

1. Brawand D, Wahli W, Kaessmann H. Loss of egg yolk genes in mammals and origin of lactation and placentation. PLoS Biol. 1989;53:33–69 [PubMed].
2. Menkhorst E, Nation A, Cui S, Selwood L. Evolution of the shell coat and yolk in amniotes: a marsupial perspective. J Exp Zool Mol Dev Evol. 2009;312B:625–38.
3. Oftedal OT. The mammary gland and its origin during synapsid evolution. J Mammary Gland Biol Neoplasia. 2002;7(3):225–52.

4. Goldmn AS. Evoluation of immune function of mammary gland and protection of the infant. Breastfeed Med. 2012;7(3):132–42. doi:10.1089/bfm.2012.0025. Epub 2012 May 11.
5. Williams P, Warwick R, Dyson M, Bannister L. Human development Gray's anatomy. 37th ed. 177, 611,612-1447-8 Churchill Livingstone; New York, 1989.
6. Gabriel A, Long JN, Maxwell GP, EDC Medscape breast embryology. Updated 25 July 2013.
7. Grossl NA. Supernumerary breast tissue: historical perspectives and clinical features. South Med J. 2000;93:29–32.
8. Loukas M, Clarke P, Tubbs RS. Accessory breasts: a historical and current perspective. Am Surg. 2007;73: 525–8.
9. Sadove AM, van Aalst JA. Congenital and acquired pediatric breast anomalies: a review of 20 years' experience. Plast Reconstr Surg. 2005;115(4): 1039–50.
10. Schmidt H. Supernumerary nipples: prevalence, size, sex and side predilection – a prospective clinical study. Eur J Pediatr. 1998;157:821–3.
11. Wieslander JB. Breastfeeding from mammary glands covered at the beginning of breast development by an expanded abdominal flap. Plast Reconstr Surg. 2012;129(4):754e–6.
12. Tapscott R. "Understanding breast "ironing": a study of the methods, motivations, and outcomes of breast flattening practices in Cameroon". Feinstein International Center (Tufts University); 2012.
13. Bayati S, Seckel BR. Inframammary crease ligament. Plast Reconstr Surg. 1995;95:501–8.
14. Garnier D, Angonin R, Foulon P, Chavoin JP, Ricbourg B, Costagliola M. The inframammary fold: myth or reality? Ann Chir Plast Esthet. 1991;36:313–9.
15. Morton DA, Foreman KB, Albertine KH, editors. Anterior thoracic wall. The big picture: gross anatomy. New York: McGraw-Hill; 2011.
16. Ramsay DT, Kent JC, Hartmann RA, Hartman PE. The anatomy of the lactating breast redefined with ultrasound imaging. Gland J Anat. 2005;206(6):525–34.
17. Muntan CD, Sundine MJ, Rink RD, Acland RD. Inframammary fold: a histologic reappraisal. Plast Reconstr Surg. 2000;105:549–56.
18. Nava M, Quattrone P, Riggio E. Focus on the breast fascial system: a new approach for inframammary fold reconstruction. Plast Reconstr Surg. 1998; 102:1034–45.
19. Jinde L, Jianliang S, et al. Anatomy and clinical significance of pectoral fascia. Plast Reconstr Surg. 2006;118(7):1557–60.
20. Schnitt SJ, Goldwyn R, Slavin SA. Mammary ducts in the areola: implication for patients undergoing reconstructive surgery of the breast. Plast Reconstr Surg. 1993;92(7):1290–3.
21. Cunningham L. The anatomy of the arteries and veins of the breast. J Surg Oncol. 1977;9:71–85.
22. Maliniac JW. Arterial blood supply of the breast. Arch Surg. 1943;47:329–43.
23. O'Dey D, Prescher A, Pallua N. Vascular reliability of nipple-areola complex-bearing pedicles: an anatomical microdissection stud. Plast Reconstr Surg. 2007; 119:1167–77.
24. Reid CR, Taylor GI. The vascular territory of the acromiothoracic axis. Br J Plast Surg. 1984;7:194–212.
25. Rosson GD, Holton LH, Silverman RP, Singh NK, Nahabedian MY. Internal mammary perforators: a cadaver study. J Reconstr Microsurg. 2005;21: 239–42.
26. Wuringer E. Refinement of the central pedicle breast reduction by application of the ligamentous suspension. Plast Reconstr Surg. 1999;103:1400–10.
27. Wuringer E, Mader N, Posche E, Holle J. Nerve and vessel supplying ligamentous suspension on the mammary gland. Plast Reconstr Surg. 1998;101:1486–93.
28. Wuringer E, Tschabitscher M. New aspects of the topographical anatomy of the mammary gland regarding its neurovascular supply along a regular ligamentous suspension. Eur J Morphol. 2002;40:181–9.
29. Batson OV. The function of the vertebral veins and their role in the spread of metastasis. Ann Surg. 1940;112(1):138–49. PMC1387927/.
30. Nakajima H, Imanishi N, Aiso S. Arterial anatomy of the nipple areola complex. Plast Reconstr Surg. 1995;96:843–5.
31. Suami H, Pan WR, Mann GB, Taylor GI. The lymphatic anatomy of the breast and its implications for sentinel lymph node biopsy: and human cadaver study. Ann Surg Oncol. 2008;15:863–71.
32. Van Deventer PV. The blood supply to the nipple-areola complex of the human mammary gland. Aesthet Plast Surg. 2004;28:393–8.
33. Estourgie SH, Nieweg OE, Olmos RA, Rutgers EJ, Kroon BB. Lymphatic drainage patterns from the breast. Ann Surg. 2004;239:232–7.
34. Munhoz AM, Aldrighi C. The influence of subfascial transaxillary breast augmentation in axillary drainage patterns and sentinel lymph node dissection. Ann Plast Surg. 2007;58(2):141–9.
35. Petrek JA, Blackwood MM. Axillary dissection: current practice and technique. Curr Probl Surg. 1995;32:259–323.
36. Romrell LJ, Bland KI. Anatomy of the breast, axilla, chest wall, and related metastatic sites. In: The breast: comprehensive management of benign and malignant diseases. Kirby I. Bland MD and Edward M. Copeland III MD (eds) 2nd ed. Philadelphia: WB Saunders Co, 2003.
37. Suami H, Shin D, Chang DW. Mapping of lymphosomes in canine forelimb: comparative anatomy between canine and humans. Plast Reconstr Surg. 2012;129(3):612–20.
38. Del Vecchyo C, Caloca Jr J, Caloca J, Gómez-Jauregui J. Evaluation of breast sensibility using dermatomal somatosensory evoked potentials. Plast Reconstr Surg. 2004;113:1975–83.
39. Farina MA, Newby BG, Alani HM. Innervation of the nipple-areola complex. Plast Reconstr Surg. 1980;66:497–501.
40. Hamdi M, Greuse M, Nemec E, Deprez C, De Mey A. Breast sensation after superior pedicle versus inferior pedicle mammaplasty: anatomical and histological evaluation. Br J Plast Surg. 2001;54:43–6.

41. Jaspars JJ, Posma AN, van Immerseel AA, Gittenberger-deGroot AC. The cutaneous innervation of the female breast and nipple-areola complex: implications for surgery. Br J Plast Surg. 1997;50:249–59.
42. Macchi V, Tiengo C, Porzionato A, Parenti A, Stecco C, Mazzoleni F, De Caro R. Medial and lateral pectoral nerves: course and branches. Clin Anat. 2007;20:157–62.
43. Terzis JK, Vincent MP, et al. Breast sensibility: a neurophysiological appraisal in the normal breast. Ann Plast Surg. 1987;19(4):318–22.
44. Robbins TH. Innervation of the nipple-areola complex. Plast Reconstr Surg. 1981;68:453.
45. Sarhadi NS, Shaw Dunn J, Lee FD, Soutar DS. An anatomical study of the nerve supply to the breast, including the nipple and areola. Br J Plast Surg. 1996;49:156–64.
46. Sarhadi NS, Shaw-Dunn J, Soutar DS. Nerve supply of the breast with special reference to the nipple and areola: Sir Astley Cooper revisited. Clin Anat. 1997;10:283–8.
47. Schlenz I, Kuzbari R, Gruber H, Holle J. The sensitivity of the nipple-areola complex: an anatomic study. Plast Reconstr Surg. 2000;105:905–9.
48. Schlenz I, Rigel S, Schemper M, Kuzbari R. Alteration of nipple and areola sensitivity by reduction mammaplasty: a prospective comparison of five techniques. Plast Reconstr Surg. 2005;115:743–51.
49. Spear SL, Hannan CM, Willey SC, Cocilovo C. Nipple -sparing mastectomy. Plast Reconstr Surg. 2009;123(6):1665–73.
50. Grim M. Ultrastructure of the ulnar portion of the contrahent muscle layer in embryonic human hand. Folia Morphol Praha. 1972;20:113–5.
51. Pillay M, Jacob SM. Bilateral presence of axillary arch muscle passing through the posterior cord of the brachial plexus. Int J Morphol. 2009;27(4):1047–50.
52. Paraskevas GK, Raikos A. Bilateral pectoral musculature malformations with concomitant vascular anomaly. Folia Morphol. 2010;69(3):187–91.
53. Poland A. Poland syndrome "deficiency of the pectoral muscles". Guys Hosp Rep. 1841;VI:191–3.
54. Spear SL, Pelletiere CV, Lee ES, Grotting JC. Anterior thoracic hypoplasia: a separate entity from Poland syndrome. Plast Reconstr Surg. 2004;113(1):69–77.
55. Akirci S, Kafa Mustafa I, Uysal M, Sendemir E. Langer's axillary arch (axillopectoral muscle): a variation of latissimus dorsi muscle a case report. Int J Anat Var. 2007;3:91–2.
56. Denti M, Facchini R, Peretti G. Partial aplasia of the pectoralis major muscle with an anomalous distal insertion: two case reports. J Pediatr Orthop. 1985;5:489–91.
57. Lama P, Potu BK, Bhat KM. Chondrohumeralis and axillary arch of Langer: a rare combination of variant muscles with unique insertion. Rom J Morphol Embryol. 2010;51(2):395–7.
58. Ucerler H, Ikiz ZA, Pinan Y. Clinical importance of the muscle arch of axilla (axillopectoral muscle Langer's axillary arch). Acta Chir Belg. 2005;105:326–8.
59. Kale SS, Hermann G, Kalimuthu R. Sternomastalis a variant of sternalis. Ann Plast Surg. 2006;56: 340–1.
60. Mehta V. Rectus thoracis bifurcalis: a new variant in the anterior chest wall musculature. Rom J Morphol Embryol. 2010;51(4):799 (Sternalis).
61. O'Neil MN, Folan-Curran J. Case report: bilateral sternalis muscles with a bilateral pectoralis major anomaly. J Anat. 1998;193:289–92 (Sternalis).
62. Pinhal-Enfield G, Varricchio P, DeFouw DO, Vasan NS. Sternalis muscle: importance of its awareness in chest imaging and clinical significance. Int J Anat Var. 2011;4:106–8.
63. Arican RY, Coskun N, Sarikcioglu L, Sindel M, Oguz N. Co-existence of the pectoralis quartus & pectoralis intermedius muscles. Morphologie. 2006;90(290):157–9.
64. Çilingir M, Malkoç C, Duman A, Eroglu S, Karacaoglan N. Microtia and pectoralis muscle agenesis. Plast Reconstr Surg. 2004;113(7):2222.
65. Clarkson P. Poland's syndactyly. Guys Hosp Rep. 1962;111:335–46.
66. Huber KM, Boyd TG, Quillo AR, Wilhelmi BJ. Implications of anomalous pectoralis muscle in reconstructive breast surgery: the oblique pectoralis anterior. Eplasty. 2012;12:e44. Epub 2012 Sep 10.
67. Loukas M, South G, Louis RG, Fogg QA, Davis T. A case of an anomalous pectoralis major muscle. Folia Morphol. 2006;65(1):100–3.
68. Rai R, Ranade AV, Prabhu LV, Prakash O, Rajanigandha V, Nayak SR. Unilateral pectoralis minimus muscle: a case report. Int J Morphol. 2008;26(1):27–9.
69. Soni S, Rath G, Suri R, Kumar H. Anomalous pectoral musculature. Anat Sci Int. 2008;83:310–3 (Pectoralis Minimus).
70. Longtaker MT, GLat PM, Colen LB, Siebert JW. Reconstruction of breast asymmetry in Poland's chest wall deformity using microvascular free flaps. Plast Reconstr Surg. 1997;99(2):429–36 [Medline].
71. Dibbell DG. Hypoplasia of the latissimus dorsi muscle complicating breast reconstruction in Poland syndrome. Ann Plast Surg. 1981;6(5):402–4 [Medline].
72. Palmer JH, Taylor GI. The vascular territories of the anterior chest wall. Br J Plast Surg. 1986;39: 287–99.

Breast Ultrasound: Diagnostic Imaging and Biopsy Techniques for the Office Practice

2

Richard E. Fine

Introduction

Breast ultrasound is not only an important breast imaging tool but also an integral part of the surgeon's management of a breast patient. The technologic advances in breast ultrasound systems over the past several decades have allowed this technology to take its place in the office setting and to be utilized for the real-time evaluation, diagnosis, and treatment of patients being seen for breast abnormalities. The modern surgeon has quickly adopted breast ultrasound as a "hands-on" technology, without deferring the performance of this important diagnostic modality to ultrasound technologists. The comfort with breast pathophysiology and a 3-dimensional intraoperative understanding of breast anatomy have also allowed for more aggressive utilization of breast ultrasound [1].

Doubts over the ability of surgeons performing both diagnostic and interventional breast ultrasound have been addressed. Whitehouse and colleagues showed a 96 % concordance between breast ultrasound performed by surgeons and radiologists [2]. Staren et al. performed 150 diagnostic ultrasounds on non-palpable, new or increasing size, mammogram-detected breast masses, with 97 patients undergoing diagnostic ultrasound only and 53 having an ultrasound-guided aspiration and/or biopsy. There were no false positives and no false negatives reported [3].

Breast sonography has been available for approximately 60 years [4]. In 1954, Wild and Reid first reported on their findings utilizing 1-dimensional, A-mode echography to visualize the human breast [5]. Dedicated equipment for breast ultrasound was not introduced until the 1970s [4]. Ultrasound technology continued to make remarkable advances, such as the availability of high-frequency, linear array, electronically focused transducers. Other advances included computer-enhanced imaging that has been directly responsible for the expanded indications for breast ultrasound that went well beyond its capacity to distinguish between a lesion's cystic and solid character [6–8]. Typical operating frequencies of 7.5–14 MHz allow the delineation of subtle characteristics to assist the clinician in determining the benign versus malignant nature of focal lesions [9–11]. Further advances now provide the ability to house the technology in smaller portable and affordable ultrasound systems, making today's ultrasound technology easily applicable to the surgeon's office setting.

Corresponding with improvements in the imaging technology and the development of portable or mobile ultrasound systems was the evolution of the spring-loaded core biopsy needles. This was quickly followed by the develop-

R.E. Fine, MD, FACS
Director of Education and Research, West Clinic Comprehensive Breast Center, 8000 Wolf River Blvd, Suite 100, Germantown, TN 38138, USA

Division of Oncology, Department of Surgery, University of Tennessee Health Science Center, College of Medicine, Memphis, TN, USA
e-mail: rfine@westclinic.com

A.I. Riker (ed.), *Breast Disease: Comprehensive Management*,
DOI 10.1007/978-1-4939-1145-5_2, © Springer Science+Business Media New York 2015

ment of the vacuum-assisted or rotating cutter biopsy devices capable of being utilized in the office setting. After assessing the probability of malignancy for a focal lesion, the need for ultrasound-guided intervention can be easily determined and performed [1]. Aspiration of a symptomatic cyst or biopsy of a highly suspicious, stellate mass can be performed with a minimally invasive ultrasound-guided approach with relative ease [1, 12–14].

The surgeon's increased comfort level with breast ultrasound as a diagnostic and intervention tool has now brought the technology into the operating room. Intraoperative ultrasound-guided localization techniques (with and without a localization device) are assisting the surgeon with both excision of non-palpable, ultrasound-visible malignant lesions and assessment of lumpectomy free margins [15–17]. Anything from percutaneous lesion removal to lesion ablation to placement of post-excision adjuvant treatments (such as brachytherapy catheters) can now be safely and effectively performed by surgeons, with the help of breast ultrasound. In fact, the interventional capability of breast ultrasound has become integral to the advancement of new technology [1].

In the mid-1990s, the national surgical community realized that surgeons seeing breast patients needed to incorporate the breast ultrasound technology into their practices. The American Society of Breast Surgeons (ASBS) and the American College of Surgeons (ACS) developed courses with hands-on workshops in order to further educate surgeons on the use of breast ultrasound. Subsequently, the ASBS developed a breast ultrasound certification program that allowed surgeons to demonstrate their ultrasound training, knowledge, and competence in utilizing breast ultrasound in the clinical setting for both diagnosis and intervention.

Scanning Techniques of Breast Ultrasound

The patient is typically positioned supine, in a contralateral oblique position with the ipsilateral arm abducted, with the hand placed above the head and a pillow positioned under the shoulder to help spread the breast evenly on the chest wall. Real-time ultrasound scanning allows for alterations in patient positioning such that patients with large, pendulous breasts may require a more decubitus position to view the lateral aspect of the breast [1]. Most often with office-based ultrasound, the surgeon performs a targeted diagnostic breast scan, concentrating upon only one-third to one-half of the breast in the region of the mammographic or clinical areas of concern [1].

In order to examine the entire breast with ultrasound, several scanning techniques have been developed. The radial scan, often referred to as "ductal echography," was first described by Teboul in 1988 [18]. By orienting the ultrasound transducer radially to the nipple-areola complex (i.e., parallel to the axis of the ducts), the normal architecture of the breast is visualized, allowing the examiner to view the full extent of the breast lobes and ducts. The standard image on the ultrasound monitor places the nipple in the upper left hand corner by convention. The radial scan begins at the nipple and moves out radially toward the periphery of the breast parenchyma. The pattern is repeated by moving around the nipple-areola complex corresponding to hours on the clock face. This way any part of the breast can be visualized with an identical anatomic orientation.

This technique is especially useful in performing whole breast scanning and may assist the neophyte in developing pattern recognition of the varying appearance of the normal breast anatomy in patients of different parity and quantity of fatty involution [1]. A more efficient method of scanning larger portions of the breast involves rotating the transducer 90° to the radial orientation and performing an anti-radial survey of the breast. This allows the scanner to cover larger portions of the breast at one time but sacrifices the anatomic orientation provided by the radial scanning technique. However, if an abnormality is visualized during an anti-radial scan, the transducer may then be rotated 90° into the radial orientation. This may be helpful in determining the extent of disease of a malignant lesion.

The transverse sweeping scan is another scanning technique utilized in a thorough examination of the breast or in searching for an abnormality with a targeted ultrasound examination. When a focal lesion is identified, it is typically documented with both a transverse and longitudinal scan (AIUM standards) [1]. Orientation of the monitor, by convention, places the patient's right on the left side of the ultrasound monitor in a transverse scan and the patient's head on the left side in a longitudinal or sagittal scan.

Scanning behind the nipple-areola complex (NAC) directly can be limited by the shadowing created due to the dense connective tissue and smooth muscle in this area. A tangential orientation of the ultrasound transducer adjacent to the areolar edge allows the retro-areolar region to be adequately visualized [1]. The surgeon may then utilize their non-scanning hand to manipulate the breast to allow the transducer face to maintain full contact with the skin, despite the tangential angle.

Sonographic Anatomy of the Breast

It is vital to become intimately familiar with the normal sonographic anatomy, including the skin, subcutaneous fat, and glandular tissue interspersed with Cooper's ligaments, as well as retroglandular fat, pectoral muscles, ribs, and pleura, in order to be proficient in both diagnostic and interventional breast ultrasound. The time-gain compensation curves are set to a uniform median-level echogenicity (gray) from the skin to the pectoral muscle [19]. The skin appears as a uniform, gray layer at the most superior aspect of the image followed by a bright white hyperechoic line which represents the interface separating the skin from the underlying subcutaneous fat below [19]. The subcutaneous tissue appears as a hypoechoic (darker) layer below the skin. Fat in the subcutaneous tissue and retromammary region or even areas of fatty involution within the breast parenchyma will have a similar echogenicity [19]. The glandular tissue below the subcutaneous fat appears as a similar echogenicity to the skin [19, 20] (Fig. 2.1).

Variation in the appearance of the glandular tissue is related to age and parity because of the amount of fatty tissue interspersed [20].

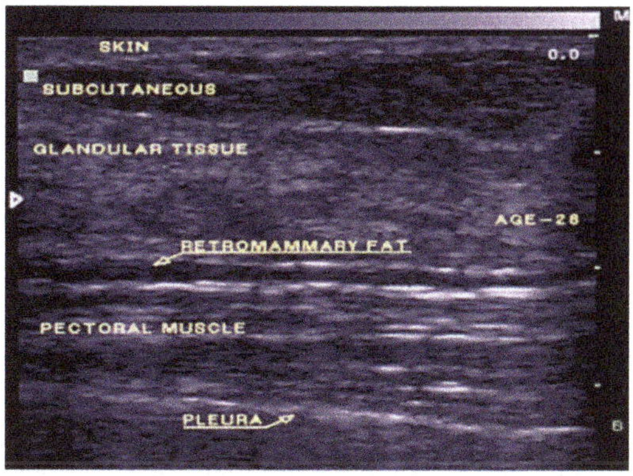

Fig. 2.1 Normal ultrasound breast anatomy in a younger patient with dense breast parenchyma

The younger patient may have very little fatty involution, and the glandular layer appears relatively uniform and dense. The postmenopausal patient with complete fatty involution may also have a uniform grayscale level of echogenicity similar to that seen with younger, dense glandular tissue. This uniform echogenic pattern may be difficult to distinguish from the glandular tissue without correlation with fatty-replaced mammogram [1, 21]. The postmenopausal breast allows the clearest depiction of the Cooper's ligaments as hyperechoic, curvilinear structures representing fibrous planes [1]. Occasionally, care must be taken to deal with an artifact of shadowing created by the convergence of Cooper's ligaments.

The partially involuted breast has a glandular appearance consisting of intermittent hypoechoic fatty lobules within dense glandular tissue. This sometimes creates the appearance of a pseudo-solid lesion that can be confirmed as a fat lobule by rotating the scan 90° and visualizing a blending of these fat lobules into the fatty parenchyma. The pectoral muscle appears as a relatively hypoechoic layer, occasionally with hyperechoic striations depending on the angle of the transducer with the muscle fibers. Again, the dynamic nature of real-time scanning allows the patient to flex the pectoral muscle for confirmation [1]. The rib appears as a hyperechoic curvilinear reflection with dense posterior shadowing. Beneath the pectoral muscle and ribs is a hyperechoic reflection that represents the pleura or interface with the lung parenchyma [19].

Sonographic Characteristics of Focal Lesions

There are a number of diagnostic criteria used to delineate the benign versus malignant characteristics of focal lesions. These criteria include margins, echogenicity, internal echo pattern, retrotumoral acoustic features, compressibility, and lateral to anterior-posterior dimension ratio [11, 20]. Margins that are smooth and well defined are used to contrast a probable benign lesion with a malignancy having jagged, indistinct margins. A solid lesion is usually hypoechoic to the surrounding glandular tissue with a homogeneous or uniform internal echo pattern more consistent with a benign abnormality [11].

When a lesion is without ultrasound echoes, it is referred to as anechoic. Though an anechoic interior is most commonly associated with a smooth-walled cyst, many malignancies are almost anechoic, but usually have a mixture of echogenicities to give a heterogeneous internal echo pattern. The internal echo pattern is one of the least specific characteristics delineating benign and malignant lesions. Complex cysts, abscesses, and other benign conditions may also have a nonhomogeneous internal echo pattern [1]. Homogeneity limits the amount of sound reflection within a focal abnormality and therefore allows greater sound transmission creating posterior enhancement, another criteria favoring a benign condition [19].

In contrast, the heterogeneity associated with malignant lesions will usually cause dense, irregular, posterior shadowing because of limited sound penetration and sound refraction. A more uniform refraction of sound, however, occurs in association with a smooth (probably benign) lesion. This type of refraction at the edges of smooth-walled lesions creates a symmetric pattern of shadowing known as bilateral edge shadowing [19]. The lateral to anterior-posterior ratio reflects the relationship of a lesion to the surrounding architecture. A malignant lesion is more likely to disrupt adjacent tissue planes growing perpendicular to the skin and muscle and therefore have an anterior-posterior dimension that is greater that the lateral dimension [1, 19]. A benign lesion grows in parallel with the tissue planes and has a lateral dimension greater that the anterior-posterior dimension.

Classification of Breast Lesions

Ultrasound characteristics of focal breast abnormalities help to place them within several categories including simple cysts, fibroadenomas (or benign fibrous nodules), indeterminate, and suspicious. Simple cysts are anechoic, well circumscribed, and thinly encapsulated, typically with posterior enhancement and often with thin edge shadows [11, 20, 22]. Fibroadenomas and benign fibrous nodules are hypoechoic, well-circumscribed lesions with a homogeneous, internal echo pattern; with a lateral to anterior-posterior dimension ratio greater than one; and with both posterior enhancement and bilateral edge shadowing [10, 11, 23]. The larger the fibroadenoma, the more likely it is to be associated with lobulations. Indeterminate lesions are usually hypoechoic with often sharp, smooth margins that may be somewhat indistinct [3, 20]. The internal echo pattern is variable and makes it difficult to distinguish the solid versus cystic nature of such lesions.

Complex cysts frequently fall into the indeterminate category. They have diffuse, low-level echoes as a result of blood, pus, or floating crystalline material and may require aspiration to distinguish them from solid lesions [3]. Movement of echoes within the lesion and compressibility may be demonstrated with real-time ultrasound imaging and, if cystic, may have posterior enhancement [1]. Suspicious breast lesions have indistinct, jagged margins; are almost anechoic; and have a heterogeneous interior, irregular posterior shadowing, and an anterior-posterior dimension greater than the lateral dimension [11, 20]. In a review of 662 consecutive patients undergoing 1,028 diagnostic breast ultrasounds, Staren et al. demonstrated an overall accuracy of greater than 90 % [17]. However, the decision to biopsy, or not biopsy, solid nodules cannot be based strictly on sonographic criteria because of these overlapping features.

Documenting Findings Using BI-RADS®

The American College of Radiology developed the BI-RADS® classification of mammographic abnormalities to improve the assessment of microcalcifications and masses. Management decisions based upon the BI-RADS® assessment have resulted in standardization of care after being incorporated into the Mammography Quality Standards Act of 1992. An ultrasound BI-RADS® classification has also been developed to better characterize sonographic breast abnormalities, including those with mammographic correlates. The need for standardization of lesion descriptors led the development of lexicons that have been incorporated into these reporting systems (Table 2.1). It is imperative to utilize this list of standard terms when describing ultrasound findings, to reduce variability among imagers and reports [24]. The ASBS has adopted the requirement for BI-RADS classification for ultrasound submissions to the ultrasound certification application.

Table 2.1 ACR breast ultrasound lexicon for BI-RADS reporting

BI-RADS®–US Lexicon	
The table below lists the terms which should be used when describing the sonographic finding. One descriptor from each category should be chosen	
Shape	Surrounding tissue
Oval	Duct changes
Round	Cooper's ligament changes
Irregular	Edema
	Architectural distortion
	Skin thickening
	Skin retraction/irregularity
Orientation	Posterior acoustic features
Parallel to skin	No features
Not parallel to skin	Enhancement
	Shadowing
	Combined pattern
Margin	Special cases
Circumscribed	Clustered microcysts
Non-circumscribed	Complicated cysts
Indistinct	Mass in or on skin
Angular	Foreign body
Microlobulated	Intramammary lymph nodes
Spiculated	Axillary lymph nodes
Lesion boundary	Calcifications
Abrupt interface	Macrocalcifications
Echogenic halo	Microcalcifications outside of a mass
	Microcalcifications within a mass
Echo pattern	Vascularity
Anechoic	Not present or not assessed
Hyperechoic	Present in lesion
Complex	Present adjacent to lesion
Hypoechoic	Increased in surrounding tissue
Isoechoic	

Adapted from ACR BI-RADS®–US Lexicon Classification Form, American College of Radiology 2003

BI-RADS®-US Assessment Categories[1]

Category 0

Incomplete:

Need Additional Imaging Evaluation: Further studies (i.e., mammography, MRI) are required before the evaluation is complete.

Category 1

Negative:

This category is for sonograms with no abnormality, such as a mass, architectural distortion, thickening of the skin, or microcalcifications. An attempt should be made to correlate the ultrasound location with the mammographic finding that necessitated the ultrasound.

Category 2

Benign Finding(s):

A report that is *negative for malignancy*. This can include benign findings such as simple cysts and intramammary lymph nodes. Fibroadenomas that have not changed in size can be included in this category.

Category 3

Probably Benign Finding: Short-interval follow-up is suggested.

This is a report that indicates a lesion that has a high chance of being benign, but does not fulfill all of the benign ultrasound characteristics. An example of this would be a solid mass with circumscribed margins, oval shape, and horizontal orientation, most likely a fibroadenoma, which would have a *less than 2 % risk of malignancy*. Generally, a 6-month follow-up is recommended.

Category 4

Suspicious Abnormality: Biopsy should be considered.

In this circumstance, the lesion is worrisome for malignancy based on the sonographic features. Lesions in this category would have an *intermediate probability of cancer, ranging from 3 to 94 %*. Category 4 can be further subdivided into a, b, or c with c being the highest risk of malignancy. However, all of these lesions require biopsy. Included in this group would be solid or cystic lesions that have some characteristics that make them suspicious, but not highly suggestive of malignancy.

Category 5

Highly Suggestive of Malignancy: Appropriate action should be taken.

The abnormality identified sonographically and placed in this category should have a *95 % or higher risk of malignancy*. These lesions require biopsy.

Category 6

Known Biopsy-Proven Malignancy

This is a lesion that has already been biopsied and proven to be cancer. An example would be on a lesion seen on ultrasound that already had undergone an MRI-guided biopsy.

[1]Adapted from ACR BI-RADS®–US American College of Radiology, 2003 [24].

Indications for Office-Based Breast Ultrasound

Though a surgeon traditionally has relied on the clinical breast examination to evaluate non-discrete palpable "lumps" or regions of nodularity, in the patient with a negative or nonspecific mammogram because of tissue density, breast ultrasound can often assist the surgeon in ruling out the presence of a focal suspicious lesion [25, 26]. By palpating the "lump" or clinical region of concern while scanning, a corresponding ridge of fibroglandular tissue can often be visualized as a homogeneous, isoechoic tissue pattern following the same contour found on physical exam [1]. When the physical examination reveals a discrete palpable abnormality, ultrasound is complementary to both the clinical and mammographic evaluation and helpful in determining the cystic versus solid nature of the lesion and directing further workup [3].

A diagnostic workup that includes breast ultrasound is very useful in evaluating mammographically indeterminate, non-palpable lesions presenting as discrete nodules, focal asymmetries, and areas of architectural distortion. Ultrasound is the primary imaging modality to establish if a discrete focal lesion on mammogram is a cystic or solid abnormality [6–8]. The determination of the fluid-filled nature of cysts as small as 2–3 mm, reaching an accuracy of 96–100 %, is easily accomplished with today's improved ultrasound technology [4, 6, 8]. With such lesions presenting as discrete nodules, ultrasound is the imaging modality of choice to differentiate cystic from solid abnormalities and also to distinguish a solid lesion's benign versus malignant nature. Areas of persistent asymmetry or architectural distortion after appropriate diagnostic focal compression mammography can be evaluated with ultrasound [4, 20, 21]. An area of asymmetry may only represent prominent fibroglandular tissue, but an underlying cystic or solid lesion may be further evaluated with ultrasound-guided intervention, depending on symptoms related to a simple cyst or the benign versus suspicious characteristics in the case of a solid lesion [1, 3, 20].

Diagnostic breast ultrasound is performed in the evaluation of younger patients [15] when mammography is less helpful and will assist the clinician in evaluating the patient who is pregnant or lactating when mammography is contraindicated [27]. The increase in water tissue density provides a favorable acoustic condition. Ultrasound may assist in the evaluation of mastitis and detection of underlying abscess formation where mammography is difficult secondary to pain and edema and may not demonstrate an abscess due to inflammation [28]. Ultrasound may guide aspiration or drainage techniques to provide nonoperative management of those ultrasound-identified breast abscesses [1, 29].

Postoperative oncologic follow-up for both mastectomy and breast conservation may be aided by evaluation with ultrasound. A palpable nodule of the chest wall may be visualized and assessed for depth of penetration, and then ultrasound may be used to guide a fine-needle aspiration or core needle biopsy for diagnosis [30]. After breast conservation surgery, there is a loss of the typical breast anatomy with an increase in tissue density that allows for evaluation and/or intervention of the lumpectomy site for evidence of recurrent disease [1]. Ultrasound is useful for postoperative follow-up for both benign and malignant diseases, including monitoring and management of seromas and hematomas [20, 30, 31].

The accuracy of intervention and tracking the pathway of a needle under real-time imaging may allow for the safe biopsy of a suspicious lesion in a patient who has undergone elective augmentation mammoplasty [32]. The axilla may be scanned for preoperative staging of the patient with a known or obvious breast cancer [1, 30]. Assessment of the axillary region for recurrent disease is aided by the enhanced imaging condition created by a decrease in fatty tissue postaxillary surgery. Ultrasound is also useful in guiding a biopsy of a pathologic-appearing lymph node in a patient with an unremarkable breast evaluation [1].

Ultrasound may assist in the workup of the patient with a pathologic nipple discharge. Considered by many radiologists to be the method of choice for evaluating nipple discharge, performing a ductogram is limited by the necessity of reproducing the discharge from a duct so that it can be successfully cannulated. Ultrasound evaluation of the ducts may be accomplished with the technique of duct echography, performed in a radial fashion, maintaining the ultrasound transducer in alignment with the ducts. By identifying a dilated, fluid-filled duct and in some cases an intraluminal filling defect or lesion responsible for the discharge, localization can be successfully performed to direct mammary duct evaluation and management [3, 20, 21]. In terms of overall cost, ultrasound is a much less expensive alternative to breast MRI in evaluating silicone breast implants for rupture or leak. Though MRI is considered by many as the standard diagnostic study of choice for identifying subtle leaks, ultrasound can often detect obvious rupture or leakage with improved cost-effective efficiency [33].

Breast ultrasound screening had historically been used more commonly in several European countries despite the prior lack of any randomized controlled trials to evaluate the impact of screening on breast cancer mortality [1, 20, 21]. Several studies have indicated that whole breast sonography as an adjunct to screening mammography may depict small, non-palpable cancers not seen on mammogram, especially when the breast tissue is dense [34, 35]. In the ACRIN 6666 trial, 2,809 women determined to be at high risk for breast cancer at 21 different site were enrolled to compare mammography screening alone to mammography plus physician-performed screening ultrasound. Berg and colleagues found that adding a single screening ultrasound found 28 % more cancers compared to mammography alone. However, the combined screening strategy led to four times the number of false positives [36]. Patients with a strong family history, a radiographically dense breast tissue, and a difficult clinical breast examination due to extensive nodularity may benefit from whole breast ultrasound [24, 25]. Whole breast ultrasound may also be useful in following the patient with multiple known sonographic lesions and to exclude multicentric malignancy when breast conservation is an option for a known malignancy [1]. Finally, ultrasound is used as the imaging modality to guide minimally invasive percutaneous aspirations, biopsies, localization procedures, and even nonoperative potentially therapeutic modalities [1, 20, 37].

Office-Based Ultrasound-Guided Intervention

Each year in the United States, women undergo an increasing number of biopsies required for the definitive diagnosis of image-detected abnormalities. Fortunately, a greater proportion of these biopsies are amenable to minimally invasive image-guided needle biopsies. The most recent International Consensus Conference on diagnosis and treatment of image-detected breast cancer once again reconfirmed that minimally invasive image-guided percutaneous breast biopsy should be the first-line intervention for both palpable and non-palpable image-detected abnormalities [38].

Image-guided percutaneous breast biopsy should eliminate the need for open surgical biopsy for diagnosis. Unfortunately, the proportion of open surgical biopsies remains high. Clark-Pearson found the average rate of open biopsy among surgeons at their institution to be 36 % [39]. This finding was disappointing as the integration of the image-guided needle biopsy approach found to be less invasive and more cost effective has been accomplished without sacrificing diagnostic accuracy [1, 37]. If image-guided needle biopsy results are benign, the patient requires no further intervention, monitored with only appropriate imaging and clinical follow-up; however, if diagnosed with breast cancer by image-guided percutaneous biopsy, the patient will proceed to definitive surgical management.

Indications for Intervention

Cysts

When diagnostic ultrasound identifies a cyst that meets all the benign criteria of a simple cyst (anechoic, smooth margins with posterior enhancement) and it is asymptomatic, no further intervention is required as there is essentially no risk of malignancy [1, 3, 37]. Enlarging, symptomatic cysts are a common indication for ultrasound-guided intervention [13, 37]. Even if palpable, direct visualization of the procedure accurately positions the needle in the lesion, ensuring complete collapse of the cyst and documenting the procedure.

Ultrasound guidance, of course, allows access to non-palpable cysts. Aspiration is easily performed with a 20–25-gauge, 1½-in. needle with either a vacutainer or syringe holder system [40]. Ultrasound-guided cyst aspiration may also resolve the issue of those indeterminate lesions that represent complex cysts (indistinct margins, heterogeneous internal echo pattern, and irregular septations). Aspiration of thick, paste-like contents, frequently associated with mammary duct ectasia, may require local anesthesia and the use of larger, 18- to 14-gauge needles [40]. Cytologic evaluation of aspirated fluid is reserved for bloody fluid or lack of cyst resolution [41].

Indeterminate Breast Abnormalities

Most patients with an indeterminate, image-detected, palpable or non-palpable breast abnormality recommended for biopsy should undergo minimally invasive image-guided percutaneous needle core biopsy. The modalities for image guidance include ultrasound, stereotactic, or MRI guidance. The choice of image guidance is dependent upon the modality of detection, the lesion type, and the tissue density of the breast parenchyma. The most common indication for ultrasound-guided percutaneous biopsy is the indeterminate or suspicious, ultrasound-visible, solid mass. However, some solid masses are better visualized on mammography because of a large fatty-replaced breast parenchyma where stereotactic guidance would be preferable.

The usual approach for the patient with mammogram-detected microcalcifications without a mass is with stereotactic-guided, percutaneous needle biopsy. However, rarely, with the advent of high-end, high-resolution ultrasound equipment, a prominent cluster of indeterminate calcifications can be biopsied with ultrasound guidance. Performing a second-look, directed ultrasound on a patient with an MRI-detected enhancing mass lesion will identify a lesion amenable to ultrasound guidance about 60 % of the time. The advantages of ultrasound guidance over other imaging modalities include patient comfort, lying supine (as opposed to prone with neck extension on the stereotactic table), and availability of ultrasound as an office-based procedure, minimizing costs and scheduling delays [1, 40, 42].

The presence of a non-palpable, solid mass is an indication for an ultrasound-guided needle core biopsy to obtain a histologic diagnosis. It is also appropriate to utilize ultrasound guidance for the solid, palpable mass according to the ASBS Position Statement on Image-Guided Percutaneous Biopsy of Palpable Breast Lesions (January 29, 2001) [43]. Without the adjunct of image guidance, the surgeon would be unable to confirm the proper penetration of the core needle through the lesion or the alignment of the tissue-sampling portion of a vacuum-assisted or rotating core device, leading to false-negative results.

The surgeon should categorize these abnormalities based on their risk of malignancy. Smooth, well-defined margins suggest that a lesion is benign, whereas irregular, indistinct margins suggest a malignancy. Heterogeneous internal echo pattern implies malignancy, while benign lesions usually display homogeneity. Posterior enhancement represents transmission of sound through the lesion related to lesion homogeneity and causes a brighter echo pattern behind the lesion, which is usually benign. The heterogeneous nature of many cancers will cause haphazard sound refraction, which leads to irregular shadowing. However, bilateral edge shadows are consistent with a smooth-walled benign lesion. Finally, benign lesions tend to be wider than they are tall (width greater than anterior-posterior diameter). In contrast, cancers tend to disrupt the adjacent normal tissue planes and appear taller than they are wide. Familiarity of these characteristics will help the surgeon anticipate the diagnosis. Any discordance between the image analysis and the pathology results will require a complete excision of the lesion [1, 40, 42].

Non-cystic lesions requiring intervention can be categorized based on their risk of malignancy [1, 17]. Hypoechoic, well-circumscribed lesions, with a homogeneous internal echo pattern, with a transverse diameter greater than its longitudinal dimension, and perhaps with posterior enhancement and bilateral edge shadowing would be considered "low-risk" lesions [3, 10, 20]. If an ultrasound-guided biopsy confirms a benign histology, the lesion may be safely monitored. For the very small (less than 5–6 mm), solid, hypoechoic lesion with completely benign features such as smooth margins, homogeneous internal echoes, bilateral edge shadows, and ellipsoid shape, ultrasound-guided needle biopsy can confirm a benign diagnosis. Others surgeons with experience in ultrasound interpretation and pathologic correlation may choose to monitor the lesion, especially with a highly compliant patient [1, 40, 42].

The "indeterminate-risk" lesions often have indistinct and lobulated yet smooth margins and a lateral to anterior-posterior dimension ratio greater than one, and often they will have heterogeneous interiors. If a surgeon cannot characterize a lesion as a simple cyst, aspiration to distinguish a complex cyst from a solid mass is required. A lesion with a mixed internal echo pattern and posterior enhancement suggests the presence of fluid versus a solid lesion, and an aspiration may be preferable, prior to a core biopsy. Another indeterminate lesion requiring intervention is the cystic-appearing lesion with a mural lesion or solid-appearing component. The risk of possible malignancy of 10–15 % must be resolved with histologic sampling [20, 21]. Only resolution of a complex cyst or a specific benign diagnosis on percutaneous needle biopsy will avoid surgical excision.

Suspicious Breast Abnormalities

The remaining "high-risk" lesions have suspicious focal ultrasound criteria such as jagged, indistinct margins, a nonhomogeneous interior, a posterior shadowing, and a lateral to anterior-posterior dimension ratio less than one, due to disruption of adjacent architectural planes. Confirmation of the malignant diagnosis obtained with ultrasound-guided biopsy in a cost-effective, efficient manner in the office setting is preferred to facilitate planning the definitive management [1, 20].

Confirmation of the histology eliminates an initial operating room procedure for diagnosis and may limit returns to the operating room for positive resection margins. Encountering positive margins is twice as frequent at definitive surgery if not preceded by an image-guided percutaneous biopsy to confirm the malignant diagnosis. Patients that may be candidates for neoadjuvant or preoperative chemotherapy will ideally be diagnosed with image-directed percutaneous biopsy. The core needle biopsy tissue provides many of the ancillary markers required for appropriate management (estrogen/progesterone receptors, Ki-67 proliferative index, and Her-2/neu status).

Pre-procedure Planning

Consistency in successful interventional ultrasound-guided procedure begins with pre-procedure information and planning. Taking an appropriate history, which includes an assessment of risk factors for breast cancer, and performing a clinical breast exam are essential. Anticoagulant medications can lead to bleeding complications, including significant hematomas. Patient anxiety related to a significant risk profile such as a strong family history might lower the threshold to perform an image-guided percutaneous biopsy on a lesion of relatively low malignant potential. The clinical breast examination correlates any palpable mass and the image-detected abnormality. The diagnostic ultrasound exam should be interpreted in complement to any additional imaging available such as mammogram or MRI. Careful evaluation of the diagnostic ultrasound performed at an outside institution may suggest lesion characteristics, such as posterior enhancement, that allows the physician to attempt a cyst aspiration and eliminate the unnecessary wasting of an expensive disposable biopsy tool for a presumed solid lesion.

The benefits and risks of an ultrasound-guided percutaneous breast biopsy are reviewed, and the patient signs an appropriate consent. The physician should emphasize to the patient that the image-guided percutaneous procedures is a diagnostic procedure and that further surgical or non-surgical intervention may still be necessary depending upon the concordance between the pathology and the imaging findings. If the benign pathology fully correlates with the ultrasound findings, then it is not necessary for the surgeon to remove the lesion, whether palpable or non-palpable. The patient must also be comfortable with the reassurance of a benign diagnosis, without removal of the suspect lesion.

An image-guided percutaneous biopsy would be inadvisable for the patient who desires complete removal of the lesion, especially when it is palpable. This is a fairly common situation in the younger patient who presents with a solid, palpable mass and has the ultrasound characteristics of a fibroadenoma. More often than not, the discussion with the patient usually ends with a desire to have the mass completely removed. It is important that the patient understands that the breast abnormality may remain on future imaging and continue to be palpable after an image-guided needle biopsy, unless percutaneous excision is planned.

Ultrasound-guided percutaneous excision is an alternative to open surgical excision for those patients who desire the removal of their lesions, especially when palpable, despite being well informed. The surgeon may accomplish percutaneous excision with vacuum-assisted biopsy devices that are capable of removing sequential core samples of tissue with a single insertion of the device into the breast. The procedure may be both therapeutic and diagnostic in a single setting. Percutaneous management of benign lesions has several benefits. In addition to avoiding the disadvantages of the surgical approach, the patient avoids the physical and emotional trauma and added cost. Further indications for percutaneous excision with ultrasound guidance include, but are not limited to, the following:

- Nonoperative potential therapy for benign lesions which may accomplish removal of image evidence and/or palpability of the lesion such as clinically apparent fibroadenomas in younger patients
- A palpable lipoma causing location-related discomfort or pain (inframammary fold)

With ultrasound-guided percutaneous excision, it should be pointed out that a small percentage of lesions would either not be successfully removed in their entirety or will again be visualized on the follow-up imaging studies. Finally, the surgeon should avoid a percutaneous image-guided biopsy if surgical excision of the target lesion were part of the definitive management. This sometimes occurs when the suspected pathology result would not be acceptable without excision, such as a subareolar lesion with or without associated nipple discharge. Complete excision would be recommended due to the possibility of a papillary lesion that is present whereby the pathologist will require the intact specimen in its entirety in order to confirm the diagnosis, while eliminating any associated atypia or a papillary carcinoma [42].

Image-Guided Minimally Invasive Breast Biopsy Devices

The physician performing the ultrasound-guided percutaneous biopsy must decide on the proper device or instrument that best accomplishes the goal of the procedure. The most important objective for any image-guided biopsy procedure is to obtain the correct diagnosis (benign versus malignant). The tools for specimen acquisition have evolved from fine-needle aspiration cytology to automated Tru-Cut® core needles providing histology. Further advancements of vacuum-assisted and rotational core technology, available with ultrasound guidance, allow for tissue acquisition with either multiple insertions of the device or a single device insertion allowing multiple tissue samples. Either approach provides adequate "sampling" capability for diagnosis for most lesions or therapeutic "removal" (by percutaneous excisional biopsy) capability for selected lesions. Understanding similarities and differences in the current technology enables the surgeon to select the most appropriate device and application.

The minimum requirement for ultrasound-guided biopsy of "indeterminate" or "high-risk" lesions is cytologic or histologic confirmation of a malignancy. Fine-needle aspiration biopsy (FNA) of solid masses has received considerable criticism, especially in the United States, related to the degree of insufficient sampling and the need for expert cytopathology [41]. Despite such criticisms, FNA is a quick and inexpensive technique to delineate benign from malignant solid breast masses. The sensitivity and specificity are affected not only by expert cytopathology evaluation but also by who is performing the FNA technique. It should be noted that many community surgeons that participate in managed care organizations may be limited to only certain choices of technique and pathology labs for specimen evaluation. Despite these limitations, in experienced hands, ultrasound-guided FNA can delineate benign from malignant solid breast masses.

Fornage and colleagues demonstrated a sensitivity of 97 % and a specificity of 91 % after evaluating 355 breast masses with ultrasound-guided FNA biopsy [12]. Gordon et al. confirmed the diagnosis of malignancy with ultrasound-guided FNA biopsy in 213 of 225 cases, yielding a sensitivity of 95 % and specificity of 92 % [44]. The majority of false-negative findings in this series (6 of 12) were lobular carcinoma, known to be difficult to diagnose with FNA due to the paucity of shed cells available for collection by aspiration. In addition to cytologic confirmation of malignancy of a "high-risk" lesion, ultrasound-guided FNA is frequently used to evaluate lesions in areas where more invasive biopsy devices may be difficult or dangerous, such as the axilla or adjacent to a breast implant [1, 32]. The diagnosis of lymph node metastasis by FNA can assist with preoperative staging, such as the consideration of neoadjuvant chemotherapy [45] or eliminating sentinel lymph node biopsy for pathologically involved lymph nodes. An adequately performed FNA provides ample cells in order to perform hormone receptor studies [46].

The limitations of FNA are essentially eliminated with the use of an automated, large-core needle biopsy, especially for "high-risk" lesions [1, 3, 20]. Histologic type and grade of a diagnosed cancer can be adequately determined with core histology, in contrast to FNA cytology which rarely provides sufficient tissue [14, 47]. Staren et al. reduced the initial false-negative rate obtained with ultrasound-guided FNA from 20 to 3.6 % using ultrasound-guided, 14-gauge core biopsies in 210 patients with a non-palpable, mammographically detected lesion [48]. There were no false positives, and no cancers were detected after a median follow-up of 18 months in the patients with a benign diagnosis.

The automated needles used to perform a core biopsy are available in a variety of lengths, gauges (12–16), and forward throw (1–2.3 cm). Some core needle devices are completely disposable, while others utilize disposable needles only within a more permanent, reusable housing device. The mechanism of tissue acquisition is similar with the automated forward movement of an inner cannula with a sampling notch. This is immediately followed by utilization of an outer sheath that cuts and samples the tissue. Two-phase firing action is accomplished under direct ultrasound visualization. The 14-gauge spring-loaded core biopsy needle has been the most common device for ultrasound-guided percutaneous biopsy device of solid lesions. It has been utilized since the mid-1990s and remains the most commonly used device for ultrasound-guided core "sampling," in particular for the larger, easily targeted suspicious masses requiring diagnosis only.

The accuracy of ultrasound needle core biopsy has been widely documented. Parker et al. found no subsequent cancers in 132 lesions with a benign diagnosis obtained by ultrasound-guided core needle biopsy [14]. Eventually, an updated report of a larger, multicenter, image-guided biopsy series (stereotactic and ultrasound guided) showed 15 false-negative cases out of 280 benign lesions diagnosed by core biopsy, with most representing a biopsy of microcalcifications [49]. The false-negative rate for ultrasound-guided needle core biopsy of solid masses was 1.4 %.

A specific benign diagnosis such as fibroadenoma, which is concordant with the radiologic imaging, does not require further intervention. The patient is placed into an appropriate follow-up protocol, such as a 6-month follow-up with mammogram and/or ultrasound [14]. A diagnosis of cancer provides the information necessary to plan definitive therapy. Once the diagnosis of breast cancer is obtained, the surgeon may alter the lumpectomy technique to improve the chances that clear pathologic margins will be obtained at the initial surgical setting. Whitten et al. achieved a tumor-free margin rate of 71 % when the initial lumpectomy followed an image-guided biopsy diagnosis. This is compared with only 35 % free margins when the initial diagnostic procedure for diagnosis was an open surgical (needle localization) biopsy [50]. Excision is necessary also for cytologic atypia, because of the significant number of cancers that are identified in association with these pathologic changes [16]. Excision of a lesion will also follow an ultrasound-guided needle core biopsy if medical judgment dictates because sample quality is inadequate or poor or there is suspected discordant pathology.

There has been an evolution of biopsy technology over the last decade in order to address both real and perceived problems associated with image-guided needle core breast biopsy tissue acquisition. Despite accurate histology with spring-loaded core needles, specimens that are more substantial, obtained with the larger, vacuum-assisted/rotational core devices, offer advantages. During the 1990s, several publications brought to light the problem of "upgrading" the diagnosis, specifically with regard to the biopsy of microcalcifications [16, 51, 52]. Stereotactically guided 14-gauge needle core biopsy was found to significantly underestimate the diagnosis of cancer. A diagnosis of atypical ductal hyperplasia (ADH) is upgraded to ductal carcinoma in situ (DCIS) on excision in 33–50 % of cases, and DCIS is upgraded to invasive carcinoma in up to 20 % of cases [16, 51, 52].

Development of the first directional, vacuum-assisted biopsy (VAB) device, Mammotome®

Breast Biopsy System (Ethicon Endo-Surgery, Inc., Cincinnati, OH), satisfied the requirement of increasing the size of the core samples obtained. Furthermore, the contiguous nature of the sampling provided a sufficient solution to the issue of diagnostic upgrading seen with stereotactic biopsy of microcalcifications. By applying suction through small holes in the notch of the probe's outer cannula, the VAB pulls the tissue down into the sampling notch. A rotating inner cannula advances forward to cut the tissue free from inside the breast. When the sampling notch is closed and the tissue captured, the inner cannula stops rotating and the front vacuum ceases.

By maintaining a constant vacuum at the back end of the inner cannula shaft, the tissue is pulled down into the inside of the biopsy probe by the reverse movement of the inner cannula. The tissue is then delivered into the collection chamber for retrieval without removing the biopsy probe from the breast. The position of the sampling notch is rotated to obtain each additional tissue core. The sampling pattern is varied in accordance with the type of lesion being sampled, the extent of sampling the operator desires, and the alignment of the lesion with the sampling notch.

In removing larger tissue samples in a more contiguous fashion, VAB technology successfully addressed the underestimation of disease [51] but also provided several other advantages. These include:

- Removal of multiple samples without the need to remove the device from the breast
- Ability to inject local anesthesia directly through the biopsy device
- Eliminating the need for pinpoint accuracy because of the ability of the vacuum to pull the lesion toward the device and the ability to directionally sample
- Ability to place a marker (clip) through the device directly into the biopsy site

There are currently two additional directional, side-cutting, VAB devices that offer the same advantages as the Mammotome®, the Automated Tissue Excision and Collection (ATEC®) Breast Biopsy and Excision System (Hologic, Inc., Bedford, MA) and the EnCor™ (Bard Biopsy Systems, Tempe, AZ).

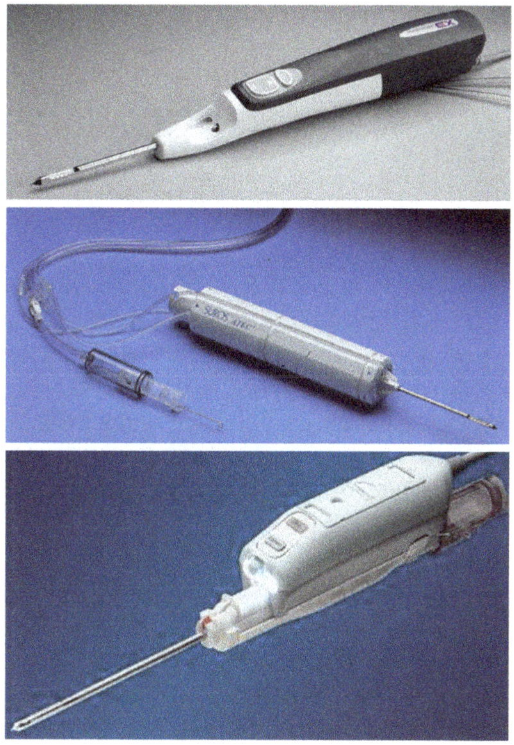

Fig. 2.2 Ultrasound-guided vacuum-assisted biopsy devices; (*top to bottom*) Mammotome® (Cincinnati, OH), the Automated Tissue Excision and Collection (ATEC®) Breast Biopsy and Excision System (Hologic, Inc., Bedford, MA), and the EnCor™ (Bard Biopsy Systems, Tempe, AZ)

Vacuum-assisted technology was subsequently adopted for ultrasound-guided biopsy procedures with similar concerns in mind, such as reducing physician error associated with multiple reinsertions and repositioning of the core biopsy needle [53–55] (Fig. 2.2). The directional capability with the ultrasound-guided VAB devices is helpful in dealing successfully with deep target lesions because the physician positions the device below the lesion and directs the sampling superiorly, away from the chest wall or an implant. Manually inserting the device without having to utilize a "firing" mechanism could help deal with the deep lesion, avoiding the risks of penetrating the pectoral muscle or implant. Compared to samples obtained with the 14-gauge, spring-loaded needle core device, the samples obtained are considerably larger.

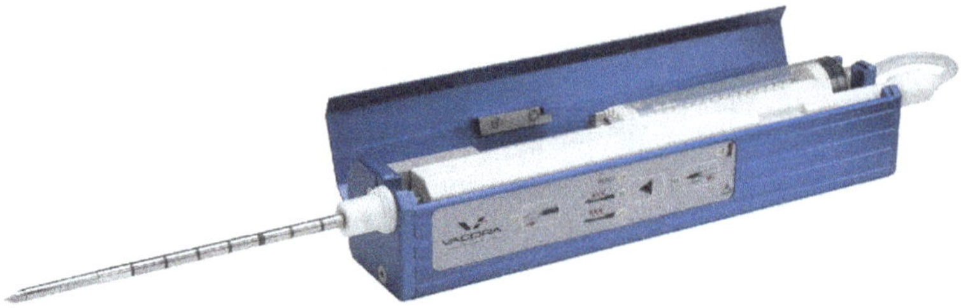

Fig. 2.3 Vacora™ Breast Biopsy System (Bard Biopsy Systems, Tempe, AZ)

Ultrasound-guided vacuum-assisted biopsy is indicated for any indeterminate ultrasound-visible, palpable or non-palpable solid mass. It may be especially helpful in obtaining a tissue diagnosis of small (<1 cm) masses that tend to be more difficult to perform with needle core biopsy. These smaller, solid lesions will more often return with a nonspecific benign diagnosis (e.g., stromal fibrosis) as opposed to fibroadenomas. By using a vacuum-assisted biopsy device to remove larger tissue samples and perhaps remove the majority of the lesion visualized, the follow-up dilemma of this mildly discordant pathology is resolved.

Other currently available devices designed to remove larger core samples, utilizing either vacuum or a rotating cutter, include EnCor 360™ (formerly the SenoCor 360; SenoRx), Celero™ spring-loaded handheld breast biopsy devices (Hologic, Inc., Bedford, MA), and Vacora™ Breast Biopsy System (Bard Biopsy Systems, Tempe, AZ) (Fig. 2.3). These devices require less capital expense than the Mammotome, ATEC, or EnCor while providing the diagnostic advantage of being able to capture larger tissue specimens. They require reinsertion for each core sample and do not generally provide percutaneous excisional capability.

An additional larger core device, utilizing a rotating cutter, the Flash™ (Encapsule Medical, Redwood City, CA), provides a single-insertion, multi-sample device in a self-contained disposable unit employing a closed collection chamber and requires no capital cost (Fig. 2.4).

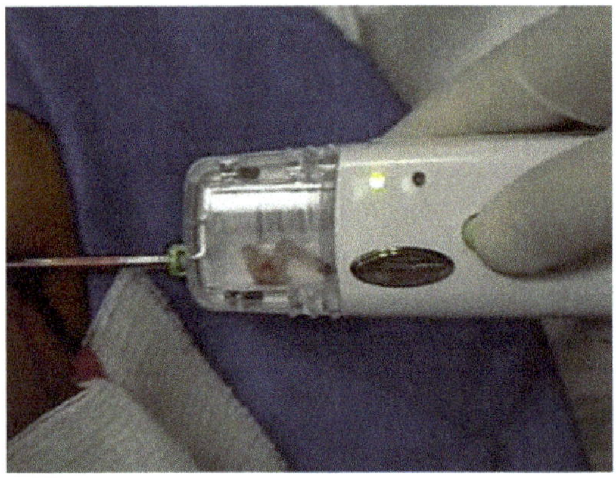

Fig. 2.4 Flash™ (Encapsule Medical, Redwood City, CA); the cores are visualized real time in the collection chamber of this single-insertion multi-sample device

The indications for ultrasound-guided VAB or rotational cutter devices are similar to those for needle core biopsy, including any indeterminate, ultrasound-visible, palpable or non-palpable solid mass. If the physicians were interested in percutaneous excision, single-insertion, multi-sample, side-cutting VAB devices would be required. These devices have successfully demonstrated their ability to remove image evidence and especially palpability of probably benign solid masses [56].

False-negative rates with the ultrasound-guided vacuum-assisted biopsy range from 0 to 2.7 % [53, 54]. The sensitivity ranges from 95 to 97 % and the specificity from 98 to 100 %, with a reported complication rate of 2–8 % (hematoma and infection) [55]. Several factors affect the success of an ultrasound-guided vacuum-assisted biopsy procedure, including less than optimal positioning of the patient, physician, and equipment along with improper positioning of the biopsy probe aperture with the lesion.

"Low"- to "intermediate"-risk lesions can be adequately addressed with the use of ultrasound-guided aspiration to resolve complex cysts and ultrasound-guided needle core biopsy or VAB for diagnosing solid masses. The majority of low- and often many intermediate-risk solid masses will turn out to be fibroadenomas or benign fibrous nodules [1, 17]. If the results of the biopsy are specific and concordant and the patient desires, the lesion can be left in place without further intervention.

Whether justified or not, many women still have concerns about leaving a benign lesion in their breast. For such patients, there are nonoperative approaches for their removal. Reasons to consider nonoperative therapy include removing the image evidence of the lesion, removing the palpability of the lesion, and avoiding histologic heterogeneity of a benign lesion with sampling [57]. With an expected benign diagnosis, devices that permit the percutaneous multi-core excision of even larger lesions are ideal when the patient wants it removed entirely. The Mammotome, ATEC, and EnCor are capable of removing all imaged evidence or palpability of a lesion (percutaneous excisional biopsy), such as a benign fibroadenoma.

Several published studies have indicated the ability of vacuum-assisted biopsy with stereotactic or ultrasound guidance to provide complete lesion removal in addition to accurate diagnosis [51, 53, 55, 56]. Fine et al. reported on the use of a vacuum-assisted handheld device with ultrasound guidance to remove low-risk palpable breast masses [56]. This was a multicenter, nonrandomized study using both the 11-gauge and 8-gauge handheld Mammotome™ (Ethicon Endo-Surgery, Cincinnati, OH) for removal of benign masses up to 3 cm in size. The initial report of 124 patients showed 88 % of the lesions had benign pathology (fibroadenomas = 70 %) with complete removal of the image lesion in the immediate post-biopsy assessment to be 99 % with the 8-gauge device and 96 % with the 11-gauge device. After further accrual to 216 patients, 73 % had no ultrasound evidence of the original mass and 98 % had no palpability of the original mass. None of the patients needed to undergo additional diagnostic or therapeutic procedures. The results of this series and others indicated that ultrasound-guided vacuum-assisted biopsy allows for diagnostic accuracy as well as therapeutic management with complete excision with regard to lesion palpability.

There are no specific studies that provide an explanation for the residual image evidence at 6 months of lesions initially considered to be completely excised at the time of the initial biopsy. It may be related to difficulty of accurately assessing complete removal at the time of biopsy secondary to tissue, fluid, and blood in the biopsy cavity. In addition, as the biopsy proceeds and the abnormality becomes smaller, the remaining pieces are difficult to visualize with real-time ultrasound. Another theory involves regrowth of these lesions from the residual tissue left behind as the excision is performed in a piecemeal fashion.

Performing Ultrasound-Guided Intervention

Positioning

Successful performance of an interventional ultrasound-guided procedure begins with proper positioning of the patient with optimization of the ultrasound machine. The patient should be positioned, as with diagnostic scanning, supine with a pillow placed under the shoulder and the ipsilateral arm raised above the head [1, 20, 40, 42]. Using a pillow under the shoulder allows the breast to disperse more evenly on the chest wall decreasing the thickness of the breast parenchyma in the region of concern. This contralateral oblique position facilitates propping the patient at an appropriate angle for access to lateral lesions. Additionally, keeping the biopsy device parallel with the pectoral muscle allows for safe access to more posterior (deeper) lesions. The position of the physician in relation to the ultrasound equipment is the key to visualization and comfort while performing a procedure. Standing directly across from the ultrasound prevents the surgeon from needing to turn their head away from the biopsy field in order to see the ultrasound monitor. It also allows for the optimal visualization of the advancing biopsy needle, along a straight line of sight down the physician's

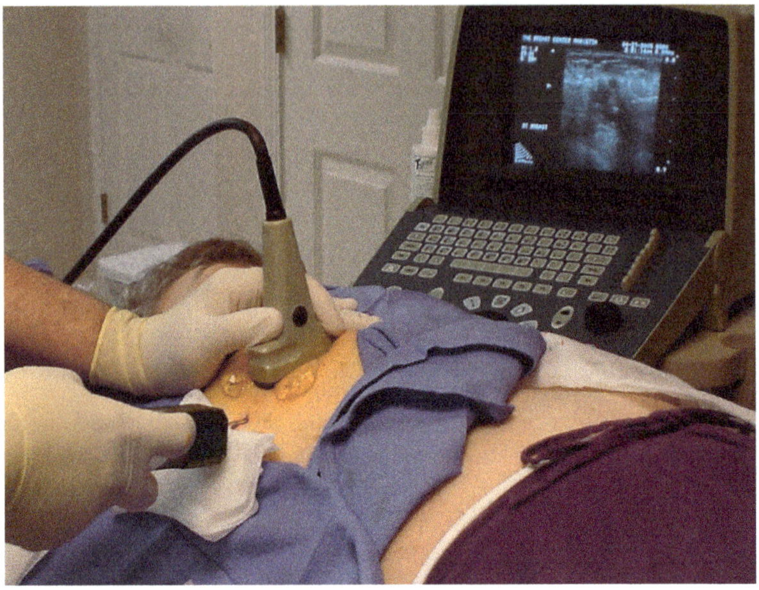

Fig. 2.5 Positioning of the physician, patient, and equipment for optimal success in ultrasound-guided intervention

arm holding the breast biopsy device, across the breast, and straight up to the ultrasound monitor (Fig. 2.5).

Optimization of the Image

To optimize the scan image, the overall gain and the time-gain compensation (TGC) must be adjusted to provide a uniform level of gray scale throughout the ultrasound image. An improper overall gain setting may alter the appearance of the internal echo pattern and limit the ability to distinguish solid from cystic lesions. The focal zone must be placed correctly at the area of concern to improve lateral resolution [19]. In preparation for intervention, the lesion of interest should be scanned in two planes at 90° angles for confirmation. Once reproduced, the lesion should be compared to the diagnostic ultrasound, especially if it was performed previously at an outside institution [6]. The lesion should be documented and measured.

Technique

Familiarity with the two basic scanning techniques (sometimes referred to as "painting" and "skiing" based upon the scanning motion utilized) is very helpful for successful intervention by identifying the portion of the lesion with the greatest diameter and moving the position of the lesion where it is visualized on the ultrasound monitor. In order to visualize the lesion at its largest diameter, the ultrasound transducer should be moved in short, stroke-like motions and perpendicular to the long axis of the transducer from one end of the lesion to the other ("painting") (Fig. 2.6). Aligning the tip of the advancing biopsy needle with the widest part of the lesion avoids veering off the edge of the lesion and allows biopsy of different portions of the lesion. To reposition the lesion along a horizontal plane from one side of the ultrasound monitor to the other, the transducer should slide along the long axis ("skiing") (Fig. 2.7). Practice with these scanning techniques allows the surgeon to become more facile at manipulating the position of the lesion to minimize the amount of breast tissue which must be traversed by the needle and to adequately sample varying portions of the lesion.

With positioning and imaging optimized and the target lesion location in the breast reestablished, the physician aligns the ultrasound transducer with its long axis oriented in a direct line between themselves and the ultrasound monitor. The approach of the biopsy device toward the target lesion will be along the long axis of the transducer. The decision for the optimal position of the entry site as well as the distance from the entry site to the transducer edge is dependent on the

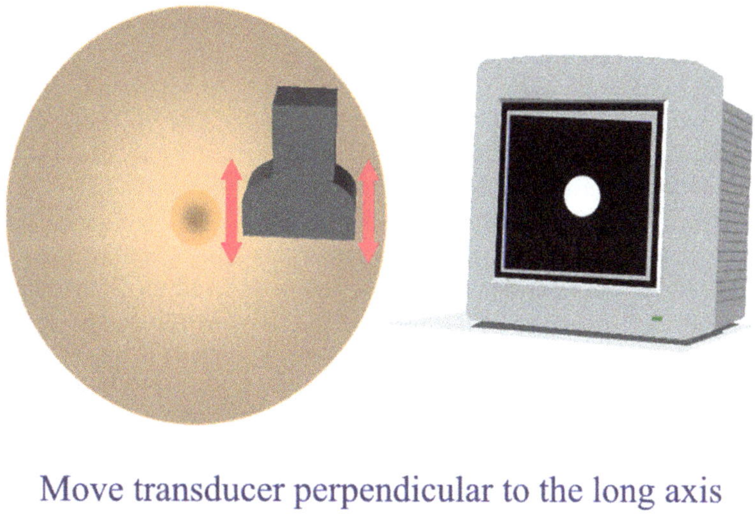

Fig. 2.6 Moving the ultrasound transducer perpendicular to its long axis allows the physician to determine the point of the lesion's greatest diameter

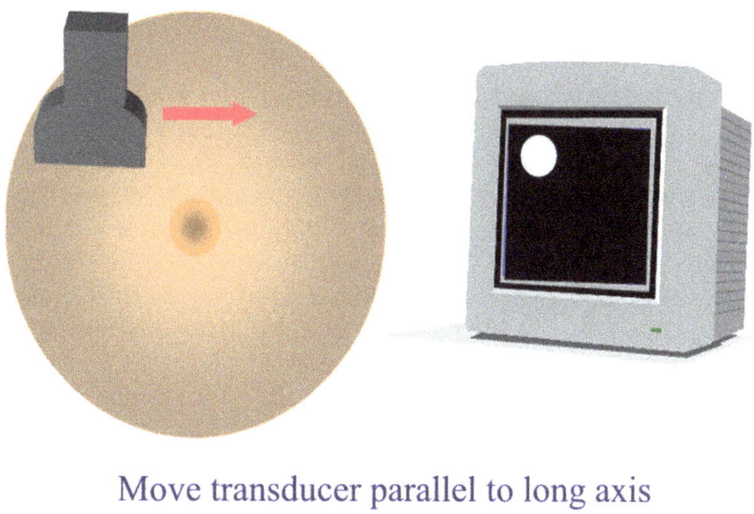

Fig. 2.7 Moving the ultrasound transducer in the same direction as its long axis allows the physician to control the position of the lesion on the monitor

type of biopsy device and the depth of the lesion. Devices that require positioning beneath the lesion and those lesions that are deeper in the breast may require an entry site further away from the transducer edge to maintain a biopsy needle/device approach that parallels the skin and pectoral muscle. This allows better visualization of the approaching biopsy device and therefore improves accuracy and safety.

Cyst Aspiration

After wiping the skin at the entrance site with an alcohol swab, a 1.5-in., 25–27-gauge needle is utilized to inject local anesthetic and raise a skin wheal. Deeper parenchymal anesthetic may be required for deeper cysts or ones suspected of containing thick fluid requiring a larger gauge needle for aspiration. Usually, a 20- or 22-gauge needle will suffice for aspiration of most cysts. The aspiration needle is guided under ultrasound guidance into the cyst, where the contents are aspirated. An attempt is made to aspirate the cyst completely, documenting the procedure with pre- and post-aspiration image documentation. The cyst fluid is discarded unless the contents are nontraumatic blood or the cyst fails to resolve with aspiration, possibly indicating a more complex process.

Fine-needle aspiration is a quick, inexpensive technique to assist in several areas of breast care management. A small gauge needle, similar to those required for simple cyst aspiration, is inserted under ultrasound guidance as previously described. The hyperechoic tip is visualized within the lesion, and then with a rapid in-and-out motion, the lesion is sampled by maintaining negative suction and until the needle hub appears to be filled with material. Image documentation of the hyperechoic needle tip within the lesion is desired. The cellular material is smeared on glass slides, fixed, and sent for cytologic interpretation [58]. Ultrasound-guided large-core needle biopsy for histologic diagnosis requires more planning than cyst aspiration or fine-needle aspiration biopsy but is still quick, minimally invasive, and cost effective and can often be performed on the initial patient evaluation [1, 40, 42].

Once the lesion requiring biopsy is visualized, the patient is appropriately positioned and the transducer is manipulated to obtain optimal positioning of the lesion on the ultrasound monitor. The skin is marked for the site of needle insertion that optimally is the shortest skin-to-lesion distance and avoiding the inner portion of the breast for cosmetic reasons [40]. A sterile or clean field is prepared. This technique is a physician's preference. There are disposable Betadine swabs available, which can be used in combination with disposable sterile towels and individual packets of sterile ultrasound gel. Others have chosen to use Betadine gel for both the antiseptic and the acoustic coupling. Alternative antiseptic solutions such as Hibiclens are available to those with an iodine allergy. A sterile ultrasound transducer cover is optional. If utilized, it is necessary to place ultrasound gel inside the cover for acoustic coupling between the transducer and the cover.

The physician then identifies the target lesion, positioning the ultrasound transducer to demonstrate the lesion's greatest diameter and minimizing the skin-to-lesion distance. The needle for injecting local anesthetic or the actual biopsy needle is inserted along the transducer's long axis, attempting to remain parallel with the transducer face. By tilting the patient, and by gently pushing the far end of the transducer into the breast, the angle of needle insertion remains parallel with the angle of the transducer allowing the needle tip (and possibly the "comet tail" of the advancing biopsy needle) to be visualized and monitored as it is placed into position. It will take some skill in order to keep the scan plane in parallel with the long axis of the transducer, which has an overall width of approximately 1–1.5 mm. The needle tip must also be maintained within this narrow scan plane as it moves forward. Attachable transducer needle guides have been useful for the beginner, but the freehand technique is quickly adopted to avoid the disadvantages of limited access to deeper lesions and the inability to deviate from the pattern of sampling the lesion [40, 42].

After appropriate sterile preparation of the breast and the transducer, local anesthetic is injected first as a skin wheal. It is then further injected along the transducer's edge and needle pathway to the lesion under direct ultrasound visualization, creating a field block around the lesion. The physician can accomplish this technique by injecting anterior and posterior to the lesion and then directing the needle superior and inferior to the lesion. Anesthetizing the breast parenchyma on the far side of the lesion, where the tip of a spring-loaded device may end its excursion, adds to patient comfort. The ability to direct the placement of local anesthesia can also be valuable in moving a superficial lesion away from the skin. It can also help in lifting a deep posterior lesion off the underlying pectoral muscle or augmentation implant capsule. This allows the needle pathway to remain parallel to the chest wall, thereby avoiding potential complications such as a pneumothorax [1, 40, 55]. This can be especially important when utilizing a biopsy device that requires placement under the target.

A small skin incision is made with an 11-blade scalpel. The size of the skin incision is a function of the biopsy device used, but usually is between 2 and 6 mm. The needle is advanced through the incision toward the lesion until the needle tip abuts against the surface of the lesion. Once inserted through the skin incision, the physician must guide the biopsy device along the long axis of the transducer, maintaining the needle in the 1–1.5-mm-thickness scan plane, constantly keeping the advancing needle tip in view on the ultrasound image (Fig. 2.8).

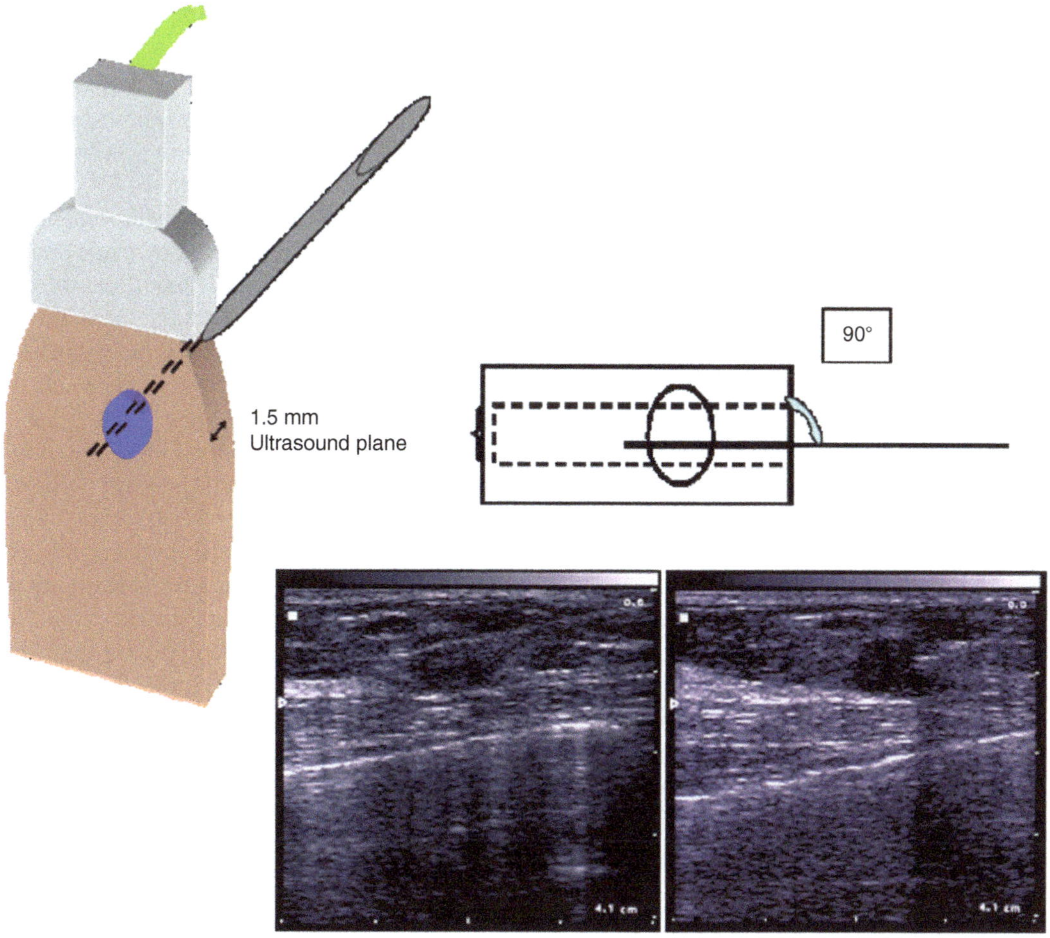

Fig. 2.8 The needle must remain within the narrow 1–1.5 mm ultrasound plane in order for it to be visualized aligned with and within the lesion on the ultrasound monitor

Maintaining the proper needle alignment within the narrow ultrasound plane is accomplished freehand allowing flexibility in the needle insertion site and angle of approach of the needle to the breast lesion [1, 40, 42]. Visualization of the needle is maximized by keeping the needle at a shallower angle and therefore parallel to the sole of the transducer. By propping the patient with a pillow laterally and by gently pushing the far end of the transducer into the breast, keeping the device parallel to the sole of the ultrasound transducer allowing better visualization of the advancing device tip, possibly even demonstrating a comet tail artifact, further confirms the biopsy device position for intervention.

Advancement of a forward cutting or coring device such as the automated Tru-Cut (ATC) device toward the target lesion under direct ultrasound visualization continues until the needle tip abuts against the lesion. When the needle position is confirmed at the front of the lesion, with image documentation, the needle-gun combination is "fired" activating the biopsy mechanism. With the ATC device, as well as other forward cutting/coring devices, lesion sampling occurs with piercing by the sampling portion of the device, followed again with post-fire image documentation. Prior to withdrawing the device to acquire the tissue sample, confirmation of the needle within the lesion is mandatory.

By scanning the ultrasound transducer in a motion perpendicular to its long axis, toward the superior end of the lesion, and then back past the portion of the lesion containing the biopsy needle toward the inferior end of the lesion, it can be assured that the needle is in the lesion. The goal is to see a portion of the lesion without a biopsy needle on either side of the scan plane containing the needle. Seeing the lesion on both sides of the device confirms that the device is inside the lesion and rules out the "image averaging" artifact that can occur when the device is immediately adjacent to the lesion. Finally, the surgeon can obtain further confirmation by turning the transducer perpendicular to the device and imaging a cross section of the device within the lesion. With this orientation, the device appears as a small bright dot within the mass.

The needle is then withdrawn and the tissue sample acquired. Rolling the tissue off the needle trough onto moistened gauze or rinsing it off in a container of saline solution is a physician's preference. The multiple insertion devices, requiring withdrawal from the breast for each tissue sample obtained, prepared (cocked) for additional sampling is reinserted into the breast through the same incision. It is important to adjust the biopsy needle tip toward different portions of the lesion to acquire an additional three to five samples and avoid a sampling error and a resulting discordant diagnosis. The number of samples required depends on the quality of the samples and the confirmation of the needle penetrating the lesion. When adequate sampling is achieved, the procedure is terminated, manual compression is applied for hemostasis, and the incision is re-approximated without suturing using Steri-Strips™ and appropriately dressed with a Tegaderm™ dressing [40]. The core samples are sent for permanent histologic diagnosis in formalin.

Ultrasound-Guided Vacuum-Assisted Biopsy

The first steps of the procedure are the same with a few exceptions. The side-cutting VAB device is again inserted along the long axis of the ultrasound transducer. It is important that it is guided underneath the lesion for sampling because the artifact created by the device would eliminate visualization of any portion of the lesion below the biopsy probe. To access underneath the lesion, especially when the lesion is in a posterior position, requires a shallow angle of insertion, which can be assisted by patient positioning (contralateral oblique), injection of local anesthetic posterior to the lesion for a lifting effect, and torquing down of the biopsy device handle as the probe approaches the underside of the lesion.

Once positioned below the lesion, the ultrasound transducer is rotated 90° to view in cross section the probe, directly below the center of the lesion. Larger amounts of local anesthetic may be needed, both for comfort and for lifting a more posterior positioned lesion off the chest wall, to allow the device to be positioned between the muscle and the lesion. Positioned beneath the lesion, rotating the ultrasound transducer 90° confirms the proper alignment of the lesion with the sampling portion of the device by being able to see the circular artifact of the device directly below the center of the lesion.

Tissue acquisition is achieved through the same mechanism of action described previously. The pattern of sampling, however, is slightly different. The sampling with the ultrasound-guided device is usually superior with a rotation of the sample notch back and forth along an arc, for example, from 10 to 2 o'clock. This pattern of sampling is, of course, altered according to the relation of the lesion's position to the vacuum-assisted biopsy probe. Following this methodology, it is especially helpful when the desire is to remove the entire image evidence of the lesion. This will avoid splitting the lesion into small fragments that become more difficult to visualize with ultrasound as the biopsy proceeds.

Intra-procedural bleeding is rarely a problem but can be minimized with injection of local anesthetic mixed with epinephrine directly through the biopsy probe and into the biopsy site. Following a VAB procedure, manual compression is applied to the breast to obtain hemostasis. The incision size is 4–6 mm, depending on the gauge of the probe (11 gauge or 8 gauge), is rarely sutured and usually re-approximated with a Steri-Strip™, and is covered with a Tegaderm™ dressing. The patient may also be sent home wrapped with a binder around the chest for patient comfort and continued pressure for hemostasis.

The goal of the ultrasound-guided percutaneous biopsy helps determine the amount of sampling for any of the devices chosen. For purely diagnostic purposes, especially confirmation of a suspicious lesion as malignant, approximately three to five good quality cores should be obtained. If the purpose of the procedure is to remove the image evidence of a solid mass that has a greater likelihood of being benign (i.e., fibroadenoma), then a vacuum-assisted biopsy device may require a much greater number of core samples. The gauge of the device may also influence the number of cores needed.

Localizing marker placement, prior to ending the procedure, is common with percutaneous image-guided biopsy. Deployment of a simple metallic marker in the center of the lesion in question will help to identify the lesion location after the patient undergoes neoadjuvant treatment. The technique of guiding the marker applicator through the biopsy incision along the long axis of the transducer follows the same ultrasound-guidance principles associated with performing the biopsy.

Removal of the image evidence of a lesion with a vacuum-assisted device, or if a small lesion is difficult to visualize after removal of multiple cores, requires a marker with ultrasound visibility characteristics. These markers serve two purposes. If the lesion requires surgical intervention for cancer or for discordance between the pathology and the radiographic interpretation, then the ultrasound-visible markers allow the surgeon to eliminate a preoperative trip for their patient to radiology for wire localization and allow them to perform their own intraoperative ultrasound localization for definitive surgery. If the ultrasound-guided percutaneous biopsy diagnosis is benign, the metallic portion of the marker remaining allows for future orientation and evaluation of the ultrasound biopsy site on mammogram. Others do not routinely utilize specialized ultrasound-visible localization markers and rely instead on the routinely ultrasound visibility of the residual VAB cavity and associated small hematoma for intraoperative localization.

The surge in large-core and VAB devices is largely based on the concept that complete removal of the imaged abnormality will be more efficacious and provide a more complete diagnosis in most patients. However, removing an abnormality in numerous pieces does not allow for optimal pathologic assessment especially in size and margin status and does not allow for specimen orientation. Newer technology under-development is evaluating the potential therapeutic effect of large, intact sampling devices. Radiofrequency devices inserted under ultrasound guidance capture the lesion as a whole intact sample, and the enclosed specimen is withdrawn through a small (10–12-mm) incision [59].

The technology of large, intact sample devices with ultrasound guidance is promising both for facilitating biopsy of breast lesions and for percutaneous removal of benign lesions. This capability provides maximal diagnostic certainty and may prove particularly helpful in removing such challenging lesions as radial scar, lesions with associated atypia (ADH, ALH), and lesions with pathologic diagnoses that are difficult without the entire lesion (papilloma, nodular adenosis, phyllodes tumor). Such success begs the question as to the role of such technology in the treatment of small, malignant breast lesions.

Another alternative to open surgery for treating fibroadenomas involves a variety of percutaneous ablation techniques using heating or cooling elements. Several potential advantages of using the cold energy of cryoablation for cell destruction have been suggested, including excellent visualization under ultrasound, anesthesia control, and minimal scarring [60, 61]. Cryoablation is performed in the office setting with an a liquid nitrogen-based treatment system using a 3.4-mm cryoprobe (IceSense 3 cryoablation system, IceCure Medical, Collierville, Tennessee). The patient is prepped, draped, and anesthetized in a manner consistent with other ultrasound-guided interventional procedures. With ultrasound guidance the cryoprobe is directed into the middle of a core biopsy proven.

The ultrasound transducer is then rotated 90° to a position perpendicular to the cryoprobe so as to confirm that the probe is centered within the lesion.

A treatment algorithm has been developed based on the fibroadenoma's size to determine the time duration of freeze cycles with intermittent thaw allowing for osmotic shifts at the cellular level so as to maximize tissue destruction [60]. The edge of the ice ball is highly echogenic, and therefore its size and proximity to the skin can be easily visualized with ultrasound [60]. Constantly monitoring the procedure with ultrasound, saline may be injected during the procedure to protect the patient's skin. The cryoprobe is removed from the patient at the end of the complete treatment cycle. Kaufman et al. reported on the treatment of 57 core biopsy samples (proven fibroadenomas) in 50 patients [60]. There was a high level of patient satisfaction and minimal complications, with lesions showing progressive shrinkage over 3–12 months.

The surgeon's direct involvement with interventional breast ultrasound has naturally led to an ever-increasing role for the use of ultrasound as an adjunct to open surgery. Ultrasound guidance may be utilized for localization of non-palpable lesions with and without localization devices. Due to limited access to ultrasound technology in the hospital or operating room, some surgeons may perform ultrasound-guided localization procedures in the office setting. However, the advanced ultrasound technology has led to the development of small, portable (even laptop style) ultrasound units with good image quality that may be taken to the operating room by the surgeon.

Traditional preoperative, mammographically guided, wire localization has a reported "miss rate" as high as 22 % [62, 63]. With the patient awake and usually upright, syncope episodes are reported in 9–20 % of pre-biopsy needle localization procedures [62]. Additionally, the patient must be scheduled in the radiology department, resulting in less flexibility for the surgeon with scheduling early morning operations, resulting in delays in the schedule as a result of a difficult localization. Other disadvantages are wire transection and dislodgement [62–64]. Thus, many have begun to replace mammographically guided wire localization with ultrasound-guided localization techniques.

The technique of performing intraoperative ultrasound for both localization and excision has been extensively described [65–67]. Traditional localization wires (Hawkins™, Bard™, Kopans™) formerly used only for mammographic or stereotactic localizations are easily inserted under direct ultrasound guidance in the operating room after the patient is in position and sedated. The wire/needle combination is guided into and through the lesion under direct ultrasound visualization. The needle is then withdrawn, allowing the barb or hook of the wire to engage the tissue just beyond the lesion's far edge so as to minimize the chance it will become dislodged during dissection. This procedure may be preceded by injection of local anesthetic under direct ultrasound visualization.

The ability to inject local anesthesia under direct visualization without the concern of obscuring the lesion is another advantage of ultrasound-guided wire localizations compared to mammographically guided needle localization [40]. This may be done immediately before surgery by the operating surgeon, thereby eliminating a trip to radiology and the resultant lack of scheduling control. The patient is on the operating table supine, which allows wire placement in accordance with the location and direction of the planned incision. If intraoperative ultrasound is not available, the same ultrasound-guided localization procedures may be performed the morning of surgery, in the office setting, with similar benefits.

Ultrasound excision without a localization device is performed using an appropriate high-frequency linear array transducer. The lesion is visualized and centered on the monitor, and the skin is marked at each end of the long axis of the transducer. After rotating 90° and maintaining the center, the skin is again marked at the ends of the transducer. The marks are connected and where they cross is the position of the lesion. The depth of the lesion is noted on the ultrasound monitor. The incision is placed appropriately close to the lesion with a greater chance for improved cosmetic results [65–68]. Consistently, the benefits of intraoperative ultrasound-guided localization and excision for both palpable and non-palpable lesions are reported including smaller excised volume and adequate margins [65–68]. The positive margins in most of these studies were related to DCIS [65–67].

Localization can be performed on any ultrasound-visible lesion requiring further evaluation or definitive management. The advantages of avoiding preoperative mammographic wire localization have recently been expanded to lesions that are traditionally considered ultrasound invisible by converting these lesions into ultrasound-visible status. An ultrasound-visible marker can be placed at the time of a stereotactic-guided breast biopsy for microcalcifications [69–71]. Several ultrasound-visible markers have become available which contain absorbable, echogenic, material plus a metallic marker [71]. The absorbable material allows ultrasound visibility for several weeks. Ultrasound-guided localization can also be performed after a stereotactic biopsy by visualizing the vacuum-assisted hematoma-filled biopsy cavity [70]. Smith et al. reported successful removal of the hematoma as long as 56 days after the biopsy [72].

Breast Tumor Ablation with Ultrasound Guidance

The management of breast disease has continued to evolve toward minimally invasive techniques as a result of an increasing number of smaller, non-palpable abnormalities identified through screening. The evaluation of percutaneous ablative techniques in the management of benign and malignant disease of the breast is consistent with this trend and offers the potential for office-based treatment with excellent cosmetic results and improved quality of life. Several clinical protocols are exploring possible treatment for small benign and malignant breast tumors, utilizing varying ablative therapy modalities, including cryoablation, radiofrequency, and interstitial laser [60, 73–76]. Ultrasound is frequently the imaging method utilized for guidance of the treatment devices, monitoring parenchymal changes, as well as follow-up of the breast for the evaluation of residual disease or recurrence. Such follow-up may include ultrasound-guided biopsy of the tissue at the periphery of the treatment zone [61]. Surgeons' involvement in ultrasound imaging for diagnosis and intervention of appropriate lesions is essential for the future advancement of breast cancer treatment.

Cryoablation for the treatment of small breast cancers utilizes the same technology described for the ablation of biopsy-proven fibroadenomas [60]. Cryotherapy began with the use of cryogens for treating skin cancers. Cryoablation of visceral tumors (liver and prostate) followed over time has provided a considerable body of basic knowledge on the biology of freezing of tumors and the potential beneficial effects [77, 78]. Tissue destruction with cold provided by the liquid nitrogen or argon gas generates an easily ultrasound-visible freeze ball helpful in measuring the treatment margins beyond the tumor edge.

In addition to ensuring adequate destruction, this allows for monitoring of the safety zone from the overlying skin. The 2-phase or double freeze-thaw cycle to a target temperature of −106 to −196 °C is required to cause crystallization within the tumor cells [61]. Rand was the first (1986) to use cryotherapy in the breast followed by mastectomy [79]. Staren et al. performed an in situ cryoablation in 1997 without surgical resection, and the patient had no evidence of recurrent disease after 7 years [77]. A pilot trial of 11 patients with small invasive breast cancers treated with cryoablation showed 90 % complete ablation in the resected specimens (7–21 days post-treatment) [78].

Radiofrequency Ablation

Radiofrequency ablation achieves cell kill through the production of heat. The 15-gauge, insulated probe is placed percutaneously into the tumor under ultrasound guidance. The electrode prongs are deployed to varying lengths to adjust for treatment volume. Frictional heat is created within the breast tissues a result of ion movement responding to the high-frequency alternating current. Temperature sensors on the prongs assist in reaching the target temperature of 95 °C in 5–7 min. The target temperature is maintained for 15 min and then followed by a cooldown period of 1 min [76, 80]. An early pilot study by Jeffrey and colleagues evaluated the success of radiofrequency ablation techniques in five patients with locally advanced breast cancer. Complete ablation was found in four of five (85 %) of the mastectomy specimens [75]. Complete ablation was also achieved by Izzo and colleagues in 96 % of 26 women with T1 and T2 invasive breast carcinomas [74].

Ultrasound is utilized in all reported radiofrequency ablation series for treatment and guiding follow-up resection with the exception of one case reported by Elliott using stereotactic guidance with clip placement and delayed surgical excision [81]. The ablation zones appear hypoechoic on ultrasound but is less distinct than the radiofrequency ablation of a hepatic metastasis. The excised tissue reveals a zone of ablation appearing firm, chalky, yellow white surrounded by a red rim (representing the outer zone of tissue destruction) [76, 80, 81].

Failure of ablation appears to be more common in patients whose tumor size is underestimated on preoperative breast imaging or those undergoing neoadjuvant chemotherapy that resulted in multifocal tumor cells remaining without visualization [61]. Despite this, Singletary et al. reported an 87 % complete ablation with reduced nicotinamide adenine dinucleotide staining (NADH) in 30 patients with T1 invasive breast cancers [80].

Laser Ablation

Another heat-activated method of tissue destruction is generated with laser. The fiberoptic probe is inserted into the center of the lesion with image guidance using a coaxial insertion technique. A temperature of 80–100 °C is maintained for 15–20 min [61, 73]. The heat is transferred in a radial fashion creating a zone of pseudo necrosis or "pseudo viability" the vaporized tissue adjacent to the laser tip and the outer ring of fat necrosis. Though on hematoxylin and eosin staining the cells in this pseudonecrotic zone appear viable, immunohistochemical and special stains confirm they are not. This outer rim may represent the limit of cancer destruction [73].

Although ultrasound can be used to localize the tumor and to insert the fiberoptic probe into the center of the tumor, the largest experience with interstitial laser therapy has utilized stereotactic guidance. Dowlatshahi has performed greater than 50 cases of laser ablation and resection over the past 7 years [61, 73]. In a series of 36 patients (34 invasive, 2 DCIS), complete ablation was demonstrated histologically in 67 %. MRI guidance has been utilized by Harms and colleagues to perform laser ablation on 12 patients with complete ablation in 100 % of tumors less than 3 cm in size [82].

Ablative technology to treat small breast cancers without surgical resection is a promising future application. Several protocols have successfully demonstrated the ability to safely and effectively destroy cancer in the breast with a number of different modalities [61, 73–82]. However, despite strict and careful patient selection, ablation has failed to reach complete ablation in all patients. Surgical positive margins must be eliminated to avoid local recurrence. Though ultrasound is extremely helpful in guiding many of these treatments, the limitation is the ability to visualize the extent of disease.

MRI may be helpful in this regard if the detection of nonspecific abnormalities can be controlled. Long-term results of ablation without resection are necessary to provide patients with a less invasive, cosmetic approach to breast cancer treatment. Questions that are yet to be answered include the ability to follow patients despite the expected posttreatment changes of fat necrosis, scarring, and "transient" residual mass that makes the physical exam more difficult and creates anxiety for the patient and the physician. Injury from these technologies such as skin burns has been dealt with by incorporating excision of the affected area into a definitive surgical treatment; therefore cosmetic results without resection are not known. Therefore, except for biopsy-proven benign disease, these techniques are not appropriate outside the setting of clinical trials.

Conclusion

This chapter has updated the role of ultrasound in the surgeon's care of benign and malignant disease of the breast. Doubts over a surgeon's capabilities in performing diagnostic and interventional breast ultrasound remain of historical significance only. Identification of asymptomatic cysts and palpable regions of fibroglandular tissue helps eliminate unnecessary intervention or biopsy. The ability to intervene with any number of tools using ultrasound guidance will eliminate most patients with complex cysts, fibroadenomas, and other benign entities from going to the operating room suite for surgical diagnosis. Low-risk, palpable and non-palpable masses can be removed percutaneously with vacuum-assisted biopsy.

When cancer, atypical, or discordant pathology requires excision for definitive management, the use of preoperative office-based or intraoperative ultrasound, with and without localization devices, has consistently facilitated excision with smaller tissue volume and a high rate of clear margins. Finally, the advancement of minimally invasive ablative technology for the treatment of benign and malignant tumors requires ultrasound for device insertion, monitoring treatment, preventing unwanted complications, and guiding both surgical and nonsurgical follow-up after ablation.

The importance of breast ultrasound education for surgeons is illustrated by the demand for didactic and hands-on courses provided by such organization as the American College of Surgeons and the American Society of Breast Surgeons. The American College of Surgeons has recently listed breast ultrasound as a requirement for general surgery residency programs. Education and training is provided to enhance expertise and clinical competency for surgeons who use diagnostic and interventional breast ultrasound in their training and practice. The American Society of Breast Surgeons has developed a breast ultrasound certification designed to ensure the highest quality in surgeons performing breast ultrasound and therefore improve the quality of care for women with breast disease.

Acknowledgments Contributing authors
Arthur Lerner, MD, FACS
Principal, TECH (Technology, Education, Consulting in Healthcare)
10428 SW Lands End Pl
Palm City, FL, 34990
William Burak, MD, FACS
Director, Advanced Breast Care
Marietta, GA
790 Church St. Suite 410
Marietta, GA, 30060
Clerical assistance
Beth Boyd, RN
Administrator, Advanced Breast Care, Marietta, GA
790 Church St. Suite 410
Marietta, GA 30060

References

1. Fine RF, Staren ED. Updates in breast ultrasound. Surg Clin N Am. 2004;84:1001–34.
2. Whitehouse PA, Baber Y, Brown G, et al. The use of ultrasound by breast surgeons in outpatients: an accurate extension of clinical diagnosis. Eur J Surg Oncol. 2001;27:611–6.
3. Staren ED. Surgical-office-based ultrasound of the breast. Am Surg. 1995;61:619–27.
4. Dempsey PJ. Breast sonography: historical perspective, clinical application, and image interpretation. Ultrasound Q. 1988;6:69.
5. Wild JJ, Reid JH. Echographic visualization of the living intact human breast. Cancer Res. 1954;14:227–82.
6. Bassett LW, Kimme-Smith C. Breast sonography. AJR Am J Roentgenol. 1991;156:449–55.
7. Jackson VP. The role of ultrasound in breast imaging. Radiology. 1990;177:305.
8. Sickles EA, Filly RA, Callen PW. Benign breast lesions: ultrasound detection and diagnosis. Radiology. 1984;151:467–70.
9. Jackson VP. Sonography of malignant breast disease. Semin Ultrasound CT MR. 1989;10:119.
10. Jackson VP, Rothchild PA, Kriepke DL, Mail JT, Holden RW. The spectrum of sonographic findings of fibroadenoma of the breast. Invest Radiol. 1986;21:34.
11. Leucht D, Madjar H. Teaching atlas of breast ultrasound. New York: Thieme Medical Publishers, Inc; 1996.
12. Fornage BD, Coan JD, David CL. Ultrasound-guided needle biopsy of the breast and other interventional procedures. Radiol Clin North Am. 1992;30(1):167–85.
13. Kopans DB, Meyer JE, Lindfors KK, et al. Breast sonography to guide cyst aspiration and wire localization of occult solid lesions. AJR Am J Roentgenol. 1984;143:489.
14. Parker SH, Jobe WE, Dennis MA, et al. Ultrasound-guided automated large core breast biopsy. Radiology. 1993;187:507.

15. Harper AP, Kelly-Fry E, Noe S. Ultrasound breast imaging – the method of choice for examine the young patient. Ultrasound Med Biol. 1981;7:231–7.
16. Liberman L, Cohen M, Dershaw D, et al. Atypical ductal hyperplasia diagnosed at stereotaxic core biopsy of breast lesions: an indication for surgical biopsy. AJR Am J Roentgenol. 1995;164:1111–3.
17. Staren ED, O'Neill TP. Surgeon-performed US: breast US. Surg Clin North Am. 1998;78:219–35.
18. Teboul M. A new concept in breast investigation: echo-histological acino-ductal 12-analysis or analytic echography. Biomed Pharmacother. 1988;42:289.
19. Staren E. Physics and principles of breast ultrasound. Am Surg. 1996;62:69.
20. Khattar S, Staren ED. Diagnostic breast ultrasound. In: Staren ED, Arrugui ME, editors. Ultrasound for the surgeon. Philadelphia: Lippincott-Raven; 1997. p. 85.
21. Stavros AT, Dennis MA. An introduction to breast ultrasound. In: Parker SH, Jobe WE, editors. Percutaneous breast biopsy. New York: Raven Press; 1993. p. 95.
22. Mendelson EB. Breast sonography. In: Rumack CM, Wilson SR, Charboneau JW, editors. Diagnostic ultrasound. St. Louis: Mosby-Year Book; 1991. p. 541.
23. Fornage BD, Lorigan JG, Andry E. Fibroadenoma of the breast: sonographic appearance. Radiology. 1989;172:671.
24. Mendelson EB, Baum JK, Berg WA, et al. BI-RADS: ultrasound. In: D'Orsi CJ, Mendelson EB, Ikeda DM, editors. Breast imaging reporting and data system: ACR BIRADS, Breast imaging atlas. 1st ed. Reston: American College of Radiology; 2003.
25. Guyer PB, Dewbury KC. Ultrasound of the breast in asymptomatic and x-ray dense breast. Clin Radiol. 1985;33:69.
26. Jackson VP, Hendrick RE, Feit SA, Kopans DB. Imaging of the radiographically dense breast. Radiology. 1993;188:297–301.
27. Hackeloer BJ, Duda V, Lauth G. Ultrasound mammography. New York: Springer; 1989.
28. Rubio IT, Henry-Tillman R, Klimberg S. Surgical use of breast ultrasound. Surg Clin North Am. 2003;83(4): 771–88.
29. Karstrup S, Nolsoe C, Braband K, et al. Ultrasonically guided percutaneous drainage of breast abscess. Acta Radiol. 1990;31:157–9.
30. Harness JK, Gittleman MA. Breast ultrasound. In: Harness JK, Wisher DB, editors. Ultrasound in surgical practice: basic principles and clinical applications. New York: Wiley-Liss; 2001. p. 159–236.
31. Mendelson EB. Evaluation of the post operative breast. Radiol Clin N Am. 1992;30:107.
32. Fornage BD, Sneige N, Singletary SE. Masses in breast with implants: diagnosis with US guided fine-needle aspiration biopsy. Radiology. 1994;191:339–42.
33. Levine RA, Collins TL. Definitive diagnosis of breast implant rupture by ultrasonography. Plast Reconstr Surg. 1991;87:1126.
34. Berg WA. Breast ultrasound – a role for screening. Semin Roentgenol. 2001;36(3):180–6.
35. Crystal P, Starno S, Shcharynski S, Koretz M. Using sonography to screen women with mammographically dense breasts. AJR Am J Roentgenol. 2003; 181(1):177–82.
36. Berg WA, et al. Combined screening with ultrasound and mammography compared to mammography alone in women at elevated risk of breast cancer: results of the first-year screen in ACRIN 6666. JAMA. 2008;299(18):2151–63.
37. Parker S, Stavros A. Interventional breast ultrasound. In: Parker S, Jobe W, editors. Percutaneous breast biopsy. New York: Raven; 1993. p. 129.
38. Silverstein MJ, et al. Image-detected breast cancer: state of the art diagnosis and treatment. J Am Coll Surg. 2005;201(4):586–97.
39. Clark-Pearson EM, et al. Quality assurance initiative at One institution for minimally invasive breast biopsy as the initial diagnostic technique. J Am Chem Soc. 2009;208(1):75–8.
40. Fine R. Image-directed breast biopsy. In: Winchester D, Winchester D, editors. Breast cancer atlas of clinical oncology. Ontario: BC Decker Inc; 2000. p. 65–88.
41. Kopans DB. Fine-needle aspiration of clinically occult breast lesions. Radiology. 1989;170:313–4.
42. Fine R. Ultrasound-guided breast percutaneous needle biopsy. In: Klimberg S, Bland K, editors. Master techniques in general surgery – breast surgery. Philadelphia: Lippincott Williams & Wilkins; 2011. p. 45–68.
43. Position statement on image-guided percutaneous biopsy of palpable breast lesions. 2001. www.breastsurgeons.org/statements
44. Gordon PB, Goldenberg SL, Chan NH. Solid breast lesions: diagnosis with US-guided fine-needle aspiration biopsy. Radiology. 1993;189:573–80.
45. Vlastos G, Fornage BD, Mirza NQ, et al. The correlation of axillary ultrasonography with histologic breast cancer downstaging after induction chemotherapy. Am J Surg. 2000;179(6):446–52.
46. Lundy J, Lozowski M, Sadri T, et al. The use of fine-needle aspirates of breast cancers to evaluate hormone-receptor status. Arch Surg. 1990;125:174.
47. Parker SH, Stavros T, Dennis MA. Needle biopsy techniques. Radiol Clin N Am. 1995;33(6):1171–86.
48. Staren ED. Ultrasound-guided biopsy of nonpalpable breast masses by surgeons. Ann Surg Oncol. 1996; 3:476.
49. Parker SH, Burbank F, Jackman RJ, et al. Percutaneous large-core breast biopsy: a multi-institutional study. Radiology. 1994;193:359–64.
50. Whitten TM, Wallace TW, Bird RE, et al. Image-guided core biopsy has advantages over needle localization biopsy for the diagnosis of nonpalpable breast cancer. Am Surg. 1997;63:1072–7.
51. Burbank F. Stereotactic breast biopsy of ADH and ductal carcinoma in-situ lesions: improved accuracy with a directional, vacuum assisted biopsy instrument. Radiology. 1997;202:843–7.
52. Philpotts LE, Lee CH, Horvath LJ, et al. Underestimation of breast cancer with 11-gauge

vacuum suction biopsy. AJR Am J Roentgenol. 2000; 175:1047–50.
53. Meloni GB, Dessole DS, Becchere MP, et al. Ultrasound-guided mammotome vacuum biopsy for the diagnosis of impalpable breast lesions. Ultrasound Obstet Gynecol. 2001;18(5):520–4.
54. Parker SH, Klaus AJ, McWey PJ, et al. Sonographically-guided directional vacuum assisted breast biopsy using a handheld device. AJR Am J Roentgenol. 2001;177:405–8.
55. Simon JR, Kalbhen CL, Cooper RA, et al. Accuracy and complications rates of US-guided vacuum-assisted core breast biopsy: initial results. Radiology. 2000;215(3):694–7.
56. Fine R, Whitworth P, Kim J, Harness J, Boyd B, Burak B. Low risk palpable breast masses removed using a vacuum-assisted hand-held device. Am J Surg. 2003;186(4):362–7.
57. Morris E, Liberman L, Trevisan S, Abramson A, Dershaw D. Histologic heterogeneity of masses at percutaneous breast biopsy. Breast J. 2002;8(4):187–91.
58. Klijanienko J, Cote JF, Thibault F, et al. Ultrasound-guided fine-needle aspiration cytology of nonpalpable breast lesions: Institut Curie's experience with 198 histologic correlated cases. Cancer. 1998;84(1):36–41.
59. Fine RE, Staren ED. Percutaneous radiofrequency-assisted excision of fibroadenomas. Am J Surg. 2006;192(4):545–7.
60. Kaufman C, Bachman B, Littrup P, White M, Carolina K, Freman-Gibb L, et al. Office-based ultrasound-guided cryoablation of breast fibroadenoma. Am J Surg. 2002;184:394–400.
61. Simmons R, Dowlatshahi K, Singletary S, Staren E. Ablative therapies for breast cancer. Contemp Surg. 2002;58:61–72.
62. Homer MJ, Smith TJ, Safaii H. Prebiopsy needle localization: methods, problems, and expected results. Radiol Clin North Am. 1992;30:139–53.
63. Norton LW, Zeligman BE, Pearlman NW. Accuracy and cost of needle localization breast biopsy. Arch Surg. 1988;123:947–50.
64. Rinassen TJ, Makarainen SI, Mattilla AI, et al. Wire localized biopsy of breast lesions: a review of 425 cases found in screening or clinical mammography. Clin Radiol. 1993;47:14–22.
65. Harlow SP, Krag DN, Ames S, et al. Intraoperative ultrasound localization to guide surgical excision of nonpalpable breast carcinoma. J Am Coll Surg. 1999;189:241–6.
66. Henry-Tillman R, Johnson AT, Smith LF, et al. Intraoperative ultrasound and other techniques to achieve negative margins. Semin Surg Oncol. 2001;20(3):206–13.
67. Paramo JC, Landeros M, McPhee MD, et al. Intraoperative ultrasound-guided excision of nonpalpable breast lesions. Breast J. 1999;5(6):389–94.
68. Smith LF, Rubio IT, Henry-Tillman R, et al. Intraoperative ultrasound-guided breast biopsy. Am J Surg. 2000;180:419–23.
69. Lechner M, Day D, Kusnick C, et al. Ultrasound visibility of a new breast biopsy marker on serial evaluations. Radiology. 2002;225(suppl):115.
70. Smith LF, Henry-Tillman R, Rubio IT, et al. Intraoperative localization after stereotactic breast biopsy without a needle. Am J Surg. 2001;182: 584–9.
71. Whaley D, Adamczyk D, Jensen E. Sonographically guided needle localization after stereotactic breast biopsy. AJR Am J Roentgenol. 2003;180:352–4.
72. Smith LF, Henry-Tillman RS, Harms S, et al. Hematoma-directed ultrasound-guided breast biopsy. Ann Surg. 2000;180(6):434–8.
73. Dowlatchahi K, Fan M, Gould V, et al. Stereotactically guided laser therapy of occult breast tumors, work in progress. Arch Surg. 2000;135(11):1345–52.
74. Izzo F, Thomas R, Delrio P, et al. Radiofrequency ablation of primary breast cancer: a pilot study in 26 patients. Cancer. 2001;92(8):2036–44.
75. Jeffrey SS, Birdwell RL, Ikeda DM, et al. Radiofrequency ablation of breast cancer: first report of an emerging technology. Arch Surg. 1999;134: 1064–8.
76. Simmons R. Ablative techniques in the treatment of benign and malignant breast disease. J Am Coll Surg. 2003;192(2):334–8.
77. Staren ED, Sabel MS, Gianakakis LM, et al. Cryosurgery of breast cancer. Arch Surg. 1997;132: 28–33.
78. Stocks L, Chang H, Kaufman C, et al. Pilot study of minimally invasive ultrasound-guided cryoablation in breast cancer. Am Soc Breast Surg. 2002 (abstract).
79. Rand R, Rand R, Eggerding F, et al. Cryolumpectomy for breast cancer: an experimental study. Cryobiology. 1985;22:307–18.
80. Singletary E, Fornage B, Sniege N, et al. Radiofrequency ablation of early-stage invasive breast tumors: an overview. Cancer J. 2002;8:177–80.
81. Elliott RL, et al. Radiofrequency ablation of a stereotactically localized nonpalpable breast carcinoma. Am Surg. 2002;68:1–5.
82. Harms SE, Cowan C, Klimberg VS, et al. Interstitial laser lumpectomy using MRI guidance as an alternative to conventional breast conservation surgery. Poster presentation, Breast Cancer Symposium. Austin; 11–15 Dec 1998.

Management of Benign Breast Disease

3

J. Michael Dixon and E. Jane Macaskill

Introduction

Over 95 % of patients who develop breast symptoms or signs have normal breasts or benign breast disease [1]. An understanding of the causes of benign breast conditions, their symptoms and their management will ensure that patients who have benign disease are treated correctly and are happy with their consultation. Benign breast disease continues to cause considerable morbidity and anxiety, and with increasing patient awareness and expectation, the number of patients seeking referral for benign breast conditions is increasing. Effective treatment includes making an accurate diagnosis followed by an adequate explanation of the condition and provision of relevant information related to both the diagnosis and how the condition is best managed.

J.M. Dixon, OBE, MD, FRCS, FRCEd, FRCP (✉)
The Edinburgh Breast Unit,
Western General Hospital, Crewe Road South,
Edinburgh EH4 2XU, Scotland, UK
e-mail: mike.dixon@ed.ac.uk

E.J. Macaskill, MBChB, MD, FRCSEd
Department of Breast Surgery,
Ninewells Hospital, Level 6,
Dundee DD1 9SY, Scotland, UK
e-mail: ejanemacaskill@nhs.net

Congenital Abnormalities

Although not diseases as such, development abnormalities of the breast can and do cause considerable anxiety and concern and are not uncommon reasons for patients to be seen by a general or breast surgeon.

Supernumerary or Accessory Breast Tissue

Accessory breast tissue is usually found in the axilla; supernumerary or accessory nipples are usually found below the breast but above the umbilicus. Accessory nipples can have underlying breast tissue, and accessory breasts in the axilla can have associated rudimentary nipples (Fig. 3.1). Accessory breast tissue can cause pain and discomfort and may only become evident during pregnancy. Reassurance is usually all that is needed. If an accessory nipple is in the bra line or an accessory breast is large, then surgery may be indicated. Excision should be reserved for those with significant symptoms because accessory nipples or breasts can be difficult to excise cosmetically. Surgery for the removal of accessory breast tissue has been reported to be associated with significant morbidity [2]. Liposuction is valuable when excising accessory breast tissue in the axilla because it helps define the planes between the accessory breast tissue and the fascia of the axilla. The best technique for excising

A.I. Riker (ed.), *Breast Disease: Comprehensive Management*,
DOI 10.1007/978-1-4939-1145-5_3, © Springer Science+Business Media New York 2015

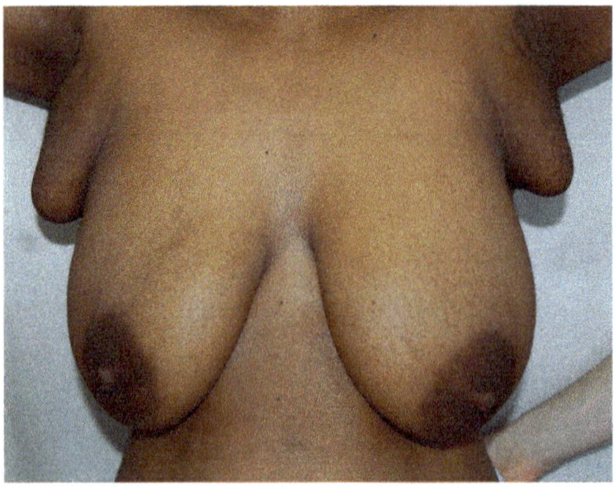

Fig. 3.1 Bilateral accessory breast tissue in axillae

accessory nipples is to excise only the skin of the nipple and adjacent areola and then to elongate the incision, medially and laterally in the skin crease lines de-epithelialising the skin medially and laterally before closure with an absorbable suture to produce a cosmetically acceptable scar.

Breast Hypoplasia

This is the failure of one breast, or rarely two breasts, to develop normally and can be congenital or acquired. Congenital causes of hypoplasia include Poland's syndrome, which is a group of conditions in which breast hypoplasia is associated with absence of, or hypoplasia of, the pectoralis major muscle, chest wall and varying degrees of syndactyly [3]. It is more common in men and is quite rare overall.

Management of Breast Hypoplasia

Treatment of hypoplasia or Poland's syndrome depends on the degree of asymmetry and deformity. For mild asymmetry, reassurance may be all that is required. If the asymmetry is marked and readily noticeable, then the smaller breast can be augmented. If there is a lack of skin over the hypoplastic breast, then tissue expansion may be required prior to permanent implant placement. Another option is to reduce the larger breast. In many, a combination of techniques involving surgery to both breasts is required in order to achieve good overall breast symmetry. Pedicled or free flaps are usually needed if there is a large defect. Fat transfer (lipomodelling) is being used increasingly as a technique to help or aid the correction of breast hypoplasia, either alone or combined with the use of breast implants [4, 5].

Hypoplasia can also be associated with tubular or tuberous breasts. This deformity is caused by a constricting ring at the base of the breast that limits vertical and horizontal growth. Management of this condition is challenging. Tissue expansion combined with radial incisions in the deep aspect of the breast can improve the shape and appearance. The large nipple-areola complex often needs to be reduced. As in other types of hypoplasia, lipomodelling is being increasingly used with acceptable cosmetic results [5].

Juvenile Hypertrophy

Some patients have excessive development of the breasts, and this may occur during puberty or at the onset of lactation and is often referred to as juvenile hypertrophy. For patients with large breasts, a reduction mammoplasty improves the significant physical and psychological problems associated with this condition [6].

Abnormalities of Normal Breast Development and Involution

Defining what represents benign disease and what is part of normal breast development and involution is challenging [7]. The breast passes through phases related to the levels of circulating hormones and how these affect the breast. There are a range of conditions that should be considered as aberrations, rather than disease, and these take place against the normal process of breast development, cyclical change and involution.

Fibroadenoma

Fibroadenoma is best classified as an aberration of normal breast development. It arises from the breast lobule including the epithelium and the associated stroma and not from a single cell [8]. Fibroadenomas are under the same hormonal control as the rest of the breast and can increase in size during pregnancy, and they become less active with involution. The activity in the stromal element defines their classification. A simple fibroadenoma contains stroma of low cellularity. There are three separate types of fibroadenoma: common fibroadenoma, giant fibroadenoma and juvenile fibroadenoma (Fig. 3.1). There is no universally accepted definition of what constitutes a giant fibroadenoma, but most consider that it should measure over 5 cm in diameter. Juvenile fibroadenomas occur in adolescent girls and sometimes undergo rapid growth, but are managed in the same way as the common fibroadenoma (Fig. 3.2).

Phyllodes Tumours

Phyllodes tumours are distinct pathologic entities. They are usually larger than fibroadenomas, occur in an older age group, have malignant potential and cannot always be differentiated from fibroadenomas clinically and on imaging. Phyllodes tumours focally can have an infiltrative margin, particularly in more aggressive forms, and phyllodes tumours range from benign (70 %) to borderline (25 %) to malignant (5 %) (Figs. 3.3, 3.4 and 3.5). About 10 % of benign phyllodes tumours recur after excision [9].

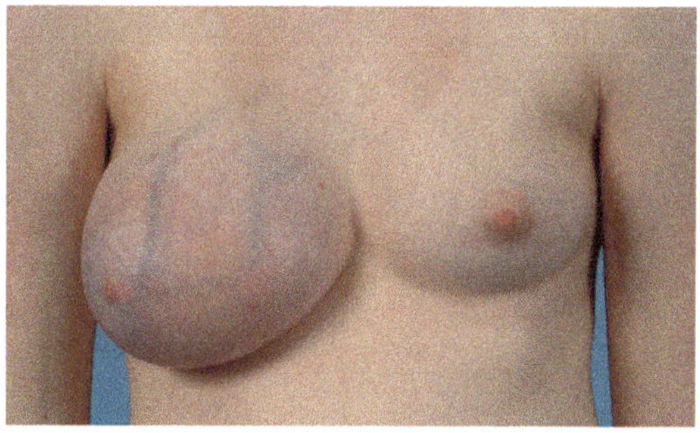

Fig. 3.2 Juvenile giant fibroadenoma (left breast)

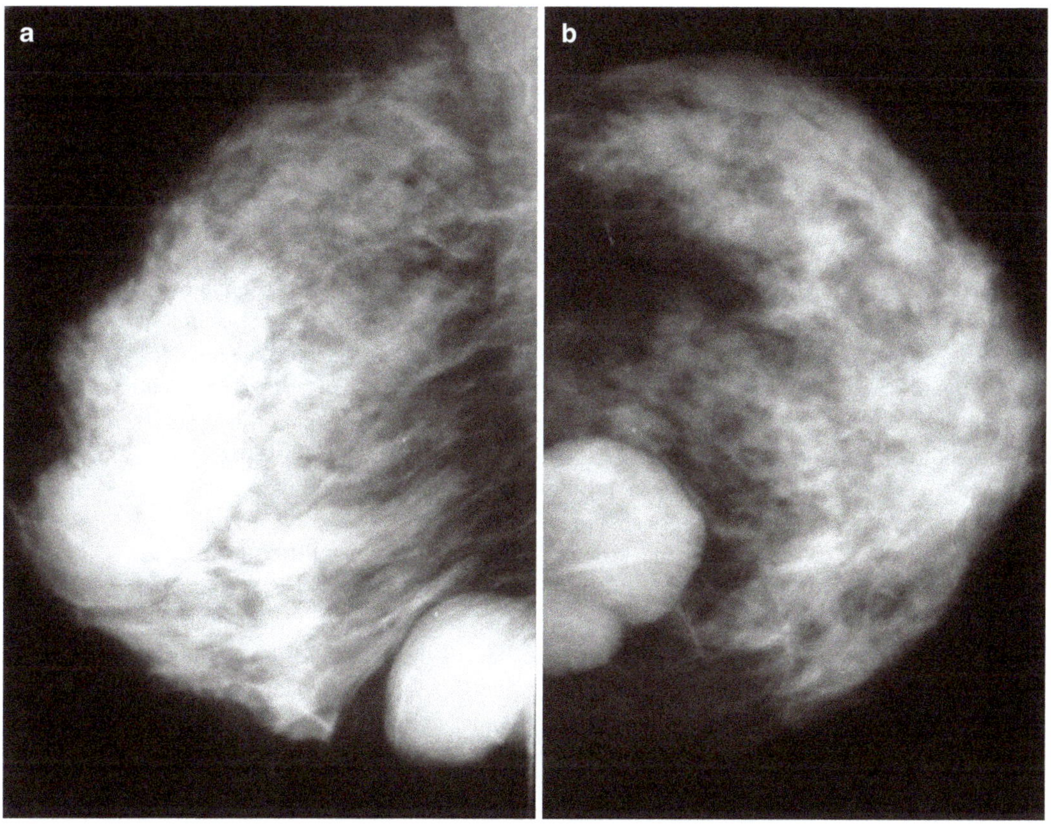

Fig. 3.3 Oblique (**a**) and craniocaudal (**b**) mammogram showing benign phyllodes tumour

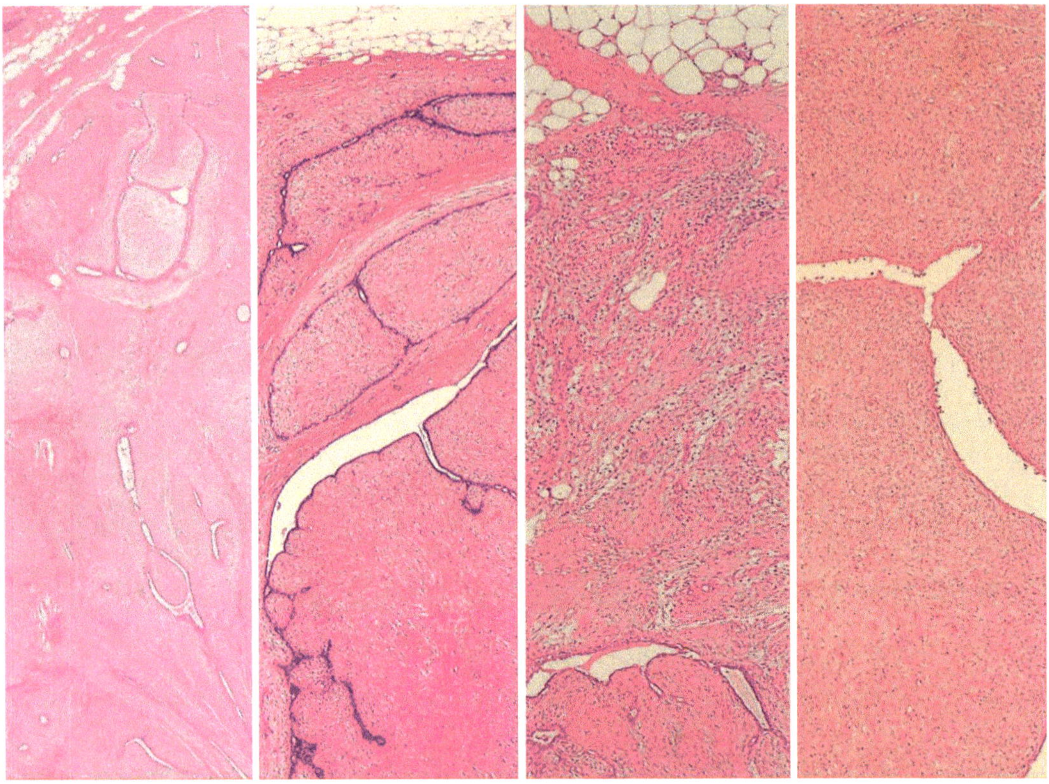

Fig. 3.4 Histology (low power) (*left–right*). (**a**) Simple fibroadenoma, (**b**) benign phyllodes, (**c**) borderline phyllodes, (**d**) malignant phyllodes

Management of a Discrete Mobile Mass in a Young Woman

A diagnosis based on imaging alone is acceptable, providing the patient is young (≤21 years old), and the lesion measures <3 cm. Otherwise, a histological diagnosis should be established by core needle biopsy. In patients with multiple fibroadenomas, two or more lesions should be sampled, and the remainder should be imaged and monitored. Any fibroadenoma over 4 cm requires full assessment by core biopsy. Multiple core biopsy passes (ideally 5–6 cores) should be performed in order to ensure that the lesion is adequately sampled and minimising potential sampling error.

Following a core biopsy pathologic diagnosis of a simple fibroadenoma, simple reassurance that the lesion is benign, with no malignant potential, is all that is required, and no further follow-up is necessary. However, excision is often performed at the request of the patient who despite this knowledge wishes the lesion to be removed. Larger lesions are usually excised first because they are often visible and symptomatic, but if they have been adequately sampled, they can be safely observed. Lesions over 5 cm are usually excised even if they are fibroadenomas on core biopsy because they are usually symptomatic, causing pain and/or discomfort. It is important to be certain that they are simple fibroadenomas and not phyllodes tumours.

How to Excise a Fibroadenoma

A cosmetic approach is recommended if a fibroadenoma is to be excised. Lesions in the lower half of the breast can be approached through an incision in the inframammary fold. Lesions in the upper half can be excised through a circumareolar incision or if near the axilla through an axillary skin crease incision.

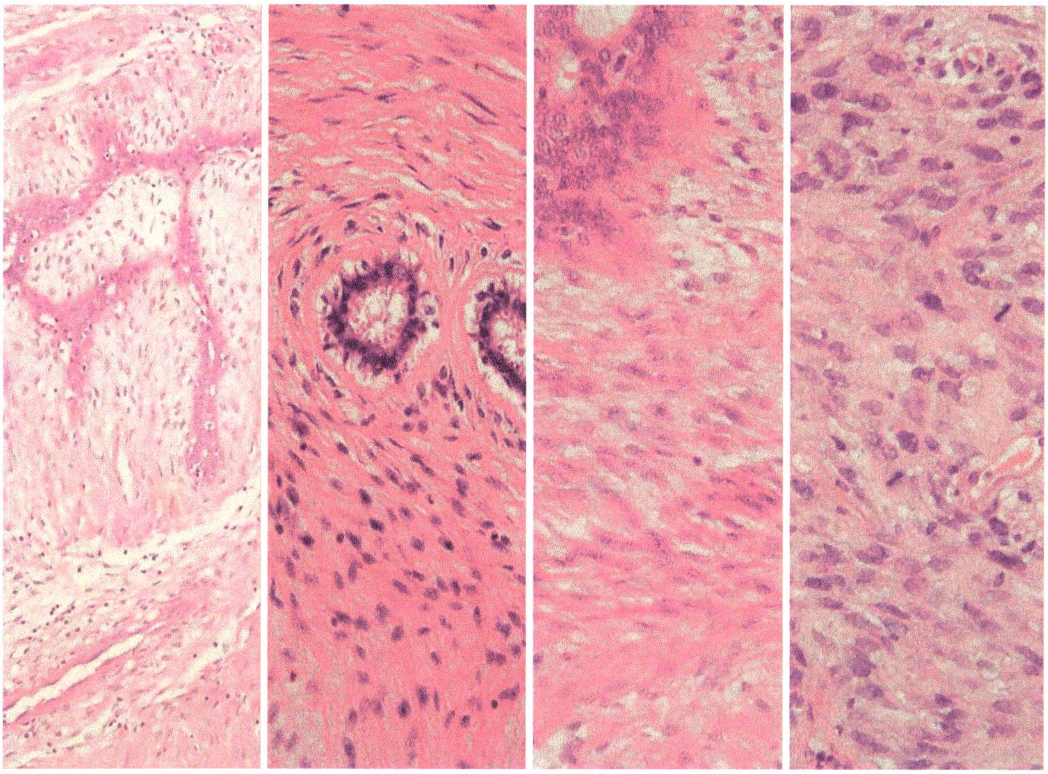

Fig. 3.5 Histology (high power) (*left–right*). (**a**) Simple fibroadenoma, (**b**) benign phyllodes, (**c**) borderline phyllodes, (**d**) malignant phyllodes

Operative Technique

If an inframammary incision is used, then the incision is taken down to the rectus abdominus muscle and pectoral major muscle. The breast is elevated from the pectoral fascia without disturbing the fascia, and the fibroadenoma is approached from behind the breast. Fibroadenomas can be enucleated, and the best way to perform this is to open the capsule with blunt dissection using a pair of Metzenbaum scissors through the posterior aspect of the breast. The scissors are aimed at the fibroadenoma and opened, and this results in opening of the breast tissue down to the capsule of the fibroadenoma. Once the capsule is reached, the scissors are pushed into the capsule and opened, and this splits the capsule. A finger can then be inserted and the fibroadenoma enucleated. It usually remains attached at the point where the blood supply enters, and at this site the fibroadenoma is adherent to the capsule. Once the fibroadenoma is fairly mobile within the capsule, it is usually possible to deliver it through the wound and divide any residual attachment to the capsule under direct vision with diathermy. The defect in the back of the breast is closed with absorbable interrupted sutures. Bleeding is rarely a problem but careful inspection of the capsule is performed, and any bleeding is stopped with diathermy. The inframammary wound is then closed carefully in layers.

If the fibroadenoma is being approached through a circumareolar incision, then having deepened the incision the plane between the subcutaneous fat and the breast fat is entered. This may be facilitated by hydrodissection using normal saline or a 1 in 500,000 adrenaline in normal saline solution. Once the breast tissue over the fibroadenoma is reached, then the tissue is opened down to the fibroadenoma using scissors pointed at the fibroadenoma with the scissors being opened to divide the overlying breast tissue, and then the capsule around the fibroadenoma is also split with scissors. Enucleation is performed with a finger, and the lesion is delivered through the tunnel into the wound and the blood supply of the fibroadenoma divided under direct vision. No sutures in the breast tissue are needed. The skin is closed in layers with absorbable sutures. Small fibroadenomas can be removed using vacuum-assisted core biopsy devices [10].

Most phyllodes tumours are benign and require total removal but do not require to be widely excised. When removing a benign phyllodes tumour, the lesion together with the capsule is excised with the aim of achieving clear margins clear (≥1 mm) of the phyllodes tumour. If following excision of an apparently simple fibroadenoma a phyllodes tumour is diagnosed and the surgeon is confident that the lesion has been excised completely, then careful follow-up, rather than re-excision, is appropriate. Borderline and malignant phyllodes may require a wider excision.

Aberrations of Cyclical Activity

Nodularity

Focal breast lumpiness is one of the most common reasons for a woman to be referred to a breast clinic. Lumpy nodular breast tissue is common. Women with a focal area of nodularity should be assessed with imaging, and providing there is no abnormality visualised on ultrasound and/or mammography, then the patient can be safely reassured. These young women with nodular breast tissue were previously considered as having fibroadenosis or fibrocystic disease, but these terms are not appropriate and should not be used because these women usually have normal breast tissue if biopsy is performed. Breast cancer can present in a young woman with asymmetrical nodularity, and if there is clinical suspicion in the face of normal imaging, then a core biopsy or fine-needle aspirate of the palpable mass should be performed.

Breast Pain

Up to 70 % of women experience breast pain at some point in their life. What women describe as breast pain can be pain that originates from the breast or is referred from adjacent areas, such as the chest wall. Breast pain is a rare symptom of breast cancer, and in one 10-year study period in Edinburgh of 8,504 patients presenting with breast pain, only 220 (2.7 %) were subsequently diagnosed as having breast cancer. During the same period 4,740 were diagnosed with breast cancer, and this means that only 4.6 % of women with breast cancer have pain as a presenting symptom [11].

Cyclical breast pain is very common and is now regarded as physiologic and not pathologic. Severe or prolonged pain is considered an aberration of normal cyclical activity.

Management of Breast Pain

It is important to differentiate between pain arising from the chest wall and true breast pain. Features suggesting that the breast pain is referred pain from the chest wall include:

- Unilateral and brought on by activity
- Very lateral or medial in the breast
- Can be reproduced by pressure on a specific area of the chest wall

Careful clinical examination is essential. A patient complaining of breast pain should have an examination lying on her side allowing the breast to fall away from the breast wall, and the underlying ribs and muscles should then be palpated. The patient should be asked to indicate if there is any localised tenderness on the palpation of the chest wall and whether the pain elicited is similar to that they normally suffer. If the patient has pain in the lower part of the breast, then the underlying chest can be checked by lifting the breast upwards with one hand while palpating the underlying chest wall with the other hand.

The mainstay of treating breast pain is reassurance that there is no serious underlying problem [12]. Lifestyle issues are important and it is not uncommon for women who spend many hours at a desk, sitting in front of a computer, to have chest wall pain. If, on examination, the pain is very localised to one specific spot on the chest wall, then infiltration of the site of the pain with a combination of prednisone (40 mg in depot form) combined with a long-acting local anaesthetic such as bupivacaine can produce long-lasting pain relief.

Pain in bed at night is a problem for many women. Wearing a soft supportive bra stops the breast pulling down on the chest wall, and this helps many women to sleep. There have been numerous studies looking at the role of caffeine, essential fatty acids, and diet as a contributing factor for breast pain. There is little evidence that activities such as cutting out caffeine, taking evening primrose oil, or transferring to a low-fat diet are beneficial [13–16].

The treatment that has been shown to have greatest efficacy in true breast pain is tamoxifen [17]. Although most commonly given for cyclical pain, it can help true noncyclical breast pain. It is best tolerated in a dosage of 10 mg a day [18]. Compared with other treatments, such as danazol, there are fewer adverse events with tamoxifen [18]. It is possible to restrict the use of tamoxifen to the luteal phase of the cycle, and this can relieve pain in up to 85 % of women [19, 20].

A variety of nonhormonal agents have been tried for breast pain. Although some studies have reported an improvement with soya milk, there is general non-compliance in studies published to date [21]. Agnus castus, a fruit extract, has been shown in one trial to improve breast pain [22]. Selective serotonin reuptake inhibitors have also been shown to improve breast pain [23].

Aberrations of Breast Involution

Palpable Breast Cysts

Approximately 7 % of women at some point in their life develop a palpable breast cyst [24]. Such cysts constitute 15 % of *a*ll discrete masses. Cysts are distended in involuted lobules and are most common in the perimenopausal period. Women generally present with a smooth, discrete breast lump that can be painful and is sometimes visible. Cysts have characteristic features on ultrasound and on mammography. Once diagnosed on imaging, simple cysts do not need to be aspirated unless they are symptomatic, complex or indeterminate. Cyst fluid should only be sent for cytology if it is blood stained, safely discarding non-bloody fluid.

After a cyst has been aspirated, the breast should be examined to check that the palpable mass has disappeared. Between 1 and 3 % of patients who have cysts in their breasts also have a carcinoma. It is therefore important that both breasts are assessed by careful clinical examination and appropriate imaging when necessary.

Management of Patients with Cysts

Following aspiration, the majority of patients require no clinical follow-up. It is only those patients who have multiple bilateral cysts who merit any further clinical follow-up. The only reason for seeing these women is that they tend to continue to develop multiple bilateral cysts and return at regular intervals to breast clinics. Regular assessment by clinical assessment and ultrasound allows them to be reassured without the need for regular re-referral. During follow-up only symptomatic cysts should be aspirated. Studies show a small but not a significant increased risk of breast cancer in women with palpable breast cysts [25].

Sclerosis

During evolution, the stroma of the breast changes and it is not uncommon to develop localised areas of excessive fibrosis or sclerosis. Pathologically, sclerosing lesions can be separated into three groups: sclerosing adenosis, radial scars, and complex sclerosing lesions. The only difference between radial scars and complex sclerosing lesions is that radial scars are small and complex sclerosing lesions are larger. Sclerosing lesions are only clinically important because they cause diagnostic problems during imaging and breast screening.

Management of Sclerosing Lesions

They are normally identified on imaging with only a few palpable on clinical examination.

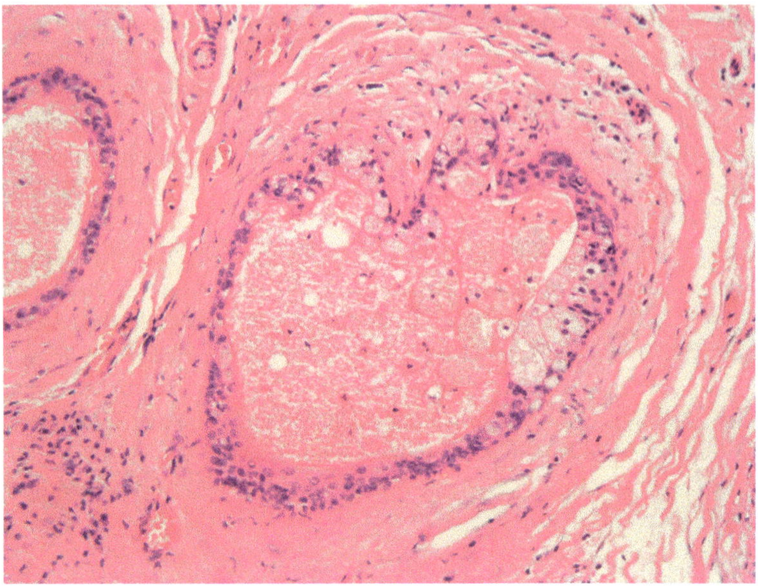

Fig. 3.6 Histology showing features of duct ectasia

A core needle biopsy should be performed. There is some concern that a standard 14-gauge core biopsy might miss a small area of DCIS in association with a radial scar or a complex sclerosing lesion. For this reason larger, vacuum-assisted core biopsy or a needle localisation excision biopsy is required to make a definitive diagnosis [26]. Debate continues as to whether all radial scars should be excised because of their association with invasive and in situ breast cancer [27].

Duct Ectasia

The major subareolar ducts dilate and shorten during ageing or involution. By the age of 70, 40 % of women have substantial duct dilatation. Some of these women develop both duct dilatation and duct shortening that manifests as nipple retraction with or without nipple discharge, and occasionally women present with a palpable periareolar mass that can be hard or doughy from the dilated ducts filled with inspissated secretion. The discharge in patients with duct ectasia is usually "cheesy" in consistency, and the nipple retraction is classically symmetrical or slit like.

Management of Duct Ectasia

Imaging can usually diagnose duct ectasia, and for patients with nipple inversion who have no suspicious features clinically or radiologically, surgery is not required. Surgery is only indicated in multiduct discharge, if it is troublesome or there is an inverted nipple and the patient wants the nipple to be everted. Duct ectasia (Fig. 3.6) should not be confused with periductal mastitis which is a separate condition [28–30]. Once cancer has been excluded, patients with duct ectasia can be reassured and do not require follow-up.

Duct Papillomas

Duct papillomas can be single or multiple. They are common and generally are considered as aberrations rather than true neoplasms as they show minimal malignant potential. The problem is that they are very common and can be visualised on imaging and are often incidental findings during screening. Core biopsy can identify that the lesion is papillary, but often cannot always exclude malignancy. More often than not, the pathologist will give this the diagnosis of a "papillary neoplasm of uncertain clinical significance", prompting removal of the lesion.

Management of Duct Papillomas

Options include observation if there is no evidence of atypia or excision (Fig. 3.7). Papillomas can be removed with vacuum-assisted core

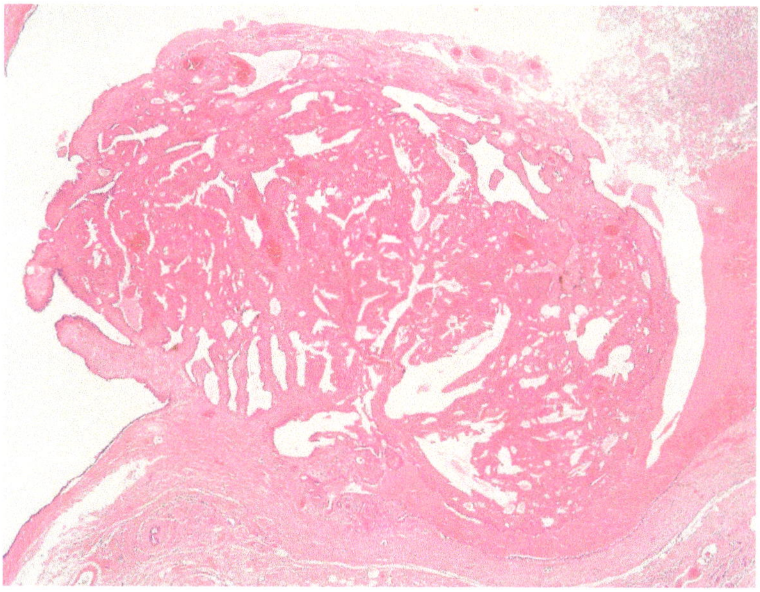

Fig. 3.7 Histology of a benign intraduct papilloma

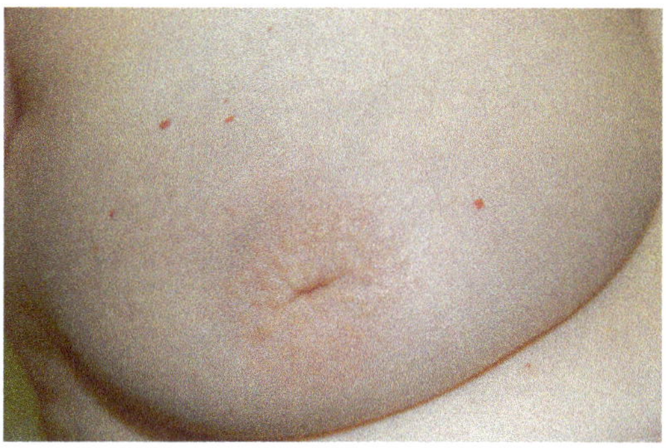

Fig. 3.8 Benign slitlike nipple inversion

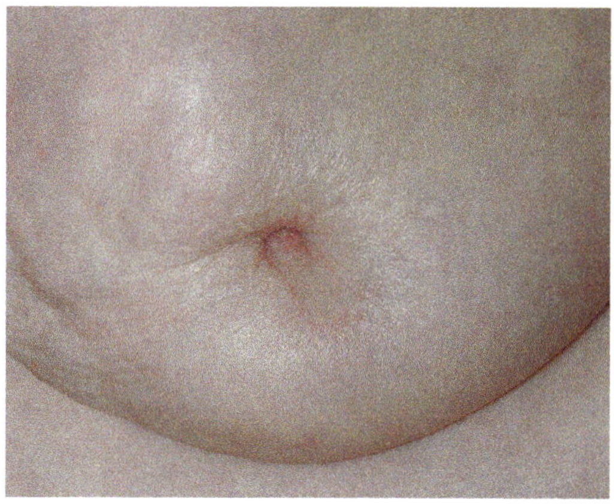

Fig. 3.9 Nipple inversion in association with malignancy

biopsy. They are often excised to exclude malignancy, but given their frequency and low rate of malignancy, there needs to be greater consideration as to whether all such lesions need to be removed [31].

Nipple Retraction

Slitlike retraction of the nipple is characteristic of benign disease (Fig. 3.8), whereas nipple inversion, when the whole nipple is pulled in, occurs in association with both breast cancer and inflammatory benign breast conditions (Fig. 3.9). For patients with congenital nipple retraction and benign acquired nipple retraction, which is unsightly and does not respond to conservative measures such as suction devices or nipple shields, surgery which may require duct division or excision is successful at everting the nipple (Fig. 3.10). Women need to be informed that duct excision can result in loss of ability to breastfeed and can result in loss of, or reduction in, nipple sensation, and occasionally some women develop nipple hypersensitivity.

Nipple Discharge

Nipple discharge accounts for approximately 5 % of all referrals to a breast clinic and is a

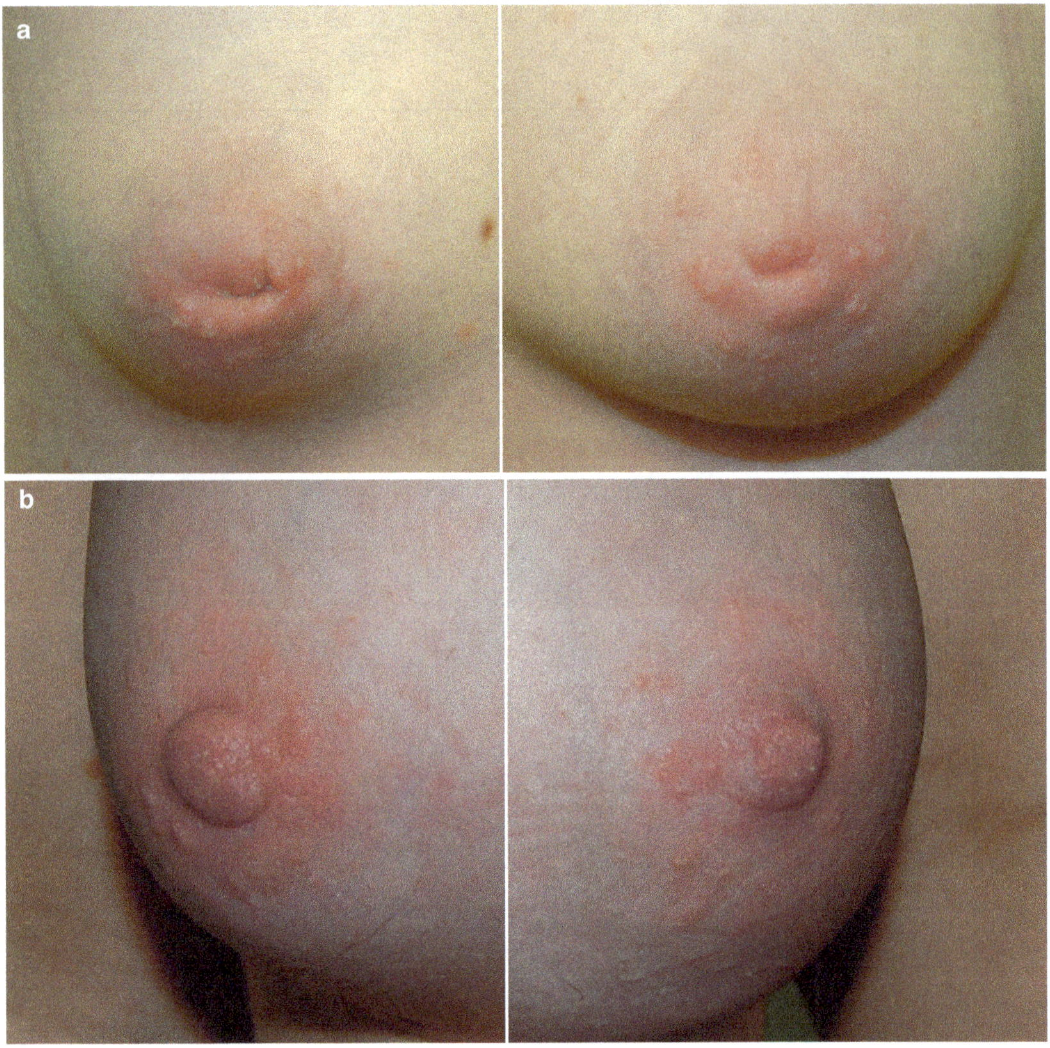

Fig. 3.10 Bilateral nipple inversion (**a**) before and (**b**) after nipple eversion surgery

frightening symptom because of the fear of cancer [32]. More than 95 % of women presenting with nipple discharge will have a benign cause [33]. Discharge associated with significant underlying pathology is spontaneous, more likely to be unilateral, arise from a single duct, be persistent (defined as more than twice a week) and be blood stained. One study found that in women with nipple discharge significant risk factors for malignancy were blood staining of the discharge (odds ratio 3.7) and spontaneous discharge (odds ratio 3.2) [34].

Investigation of Nipple Discharge

Physical examination should include application of firm pressure around the areola as the presence of a dilated duct will result in the production of discharge through the nipple (Fig. 3.11). The nipple should also be squeezed with firm digital pressure, and if fluid is expressed, then the site and character of the discharge recorded. Age is an important predictor of malignancy, and in one study 3 % of patients younger than 40, 10 % of patients between the ages of 40 and 60 and 32 % of women older than 60 years of age who had nipple discharge as their only symptom were found to have cancer [35]. Mammography has a low sensitivity of only approximately two thirds in women with nipple discharge [36, 37]. Ultrasound can identify visible lesions within the breast ducts including papillomas [38]. Imaging the ductal tree by ductography or galactography can identify intraductal lesions, but this investigation has a sensitivity of only 60 % for malignancy [33, 39]. Nipple cytology, ductoscopy and ductal lavage have a role in routine assessment of nipple discharge [40–44]. Of these techniques, ductoscopy is the most accurate but takes longer than 6 months to learn and the equipment is costly [45].

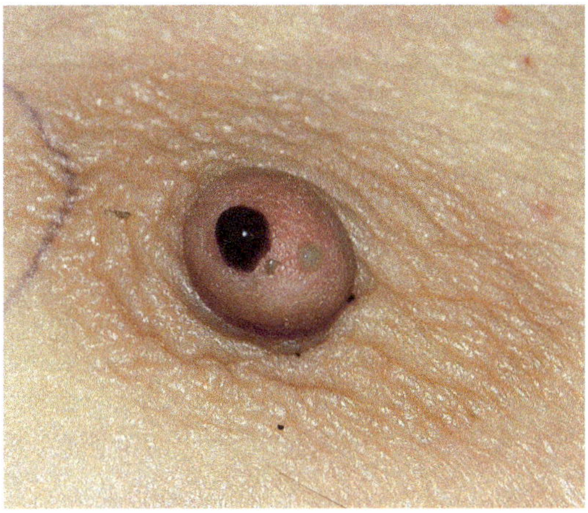

Fig. 3.11 Example of nipple physiological multiduct, multicolour discharge

Management of Nipple Discharge (Fig. 3.12)
If clinical examination demonstrates a mass lesion visible on mammography or ultrasonography, then image-guided core biopsy of this lesion should be performed and the patient managed appropriately [38]. Otherwise, if no abnormalities are found on clinical examination, surgery is indicated for spontaneous discharge from a single duct that has one or more of the following characteristics:

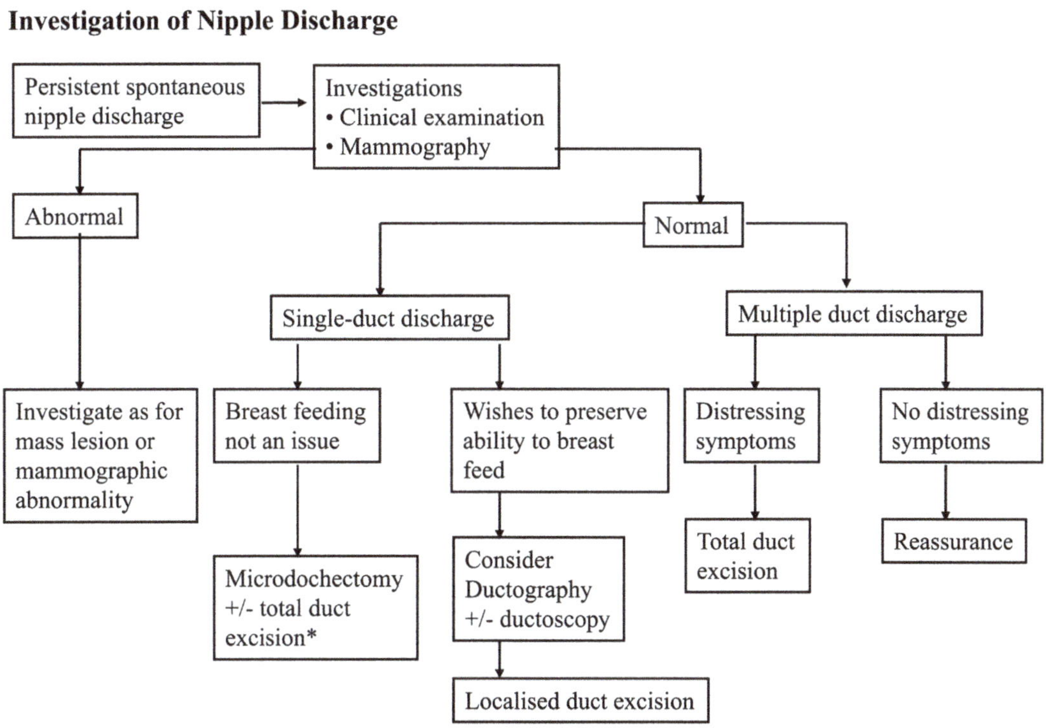

*Some surgeons prefer total duct excision in women >45 to reduce incidence of discharge from other ducts

Fig. 3.12 Flow diagram for investigation of nipple discharge

- Blood stained.
- Persistent and stains clothes.
- Associated with a mass.
- New development in a woman of over 50 years of age.
- The discharge is not thick or cheesy.

Discharge from multiple ducts normally only requires surgery when it causes distressing symptoms.

Options for surgery for single-duct discharge include microdochectomy or total duct excision. Current evidence suggests that total duct excision is more effective than microdochectomy at establishing a specific diagnosis and has a lower chance of missing any malignancy that is present [46]. For this reason, many units perform total duct excision in women over the age of 45 and only perform microdochectomy in younger women [47].

Microdochectomy

Microdochectomy can be performed through a circumareolar or radial incision. The discharging duct is cannulated either with a probe or a blunt-ended needle, through which methylene blue can be injected. Both techniques allow the involved duct to be identified underneath the nipple through the skin incision. The discharging duct, once it has been identified, is dissected distally into the breast over a distance of about 5 cm. Almost all significant disease that causes nipple discharge involves the proximal 5 cm [44, 48]. Following excision of the involved duct, the remaining distal duct in the breast should be inspected, and if there is a visible dilated duct passing into the breast, then further tissue can be excised, or the duct opened and any visible lesion in the duct removed. This is because some DCIS lesions develop at some distance from the nipple, and these produce nipple discharge, but can be missed on microdochectomy. They are diagnosed only if the distal ducts are inspected and excised if abnormal.

Total Duct Excision

Total duct excision is best performed through a circumareolar incision based at 6 o'clock. If the operation is being performed for periductal mastitis, then the patient should receive perioperative and postoperative appropriate antibiotic therapy such as amoxicillin-clavulanic acid or a combination of erythromycin and metronidazole hydrochloride. Having deepened the incision, dissection continues towards the nipple. It is usually better to use scissors or a knife near the nipple rather than cautery. Dissection with Metzenbaum scissors is continued under the areola down either side of the major ducts. Curved tissue forceps are then passed around the ducts, and all the ducts that have been encircled are delivered into the wound. Having secured the distal ducts with tissue forceps, they are then divided from the underside of the nipple.

If a total duct excision is being performed for periductal mastitis, it is important to excise all the ducts up to the nipple skin [49]. If the surgery is being performed for nipple inversion, then the ducts can be simply divided. Otherwise, approximately 2–5 cm of ducts are excised [50]. It is often useful to close any defect in the breast with absorbable sutures. If the nipple was inverted prior to surgery, then it is important to evert the nipple before wound closure, and this may involve dividing any scar tissue that is distorting the nipple. The nipple may need to be squeezed between the thumb and index finger to break down any adhesions to maintain eversion. Sutures are rarely if ever required to maintain eversion because if the nipple does not remain everted without sutures, then it will invert even if sutures are placed. No drains are needed and the wound is closed in layers with absorbable sutures. Patients should be warned before surgery that this operation will reduce nipple sensitivity in up to 40 % of women [49].

Benign Disease in Men

Gynecomastia

Gynecomastia is the growth of breast tissue in males to any extent. It is entirely benign and usually reversible. It is seen most frequently during puberty and old age. In boys aged 10–16 years of age, between 30 and 60 % have breast enlargement, and this usually requires no treatment as 80 % of this breast enlargement resolves spontaneously within 2 years.

Surgery for gynecomastia is not straightforward and should be performed by an experienced surgeon. Embarrassment and persistent enlargement of the breast tissue are both indications for surgery.

Gynecomastia commonly affects older men between the ages of 60 and 80 (Fig. 3.13). In the majority, it does not seem to be associated with any significant endocrine abnormality [51, 52]. There are a variety of specific causes including several classes of medications. A careful alcohol and drug history and an examination often reveal the cause.

Patients with recent progressive breast enlargement without any easily identifiable cause require a hormonal profile and blood tests to exclude a metabolic cause. Mammography and ultrasound can differentiate between breast enlargement due to fat or gynecomastia and can identify malignancy if this is suspected. Breast cancer usually presents as a firm lump that is eccentric, whereas gynecomastia is concentric. If imaging is suspicious, then core biopsy should be performed.

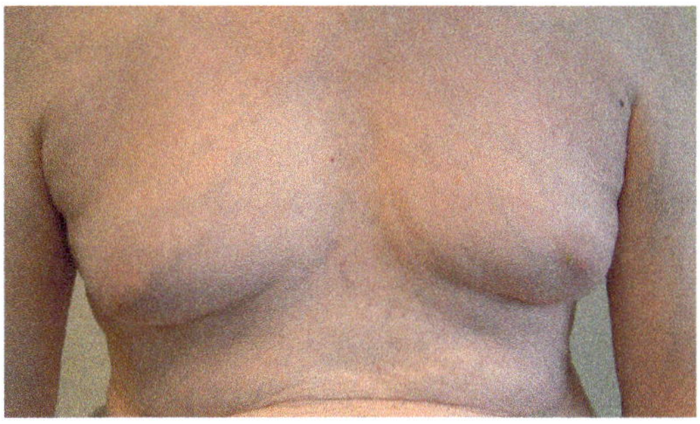

Fig. 3.13 Bilateral senescent gynecomastia

Management of Gynecomastia

In drug-related gynecomastia, withdrawal of the drug or change to an alterative treatment should be considered. Gynecomastia is seen in bodybuilders who take anabolic steroids, and some of these have learned that by taking tamoxifen, they can counteract these symptoms. Bodybuilders should be encouraged to reduce or stop steroids. In young men, gynecomastia is seen in both heavy beer and lager drinkers and in young men who smoke cannabis. There are phytoestrogens in beer and lager; cannabis is also estrogenic in its action.

In patients with symptomatic gynecomastia, both tamoxifen and danazol improve symptoms, but recurrence when the drug stops can be a problem [53, 54]. Tamoxifen at a dose of 10 mg is effective and produces less side effects than 20 mg. Surgery for gynecomastia is not straightforward and should normally be performed by experienced breast surgeons or plastic surgeons. It often involves a combination of excision of breast tissue and liposuction occasionally with removal of overlying skin [55–57] (Fig. 3.14).

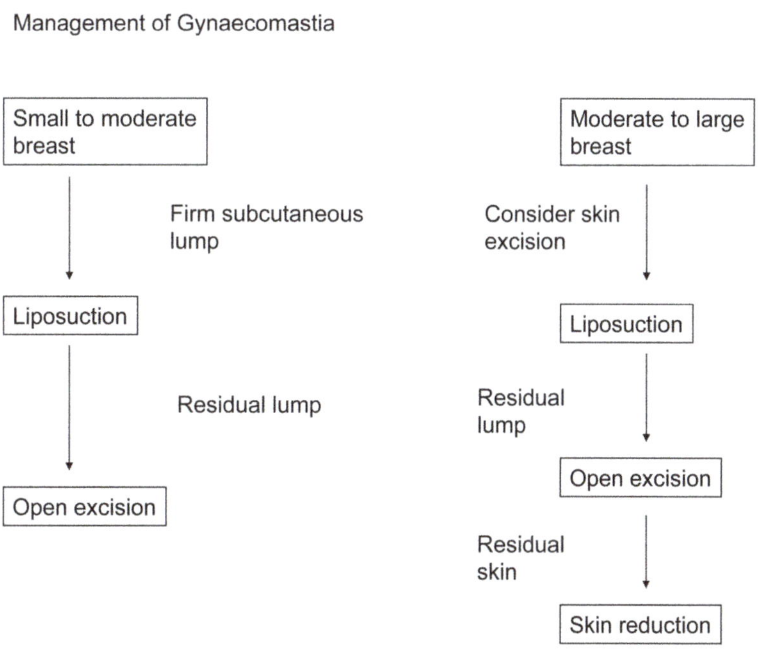

Fig. 3.14 Algorithm for the management of gynecomastia

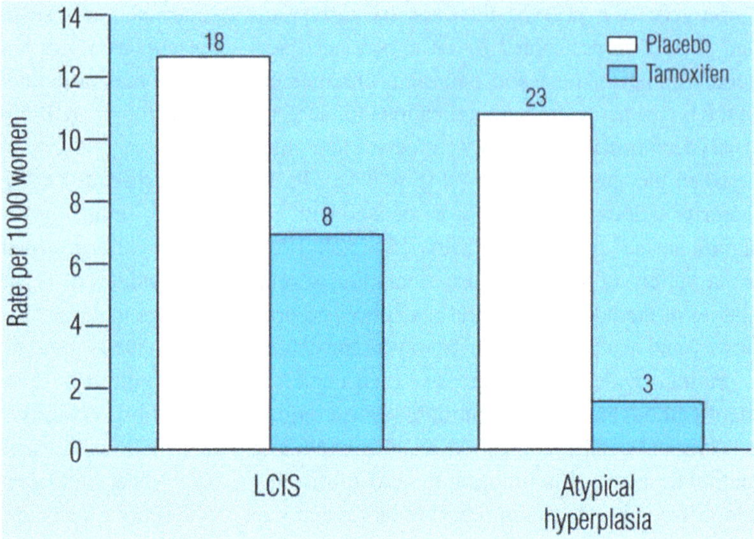

Fig. 3.15 Results of chemoprevention for atypical ductal hyperplasia and lobular intraepithelial neoplasia from the NSABP study

Benign Neoplasms and Proliferations

Epithelial Hyperplasia

This is an increase in the number of cells lining the terminal duct lobular unit. Previously called epitheliosis or papillomatosis, these terms are no longer in common use. The degree of hyperplasia can be graded as mild, moderate or severe. Atypical hyperplasia is diagnosed if the hyperplastic cells also show cellular atypia. Atypical hyperplasia is one of the few benign conditions that are associated with a significantly increased risk of breast cancer. The absolute risk of breast cancer in women with atypical hyperplasia who do not have a first-degree relative with breast cancer is about 8 % at 10 years [58]. However, in women who do have a first-degree relative with breast cancer, the risk increases to 20–25 % at 15 years [58]. Hyperplasia can consist of cells with so-called "ductal" or "lobular" morphology. Atypical hyperplasia of lobular type is now classified together with lobular carcinoma in situ as a single entity called lobular intraepithelial neoplasia.

Management of Atypical Hyperplasia and Lobular Intraepithelial Neoplasia

Options include regular screening, breast screening with annual mammography or chemoprevention. Tamoxifen reduced the risk of breast cancer by 87 % in women with atypical hyperplasia and 56 % in LCIS (Fig. 3.15). Patients with atypical hyperplasia of ductal type are at increased risk of developing breast cancer in the same breast, whereas patients with lobular intraepithelial neoplasia are at risk of developing breast cancer in either breast.

Breast Infection

Breast infection is now less common that it used to be. Breast infection can be subdivided into lactational, non-lactational and postsurgical. The skin overlying the breast can also become infected

Table 3.1 Organisms responsible for different types of breast infection and appropriate antibiotics

Type of infection	Organism	No penicillin allergy	Penicillin allergy
Neonatal	*Staphylococcus aureus* (rarely *Escherichia coli*)	Flucloxacillin (500 mg four times daily)	Erythromycin (500 mg twice daily)
Lactational	*S. aureus* (rarely *S. epidermidis* and streptococci)	Flucloxacillin (500 mg four times daily)	Erythromycin (500 mg twice daily)
Skin associated	*S. aureus* (500 mg four times daily)	Flucloxacillin (500 mg twice daily)	Erythromycin (500 mg twice daily)
Non-lactating	*S. aureus*, enterococci, anaerobic streptococci, *Bacteroides* spp.	Co-amoxiclav (375 mg three times daily)	Combination of erythromycin (500 mg twice daily) with metronidazole (200 mg three times daily)

either primarily or secondarily to an existing lesion such as an epidermoid cyst or as a consequence of a more generalised skin condition such as hidradenitis suppurativa. Breast infection is also occasionally seen in neonates. The organisms responsible for breast infection and the most appropriate antibiotics with activity against these organisms are summarised in Table 3.1 [59].

Lactational Infection

This is most commonly seen during the first pregnancy and in the first 6 weeks of breastfeeding but can also occur during weaning. The first stage in the development of breast infection is usually a cracked nipple or skin abrasion due to nipple trauma from breast feeding. This produces oedema of the subareolar ducts and poor milk drainage. A consequence of nipple maceration is an increased number of organisms on the skin, and together with a poorly draining segment, the milk becomes infected. The most common causal organism is *Staphylococcus aureus*, but *Staphylococcus epidermidis* can sometimes be the cause.

Symptoms include pain, erythema, swelling, tenderness and occasionally systemic signs of infection. A fluctuant mass with overlying shiny red skin is the classic feature of a breast abscess, but the clinical signs are usually more subtle consisting of erythema overlying a tender wooden area of breast tissue. Enlarged lymph nodes are not usually a feature, although occasionally patients can be toxic with pyrexia, tachycardia and a raised white count.

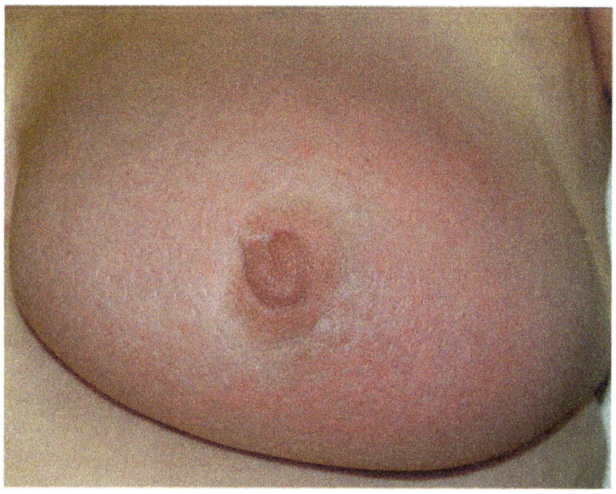

Fig. 3.16 Inflammatory breast cancer mimicking cellulitis

Management of Lactational Infection

In the early stages, antibiotics and promotion of breast feeding is usually effective at resolving the infection. Appropriate antibiotics for treating different infections are listed in Table 3.1. Tetracycline, ciprofloxacin and chloramphenicol should not be used as they can potentially harm the baby [60]. A patient whose condition does not improve rapidly within a few days of starting an appropriate antibiotic should have ultrasonography performed. Inflammatory cancers can sometimes be difficult to differentiate from breast infections (Fig. 3.16).

How I Do It: Management of Breast Abscesses

If an abscess is evident on ultrasound (Fig. 3.17a), then management depends on the state of the overlying skin. If the skin is not thinned or necrotic, then the abscess should be aspirated to dryness under ultrasound guidance. One percent lidocaine with 1 in 200,000 adrenaline is injected into the normal skin some distance away from the abscess and injected into the breast parenchyma up to the edge of the abscess. A long needle (spinal needle) may be required if the abscess is deep in the breast to ensure the whole length of the needle track is anaesthetised. Either using the

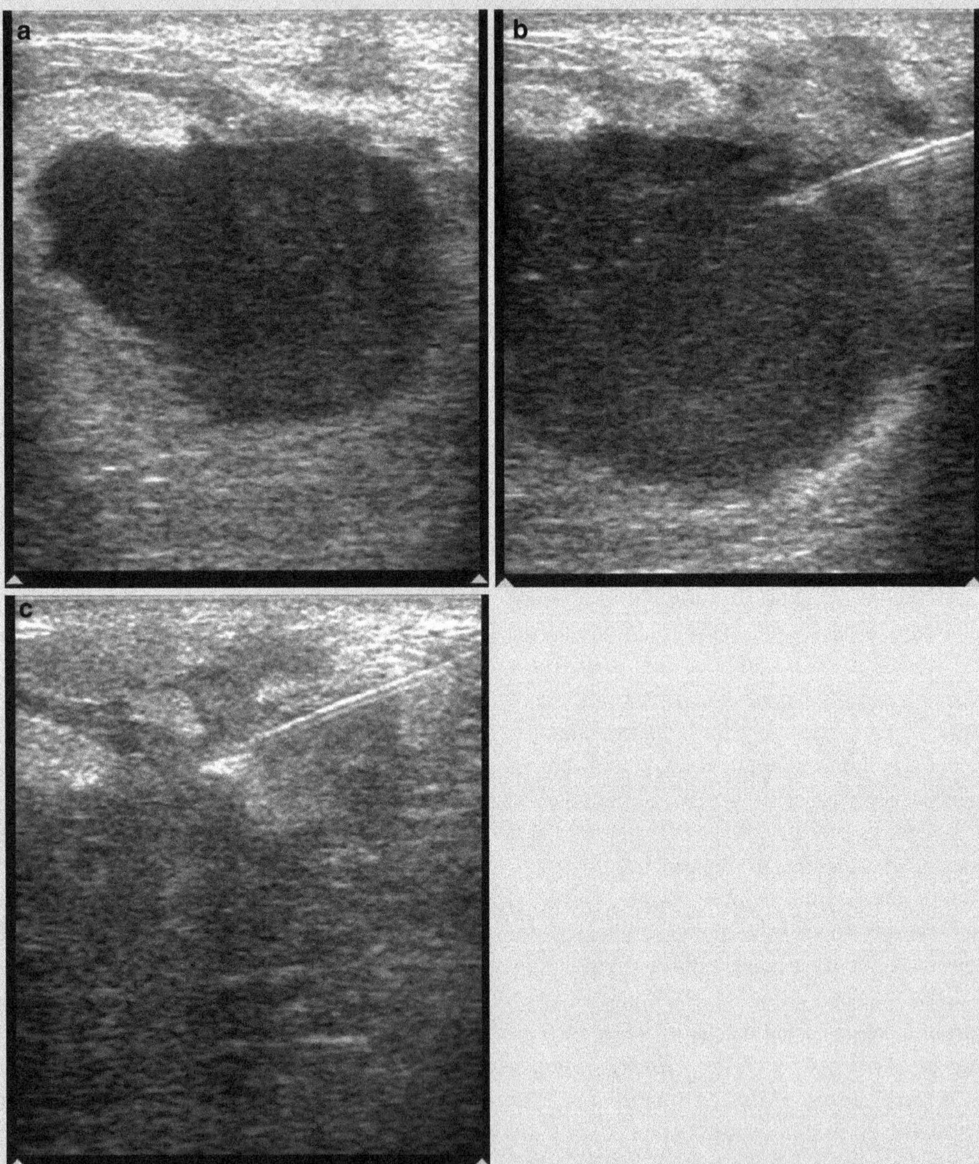

Fig. 3.17 (**a**) Ultrasound of lactating breast abscess. (**b**) Ultrasound of lactating breast abscess with needle in abscess. (**c**) Ultrasound of lactating breast abscess post aspiration

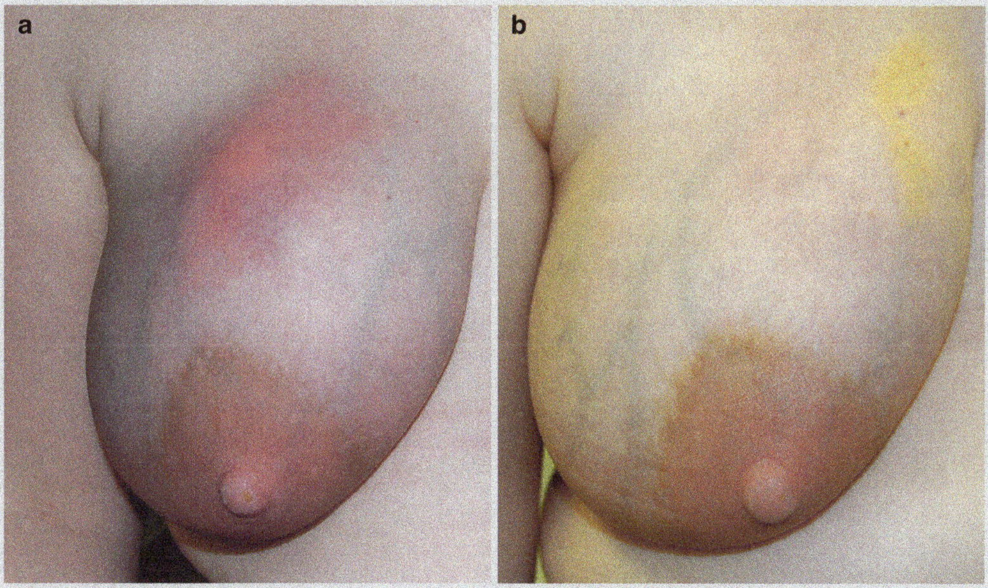

Fig. 3.18 Lactating abscess (**a**) pre- and (**b**) posttreatment with needle aspiration

same needle or using a larger needle, local anaesthetic with adrenaline is then irrigated into and out of the abscess cavity until the fluid aspirated comes back clear (Fig. 3.17b). The local anaesthetic has two roles; first it reduces pain and, second, it dilutes out any thick pus and allows this to be aspirated. The adrenaline reduces bleeding and allows greater volumes of local anaesthetic to be used. As most of the anaesthetic irrigated into the cavity is re-aspirated, large volumes can be used safely. Once the fluid comes back clear, then the abscess is aspirated to dryness (Fig. 3.17c). The patient is then reviewed in 48–72 h. A combination of aspiration every 2 or 3 days and oral antibiotics is effective at resolving most breast abscesses (Fig. 3.18a, b) [59–61]. Characteristically, the fluid aspirated changes over a week from pus to serous fluid and then to milk.

If the skin overlying the abscess is thinned (Fig. 3.19a) and pus is visible on ultrasound close to the skin, then the lidocaine and adrenaline are injected directly into the thinned skin over the abscess with a 23- or 25-gauge needle (Fig. 3.19b). A small stab incision is then made 5–10 min later into the anaesthetised skin (Fig. 3.19c). Through this small incision, pus is drained (Fig. 3.19d) and the cavity is irrigated with local anaesthetic solution (Fig. 3.19e). Irrigation is continued until all pus has been drained (Fig. 3.19f). The incision can be kept open with a small piece of Kaltostat, but the abscess should not be packed. A dry dressing is then placed over the Kaltostat to collect any fluid that drains from the abscess cavity. The patient is reviewed 2–3 days later and the cavity irrigated every 2–3 days with saline or local anaesthetic until resolution. Few if any lactational abscesses require drainage under general anaesthesia. The use of drains and packing of any breast abscess is unnecessary. Breastfeeding should continue if possible because the infant is not harmed by the bacteria in the milk nor the antibiotics, and continuing to breastfeed promotes abscess resolution. There are some women who have multiple areas of breast infection and who are exhausted by breastfeeding, in whom consideration should be given to stopping breastfeeding and halting milk flow. Stopping milk production is achieved by prescribing cabergoline 2.5 mcg given twice a day for 2 days.

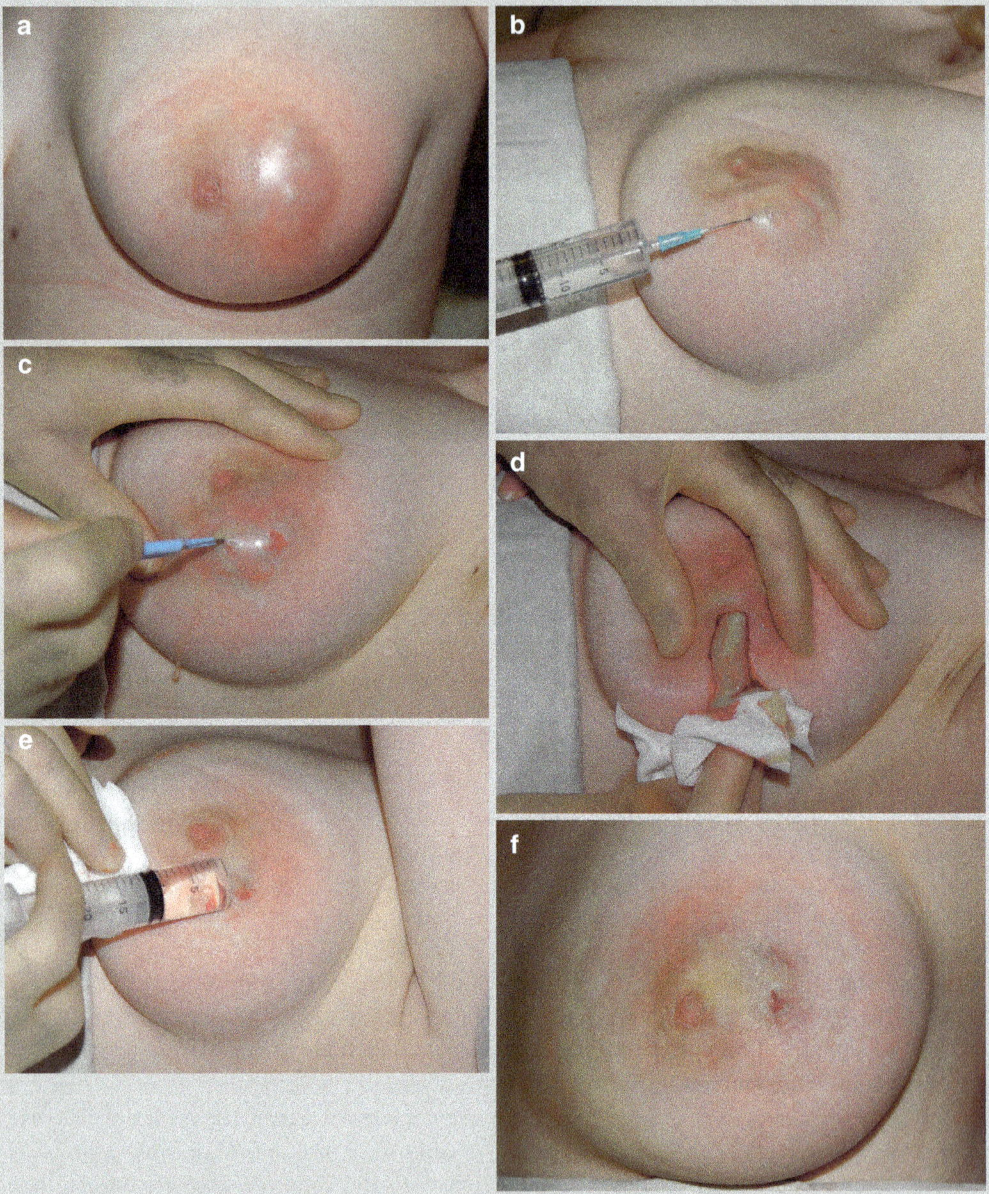

Fig. 3.19 (**a**) Non-lactating abscess with shiny overlying skin (left breast). (**b**) Infiltration of 1 % lidocaine + 1 in 200,000 adrenaline into skin. (**c**) Incision through skin overlying the abscess. (**d**) Pus draining from abscess. (**e**) Irrigation of abscess cavity with local anaesthetic solution. (**f**) Abscess post incision and drainage

Non-lactational Infection

Central or Periareolar Infection

Periareolar infection is most commonly seen in young women with a mean age of 32 years, and most are cigarette smokers [62]. The reason patients get periareolar infection is as a consequence of infection of areas of periductal mastitis [59, 63]. This condition has been confused with, and called, duct ectasia, but duct ectasia is a separate condition affecting older women and is characterised by subareolar duct dilatation and less pronounced and less active periductal inflammation [30]. Current evidence suggests that smoking is the most important factor in the aetiology of periductal mastitis: about 90 % of women who get periductal mastitis, or its complications, smoke cigarettes; this compares with 38 % of the same age group in the general population [64]. Substance in cigarette smoke may either directly or indirectly damage the wall of the subareolar breast ducts. Aerobic or anaerobic organisms then infect these damaged tissues [65].

In North America, a widely held view is that periductal mastitis is due to duct obstruction by squamous metaplasia that is seen commonly in this condition. All ducts in non-lactating women are plugged with keratin, so duct obstruction is not important, and the squamous metaplasia seen in periductal mastitis is likely to be a consequence of chronic infection, rather than the cause of it. Initial presentation of periductal mastitis may be with periareolar inflammation (with or without an associated mass) or with an established abscess (Fig. 3.20). Associated features include central breast pain, nipple retraction at the site of the diseased duct and purulent nipple discharge. The organisms responsible for periductal mastitis and periareolar infection are different to those in lactational infection and often include anaerobes (Table 3.1). Periareolar infection should initially be treated by antibiotics, but if this does not settle, an ultrasound should be performed. Any abscess should be treated by aspiration and mini-incision and drainage as with lactational infection. Periareolar inflammation tends to be recurrent because incision and drainage or aspiration of any abscess does not remove the underlying cause of the periductal mastitis.

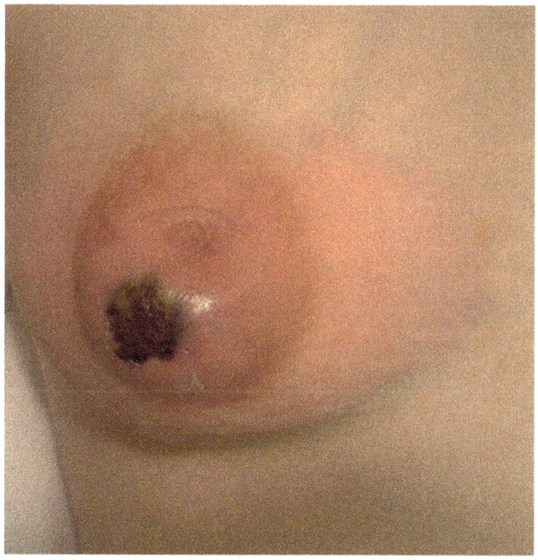

Fig. 3.20 Periareolar non-lactating abscess (right breast) with skin necrosis requiring incision and drainage

Mammary Duct Fistulae

A mammary duct fistula is a communication between the skin usually and the periareolar region and a major subareolar duct [59]. They are seen to develop most commonly after incision and drainage of a non-lactational abscess, although they can also occur following spontaneous discharge of a periareolar inflammatory mass or following biopsy of an area of periductal mastitis [66].

Management of Mammary Duct Fistula

Management of mammary duct fistula consists of either opening up the fistula tract or excising it [66, 67]. Fistula operations are best performed under general anaesthetic. A probe is passed along the fistula either from its opening through the nipple or through the opening at the areolar margin. The simplest procedure is to simply cut

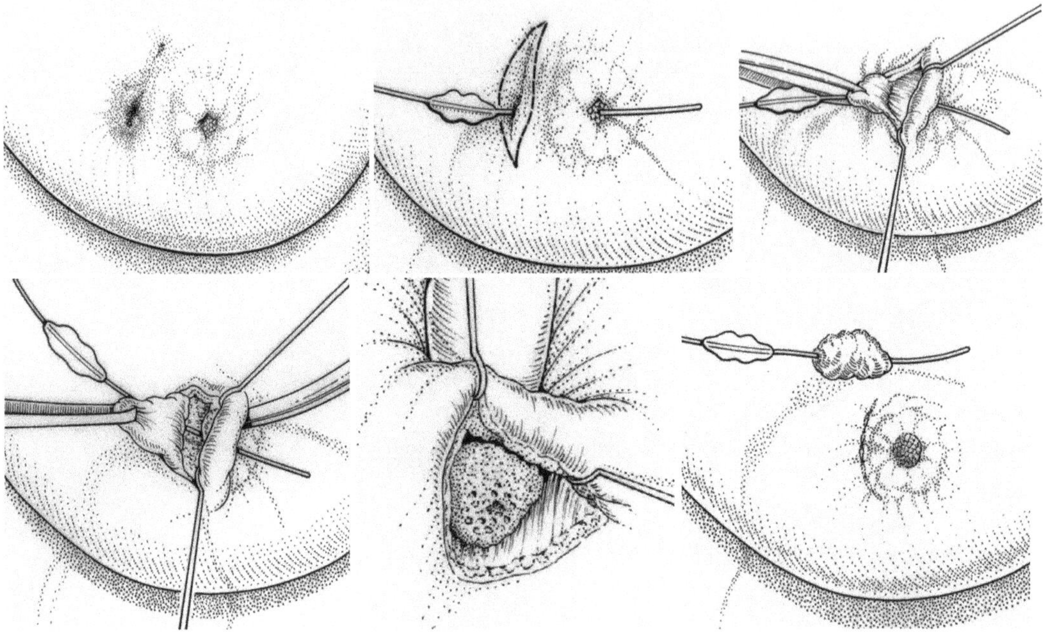

Fig. 3.21 Diagrammatic illustration of the steps involved in excision of a mammary duct fistula performed through a circumareolar incision with primary wound closure under antibiotic cover [67]

down onto the fistula probe (fistulotomy). This is the operation as described by Atkins [67] and is effective but tends to leave an ugly scar. Another option is to excise the skin over the fistula probe and excise the whole of the fistula tract (fistulectomy). This is achieved by deepening the incision underneath the fistula probe to ensure the entire fistula tract is removed. This is usually successful but leaves a poor cosmetic outcome. An alternative is to make a periareolar incision incorporating the exit site of the fistula at the areolar margin (Fig. 3.21) [68]. The incision is deepened and the skin anterior to the fistula probe on the areola is lifted off and left intact and dissection continued under the skin to excise the tract incorporating all the granulation lined fistula tract up to the nipple. It is important to excise the entire fistula directly up to the nipple skin.

This is a more technically demanding operation than simple fistulotomy or fistulectomy, and to excise the whole of the fistula usually requires a total duct excision, with excision of all the ducts up to the back of the nipple skin. Excision of the whole of the diseased duct usually leaves a small hole in the nipple skin at the site of the affected duct. This does not need to be closed and no deep sutures are required. The circumareolar wound is closed in layers with absorbable sutures. As fistulae are infected the operation should be covered by peri-antibiotics (Table 3.1), and if the wound has been closed, then the patient should be given 5 days of post-operative antibiotics.

Peripheral Non-lactating Abscesses

Peripheral non-lactating abscesses are less common than periareolar abscesses, and although they have been reported to be associated with conditions such as rheumatoid arthritis, diabetes, steroid treatment and trauma in the majority, there is no obvious cause [69] (Fig. 3.22). *Staphylococcus aureus* is most commonly responsible. Peripheral abscesses are treated by aspiration or incision and drainage as for other breast abscesses.

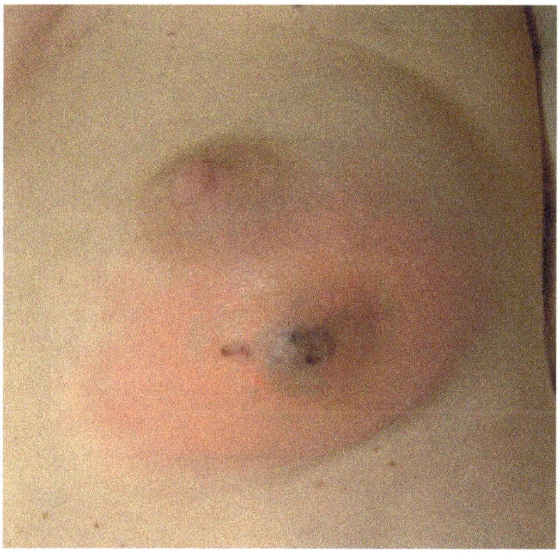

Fig. 3.22 Peripheral breast abscess with thinned overlying skin

Skin-Associated Infection

Cellulitis

Cellulitis is an uncommon infection in the breast and can be difficult to distinguish from inflammatory breast cancer or benign erythematous conditions of the breast. Pain is a prominent feature of breast cellulitis and is associated with erythema, swelling, and warmth. Treatment is with antibiotics Table 3.1.

Eczema

Patients with eczema involving the skin overlying the breast may develop secondary cellulitis. Appropriate treatments for the eczema reduce recurrence of the cellulitis.

Epidermoid Cysts

Epidermoid cysts are discrete nodules that often are referred to as sebaceous cysts, but there is no sebaceous component. These cysts are common within the skin of the breast and can become infected, forming local abscesses that require mini incision and drainage.

Hidradenitis Suppurativa

Hidradenitis suppurativa is a condition that affects the apocrine sweat glands and can result in recurrent infection and abscess formation of the skin of the lower half of the breast as well as the axilla [59, 70–73]. Treatment of hidradenitis suppurativa involves stopping smoking and keeping the area of skin as clean and dry and possible. A variety of drug treatments have been tried and are partially effective. Excision and skin grafting has a success rate of up to 50 %.

Intertrigo

Intertrigo is inflamed skin in the inframammary folds, and this is usually due to the skin becoming moist and macerated [74, 75]. This is a recurrent problem in women with large ptotic breasts that make contact with the chest wall. Fungi play no aetiological role in this condition. The primary management of intertrigo is to educate the patient about keeping the area as clean and dry as possible. The skin should be washed gently two times a day with simple soap, a mild cleansing solution or hypoallergenic skin wipes and then dabbed dry with a towel or dried with a hair dryer at a low setting [74, 75]. Preventive measures include wearing cotton against the skin and keeping the skin dry and clean. Steroids and antifungal creams should be avoided.

Piercing

Nipple rings can result in subareolar breast abscess and recurrent nipple infections, particularly in smokers (Fig. 3.23). Nipple piercing is a significant risk factor for a subareolar breast abscess (objective risk (OR) 20 [95 % CI 2.01–204.28]) as is smoking (OR 11 [95 % CI 4.41–29.94]) [76].

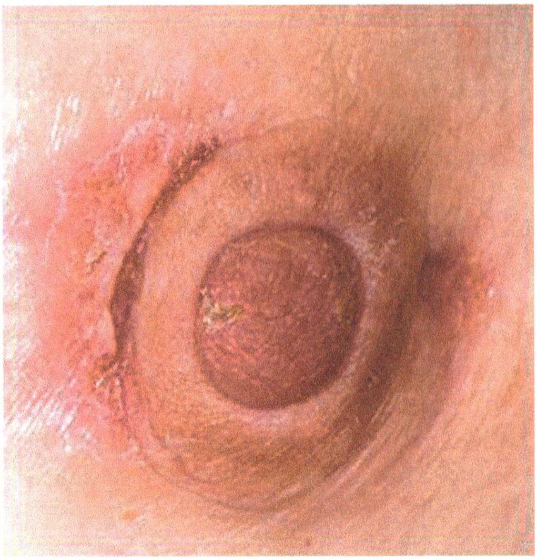

Fig. 3.23 Infection resulting from nipple piercing (piercing removed) with scars of abscess drainage

Other Rare Infections

Tuberculosis is rare in Western countries but the breast can be the primary site [59, 60].

Granulomatous Lobular Mastitis

Granulomatous lobular mastitis is characterised by noncaseating granulomata and microabscesses confined to the breast lobule [77, 78]. It can present as a firm mass which may be indistinguishable from breast cancer or multiple and sometimes recurrent abscesses (Fig. 3.24). Occasionally skin ulceration is seen. It is most common in young women who have a history of breast feeding although not all women who develop this condition are parous [79]. Its exact cause is not

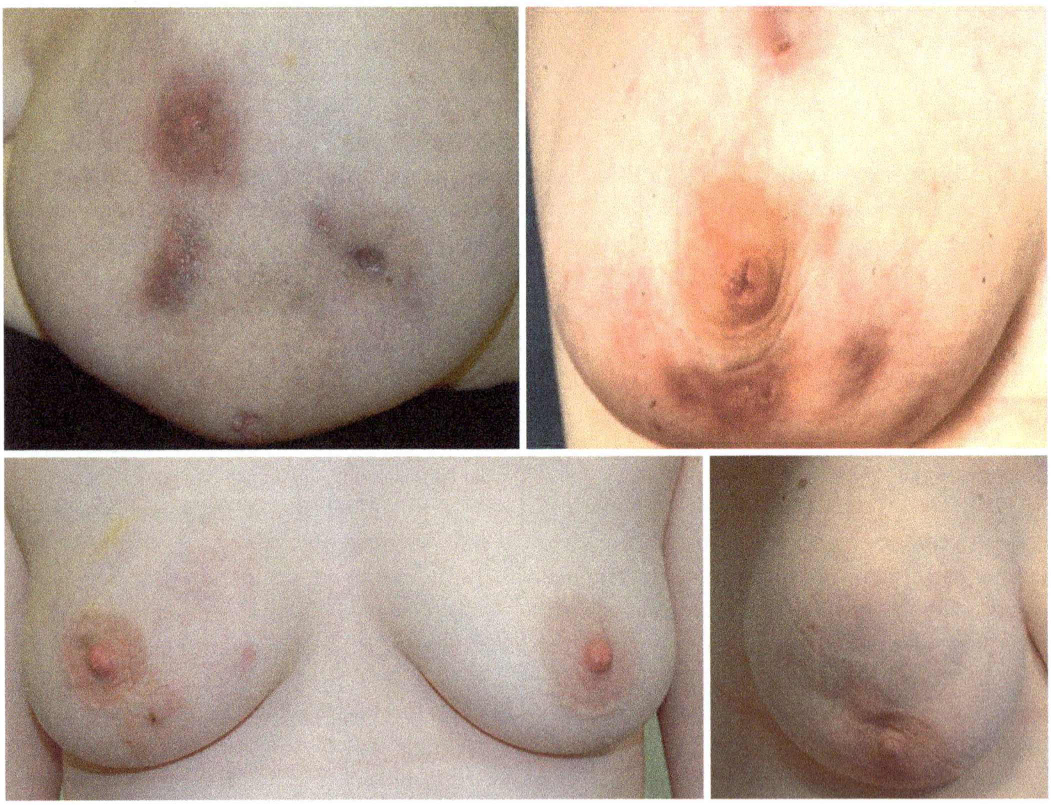

Fig. 3.24 Spectrum of granulomatous lobular mastitis with overlying skin changes and swelling and distortion that can be seen in this condition

clear and different aetiologies including hyperprolactinemia and corynebacterium have been suggested as having an aetiological role, but there is no real evidence that they are the underlying cause.

Management of Granulomatous Lobular Mastitis

Current treatment involves establishing a diagnosis preferably with a core biopsy and observation. There is a strong tendency for this condition to recur even if it is excised. Steroids have been tried but without consistent success [78]. More recently, methotrexate has been proposed as a treatment, but this may work simply as an immunosuppressant, and whether it alters the course of the disease is not clear [80].

Breast Infection After Surgery

Rates of breast infection after surgery vary in relation to the extent of the surgery and the preoperative risk factors including smoking, obesity and the presence of diabetes. Rates of over 10 % are seen after mastectomy and axillary lymph node dissection [81]. Preoperative antibiotics reduce the risk of infection by approximately 36 %, and therefore these should be administered to the majority of patients undergoing breast surgical operations [82].

Other Benign Breast Conditions

Galactorrhea

Galactorrhea is copious bilateral milky discharge not associated with pregnancy or breastfeeding [83]. Prolactin levels are usually, but not always, raised. A careful drug history should be taken as a variety of agents, particularly psychotropic agents, can cause hyperprolactinaemia. In the absence of a relevant drug cause, a search for a pituitary tumour should be instituted in a patient with a raised prolactin greater than 1,000 IU/l.

Lipomas

Lipomas are soft, lobulated radiolucent lesions and they need to be differentiated from pseudolipomas which are soft masses that can be felt around breast cancers caused by indrawing of surrounding fat by the cancer. Ultrasound and mammography are helpful in establishing the diagnosis. Lipomas only need to be excised if they are troublesome.

Nipple Adenoma

Nipple adenoma is an ulcerated lesion of the nipple that can either present as a lump in the nipple or nipple discharge (Fig. 3.25). Treatment is by wide excision and it is usually possible to save the nipple. Recurrence is seen if the lesion is not completely excised.

Hematoma

Hematomas most commonly follow trauma, such as road traffic accident, but can occur after core biopsy, fine-needle aspiration cytology or open biopsy. In extremely unusual circumstances a breast cancer can present as a spontaneous hematoma.

Fat Necrosis

Fat necrosis is common. It is often called traumatic fat necrosis although there is only a history of trauma in around 40 % of cases. Fat necrosis can be difficult to differentiate from malignancy. Imaging usually suggests the diagnosis. Core biopsy features are characteristic, and such areas rarely need to be excised.

Mondor's Disease

Mondor's Disease is thrombosis of the superficial veins of the breast. The thoracoepigastric vein is

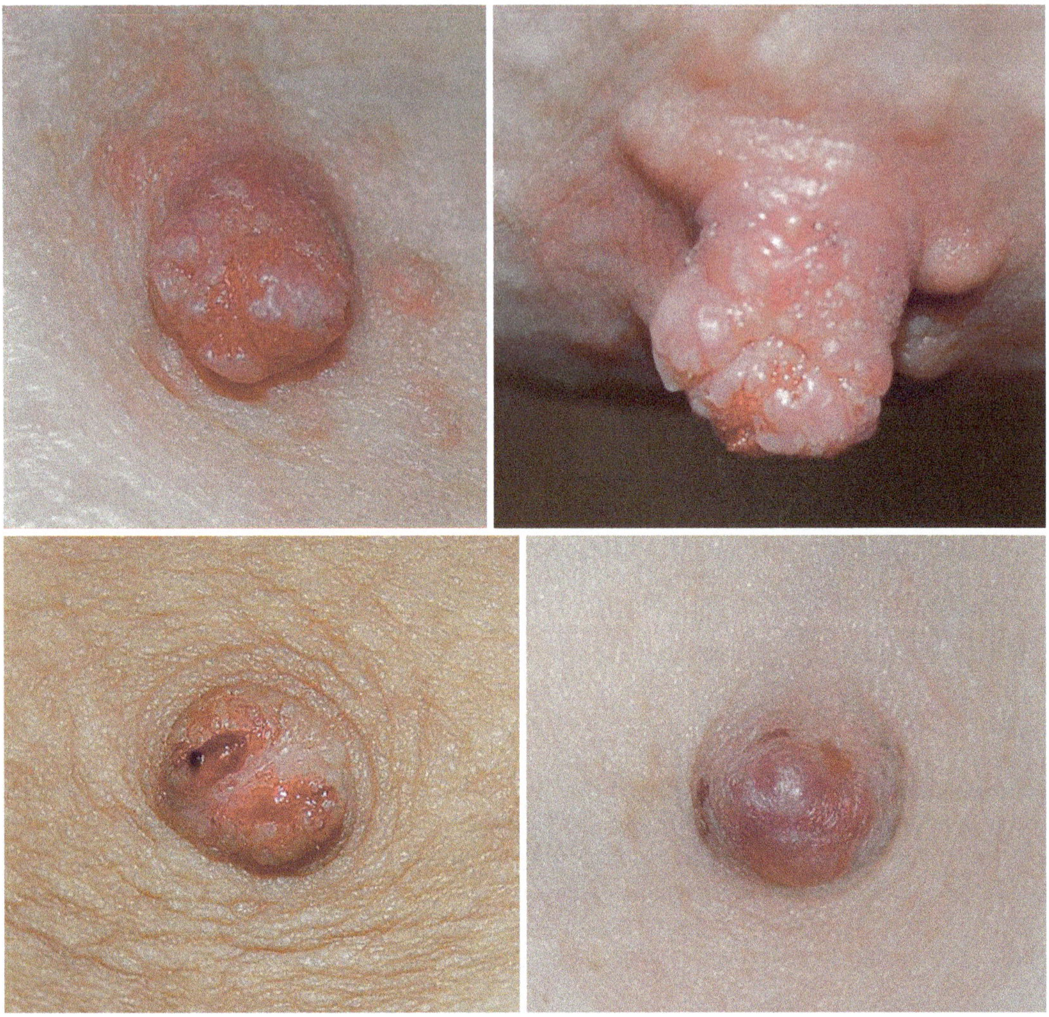

Fig. 3.25 Examples of nipple adenomas

the most common site. It is seen after surgery or trauma although it can occur spontaneously. It is often painful and tender to touch. Other than analgesia, no specific treatment is required.

Hamartoma

Hamartomas, otherwise known as fibroadenolipomas, are quite common. They present as a discrete mass and are often misinterpreted clinically and on ultrasound as fibroadenomas. It is important for clinicians when biopsying lesions likely to be hamartomas to inform the pathologist of the suspicion the lesion may be a hamartoma; otherwise, the core biopsy may be reported as showing normal breast tissue, and thus the suspicion may be the lesion has been missed. The pathology of hamartomas is subtle and includes normal breast tissue elements in a disorganised manner.

Enlarged Montgomery's Tubercles

Montgomery's Tubercles are blind ending ducts in the areola. Secretions can become inspissated and they can develop into a lump in the areolar skin. They only need to be excised if troublesome.

Para Areola Cysts

Para areola cysts are rare but are seen in pubertal and post-pubertal teenagers (13–16 years). They present as discrete superficial masses at the areola margin. They can often be seen through the skin and contain green or blue/black fluid. Because the fluid can be inspissated, they can sometimes be interpreted on ultrasound as solid. Once a diagnosis has been established, they do not need treatment as they usually resolve, but if the lesion is large, it can be aspirated.

Morphoea

Morphoea is a form of localised scleroderma of the breast and presents as a thickened, white oedematous area of the skin. It can result in distortion of the breast contour and is most common in women who have had radiotherapy after breast conserving surgery [84]. Treatment is symptomatic with local chemotherapeutic creams if there is significant a degree of inflammatory change.

Arteritis and Aneurysm

Patients with generalised vascular disease can develop localised vasculitis of the breast. Aneurysmal dilatation of arteries in the breast has also been reported [85].

Sarcoidosis

Patients with sarcoid can present with a single or multiple masses within the breast. Although it can be the first presentation of sarcoid, it is more common in patients with disease elsewhere.

Granular Cell Tumours

Granular cell tumours are uncommon benign neoplasms that originate from Schwann cells or peripheral nerves in the breast. About 6 % of all granular tumours involve the breast [86]. They are benign and treatment is by excision.

Diabetic Mastopathy

Diabetic mastopathy is a form of breast sclerosis occurring in premenopausal women and occasionally men with type 1 diabetes [87]. It can present clinically as one or more hard masses which are indistinguishable from malignancy. Core biopsy establishes the diagnosis.

References

1. Thrush S, Sayer G, Scott-Coombes D, et al. Is the grading of referrals to a specialist breast unit appropriate or effective? Br Med J. 2002;324:1279.
2. Down S, Barr L, Baildam AD, et al. Management of accessory breast tissue in the axilla. Br J Surg. 2003;90:1213–4.
3. Nerakha GJ. In: Gallager HS, Leis HP, Synderman RK, et al., editors. The breast. St. Louis: Mosby; 1978. p. 442–51.
4. Pinsolle V, Chichery A, Grolleau JL, et al. Autologous fat injection in Poland's syndrome. J Plast Reconstr Aesthet Surg. 2008;61(7):784–91.
5. Delay E, Garson S, Tousson G, Sinna R. Fat injection to the breasts: technique, results and indications based on 880 procedures over 10 years. Aesthet Surg J. 2009;29:360–76.
6. Hall-Findlay EJ. Vertical breast reduction using the superomedial pedicle. In: Speark SL, editor. Surgery of the breast, principles and art. Philadelphia: Lippincott Williams and Wilkins; 2006. p. 1072–92.
7. Hughes LE, Mansel RE, Webster DJ. Aberrations of normal development and involution (ANDI): a new perspective on pathogenesis and nomenclature of benign breast disorders. Lancet. 1987;2:1316–9.
8. World Health Organisation. Histological typing of breast tumours. 2nd ed. Geneva: WHO; 1981.
9. Guillot E, Couturaud B, Reyal F. Management of phyllodes breast tumors. Breast J. 2011;17(2):129–37.
10. Sperber F, Blank A, Metser U, et al. Diagnosis and treatment of breast fibroadenomas by ultrasound guided vacuum-assisted biopsy. Arch Surg. 2003;138:796–800.
11. Mansel RE. ABC of breast diseases: breast pain. Br Med J. 1994;309:866–8.
12. Barros AC, Mottola J, Ruiz CA, et al. Reassurance in the treatment of mastalgia. Breast J. 1999;5:162–5.
13. Khoo SK, Munro C, Battistutta D. Evening primrose oil and treatment of premenstrual syndrome. Med J Aust. 1990;153:189–92.

14. Blommers J, de Lange-De Klerk ES, Kuik DJ, et al. Evening primrose oil and fish oil for severe chronic mastalgia: a randomised, double blind controlled trial. Am J Obstet Gynecol. 2002;187:1389–94.
15. Pashby NH, Mansel RE, Hughes LE, et al. A clinical trial of evening primrose oil in mastalgia. Br J Surg. 1981;68:801–24.
16. Boyd NF, McGuire V, Shannon P, et al. Effect of a low-fat high-carbohydrate diet on symptoms of clinical mastopathy. Lancet. 1988;2:128–32.
17. Fentiman IS, Caleffi M, Brame K, et al. Double blind controlled trial of tamoxifen therapy for mastalgia. Lancet. 1986;1:287–8.
18. Kontostolis E, Stefanidis K, Navrozoglou I, et al. Comparison of tamoxifen with danazol for treatment of cyclical mastalgia. Gynecol Endocrinol. 1997;11: 393–7.
19. GEMB Group Argentine. Tamoxifen therapy for cyclical mastalgia: dose randomised trial. Breast. 1997;5:212–3.
20. O'Brien PM, Abukhalil IE. Randomised controlled trial of the management of premenstrual syndrome and premenstrual mastalgia using luteal phase-only danazol. Am J Obstet Gynecol. 1999;180:18–23.
21. McFayden IJ, Chetty U, Setchell KDR, et al. A randomized double blind crossover trial of soya protein for the treatment of cyclical breast pain. Breast. 2000;9:271–6.
22. Halaska M, Raus K, Beles P, et al. Treatment of cyclical mastodynia using an extract of Vitex agnus castus: results of a double blind comparison with a placebo. Ceska Gynecol. 1998;63:388–92.
23. Eriksson E. Serotonin reuptake inhibitors for the treatment of premenstrual dysphoria. Int Clin Psychopharmacol. 1999;14 Suppl 2:S27–33.
24. Haagenson CD. Diseases of the breast. 3rd ed. Philadelphia: WB Saunders; 1986.
25. Dixon JM, McDonald C, Elton RA, Miller WR, on behalf of the Edinburgh Breast Group. Risk of breast cancer in women with palpable breast cysts: a prospective study. Lancet. 1999;353:1742–5.
26. Brenner RJ, Jackman RJ, Parker SH, et al. Percutaneous core needle biopsy of radial scars of the breast: when is excision necessary? Am J Roentgenol. 2002;179(5):1179–84.
27. Andacoglu O, Kanbour-Shakir A, Teh YC, et al. Rationale of excisional biopsy after the diagnosis of benign radial scar on core biopsy: a single institutional outcome analysis. Am J Clin Oncol. 2013;36(1):7–11.
28. Bonser GM, Dossett JA, Jull JW. Human and experimental breast cancer. London: Pitman Medical; 1961. p. 237.
29. Dixon JM. Periductal mastitis/duct ectasia. World J Surg. 1989;13:715.
30. Dixon JM, Ravi Sekar O, Chetty U, et al. Periductal mastitis and duct ectasia: different conditions with different aetiologies. Br J Surg. 1996;83:820.
31. Bennett LE, Ghate SV, Bentley R, et al. Is surgical excision of core biopsy proven benign papillomas of the breast necessary? Acad Radiol. 2010;17(5):553–7.
32. Dixon JM, Mansel RE. Symptoms, assessment and guidelines for referral. ABC of breast diseases. BMJ. 1994;309:722.
33. Ambrogetti D, Berni D, Catarzi S, et al. The role of ductal galactography in the differential diagnosis of breast carcinoma. Radiol Med (Torino). 1996;91:198.
34. Morrogh M, Park A, Elkin EB, et al. Lessons learned from 416 cases of nipple discharge of the breast. Am J Surg. 2010;200(1):73–80.
35. Selzer MH, Perloff LJ, Kelley RI, et al. Significance of age in patients with nipple discharge. Surg Gynecol Obstet. 1970;131:519.
36. Simmons R, Adamovich T, Brennan M, et al. Nonsurgical evaluation of pathologic nipple discharge. Ann Surg Oncol. 2003;10:113–6.
37. Pisano ED, Gatsonis C, Hendrick E, et al. The Digital Mammographic Imaging Screening Trial (DMIST) Investigators Group. Diagnostic performance of digital versus film mammography for breast-cancer. N Engl J Med. 2005;353(17):1773–83.
38. Cabioglu N, Hunt KK, Singletary SE, et al. Surgical decision making and factors determining a diagnosis of breast cancer in women presenting with nipple discharge. J Am Coll Surg. 2003;196:354–64.
39. King BL, Love SM, Rochman S, et al. The fourth international symposium on the intraductal approach to breast cancer, Santa Barbara, California. Breast Cancer Res. 2005;7(5):198–204.
40. Dooley WS. Routine operative breast endoscopy for bloody nipple discharge. Ann Surg Oncol. 2002;9: 920–3.
41. Matsunaga T, Ohta D, Misaka T, et al. A utility of ductography and fibreoptic ductoscopy for patients with nipple discharge. Breast Cancer Res Treat. 2001;70:103–8.
42. Shen KW, Wu J, Lu JS, et al. Fiberoptic ductoscopy for breast cancer patients with nipple discharge. Surg Endosc. 2001;15:1340–5.
43. Khan SA, Baird C, Staradub VL, et al. Ductal lavage and ductoscopy: the opportunities and the limitations. Clin Breast Cancer. 2002;3:185–95.
44. Van Zee KJ, Ortega Perez G, Minnard E, et al. Preoperative galactography increases the diagnostic yield of major duct excision for nipple discharge. Cancer. 1998;82:1874.
45. Simpson JS, Connolly EM, Leong WL, et al. Mammary ductoscopy in the evaluation and treatment of pathologic nipple discharge: a Canadian experience. Can J Surg. 2009;52(6):E245–8.
46. Sharma R, Dietz J, Wright H, et al. Comparative analysis of minimally invasive microductectomy versus major duct excision in patients with pathologic nipple discharge. Surgery. 2005;138:591–6.
47. Hughes LE, Mansel RE, Webster DJT. Nipple discharge. In: Hughes LE, Mansel RE, Webster DJT, editors. Benign disorders and diseases of the breast: concepts and clinical management. 2nd ed. London: WB Saunders; 2000. p. 171.
48. Oyama T, Koerner FC. Noninvasive papillary proliferations. Semin Diagn Pathol. 2004;21:32–41.

49. Dixon JM, Kohlhardt SR, Dillon P. Total duct excision. Breast. 1998;7:216.
50. Kalbhen CL, Kezdi-Rogus PC, Dowling MP, et al. Mammography in the evaluation of nipple inversion. AJR Am J Roentgenol. 1998;170:117.
51. Carlson HE. Gynecomastia. N Engl J Med. 1980; 303:795–9.
52. Ismail AA, Barth JH. Endocrinology of gynaecomastia. Ann Clin Biochem. 2001;38:596–607.
53. Jones DJ, Holt SD, Surtees P, et al. A comparison of danazol and placebo in the treatment of adult idiopathic gynecomastia: results of a prospective study in 55 patients. Ann R Coll Surg Engl. 1990;72:296–8.
54. Khan HN, Blamey RW. Endocrine treatment of physiological gynaecomastia. Br Med J. 2003;327:301–2.
55. Wray Jr RC, Hoopes JE, Davis GM. Correction of extreme gynaecomastia. Br J Plast Surg. 1974;27:39–41.
56. Samdal F, Kleppe G, Amland PF, et al. Surgical treatment of gynaecomastia. Five years' experience with liposuction. Scand J Plast Reconstr Surg Hand Surg. 1994;28:123–30.
57. Fruhstorfer BH, Malata CM. A systematic approach to the surgical treatment of gynaecomastia. Br J Plast Surg. 2003;56:237–46.
58. Sestak I, Cuzick J, Evans G, Kwong A. Prevention of breast cancer. In: Dixon JM, editor. ABC of breast disease. 4th ed. Oxford: Wiley-Blackwell; 2012.
59. Dixon JM. Breast infection: ABC of breast diseases. BMJ. 1994;309:946.
60. Hughes LE, Mansel RE, Webster DJT. Infections of the breast. In: Hughes LE, Mansel RE, Webster DJT, editors. Benign disorders and diseases of the breast: concepts and clinical management. 2nd ed. London: WB Saunders; 2000. p. 187.
61. Dixon JM. Repeated aspiration of breast abscesses in lactating women. BMJ. 1988;297:1517.
62. Schafer P, Furrer C, Merillod B. An association between smoking with recurrent subareolar breast abscess. Int J Epidemiol. 1988;17:810–3.
63. Dixon JM. Periductal mastitis and duct ectasia: an update. Breast. 1998;7:128.
64. Bundred NJ, Dover MS, Aluwihare N, et al. Smoking and periductal mastitis. BMJ. 1993;307:772.
65. Bundred NJ. Surgical management of periductal mastitis. Breast. 1988;7:79.
66. Bundred NJ, Dixon JM, Chetty U, et al. Mammillary fistula. Br J Surg. 1987;74:466.
67. Atkins HJB. Mammillary fistula. BMJ. 1955;2:1473.
68. Dixon JM, Thompson AM. Effective surgical treatment for mammillary fistula. Br J Surg. 1991;78:1185.
69. Rogers K. Breast abscess and problems with lactation. In: Smallwood JA, Taylor I, editors. Benign breast disease. London: Edward Arnold; 1990. p. 96.
70. Attar KH, Waghorn D, Lyons M, et al. Rare species of actinomyces as causative pathogens in breast abscess. Breast J. 2007;13:501–5.
71. Wilson JP, Massoll N, Marshall J, et al. Idiopathic granulomatous mastitis: in search of a therapeutic paradigm. Am Surg. 2007;73:798.
72. Alikhan A, Lynch PJ, Eisen DB. Hidradenitis suppurativa: a comprehensive review. J Am Acad Dermatol. 2009;60:539.
73. Buimer MG, Wobbes T, Klinkenbijl JH. Hidradenitis suppurativa. Br J Surg. 2009;96:350.
74. Janniger CK, Schwartz RA, Szepietowski JC, Reich A. Intertrigo and common secondary skin infections. Am Fam Physician. 2005;72:833.
75. Mistiaen P, Poot E, Hickox S, et al. Preventing and treating intertrigo in the large skin folds of adults: a literature overview. Dermatol Nurs. 2004; 16:43.
76. Gollapalli V, Liao J, Dudakovic A, et al. Risk factors for development and recurrence of primary breast abscesses. J Am Coll Surg. 2010;211:41.
77. Going JJ, Anderson TJ, Wilkinson S, et al. Granulomatous lobular mastitis. J Clin Pathol. 1987;40:535.
78. Howell JD, Barker F, Gazet J-C. Granulomatous lobular mastitis: report of a further two cases and a comprehensive literature review. Breast. 1994;3:119.
79. Al-Khaffaf B, Knox F, Bundred NJ. Idiopathic granulomatous mastitis: a 25-year experience. J Am Coll Surg. 2008;206:269–73.
80. Akbulut S, Yilmaz D, Bakir S. Methotrexate in the management of idiopathic granulomatous mastitis: review of 108 published cases and reports of four cases. Breast J. 2011;17(6):661–8.
81. Olsen MA, Chu-Ongsakul S, Brandt KE, et al. Hospital-associated costs due to surgical site infection after breast surgery. Arch Surg. 2008;143(1): 53–60.
82. Sajid MS, Hutson K, Akhter N, et al. An updated meta-analysis on the effectiveness of preoperative prophylactic antibiotics in patients undergoing breast surgical procedures. Breast J. 2012;18(4):312–7.
83. Kleinberg D, Noel G, Frantz A. Galactorrhoea: a study of 235 cases including 48 with pituitary tumors. N Engl J Med. 1977;296:589.
84. Csuka ME, Kushi J. Generalized morphea after breast cancer radiation therapy. Case Rep Rheumatol. 2011;Article ID 951948: 4 p.
85. Dehn TC, Lee EC. Aneurysm presenting as a breast mass. Br Med J (Clin Res Ed). 1986;292(6530): 1240.
86. Adeniran A, Al-Ahmadie H, Mahoney MC, Robinson-Smith TM. Granular cell tumor of the breast: a series of 17 cases and review of the literature. Breast J. 2004;10(6):528–31.
87. Kudva YC, Reynolds CA, O'Brien T, et al. Mastopathy and diabetes. Curr Diabetes Rep. 2003;3:56–9.

Management of Breast Pain

4

Julia A. Files, Summer V. Allen, and Sandhya Pruthi

Abbreviations

CM	Cyclic mastalgia
EP	Extramammary pain
NCM	Noncyclic mastalgia

Introduction

Breast pain, or mastalgia, is one of the most common breast disorders affecting women worldwide. Although some studies have suggested that up to 70 % of women in Western societies experience breast pain in their lifetime, few experience symptoms severe enough to seek care for evaluation and treatment [1, 2]. Additionally, the prevalence is greatly influenced by the overall population being studied and the definitions used by the investigators. Although a common condition, the etiology of mastalgia remains quite enigmatic, also occurring in men but much more limited in terms of incidence as compared to females [3–5].

In a retrospective cohort study involving 2,400 women aged 40–69 who were enrolled in a health maintenance organization, breast pain was the most common breast symptom prompting evaluation, accounting for almost half (47 %) of all breast-related visits [6]. A second study of 1,171 women who answered a questionnaire on breast pain found that 69 % of women experienced premenstrual breast pain, noting that it impacted sexual activity (48 %), physical activity (37 %), social activity (12 %), and work or school activity (8 %) [7].

Pain of extramammary origin may often be perceived as breast pain. The differential diagnosis for pain perceived as emanating from the breasts is broad and should be considered in any patient presenting with the chief complaint of mastalgia (Table 4.1). The definition of breast pain is further classified as cyclic (breast pain that occurs in relationship to the menstrual cycle) and noncyclic (breast pain not associated with the menstrual cycle) [3]. Herein, we will review the etiology, diagnosis, management, and prevention of cyclic and noncyclic breast pain.

Cyclic Mastalgia

Clinical Features

Cyclic mastalgia is defined as breast pain of moderate-to-severe intensity, lasting ≥7 days and, because it demonstrates a relationship to

J.A. Files, MD (✉)
Division of Women's Health Internal Medicine, Mayo Clinic in Arizona, 13737 North 92nd Street, Scottsdale, AZ 85260, USA
e-mail: files.julia@mayo.edu

S.V. Allen, MD
Department of Family Medicine, Mayo Clinic, 200 First Street SW, Rochester, MN 55905, USA
e-mail: allen.summer@mayo.edu

S. Pruthi, MD
General Internal Medicine, Mayo Clinic, 200 First Street SW, Rochester, MN 55905, USA
e-mail: pruthi.sandhya@mayo.edu

A.I. Riker (ed.), *Breast Disease: Comprehensive Management*,
DOI 10.1007/978-1-4939-1145-5_4, © Springer Science+Business Media New York 2015

Table 4.1 Differential diagnosis of mastalgia

Location	Differential diagnosis
Breast-related	Mastalgia
	Cyclic mastalgia
	Noncyclic mastalgia
	Mastitis
	Breast trauma
	Thrombophlebitis/Mondor's disease
	Cysts
	Benign breast tumors
	Breast cancer
Musculoskeletal	Chest wall pain (intercostal muscle strain/tear)
	Tietze syndrome/costochondritis
	Chest wall trauma/rib fracture or contusion
	Fibromyalgia
	Cervical radiculopathy
	Shoulder pain
	Herpes zoster
Miscellaneous causes	Coronary artery disease/angina
	Pericarditis
	Pulmonary embolus
	Pleurisy
	Gastroesophageal reflux/esophageal spasm
	Peptic ulcer disease
	Cholelithiasis/cholecystitis
	Sickle cell anemia
	Psychological
	Pregnancy
	Medication (see Table 4.2)

Adapted from Smith et al. [3]

the menstrual cycle, occurring in premenopausal women [7]. Typically, it follows a course of relapse and remission, often confused with premenstrual breast pain. However, premenstrual breast tenderness is a normal physiologic response that occurs about 2–3 days before the onset of menstrual flow. In this context, breast symptoms are mild to moderate, most often bilateral, associated with swelling and tenderness, and self-limited [7].

Symptoms of cyclic mastalgia are usually most significant during the luteal phase of the menstrual cycle and may involve one or both breasts. The pain often resolves with the onset of the menstrual cycle, but a low level of pain may persist throughout the month with luteal phase intensification [3]. Most patients report a dull or aching sensation in the breasts, rarely reporting a sharp or stabbing nature to the pain. Women with cyclic mastalgia frequently experience the onset of symptoms in the third or fourth decade of life with almost half demonstrating resolution with the cessation of menses (menopause) [8].

Etiology

A number of theories of causality for cyclic mastalgia have been proposed, but no specific etiology has been determined. In spite of the association with menstrual cyclicity, cyclic mastalgia has not been shown to correlate with specific changes in hormonal levels (i.e., estrogen, progesterone, prolactin) in studies comparing women with and without symptoms [9]. Although an intriguing hypothesis, fluid retention has not been shown to cause cyclic mastalgia. In a study by Preece et al., total body water was measured early and late in the menstrual cycle for women with breast pain and in asymptomatic women, with no apparent correlation identified [10]. Histopathological changes of fibrocystic breast disease can be found in women with and without cyclic mastalgia. Additionally, no nutritional, inflammatory, or psychiatric associations have been substantiated based upon the current literature [3].

Noncyclic Mastalgia

Clinical Features

Noncyclic mastalgia has no clear association with a woman's menstrual cycle and can be intermittent or constant. Pain associated with noncyclic mastalgia may often localize to a specific quadrant of one breast, but it may also be diffuse and similar to that of cyclic mastalgia [11]. In contrast to cyclic mastalgia, noncyclic mastalgia is often a condition of the postmenopausal years, most commonly occurring in the fourth or fifth decade. Although less common than cyclic mastalgia, it still accounts for 31 % of women presenting with breast pain to some mastalgia clinics [8]. It can occur before, at, or after menopause and for some women may be even more problematic than cyclic mastalgia as the inciting event or cause for resolution can remain a mystery.

Etiology

The majority of noncyclic breast pain is of idiopathic origin, while a minority of patients can attribute their symptoms to anatomical changes resulting from pregnancy, mastitis, or trauma. Noncyclic breast pain is less likely due to thrombophlebitis, macrocysts, benign tumors, cancer, or medications. A number of medications however have been shown to have an association with breast pain. Awareness of this association allows for appropriate patient counseling prior to the institution of therapy (Table 4.2).

Recently, duct ectasia has been proposed as a cause for noncyclic mastalgia. An ultrasound study comparing maximum mean width of milk ducts in asymptomatic women and women with cyclic and noncyclic mastalgia found a significant increase in maximum mean width of milk ducts in women with both types of pain. Pain intensity correlated with ductal width [12]. It is also suggested that the dilatation of the ducts with stagnant secretions leads to periductal inflammation (periductal mastitis which may be subclinical). The pain is often described as a throbbing sensation, and nipple retraction and purulent nipple discharge may also occur. A short course of antibiotics may be considered as the first line of treatment, and if no improvement occurs, surgical management should be considered [13].

Table 4.2 Medications associated with breast pain in women

Categories	Medications
Hormonal medications	Estrogens
	Progestogens
	Combination medication
	Oral contraceptives
	Menopausal hormone therapy
	Diethylstilbestrol
	Clomiphene
	Cyproterone
Antidepressant, antipsychotic, and anxiolytic medications	Sertraline (and other serotonin reuptake inhibitors)
	Venlafaxine
	Mirtazapine
	Chlordiazepoxide
	Amitriptyline[a]
	Doxepin[a]
	Haloperidol (and other antipsychotic agents)
Antihypertensive and cardiac medications	Spironolactone[a]
	Methyldopa
	Minoxidil
	Digoxin[a]
	Reserpine[a]
Antimicrobial agents	Ketoconazole[a]
	Metronidazole[a]
Miscellaneous agents	Cimetidine[a]
	Cyclosporine
	Domperidone
	Penicillamine
	Methadone[a]
	Carboprost, dinoprostone (and other prostaglandins)
	Estramustine

Adapted from Smith et al. [3]
Information obtained from MEDLINE, MICROMEDEX, and discussion with breast specialists and pharmacists
[a]Medications causing galactorrhea and gynecomastia and believed to be associated with breast pain. Other medications (not listed) also may be associated with breast pain and should be considered according to clinical circumstances

Clinical Impact

Cyclic and noncyclic mastalgias significantly impact quality of life for many women. A study by Davies et al. demonstrated a negative impact on sexual relations in 28 % of women with cyclic mastalgia and 20 % with noncyclic mastalgia, for women reporting moderate-to-severe pain [8]. Clinical complaints of mastalgia often lead to further evaluation. In a health maintenance organization cohort study evaluating the outcome of breast symptom episodes, further evaluation was recommended for 391 (73 %) episodes, which included a surgical consultation (38 %), return for repeat examination (23 %), and diagnostic studies including mammography (30 %), fine-needle aspiration (8 %), biopsy (4 %), and ultrasonography (1 %) [6]. Significant resources are utilized in the ensuing workup leading to an increase in health-care costs.

Interestingly, in a study of 1,200 female veterans, those with frequent mastalgia (defined as ≥ weekly) compared to women without mastalgia were more likely to experience the following: panic disorder (odds ratio [OR] 7.1, 95 % CI 3.9–12.8), posttraumatic stress disorder (OR 5.2, 95 % CI 3.2–8.4), chronic pelvic pain (OR 5.4, 95 % CI 2.7–10.5), major depression (OR 4.2, 95 % CI 2.6–6.9), fibromyalgia (OR 3.9, 95 % CI 2.1–7.4), domestic violence (OR 3.1, 95 % CI 1.9–5.0), irritable bowel syndrome (OR 2.8, 95 % CI 1.6–4.8), eating disorder (OR 2.6, 95 % CI 1.5–4.7), or alcohol misuse (OR 1.8, 95 % CI 1.1–2.8) [14]. This study highlights the need to consider comorbidities in patients presenting with a chief complaint of mastalgia.

Women with cyclic and noncyclic mastalgia often express concerns about the association of pain with breast cancer. However, pain as a presenting symptom, or the only symptom, of breast cancer is a relatively rare occurrence, reported as a presenting symptom in only 5–18 % of breast cancers [2]. Studies of the association of mastalgia and breast cancer have shown conflicting results. A potential association between breast pain and cyclic mastalgia has been identified in premenopausal women with early-stage breast cancer and breast pain. In a cohort study of 247 French women with benign breast disease (and free of any hormonal treatment), the OR for breast cancer was 1.35 (95 % CI 1.01–1.83) for women with any cyclic pain compared to 3.32 for women with symptoms rated as severe when compared to controls. With a mean follow-up of 16 ± 5 years, a total of 22 breast cancers were found. Utilizing the Cox model, the corresponding relative risk for 37 months of cyclical mastalgia was 5.31 % (95 % CI 1.92–14.72) [15]. Results in these studies may have been influenced by bias in reporting, as women with breast cancer may have a higher rate of reporting symptoms. A larger study of 5,463 women seen in a breast care center demonstrated that breast pain was associated with a decreased risk of breast cancer [16]. Clearly, further study is needed to clarify this possible association.

Clinical Evaluation

An approach to evaluating the patient presenting with breast pain entails a thorough history and physical examination. Identifying the onset, quality, and duration of pain, as well as aggravating and alleviating factors or association with a mass or inflammation, can aid in differentiating the etiology of breast pain. Assessing pain severity using a standardized pain scale, such as the Likert scale of 1–10, and documenting the change in severity over time will guide treatment recommendations with both non-pharmacologic and pharmacologic treatment options (Table 4.3).

Although known risk factors for breast cancer include reproductive history, family history, personal breast cancer, or a prior precancerous breast lesion, the presence or absence of these factors should not detract from a thorough evaluation of breast pain in order to exclude malignancy or other benign etiologies. Various medications including hormonal preparations and antidepressants and antihypertensive medications have been associated with breast pain (Table 4.2). Discontinuation, taking a drug holiday, or switching to a different dose or formulation may be indicated in the management of breast pain.

Physical Examination

The diagnostic clinical breast examination entails inspection and palpation performed in the seated or supine position, sometimes both. It is helpful to visualize both breasts at the same time to allow for comparison of size and symmetry and to assess for presence of erythema, skin dimpling (peau d'orange), nipple changes (inversion or discharge), and distortion of the breast architecture.

Table 4.3 Historical factors to elicit in the clinical evaluation of breast pain

History	Differentiating features	Cyclic mastalgia (CM) versus noncyclic mastalgia (NCM) or extramammary pain (EP)
Location	Unilateral and localized	NCM
	Bilateral and generalized	CM
Duration	Acute (<month), subacute (1–6 months), or chronic (<6 months)	CM or NCM or EP
Severity	Likert pain scale 1–10	
Quality of pain	Burning or aching sensation	NCM
	Dull or heavy sensation	CM
Exacerbating or alleviating factors	Relationship to physical activity or activities of daily living (sleep)	NCM or CM
	Initiation of new medication	NCM
	Caffeinated beverage use	NCM
Associated factors	Palpable breast mass, erythema, nipple discharge, or skin changes	NCM
	Chest wall pain	EP
Reproductive factors	Relationship to menstrual cycle	CM
	Pregnancy	NCM
Medications	See Table 4.2	

Palpation of the entire breast including the nipple areolar complex and regional lymph nodes should be performed on all patients. Tenderness may localize to discrete areas in the breast and may be generalized or of extramammary etiology. Having the patient bend over or lie on their side to allow the breast tissue to fall away from the pectoralis muscle and chest wall can help differentiate pain emanating from the breast versus the chest wall [9]. The finding of a discrete mass or localized area of pain should be further evaluated with diagnostic imaging including ultrasound and mammogram.

Diagnostic Evaluation

The diagnostic workup of breast pain can be challenging, with the determination of the ideal imaging study often dependent upon the clinical findings and patient age. In a patient younger than 30, the sensitivity of diagnostic mammography is markedly decreased due to the overall increased density of the young breast. Therefore, if no mass is palpated in association with localized breast pain, we proceed first with a targeted ultrasound as the preferred initial modality for imaging the breast tissue. Mammography may be added depending on the clinical context and perceived individual risk. Patients older than 30 should undergo diagnostic mammography in addition to a focused ultrasound. Diffuse pain without a palpable mass is further categorized into cyclic versus noncyclic etiologies, with patients older than 30 with noncyclic pain undergoing diagnostic mammography first. A reasonable treatment algorithm provides a typical approach to the patient with breast pain (Fig. 4.1).

Irrespective of age, if a palpable mass is clearly found on clinical examination, this will require both a diagnostic mammogram and ultrasound. If clinical suspicion is high for malignancy and diagnostic imaging is negative, referral to a surgeon for consideration of biopsy of the palpable finding is recommended. Masses that are palpable but located deep within the breast tissue are very challenging and may require an open biopsy rather than biopsy in an outpatient setting. If clinical suspicion is low for malignancy and diagnostic imaging is negative, short-term follow-up with reexamination and consideration of additional imaging if the area of concern has changed is recommended. Depending on available resources, MRI may be utilized; however, the utility of diagnostic MRI in this setting is not yet fully defined and may offer a low yield of a cancer diagnosis [17]. In situations where the mass is visible on MRI, consideration could be given to an MRI-guided biopsy.

Smith et al. reported that the yield of either mammography or ultrasound in the context of a

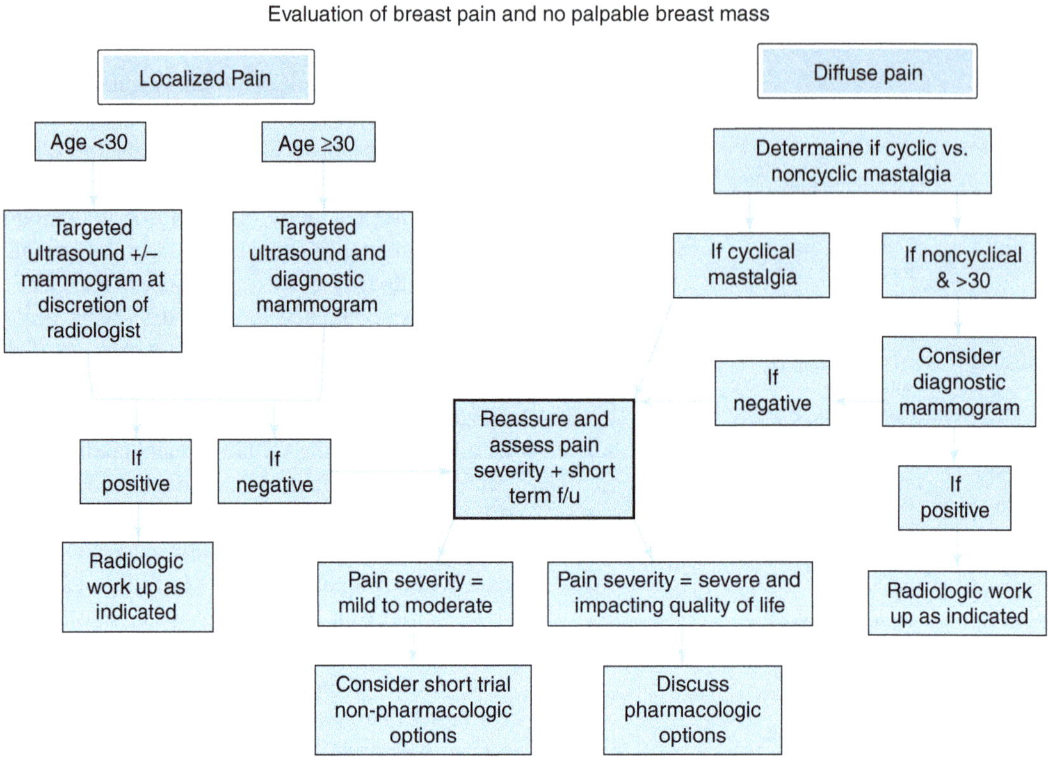

Fig. 4.1 Algorithm: evaluation of breast pain and no palpable breast mass

presenting symptom of breast pain was low for detecting a breast malignancy [3]. Ultrasound is most often ordered as a first-line imaging study primarily to exclude a focal or discrete mass. A study of 110 directed ultrasonographic exams performed for focal breast pain showed no breast cancer, with a benign finding identified at the site of the pain in 18/110 (%) patients [18]. There are no specific laboratory hormonal tests to assist in the evaluation of breast pain other than a pregnancy test if clinically indicated in a woman of reproductive age.

For those patients who are found to have either cyclic or noncyclic mastalgia with negative imaging studies, a short trial of non-pharmacologic therapies may be the logical first step for mild-to-moderate pain. For patients with pain that is clearly impacting their daily quality of life, consideration can be given to pursuing pharmacologic measures as a first-line intervention.

Management Options

The treatment of breast pain requires an individualized approach with careful consideration and understanding of the patient's concerns and its impact upon their quality of life. Often, reassurance that no serious problem underlies the pain is the only intervention required. A minority of women, once reassured, will still require treatment in order to decrease or alleviate symptoms related to the anxiety and uncertainty associated with this often new symptom [19, 20]. Assessing the efficacy of treatment strategies is often clinically challenging as the symptoms may wax and wane, often self-limited. Further complicating the evaluation of therapeutic response is the robust placebo response reported in a number of studies, ranging from 10 to 40 % [21, 22]. Encouraging the use of a symptom diary utilizing a pain scale aids in the choice of therapeutic modalities and the evaluation of efficacy.

Non-pharmacologic Therapies

A number of non-pharmacologic options should first be considered as the initial treatment for both the prevention and treatment of breast pain. These include physical measures, relaxation training, dietary changes, and nutritional supplements. Although evidence-based research on the therapeutic value of these measures is limited, a trial of 3–6 months can certainly be considered, followed by reassessment. It is both reasonable and appropriate to counsel patients presenting with breast pain of mild-to-moderate intensity to try these non-pharmacologic approaches, particularly if the symptoms are interfering with their quality of life.

Physical Measures

Approximately 70 % of women wear a brassiere that does not provide adequate support, is improperly fitted, or has underwiring [23]. For both cyclic and noncyclic breast pain, wearing a well-fitted bra during the day and a soft supporting bra while sleeping can result in an improvement of breast pain. A prospective study comparing danazol to wearing a sports brassiere demonstrated an 85 % relief of symptoms among patients instructed to wear sports brassieres compared to only 58 % relief of symptoms in the group who received danazol [24]. A well-fitted brassiere worn during exercise provides support to Cooper's ligaments which can be impacted by the amplitude of movement especially with activities that involve breast motion (running, aerobics, and walking) [25].

Relaxation Training

There is good evidence regarding the impact of psychological factors and stress as contributors to breast pain, and so, it is important to obtain this as part of the history when evaluating a patient with breast pain. A small study of premenopausal women reporting severe cyclic mastalgia demonstrated higher levels of anxiety and depression compared with women with no symptoms [26]. A psychological assessment may be important to screen for depression, with an appropriate psychological referral considered for further psychiatric consultation and possible intervention. In the circumstance where patients report a high level of stress but are not clinically depressed, implementation of relaxation training into a patient's daily lifestyle may be able to avert psychological distress and possibly prevent breast pain. A study evaluating the use of an audiocassette that discusses progressive muscular relaxation over a 4-week period demonstrated that 61 % of women reported relief of breast pain compared to those who did not use the audiocassette [27].

Dietary Changes

Historically, women have often been counseled to avoid caffeine-containing foods such as coffee, tea, and chocolate as a strategy to decrease or prevent breast pain. However, the data on methylxanthine avoidance (specifically caffeine) has been conflicting.

There have been several trials showing that a caffeine-free diet did not impact symptoms of breast pain [28, 29]. It is postulated that breast pain may be influenced through the effects of caffeine on endogenous hormone levels. Caffeine intake has been found to be associated with altered hormone levels such as elevated plasma estrone, decreased testosterone, and increased sex hormone-binding globulin [30]. A randomized trial assessing caffeine intake and the relationship to fibrocystic changes and nodularity has shown improvement in breast nodularity, but not necessarily a decrease in breast discomfort [31]. For women who do consume moderate-to-heavy caffeine, it is reasonable to discuss reduction of caffeine intake as a preventive intervention.

Nutritional Supplements

The evidence evaluating herbal therapies such as vitamin E and evening primrose oil for management of moderate-to-severe breast pain has been equivocal. The mechanism of action for vitamin E is primarily through an antioxidant effect and inhibition of the hormonal influence on breast receptors [32, 33]. Evening primrose oil, a nutritional supplement that contains gamma linolenic acid, is speculated to reduce breast sensitivity in women who have a dietary deficiency of gamma linolenic acid [34]. A meta-analysis comparing several pharmacologic therapies versus evening oil of primrose was conducted. In this study, the authors included three randomized placebo-controlled trials of evening primrose oil with the outcomes presented as a mean pain score. The results demonstrated that evening primrose oil compared to placebo showed no benefit in improving the pain score [35].

A small pilot study in premenopausal women was conducted to compare vitamin E alone, evening primrose oil alone versus combining vitamin E with evening primrose oil, and a placebo group for cyclic mastalgia over a 6-month period. The dose of the vitamin E was 400 IU three times per day and evening primrose oil 3,000 IU three times per day. This study demonstrated a trend to improvement in breast pain in all three arms when compared to placebo [36]. A randomized placebo-controlled study of vitamin E 200 IU twice a day versus placebo for cyclic mastalgia demonstrated improvement after two months of treatment, with no additional benefit after 4 months of usage among premenstrual women [32].

Dietary flaxseed is another supplement that has been examined in a randomized placebo-controlled fashion for its effect on cyclic mastalgia. Flaxseed muffins containing 25 g daily consumed for up to four menstrual cycles compared to placebo resulted in a significantly greater degree in breast pain improvement compared to the placebo group and was associated with minimal side-effects [37].

In general, women presenting with mild-to-moderate pain are often more inclined and receptive to a short trial of an herbal supplement before pursuing pharmacologic therapy. The herbal preparations are often better tolerated and considered to be a safe alternative to pharmacologic therapies. Following a short therapeutic trial, follow-up visit and reassessment are prudent, and if no improvement is reported, then the supplement should be discontinued.

Pharmacologic Therapies

In patients who fail to respond to non-pharmacologic measures, consideration should be given to a trial of pharmacologic interventions. First-line interventions for the treatment of breast pain that is related to medication use should include dose and delivery modifications. Postmenopausal hormone therapy has been shown to be associated with breast pain, and the reduction of the estrogen dose may provide a decrease in symptoms [38, 39].

Oral contraceptives may also be associated with breast pain although pain may resolve after completion of a few cycles [2]. If pain persists, a trial of another agent with a lower dose of estrogen may alleviate symptoms. Conversely, oral contraceptives may be used to alleviate symptoms that are related to the cyclicity of the menstrual cycle. Studies evaluating the risk of breast pain in oral contraceptives that contain very low doses of estrogen (ethinyl estradiol 20 mcg) have shown no increased risk when compared with placebo [40]. In women with persistent pain despite a trial of low-dose estrogen preparations, a trial of progestin-only pills or long-acting parenteral progestins may provide relief while still providing adequate contraceptive effect [41].

Danazol

Danazol is the only US Food and Drug Administration-approved medication available for the treatment of breast pain or mastalgia. In numerous clinical trials, 59–92 % of women treated with danazol reported relief of breast pain [42–55]. Unfortunately, side effects limit the use of danazol, and although dose-related, they are significant enough to cause discontinuation in as many as 15 % of patients. Possible side effects include acne, voice changes, male pattern hair loss, weight gain, mood disturbances, and menstrual irregularity [22]. Luteal phase-only administration of danazol has been shown to provide symptom relief without an increase in side effects when compared to placebo [53, 54].

Dopamine Agonists

Dopamine agonists have shown promising results for the treatment of breast pain with several studies documenting a significant decrease in breast pain in treated patients [56, 57]. The mechanism underlying the efficacy may relate to the impact of dopamine agonists on prolactin secretion. A number of studies have documented the presence of thyrotropin-induced increases in prolactin occurring in women with mastalgia [58, 59]. Bromocriptine has shown efficacy ranging from 47 to 88 % of women studied, but its use is also limited by its side effect profile (GI upset, headache, fatigue). Interestingly, clinical improvement of mastalgia may persist despite discontinuation of bromocriptine [60].

Selective Estrogen Receptor Modulators

The selective estrogen receptor modulators (SERMS) are used in the treatment and prevention of breast cancer. Tamoxifen has been studied in cyclic and noncyclic mastalgia and has demonstrated efficacy in pain reduction with studies revealing a decrease in pain in cyclic mastalgia ranging from 71 to 96 % of women treated and in 56 % of those treated who had noncyclic mastalgia. A number of controlled trials have been conducted assessing the efficacy of treatment with tamoxifen [61–67].

When considering the use of tamoxifen for mastalgia, the risk of side effects must be factored into the decision. Although effective, the risk of significant adverse side effects often outweighs the benefits especially in mild-to-moderate pain. We recommend that tamoxifen be reserved for the treatment of symptoms that are moderate to severe in intensity and have failed more conservative measures. The dose of the tamoxifen used for management of breast pain ranges from 10 to 20 mg per day. Raloxifene, another SERM, has not been specifically studied for efficacy in the treatment of mastalgia (Table 4.4 [61–67]).

Gonadotropin-Releasing Hormone Agonists

The administration of gonadotropin-releasing hormone agonists results in the suppression of pituitary ovarian hormone production. In estrogen-deficient states, women experience improvement in breast pain but experience significant symptoms resulting from the lack of estrogen. Although promising for treatment efficacy, these agents can only be used short term and must be further evaluated to assess their role in the ongoing treatment of mastalgia [3, 68].

Simple analgesics such as nonsteroidal anti-inflammatories or acetaminophen often provide adequate therapy for the treatment of mild-to-moderate breast discomfort and can be recommended for use during periods of pain intensification. They should be considered as first-line therapy and may be used in addition to other agents.

Finally, there is no role for surgical management as a preventive therapy of cyclic or noncyclic mastalgia. For a majority of women, the reassurance that the breast pain is not due to malignancy is often the most effective therapy and uniformly well received [3].

Table 4.4 Clinical trials of tamoxifen for treatment of mastalgia

	No. (%) of subjects responding to intervention					
	Tamoxifen					
Study	10 mg	20 mg	Danazol	Bromocriptine	Placebo	Comments
Fentiman et al. [61]	NE	22/31 (71)	NE	NE	11/29 (38)	Randomized double-blind trial of daily tamoxifen or placebo in 60 subjects with cyclic or noncyclic pain; response (≥50 % decrease in mean pain score) at 3 months. Significant difference between groups ($P<0.025$); 6 in each group stopped study due to adverse effects
Powles et al. [62]	NE	22/25 (88)	20/25 (80)	NE	NE	Randomized trial of tamoxifen 20 mg/d and danazol 100 mg twice daily; agents were of equal efficacy ($P>0.10$), but fewer adverse effects were noted with tamoxifen ($P<0.01$)
Messinis and Lolis [63]	16/18 (89)	NE	NE	NE	6/16 (38)	Randomized trial of tamoxifen or placebo administered from days 5 to 24 for 6 consecutive menstrual cycles; significant difference between groups ($P<0.0001$)
Fentiman, et al. [64]	26/29 (90)	24/28 (86)	NE	NE	NE	Randomized double-blind trial of 10 or 20 mg of tamoxifen daily for 3 or 6 months. Each dosage and duration equally effective[a]; fewer adverse effects in 10 mg compared with 20-mg group (21 % vs 64 %; $P<0.0001$)
GEBM [65]	127/155 (82)	107/142 (75)	NE	NE	NE	Randomized trial of 10 or 20 mg of tamoxifen from days 15 to 25 of menstrual cycle; doses equally effective ($P=$NS) with fewer adverse effects[b] in 10-mg group ($P<0.05$)
Sandrucci et al. [66]	18/20 (90)	NE	NE	16/18 (89)	NE	Randomized, blind trial of tamoxifen 10 mg from days 15 to 25 of menstrual cycle or bromocriptine 7.5 mg/d; agents equally effective ($P=$NS); adverse effects reported as mild and similar
Kontostolis et al. [67]	23/32 (72)	NE	21/32 (66)	NE	11/29 (38)	Randomized trial of tamoxifen 10 mg from days 5 to 24 of menstrual cycle, danazol 100 mg twice daily, or placebo for 6 months. Tamoxifen was more effective than danazol ($P<0.001$), but both were more effective than placebo ($P<0.035$, $P<0.011$, respectively)

Adapted from Smith et al. [3]

GEMB Grupo de Estudio de Mastopatias Benignas, *NE* not evaluated in the study

[a]Relapse occurred in 48 and 39 % of subjects in 10- and 20-mg group at 3 months median time after treatment

[b]Hot flashes, gastrointestinal discomfort, vaginal discharge, ankle edema, and menorrhagia

Conclusion

Breast pain is a very common complaint in women, affecting up to 70 % of women in Western societies during their lifetime. Although frequently concerning and anxiety-producing, it is rarely associated with breast cancer. Simple reassurance is often the only therapy required to alleviate concern and to mitigate pain intensity. If education and reassurance fail to achieve adequate symptom relief, a number of non-pharmacologic and pharmacologic measures have demonstrated efficacy. Selection of a specific agent must be guided by patient expectation, side effect profile, and severity of symptoms. Ongoing follow-up is necessary as mastalgia often resolves allowing for discontinuation of therapy. Spontaneous remission can occur and therapeutic interventions can lead to long-lasting resolution of symptoms. Further study is needed to assess newer agents for efficacy.

References

1. Leinster SJ, Whitehouse GH, Walsh PV. Cyclical mastalgia: clinical and mammographic observations in a screened population. Br J Surg. 1987;74(3):220–2.
2. Rosolowich V, Saettler E, Szuck B, Lea RH, Levesque P, Weisberg F, et al. Mastalgia. J Obstet Gynaecol Can. 2006;28(1):49–71; quiz 58–60, 72–4.
3. Smith RL, Pruthi S, Fitzpatrick LA. Evaluation and management of breast pain. Mayo Clin Proc. 2004;79(3):353–72.
4. Pitt B, Zannad F, Remme WJ, Cody R, Castaigne A, Perez A, et al. The effect of spironolactone on morbidity and mortality in patients with severe heart failure. Randomized Aldactone Evaluation Study Investigators. N Engl J Med. 1999;341(10):709–17.
5. Braunstein G. Gynecomastia. In: Harris J, Lippman M, Morrow M, Hellman S, editors. Diseases of the breast. Philadelphia: Lippincott-Raven; 1996. p. 54–60.
6. Barton MB, Elmore JG, Fletcher SW. Breast symptoms among women enrolled in a health maintenance organization: frequency, evaluation, and outcome. Ann Intern Med. 1999;130(8):651–7.
7. Ader DN, Browne MW. Prevalence and impact of cyclic mastalgia in a United States clinic-based sample. Am J Obstet Gynecol. 1997;177(1):126–32.
8. Davies EL, Gateley CA, Miers M, Mansel RE. The long-term course of mastalgia. J R Soc Med. 1998;91(9):462–4.
9. Miltenburg DM, Speights Jr VO. Benign breast disease. Obstet Gynecol Clin North Am. 2008;35(2):285–300, ix.
10. Preece PE, Richards AR, Owen GM, Hughes LE. Mastalgia and total body water. Br Med J. 1975;4(5995):498–500.
11. Mansel RE. ABC of breast diseases. Breast pain. BMJ. 1994;309(6958):866–8.
12. Peters F, Diemer P, Mecks O, Behnken LL. Severity of mastalgia in relation to milk duct dilatation. Obstet Gynecol. 2003;101(1):54–60.
13. Dixon JM. Periductal mastitis/duct ectasia. World J Surg. 1989;13(6):715–20.
14. Johnson KM, Bradley KA, Bush K, Gardella C, Dobie DJ, Laya MB. Frequency of mastalgia among women veterans. Association with psychiatric conditions and unexplained pain syndromes. J Gen Intern Med. 2006;21 Suppl 3:S70–5.
15. Plu-Bureau G, Le MG, Sitruk-Ware R, Thalabard JC. Cyclical mastalgia and breast cancer risk: results of a French cohort study. Cancer Epidemiol Biomarkers Prev. 2006;15(6):1229–31.
16. Khan SA, Apkarian AV. Mastalgia and breast cancer: a protective association? Cancer Detect Prev. 2002;26(3):192–6 [Erratum in Cancer Detect Prev. 2003;27(1):82].
17. Olsen ML, Morton M, Stan D, Pruthi S. Is there a role for magnetic resonance imaging in diagnosing palpable breast masses when mammogram and ultrasound are negative? J Womens Health. 2012;21(11):1149–54.
18. Leung JW, Kornguth PJ, Gotway MB. Utility of targeted sonography in the evaluation of focal breast pain. J Ultrasound Med. 2002;21(5):521–6; quiz 8–9.
19. Klimberg V. Etiology and management of breast pain. In: Harris J, Lippman M, Morrow M, Hellman S, editors. Diseases of the breast. Philadelphia: Lippincott-Raven; 1996. p. 99–106.
20. Millet AV, Dirbas FM. Clinical management of breast pain: a review. Obstet Gynecol Surv. 2002;57(7):451–61.
21. Maddox PR, Mansel RE. Management of breast pain and nodularity. World J Surg. 1989;13(6):699–705.
22. Gateley CA, Mansel RE. Management of cyclical breast pain. Br J Hosp Med. 1990;43(5):330–2.
23. BeLieu RM. Mastodynia. Obstet Gynecol Clin North Am. 1994;21(3):461–77.
24. Hadi MS. Sports brassiere: is it a solution for mastalgia? Breast J. 2000;6(6):407–9.
25. Mason BR, Page KA, Fallon K. An analysis of movement and discomfort of the female breast during exercise and the effects of breast support in three cases. J Sci Med Sport. 1999;2(2):134–44.
26. Downey H, Deadman J, Davis C, Leinster S. Psychological characteristics of women with cyclical mastalgia. Breast Dis. 1993;6:99–105.
27. Fox H, Walker LG, Heys SD, Ah-See AK, Eremin O. Are patients with mastalgia anxious, and does relaxation therapy help? Breast. 1997;6(3):138–42.
28. Allen SS, Froberg DG. The effect of decreased caffeine consumption on benign proliferative breast disease: a randomized clinical trial. Surgery. 1987;101(6):720–30.
29. Lubin F, Ron E, Wax Y, Black M, Funaro M, Shitrit A. A case-control study of caffeine and methylxanthines in benign breast disease. JAMA. 1985;253(16):2388–92.
30. Ferrini RL, Barrett-Connor E. Caffeine intake and endogenous sex steroid levels in postmenopausal women. The Rancho Bernardo Study. Am J Epidemiol. 1996;144(7):642–4.
31. Ernster VL, Mason L, Goodson 3rd WH, Sickles EA, Sacks ST, Selvin S, et al. Effects of caffeine-free diet on benign breast disease: a randomized trial. Surgery. 1982;91(3):263–7.
32. Parsay S, Olfati F, Nahidi S. Therapeutic effects of vitamin E on cyclic mastalgia. Breast J. 2009;15(5):510–4.

33. Meyer EC, Sommers DK, Reitz CJ, Mentis H. Vitamin E and benign breast disease. Surgery. 1990;107(5):549–51.
34. Gateley CA, Maddox PR, Pritchard GA, Sheridan W, Harrison BJ, Pye JK, et al. Plasma fatty acid profiles in benign breast disorders. Br J Surg. 1992;79(5):407–9.
35. Srivastava A, Mansel RE, Arvind N, Prasad K, Dhar A, Chabra A. Evidence-based management of Mastalgia: a meta-analysis of randomised trials. Breast. 2007;16(5):503–12.
36. Pruthi S, Wahner-Roedler DL, Torkelson CJ, Cha SS, Thicke LS, Hazelton JH, et al. Vitamin E and evening primrose oil for management of cyclical mastalgia: a randomized pilot study. Altern Med Rev. 2010;15(1):59–67.
37. Goss P, Li T, Theriault M, Pinto S, Thompson L. Effects of dietary flaxseed in women with cyclical mastalgia [Abstract]. Breast Cancer Res Treat. 2000;64(1):49.
38. Speroff L, Rowan J, Symons J, Genant H, Wilborn W. The comparative effect on bone density, endometrium, and lipids of continuous hormones as replacement therapy (CHART study). A randomized controlled trial. JAMA. 1996;276(17):1397–403.
39. Crandall CJ, Aragaki AK, Cauley JA, McTiernan A, Manson JE, Anderson G, et al. Breast tenderness and breast cancer risk in the estrogen plus progestin and estrogen-alone women's health initiative clinical trials. Breast Cancer Res Treat. 2012;132(1):275–85.
40. Coney P, Washenik K, Langley RG, DiGiovanna JJ, Harrison DD. Weight change and adverse event incidence with a low-dose oral contraceptive: two randomized, placebo-controlled trials. Contraception. 2001;63(6):297–302.
41. Euhus DM, Uyehara C. Influence of parenteral progesterones on the prevalence and severity of mastalgia in premenopausal women: a multi-institutional cross-sectional study. J Am Coll Surg. 1997;184(6):596–604.
42. Mansel RE, Wisbey JR, Hughes LE. Controlled trial of the antigonadotropin danazol in painful nodular benign breast disease. Lancet. 1982;1(8278):928–30.
43. Ramsey-Stewart G. The treatment of symptomatic benign breast disease with danazol. Aust N Z J Obstet Gynaecol. 1988;28(4):299–304.
44. Watts JF, Butt WR, Logan Edwards R. A clinical trial using danazol for the treatment of premenstrual tension. Br J Obstet Gynaecol. 1987;94(1):30–4.
45. O'Brien PM, Abukhalil IE. Randomized controlled trial of the management of premenstrual syndrome and premenstrual mastalgia using luteal phase-only danazol. Am J Obstet Gynecol. 1999;180(1 Pt 1):18–23.
46. Gorins A, Perret F, Tournant B, Rogier C, Lipszyc J. A French double-blind crossover study (danazol versus placebo) in the treatment of severe fibrocystic breast disease. Eur J Gynaecol Oncol. 1984;5(2):85–9.
47. Sutton GL, O'Malley VP. Treatment of cyclical mastalgia with low dose short term danazol. Br J Clin Pract. 1986;40(2):68–70.
48. Peters F, Reck G, Zimmermann G, Breckwoldt M. The effect of danazol on the pituitary function, thyroid function, and mastodynia. Arch Gynecol. 1980;230(1):3–8.
49. Baker HW, Snedecor PA. Clinical trial of danazol for benign breast disease. Am Surg. 1979;45(11):727–9.
50. Greenblatt B, Ben-Nun I. Danazol in the treatment of mammary dysplasia. Drugs. 1980;19(5):349–55.
51. Doberl A, Tobiassen T, Rasmussen T. Treatment of recurrent cyclical mastodynia in patients with fibrocystic breast disease. A double-blind placebo-controlled study–the Hjorring project. Acta Obstet Gynecol Scand Suppl. 1984;123:177–84.
52. Tobiassen T, Rasmussen T, Doberl A, Rannevik G. Danazol treatment of severely symptomatic fibrocystic breast disease and long-term follow-up–the Hjorring project. Acta Obstet Gynecol Scand Suppl. 1984;123:159–76.
53. Maddox PR, Harrison BJ, Mansel RE. Low-dose danazol for mastalgia. Br J Clin Pract Suppl. 1989;68:43–7; discussion 9–53.
54. Harrison BJ, Maddox PR, Mansel RE. Maintenance therapy of cyclical mastalgia using low-dose danazol. J R Coll Surg Edinb. 1989;34(2):79–81.
55. Ouimet-Oliva D, Van Campenhout J, Hebert G, Ladouceur J. Effect of danazol on the radiographic density of breast parenchyma. J Can Assoc Radiol. 1981;32(3):159–61.
56. Kaleli S, Aydin Y, Erel CT, Colgar U. Symptomatic treatment of premenstrual mastalgia in premenopausal women with lisuride maleate: a double-blind placebo-controlled randomized study. Fertil Steril. 2001;75(4):718–23.
57. Ioannidou-Mouzaka L, Niagassas M, Galanos A, Kalovidouris A. Pilot study on the treatment of cyclical mastodynia with Quinagolide. Eur J Gynaecol Oncol. 1999;20(2):117–21.
58. Kumar S, Mansel RE, Scanlon MF, Hughes LE, Edwards CA, Woodhead JS, et al. Altered responses of prolactin, luteinizing hormone and follicle stimulating hormone secretion to thyrotrophin releasing hormone/gonadotrophin releasing hormone stimulation in cyclical mastalgia. Br J Surg. 1984;71(11):870–3.
59. Kumar S, Mansel RE, Hughes LE, Woodhead JS, Edwards CA, Scanlon MF, et al. Prolactin response to thyrotropin-releasing hormone stimulation and dopaminergic inhibition in benign breast disease. Cancer. 1984;53(6):1311–5.
60. Mansel RE, Dogliotti L. European multicentre trial of bromocriptine in cyclical mastalgia. Lancet. 1990;335(8683):190–3.
61. Fentiman IS, Caleffi M, Brame K, Chaudary MA, Hayward JL. Double-blind controlled trial of tamoxifen therapy for mastalgia. Lancet. 1986;1(8476):287–8.
62. Powles TJ, Ford HT, Gazet J-C. A randomised trial to compare tamoxifen with danazol for treatment of benign mammary dysplasia. Breast Dis (Senologia). 1987;1987(2):1–5.

63. Messinis IE, Lolis D. Treatment of premenstrual mastalgia with tamoxifen. Acta Obstet Gynecol Scand. 1988;67(4):307–9.
64. Fentiman IS, Caleffi M, Hamed H, Chaudary MA. Dosage and duration of tamoxifen treatment for mastalgia: a controlled trial. Br J Surg. 1988;75(9):845–6.
65. GEMB Group (Grupo de Estudio de Mastopatias Benignas) Argentine. Tamoxifen therapy for cyclical mastalgia: dose randomised trial. Breast. 1997;5:212–3.
66. Sandrucci S, Mussa A, Festa V. Comparison of tamoxifen and bromocriptine in management of fibrocystic breast disease: a randomized blind study. Ann N Y Acad Sci. 1990;586:626–8.
67. Kontostolis E, Stefanidis K, Navrozoglou I, Lolis D. Comparison of tamoxifen with danazol for treatment of cyclical mastalgia. Gynecol Endocrinol. 1997;11(6):393–7.
68. Hamed H, Caleffi M, Chaudary MA, Fentiman IS. LHRH analogue for treatment of recurrent and refractory mastalgia. Ann R Coll Surg Engl. 1990;72(4):221–4.

5 Management of the High-Risk Breast Lesion

Jared Linebarger, Jon Zellmer, and Monica Rizzo

Introduction

The clinical management of high-risk breast lesions is intellectually challenging, continually evolving over time and occasionally controversial. The evaluation of all breast conditions begins with a thorough history and physical exam, appropriate breast imaging, and cytologic or histologic evaluation when indicated. Percutaneous core needle biopsy (CNB) has become the diagnostic modality of choice for both palpable and non-palpable breast lesions when histologic assessment is desired [1–3]. In the treatment of breast cancer, preoperative diagnosis by CNB offers many advantages over open surgical biopsy. CNB provides preoperative clinical staging and tumor marker assessment, enables discussion of neoadjuvant options, and increases the rate of breast-conserving therapy. Yet, the majority of image-detected breast lesions are benign, and most patients who undergo a breast biopsy will not have a diagnosis of malignancy. When there is concordance among clinical history, physical examination, imaging, and needle biopsy pathology, CNB may obviate the need for surgery to prevent under- and overtreatment of patients. However, some CNB findings are considered "borderline" because the CNB reveals a nonmalignant diagnosis, but cancer might be present at the biopsy site, implying a sampling error. The management of these high-risk lesions may be variable among practitioners, and a need for consensus in management of many of these lesions exists. In a position statement in 2011, the American Society of Breast Surgeons (ASBrS) defined a subset of benign and borderline breast lesions discovered on CNB that are associated with an upgrade in diagnosis to malignancy when CNB is followed by surgical excisional biopsy.

These lesions will be described in this chapter and include:

- Atypical ductal hyperplasia (ADH)
- Lobular neoplasia (lobular carcinoma in situ and atypical lobular hyperplasia)
- Columnar cell lesions (hyperplasia or flat epithelial atypia)
- Papillary lesions
- Radial scar (complex sclerosing lesions)
- Fibroepithelial lesion (with or without cellular stroma)

J. Linebarger, MD
Department of General Surgery, Gundersen Health System, La Crosse, WI, USA

Norma J Vinger Center for Breast Care (NJVCBC), La Crosse, WI, USA
e-mail: jhlineba@gundluth.org

J. Zellmer, MD
Department of Medical Education, Gundersen Lutheran Medical Foundation (GLMF), La Crosse, WI, USA
e-mail: jdzellme@gundluth.org

M. Rizzo, MD, FACS (✉)
Division of Surgical Oncology, Department of Surgery, Emory University School of Medicine, Winship Cancer Institute, 550 Peachtree Street, 9th floor, Atlanta, GA 30308, USA
e-mail: monica.rizzo@emory.edu

A.I. Riker (ed.), *Breast Disease: Comprehensive Management*,
DOI 10.1007/978-1-4939-1145-5_5,

- Mucocele-like lesion
- Spindle cell lesion

The upgrade rate to ductal carcinoma in situ (DCIS) or invasive ductal carcinoma (IDC) when a borderline breast lesion in diagnosed on CNB is summarized in Table 5.1.

Patient counseling following identification of a borderline breast lesion must take into account an assessment of concordance between the clinical suspicion and CNB result, an estimation of the risk and implications of associated lesions of greater clinical significance (such as malignancy), and knowledge of the natural history of the specific high-risk lesion identified. The Gail risk model, along with other risk assessment models, has been increasingly used to estimate future breast cancer risk based on the results of breast biopsy [21, 22]. Utilizing the Gail model in clinical trial enrollment, the NSABP P-1 study first showed a significant reduction in the incidence of breast cancer in women at higher risk, including those with ADH and lobular neoplasia, when tamoxifen therapy was administered. Subsequently, risk assessment along with individual care plans for borderline breast lesions has become standard of care [23, 24]. In the clinical management of borderline breast lesions today, risk assessment assists in informing appropriate follow-up, prevention, and screening discussions, including the use of breast MRI [25]. When these high-risk lesions are identified by CNB, management may include structured observation, repeat CNB, or surgical excision, and the chosen care pathway must represent a practice of informed discussion with the patient and shared decision-making.

Table 5.1 Summary of the upgrade rate (%) to ductal carcinoma in situ (DCIS) or invasive ductal cancer (IDC) or invasive lobular carcinoma (ILC) when a borderline breast lesion is diagnosed on core needle biopsy (CNB) and followed by surgical excision

Borderline breast lesio(ns diagnosed on core needle biopsy	Upgrade to malignancy DCIS (%)	Upgrade to malignancy IDC (%)	Increase relative risk of breast ca
ADH [4–7]	30–40	20	4–6
Lobular neoplasia			
ALH [8, 9]	20*		4–5
LCIS [8, 9]	30*		8–12
pLCIS [8, 10, 11]		40–60 (ILC)	
Columnar cell lesions			
CCH with atypia [4, 5, 12]	25–33*		
FEA [13, 14]	9–15*		
Papillary breast lesion			
Intraductal papilloma (IDP) [15]	8*		
Radial scar [10, 16, 17]	5–9*		1.8–3
Mucocele-like lesions [18–20]	18–30**		

ADH atypical ductal hyperplasia, *ALH* atypical lobular hyperplasia, *LCIS* lobular carcinoma in situ, *pLCIS* pleomorphic lobular carcinoma in situ, *CCH* columnar cell hyperplasia, *FEA* flat epithelial atypia
The numbers in superscript in the first column indicate the bibliographic reference. The asterisk sign * indicates the % of upgrade to DCIS and IDC combined. ** includes also the % of upgrade to ADH

Atypical Ductal Hyperplasia (ADH)

Atypical ductal hyperplasia (ADH) is described as a breast lesion involving the epithelial cells within the ductal system that is felt to be not only a precursor on the continuum from normal breast tissue to breast carcinoma but also a risk factor for future breast cancer. The model for a linear progression from hyperplasia to invasive breast carcinoma was initially described by Wellings and Jensen [26]. This model proposes a natural progression along a histologic continuum through an accumulation of molecular changes, ultimately resulting in an invasive phenotype. Flat epithelial atypia (FEA), ADH, and DCIS are accepted as the non-obligate precursors to invasive ductal carcinoma. This model is supported by morphologic, immunohistochemical, and transcriptional profiling data [27]. For example, ADH is described as a ductal epithelial lesion containing some, but not all, of the features of DCIS. A diagnosis of ADH on CNB is complicated by its similar

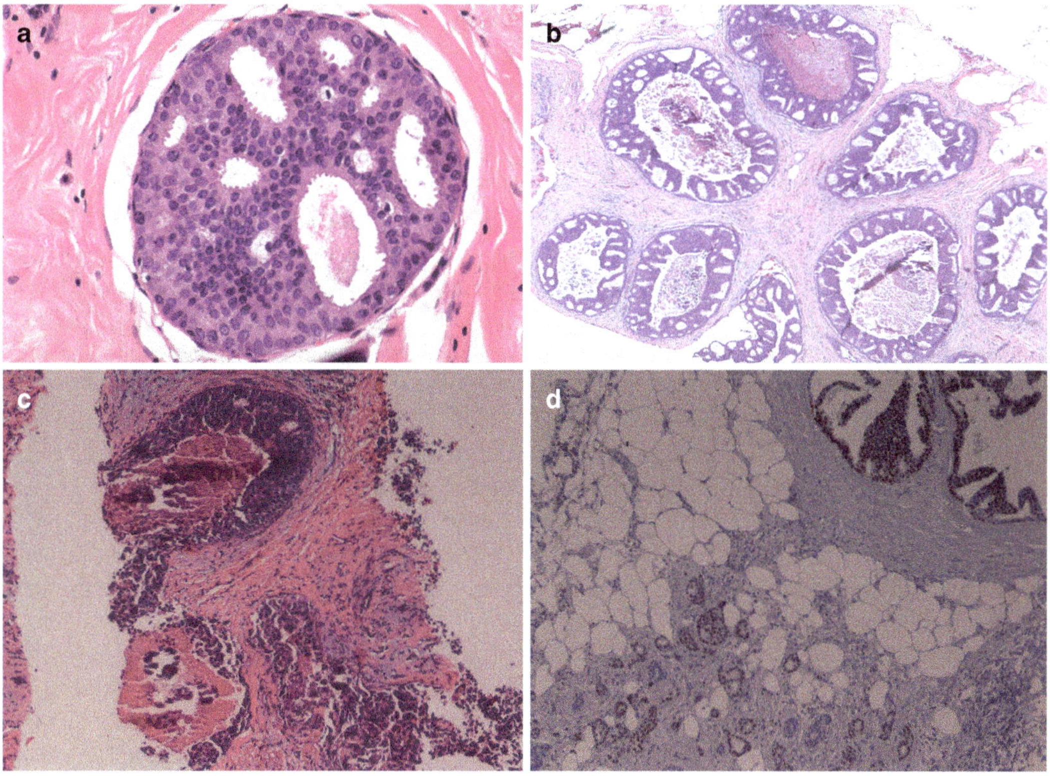

Fig. 5.1 (**a**) Single duct with monotonous, atypical, but uniform epithelial cells which partially or completely fill the ductal spaces with maximal dimension of 2 mm consistent with ADH. If more ducts like this present or expanded duct measures more than 2 mm, then it qualifies as low-grade cribriform DCIS. (**b**, **c**) DCIS with central comedo necrosis and calcification in the middle, in purple. (**d**) Cribriform DCIS (upper right) and invasive ductal carcinoma both strongly positive with nuclear estrogen receptor (Courtesy of Marina Mosunjac, MD Emory University Atlanta)

appearance to low-grade DCIS, with only quantitative differences.

Typically, ADH is detected by screening mammography as microcalcifications in an asymptomatic patient, and ADH represents 10 % of radiographically detected lesions [4]. Morphologically, a diagnosis of ADH requires atypical but uniform epithelial cells which partially or completely fill the ductal spaces, with a maximal dimension of 2 mm for each focus, distinguishing it from low-grade DCIS [5, 10, 28] (Fig. 5.1a, b). Due to the limited tissue sampling with CNB and the varied benign and malignant lesions associated with ADH, a diagnosis of ADH by CNB has a well-recognized potential for coexistent DCIS or invasive cancer that is related to sampling size [28] (Fig. 5.1c, d). Furthermore, FEA, ADH, and DCIS have been shown to display similar genetic alterations and chromosomal aberrations, such as loss of 16q, and progression to invasive cancer has been proposed to occur along potentially multiple such pathways through the acquisition of genetic alterations under selective pressure [27]. As a result, ADH is commonly found to be coexistent in the setting of other high-risk breast lesions as well as DCIS and invasive carcinoma [5, 10, 28].

At the same time, ADH also represents a marker for elevated risk of future cancer. Even in the absence of synchronous associated malignancy, a diagnosis of ADH incurs at least a four to five times relative risk of subsequent breast cancer diagnosis, perhaps as high as sixfold in premenopausal women [6]. This increased risk is evident in both the ipsilateral and contralateral breast [4, 7]. When malignancy is found in a surgical excision following a CNB diagnosis of ADH, an "upgrade" in diagnosis is said to have occurred. A wide range of upgrade percentages have been reported in the literature, with rates as low as 4 % and as high as 87 % [5]. One of largest recent retrospective studies looking at 422 CNB diagnoses of ADH reported an upgrade percentage of 31.3 %, with the majority upgrading to DCIS (22.7 %) [7].

Additionally, the presence of multiple radiographic foci of ADH has been shown to increase the rate of associated malignancy identified if excisional biopsy is subsequently performed (7 % for 1–2 foci vs. 39 % for >2 foci) [4]. In addition to discussion of the risk of concurrent malignancy, management of ADH must also include an estimation of the implied relative risk for future diagnosis of breast cancer. Lifestyle modifications, including avoiding risk factors such as prolonged use of hormone replacement therapy and increasing protective factors such as low fat diet and exercise, are believed to impart a modest risk reduction for development of future breast cancer. The original report of the breast cancer prevention trial, NSABP P-1, in 1998 [23] established the efficacy of tamoxifen use in reducing the risk of future breast cancer in patients with above-average risk by almost 50 %. Importantly, ADH patients in this trial received the most benefit, reducing risk of cancer by 86 %. Meanwhile, prophylactic surgery for the diagnosis of ADH alone is controversial [29, 30]. In summary, when ADH is identified by CNB, excision should be strongly considered in order to evaluate for coexistent malignancy. When malignancy is not identified following excision, informed discussion should include an estimation of future risk of malignancy as well as an acceptable plan for surveillance and risk reduction, including lifestyle modifications and chemoprevention with hormonal therapy.

Lobular Neoplasia: Atypical Lobular Hyperplasia (ALH) and Lobular Carcinoma In Situ (LCIS)

Lobular proliferative lesions include atypical lobular hyperplasia (ALH) and lobular carcinoma in situ (LCIS). LCIS was first describe by Ewing in 1919, and later the term lobular neoplasia (LN) was coined by Haagensen in 1978 to encompass both ALH and LCIS [31]; however, the term has not gained universal acceptance. Linear progression models for lobular breast changes are less well studied than their ductal counterpart, although some recent genetic and molecular studies have displayed similar genetic changes in ALH and LCIS with both IDC and invasive lobular carcinoma (ILC) [27]. LN represents a continuum from ALH to pleomorphic LCIS (pLCIS), the most aggressive subtype of LCIS [8]. LN is characterized by atypical epithelial cells with intraepithelial lobular proliferation of terminal duct-lobular units with differing degrees of filling and atypia. ALH and LCIS can be distinguished by the amount of acini involvement. LCIS is diagnosed by acini involvement of more than half with no central lumina where ALH has less than half of the acini affected [8, 10] (Fig. 5.2a, b). When unable to differentiate ductal versus lobular features, particularly important in the pleomorphic variant, the cellular adhesion molecule E-cadherin is utilized. Negativity for E-cadherin is a hallmark molecular feature of lobular histology (Fig. 5.2c, d).

Pleomorphic LCIS, which can be thought of as a separate entity due to its aggressive natural history, is distinguished by its approximately four-times larger nuclei and significant nuclear pleomorphism. Although LCIS and pLCIS are normally ER/PR positive (pLCIS can be negative), and E-cadherin negative, pLCIS may show HER2 overexpression, p53 positivity, and an elevated Ki67 index compared with LCIS. pLCIS also shows similarities to DCIS with occasional chromosomal deletions and ontogenesis. These features have significant implications when evaluating upgrade percentage and breast cancer risk with pLCIS, which is universally considered as a precursor lesion to breast cancer [8, 10]. LN is typically an incidental diagnosis without specific physical exam or radiographic findings, although it may be associated with microcalcifications in the pLCIS subtype. When LN is diagnosed, up to 85 % are multicentric and 50 % are multifocal, with up to one third with LN identified in the contralateral breast [4, 10].

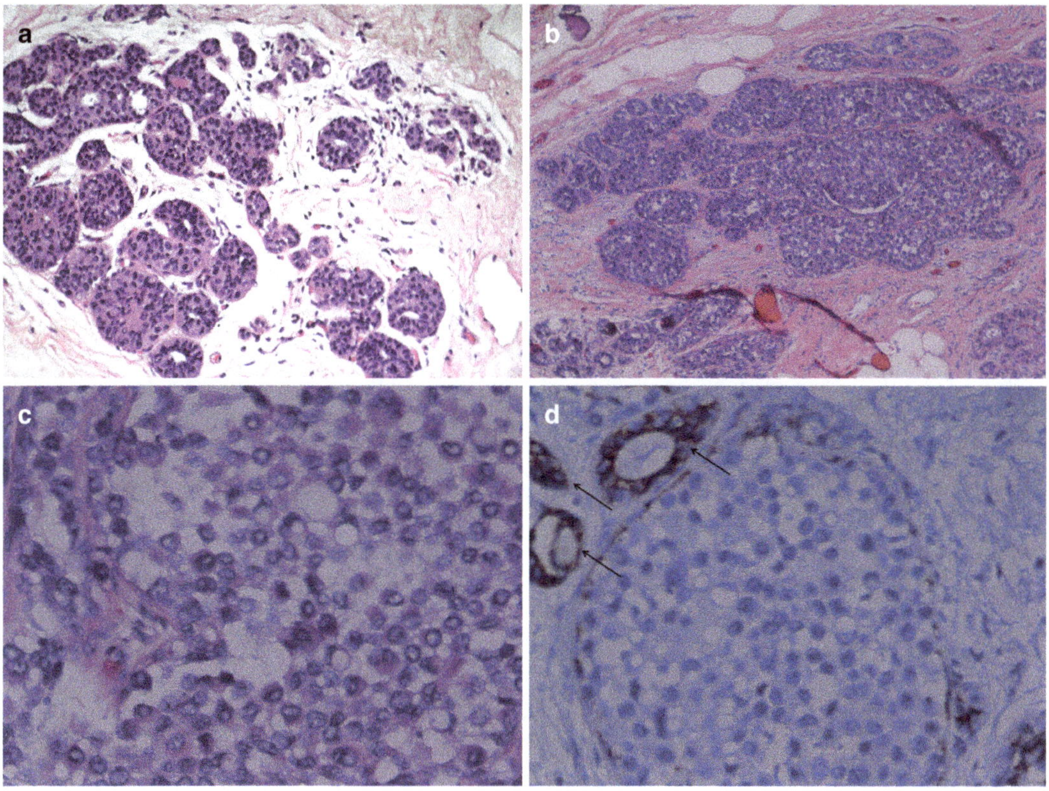

Fig. 5.2 (**a**) Atypical lobular hyperplasia ALH with mildly expanded lobules with monotonous smaller cells, not enough for LCIS. (**b**) Lobular carcinoma in situ. Extended lobules filled with small dyscohesive uniform cells. There is a feel of "bag of marbles," and if you were to turn the slide upside down, the marbles would fall out, different from DCIS where cells usually are more tightly packed. (**c**) Lobular carcinoma in situ: at higher power, the dyscohesiveness of the LCIS cells. (**d**) E-cadherin, membranous stain, not staining LCIS but staining adjacent ducts (Courtesy of Marina Mosunjac, MD Emory University Atlanta)

LN has classically been considered a marker of future breast cancer risk, and not a precursor lesion, and management is still somewhat controversial, particularly in cases without a radiographic abnormality. The average age for the diagnosis of LN is between 44 and 47 years. It is 12 times more common in white than black patients [32]. The relative risk for the development of breast cancer in a patient diagnosed with LN is four- to fivefold for ALH and about eight- to ninefold for LCIS [9]. With LCIS, the cumulative risk of ipsilateral and contralateral breast cancer is similar (18 % and 14 %, respectively) with 40 % being ILC and 60 % IDC [11]. When excised, an upgrade in diagnosis from LN to malignancy is reported to occur at rates ranging from 0 to 50 % [8]. This wide range is likely related to the limited radiographic findings, variable indications for excision, and inherent differences between the subtypes of LN. A recent meta-analysis of over 1,200 LN patients displayed upgrade percentages of 19 % of the ALH cases, 32 % of the LCIS cases, and 41 % (40–60 % in the literature) of the pLCIS cases [8].

Management of LN diagnosed by CNB must start with an assessment of clinical and pathologic concordance, as the diagnosis of LN often is not related to the underlying clinical findings. LN typically presents with limited suggestive history or exam and imaging findings (excluding the pLCIS subtype), indicating a need to consider the possibility of misdiagnosis following CNB and the possibility for alternative diagnoses following any proposed excision. Management of pLCIS is unique from management of LN in general. Due to its high associated underlying risk of invasive lobular carcinoma of about 40–60 %, it is considered a precursor lesion, and excision with negative margins should be recommended in all patients when seen on CNB.

For the remaining LN lesions, surveillance may be appropriate when another concordant benign pathologic lesion, such as a fibroadenoma, is identified in the CNB specimen. Repeat biopsy or surgical excision may be considered appropriate in the setting of clinical-pathologic discordance, identification of another associated high-risk lesion, or presence of unusual histologic features such as mitoses or necrosis. In such instances, underlying DCIS and invasive carcinoma are more likely to be identified [5]. Compared to the general population, ALH carries 4- to 5-fold and LCIS 8- to 12-fold greater lifetime risk of developing invasive cancer [33, 34]. When ALH or LCIS is diagnosed, an informed discussion must also include an established plan for surveillance, including possible MRI, lifestyle modifications, chemoprevention with hormonal therapy, and bilateral prophylactic mastectomy.

Columnar Cell Lesions: Flat Epithelial Atypia and Columnar Cell Hyperplasia with Atypia

Columnar cell lesions (CCLs) were first described in the literature in 1979 [35, 36] as "monomorphic clinging carcinoma in situ," and the term flat epithelial atypia (FEA) was more recently recognized by the World Health Organization to describe CCLs with atypia. The overall incidence of finding CCLs by CNB has been increasing recently with a current prevalence of 3.7–10 % [13]. CCLs are not normally diagnosed on physical exam, but radiographically they can be associated with pleomorphic calcifications [4]. Histologically, CCLs are characterized by enlarged terminal ductal-lobular units with dilated acini lined with columnar cells and with associated apical snouts. Columnar cells are epithelial cells that are columnar in shape, giving them their name (Fig. 5.3a, b). Elongated nuclei and intraluminal secretions are also noted. Cytologically, CCLs are composed of similar progenitor cells to ADH and DCIS and include a spectrum of lesions, including columnar cell change (CCC), columnar cell hyperplasia (CCH), and FEA. As previously discussed, these lesions, particularly FEA, are felt to be early in the spectrum from normal breast tissue to carcinoma. CCC is distinguished by having only two layers of cells, without atypia, lining the ductal components, while CCH exhibits greater than 2 layers of cells, and FEA displays associated atypia (Fig. 5.4a, b).

A grading system (low, medium, high) has been proposed to describe the degree of atypia noted [10, 13]. ADH is distinguished from columnar cell lesions (CCLs) by the degree of cytonuclear atypia and abnormal architecture [13]. The majority of CCLs display ER/PR positivity. While considered benign lesions, CCLs have a known association with other high-risk benign lesions and malignancy. The diagnosis of CCLs may possibly represent a risk factor for and/or early precursor to carcinoma, although this is yet to be proven [5, 13, 27]. When excised, CCLs with atypia are found to occur concurrently with other high-risk benign lesions 25–33 % of the time, with associated ALH and ADH being identified at a rate of 5 and 3.5 %, respectively [4, 5, 12].

Additionally, the reported rate of upgrade in diagnosis to in situ or invasive cancer following excisional biopsy for CCLs has been reported at rates ranging from 0 to 26 %. These rates have been shown to be significantly higher for CCH (20 %) and FEA (9 %) when compared to CCC; however, the true rate of associated malignancy is difficult to estimate, as many lesions are managed without excision [13, 14]. In practice, the management of CCH and FEA often differs from the management of CCC based on the described disparity in associated risk. Surgical excision should be presented as the preferred management whenever CNB of a breast lesion yields a diagnosis of CCH or FEA. Occasionally, continued surveillance is also discussed with patients in the setting of

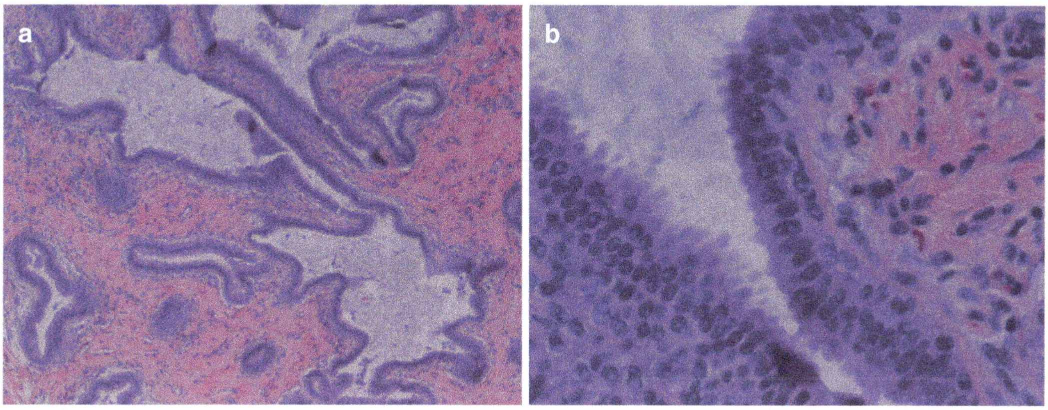

Fig. 5.3 (**a**, **b**) Columnar cell lesions are characterized by enlarged terminal ductal-lobular units with dilated acini lined with columnar cells and with associated apical snouts. Columnar cells are epithelial cells that are columnar in shape, giving them their name (Courtesy of Marina Mosunjac, MD Emory University Atlanta)

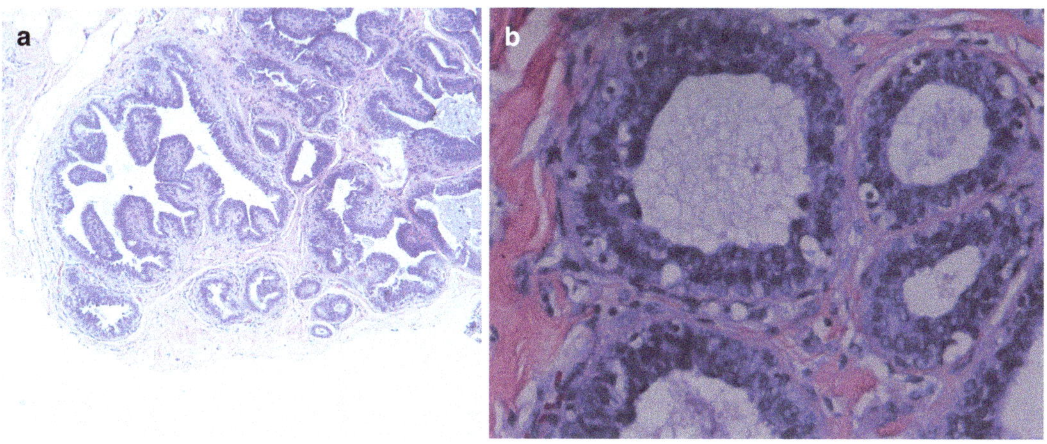

Fig. 5.4 (**a**) Columnar cell hyperplasia. Cysts lined by orderly columnar cells with minimal atypia. (**b**) Flat epithelial atypia (FEA) cysts lined by pseudostratified slightly disordered larger atypical cells (Courtesy of Marina Mosunjac, MD Emory University Atlanta)

an informed discussion. Interval clinical and imaging follow-up is more often practiced following a CNB diagnosis of CCC.

Papillary Lesions

Papillary breast lesions (PBLs) span a wide pathologic spectrum ranging from benign to malignant and include intraductal papilloma (IDP), atypical papilloma, intracystic papillary carcinoma, and invasive papillary carcinoma. PBLs present with a diverse clinical behavior and radiographic presentation. Radiographically, PBLs can present as architectural distortion, asymmetric density, and occasionally a palpable breast mass with or without associated microcalcifications, or microcalcifications alone. However, mammography and ultrasonography cannot reliably distinguish benign from malignant PBLs [37]. The hallmark of PBLs is the formation of papillary structures composed of two layers of cells, one epithelial and one myoepithelial, on a fibrovascular core (Fig. 5.5a–c). Distinguishing among the spectrum of papillary lesions, such as an atypical papilloma versus DCIS arising within a papilloma, can be very challenging for the pathologist. Additionally, other proliferative lesions can

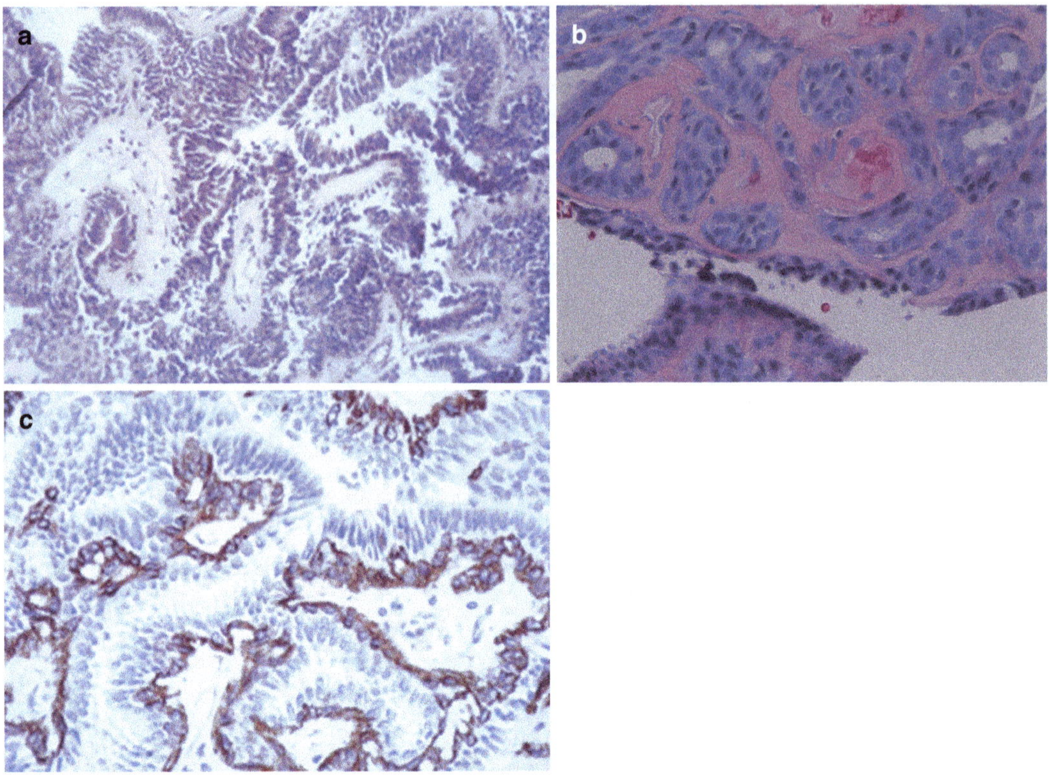

Fig. 5.5 (**a**, **b**) Benign intraductal papilloma (IDP) of the breast showing fibrovascular cores lined by two distinct layers of cells, myoepithelial cells and ductal cells. (**c**) Calponin stain (×400) specifically delineates myoepithelial cells in a benign IDP (Courtesy of Marina Mosunjac, MD Emory University Atlanta)

be present at the periphery of the suspicious mass or area, further complicating the diagnosis.

Moreover, the accurate diagnosis on CNB can be difficult because of fragmentation, limited material, sampling error, or presence of other nonneoplastic proliferations, such as florid papillomatosis, radial sclerosing lesions (RSLs), and micropapillary hyperplasia [10]. Yet, as percutaneous stereotactic or ultrasound-guided CNB has been used increasingly in the diagnosis of clinically occult and palpable breast lesions, recent data have suggested that benign papillary lesions (mainly IDPs) can be diagnosed accurately by CNB [38, 39]. In spite of the inherent limitations of CNB, papillary lesions account for approximately 5–10 % of all CNBs, and the subsequent decision about clinical treatment is now based largely on the CNB diagnosis [40, 41].

A number of studies have been published on the management of atypical papillary lesions, inclusive of IDP with atypia or IDP with associated ADH, with most recommending surgical excision based upon the increased risk of associated DCIS and invasive carcinoma [37, 40–42]. In contrast to atypical papillary lesions, the management of benign IDP remains controversial, with no clear consensus on the optimal approach to management. The reported incidence of finding a more advanced lesion (ADH, DCIS, and invasive carcinoma) on follow-up excisional biopsy after the diagnosis of benign IDP on CNB ranges from 0 to 25 % [43]. In one retrospective review [44] of 276 consecutive cases of IDP undergoing surgical excision, there was a clear higher rate of upgrade in diagnosis to DCIS/IDC when compared to isolated IDP, 33 %/5 % vs. 8 %/1 %, respectively. For isolated IDP, an 18 % upgrade in diagnosis to ADH was also noted. Therefore, even when CNB demonstrated benign IDP, an upgrade in diagnosis to a lesion of greater clinical significance was demonstrated 27 % of the time following excisional biopsy [44]. While the clinical significance of identifying IDC/DCIS is appreciated, an upgrade in diagnosis to a benign lesion such as ADH can have significant patient management implications. Surgical excision is the current recommendation considered as optimal management for all breast papillary lesions identified on CNB.

Radial Sclerosing Lesions: Radial Scar and Complex Sclerosing Lesions

Radial sclerosing lesions (RSLs) of the breast are a group of benign, stellate-appearing breast lesions, with the incidence of radial scars identified on CNB ranging from 4 to 26 %. These lesions have been referred to by several different names, including scleroelastotic lesion, indurative mastopathy, nonencapsulated sclerosing lesion, and sclerosing papillary proliferation [45]. RSLs are often categorized by size as either radial scar (<1 cm) or complex sclerosing lesion (>1 cm). These lesions can have a clinical and radiologic presentation as well as gross pathologic appearance resembling that of carcinoma [10]. Typically, patients diagnosed with RSLs have no particular exam or imaging findings, and RSL is often an incidental finding on CNB biopsy for another concordant abnormality. However, patients may also present with a palpable breast mass. Mammographic findings, when present, usually display a spiculated lesion with dense radiolucent cores and thin spicules radiating out from the core, which can be nearly impossible to distinguish from carcinoma [15, 46] (Fig. 5.6a, b). Histologically, RSL are characterized by fibroelastotic cores with ducts and lobules radiating centrifugally with typical or atypical epithelial proliferative changes or cysts [10, 15, 45].

The clinical significance of RSLs lies in both the implicit associated increase risk of developing breast cancer in the future and the associated risk of concurrent malignancy. The relative risk increase imparted by a diagnosis of RSL ranges from 1.8 to 3 [47, 48], and a diagnosis of associated malignancy following excision has been reported at a rate of 0–40 % [10]. Due to the similarities in clinical appearance to carcinoma and the potential risk of associated breast cancer, RSLs have traditionally been treated with excisional biopsy. The more recent literature showing percutaneous underestimation rates of malignancy in the 5–9 % range makes management more complex, with options for surveillance seeming more acceptable, particularly in higher operative risk or multiply-comorbid patients [15, 46]. The absence of cytologic atypia, increased number of cores taken at the time of CNB, and extensive sampling with vacuum-assisted needle biopsy have all been described as methods to identify patients that may safely be monitored. However, no clear clinical radiographic predictors have been identified to determine lesions at increased risk for associated malignancy, and surgical excision recommendations should be made independent of imaging findings [45]. For most patients of acceptable operative risk, optimal management continues to be complete surgical excision.

Fibroepithelial Lesions with Cellular Stroma

Fibroepithelial tumors of the breast represent a varied group of lesions containing both mesenchymal and epithelial components. The epithelial elements contain Ck5/14-positive progenitor cells with their glandular and myoepithelial progeny, whereas the stromal component shows vimentin/CD34 positivity with potential for multi-lineage differentiation as seen in spindle cell lesions of the breast [16, 17]. The proliferation of fibroepithelial elements along divergent pathways gives rise to fibroadenomas, phyllodes tumors, sclerosing lobular hyperplasia, and hamartomas.

Fibroadenoma is the most common benign breast tumor and clinically presents as a palpable mass or as an abnormal imaging finding. Lesions may be identified in women at any age, typically presenting during early adolescence, with a mean age of 30 at presentation. Multiple

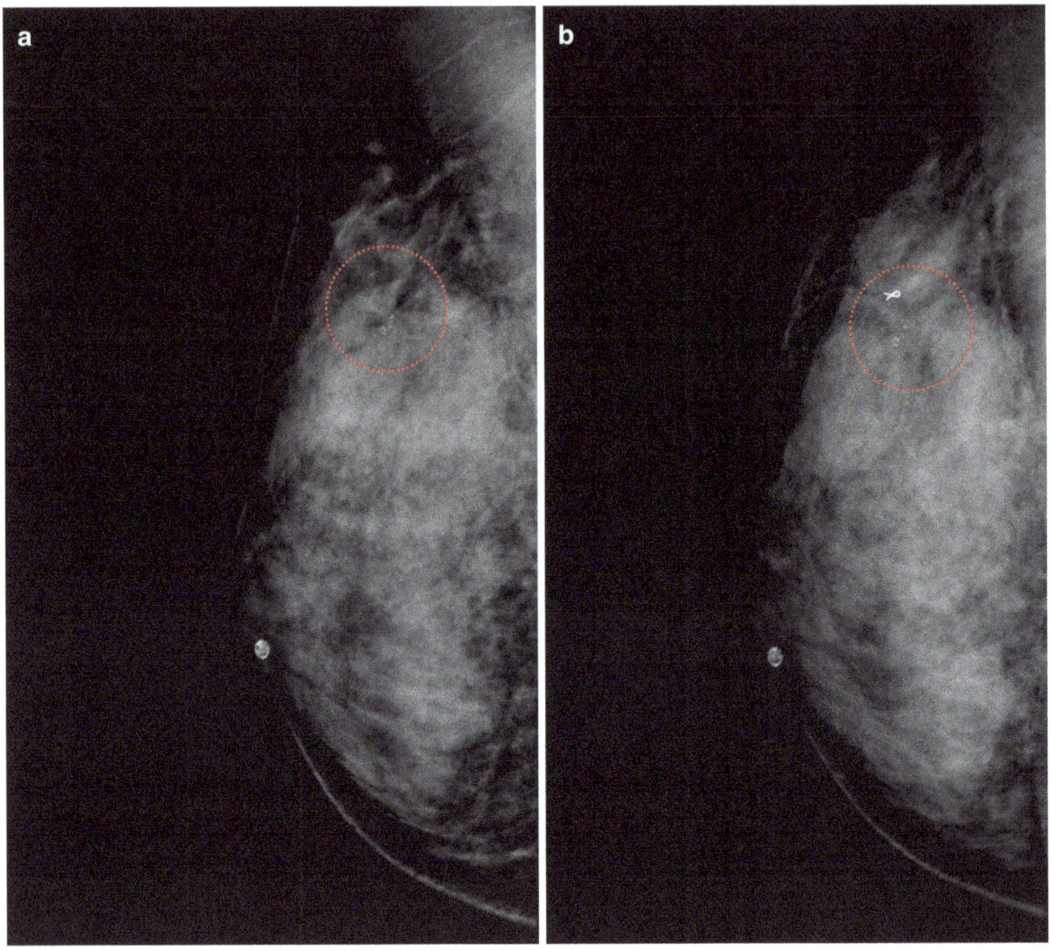

Fig. 5.6 Forty-three-year-old asymptomatic female presenting with an abnormal screening mammogram showing architectural distortion (*circle*) with radiating spicules (**a**). She underwent ultrasound-guided core needle biopsy with clip placement. Pathology from the core needle biopsy showed a radial scar (**b**) (Courtesy Dr Michael Cohen Emory University Atlanta)

fibroadenomas can be identified at presentation approximately 15 % of the time. When palpable, fibroadenomas are typically small, smooth, mobile, and firm or rubbery masses with >90 % smaller than 4 cm. Fibroadenomas may develop into very large masses particularly in adolescent girls and young women, often called juvenile giant fibroadenomas (Fig. 5.7a, b) [49]. On mammography, fibroadenomas appear as well-defined round, oval, or lobulated masses, which may be calcified. On ultrasound, fibroadenomas are well-circumscribed, uniform hypoechoic or isoechoic ovoid masses, and the lesions are typically wider than tall with a well-demarcated margin [50].

Fibroadenomas arise from the epithelium and stroma of the terminal duct-lobular unit, with pathologic findings typically revealing well-defined borders consisting of elongated ducts lined with two layers of epithelium and situated in a stroma with low cellularity. When the diagnosis is made by CNB, a decision must be made whether to monitor or excise the lesion. In rare cases, fibroadenomas can progress in both epithelial and stromal directions to malignant tumors [51]. However, most fibroadenomas tend to be self-limited or even regress, and it is not necessary to remove them all, while percutaneous excisional or ablative treatment may be appropriate in select patients as defined recently by the ASBrS. Size

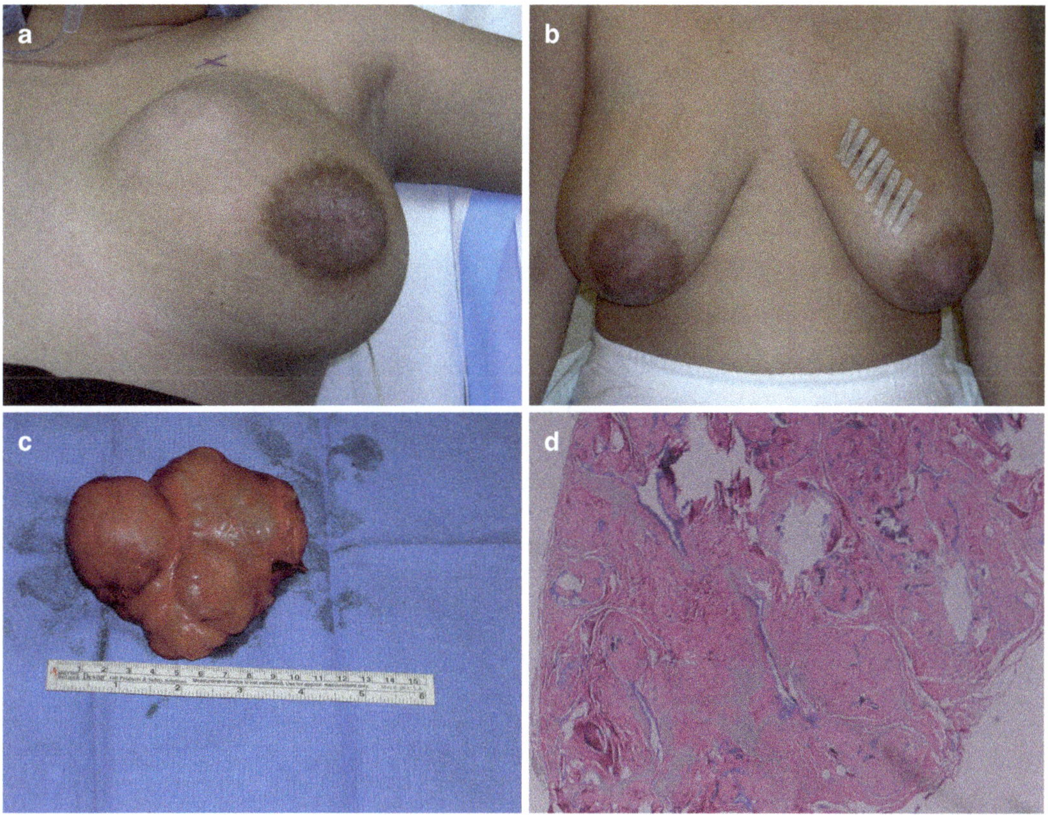

Fig. 5.7 Juvenile giant fibroadenoma of the breast. (**a**) Eighteen-year-old female at presentation. (**b**) One week after surgery. (**c**) Surgical specimen 12×11×8 cm. (**d**) Microscopically, the fibroadenoma showed mainly a hyalinized component (Courtesy of Monica Rizzo, MD and Marina Mosunjac, MD Emory University Atlanta)

(greater than 2.0–2.5 cm), growth, symptoms, positive family history, discordance, and age (greater than 35 years) are reasonable indications for surgical excision. It should be discussed that there is a potential for upgrade in the final pathologic diagnosis to a phyllodes tumor, in situ, or even invasive carcinoma in rare instances [51].

Phyllodes tumor is an exceedingly rare lesion with an estimated incidence of 2.1 per million women. Presentation typically occurs between the ages of 45 and 49, typically about 15 years later in age compared to fibroadenomas [52]. The presentation of a phyllodes tumor is clinically indistinguishable from that of a fibroadenoma [53]. Phyllodes tumor is felt to arise from the perilobular-periductal stroma. Microscopically, a circumscribed lesion with mixed epithelial and mesenchymal components is seen with a double-layered epithelial component and overgrowth of a hypercellular stromal component. FNA and CNB typically cannot discriminate between fibroadenoma and phyllodes tumor; however, the diagnosis may be suggested [54, 55]. Several systems for grading of phyllodes tumors exist, and while many authors use a three-tiered system to distinguish between benign, borderline, and malignant cases, others omit the intermediate category [56, 57].

A benign phyllodes tumor is characterized as having few mitoses in a high-power field (HPF), <2 per 10 HPF; no more than mild atypia, and no stromal overgrowth. Borderline phyllodes tumor has 2–5 mitoses per 10 HPF, more atypia with no stromal overgrowth. Malignant phyllodes tumor has marked atypia, more than 10 mitoses per HPF and stromal overgrowth (Fig. 5.8a, b). The grading system reflects the clinical behavior, with local recurrence and rare metastases noted in benign cases and distant metastases more common in

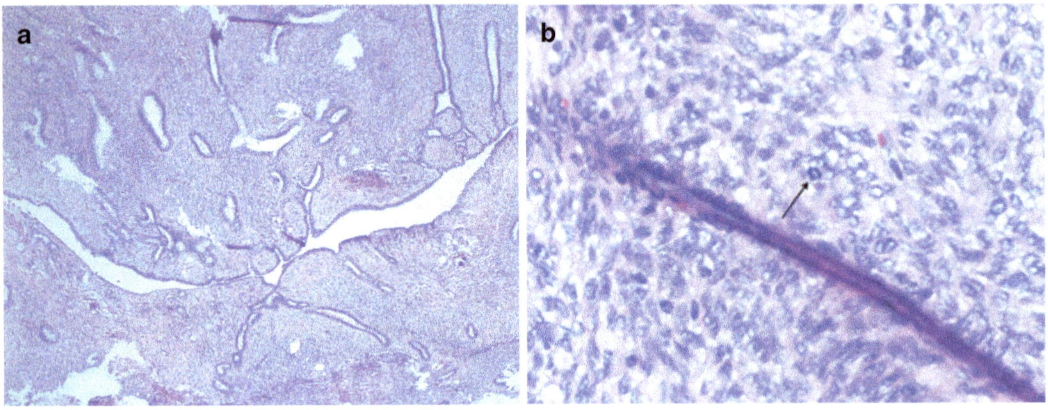

Fig. 5.8 (**a**) Phyllodes tumor. Ducts embedded into hypercellular stroma. (**b**) Stroma contains mitoses (*arrows*) (Courtesy of Marina Mosunjac, MD Emory University Atlanta)

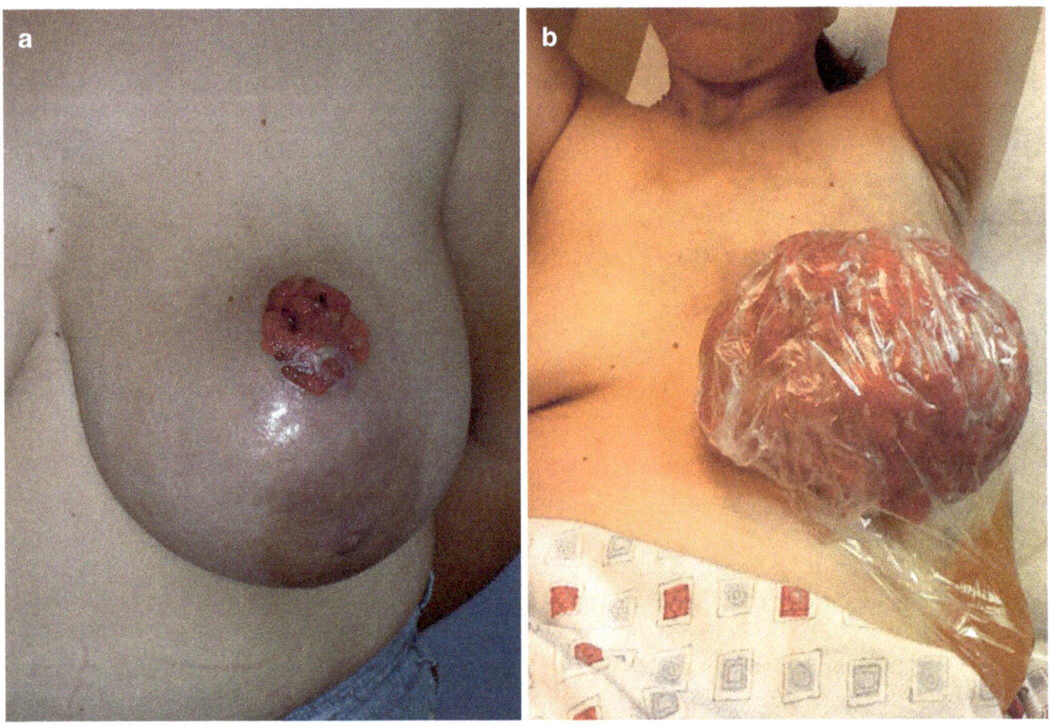

Fig. 5.9 Malignant phyllodes tumor. The patient refused surgical treatment when originally diagnosed (**a**). She developed a large ulcerated growth over 3 years (**b**) (Courtesy of Monica Rizzo, MD Emory University Atlanta)

malignant cases. When phyllodes tumor is diagnosed by CNB, the ability to differentiate benign, intermediate, and malignant lesions is unreliable [56]. Wide local excision with the intent of removing >1 cm margins is the preferred treatment of a phyllodes tumor (Fig. 5.9a, b). There is a relatively high incidence of local recurrence, reported from 8 to 46 % in cases of positive surgical margins [57]. Often, the diagnosis of phyllodes tumor is not made until excisional biopsy has been performed. When excising a fibroadenoma, removal of a rim of normal breast tissue around the lesion is acceptable, in case an upgrade in diagnosis to a phyllodes tumor does occur.

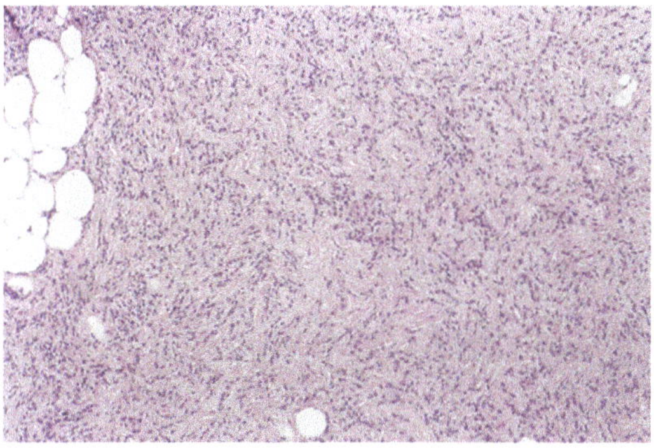

Fig. 5.10 Breast hamartoma. Microscopically, the tumor shows fibrous stroma with scattered ductal elements and adipose tissue on the left without any lobular units (Courtesy of Marina Mosunjac, MD Emory University Atlanta)

Hamartomas and sclerosing lobular hyperplasia are rare benign fibroepithelial lesions with a nonspecific presentation that may be suspicious for fibroadenoma clinically and radiographically [58, 59]. While hamartomas are typically benign, malignant transformation has been rarely reported (Fig. 5.10). Hamartomas can occur at any age but are more common between the ages of 30 and 50 [60]. Diagnosis of hamartoma on CNB is problematic, with CNB results usually revealing benign breast tissue. Excisional biopsy to completely remove the lesion typically results in a very low local recurrence rate. However, they can be seen in high frequency in Cowden's syndrome and suggest an elevated lifetime risk of breast cancer [61]. Sclerosing lobular hyperplasia can be difficult to distinguish from fibroadenoma by needle biopsy, and excisional biopsy may be recommended for reasons identical to those considered in recommending excision of fibroadenoma. While the lesion itself is benign and does not require excision, the diagnosis often is only made upon complete surgical removal [59].

Mucocele-Like Lesions

Mucocele-like tumors of the breast were originally described by Rosen in 1986 [62] as an uncommon benign cystic lesion containing abundant mucin with extravasation into the surrounding stroma. Histologically, these lesions are difficult to distinguish from colloid carcinoma on fine-needle aspiration. At gross inspection, mucocele-like tumors are multicystic or multi-loculated, with multiple cysts in fibrous stroma seen by microscopy. Mucocele-like lesions of the breast may be identified on breast self-exam or on clinical exam as a palpable mass. Mammographically, they are identified in the setting of indeterminate microcalcifications, from dystrophic calcification of the mucin pool, or as a nodule. Sonographically, they appear to be hypoechoic lesions resembling complex cysts, and multiple oval or tubular structures with low-level internal acoustic echoes may be seen along with calcified or non-calcified mural nodules [63, 64] (Fig. 5.11a, b).

While originally reported as a benign lesion, a high incidence of associated ADH and carcinoma has subsequently been reported [65–67]. Weaver et al. postulated the existence of a pathologic continuum of mucinous breast lesions spanning the spectrum from benign mucocele-like tumor to invasive mucinous carcinoma. They examined a series of 23 consecutive invasive mucinous carcinomas of the breast for the association with intermediate mucinous lesions. The associated intermediate lesions included mucin-filled ducts (MFD) with unremarkable epithelium (65 %), MFD with typical ductal hyperplasia (39 %), MFD with atypical ductal hyperplasia (22 %), and MFD with intraductal carcinoma (57 %) [67]. The potential to reliably differentiate benign mucocele-like lesions from those with associated ADH or carcinoma based on imaging is unclear and continues to be studied [64, 68, 69]. When mucocele-like lesions are diagnosed on CNB, a high rate of upgrade in diagnosis to ADH or carcinoma continues to be reported in the literature, ranging from 18 to 30 % [69–71]. Due to concerns for sampling error, the high rate of coexistent lesions, and the unclear natural history, surgical excision following CNB diagnosis of a benign mucocele-like lesion of the breast represents optimal management.

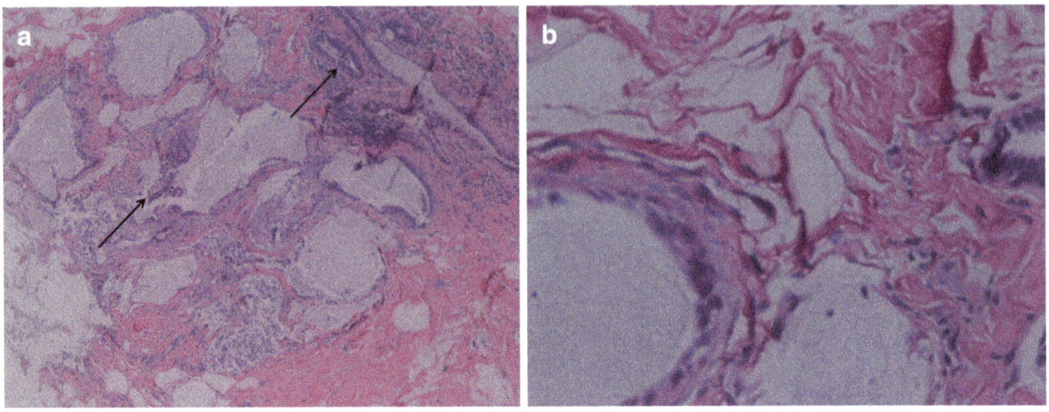

Fig. 5.11 (**a**) Mucocele-like lesion: large mucin-filled cysts focally disrupted and adjacent cysts with columnar cell change (*arrows*). (**b**) High power of mucocele-like lesion (Courtesy of Marina Mosunjac, MD Emory University Atlanta)

Spindle Cell Lesions

While epithelial and fibroepithelial lesions comprise most of the proliferations arising within the breast, a diverse group of lesions displaying a predominantly monomorphic proliferation of spindle cells has been described as well. As with fibroepithelial lesions of the breast, such as fibroadenomas and phyllodes tumors, the putative precursor of these lesions is the uncommitted vimentin+/CD34+ fibroblast of the mammary stroma. It is capable of divergent mesenchymal differentiation, and the clinical behavior of these lesions can span a wide spectrum from benign to malignant [18, 19, 72].

Benign spindle cell tumors (BSCTs) of the mammary stroma were first described by Toker in 1981, [20] though consensus on the current nomenclature occurred much later. In the initial report of four cases, Toker et al. described the histologic relationship of these tumors to benign spindle cell lipomas, as well as the benign clinical history following complete excision [20]. A cytologically diverse population of fibroblasts, myofibroblasts, smooth muscle cells, and undifferentiated mesenchymal cells was noted, and the possibility of a common mesenchymal precursor was suggested [20]. Numerous case reports subsequently emerged in the literature, describing different unique benign spindle cell lesions of the breast with varied histologic and immunophenotypical permutations. Furthermore, these variations were noted not only among different tumors but also seen within the same tumor. Consequently, a multitude of designations, often used interchangeably, emerged in the literature to describe these benign monomorphic proliferations of bland-looking spindle cell lesions of the breast [17, 18, 73–76] including spindle cell lipoma, myofibroblastoma, solitary fibrous tumor, myogenic stromal tumor, and atypical variant of leiomyoma. A continuous morphologic and immunophenotypical spectrum resulting in lesions of subtle variable heterogeneity has been described, and the term "benign spindle cell tumor (BSCT) of the mammary stroma" has been advocated to cover the entire continuum of such lesions.

BSCTs of the mammary stroma have been divided into four main categories by light microscopy and immunocytochemistry: fibroblastic (benign spindle cell tumor NOS, benign spindle cell tumor with adipocyte component, solitary fibrous tumor), myofibroblastic (myofibroblastoma, leiomyoma), fibrohistiocytic (benign fibrous histiocytoma), and mixed tumors (components of the above) [18]. They clinically present as a one-sided, rounded, well-circumscribed, and slowly enlarging lesion during the course of several months. Mammography usually reveals a well-defined, ovoid dense mass in the absence of microcalcifications, although irregular

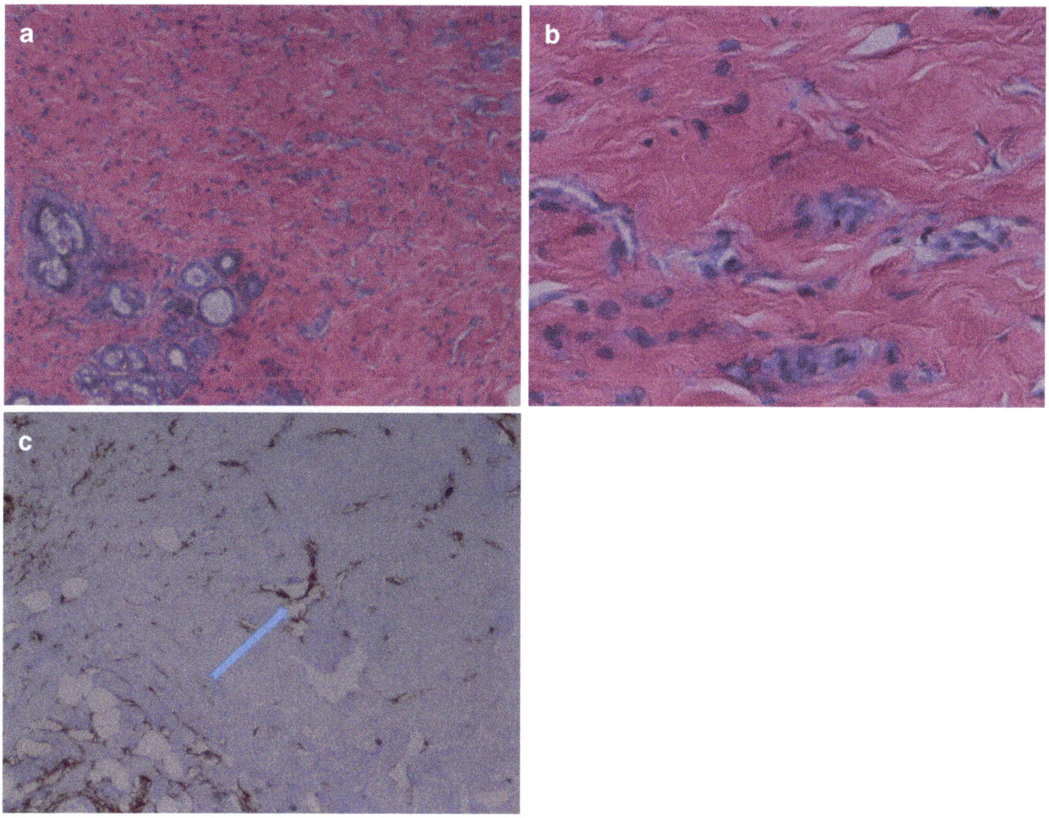

Fig. 5.12 Pseudoangiomatous stromal hyperplasia (PASH) consists of anastomosing slit-like spaces lined by myofibroblasts with intervening band-like segments of eosinophilic hyalinized stroma. Dense fibrotic (*pink*) tissue with slit-like (*white*) cracks and small vessels. (**a**, **b**) The spindle cell component is positive for CD34 (**c**, *arrow*) (Courtesy of Marina Mosunjac, MD Emory University Atlanta)

margins can infrequently be seen. Ultrasound findings may include a homogeneously solid and hypoechoic mass, with or without increased vascularity on Doppler sonogram [17].

By definition, BSCTs of the mammary stroma have a benign clinical course following surgical excision [17, 20]. However, the natural history of BSCTs observed following a diagnosis by CNB and rates of upgrade in diagnosis to a lesion of greater clinical significance are lacking in the literature. Toker et al. was the first to emphasize the importance of differentiating BSCT of the mammary stroma from other bland-looking monomorphic spindle cell lesions of the breast [20]. The differential diagnosis includes other benign but low-grade tumors and tumorlike lesions: pseudoangiomatous stromal hyperplasia (PASH), nodular fasciitis, primary mammary fibromatosis (PMF), and inflammatory myofibroblastic tumor (IMF).

PASH was first described by Vuitch et al. in 1986 [77] and was subsequently recognized as a common occurrence, found in one retrospective review in 23 % of biopsy and mastectomy specimens [78]. The age of diagnosis ranges from the late teens to the mid-50s. Microscopically, PASH consists of anastomosing slit-like spaces lined by myofibroblasts with intervening band-like segments of eosinophilic hyalinized stroma. The spindle cell component is positive for CD34 and vimentin, with morphology reminiscent of myofibroblastoma, and the absence of atypia or mitoses in the lobules and ducts helps to differentiate from borderline fibroepithelial lesions [19] (Fig. 5.12a–c). Infrequently, PASH may form a mass ("tumoral PASH") that is generally non-tender, circumscribed, and nonencapsulated, and imaging findings may be concerning for malignancy [79].

Typically, tumoral PASH presents as a small lesion; however, tumors up to 12 cm and occupying much of the breast have been reported [80]. PASH is not recognized as being associated with synchronous malignancy, a premalignant lesion, or a pathologic finding suggestive of a higher risk of future malignancy [81]. No treatment is generally recommended for PASH unless it forms a mass, and the purpose of excision is generally to differentiate from fibroepithelial or spindle cell neoplasms. A selective approach to surgical excision is felt to be appropriate for enlarging or symptomatic lesions. Recurrence in the ipsilateral or contralateral breast is reported but rarely occurs [82].

Nodular fasciitis is a rare spindle cell lesion of the breast parenchyma or subcutaneous tissue that presents as an unencapsulated mass with expansile growth that typically displaces the adjacent ducts and lobules. This growth pattern may mimic invasion into the adjacent tissue, and the radiographic findings, which usually mimic that of a fibroadenoma, may also simulate invasive carcinoma. Microscopically, the spindle cells are arranged in short fascicles, and an inflammatory component is noted with microcystic degeneration and extravasated erythrocytes [18, 19]. The natural history of nodular fasciitis is not well understood, since most lesions are treated with excision; however, regression after FNA biopsy has been reported [83]. Nevertheless, excision is typically recommended to rule out lesions of greater clinical significance such as fibromatosis, metaplastic spindle cell carcinoma, fibromatosis-like carcinoma, and low-grade sarcoma. Rare local recurrence has been reported [18].

Primary mammary fibromatosis (PMF) is a spindle cell tumor identical to desmoid tumors occurring at other anatomic sites and is sometimes seen in association with familial adenomatous polyposis and Gardner's syndromes [84, 85]. The lesions almost always present as a firm, palpable, painless mass that often causes retraction of the skin or nipple, and the clinical presentation often mimics invasive carcinoma [19, 86]. Infrequently, the lesions may be initially detected by mammography, [87] which normally displays a stellate or spiculated tumor indistinguishable from carcinoma but devoid of calcifications [88]. Like desmoid tumors elsewhere, previous trauma has often been described at the site of mammary fibromatosis in some patients, but the incidence is infrequent for mammary lesions and the role of trauma or previous surgery in the pathogenesis is considered controversial [19, 86]. PMF may be diagnosed by CNB, and the histologic findings consist of spindle cells arranged in long and sweeping fascicles with variable amounts of fibrous stroma and an infiltrative pattern. While a benign lesion, PMF is locally aggressive and wide excision with negative margins is the optimal management [19, 86]. Local recurrence is more common in younger women and, in cases with positive margins, usually occurs within 3 years and may be disfiguring, be difficult to control, and spread to the chest wall. The role of sulindac or tamoxifen remains unclear in the management of PMF [86].

Inflammatory myofibroblastic tumor (IMT), also known as inflammatory pseudotumor of the breast, is a very rare low-grade spindle cell lesion of the breast that clinically and radiographically may mimic cancer. The lesion was first described by Pettinato et al. in 1988 as an extrapulmonary presentation of plasma cell granuloma of the breast [89]. Like other benign spindle cell lesions of the breast, IMT typically presents as a painless palpable breast mass. Mammographic findings may be suggestive of malignancy and include a high-density mass with irregular, spiculated margins and devoid of calcifications. Sonography typically shows a hypoechoic and heterogeneous solid mass with irregular margins [30, 90]. The benign diagnosis may be suggested on CNB and confirmed on excisional biopsy [89]. Histologic evaluation shows spindle to oval cells in a myxoid to fibrous keloid-like stroma with a marked component of plasma cells, lymphocytes, and eosinophils [18, 89, 90]. While benign, local recurrence and malignant transformation may occur, thus wide local excision is the optimal management [18, 30, 90].

Conclusion

The identification of a high-risk or borderline breast lesion on CNB may have implications regarding future breast cancer risk, screening and surveillance, breast cancer prevention, and surgery. The current lack of a consensus regarding the optimal management of many of the high-risk lesions continues to manifest itself in the medical literature. The position statement published by the American Society of Breast Surgeons in 2011 regarding the management of high-risk breast lesions and NCCN guidelines for "breast cancer screening and diagnosis" offer valuable advice in the management of these lesions. Repeat percutaneous CNB, surgical excision, and surveillance are all acceptable clinical management options in the appropriate clinical scenarios, and the relative merits of each alternative must be considered on a unique case-by-case basis. A multidisciplinary approach is optimal, and discussion of lesion associated risk and individual estimated risk is appropriate. Ultimately, clinical management must account for patient preferences, informed discussion, and shared decision-making between the patient and breast care providers.

References

1. Silverstein MJ, Recht A, Lagios MD, et al. Special report: consensus conference III. Image-detected breast cancer: state-of-the-art diagnosis and treatment. J Am Coll Surg. 2009;209(4):504–20.
2. Silverstein M. Where's the outrage? J Am Coll Surg. 2009;208(1):78–9.
3. Linebarger JH, Landercasper J, Ellis RL, et al. Core needle biopsy rate for new cancer diagnosis in an interdisciplinary breast center: evaluation of quality of care 2007–2008. Ann Surg. 2012;255(1):38–43.
4. Neal L, Tortorelli CL, Nassar A. Clinician's guide to imaging and pathologic findings in benign breast disease. Mayo Clin Proc. 2010;85(3):274–9.
5. Corben AD, Edelweiss M, Brogi E. Challenges in the interpretation of breast core biopsies. Breast J. 2010;16 Suppl 1:S5–9.
6. Pinder SE, Ellis IO. The diagnosis and management of pre-invasive breast disease: ductal carcinoma in situ (DCIS) and atypical ductal hyperplasia (ADH)–current definitions and classification. Breast Cancer Res. 2003;5(5):254–7.
7. Deshaies I, Provencher L, Jacob S, et al. Factors associated with upgrading to malignancy at surgery of atypical ductal hyperplasia diagnosed on core biopsy. Breast. 2011;20(1):50–5.
8. Hussain M, Cunnick GH. Management of lobular carcinoma in-situ and atypical lobular hyperplasia of the breast–a review. Eur J Surg Oncol. 2011;37(4):279–89.
9. O'Malley FP. Lobular neoplasia: morphology, biological potential and management in core biopsies. Mod Pathol. 2010;23 Suppl 2:S14–25.
10. Masood S, Rosa M. Borderline breast lesions: diagnostic challenges and clinical implications. Adv Anat Pathol. 2011;18(3):190–8.
11. Fentiman IS. 8. The dilemma of in situ carcinoma of the breast. Int J Clin Pract. 2001;55(10):680–3.
12. Verschuur-Maes AH, van Deurzen CH, Monninkhof EM, van Diest PJ. Columnar cell lesions on breast needle biopsies: is surgical excision necessary? A systematic review. Ann Surg. 2012;255(2):259–65.
13. Sudarshan M, Meguerditchian AN, Mesurolle B, Meterissian S. Flat epithelial atypia of the breast: characteristics and behaviors. Am J Surg. 2011;201(2):245–50.
14. Verschuur-Maes AH, de Bruin PC, van Diest PJ. Epigenetic progression of columnar cell lesions of the breast to invasive breast cancer. Breast Cancer Res Treat. 2012;136(3):705–15.
15. Bianchi S, Giannotti E, Vanzi E, et al. Radial scar without associated atypical epithelial proliferation on image-guided 14-gauge needle core biopsy: analysis of 49 cases from a single-centre and review of the literature. Breast. 2012;21(2):159–64.
16. Moore T, Lee AH. Expression of CD34 and bcl-2 in phyllodes tumours, fibroadenomas and spindle cell lesions of the breast. Histopathology. 2001;38(1):62–7.
17. Magro G, Bisceglia M, Michal M, Eusebi V. Spindle cell lipoma-like tumor, solitary fibrous tumor and myofibroblastoma of the breast: a clinico-pathological analysis of 13 cases in favor of a unifying histogenetic concept. Virchows Arch. 2002;440(3):249–60.
18. Magro G, Michal M, Bisceglia M. Benign spindle cell tumors of the mammary stroma: diagnostic criteria, classification, and histogenesis. Pathol Res Pract. 2001;197(7):453–66.
19. Brogi E. Benign and malignant spindle cell lesions of the breast. Semin Diagn Pathol. 2004;21(1):57–64.
20. Toker C, Tang CK, Whitely JF, Berkheiser SW, Rachman R. Benign spindle cell breast tumor. Cancer. 1981;48(7):1615–22.
21. Gail MH, Brinton LA, Byar DP, et al. Projecting individualized probabilities of developing breast cancer for white females who are being examined annually. J Natl Cancer Inst. 1989;81(24):1879–86.
22. Costantino JP, Gail MH, Pee D, et al. Validation studies for models projecting the risk of invasive and total breast cancer incidence. J Natl Cancer Inst. 1999;91(18):1541–8.

23. Fisher B, Costantino JP, Wickerham DL, et al. Tamoxifen for prevention of breast cancer: report of the National Surgical Adjuvant Breast and Bowel Project P-1 Study. J Natl Cancer Inst. 1998;90(18):1371–88.
24. Fisher B, Costantino JP, Wickerham DL, et al. Tamoxifen for the prevention of breast cancer: current status of the National Surgical Adjuvant Breast and Bowel Project P-1 study. J Natl Cancer Inst. 2005;97(22):1652–62.
25. Rockhill B, Spiegelman D, Byrne C, Hunter DJ, Colditz GA. Validation of the Gail et al. model of breast cancer risk prediction and implications for chemoprevention. J Natl Cancer Inst. 2001;93(5):358–66.
26. Wellings SR, Jensen HM, Marcum RG. An atlas of subgross pathology of the human breast with special reference to possible precancerous lesions. J Natl Cancer Inst. 1975;55(2):231–73.
27. Bombonati A, Sgroi DC. The molecular pathology of breast cancer progression. J Pathol. 2011;223(2):307–17.
28. Krishnamurthy S, Bevers T, Kuerer H, Yang WT. Multidisciplinary considerations in the management of high-risk breast lesions. AJR Am J Roentgenol. 2012;198(2):W132–40.
29. Wood WC. Should the use of contralateral prophylactic mastectomy be increasing as it is? Breast. 2009;18 Suppl 3:S93–5.
30. Haj M, Weiss M, Loberant N, Cohen I. Inflammatory pseudotumor of the breast: case report and literature review. Breast J. 2003;9(5):423–5.
31. Haagensen CD, Lane N, Lattes R, Bodian C. Lobular neoplasia (so-called lobular carcinoma in situ) of the breast. Cancer. 1978;42(2):737–69.
32. Rosner D, Bedwani RN, Vana J, Baker HW, Murphy GP. Noninvasive breast carcinoma: results of a national survey by the American College of Surgeons. Ann Surg. 1980;192(2):139–47.
33. Page DL, Dupont WD, Rogers LW, Rados MS. Atypical hyperplastic lesions of the female breast. A long-term follow-up study. Cancer. 1985;55(11):2698–708.
34. McLaren BK, Schuyler PA, Sanders ME, et al. Excellent survival, cancer type, and Nottingham grade after atypical lobular hyperplasia on initial breast biopsy. Cancer. 2006;107(6):1227–33.
35. Martinez V, Azzopardi JG. Invasive lobular carcinoma of the breast: incidence and variants. Histopathology. 1979;3(6):467–88.
36. Azzopardi JG, Ahmed A, Millis RR. Problems in breast pathology. Major Probl Pathol. 1979;11:i–xvi, 1–466.
37. Jacobs TW, Connolly JL, Schnitt SJ. Nonmalignant lesions in breast core needle biopsies: to excise or not to excise? Am J Surg Pathol. 2002;26(9):1095–110.
38. Agoff SN, Lawton TJ. Papillary lesions of the breast with and without atypical ductal hyperplasia: can we accurately predict benign behavior from core needle biopsy? Am J Clin Pathol. 2004;122(3):440–3.
39. Ivan D, Selinko V, Sahin AA, Sneige N, Middleton LP. Accuracy of core needle biopsy diagnosis in assessing papillary breast lesions: histologic predictors of malignancy. Mod Pathol. 2004;17(2):165–71.
40. Irfan K, Brem RF. Surgical and mammographic follow-up of papillary lesions and atypical lobular hyperplasia diagnosed with stereotactic vacuum-assisted biopsy. Breast J. 2002;8(4):230–3.
41. MacGrogan G, Tavassoli FA. Central atypical papillomas of the breast: a clinicopathological study of 119 cases. Virchows Arch. 2003;443(5):609–17.
42. Kil WH, Cho EY, Kim JH, Nam SJ, Yang JH. Is surgical excision necessary in benign papillary lesions initially diagnosed at core biopsy? Breast. 2008;17(3):258–62.
43. Rizzo M, Lund MJ, Oprea G, Schniederjan M, Wood WC, Mosunjac M. Surgical follow-up and clinical presentation of 142 breast papillary lesions diagnosed by ultrasound-guided core-needle biopsy. Ann Surg Oncol. 2008;15(4):1040–7.
44. Rizzo M, Linebarger J, Lowe MC, et al. Management of papillary breast lesions diagnosed on core-needle biopsy: clinical pathologic and radiologic analysis of 276 cases with surgical follow-up. J Am Coll Surg. 2012;214(3):280–7.
45. Linda A, Zuiani C, Furlan A, et al. Radial scars without atypia diagnosed at imaging-guided needle biopsy: how often is associated malignancy found at subsequent surgical excision, and do mammography and sonography predict which lesions are malignant? AJR Am J Roentgenol. 2010;194(4):1146–51.
46. Sohn VY, Causey MW, Steele SR, Keylock JB, Brown TA. The treatment of radial scars in the modern era–surgical excision is not required. Am Surg. 2010;76(5):522–5.
47. Sanders ME, Page DL, Simpson JF, Schuyler PA, Dale Plummer W, Dupont WD. Interdependence of radial scar and proliferative disease with respect to invasive breast carcinoma risk in patients with benign breast biopsies. Cancer. 2006;106(7):1453–61.
48. Jacobs TW, Byrne C, Colditz G, Connolly JL, Schnitt SJ. Radial scars in benign breast-biopsy specimens and the risk of breast cancer. N Engl J Med. 1999;340(6):430–6.
49. Wechselberger G, Schoeller T, Piza-Katzer H. Juvenile fibroadenoma of the breast. Surgery. 2002;132(1):106–7.
50. Goel NB, Knight TE, Pandey S, Riddick-Young M, de Paredes ES, Trivedi A. Fibrous lesions of the breast: imaging-pathologic correlation. Radiographics. 2005;25(6):1547–59.
51. Kuijper A, Buerger H, Simon R, et al. Analysis of the progression of fibroepithelial tumours of the breast by PCR-based clonality assay. J Pathol. 2002;197(5):575–81.
52. Bernstein L, Deapen D, Ross RK. The descriptive epidemiology of malignant cystosarcoma phyllodes tumors of the breast. Cancer. 1993;71(10):3020–4.

53. Cohn-Cedermark G, Rutqvist LE, Rosendahl I, Silfversward C. Prognostic factors in cystosarcoma phyllodes. A clinicopathologic study of 77 patients. Cancer. 1991;68(9):2017–22.
54. Norris HJ, Taylor HB. Relationship of histologic features to behavior of cystosarcoma phyllodes. Analysis of ninety-four cases. Cancer. 1967;20(12):2090–9.
55. Moffat CJ, Pinder SE, Dixon AR, Elston CW, Blamey RW, Ellis IO. Phyllodes tumours of the breast: a clinicopathological review of thirty-two cases. Histopathology. 1995;27(3):205–18.
56. Choi J, Koo JS. Comparative study of histological features between core needle biopsy and surgical excision in phyllodes tumor. Pathol Int. 2012;62(2):120–6.
57. Taira N, Takabatake D, Aogi K, et al. Phyllodes tumor of the breast: stromal overgrowth and histological classification are useful prognosis-predictive factors for local recurrence in patients with a positive surgical margin. Jpn J Clin Oncol. 2007;37(10):730–6.
58. Wahner-Roedler DL, Sebo TJ, Gisvold JJ. Hamartomas of the breast: clinical, radiologic, and pathologic manifestations. Breast J. 2001;7(2):101–5.
59. Panikar N, Agarwal S. Sclerosing lobular hyperplasia of the breast: fine-needle aspiration cytology findings–a case report. Diagn Cytopathol. 2004;31(5):340–1.
60. Fisher CJ, Hanby AM, Robinson L, Millis RR. Mammary hamartoma–a review of 35 cases. Histopathology. 1992;20(2):99–106.
61. Anani PA, Hessler C. Breast hamartoma with invasive ductal carcinoma. Report of two cases and review of the literature. Pathol Res Pract. 1996;192(12):1187–94.
62. Rosen PP. Mucocele-like tumors of the breast. Am J Surg Pathol. 1986;10(7):464–9.
63. Glazebrook K, Reynolds C. Original report. Mucocele-like tumors of the breast: mammographic and sonographic appearances. AJR Am J Roentgenol. 2003;180(4):949–54.
64. Kim SM, Kim HH, Kang DK, et al. Mucocele-like tumors of the breast as cystic lesions: sonographic-pathologic correlation. AJR Am J Roentgenol. 2011;196(6):1424–30.
65. Fisher CJ, Millis RR. A mucocoele-like tumour of the breast associated with both atypical ductal hyperplasia and mucoid carcinoma. Histopathology. 1992;21(1):69–71.
66. Hamele-Bena D, Cranor ML, Rosen PP. Mammary mucocele-like lesions. Benign and malignant. Am J Surg Pathol. 1996;20(9):1081–5.
67. Weaver MG, Abdul-Karim FW, al-Kaisi N. Mucinous lesions of the breast. A pathological continuum. Pathol Res Pract. 1993;189(8):873–6.
68. Kim JY, Han BK, Choe YH, Ko YH. Benign and malignant mucocele-like tumors of the breast: mammographic and sonographic appearances. AJR Am J Roentgenol. 2005;185(5):1310–6.
69. Jaffer S, Bleiweiss IJ, Nagi CS. Benign mucocele-like lesions of the breast: revisited. Mod Pathol. 2011;24(5):683–7.
70. Leibman AJ, Staeger CN, Charney DA. Mucocelelike lesions of the breast: mammographic findings with pathologic correlation. AJR Am J Roentgenol. 2006;186(5):1356–60.
71. Carder PJ, Murphy CE, Liston JC. Surgical excision is warranted following a core biopsy diagnosis of mucocoele-like lesion of the breast. Histopathology. 2004;45(2):148–54.
72. Al-Nafussi A. Spindle cell tumours of the breast: practical approach to diagnosis. Histopathology. 1999;35(1):1–13.
73. Chan KW, Ghadially FN, Alagaratnam TT. Benign spindle cell tumour of breast–a variant of spindled cell lipoma or fibroma of breast? Pathology. 1984;16(3):331–6.
74. Begin LR. Intracisternal microtubular aggregates in classic (non chondroid) chordoma. J Submicrosc Cytol Pathol. 1995;27(3):295–301.
75. Damiani S, Miettinen M, Peterse JL, Eusebi V. Solitary fibrous tumour (myofibroblastoma) of the breast. Virchows Arch. 1994;425(1):89–92.
76. Eyden BP, Shanks JH, Ioachim E, Ali HH, Christensen L, Howat AJ. Myofibroblastoma of breast: evidence favoring smooth-muscle rather than myofibroblastic differentiation. Ultrastruct Pathol. 1999;23(4):249–57.
77. Vuitch MF, Rosen PP, Erlandson RA. Pseudoangiomatous hyperplasia of mammary stroma. Hum Pathol. 1986;17(2):185–91.
78. Ibrahim RE, Sciotto CG, Weidner N. Pseudoangiomatous hyperplasia of mammary stroma. Some observations regarding its clinicopathologic spectrum. Cancer. 1989;63(6):1154–60.
79. Wieman SM, Landercasper J, Johnson JM, et al. Tumoral pseudoangiomatous stromal hyperplasia of the breast. Am Surg. 2008;74(12):1211–4.
80. Gow KW, Mayfield JK, Lloyd D, Shehata BM. Pseudoangiomatous stromal hyperplasia of the breast in two adolescent females. Am Surg. 2004;70(7):605–8.
81. Degnim AC, Frost MH, Radisky DC, et al. Pseudoangiomatous stromal hyperplasia and breast cancer risk. Ann Surg Oncol. 2010;17(12):3269–77.
82. Powell CM, Cranor ML, Rosen PP. Pseudoangiomatous stromal hyperplasia (PASH). A mammary stromal tumor with myofibroblastic differentiation. Am J Surg Pathol. 1995;19(3):270–7.
83. Stanley MW, Skoog L, Tani EM, Horwitz CA. Nodular fasciitis: spontaneous resolution following diagnosis by fine-needle aspiration. Diagn Cytopathol. 1993;9(3):322–4.
84. Haggitt RC, Booth JL. Bilateral fibromatosis of the breast in Gardner's syndrome. Cancer. 1970;25(1):161–6.
85. Abraham SC, Reynolds C, Lee JH, et al. Fibromatosis of the breast and mutations involving the APC/beta-catenin pathway. Hum Pathol. 2002;33(1):39–46.

86. Rosen PP, Ernsberger D. Mammary fibromatosis. A benign spindle-cell tumor with significant risk for local recurrence. Cancer. 1989;63(7):1363–9.
87. el-Naggar A, Abdul-Karim FW, Marshalleck JJ, Sorensen K. Fine-needle aspiration of fibromatosis of the breast. Diagn Cytopathol. 1987;3(4):320–2.
88. Cederlund CG, Gustavsson S, Linell F, Moquist-Olsson I, Andersson I. Fibromatosis of the breast mimicking carcinoma at mammography. Br J Radiol. 1984;57(673):98–101.
89. Pettinato G, Manivel JC, Insabato L, De Chiara A, Petrella G. Plasma cell granuloma (inflammatory pseudotumor) of the breast. Am J Clin Pathol. 1988;90(5):627–32.
90. Sari A, Yigit S, Peker Y, Morgul Y, Coskun G, Cin N. Inflammatory pseudotumor of the breast. Breast J. 2011;17(3):312–4.

Website Cited in this Chapter

Concordance assessment of image-guided breast biopsies and management of borderline or high-risk lesions. https://www.breastsurgeons.org/statements/index.php. Approved 15 Aug 2011.
Management of fibroadenomas of the breast. https://www.breastsurgeons.org/statements/index.php. Revised 29 Apr 2008
https://www.nccn.org/professionals/physician_gls/f_guidelines.asp#breast_screening

Current Management of Nipple Discharge

6

Richard J. Gray and Barbara A. Pockaj

Background and Pathophysiology

Nipple discharge is a relatively common complaint, with a reported incidence of 2–5 % [1] and occurring among 10–50 % of patients with benign breast disease [1, 2]. Typically, the primary concern and initial fear of patients who experience nipple discharge is whether it is due to an underlying breast cancer. The risk of carcinoma among those with nipple discharge has been reported to be between 6 and 21 % [2–10], with some reports including only those patients undergoing an operation, while others do not [3, 7–10]. Nipple discharge can be separated into categories of normal milk production (lactation), galactorrhea (physiologic nipple discharge), or pathologic nipple discharge based on the characteristics of presentation [11].

Lactation occurs as early as the second trimester of pregnancy and can continue for up to 2 years after delivery or cessation of breastfeeding [12]. Lactating women may also have occult or gross blood within their discharge, due to the delicate capillary networks in the developing epithelium [13–15]. Galactorrhea is manifested as bilateral milky nipple discharge involving multiple ducts not associated with pregnancy or recent breastfeeding. Galactorrhea is frequently caused by hyperprolactinemia, which may be secondary to medications, endocrine tumors (i.e., pituitary adenoma), endocrine abnormalities, or a variety of other medical conditions [16].

Pathologic nipple discharge is characterized by a unilateral, spontaneous, persistent discharge from a single duct. Pathologic discharge is not necessarily caused by an underlying carcinoma, and in fact, most pathologic nipple discharge is a result of a periductal mastitis, duct ectasia, or benign intraductal papilloma. Periductal mastitis typically produces multicolored, sticky discharge. Duct ectasia is the result of increased glandular secretions by the lactiferous ducts and results in multi-duct, colored discharge that can often be bilateral. Intraductal papilloma generally produces serous or bloody discharge from a single duct. Other related nipple abnormalities that the clinician should be aware of that can produce symptoms perceived by patients as nipple discharge include Paget's disease of the nipple and subareolar abscess.

The difficulty in managing nipple discharge is that the risk of carcinoma, despite being low [1, 17], cannot be eliminated without surgical duct excision and histologic confirmation. Thus, duct excision in all patients with pathologic nipple discharge has been widely recommended [6, 8, 9, 11, 18, 19]. In addition, although the risk of carcinoma has been reported to be as high as 21 %, most studies examining the risk of underlying carcinoma include only those patients referred to departments of surgery, specialty breast centers [4–6, 20] or

R.J. Gray, MD (✉) • B.A. Pockaj, MD
Department of Surgery, Mayo Clinic Arizona, 5777 E. Mayo Blvd., Phoenix, AZ 85054, USA
e-mail: gray.richard@mayo.edu; pockaj.barbara@mayo.edu

A.I. Riker (ed.), *Breast Disease: Comprehensive Management*,
DOI 10.1007/978-1-4939-1145-5_6, © Springer Science+Business Media New York 2015

those patients who underwent duct excision [7–10]. In a broader population of women with nipple discharge, the rate of underlying carcinoma was found to be only 3 % [17], with referral patterns and selection bias likely playing a significant role in the reported incidence of carcinoma among women with nipple discharge. Patients presenting with nipple discharge represent only 1 % of patients with DCIS and <1 % of those with invasive breast carcinoma [17].

Diagnostic Approach to Nipple Discharge

Our current approach to the evaluation and management of patients with nipple discharge is summarized in Fig. 6.1. History taking and physical examination are the first important steps. Older age predicts a higher risk of carcinoma [17, 8, 20] while a personal and family history of breast cancer is not predictive of an underlying cancer etiology [8]. Recent onset of amenorrhea or other symptoms of hypogonadism (hot flashes, vaginal dryness) should prompt consideration of hyperprolactinemia.

The characteristics of the discharge should be obtained and recorded in detail with an attempt to categorize whether it is due to lactation, galactorrhea, or pathologic discharge. The clinician should be sure to understand if the discharge is spontaneous or induced, unilateral or bilateral, the characteristics of the discharged fluid (including volume), the frequency of the discharge, and whether the patient is stimulating his or her nipple to examine for discharge. This latter factor is important as regular self-examination for discharge can produce ongoing, even spontaneous, discharge. Regular self-examination or other forms of breast stimulation can repress the secretion of hypothalamic prolactin inhibitory factor, resulting in hyperprolactinemia and galactorrhea [16].

The physical examination should include careful inspection of the breast skin, nipple, and areola as well as palpation of all the breast parenchyma, including the subareolar tissue and the regional lymph nodes. Care should be taken to examine the nipple for evidence of a central horizontal crease that is associated with duct ectasia, an entity which can also produce nipple discharge. Careful pressure can be exerted at the areolar margin circumferentially to examine for discharge. The discharged fluid can then be inspected for origin from a single or multiple ducts, color, and texture (thin, thick, sticky, etc.).

Hemoccult testing of the discharge is not usually performed, as both serous and bloody discharge can be associated with an underlying breast carcinoma [9, 20]. Cytologic analysis is not regularly performed, as the results of such studies are neither sensitive nor specific for an underlying breast cancer [9, 20–23]. Among patients with biopsy proven carcinoma, 29 % of cytology specimens of the discharge have been reported to show no evidence of carcinoma or atypia [24]. If the patient is found to have subareolar tenderness and periareolar erythema with purulent nipple discharge, this is consistent with a subareolar abscess rather than true nipple discharge. These patients are obviously approached differently and should be treated with an appropriate combination of antibiotics and possible incision and drainage and/or an excision of the subareolar major ducts [25].

Imaging and Laboratory Investigations in Nipple Discharge

There are no radiologic studies that are essential, except for routine screening mammography, when the history and physical examination reveals that the discharge has characteristically benign features (Fig. 6.1). Patients with lactation discharge need no further evaluation, including those with occult or gross blood in the discharged milk. Patients with galactorrhea need no further evaluation for breast carcinoma, but should be evaluated for an underlying cause of hyperprolactinemia including a careful review of medications, review of the patient's history for possible causes of neurogenic stimulation of the nipple-areola complex that would represses the secretion of hypothalamic prolactin inhibitory factor, and review of the history and physical examination for signs or symptoms of pituitary adenoma [16]. One may then perform laboratory

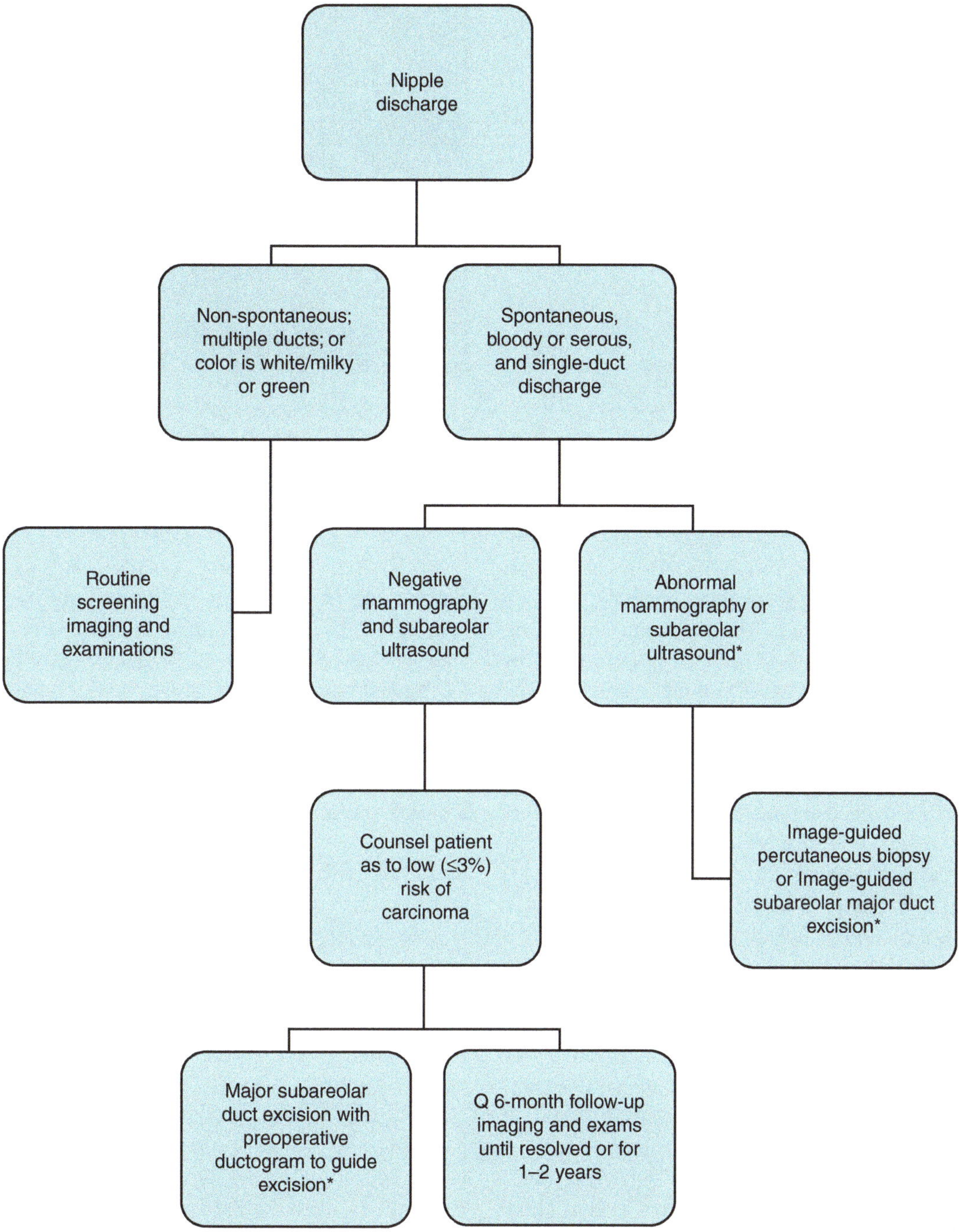

Fig. 6.1 Algorithm for the management of nipple discharge. *If patient plans future breastfeeding, selective duct excision is preferred over major duct excision

workup of the galactorrhea with serum prolactin levels, though the serum prolactin concentration is normal in nearly half of women who present with galactorrhea [26]. Galactorrhea in the absence of hyperprolactinemia is usually not the result of any ongoing disease process.

Table 6.1 Comparative rates of carcinoma risk

Characteristic	Carcinoma rates (%)	*p*
Age ≥50 vs. <50 years	6 % vs. 0 %	0.02
Unilateral vs. bilateral discharge	4 % vs. 2 %	0.49
Spontaneous vs. non-spontaneous	5 % vs. 0 %	0.13
Serous/bloody vs. other discharge	5 % vs. 0 %	0.10
Abnormal vs. normal mammogram	38 % vs. 3 %	<0.01
Abnormal vs. normal ultrasound	12 % vs. 1 %	<0.01
Abnormal vs. normal ductogram	6 % vs. 0 %	0.64

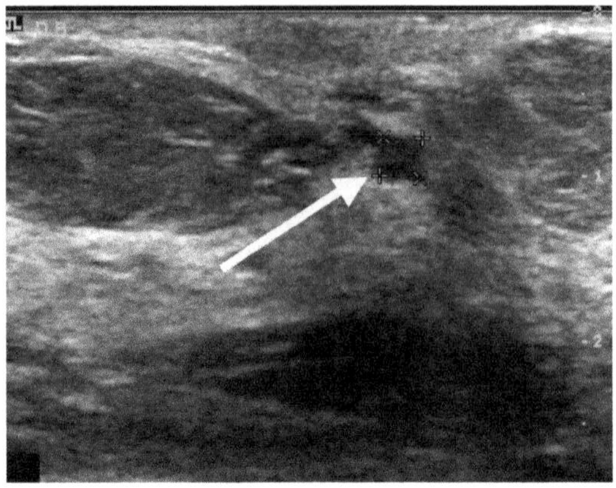

Fig. 6.2 Subareolar ultrasound demonstrating a 0.35 cm intraductal lesion (*arrow*) in a patient subsequently found to have ductal carcinoma in situ upon subareolar duct excision

For those patients with pathologic nipple discharge and without clearly benign features (Fig. 6.1), we proceed to diagnostic mammography (for those 30 years of age and older) and subareolar ultrasound. These imaging modalities have been reported to be able to separate patients with a high risk of underlying carcinoma from those with a low risk (Table 6.1) [17, 6, 8, 9, 11, 20, 27]. The risk of carcinoma with pathologic nipple discharge and an abnormal mammogram, while an uncommon scenario, is as high as 60 %, and the risk with an abnormal ultrasound but normal mammogram is 7 % (Fig. 6.2, Table 6.2) [17].

Ductography can be helpful in the evaluation of pathologic nipple discharge, though the use of subareolar ultrasound in skilled hands greatly minimizes the additional diagnostic yield of ductography. At our institution, we seldom use ductography as a diagnostic tool but rather to provide a "roadmap" as needed for subareolar duct excision once a decision has been made to perform this operation (Fig. 6.1). The primary benefit of ductography is to localize the lesion, especially in the case of multiple and peripheral lesions [4, 20, 28–32]. This allows radiologic guidance, such as wire or radioactive seed localization [33], to be used to direct the major duct excision and be certain that the area/lesion is completely resected.

Of note, ductography has been reported to miss as many as 20 % of ductal lesions, including those of a benign nature [4]. Although the negative predictive value is relatively high (82–91 %) [4, 9, 20, 31], it is still not sensitive enough to exclude the possibility of malignancy. In one series of 163 patients, ductography was associated with a sensitivity of 76 %, a specificity of 11 %, and a positive predictive value of only 19 % [34]. Such performance of this test makes it difficult to justify regularly subjecting patients to a sometimes painful procedure if reliable subareolar ultrasound is available.

The role of ductoscopy in nipple discharge remains to be defined. While this procedure holds some promise, the presence of cancer has been reported to predict unsuccessful ductal cannulation with the ductoscope [27]. Ductoscopy-guided excision, like ductograpy-guided excision, has been reported to increase the yield of atypia or carcinoma in at least one series [35]. Among 114 women in which half the patients were evaluated with ductoscopic guidance and half with surgery alone, the yield of pathologic diagnoses did not significantly differ between the groups [35]. In addition, ductoscopy was technically unsuccessful in 13 % of patients [35]. Currently, we believe that ductoscopy adds little diagnostic value in nipple discharge, with further refinements in instrumentation and technique possibly increasing its usefulness in the future.

While breast MRI may be better than conventional imaging at detecting occult malignancies among patients with nipple discharge [36], others

Table 6.2 Cancer risk by clinical scenario

Clinical scenario[a] – nipple discharge with	N	Risk of carcinoma (%)	Risk in other reports
All patients with nipple discharge	204	3	6–21 % [1–6, 13]
Nipple discharge, underwent biopsy	75	9	
Non-spontaneous discharge	49	0	
Bilateral discharge	52	2	
Unilateral, spontaneous, serous discharge from single duct	49	4	
Unilateral, spontaneous, bloody discharge from single duct	60	7	
Unilateral bloody/serous discharge, single duct, and negative mammogram	106	3	3 % [11]
Unilateral bloody/serous discharge, single duct, negative mammogram and negative ultrasound[b]	57	0	3 % [1]
Unilateral bloody/serous discharge, single duct, negative mammogram and abnormal ultrasound	30	7	
Unilateral bloody/serous discharge, single duct, and abnormal mammogram	5	60	13 % [11]

[a]Some patients' characteristics overlap categories

[b]One patient with carcinoma had *bilateral* discharge and a negative mammogram and ultrasound, but she had undergone wire-localized, bilateral subareolar duct excisions 6 months prior at another institution

studies show that most papillomas are MRI-occult which may predict limited sensitivity for otherwise-occult malignancy [37]. In a series of 52 patients with suspicious nipple discharge who were studied with a breast MRI, the sensitivity and specificity for malignancy were 77 and 62 %, respectively [34]. The positive predictive value of MRI in this series was 56 % and the negative predictive value 87 %. Given the low pretest probability of underlying carcinoma for women with nipple discharge, the relatively limited specificity of breast MRI would be expected to produce a significant rate of false positive findings. This combined with the cost of breast MRI makes its current value in this entity limited.

Decision-Making for Biopsy and Subareolar Duct Excision

Once the history and physical examination has eliminated patients with characteristically benign discharge and a normal mammogram and subareolar ultrasound have been obtained, the risk of carcinoma is low. The rate of carcinoma in a 57-patient cohort with these characteristics who underwent subareolar duct excision was 0 % with another 124 patients having no carcinoma with 2-year median follow-up [17]. Other studies have reported an ~3 % risk of carcinoma with a normal physical examination, normal mammogram, and normal ultrasound [20]. When counseled about these low risk levels, most patients choose close clinical follow-up rather than subareolar duct excision.

If patients choose close clinical follow-up, it is appropriate to perform physical examination and subareolar ultrasound every 6 months for 1–2 years or until the discharge resolves, whichever comes first (Fig. 6.1). Many women choose subareolar duct excision for symptom relief if their discharge persists for 1 year or more, regardless of the low risk of underlying carcinoma. The median duration of benign discharge has been reported to be 12 months [20], but nipple discharge has been present in some patients for up to 40 years [17].

For those patients who have an imaging abnormality or who choose to undergo diagnostic subareolar duct excision, a major duct excision is preferable if she does not plan future breastfeeding. Major duct excision has been reported to detect a higher percentage of occult carcinoma than microdochotomy [10], result in fewer patients requiring repeat duct excision [10], and is associated with a 0 % rate of breast cancer diagnosis over the subsequent 5 years [18]. Unless the targeted lesion is identified by mammogram or ultrasound and is within 2 cm of the nipple, ductography should be considered to identify the position of the lesion with precision. If the lesion is identified by mammography, sonography, or ductography and is greater than 2 cm from the nipple, radiologic localization is appropriate to precisely and effectively resect the offending lesion. For other patients, cannulation of the offending duct with a lacrimal probe intraoperatively is frequently used to guide the excision.

In a series of 192 patients evaluated and treated at our institution utilizing a defined algorithm (Fig. 6.1), 66 % of patients chose to undergo close clinical follow-up rather than subareolar duct excision, including 88 % who did not have an abnormality on mammography or sonography. All patients with carcinoma were found to have an imaging abnormality. Of the patients followed clinically, 20 % eventually chose to have subareolar duct excision due to persistent discharge. Among patients not undergoing subareolar duct excision, 81 % had spontaneous resolution of their nipple discharge.

Conclusion

In conclusion, using a systematic approach to nipple discharge allows the clinician to stratify patients with pathologic nipple discharge into low- and high-risk groups. Low-risk patients can be safely offered close clinical follow-up rather than subjecting all patients with pathologic discharge to operative intervention and additional expensive tests. Patients that are provided with risk-stratification data usually choose to avoid operative intervention when they are found to be at low risk, though 20 % will eventually choose surgery for their persistent symptoms.

References

1. Gulay H, Bora S, Kilicturgay S, et al. Management of nipple discharge. J Am Coll Surg. 1994;178(5):471–4.
2. Newman HF, Klein M, Northrup JD, et al. Nipple discharge. Frequency and pathogenesis in an ambulatory population. N Y State J Med. 1983;83(7):928–33.
3. Murad TM, Contesso G, Mouriesse H. Nipple discharge from the breast. Ann Surg. 1982;195(3):259–64.
4. Dawes LG, Bowen C, Venta LA, Morrow M. Ductography for nipple discharge: no replacement for ductal excision. Surgery. 1998;124(4):685–91.
5. Florio MG, Manganaro T, Pollicino A, et al. Surgical approach to nipple discharge: a ten-year experience. J Surg Oncol. 1999;71(4):235–8.
6. King TA, Carter KM, Bolton JS, Fuhrman GM. A simple approach to nipple discharge. Am Surg. 2000;66(10):960–5; discussion 965–6.
7. Locker AP, Galea MH, Ellis IO, et al. Microdochectomy for single-duct discharge from the nipple. Br J Surg. 1988;75(7):700–1.
8. Adepoju LJ, Chun J, El-Tamer M, et al. The value of clinical characteristics and breast-imaging studies in predicting a histopathologic diagnosis of cancer or high-risk lesion in patients with spontaneous nipple discharge. Am J Surg. 2005;190(4):644–6.
9. Simmons R, Adamovich T, Brennan M, et al. Nonsurgical evaluation of pathologic nipple discharge. Ann Surg Oncol. 2003;10(2):113–6.
10. Sharma R, Dietz J, Wright H, et al. Comparative analysis of minimally invasive microductectomy versus major duct excision in patients with pathologic nipple discharge. Surgery. 2005;138(4):591–6; discussion 596–7.
11. Sakorafas GH. Nipple discharge: current diagnostic and therapeutic approaches. Cancer Treat Rev. 2001; 27(5):275–82.
12. Isaacs JH. Other nipple discharge. Clin Obstet Gynecol. 1994;37(4):898–902.
13. Kline TS, Lash S. Nipple secretion in pregnancy. A cytologic and histologic study. Am J Clin Pathol. 1962;37:626–32.
14. Scott-Conner CE, Schorr SJ. The diagnosis and management of breast problems during pregnancy and lactation. Am J Surg. 1995;170(4):401.
15. Lafreniere R. Bloody nipple discharge during pregnancy: a rationale for conservative treatment. J Surg Oncol. 1990;43(4):228.
16. Leung AK, Pacaud D. Diagnosis and management of galactorrhea. Am Fam Physician. 2004;70(3):543.
17. Gray RJ, Pockaj BA, Karstaedt PJ. Navigating murky waters: a modern treatment algorithm for nipple discharge. Am J Surg. 2007;194(6):850–5.
18. Nelson RS, Hoehn JL. Twenty-year outcome following central duct resection for bloody nipple discharge. Ann Surg. 2006;243(4):522–4.
19. Sauter ER, Schlatter L, Lininger J, Hewett JE. The association of bloody nipple discharge with breast pathology. Surgery. 2004;136(4):780–5.
20. Cabioglu N, Hunt KK, Singletary SE, et al. Surgical decision making and factors determining a diagnosis of breast carcinoma in women presenting with nipple discharge. J Am Coll Surg. 2003;196(3):354–64.
21. Ito Y, Tamaki Y, Nakano Y, et al. Nonpalpable breast cancer with nipple discharge: how should it be treated? Anticancer Res. 1997;17(1B):791–4.

22. Ambrogetti D, Berni D, Catarzi S, Ciatto S. The role of ductal galactography in the differential diagnosis of breast carcinoma. Radiol Med (Torino). 1996;91(3): 198–201.
23. Sessa M, Cerroni L, Bertolotti A. Proliferative pathology of the mammary ducts. Diagnostic value of ductogalactography and cytologic correlations. Radiol Med (Torino). 1991;81(5):597–600.
24. Das DK, Al-Ayadhy B, Ajrawi MT, et al. Cytodiagnosis of nipple discharge: a study of 602 samples from 484 cases. Diagn Cytopathol. 2001; 25(1):25–37.
25. Li S, Grant CS, Degnim A, Donohue J. Surgical management of recurrent subareolar breast abscesses: Mayo Clinic experience. Am J Surg. 2006;192(4): 528–9.
26. Kleinberg DL, Noel GL, Frantz AG. Galactorrhea: a study of 235 cases, including 48 with pituitary tumors. N Engl J Med. 1977;296(11):589.
27. Dietz JR, Crowe JP, Grundfest S. Directed duct excision by using mammary ductoscopy in patients with pathologic nipple discharge. Surgery. 2002;132(4): 582–7; discussion 587–8.
28. Baker KS, Davey DD, Stelling CB. Ductal abnormalities detected with galactography: frequency of adequate excisional biopsy. AJR Am J Roentgenol. 1994; 162(4):821–4.
29. Cardenosa G, Doudna C, Eklund GW. Ductography of the breast: technique and findings. AJR Am J Roentgenol. 1994;162(5):1081–7.
30. Rongione AJ, Evans BD, Kling KM, McFadden DW. Ductography is a useful technique in evaluation of abnormal nipple discharge. Am Surg. 1996;62(10):785–8.
31. Dinkel HP, Trusen A, Gassel AM, et al. Predictive value of galactographic patterns for benign and malignant neoplasms of the breast in patients with nipple discharge. Br J Radiol. 2000;73(871):706–14.
32. Van Zee KJ, Ortega Perez G, Minnard E, Cohen MA. Preoperative galactography increases the diagnostic yield of major duct excision for nipple discharge. Cancer. 1998;82(10):1874–80.
33. Gray RJ, Pockaj BA, Karstaedt PJ, Roarke MC. Radioactive seed localization of nonpalpable breast lesions is better than wire localization. Am J Surg. 2004;188(4):377–80.
34. Morrogh M, Morris EA, Liberman L, Borgen PI, King TA. The predictive value of ductography and magnetic resonance imaging in the management of nipple discharge. Ann Surg Oncol. 2007;14(12):3369.
35. Moncrief RM, Nayar R, Diaz LK, et al. A comparison of ductoscopy-guided and conventional surgical excision in women with spontaneous nipple discharge. Ann Surg. 2005;241(4):575–81.
36. Rovno HD, Siegelman ES, Reynolds C, et al. Solitary intraductal papilloma: findings at MR imaging and MR galactography. AJR Am J Roentgenol. 1999;172(1): 151–5.
37. Orel SG, Dougherty CS, Reynolds C, et al. MR imaging in patients with nipple discharge: initial experience. Radiology. 2000;216(1):248–54.

The Initial Consultation: Malignant Disease

7

Barbara L. Krueger and Adam I. Riker

The essential components of the initial consultation with the breast surgeon involves a thorough history and physical exam, review of systems, personal evaluation of all imaging studies, and a second opinion review of all pathology slides that originate from outside of the home institution. A pre-treatment up-to-date clinical stage should be established utilizing current NCCN treatment guidelines [1]. Based on the information gathered above, decisions regarding genetic testing, potential further imaging looking for further extent of both local and distant disease may alter the surgical plan significantly. The determination of primary tumor characteristics and apparent extent of disease may impact the decision of a neo-adjuvant approach to therapy. Clinical trials are certainly discussed when available for those patients that may meet eligibility criteria. Whenever possible, patients should be managed utilizing a multidisciplinary approach that involves the major disciplines of therapy, mainly, radiation, medical, and surgical oncology. This approach has been examined in several studies that have validated the utility of the multidisciplinary approach to the evaluation and treatment of breast cancer [2–4]. This chapter addresses the initial office evaluation, evaluation of locoregional and distant disease, and areas of special consideration for the patient with breast cancer.

B.L. Krueger, MD, FACS (✉)
Breast Cancer Program, Advocate Cancer Institute, Advocate Christ Medical Center, 4400 West 95th Street, Suite 107 POB 408, Oak Lawn, IL 60453, USA
e-mail: bkrueger333@comcast.net, barbara.krueger@advocatehealth.com

A.I. Riker, MD, FACS
Advocate Center for Breast Health, Advocate Cancer Institute, Advocate Christ Medical Center, 4400 West 95th Street, Suite 107 POB 408, Oak Lawn, IL 60453, USA
e-mail: adam.riker@advocatehealth.com

Initial Office Visit

It is important to note that establishing a rapport and a sense of partnership with the patient at the initial consultation improves communication, patient-physician relationships, and may importantly influence health outcomes [5]. Employing a participatory style that clearly involves the patients in the decision-making process will greatly enhance the overall level of trust and confidence with their surgeon as well as the health-related quality of life [6]. Involving other family members and significant partners in this process is strongly encouraged, with their participation central to the development of transparency in the discussions of treatment options. It further assists to have an extra "set of ears" to hear the discussion, as the patient may not be fully able to take in such a large amount of information at one sitting.

History and Review of Systems

An accurate and complete history of present illness; review of systems, past medical history, and past surgical history; and review of medications

A.I. Riker (ed.), *Breast Disease: Comprehensive Management*,
DOI 10.1007/978-1-4939-1145-5_7, © Springer Science+Business Media New York 2015

including supplements and herbals, allergies, menstrual history, parity, use of hormones, and use of alcohol, tobacco, and drugs should be obtained at the initial encounter. A detailed family history of breast, ovarian, and other cancers is necessary and should also include the ages at which the relatives were diagnosed, if possible. This information is central to the decision as to whether the patients may meet criteria for subsequent genetic counseling and testing for possible associated gene mutations that may put such patients at high risk for the development of future cancers. An example of the intake form utilized within our multidisciplinary breast oncology clinic is given in (Fig. 7.1).

The history of present illness should note the means of how the cancer was initially identified, such as a palpable mass, an abnormality identified on a screening mammogram, nipple discharge, or the development of focal pain. Of course, it is important to obtain all outside imaging studies, with a personal review of such studies by both the treating surgeon and institutional breast radiologist. Tumor characterization, overall diameter, and clinical stage should be documented, with further evaluation of other imaging abnormalities that may not have been identified on the initial studies.

A thorough physical exam of the breasts and regional nodal basins should be performed [7]. If possible, evaluation of the regional nodal basin with ultrasound has been found to be helpful in the identification of suspicious-appearing lymph nodes that may require further evaluation and possible ultrasound-guided biopsy. Such information has clinical implications on the role, or lack thereof, for performing a sentinel node biopsy in the face of known nodal metastases [8, 9]. Accurate past medical and surgical histories are also important to obtain beforehand, as part of the general well-being of the patient and associated comorbidities that may potentially affect (alter) surgical, radiation, and medical oncology recommendations. A few such examples may be a previous history of mantle radiation for lymphoma or radiation for lung cancer, history of scleroderma, or connective tissue disorder that may prohibit or limit the use of radiation therapy.

A comprehensive history of current medications, including supplements and herbal medications, should be documented. Ideally, patients should bring their medication to the initial visit to avoid errors in the names of the drug or dosage. Allergies should also be identified, not only to medications, but also food, topicals, latex, and environmental substances. The review of systems is particularly important to identify possible coexisting conditions, second primary cancers, and findings suspicious for distant disease. A thorough menstrual and reproductive history should be obtained along with a history of hormone use such as oral contraceptives, impregnated intrauterine devices, depot contraception, hormone replacement therapy, and fertility drugs. It is also important to remember that cast menstrual period (CMP) is not an accurate reflection of menopausal state if a woman has had a hysterectomy without oophorectomy or has undergone a uterine ablation procedure. Ovarian function dictates endocrine therapy choices in hormone receptor-positive tumors and should be evaluated with FSH levels if any question exists [10].

A thorough family history of cancer is necessary to assess the risk of developing a genetically associated breast cancer. All types of cancer should be included, along with age at diagnosis, bilateral disease (where appropriate), and whether the family member experienced a recurrence of their cancer. A history of cigarette use, alcohol consumption, and recreational drug use should also be documented. All imaging studies should undergo a second opinion by your own department of breast radiology. Changes in interpretation of imaging studies and pathology findings can result in significant changes in the overall treatment plan [1, 4, 11, 12]. All outside pathology should also be obtained for second opinion by your institute's breast pathologists in order to insure that the pathologic diagnosis is accurate and that the receptors, ER/PR and HER2-neu, are assessed at a minimum [13].

Evaluation of Local Disease Extent

It seems fairly intuitive that all patients who initially present with a diagnosis of breast cancer should undergo diagnostic mammography and ultrasound as indicated. As previously mentioned, ultrasound evaluation with biopsy of local nodal basins can be a valuable adjunct in establishing if

PROGRESS NOTE GENERAL SURGERY – BREAST HEALTH	AFFIX PATIENT LABEL

Barbara Krueger, M.D. OTHER PROVIDER______________________

Referred by______________________ Date of Exam__________

CHIEF COMPLAINT

____

____

MARITAL STATUS S M W D S

HISTORY OF PRESENT ILLNESS

____

PAST MEDICAL HISTORY (update) **Reviewed prior History dated:**__________

Surgeries:______________________

Medical:______________________

Medications:______________________

Allergies:______________________

☐ **Patient verbalized understanding / All questions answered**

FAMILY HISTORY ☐ **Instruction Booklet Given**

____

ROS:

Other Skin	☐ Negative	☐ Other__________
Neurological	☐ Negative	☐ Other__________
Psychiatric	☐ Negative	☐ Other__________
Endocrine	☐ Negative	☐ Other__________
Genitourinary	☐ Negative	☐ Other__________
Sexual Function	☐ Abnormal	☐ Other__________
Hemato/Lymph	☐ Negative	☐ Other__________
Allergy/Immunol	☐ Negative	☐ Other__________
Constitutional	☐ Negative	☐ Other__________
Eyes	☐ Negative	☐ Other__________
ENT/Mouth	☐ Negative	☐ Other__________
Cardiovascular	☐ Negative	☐ Other__________
Respratory	☐ Negative	☐ Other__________
GI	☐ Negative	☐ Other__________
Musculoskeletal	☐ Negative	☐ Other__________

G_____ P_____ Ab_____ 1st Birth_____ Breast Feed_____

Menses_____ LMP_____ OCP_____ HRT_____

HABITS Smoking_____ CIG/Day_____yrs. Alcohol_____oz/wk Street Drugs__________

PERFORMANCE STATUS CODE

ECOG (or Zubrod) SCALE		KARNOFSKY SCORE
0	Asymptomatic and fully active	100%
1	Symptomatic; fully ambulatory; restricted in physical strenuous activity	80-90%
2	Symptomatic; ambulatory; capable of self-care; more than 50% of waking hours are spent out of bed	60-70%
3	Symptomatic; limited self-care; spends more than 50% of time in bed, but not bedridden	40-50%
4	Completely disabled; no self-care; bedridden	20-30%

Fig. 7.1 (**a**, **b**) The Advocate Christ Medical Center's multidisciplinary oncology breast clinic's intake form

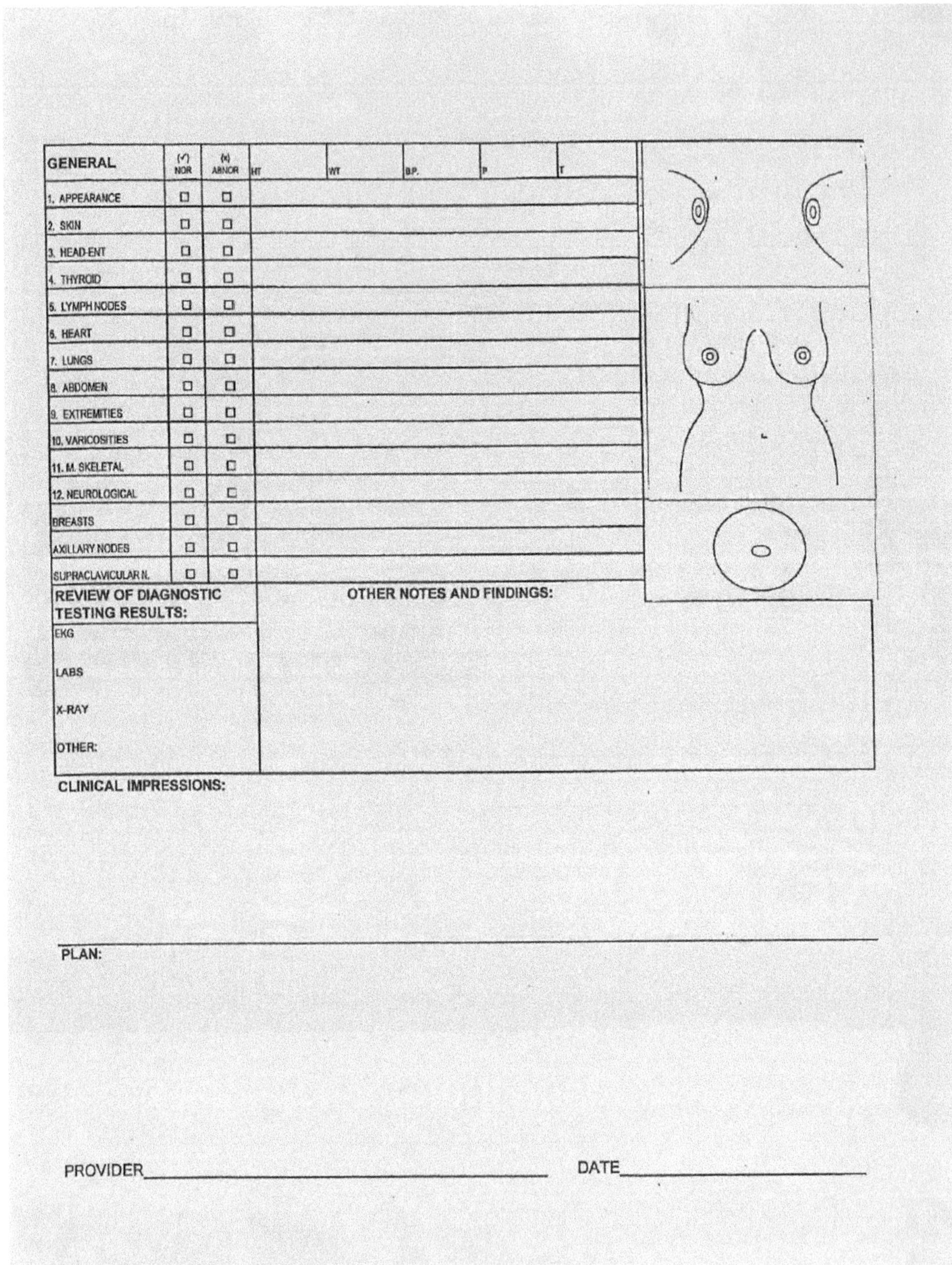

GENERAL	(✓) NOR	(x) ABNOR	HT	WT	B.P.	P	T
1. APPEARANCE	☐	☐					
2. SKIN	☐	☐					
3. HEAD-ENT	☐	☐					
4. THYROID	☐	☐					
5. LYMPH NODES	☐	☐					
6. HEART	☐	☐					
7. LUNGS	☐	☐					
8. ABDOMEN	☐	☐					
9. EXTREMITIES	☐	☐					
10. VARICOSITIES	☐	☐					
11. M. SKELETAL	☐	☐					
12. NEUROLOGICAL	☐	☐					
BREASTS	☐	☐					
AXILLARY NODES	☐	☐					
SUPRACLAVICULAR N.	☐	☐					

REVIEW OF DIAGNOSTIC TESTING RESULTS:

EKG

LABS

X-RAY

OTHER:

OTHER NOTES AND FINDINGS:

CLINICAL IMPRESSIONS:

PLAN:

PROVIDER__________ DATE__________

Fig. 7.1 (continued)

there is any possibility of locoregional involvement. The decision to perform further imaging prior to the operation interventional is at the surgeon's discretion, determined on need with each patient. The use of MRI or PEM technology should be critically applied, both in whom it should be used for and under what clinical circumstances. Mammographically, occult tumors, nodal metastases with an occult primary lesion, dense breast tissue, and unclear delineation of the primary tumor on mammography or ultrasound are all clinically reasonable situations where further evaluation of the breast with MRI or PEM may be appropriate. Breast MRI, in particular, is very useful for the surveillance of high-risk BRCA-positive patients and in the setting of neoadjuvant systemic therapy in order to evaluate the disease response [1, 13–18].

Evaluation of Distant Disease

The routine screening for distant disease in an asymptomatic patient with early-stage breast cancer is not indicated nor recommended [1, 19–21]. Overall, fewer than 6 % of patients will present with metastatic disease (stage 4) at their initial diagnosis [22, 23]. The NCCN treatment guidelines recommend additional studies for clinical stage I and IIB disease only if there are signs or symptoms that may raise the clinical suspicion of metastatic involvement, such as bone pain, or recent onset of headaches or vision changes. For patients with stage III breast cancer, the incidence of distant metastases at the time of diagnosis ranges from 8 % to 14 %, with the predominant site of metastatic disease found in the bone [20, 21, 23].

The presence of distant metastases in patients with locally advanced or symptomatic early-stage breast cancers may result in a significant change in the initial treatment strategy. An initial operative strategy may not be the best approach in the face of metastatic disease, with an initial systemic therapy approach with chemotherapy indicated. Systemic therapy considerations may also be altered, as endocrine therapy may be preferred over chemotherapy in hormone receptor-positive breast cancer. The most common, but not exclusive, sites of metastases for breast cancer are the bone, liver, lung, and brain. Early intervention in cases of potentially catastrophic and debilitating sequelae of distant metastases may improve quality of life in these patients. Table 7.1 outlines potential oncologic emergencies associated with metastatic breast cancer. There are many signs and symptoms that the patient may manifest, with pain the most common symptom identified (Table 7.2). The most common laboratory abnormalities are also listed in the face of metastatic disease (Table 7.3).

Table 7.1 Oncologic emergencies

Condition	Symptom	Morbidity
Spinal cord compression	Back pain, leg weakness	Paralysis
Bone metastases	Bone pain	Pathologic fracture
Superior vena cava syndrome	Face/neck swelling	Dyspnea, trochlea compression

Table 7.2 Potential symptoms of metastatic disease

Symptoms	Site
Pain	Bone, visceral
Leg weakness	Spinal cord
Jaundice	Liver
Dyspnea, cough	Lung, SVC syndrome, pleural effusion
Headache Seizure Vision changes Weakness Confusion	CNS involvement

Table 7.3 Serum abnormalities associated with metastatic disease

Serum value	Site of concern
Elevated alkaline phosphatase	Bone/liver
Elevated liver function tests	Liver
Hypercalcemia	Bone/paraneoplastic syndrome
Anemia thrombocytopenia	Bone marrow

Fertility

The incidence of breast cancer in women under the age of 40 is estimated to be about 1 in 200 [24], or 6–7 % of all breast cancers. For this group of young women, premature menopause, infertility, and the likely prolonged use of endocrine therapy and its affect upon fertility are all major concerns for those who wish to conceive in the face of breast cancer [25]. Fertility preservation should be addressed and, whenever possible, the patient referred to an oncofertility specialist [24]. Retrospective cohort studies have shown that there is no significant difference in cancer outcomes between cancer survivors who become pregnant after diagnosis and those who did not. Interestingly, many suggested a protective effect post-pregnancy [26].

Male Breast Cancer

The initial evaluation of a male with breast cancer parallels that of females [22]. One percent of breast cancer cases occur in males, with an incidence in the general population of approximately 1 per 100,000. It is important to note that males with breast cancer should be referred for genetic evaluation as several studies have shown an associated risk of BRCA2 gene mutation in up to 15 % of males [22, 27]. Young males with breast cancer should also be referred to reproductive specialists [28, 29].

Pregnancy

A patient who develops breast cancer during pregnancy presents several challenges for the proper sequence of treatment related to the gestational age of the fetus. The incidence of breast cancer in pregnancy is 0.2–3.8 % and occurs at a median gestational age of 20–22 weeks [22, 30]. Initial evaluation of locoregional disease should include physical exam, mammography with shielding of the abdomen, and ultrasound of the breast and nodal basins [22, 31]. Obtaining a breast MRI is problematic from the standpoint of accuracy and uncertainty concerning the safety of intravenous gadolinium during pregnancy [22, 32]. Distant disease evaluation is often limited due to concerns related to the radiation dose associated with each study. An initial chest x-ray with abdominal shielding may be helpful, with some basic blood work appropriate, such as a complete blood count and liver and renal function [22, 32]. Ultrasound may be both useful and safe in the surveillance of the liver if initial studies are found to be elevated or abnormal [32]. Appropriate treatment of a pregnant woman with breast cancer results in equivalent survival when compared to non-pregnant women [22, 30, 31]. A multidisciplinary approach involving maternal fetal medicine is essential to optimize outcome for both the mother and fetus [22, 31, 33].

Final Comment

The initial evaluation of a patient with newly diagnosed breast cancer should be conducted using a multidisciplinary approach. This collaborative effort allows for a comprehensive review of all imaging and pathology. The team approach of medical, surgical, and radiation oncology is key to provide a consensus of treatment options for the patient, allowing for the optimal quality and efficiency of the individualized treatment plan [2–4]. The appropriate clinical trials should always be offered to those willing to participate and meet the specific eligibility criteria for that trial [1]. The surgeon is central to the initial conversation and discussion with the patient, providing a complete overview of what lies ahead in their overall treatment.

References

1. National Comprehensive Cancer Network (NCCN) Guidelines. Clinical factors in diagnosis and staging of newly diagnosed breast cancer. www.NCCN.org/patients. Accessed Mar 2013.
2. Pruthi S, Brandt KR, Degnim AC, Goetz MP, Perez EA, Reynolds CA, et al. A multidisciplinary approach to the management of breast cancer. Part 1 – prevention and diagnosis. Mayo Clin Proc. 2007;82(8):999–1012.
3. Pruthi S, Boughey JC, Brandt KR, Degnim AC, Dy GK, Goetz MP, et al. A multidisciplinary approach to the management of breast cancer. Part 2 – therapeutic considerations. Mayo Clin Proc. 2007;82(9):1131–40.
4. Newman EA, Guest AB, Helvie MA, Roubidoux MA, Chang AE, Kleer CG, et al. Changes in surgical management resulting from case review at a breast cancer multidisciplinary tumor board. Cancer. 2006;107(10):2346–51.
5. Kaplan SH, Greenfield S, Ware JE. Assessing the effects of physician-patient interaction on the outcome of chronic disease. Med Care. 1989;27(3):S110–27.

6. Arora NK, Weaver KE, Clayman ML, Oakley-Girvan I, Potosky A, et al. Physicians' decision-making style and psychosocial outcomes among cancer survivors. Patient Educ Couns. 2009;77(3):404–12.
7. Powell RW. Breast examination. Clinical methods. NCBI bookshop. Chapter 176. In: Breast examination. #1 Clinical methods. The history, physical, and laboratory examination. Boston: Butterworth Publishing; 1990. pp. 822–6.
8. Leenders MWH, Broeders M, Croese C, Richir MC, Go HLS, Langenhorst BL, et al. Ultrasound and fine needle aspiration cytology of axillary lymph nodes in breast cancer: to do or not to do? Breast J. 2012;21(4):578–83.
9. Caretta-Weyer H, Sisney GA, Beckman C, et al. Impact of axillary ultrasound and core needle biopsy on the utility of intraoperative frozen section analysis and treatment decision making in women with invasive breast cancer. Am J Surg. 2012;204(3):308–14.
10. Butler L, Santoro N. The reproductive endocrinology of the menopausal transition. Steroids. 2011;76(7):627–35.
11. Shuster TD, Girshovich L, Whitney TM, Hughes KS. Multidisciplinary care for patients with breast cancer. Surg Clin North Am. 2000;80(2):505–33.
12. Rakovitch E, Mihai A, Pignol JP, Hanna W, Kwinter J, Chartier C, et al. Is expert breast pathology assessment necessary for the management of ductal carcinoma in situ? Breast Cancer Res Treat. 2004;87(3):265–72.
13. Harris L, Fritsche K, Mennel R, Norton L, Ravdin P, Taube S, et al. American Society of Clinical Oncology 2007 update of recommendations for use of tumor markers in breast cancer. J Clin Oncol. 2007;25(33):5287–311.
14. Ha GW, Yi MS, Lee BK, Youn HJ, Jung SH. Clinical outcome of magnetic resonance imaging detected additional lesions in breast cancer patient. J Breast Cancer. 2011;14(3):213–8.
15. Houssami N, Hayes DF. Review of preoperative magnetic resonance imaging in breast cancer: should MRI be performed on all women with newly diagnosed early stage breast cancer? CA Cancer J Clin. 2009;59(5):290–302.
16. Houssami N, Turner R, Morrow M. Preoperative magnetic resonance imaging in breast cancer: meta-analysis of surgical outcomes. Ann Surg. 2013;257(2):249–55.
17. Marcos de Paz LM, Tejerina Bernal A, Arranza Merino ML, Calvo de Juan V. Breast MR imaging changes after neoadjuvant chemotherapy: correlation with molecular subtypes. Radiologia. 2012;54(5):442–8.
18. Chen JH, Feig BA, Hsiang DJ, Butler JA, Mehta RS, Bahri S, et al. Impact of MRI evaluated neoadjuvant chemotherapy response on change of surgical recommendations in breast cancer. Ann Surg. 2009;249(3):448–54.
19. Güth U, Vetter M, Huang DJ, Heinzelmann-Schwarz V. Staging for distant metastases in operable breast cancer: a suggested expansion of the ESMO guideline recommendation for staging imaging of node-negative hormone receptor-negative disease. Ann Oncol. 2013;24(2):555–7.
20. Myers R, Johnston M, Pritchard K, Levine M, Oliver T, et al. Baseline staging tests in primary breast cancer: a practice guideline. Can Med Assoc J. 2001;164:1439–44.
21. Puglisi F, Follador A, Minisini AM, Cardellino GG, Russo S, Andreetta C, et al. Baseline staging tests after a new diagnosis of breast cancer; further evidence of their limited indications. Ann Oncol. 2005;16:263.
22. Gold J, Winer ED. Chapter 76: Chemotherapy for metastatic breast cancer. In: Copeland EM, editor. The breast: comprehensive management of benign and malignant diseases. Bland: Elsevier; 2013.
23. Ravaioli A, Pasini G, Polselli A, Papi M, Tassinari D, Arcangeli V, et al. Staging of breast cancer: new recommended standard procedure. Breast Cancer Res Treat. 2002;72:53.
24. Moffat R, de Geyter C, Myrick ME, Schmid SM, Sattman C, Tschudin S, et al. Young women with breast cancer: how many are actually candidates for fertility preservation? Arch Gynecol Obstet. 2012;286(6):1521–7.
25. Christinat A, Pagani O. Fertility after breast cancer. Maturitas. 2012;73(3):191–6.
26. Litton JK. Breast cancer and fertility. Curr Treat Options Oncol. 2012;13(2):137–45.
27. Ottini L, Masala G, D'Amico C, Mancini B, Saieva C, Aceto G, et al. BRCA1 and BRCA2 mutation status and tumor characteristics in male breast cancer: a population based study in Italy. Cancer Res. 2003;63(2):342–7.
28. Trost LW, Brannigan RE. Oncofertility and the male cancer patient. Curr Treat Options Oncol. 2012;13(2):146–60.
29. Loren AW, Mangu PB, Beck LN, Brennan L, Magdalinski AJ, Partridge AH, et al. Fertility preservation for patients with cancer: American Society of Clinical Oncology clinical practice guideline update. J Clin Oncol. 2013;31(19):2500–10.
30. Loibl S, Han SN, von Minckwitz G, Bontenbal M, Ring A, Giermek J, et al. Treatment of breast cancer during pregnancy: an observational study. Lancet Oncol. 2012;13(9):887–96.
31. Cardoso F, Loibl S, Pagani O, Graziottin A, Panizza P, Martincich L, et al. The European Society of Breast Cancer Specialists recommendations for the management of young women with breast cancer. Eur J Cancer. 2012;48(18):3355–77.
32. Berry DL, Theriault RL, Holmes FA, Parisi VM, Booser DJ, Singletary SE, et al. Management of breast cancer during pregnancy using a standardized protocol. J Clin Oncol. 1999;17(3):855–61.
33. Meisel JL, Economy KE, Calvillo KZ, Schapira L, Tung NM, Gelber S, et al. Contemporary multidisciplinary treatment of pregnancy associated breast cancer. Springerplus. 2013;2(1):297.

The Emerging Role of Prophylactic Mastectomy

8

Pamela R. Portschy and Todd M. Tuttle

Introduction

Selected high-risk women without breast cancer choose to undergo bilateral prophylactic mastectomy (BPM) to reduce their risk of developing breast cancer. In addition, an increasing proportion of patients with unilateral breast cancer choose contralateral prophylactic mastectomy (CPM) to prevent cancer in the contralateral breast. The purpose of this chapter is to review the indications, outcomes, and trends in the use of BPM. We will also review the trends in CPM use, the potential reasons for the observed trends, and the outcomes after CPM.

Bilateral Prophylactic Mastectomy

Indications

The Society of Surgical Oncology issued a position statement in 2007 regarding indications for prophylactic mastectomy among healthy women without breast cancer [1]. In this statement, potential indications for BPM include the presence of BRCA gene mutations or other susceptibility genes, strong family history without genetic mutation, and histologic risk factors (atypical ductal hyperplasia (ADH), atypical lobular hyperplasia, or lobular carcinoma in situ (LCIS)). Although ADH and LCIS are associated with an increased risk of breast cancer, surgical risk reduction is not frequently performed for these indications alone. Current National Comprehensive Cancer Network (NCCN) guidelines state that risk-reduction mastectomy is not recommended for most women with LCIS without additional risk factors [2]. Bilateral prophylactic mastectomy should also be discussed for other high-risk groups including women treated with mantle radiation (particularly at a young age) for Hodgkin's lymphomas and those with non-BRCA hereditary breast cancer syndromes (Cowden, Li-Fraumeni).

Importantly, many women without breast cancer substantially overestimate their risk of developing breast cancer in the future. In one study of 200 women without breast cancer, respondents overestimated their probability of dying from breast cancer within 10 years by more than 20-fold as compared to the probabilities derived from utilizing the Gail model [3]. In a survey study of patients participating in chemoprevention trials, the mean lifetime calculated risk using the Gail model was 15 %; however, the median risk perceived by patients was 50 % [4]. After an educational intervention, the median perceived risk declined to 25 %. Thus, physicians should provide patients with accurate estimates of breast cancer risk in discussing management strategies.

P.R. Portschy, MD (✉) • T.M. Tuttle, MD
Department of Surgical Oncology,
University of Minnesota,
420 Delaware Street SE MMC 195,
Minneapolis, MN 55455, USA
e-mail: ports001@umn.edu; tuttl006@umn.edu

A.I. Riker (ed.), *Breast Disease: Comprehensive Management*,
DOI 10.1007/978-1-4939-1145-5_8, © Springer Science+Business Media New York 2015

Results After BPM

Several studies have demonstrated that BPM reduces the risk of breast cancer in moderate- to high-risk women, including those with BRCA mutations [5–8]. Hartmann et al. conducted a retrospective review of all women with a family history of breast cancer that underwent BPM at the Mayo Clinic between 1963 and 1990 [5]. Using the Gail model and sisters of patients as controls, the authors determined the expected number of breast cancers in both moderate- and high-risk groups. In the moderate-risk group, 37.4 cancers were expected but only four occurred, a risk reduction of 89.5 %. In the high-risk group, a risk reduction of 90 % was observed. Other studies have demonstrated that the risk reduction is about 90 % after BPM for patients with BRCA mutations [6]. A Cochrane review published in 2010 reported that BPM studies have demonstrated reductions in breast cancer incidence and mortality after BPM, particularly for those with BRCA 1/2 gene mutations [7]. Using Markov modeling, Schrag et al. estimated that an average 30-year-old woman who carries a BRCA 1/2 mutation would gain an additional 2.9–5.3 years of life expectancy from undergoing prophylactic mastectomy [9].

Surgical Options

The three main options for surgical risk reduction are bilateral simple mastectomy without immediate reconstruction, bilateral skin-sparing mastectomy with immediate reconstruction, and bilateral nipple-sparing mastectomy with immediate reconstruction. Surgical complications from bilateral skin-sparing mastectomy occur in about 20 % of patients, with the most common complications reported are wound infection, flap necrosis, and partial or complete loss of reconstruction. In addition, Zion et al. reported that unanticipated operations occur in about half of patients within 14 years after BPM plus immediate reconstruction; the most common complications were implant related [10].

An increasing number of patients are choosing to undergo surgical risk reduction with bilateral nipple-sparing mastectomies (NSM). Ideal candidates for NSM are younger patients, nonsmokers, and nonobese patients. Generally, NSMs are performed with either a radial or inframammary incision. Ductal tissue beneath the nipple is excised and submitted to pathology separately. If DCIS or invasive cancer is identified in this tissue, then the nipple-areolar complex is excised. The cosmetic outcomes after nipple-sparing mastectomy and reconstruction are excellent, with very high patient satisfaction with this procedure. Nipple necrosis can occur in about 5 % of patients. The occurrence of cancer in the nipple-areolar complex after NSM is extremely rare.

Patient Satisfaction

Despite the potential complications and requirements for unanticipated surgery, most patients are satisfied with their decision to undergo BPM. In a survey study of high-risk patients who underwent BPM, Geiger et al. reported that 84 % were satisfied with their decision [11]. In another study, Altschuler et al. evaluated the psychosocial response and satisfaction in women following prophylactic mastectomy [12]. The authors concluded that although most patients were satisfied with their decision to undergo risk-reducing surgery, some patients expressed more negative impressions of their procedures [12].

A recent study examined the impact of body image and sexual and partner relationship satisfaction in 48 healthy BRCA 1/2 mutation carriers after undergoing BPM with breast reconstruction [13]. The authors reported that sexual relationship satisfaction and body image tended to be lower compared to baseline. After a median follow-up of 21 months, 37 % of women reported that their breasts felt unpleasant, 29 % were unsatisfied with breast appearance, and 21 % felt embarrassed of their naked body. The authors concluded that the psychosocial impact of BPM with reconstruction should not be underestimated [13]. Thus, it is vitally important to a very thorough and detailed discussion with all patients considering BPM, as to the irreversibility of their decision and the subsequent possibly negative impact upon both psychosocial aspects and well-being.

Trends

Since most state and national cancer databases do not collect information on healthy women without breast cancer, precise determination of the national trends of BPM use is difficult. A recently published study from McLaughlin et al. utilized New York state cancer registry to study trends of prophylactic mastectomy from 1995 to 2005 [14]. This study included 1,196 women who underwent BPM and had no history of breast cancer. McLaughlin et al. found that BPM was uncommonly performed, and the BPM rates increased only slightly during the study period. The authors are not aware of any other published studies using either state or national databases reporting BPM use and trends. Nevertheless, we conjecture that BPM rates have likely increased in the United States secondary to increased awareness of genetic breast cancer, increased genetic testing, and improvements in mastectomy and reconstruction techniques.

Conclusions

Bilateral prophylactic mastectomy reduces the incidence of breast cancer in moderate- and high-risk women and may reduce breast cancer mortality among carriers of BRCA gene mutations. Nevertheless, BPM is a major operation, is irreversible, and is not without risk. Patients must clearly understand all of the potential risks associated with BPM before proceeding with this operation. Many patients substantially overestimate their risk of developing breast cancer, with patient education again key in having them understand the true actual risks involved. Overall, patients are satisfied with their decision to undergo risk-reduction surgery, but physicians must provide accurate education and counseling to ensure that risk-reducing surgery is performed in the most appropriate setting, for the right reasons and with realistic expectations of the cosmetic outcomes. Alternative strategies for managing high-risk patients include rigorous surveillance (clinical breast examinations, mammography, and potentially breast MRI), endocrine prevention, and lifestyle changes.

Contralateral Prophylactic Mastectomy

Trends

Contralateral prophylactic mastectomy is the removal of the normal intact breast among women with unilateral breast cancer. The Surveillance Epidemiology and End Results (SEER) registry began coding CPM in 1998. At that time, the proportion of patients who underwent CPM in the United States was less than 2 %. However, the CPM rate among all surgically treated patients with invasive breast cancer increased by 150 % from 1998 to 2003 in the United States [15]. Among mastectomy patients, the CPM rate increased 162 % from 1998 to 2003. These trends were observed for all cancer stages and continued to increase at the end of the study period with no plateau. Although significant geographic variations were observed between different SEER registries, no general geographic trends were identified. Similar findings were observed in the SEER database among patients with ductal carcinoma in situ (DCIS) [16].

Other studies using different databases have confirmed these findings. Using the American College of Surgeons' National Cancer Data Base (NCDB), Yao et al. reported similar increases in CPM rates from 1998 to 2007, with the rates still increasing at the end of the study period in 2007 [17]. In a similar study using the New York State Cancer Registry, McLaughlin et al. reported that CPM use more than doubled from 1995 to 2005 [14]. Single-institutional studies have also demonstrated marked increases in CPM rates [18–20].

In contrast, similar trends have not been observed in Europe. In a single-center study from Switzerland, Güth et al. reported that the CPM rates at an academic surgery center did not

Table 8.1 Factors associated with contralateral prophylactic mastectomy use

Patient	
	Young age
	White race
	Private insurance
	Family history of breast cancer
Tumor	
	Infiltrating lobular histology
	Multicentric disease
	Tumor size
Treatment	
	BRCA testing
	MRI
	Breast reconstruction
	Facility type

increase from 1995 to 2009 [21]. The authors concluded that the increased use of CPM was a "trend made in the USA." A similar study by Metcalfe et al. also supports this viewpoint, examining an international registry of women with unilateral breast cancer and BRCA mutation. They report that 49 % of women in the United States underwent CPM, compared to a much lower rate among women from Europe and Israel of only 10 % or less [22].

The factors associated with the decision for CPM appear to be multifactorial (Table 8.1). Younger women are much more likely to receive CPM [15, 17]; other factors such as white race, higher education level, private health insurance, and family history of breast cancer are also associated with higher CPM rates [15, 17, 18, 20]. In the SEER study, the presence of infiltrating lobular histology was one of the strongest predictors of CPM [15]. Yet, population-based studies indicate that the risk of contralateral breast cancer is not significantly increased for infiltrating lobular histology as compared with infiltrating ductal histology [23]. Multicentric breast cancer has also been associated with higher CPM rates [24]. BRCA testing is significantly associated with CPM, even among patients who do not have BRCA mutations. In one single-center study, the CPM rate was 40 % among those patients who tested negative for mutations [25]. Several studies have reported that preoperative MRI is associated with CPM [18, 20, 24]. Patients treated at comprehensive cancer programs or teaching facilities are more likely to receive CPM [17].

Reasons for Increased CPM Rates

This trend towards more aggressive breast cancer surgery is curious and appears somewhat counterintuitive in the modern era of minimally invasive surgery. The following section of this chapter is largely speculative because the exact reasons for increased CPM rates in the United States are really unknown. However, many factors are likely to contribute to the increased use of CPM. Public awareness of genetic breast cancer and increased BRCA testing may partially explain these observations. Improvements in mastectomy (including skin-sparing and nipple-sparing mastectomy) and reconstruction techniques and access to plastic surgeons who specialize in breast reconstruction probably contribute to increased CPM rates. Moreover, symmetric reconstruction is often easier to achieve after bilateral mastectomy as compared to unilateral mastectomy. Additionally, the native and reconstructed breast age differently, so symmetric outcomes may diminish over time.

Several studies have reported that preoperative breast MRI is associated with higher CPM rates [18, 20]. The proposed explanation is that MRI findings introduce concern about the opposite breast. For example, a patient is diagnosed with a unilateral breast cancer, and clinical breast examination and mammography of the contralateral breast are normal. The patient is an ideal candidate for breast-conserving treatment. However, an MRI is obtained which demonstrates an occult indeterminate lesion in the contralateral breast. Next, the patient undergoes a second-look (targeted) ultrasound to characterize this MRI finding. The ultrasound imaging is normal, so she gets called back again for an MRI-guided biopsy, which is negative for cancer. However, the patient decides to have bilateral mastectomy to avoid this stressful scenario again. Preoperative breast MRI probably contributes to increased CPM rates, but the initial observed CPM trends in the United States preceded the widespread use of breast MRI [15, 17].

Obesity rates in the United States have markedly increased over the past two decades. An obese woman with large breasts may encounter symmetry and balance problems after unilateral mastectomy without reconstruction. Additionally, the plastic surgeon may have technical challenges in achieving a symmetric reconstruction after unilateral mastectomy for an obese woman with large, pendulous breasts. For some women, bilateral mastectomy with or without reconstruction may provide effective local breast cancer treatment, avoid future radiographic surveillance, and may relieve the chronic symptoms often associated with macromastia. Nevertheless, it is not known with certainty whether increasing obesity rates in the United States are contributing to current CPM trends.

Another possible explanation for the increased CPM rates is that some patients may considerably overestimate their risk of contralateral breast cancer. Previous studies have reported that women with early breast cancer markedly overestimate their risk of recurrence [26]. In a recent survey of 350 mastectomy patients, Han et al. reported that the most common reason for CPM was worry about contralateral breast cancer [27]. However, the rates of metachronous contralateral breast cancer have declined in the United States in recent decades [28]. The increased use of adjuvant therapies likely explains these findings.

The Early Breast Cancer Trialists' Collaborative Group recently updated their meta-analyses and reported that the annual rate of contralateral breast cancer was about 0.4 % for patients with estrogen receptor-positive breast cancer treated with tamoxifen [29]. The annual rate of contralateral breast cancer was about 0.5 % for patients with estrogen receptor-negative breast cancer. Thus, the 10-year cumulative risk of contralateral breast cancer is about 4–5 %. Abbott et al. recently published the results of a prospective single-center study designed to determine a patients perceived risk of contralateral breast cancer [30]. Patients completed a standardized survey prior to surgical consultation and were asked to estimate their risk of contralateral breast cancer. Patients substantially overestimated their 10-year cumulative risk of contralateral breast cancer, with a mean perceived risk of 31.4 %.

Moreover, some patients may overestimate the oncologic benefits of CPM. In a review of open-ended comments from women who underwent CPM, Altschuler et al. recorded comments such as "I do not worry about recurrence" and I am "free of worries about breast cancer" [12]. Such comments suggest a true lack of understanding as to the benefits of CPM, since removal of the normal contralateral breast does not treat systemic metastases from the known ipsilateral breast cancer.

Outcomes After CPM

Several studies have demonstrated that CPM is effective in reducing the risk of contralateral breast cancer. In a study of 745 breast cancer patients with a family history of breast cancer, McDonnell et al. reported that CPM reduced the incidence of contralateral breast cancer by more than 90 % [31]. In a retrospective study of 239 patients, Goldflam et al. reported that only one contralateral breast cancer (0.4 %) developed after CPM [8]. Depending upon the statistical methods used, CPM reduces the risk of contralateral breast cancer by about 90 %.

However, the effectiveness of CPM in reducing breast cancer mortality is not as clear. The only plausible way that CPM improves breast cancer survival is by reducing the risk of a potentially fatal contralateral breast cancer. A recent survival analysis of the SEER database included patients with unilateral breast cancer diagnosed between 1998 and 2003 [32]. The authors concluded that CPM is associated with a small improvement (4.8 %) in 5-year breast-cancer-specific survival rates for young women with early-stage estrogen receptor-negative breast cancer.

Of note, the cumulative incidence of contralateral breast cancer was less than 1 % in this study; therefore, the apparent survival benefit is most likely due to selection bias. In a retrospective single-center study, Boughey et al. reported that CPM was associated with improved overall survival and disease free survival rates [33]. However, a recent Cochrane review of published CPM studies concluded that there is insufficient evidence at the present time that CPM improves overall survival [7].

Despite the results of retrospective or cancer registry studies, CPM is not likely to improve breast cancer survival rates for patients who do not have BRCA mutations. For these patients, the 10-year cumulative risk of contralateral breast cancer is about 4–5 %; most metachronous contralateral breast cancers are stage I or IIA with a 10-year mortality rate of about 10–20 %. Thus, the 20-year mortality rate from a contralateral breast cancer is about 1 % or less. In addition, many patients die from systemic metastases from their known ipsilateral breast cancer or from other causes during 20-year follow-up. Finally, CPM does not prevent all contralateral breast cancers. Thus, CPM will likely not decrease breast cancer mortality rates for most breast cancer patients without BRCA mutations.

On the other hand, for patients with BRCA-associated unilateral breast cancer, the annual risk of contralateral breast cancer is about 4 % per year with a cumulative 10-year risk of contralateral breast cancer of about 40 % [34]. Thus, the possibility of developing a potentially fatal contralateral breast cancer is substantially higher among breast cancer patients with a BRCA mutation. The relative risk reduction of CPM is similar for patients with and without BRCA mutations. Using Markov modeling, Schrag et al. estimated that CPM would increase life expectancy by 0.6–2.1 years for a 30-year-old patient with a BRCA mutation [35]. Clearly, randomized trials comparing CPM versus no CPM for either selected (BRCA mutations) or heterogenous patients are not feasible.

Contralateral prophylactic mastectomy is an irreversible procedure and is not without risks. Some of the more severe potential complications after CPM may significantly delay recommended adjuvant therapy, such as chemotherapy. Complications that require additional surgical procedures and subsequent loss of reconstruction must be considered and thoroughly discussed with all patients. The overall complication rate after bilateral mastectomy and reconstruction is about 20 % [8]. About half of the complications are secondary to the prophylactic mastectomy. Even without complications, these operations are relatively lengthy (often 5–6 h) and require 2–3 days of inpatient hospital care, drainage catheters, and about 3–4 weeks of overall recovery.

Despite potential risks and complications, most patients are satisfied with their decision to undergo CPM. The greatest reported benefit contributing to patient satisfaction is a reduction in breast cancer-related concerns. Frost et al. reported that 83 % of patients were either satisfied or very satisfied with their decision to undergo CPM at a mean of 10 years after surgery [36]. Some women have negative psychosocial outcomes following CPM, most often related to high levels of psychological distress, sexual function, and body image or poor cosmetic outcome [12]. Montgomery et al. reported that the most common reasons for regret after CPM were a poor cosmetic outcome and diminished sense of sexuality [37].

Alternatives to CPM

Patients with unilateral breast cancer have several nonoperative options that are less invasive than CPM. Surveillance with clinical breast examination, mammography, and potentially breast MRI may detect cancers at earlier stages. Several prospective randomized trials have demonstrated that tamoxifen, given as an adjuvant therapy for estrogen receptor-positive breast cancer, significantly reduces the rate of contralateral breast cancer. In the National Surgical Adjuvant Breast and Bowel Project (NSABP) B-14 study, 2,892 women with node-negative, estrogen receptor-positive breast tumors were randomly assigned to either tamoxifen (20 mg/d) or placebo for at least 5 years [38]. After an average follow-up of 53 months, 55 contralateral breast cancers developed in placebo-treated women and 28 developed in the tamoxifen-treated women ($p=0.001$). Aromatase inhibitors also reduce the risk of contralateral breast cancer as much as, or even more than, tamoxifen [39]. The ATAC (Arimidex, Tamoxifen Alone or in Combination) Trial demonstrated that anastrozole was superior to tamoxifen in preventing contralateral breast cancer in postmenopausal women. Ovarian ablation and cytotoxic chemotherapy also reduce the risk of contralateral breast cancer [40].

Conclusions

Increasingly, more patients in the United States with invasive breast cancer and DCIS undergo CPM to prevent contralateral breast cancer. Patient, tumor, and treatment factors are associated with increased use of CPM. It appears that CPM does reduce the risk of contralateral breast cancer, but does not impact upon breast cancer survival rates. Controversy exists about whether the physician or patient should initiate the discussion of CPM. If a patient appropriately chooses breast-conserving surgery, then CPM is not a relevant treatment. For patients who undergo mastectomy, CPM may be a reasonable option, particularly if a patient has a BRCA mutation, strong family history, is obese, or if imaging of the contralateral breast is difficult. Recent studies have demonstrated that many patients are not well informed about the risk of contralateral breast cancer or the benefits of CPM. Physicians need to provide breast cancer patients with accurate information on the true risk of contralateral breast cancer based upon current data, as well as the risks and benefits of CPM. In addition, physicians should encourage appropriate patients to consider less drastic options (e.g. endocrine therapy) to reduce the risk of contralateral breast cancer.

Presently, there has been no study that has prospectively evaluated the complex decision-making processes that lead to CPM. Future research should include development of models and instruments to elucidate these processes. It is clear that the surgeon's role and influence in choice of breast cancer surgery plays a central and critical role in the resulting decision for CPM. Finally, decision aids and improved educational material should be developed for breast cancer patients and physicians.

References

1. Guiliano AE, Boolbol S, Degnim A, et al. Society of Surgical Oncology: position statement on prophylactic mastectomy. Ann Surg Oncol. 2007;14:2425–7.
2. www.nccn.org v1. 2012. Accessed 31 Dec 2012.
3. Black WC, Nease Jr RF, Tosteson AN. Perceptions of breast cancer risk and screening effectiveness in women younger than 50 years of age. J Natl Cancer Inst. 1995;87:720–31.
4. Alexander NE, Ross J, Sumner W, Nease Jr RF, et al. The effect of an educational intervention on the perceived risk of breast cancer. J Gen Intern Med. 1996;11(2):92–7.
5. Hartmann LC, Schaid DJ, Woods JE, et al. Efficacy of bilateral prophylactic mastectomy in women with a family history of breast cancer. NEJM. 1999;340:77–84.
6. Rebbeck TR, Freibel T, Lynch HT, et al. Bilateral prophylactic mastectomy reduces breast cancer risk in BRCA1 and BRCA2 mutation carriers: the PROSE Study Group. J Clin Oncol. 2004;22:1055–62.
7. Lostumbo L, Carbine N, Wallace J, et al. Prophylactic mastectomy for the prevention of breast cancer. Cochrane Database Syst Rev. 2004;(4):CD002748.
8. Goldflam K, Hunt KK, Gershenwald JE, et al. Contralateral prophylactic mastectomy. Predictors of significant histologic findings. Cancer. 2004;101:1977–86.
9. Schrag D, Kuntz KM, Garber JE, et al. Decision analysis—effects of prophylactic mastectomy and oophorectomy on life expectancy among women with BRCA 1 or BRCA 2 mutations. N Engl J Med. 1997;336(20):1465–71.
10. Zion SM, Slevak JM, Sellers TA, et al. Reoperations after prophylactic mastectomy with or without implant reconstruction. Cancer. 2003;98(10):2152–60.
11. Geiger AM, Nekhlyudov L, Herrinton LJ, et al. Quality of life after bilateral prophylactic mastectomy. Ann Surg Oncol. 2007;14(2):686–94.
12. Altschuler A, Nekhlyudov L, Rolnick S, et al. Positive, negative, and disparate–women's differing long-term psychosocial experiences of bilateral or contralateral prophylactic mastectomy. Breast J. 2008;14:25–32.
13. Gopie JP, Mureau MA, Seynaeve C, et al. Body image issues after bilateral prophylactic mastectomy with breast reconstruction in healthy women at risk for hereditary breast cancer. Familial Cancer. 2013;12(3):479–87.
14. McLaughlin CC, Lillquist PP, Edge SB. Surveillance of prophylactic mastectomy: trends in use from 1995 through 2005. Cancer. 2009;115:5404–12.
15. Tuttle TM, Habermann EB, Grund EH, et al. Increasing use of contralateral prophylactic mastectomy for breast cancer patients: a trend toward more aggressive surgical treatment. J Clin Oncol. 2007;25:5203–9.
16. Tuttle TM, Jarosek S, Habermann E, et al. Increasing rates of contralateral prophylactic mastectomy among

patients with ductal carcinoma in situ. J Clin Oncol. 2009;27:1362–7.
17. Yao K, Stewart AK, Winchester DJ, Winchester DP. Trends in contralateral prophylactic mastectomy for unilateral cancer: a report from the National Cancer Data Base, 1998–2007. Ann Surg Oncol. 2010;17(10):2554–62.
18. Sorbero ME, Dick AW, Burke Beckjord E, et al. Diagnostic breast magnetic resonance imaging and contralateral prophylactic mastectomy. Ann Surg Oncol. 2009;16:1597–605.
19. Jones NB, Wilson J, Kotur L, et al. Contralateral prophylactic mastectomy for unilateral breast cancer: an increasing trend at a single institution. Ann Surg Oncol. 2009;16:2691–6.
20. King TA, Sakr R, Patil S, et al. Clinical management factors contribute to the decision for contralateral prophylactic mastectomy. J Clin Oncol. 2011;29(16):2158–64.
21. Güth U, Myrick ME, Viehl CT, et al. Increasing rates of contralateral prophylactic mastectomy-a trend made in USA? Eur J Surg Oncol. 2012;38:296–301.
22. Metcalfe KA, Lubinski J, Ghadirian P, Hereditary Breast Cancer Clinical Study Group, et al. Predictors of contralateral prophylactic mastectomy in women with a BRCA1 or BRCA2 mutation: the Hereditary Breast Cancer Clinical Study Group. J Clin Oncol. 2008;26:1093–7.
23. Gao X, Fisher SG, Emami B. Risk of second primary cancer in the contralateral breast in women treated for early-stage breast cancer: a population-based study. Int J Radiat Oncol Biol Phys. 2003;56:1038–45.
24. Stucky CC, Gray RJ, Wasif N, et al. Increase in contralateral prophylactic mastectomy: echoes of a bygone era? Surgical trends for unilateral breast cancer. Ann Surg Oncol. 2010;17 Suppl 3:330–7.
25. Yi M, Hunt KK, Arun BK, et al. Factors affecting the decision of breast cancer patients to undergo contralateral prophylactic mastectomy. Cancer Prev Res. 2010;3(8):1026–34.
26. Rakovitch E, Franssen E, Kim J, et al. A comparison of risk perception and psychological morbidity in women with ductal carcinoma in situ and early invasive breast cancer. Breast Cancer Res Treat. 2003;77:285–93.
27. Han E, Johnson N, Glissmeyer M, et al. Increasing incidence of bilateral mastectomies: the patient perspective. Am J Surg. 2011;201(5):615–8.
28. Nichols HB, Berrington de González A, et al. Declining incidence of contralateral breast cancer in the United States from 1975 to 2006. J Clin Oncol. 2011;29(12):1564–9.
29. Early Breast Cancer Trialists' Collaborative Group (EBCTCG), Davies C, Godwin J, Gray R, et al. Relevance of breast cancer hormone receptors and other factors to the efficacy of adjuvant tamoxifen: patient-level meta-analysis of randomised trials. Lancet. 2011;378(9793):771–84.
30. Abbott E, Rueth N, Pappas-Varco S, et al. Perceptions of contralateral breast cancer: an overestimation of risk. Ann Surg Oncol. 2011;18:3129–36.
31. McDonnell SK, Schaid DJ, Myers JL, et al. Efficacy of contralateral prophylactic mastectomy in women with a personal and family history of breast cancer. J Clin Oncol. 2001;19:3938–43.
32. Bedrosian I, Hu CY, Chang GJ. Population-based study of contralateral prophylactic mastectomy and survival outcomes of breast cancer patients. J Natl Cancer Inst. 2010;102(6):401–9.
33. Boughey JC, Hoskin TL, Degnim AC, et al. Contralateral prophylactic mastectomy is associated with a survival advantage in high-risk women with a personal history of breast cancer. Ann Surg Oncol. 2010;17(10):2702–9.
34. Metcalfe K, Lynch HT, Ghadirian P, et al. Contralateral breast cancer in BRCA1 and BRCA2 mutation carriers. J Clin Oncol. 2004;22:2328–35.
35. Schrag D, Kuntz KM, Garber JE, et al. Life expectancy gains from cancer prevention strategies for women with breast cancer and BRCA1 or BRCA2 mutations. JAMA. 2000;283:617–24.
36. Frost MH, Slezak JM, Tran NV, et al. Satisfaction after contralateral prophylactic mastectomy: the significance of mastectomy type, reconstructive complications, and body appearance. J Clin Oncol. 2005;23:7849–56.
37. Montgomery LL, Tran KN, Heelan MC, et al. Issues of regret in women with contralateral prophylactic mastectomies. Ann Surg Oncol. 1999;6:546–52.
38. Fisher B, Redmond C. New perspective on cancer of the contralateral breast: a marker for assessing tamoxifen as a preventive agent. J Natl Cancer Inst. 1991;83:1278–80.
39. Baum M, Budzar AU, Cuzick J, et al. Anastrozole alone or in combination with tamoxifen versus tamoxifen alone for adjuvant treatment of postmenopausal women with early breast cancer: first results of the ATAC randomised trial. Lancet. 2002;359:2131–9.
40. Tamoxifen for early breast cancer: an overview of the randomised trials. Early Breast Cancer Trialists' Collaborative Group. Lancet. 1998;351:1451–67.

Genetically Based Breast Cancer: Risk Assessment, Counseling, and Testing

9

Mary B. Daly and Andrea Forman

Abbreviations

ACS	American Cancer Society
AJ	Ashkenazi Jews
ASCO	American Society of Clinical Oncology
ER+	Estrogen receptor positive
FDA	Food and Drug Administration
FLB	First live birth
HBOC	Hereditary breast-ovarian cancer
HDGC	Hereditary diffuse gastric cancer
HRT	Hormone replacement therapy
LCIS	Lobular carcinoma in situ
LFS	Li-Fraumeni syndrome
NCCN	National Comprehensive Cancer Network
NSGC	National Society of Genetic Counselors
OC	Oral contraceptives
PGD	Preimplantation genetic diagnosis
PJS	Peutz-Jeghers syndrome
RRM	Risk-reducing mastectomy
RRSO	Risk-reducing salpingo-oophorectomy
SCTATs	Sex cord tumors with annular tubules
SEER	Surveillance, Epidemiology, and End Results
US	United States
USPSTF	United States Preventive Services Task Force
VUS	Variants of uncertain significance

M.B. Daly, MD, PhD (✉) • A. Forman, MS, CGC
Department of Clinical Genetics,
Fox Chase Cancer Center, 333 Cottman Avenue,
Philadelphia, PA 19111, USA
e-mail: mary.daly@fccc.edu;
andrea.forman@fccc.edu

Introduction

The focus of this chapter is to provide the evidence for a genetic basis of breast cancer and the expanding availability of genetic risk assessment services in the clinical setting. First, we present an overview of the traditional risk factors that are associated with an increased risk for the development of breast cancer. We will then focus on the growing body of data describing the genetic patterns of breast cancer. Lastly, we will discuss the role of genetic risk evaluation, counseling, and testing for inherited breast cancer risk, including the provision of appropriate risk management options.

Epidemiology of Breast Cancer

Breast cancer remains the most common cause of cancer among women both in the United States (US) and globally. It is the leading cause of cancer deaths among females worldwide accounting for 458,400 deaths and the second leading cause of death due to cancer among women in the US, with approximately 40,030 deaths expected per year [1, 2]. After decades of increasing incidence rates among women in the USA, data from the Surveillance, Epidemiology, and End Results

A.I. Riker (ed.), *Breast Disease: Comprehensive Management*,
DOI 10.1007/978-1-4939-1145-5_9, © Springer Science+Business Media New York 2015

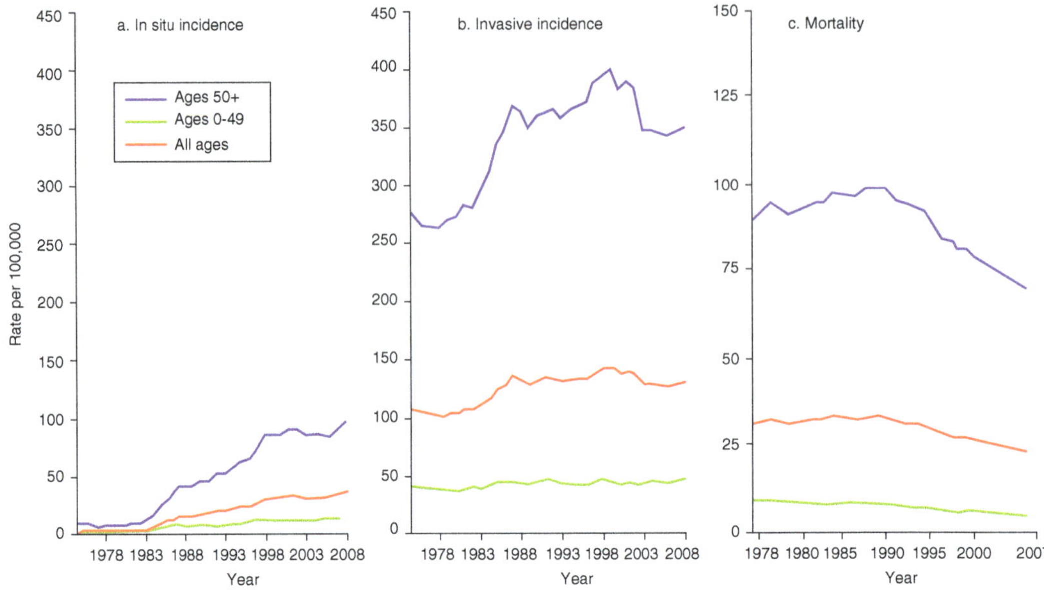

Fig. 9.1 Incidence and mortality rates of female breast cancer by age, United States, 1975–2008 (*Source*: SEER 2012 [5])

(SEER) program indicate an overall plateau in rates of new cases between 2000 and 2009 [3] and a shift in stage from regional and distant stages to more localized disease. Over the same period of time, breast cancer death rates have declined on average 2.2 % per year [4] (see Fig. 9.1).

Despite these recent promising trends, breast cancer represents a significant personal and societal burden that affects many women in the prime of their lives, accounting for a large portion of the oncology health-care budget. A long history of classical epidemiologic studies, now coupled with new information emerging from the field of molecular genetics, is beginning to elucidate the basic mechanisms of breast carcinogenesis and enable the development of novel prevention, detection, and treatment strategies.

Age

The risk of developing breast cancer increases throughout a woman's lifetime, with it being relatively rare in younger women. Rates increase rapidly until age 50 and then continue to rise at a slower pace [6]. Despite the lower rates for young, premenopausal women that are less than 35 years old, they are more likely to be carriers of a breast cancer susceptibility gene. They also present with higher-grade tumors, a more advanced stage, and have a more biologically aggressive form of the disease, resulting in decreased disease-free and overall survival rates [7, 8]. The overall association of breast cancer incidence with increasing age is consistent with a stochastic model of breast cancer, wherein a progressive series of genetic changes within the cell lead to cancer initiation. It is becoming increasingly clear that these genetic changes are the result of a multitude of risk-related factors.

Race/Ethnicity

There are striking racial/ethnic differences in both the incidence and mortality rates for breast cancer. The incidence rates are highest for Caucasian women; lowest for Hispanic, Native American, and Asian American/Pacific Islanders; and intermediate for African-American women (see Fig. 9.2). However, despite having lower incidence rates than Caucasian women, African-American women have the highest death rates

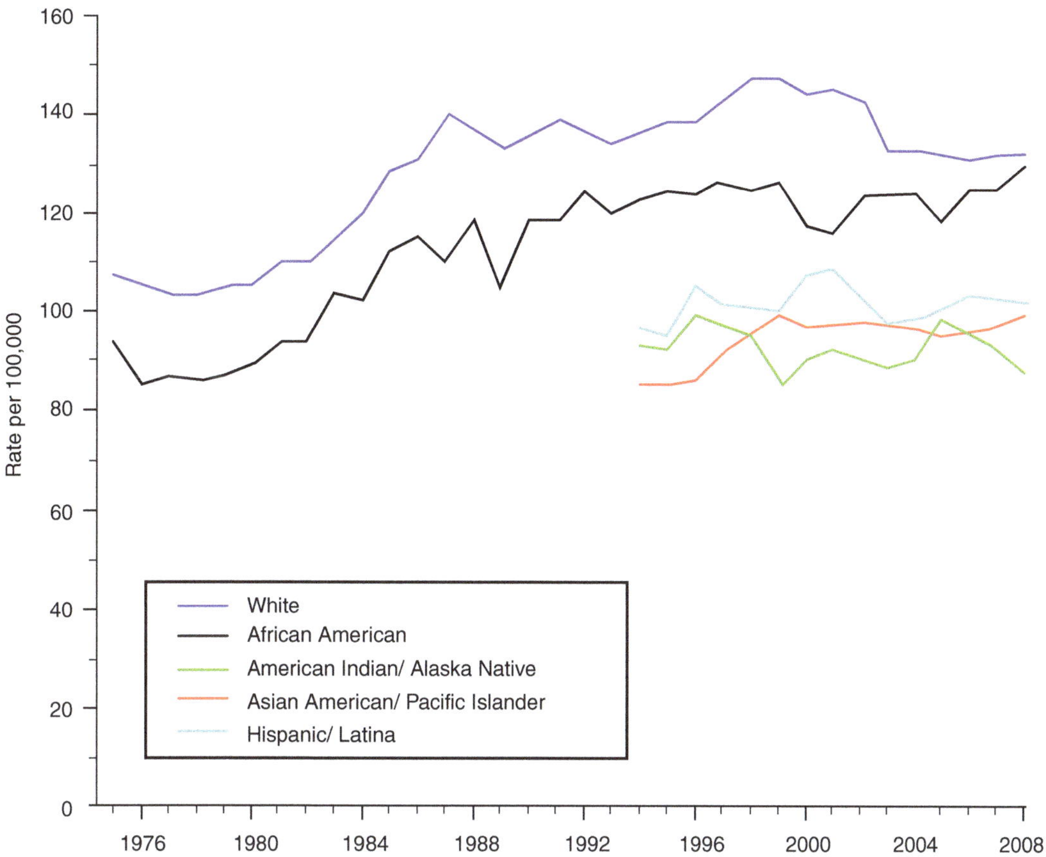

Fig. 9.2 Trends in female breast cancer incidence rates by race and ethnicity, 1975–2008 (*Source*: SEER 2012 [5])

(see Fig. 9.3). Potential explanations for the discrepancies in rates among ethnic groups include environmental, societal, hormonal, and biological factors. Epidemiologic studies have consistently noted increased rates of breast cancer among Jewish women, an observation which is most likely explained by the recent identification of mutations in the *BRCA1/2* genes which are more prevalent among individuals of Ashkenazi Jewish descent [9].

Country of Origin

The international patterns of breast cancer incidence reveal higher rates for Western, industrialized nations and lower rates for less industrialized and Asian countries (see Fig. 9.4). Furthermore, breast cancer incidence rates increase in migrants as they move from low-risk to high-risk countries [11]. These significant differences are thought to be attributable to variations in risk factors that are important in the etiology of the disease, such as reproductive practices, diet, differences in the availability of screening services [1], and perhaps genetic heterogeneity. While the long-term trend in increasing mortality rates for breast cancer has begun to be reversed in some countries, the trend is not universal, with mortality rates continuing to rise in India, South Korea, and Uganda [1]. Even within the US, there is significant geographic diversity in breast cancer rates, with mortality rates declining in the majority of states but stable in the South and the Western states [4]. Most of this variation is thought to be due to regional differences in breast cancer risk factors and variations in screening prevalence.

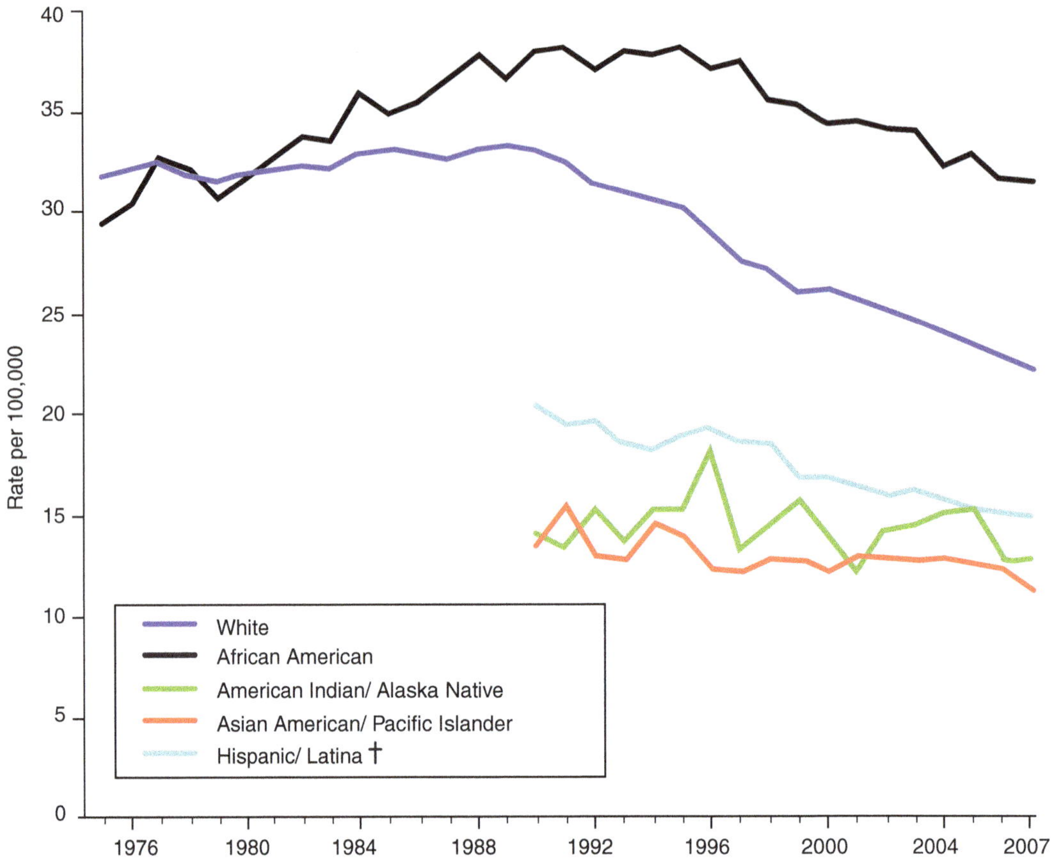

Fig. 9.3 Trends in female breast cancer death rates by race and ethnicity, 1975–2007 (*Source*: SEER 2011 [4])

Benign Breast Disease

Fibrocystic breast disease has often been cited as a risk factor for subsequent breast cancer. However, careful evaluation of histologic patterns of benign breast disease has identified those groups in whom the risk is truly elevated. In the largest retrospective cohort study published, Dupont and Page [12] reevaluated over 10,000 consecutive biopsies performed over a two-decade time period, correlating histologic patterns with the subsequent incidence of breast cancer. Women undergoing breast biopsies, whose tissue showed no evidence of proliferation, had no increase in the relative risk of breast cancer. Risk increased from 1.4 to 4.4 with the degree of proliferation and atypia seen in the biopsy specimen.

There also appeared to be an interaction between the presence of proliferative breast disease and family and reproductive history, with relative risk increasing to as high as eightfold in the setting of a positive family history, nulliparity, or late age at first birth. This further suggests that the proliferative process itself is affected by other risk factors [12]. They also identified sclerosing adenosis and fibroadenomas as an independent risk factor for invasive disease, with relative risks in the 1.5–2.0 range [13, 14]. Confirmatory evidence of these findings comes from the prospective Nurses' Health Study in which a prior diagnosis of atypical ductal hyperplasia or atypical lobular hyperplasia conferred an odds ratio of subsequent breast cancer of 2.4 and 5.3, respectively [15].

Lobular carcinoma in situ (LCIS) is the most common benign lesion to present as a multicentric and/or bilateral process and is often associated with sclerosing adenosis, stromal fibrosis, fat necrosis, duct ectasia, and fibroadenoma [16].

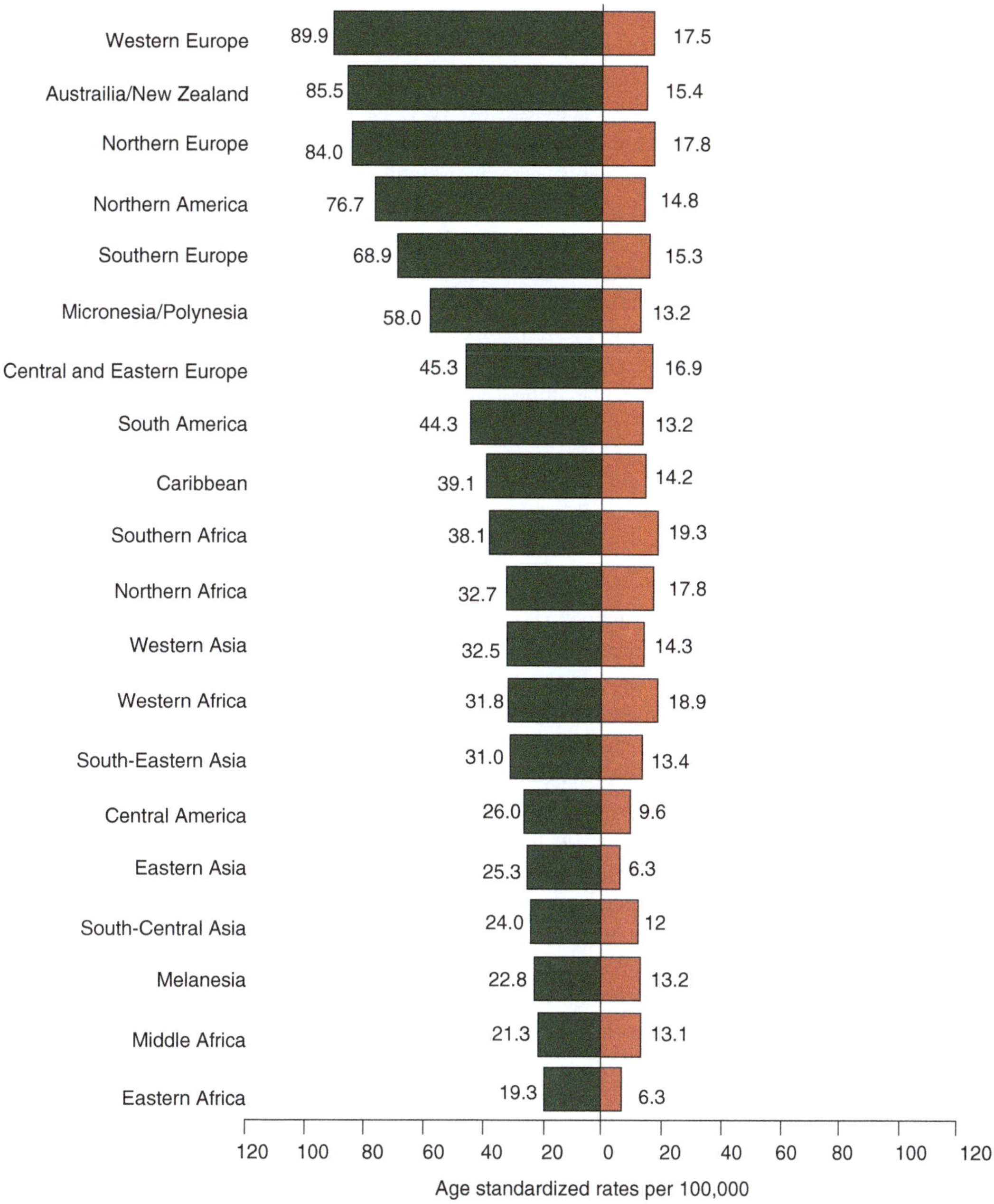

Fig. 9.4 Age-standardized breast cancer incidence and mortality rates by world area (*Source*: GLOBOCAN 2010 [10])

A diagnosis of LCIS increases the risk of subsequent breast cancer in either breast by a factor of 4–9 times the general population and is thought to be a marker of proliferation rather than a premalignant lesion itself [17]. The excess risk is highest for women who develop LCIS before the age of 40 years old [18].

Mammographic Density

The current data suggests an independent association between the degree of breast density seen on mammography and the risk for breast cancer. The increased relative risk for breast cancer ranges from 1.5 to sixfold among women in whom 75 % of the breast appears dense. Breast density is greatest in younger women; decreases with age, menopause, and pregnancies; and is thought to be a marker of proliferative activity [19, 20]. There also appears to be an additive effect of breast density and hormone exposure, with breast cancer risk higher among premenopausal women who have taken oral contraceptives (OC) and among postmenopausal women who took combined estrogen and progesterone hormone replacement therapy (HRT) [21, 22]. Breast density appears to be a heritable trait, with inherited factors accounting for 63 % of the variance [19].

Reproductive Risk Factors

One of the most consistent epidemiologic observations is the association of reproductive factors with the subsequent risk of breast cancer. One of the first observations noted an increased risk of developing breast cancer among nulliparous women. Not only was it noted that parous women had a decreased risk for breast cancer, but it was also observed that the degree of protection afforded by pregnancy depends on the age at the time of the first live birth (FLB), with the greatest protection seen among women whose FLB occurred before age 20 years [23]. In fact, when the FLB is delayed to age 35 or older, the risk for breast cancer equals, or exceeds, that of a nulliparous woman. The addition of subsequent pregnancies and/or lactation among young women adds additional protection. By causing breast epithelial cells to become fully differentiated and mature and less likely to undergo further mitoses, an early full-term pregnancy is thought to protect the cells from subsequent genotoxic events which may initiate the carcinogenic process.

An alternative hypothesis may be that pregnancy modifies age-related changes in plasma hormone levels [24, 25]. The total length of menstruation during a woman's lifetime contributes to their overall risk. Both early age at menarche and late age at menopause are associated with an increased risk [26]. On the other hand, the risk for breast cancer is significantly decreased among women undergoing surgical oophorectomy, particularly if the surgery is performed before age 40 years [27]. The relevance of these findings appears to be related to the overall length of ovarian activity and the duration of exposure to ovarian hormones in the promotion of breast cancer.

An increased risk of breast cancer among postmenopausal women has been associated with the use of HRT. The Women's Health Initiative examined postmenopausal women and randomized them to receive conjugated equine estrogen and medroxyprogesterone acetate versus placebo. The HRT group experienced significantly more cases of invasive breast cancer compared to the control group, HR 1.25 (CI 1.07–1.46), and were significantly more likely to present with lymph node-positive disease, HR 1.78 (CI 1.23–2.58). There were also significantly more deaths from breast cancer in the HRT group, HR 1.96 (CI 1.00–4.04) [28]. The resultant decline in use of HRT is thought to, in part, account for the decrease in breast cancer incidence seen in subsequent years.

Although the complex set of interactions which determine breast cancer risk are not fully known, there is a significant body of data linking factors associated with reproductive hormones to breast cancer incidence. This has led to the proposal that endogenous sex hormones are major determinants of breast cancer risk and that the role of other factors, including genetic polymorphisms, environmental exposures, and lifestyle events, may be in the modulation or metabolism of estrogen, progesterone, and/or androgenic hormones. Furthermore, this suggests that there is differential susceptibility of breast tissue to the adverse effects of hormone exposure, with the highest vulnerability found among less differentiated cells during periods of rapid growth. The lowest vulnerability is seen in cells which have undergone complete maturation during a full-term pregnancy. In this model, the initiation of cancer is seen as a multifactorial event, depending on the stage of development of the breast, the hormonal environment, the genetic susceptibility, and the presence or absence of modifying factors [29, 30].

Radiation Exposure

Epidemiologic studies have linked diagnostic and therapeutic ionizing radiation to subsequent breast cancer risk. Repeated diagnostic radiology procedures among adolescents and young women, for example, monitored for scoliosis or tuberculosis, have been associated with an increased risk for breast cancer that persists for decades after exposure [31]. Rates of breast cancer risk are also increased among women exposed to thymic radiation during infancy [32]. Perhaps the strongest radiation-associated risk for breast cancer is seen in women treated with chest radiation (mantle) for Hodgkin's lymphoma. Among women treated before age 30 years, the risk for breast cancer is six times greater than that of the general population. Survivors of Hodgkin's lymphoma are also more likely to experience contralateral breast cancers [33]. The degree of risk has been demonstrated to vary by age at treatment, time since diagnosis, and radiation dose [34].

Physical Activity

Both case-control and prospective studies have identified an inverse relationship between physical activity and breast cancer incidence. Reports of the risk reduction associated with moderate physical activity range from 15 to 40 %, and the effect is seen for both invasive and in situ breast cancer and among several ethnic groups [35, 36]. Several biological mechanisms have been proposed, including decreased body fat, decreased exposure to ovarian hormones, and decreased fasting insulin levels [37, 38].

Obesity

Obesity has been linked to an increased risk for breast cancer in both retrospective and prospective studies. The association of obesity with breast cancer risk is seen in Caucasian, African-American, and Asian women [39, 40]. The increased risk is best established among postmenopausal women, likely related to the interactions among cytokines, growth factors, inflammatory pathways, and steroid hormones [41].

Alcohol

Several studies have revealed an association between alcohol consumption and breast cancer risk [42, 43]. The relative risk increases with increasing intake of alcohol [44] (see Fig. 9.5). The risk appears to be greater among women taking hormone therapy and is confined to breast cancers that express estrogen receptors, suggesting an interaction between alcohol and hormone pathways [45–47]. Alternative hypotheses are that alcohol is acting as a cumulative carcinogen and/or a tumor promoter [48].

Genetic Risk Factors

The basis of most, if not all, cancers involve one or more mutations in genes that are involved in the regulation of cell growth and/or DNA repair. Most cancer-related mutations are sporadic, i.e., they are acquired during the life of the individual and occur only in the tumor cells. However, the observation of familial clustering of certain cancers has led to the identification of a number of heritable forms of cancer in which the mutated gene is passed on from parent to child. We have now found several such genes that help to explain the clustering of breast cancer with other malignancies within family members. These hereditary breast cancer syndromes account for 5–10% of all breast cancer (see Table 9.1). They all share several features, including a Mendelian inheritance pattern, vertical transmission from both maternal and paternal lines, early age at onset, multiple primaries, and a high penetrance.

Mutations in the *BRCA1* and *BRCA2* genes account for the majority of hereditary breast cancer. In addition to breast cancer, individuals with *BRCA1/2* mutations are at an increased risk for cancer of the ovary and fallopian tubes, high-grade prostate cancer, male breast cancer, melanoma, and pancreatic cancer. Of the several

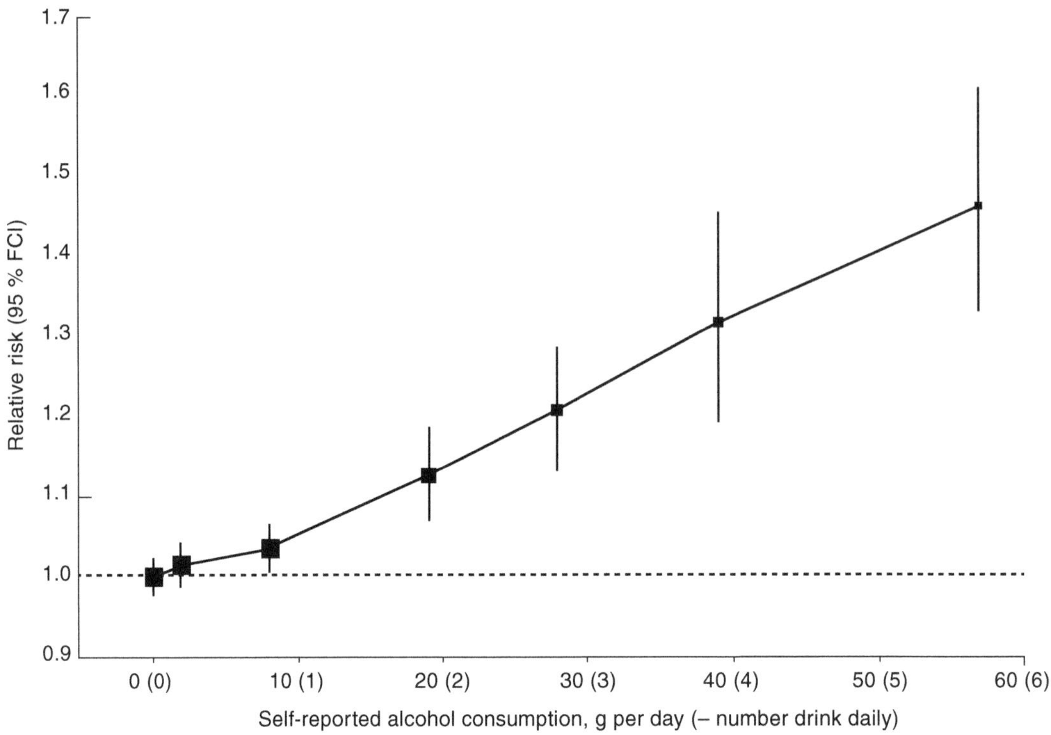

Fig. 9.5 Relative risk of breast cancer in relation to reported intake of alcohol [24, 44]

Table 9.1 Inherited breast cancer syndromes for which clinical testing is available

Syndrome	Involved gene(s)	Associated cancers
Hereditary breast-ovarian cancer (HBOC) syndrome	*BRCA1* at 17q21, *BRCA2* at 13q12	Breast, ovary, prostate, pancreas, melanoma
Cowden syndrome	*PTEN* at 10q23	Breast, uterus, thyroid, kidney, melanoma, glioblastoma
Li-Fraumeni syndrome	*TP53* at 17p13.1	Sarcoma, breast cancer, leukemia, adrenocortical cancer, brain cancer
Diffuse gastric cancer syndrome	*CDH1* at 16q22.1	Diffuse gastric cancer, lobular breast cancer
Peutz-Jeghers syndrome	*STK11* at 19p13.3	Colon, breast, pancreas, uterus, lung, testis, and ovarian cancer

hundred mutations described for the *BRCA1/2* genes, most lead to a frameshift resulting in a missing or nonfunctional protein. These genes are known to be associated with a role as a "gatekeeper," characterized by interactions with other genes in the regulation of the cell cycle and DNA repair [49].

The frequency of mutations in the *BRCA1/2* genes in the general population has been estimated to range from 1 in 400 to 1 in 800. Carrier rates are not distributed evenly, however, and tend to concentrate in families with multiple cases of breast and/or ovarian cancer. *BRCA1* and *BRCA2* also share differential prevalence rates in certain ethnic groups. Most notably, three specific mutations, the 185delAG mutation and the 5382insC mutation on *BRCA1* and the 6174delT mutation on *BRCA2*, have been found to be common among Ashkenazi Jews (AJ). The frequency of these three mutations approximates 1 in 40 in this population and accounts for up to 25 % of all AJ families with early-onset breast cancer and up to 90 % with both breast and ovarian cancer [9, 50]. Additional "founder effects" have been described in other populations.

The actual expression of disease in gene mutation carriers is known as the penetrance. Breast and ovarian cancer are the predominant cancers seen with *BRCA1/2* mutations. The estimated risk for breast cancer by age 70 years is 47–66% for *BRCA1* carriers and 40–57% for *BRCA2* carriers. Ovarian cancer risk is estimated to be 35–46% for *BRCA1* carriers and from 13 to 23 % among *BRCA2* carriers [51, 52]. Among female *BRCA1* and *BRCA2* carriers who have already developed a primary breast cancer, estimates for a second contralateral breast cancer range from 39 to 56 %. Risks are higher among women whose first diagnosis was before age 40 and for women with *BRCA1* mutations [53]. It is not known whether specific mutations within each gene confer differential rates of penetrance or what other genetic, environmental, or lifestyle factors may interact with the presence of a mutation to determine expressivity, thus making precise penetrance estimates in individuals somewhat difficult.

The phenotypic expression of *BRCA1/2* breast cancer includes distinctive pathologic features. Breast cancers associated with the *BRCA1* gene are typically estrogen receptor, progesterone receptor, and Her2/neu negative (triple negative), conferring an overall more aggressive disease course [54–56]. Sixty-nine percent of breast cancers arising in *BRCA1* carriers are triple negative [54]. The prevalence of *BRCA1* mutations among women with triple-negative disease has been reported to range from 11 to 35 % [57]. The phenotype for *BRCA2*-related tumors appears to be more heterogeneous and may include an excess of lobular histology [56].

Li-Fraumeni Syndrome

Breast cancer is also a component of the rare Li-Fraumeni syndrome (LFS) in which germline mutations of the *TP53* gene on chromosome 17p have been documented. This syndrome is characterized by premenopausal breast cancer in combination with childhood sarcoma, brain tumors, leukemia and lymphoma, lung cancer, colon cancer, and adrenocortical carcinoma [58]. Individuals with LFS often develop multiple primary cancers [59]. A germline mutation in the *TP53* gene has been identified in over 50 % of families exhibiting this syndrome, and inheritance is autosomal dominant with a penetrance of at least 50 % by age 50 [60].

Cowden Syndrome

One of the more than 50 cancer-related genodermatoses, Cowden syndrome is characterized by an excess of breast cancer, gastrointestinal malignancies, genitourinary malignancies, and thyroid disease (both benign and malignant). Skin manifestations include multiple trichilemmomas, oral fibromas and papillomas, and acral, palmar, and plantar keratoses. Germline mutations in *PTEN*, a protein tyrosine phosphatase with homology to tensin, located on chromosome 10q23, are responsible for this syndrome. Loss of heterozygosity observed in a high proportion of related cancers suggests that *PTEN* functions as a tumor suppressor gene. Its defined enzymatic function indicates a role in maintenance of the control of cell proliferation. Disruption of *PTEN* appears to occur late in tumorigenesis and may act as a regulatory molecule of cytoskeletal function. The lifetime risk of breast cancer in women with *PTEN* mutations is estimated at 25–50%, with a characteristic early age of onset [61].

Peutz-Jeghers Syndrome

Peutz-Jeghers syndrome (PJS) is characterized by gastrointestinal polyposis, particularly hamartomatous polyps, and melanocytic macules on the lips and perioral and buccal tissues [62, 63]. Although the most common cancers in PJS are gastrointestinal, the cumulative risk of breast cancer is 35–54% [63, 64]. Additional cancer risks include pancreatic and ovarian cancers as well as ovarian sex cord tumors with annular tubules (SCTATs) and mucinous tumors of the ovaries and fallopian tubes and Sertoli cell tumors of the testes [65, 66]. Germline mutations in the *STK11* gene on chromosome 10p have been identified in the majority of PJS families [63, 67].

Hereditary Diffuse Gastric Syndrome

Hereditary diffuse gastric cancer (HDGC), which arises from mutations in the *CDH1* gene, is associated with an increased risk of lobular breast cancer, with lifetime risks as high as 52 % and an average age of onset of 53 years old [68]. HDGC is unique in the predominant lobular pathology of the breast cancer occurrences as well as the diffuse nature of the gastric cancer cases. The risk for diffuse gastric cancer is >80 % in *CDH1* gene carriers [69]. Loss of the E-cadherin protein causes the tumor cells to infiltrate the mucosa of the stomach, causing thickening and rigidity of the gastric wall, called *linitis plastica*, and malignant cells often have a signet ring appearance [70].

Lower-Penetrance Genes

In addition to the rare but highly penetrant genes described above, there is growing evidence that more common, but less penetrant, genes may account for a significant proportion of hereditary breast cancer. Both candidate gene and genome-wide searches have been used to identify low-penetrance polymorphisms that alone or in combination are associated with breast cancer. The identification and location of these breast cancer genes will ultimately permit further investigation of the precise role they play in cancer progression and will allow us to determine the percentage of total breast cancer caused by the inheritance of mutant genes. This, in turn, will ultimately enrich our understanding of all breast cancer, sporadic as well as hereditary, and will improve the identification of high-risk individuals.

Genetic Counseling for Breast/Ovarian Cancer

The technologic developments that have facilitated the location and isolation of cancer susceptibility genes have integrated the fields of oncology, cancer prevention, genetics, and counseling. This, in turn, has helped to create a new subspecialty of cancer risk counseling with an emphasis on the communication of risk information based on personal and family histories. The National Society of Genetic Counselors (NSGC) defines genetic counseling as the process of helping people understand and adapt to the medical, psychological, and familial implications of genetic contributions to disease [71]. Genetic counseling for cancer, also known as cancer risk assessment, is the important process of differentiating patients at low, moderate, or high risk for cancer and identifying appropriate patients for genetic testing of known hereditary cancer syndromes.

The specific goals of the counseling process are to (1) provide accurate information on the genetic, biologic, and environmental factors related to the individual's risk of cancer; (2) provide a sufficient understanding of the genetic basis of breast and ovarian cancer to assist in decisions regarding genetic testing; (3) provide a realistic assessment of personal risk both for the genetic syndrome and for the disease(s) itself; (4) formulate appropriate options and recommendations for prevention and screening; and (5) offer psychosocial support, appropriate to a family's culture, to facilitate adjustment to an altered-risk perception and promote adherence to the recommended actions. Using personal and family histories, risk models, and molecular and tumor testing, a counselor can help to identify patients at the highest risks for cancer [72]. As only 5–10% of cancer cases have a hereditary component, risk assessment can serve as a "gatekeeper" that identifies those patients most appropriate for high-cost genetic tests, ensuring tests and services are being utilized in a suitable manner. The session can also educate patients who are not appropriate for genetic testing but who still may have increased risks for cancer [73].

Target Population

With the growing awareness of the familial nature of breast cancer, increasing numbers of family members of women diagnosed with breast cancer are seeking information and advice about the disease, their potential risk, and available risk-reducing options. Women who seek counseling are often highly motivated by a personal experience with cancer in their family and by concern for the risks faced by themselves and their close relatives. As physicians become more aware of the importance of family history in determining a woman's risk for breast cancer, they are increasingly referring their patients for cancer risk counseling. Even those individuals who are not candidates for genetic testing will benefit from having a realistic estimate of their cancer risk. In addition to providing risk information and risk counseling to the individual concerned about her risk for cancer, the process often has wide-reaching implications for the family and may ultimately extend to include additional family members.

The Counseling Team

Historically, the medical genetic counseling team has consisted of a medical geneticist, a genetic counselor, and, to a lesser extent, the referring primary care physician. As the field of genetic counseling has expanded to include adult diseases such as cancer, other disciplines, including oncology, gynecology, molecular genetics, social work, and psychology, have joined the team in order to provide the multidisciplinary approach needed.

There is also a growing interest in genetics on the part of nurses, many of whom are beginning to seek specialized training in the field. Genetic counselors and nurses trained in genetics are now increasingly delivering medical and genetic risk information about familial forms of cancer and counseling individuals and families about disease risk and management. Originally, cancer risk counseling programs were mainly situated in cancer centers and academic institutions, but these services are expanding to community hospitals, worksites, and health centers where they are often one component of a more broad-based health promotion program.

Table 9.2 Components of information gathering

Establishment of needs, concerns, questions, priorities
Assessment of psychosocial dimensions
Personal medical history
Detailed family history
Personal risk factor profile
Personal screening and health behavior history

Risk Assessment

The genetic counseling process begins with the collection of several components of information. The first step in evaluating a woman's risk for breast cancer is to evaluate her worries, questions, concerns, beliefs, and reasons for seeking counseling to guarantee that personal needs and priorities will be met in the counseling process. It is important at this early stage of counseling to establish a mutual trust and to negotiate a mutually agreeable agenda between the counselor and the individual seeking counseling. The counselor attempts to assess whether the individual's expectations of cancer risk counseling are realistic. An exploration of the patient's current knowledge of genetics, beliefs about the causes of cancer, and experiences with cancer can help to guide and personalize the session and ensure the clinician tailors their information for the patient. Throughout the course of the counseling process, the potential for psychological impact should be assessed and addressed. This includes evaluating for depression or anxiety, patient coping mechanisms and resilience, and available support systems (see Table 9.2). If necessary, referrals to mental health-care professionals should be provided [63].

Family and Personal Health History

An expanded family pedigree that includes first-, second-, and third-degree relatives (parents, siblings, children, half-siblings, aunts, uncles, grandparents, cousins, etc.) using standard human pedigree nomenclature [74] begins the process of estimating cancer hereditary risks. Both maternal and paternal history should be evaluated for types of cancer, bilaterality, pathol-

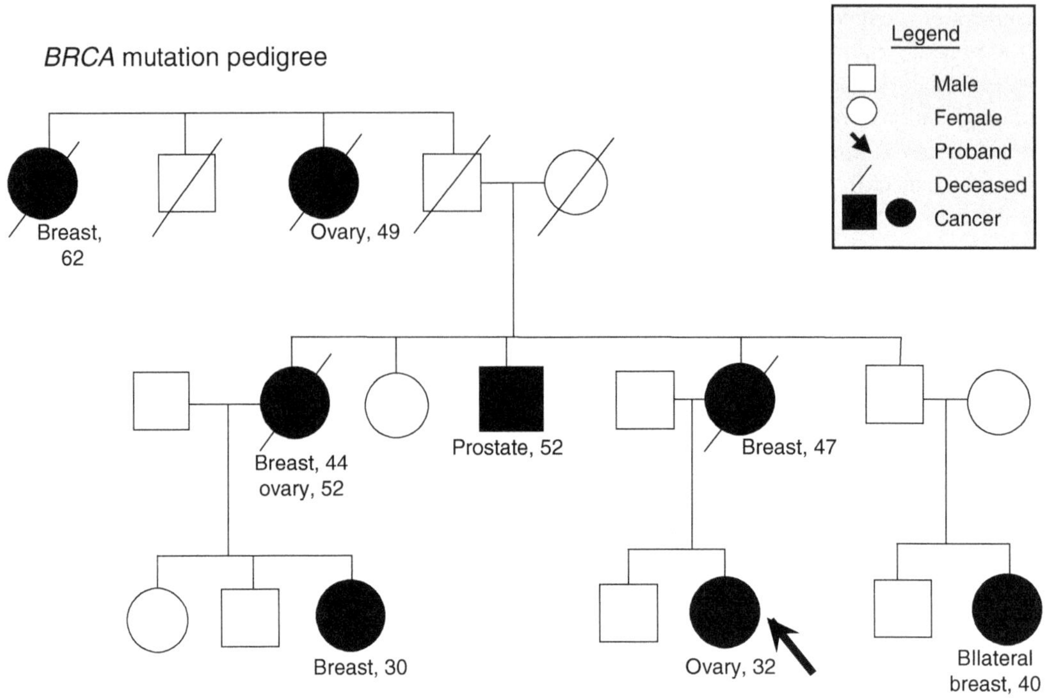

Fig. 9.6 *BRCA* mutation pedigree with standard nomenclature

ogy, ages at diagnosis and/or death, and history of risk-reducing steps, such as chemoprevention or surgeries [75]. Ancestry/ethnicity and consanguinity information are also important when calculating likelihood of a genetic risk, because specific mutations (i.e., founder mutations) occur with increased frequency in certain populations.

It is important to include all relatives, both affected and unaffected, in the family history in order to judge the degree of penetrance of the disease. In the case of hereditary breast cancer, it is also important to document cases of ovarian and other cancers in the family. Limitations to family history, such as small family size, unknown history and adoption, early deaths precluding the possibility of developing adult-onset diseases, prophylactic surgeries which remove an organ from subsequent risk of cancer, or few family members of the gender most affected by the cancer syndrome risks, e.g., few women in a family at risk for hereditary breast ovarian cancer (HBOC) syndrome, can challenge the clinician's ability to estimate hereditary risk [76]. Reported family histories may be inaccurate, and confirming documentation, such as pathology reports, should be obtained when possible [77, 78].

Family history data is then graphically represented on a pedigree, which follows standard nomenclature to illustrate family relationships and disease information in graphical format (Fig. 9.6). The hallmarks of features of a family history which suggest a hereditary pattern include multiple cancers in close relatives, multiple cancers in a single individual, multiple cancers across generations, early age of onset of cancer, bilateral cancer in paired organs (e.g., breast), the presence of precursor lesions known to be associated with the cancer phenotype, and ancestry [72] (see Table 9.3).

The patient's personal medical history should also be ascertained at this time, including prior medical conditions, cancer diagnoses, and treatments. Additional information about carcinogen exposure, reproductive history, hormone use, lifestyle factors, and previous breast biopsy history will influence estimates of cancer risk. A record of past cancer screening practices establishes a history of health promotion behavior and

Table 9.3 Features of hereditary cancers

Multiple cancers in close relatives
Multiple cancers in a single individual
Multiple cancers across generations
Early age of onset of cancer
Bilateral cancer in paired organs (e.g., breast)
The presence of precursor lesions known to be associated with the cancer phenotype (e.g., multiple polyps in hereditary colon cancer)

will help guide the counselor in making reasonable and appropriate health recommendations. Physical findings associated with a hereditary breast cancer syndrome can also be evaluated during the risk assessment session [75]. In the absence of a clinician qualified to evaluate physical features, appropriate referrals to specialists should be made, e.g., dermatologic assessment of features of Cowden syndrome [61]. Beyond the data obtained during the creation of the family tree, this process allows the clinician to assess the client's emotional state, become aware of family dynamics and level of support, and set the tone for the session [79]. This part of the session can also provide information about a patient's perception of risk, which may be influenced by cultural and ethnic identity, family interaction, personal experience with the condition, and spirituality [79].

Risk Communication

The objective of risk communication is to provide patients with accurate information to help them understand and interpret their risk in order to make informed decisions about genetic testing and/or medical management [63]. Risk communication is particularly challenging in cancer genetic counseling due to the sheer number of different risks being shared with the patient (see Table 9.4).

Care should be taken in presenting risk information so that patients are not confused about risk estimates. Presenting risk in a genetic counseling session is complicated not only by the diversity of risks discussed but by the frequent lack of straightforward values. There are various ways to present risk, such as numerical, verbal, or visual, as well as many types of values, such as percentages, proportions, or ranges. Often, more than one approach is necessary to fully inform the patient [80]. The counselor starts with what the patient knows, provides both qualitative and quantitative data, presents both sides of the risk figures, and stresses that these numbers do not guarantee outcome. Focusing on the most relevant facts and figures, keeping language simple, and using visual aids will increase patient comprehension [63, 79].

Table 9.4 Risk communication

Cancer risks based on family history alone
Cancer risks associated with carrying a gene mutation
Risk the patient or family will test positive for a hereditary cancer syndrome
Risk that other family members could carry the same genetic mutation if the patient tests positive
Risks, benefits, and limitations of genetic testing
Risks, benefits, and limitations of cancer surveillance and risk-reduction options
Risk of a de novo mutation in the absence of family history
Risk of receiving an unclear or inconclusive test result

Using the combination of family and personal medical history as a guide, the counselor then considers whether genetic testing is appropriate for the patient and which hereditary breast cancer syndrome is most likely. The majority of families will represent the effect of a combination of multiple genetic and environmental factors that interact to increase cancer risk to a moderate degree. Counselors often use empirical approaches based on epidemiologic data that provide age-specific risks of cancer that can incorporate several pertinent risk factors. For some cancers, these empirical data have been integrated into mathematical models that can predict cumulative risk estimates of developing a cancer over a defined time period.

The Gail model, for example, predicts breast cancer risk from age 35 to 80 years, using a model that includes current age, age at menarche, age at first live birth, number of first-degree relatives with breast cancer, and number of breast biopsies [81]. It has been validated with data from the Breast Cancer Prevention Trial [82] and is most accurate in predicting breast cancer among women who are being screened with regular mammograms [83]. This model is now available online from the National Cancer Institute [84].

Genetic Testing

For those families exhibiting the features of hereditary breast cancer, quantitative risk of carrying a *BRCA1* or *BRCA2* gene mutation can be found by utilizing BRCAPRO, Tyrer-Cuzick, or BOADICEA models. Penn II, a web-based model, and the Myriad prevalence tables also provide numerical probabilities of carrying a *BRCA1* or *BRCA2* mutation, while the Couch model only provides risk of carrying a mutation in the *BRCA1* gene [85–90]. Each has its own limitations, which have been reviewed in detail elsewhere [91, 92]. All of these models are used mainly as an adjunct to the information obtained from the family history.

Guidelines for testing have been established by several groups including the NCCN, ASCO, and the US Preventive Services Task Force (USPSTF) to identify families who are candidates for genetic testing. With these guidelines as a reference, the counselor presents the benefits of testing and confirms that the testing is voluntary and that the patient or her proxy can provide informed consent [72]. Once genetic testing has been deemed appropriate, the next step is identifying which test to order and for which family member. The most appropriate person to test is a family member affected by a syndrome-related cancer, preferably the one with the strongest suggestion of risk, such as early age of onset or bilaterality.

If affected family members are unavailable for testing, due to death or unwillingness, then unaffected family members can pursue testing [75]. Individuals under the age of 18 are generally not appropriate for genetic testing of hereditary breast cancer syndromes as medical management will not be influenced at these younger ages. Exceptions include families suggestive of cancer syndromes with known risks for cancers occurring in childhood, such as the Li-Fraumeni syndrome. Delaying genetic testing also allows the testing decision to be made by the individual at legal adulthood and with full autonomy [63, 93, 94].

Members of ethnic groups with known founder mutations, such as AJ individuals, should be offered testing for these founder mutations with the possibility of further testing of more rare mutations in the same or other genes if they meet additional guidelines [94]. It is important to note that, in the case of individuals of maternal and paternal AJ ancestry, testing for all three founder mutations is recommended even when one of these mutations have already been identified in the family [94]. This is due to the higher than average rate of these founder mutations occurring in this population [9].

Patients in families where a cancer syndrome gene mutation has already been identified should typically first be offered single-site analysis for the known gene mutation, with the possibility of additional mutation analysis only if the family history suggests the additional hereditary risk, e.g., a history on the opposite side of the family. For appropriate individuals with no previous testing in the family and no specific founder mutation testing indicated, genetic testing should include comprehensive DNA sequencing as well as genomic rearrangement, also called deletion/duplication analysis [79, 94].

Before making an informed decision about testing, patients must be aware of the possible outcomes associated with genetic testing. The NCCN divides genetic test results into four categories: true positive, true negative, indeterminate (uninformative negative), and inconclusive (variants of uncertain significance or VUS) (see Table 9.5). A positive test result indicates the presence of a pathogenic mutation known to increase the risk for cancer associated with the hereditary syndrome. Patients positive for a pathogenic mutation are generally given recommendations based on professional guidelines, such as NCCN and USPSTF [75, 95], which often include high-risk screening and risk-reduction options. First-degree relatives, i.e., children and siblings, are at 50 % risk of carrying the same mutation and are recommended to undergo genetic risk assessment and consider the option of testing for the known mutation. Additional rel-

Table 9.5 Types of genetic test results and their Implications

Result	Interpretation	Medical management	Family implications
True positive	Found to carry an alteration in a known cancer-predisposing gene	Follow hereditary risk guidelines outlined by professional groups such as NCCN and USPSTF	Recommend genetic risk assessment and testing of known alteration for at-risk family members
True negative	Not a carrier of a known alteration previously found in a family member	Follow general population recommendations and tailor based on personal risk factors	Recommend genetic risk assessment and testing of known alteration for at-risk family members
Indeterminate (uninformative negative)	No alteration is identified and none is known in another family member	Tailor based on personal and family history of cancer and known risk factors	Additional testing only for appropriate family members, particularly those affected by cancer
Inconclusive (variants of uncertain significance [VUS])	An alteration has been found but the clinical significance is currently unknown	Tailor based on personal and family history of cancer and known risk factors	Consider additional testing for appropriate family members on a research basis

atives may also be candidates for risk assessment and testing and should be informed of the mutation identified in the family. Family members are likely to have insurance coverage for single-site testing for the familial mutation, whether or not they are affected by cancer [72, 79].

Genetic test results can influence reproductive choices. A discussion of options regarding preimplantation genetic diagnosis (PGD), assisted reproduction, and prenatal testing is appropriate for patients who are concerned about the transmission of a mutation to their offspring [94]. Studies suggest that the majority of women at high risk of HBOC feel that PGD is an acceptable option to offer patients (75 %) even though fewer reported that they would consider PGD themselves (37.5 %) [96–97].

True-negative patients do not carry the previously identified familial mutation, and their risk for cancer is generally comparable with that of the general population. Medical management recommendations are similar to the general population or based on personal risk factors such as prior biopsy history [94, 98]. Patients should understand that an individual with a true-negative result can still develop cancer, and it does not rule out the possibility of the familial mutation being present in a sibling or other at-risk family members. However, the true-negative patient cannot pass the familial mutation on to his/her children [79].

An indeterminate result, also called uninformative negative, is one in which no mutation is identified within the genes tested. While an indeterminate result decreases the likelihood that a patient has an inherited risk for cancer, it does not remove this risk entirely due to the possibility of other genes not detectable by the current technology. Ideally, genetic testing should be performed on the family member deemed "most likely" to carry a gene mutation due to her personal history of early-onset, bilateral, or otherwise suggested cancer diagnosis. However, additional affected family members or first-degree relatives of an affected family member may produce informative test results [94]. Of note, patients with no mutation detected are not at risk for passing on a detectable mutation to their children. Indeterminate patients are often challenging to provide recommendations for, as their care should be individualized based on personal and family history [94]. In families strongly suggestive of a hereditary cancer syndrome, it is particularly important that a patient not be falsely reassured if no mutations are detected and informed that she may still be a candidate for additional high-risk screening or risk-reducing options [72, 79].

Variants of uncertain significance (VUS) are a particularly important limitation to genetic testing for which patients must be aware [79, 93]. A VUS is unable to be characterized as either a pathogenic mutation or a benign polymorphism that does not influence cancer risk, i.e., a VUS is neither positive nor negative. The ambiguous nature of these results can be confusing to patients, who may find it difficult to accept that a change within the gene might not increase the risk for cancer [99–100]. Patients who are making time-sensitive decisions regarding treatment and medical management may find these results particularly distressing and may even pursue unnecessary surgeries [93, 100, 101].

Given the challenge in interpreting a VUS result, medical management should be tailored based upon personal and medical history [73, 75, 79, 94, 100]. VUS results should not lead to clinical testing of other family members, unless the family member already meets criteria for genetic testing based on personal and family history. Testing of such family members may provide additional information including the possibility of discovering a previously unidentified deleterious mutation. Appropriate family members may be asked to contribute samples for research purposes that may or may not lead to clarification of the results [72, 79]. Studies have suggested that consultations with knowledgeable cancer risk providers can reduce adverse outcomes [99].

Prior to genetic testing, a patient should provide voluntary informed consent. Several states require informed consent be obtained before genetic tests can be ordered, with this responsibility falling upon the ordering clinician [72, 102]. Many molecular laboratories have informed consent documents and require a signature from the ordering clinician acknowledging that patients have been provided the necessary information and resources to give consent. Elements of informed consent have been reviewed in detail by ASCO [93]. The consent process should include a review of the specific test being performed; possible outcomes; the risks, benefits, and limitations of testing; implications for the patient and family members; alternatives to testing; and the plan for disclosure of results and follow-up [72]. Any remaining questions or concerns should be elicited and answered at this time.

Posttest Counseling

Disclosure of results can be complex whether they are positive, uninformative, or inconclusive as risks and recommendations need to be tailored for each individual and family. The plan for test result disclosure should be made in advance so the patient will know how results will be disclosed (face to face or by telephone), when to expect the results, and who will be present at the disclosure. Once the patient has confirmed that she is ready to hear the results, results disclosure should take place early in the conversation and with direct and clear language. The consultation should include explanation of the test results, modified risk assessment based on the results and family history, and a discussion of other family members who could consider further testing [72, 79].

Psychological assessment remains crucial throughout the disclosure session. Patients can have a variety of emotional responses, from relief, sadness, anger, or worry, and they should be given time to react and process the information [79]. While test results can illicit strong emotional reactions, studies have shown that patients who test positive tend to adjust well to the news and that additional interventions are often not necessary [63, 103]. Significant baseline depression, other life stressors, and results that are unexpected may contribute to greater distress [79] as can personal and family histories of cancer [104, 105].

It may be recommended that other family members undergo testing, either to help clarify the interpretation of the patient's results or because a mutation has been identified and other family members are at risk to carry the same alteration. In the case of a known mutation, it is particularly important to educate the patient on the importance of sharing these results with at-risk family members. The clinician can help to facilitate family communications with educational materials and referrals that the patient can then pass on to relatives. In addition to an explanation of the results and implications for family members, patients will need to receive tailored medical management recommendations.

Patients with an indeterminate or inconclusive test result may still have elevated risks for cancer and should receive screening and prevention recommendations based on their personal and family history of cancer and other risk factors [94]. Additional genetic testing may be recommended, as needed. Patients who are found to carry a pathogenic mutation can be provided medical management guidelines from consensus statements such as NCCN, American Cancer Society (ACS), and USPSTF [79]. Once tailored medical management is reviewed for the patient and at-risk family members, the patient should be provided with referrals to specialists, copies of genetic test results, and a summary document of results and recommendations [79].

Effectiveness of Cancer Risk Counseling

Several studies have attempted to assess the effectiveness and efficacy of genetic counseling. Utilization of genetic counseling services is associated with higher socioeconomic status and educational level and, in the setting of prenatal genetic conditions, with intention to have children [106]. Understanding and retention of the information received have been found to be higher among individuals who are self-referred, those with higher educational levels, and those families at higher-risk levels. Multiple counseling sessions have been shown to boost understanding and information retention [107]. Another consistent observation has been that while important, the information obtained at a genetic counseling session is not the only factor contributing to risk-related decisions. Rather, perception of risk is a concept formed over a person's lifetime and is a result of internalizing personal experiences and beliefs. Decisions made in the genetic counseling setting therefore reflect a complicated interplay of expectations, emotions, and value judgments. As a result, the genetic counselor is likely to be most successful when the information shared during genetic counseling is provided in the context of the patient's personal orientation and belief system.

Risk Management Strategies

A primary motivation for seeking cancer risk counseling is to identify ways to reduce or delay the risk of developing breast/ovarian cancer or to improve the possibility of detecting it at an early curable stage. Individuals who seek these services clearly want recommendations for the medical management of their risk from their providers. By achieving a reliable estimate of cancer risk, either by considering personal and family history or by performing genetic testing, the cancer risk counselor, working with the medical team, can provide primary and secondary prevention strategies to the individual. Recommendations fall into four general categories: increased screening, pharmacologic interventions (chemoprevention), surgical prophylaxis, and lifestyle changes.

Screening recommendations for women with a hereditary breast cancer syndrome are based on the high risk of breast cancer and the potential for early age of onset. For these women, screening is recommended to start at age 25 years. The sensitivity of mammography is reduced in young women who tend to have denser breasts. Several studies of women with *BRCA1/2* mutations have shown an improved detection rate when both MRI and mammograms are performed annually [108]. On the basis of this data, the ACS has recommended the addition of breast MRI to annual mammogram for women who are carriers of breast cancer susceptibility genes and/or those with a risk of breast cancer of 20–25% or greater, as determined by an empiric risk model that is based on family history [109]. Men with a *BRCA1/2* mutation are recommended to perform breast self-exam and to have a clinical breast exam twice yearly. To date, there is no effective screening modality to detect early stage ovarian cancer.

Based on randomized control clinical trials showing a 50 % reduction in ER+ breast cancer with a 5-year course of either tamoxifen or raloxifene [110, 111], both drugs have been approved by the Food and Drug Administration (FDA) for the prevention of breast cancer among women at increased risk of breast cancer as determined by the Gail model. However, there have not been any such trials that have looked at the efficacy of these drugs specifically among women with *BRCA1/2* mutations. A thorough discussion with the patient is crucial for them to understand their risks and potential benefits of such therapy in light of a clear lack of convincing data. Long-term use of oral contraceptives has been shown in retrospective case-control studies to reduce the risk of ovarian cancer by 40–50%. This protection has been demonstrated in both average-risk women and women with a *BRCA1/2* mutation and increases with longer duration of use [112].

Risk-reducing mastectomy (RRM) has been shown to reduce the risk of breast cancer in *BRCA1/2*-positive women by up to 90 % [113]. Patient agreeance of this option depends upon many factors, such as ethnicity and culture, geography, health-care availability, and most importantly the recommendations of the providing physician. Mutation carriers newly diagnosed with breast cancer are the most likely group to choose this option given the high rate of subsequent contralateral cancer. A variety of options for breast reconstruction are available in this setting for women choosing RRM.

Due to the lack of effective screening tools for identifying ovarian cancer, women with a *BRCA1/2* mutation are recommended to undergo risk-reducing salpingo-oophorectomy (RRSO) after childbearing is complete or at age 35–40 years old [75]. A meta-analysis of ten studies showed that RRSO among mutation carriers resulted in an 80 % reduction in the risk of ovarian cancer [114]. Occult cancers, primarily in the fallopian tubes, have been found at the time of prophylactic oophorectomy in 2–3% of women undergoing the procedure. In addition, there is a 1–4.3 % risk of subsequent primary peritoneal carcinoma [114, 115].

The introduction of RRSO for prophylaxis among mutation carriers has led to a new understanding of the origin of ovarian cancer. Careful histopathologic examination of the fallopian tubes removed at the time of RRSO has identified a high percentage of dysplastic and hyperplastic lesions that are thought to represent premalignant changes in the fimbriated end of the fallopian tube. As a result, there is a growing consensus that the origin of most, if not all, serous ovarian tumors among *BRCA1/2* mutation carriers is the distal segment of the fallopian tube, not the surface epithelium of the ovary [116, 117]. Serious consideration is being given to performing bilateral salpingectomy as an interim measure to preserve ovarian function until the time of natural menopause [118].

RRSO also reduces the risk of breast cancer by approximately 50 % [27, 117]. In addition to reducing the risk of breast/ovarian cancer, there is evidence that both prophylactic mastectomy and prophylactic oophorectomy confer an overall survival advantage [119].

There is intense interest on the part of high-risk individuals to learn about opportunities to reduce their cancer risk by changes in diet, exercise, or other lifestyle modifications that may minimize their exposure to carcinogens. Preliminary data suggests, for instance, that the use of exogenous estrogens, including oral contraceptives and estrogen replacement, may confer an increased risk for breast cancer among women with a hereditary predisposition [120] and that limiting exposure to these agents may be beneficial. The exact role of diet and exercise remains elusive for most cancers although recommendations can be made on the basis of general health and ideal weight maintenance.

Conclusion

A great deal of progress has been made in our understanding of the underlying etiology of breast cancer. Scientific advances, particularly in the field of genetics, have made it possible to better define risk for ovarian cancer and to target cancer prevention and control strategies. Long-term follow-up of mutation carriers will help to explore the spectrum of cancer risk, the clinical course of hereditary ovarian cancer, and response to treatment. Women are becoming increasingly aware of the role of family history in defining their own personal risk and are seeking information and recommendations for risk reduction. The creation of multidisciplinary teams of health professionals to provide risk education, assessment, and counseling will complement the care of the ovarian cancer patient and may ultimately result in reductions in breast cancer morbidity and mortality.

References

1. Jemal A, Bray F, Center MM, Ferlay J, Ward E, Forman D. Global cancer statistics. CA Cancer J Clin. 2011;61:69–90.
2. Siegel R, Naishadham D, Jemal A. Cancer Statistics, 2013. CA Cancer J Clin. 2013;63:11–30.
3. Jemal A, Dimard EP, Dorell C, Noone A, Markowitz LE, Kohler B, et al. Annual report to the nation on the status of cancer, 1975–2009, featuring the burden and trends in human papillomavirus (HPV)-associated cancers and HPV vaccination coverage levels. JNCI. 2013;105(3):175–201.
4. DeSantis C, Siegel R, Bandi P, Jemal A. Breast cancer statistics, 2011. CA Cancer J Clin. 2011;61:409–18.
5. Howlader N, Noone AM, Krapcho M, Neyman N, Aminou R, Altekruse SF, et al. SEER cancer statistics review, 1975–2009 (Vintage 2009 Populations). Bethesda: National Cancer Institute; 2012. http://seer.cancer.gov/csr/1975_2009_pops09/, based on November 2011 SEER data submission, posted to the SEER web site.
6. Anderson WF, Pfeiffer RM, Dores GM, Sherman ME. Comparison of age distribution patterns for different histopathologic types of breast carcinoma. Cancer Epidemiol Biomarkers Prev. 2006;15(10):1899–905.
7. De La Rochefordiere A, Asselain B, Campana F, Scholl S, Fenton J, Vilcoq J, et al. Age as prognostic factor in premenopausal breast carcinoma. Lancet. 1993;341(8852):1039–43.
8. Winchester D, Osteen R, Menck H. The national cancer data base report on breast carcinoma characteristics and outcome in relation to age. Cancer. 1996;78:1838–43.
9. Struewing JP, Hartge P, Wacholder S, Baker SM, Berlin M, McAdams M, et al. The risk of cancer associated with specific mutations of *BRCA1* and *BRCA2* among Ashkenazi Jews. N Engl J Med. 1997;336:1401–8.
10. Ferlay J, Shin HR, Bray F, Forman D, Mathers C, Parkin DM. GLOBOCAN 2008 v2.0, cancer incidence and mortality worldwide: IARC cancer base no. 10 [Internet]. Lyon: International Agency for Research on Cancer; 2010. Available from: http://globocan.iarc.fr.
11. Berg J. Clinical implications of risk factors for breast cancer. Cancer. 1984;53:589–91. 2013;(2):155–63.
12. Dupont W, Page D. Breast cancer risk associated with proliferative disease, age at first birth, and a family history of breast cancer. Am J Epidemiol. 1987;125:769–79.
13. Dupont W, Page D, Parl D, Vneneak-Jones C, Plummer W, Rados M, et al. Long-term risk of breast cancer in women with fibroadenomas. NEJM. 1994;331:10–5.
14. Jensen RA, Page DL, Dupont WD, Rogers LW. Invasive breast cancer risk in women with sclerosing adenosis. Cancer. 1989;64(10):1977–83.
15. Marshall L, Hunter D, Connolly J, Schnitt S, Byrne C, London S, et al. Risk of breast cancer associated with atypical hyperplasia of lobular and ductal types. Cancer Epidemiol Biomarkers Prev. 1997;6:297–301.
16. Osborne M, Hoda S. Current management of lobular carcinoma in situ of the breast. Oncology. 1994;8(2):45–9.
17. Hutter R. Lobular carcinoma in situ. CA Cancer J Clin. 1982;32(4):231–2.
18. Bodian C, Perzin K, Lattes R. Lobular neoplasia, long term risk of breast cancer and relation to other factors. Cancer. 1996;78:1024–34.
19. Boyd NF, Rommens JM, Vogt K, Lee V, Hopper JL, Yaffe MJ, et al. Mammographic breast density as an intermediate phenotype for breast cancer. Lancet Oncol. 2005;6:798–808.
20. McCormack VA, dos Santos Silva I. Breast density and parenchymal patterns as markers of breast cancer risk: a meta-analysis. Cancer Epidemiol Biomarkers Prev. 2006;15(6):1159–69.
21. Boyd NF, Melnichouk O, Martin LJ, Hislop G, Chiarelli AM, Yaffe MJ, et al. Mammographic density, response to hormones, and breast cancer risk. J Clin Oncol. 2011;29:2985–92.
22. Kerlikowske K, Cook AJ, Buist DSM, Cummings SR, Vachon C, Vacek P, et al. Breast cancer risk by breast density, menopause, and postmenopausal hormone therapy use. J Clin Oncol. 2010;28:3830–7.
23. Dearth RK, Delgado DA, Hiney JK, Pathiraja T, Oesterreich S, Medina D, et al. Parity-induced decrease in systemic growth hormone alters mammary gland signaling: a potential role in pregnancy protection from breast cancer. Cancer Prev Res. 2010;3(3):312–21.
24. Collaborative Group on Hormonal Factors in Breast Cancer. Breast cancer and breastfeeding: collaborative reanalysis of individual data from 47 epidemiological studies in 30 countries, including 50,302 women with breast cancer and 96,973 women without the disease. Lancet. 2002;360(9328):187–95.
25. Russo J, Balogh GA, Russo IH. Full-term pregnancy induces a specific genomic signature in the human breast. Cancer Epidemiol Biomarkers Prev. 2008;17(1):51–66.
26. Titus-Ernstoff L, Longnecker MP, Newcomb PA, Dain B, Greenberg ER, Mittendorf R, et al. Menstrual factors in relation to breast cancer risk. Cancer Epidemiol Biomarkers Prev. 1998;7:783–9.
27. Eisen A, Lubinski J, Klijn J, Moller P, Lynch HT, Offit K, et al. Breast cancer risk following bilateral oophorectomy in BRCA1 and BRCA2 mutation carriers: an international case-control study. J Clin Oncol. 2005;23:7491–6.
28. Chlebowski RT, Anderson GL, Gass M, Lane DS, Aragaki AK, Kuller LH, et al. Estrogen plus proges-

tin and breast cancer incidence and mortality in postmenopausal women. JAMA. 2010;304(15):1684–92.
29. Russo IH, Russo J. Hormonal approach to breast cancer prevention. J Cell Biochem Suppl. 2000;34:1–6.
30. Russo IH, Russo J. Pregnancy-induced changes in breast cancer risk. J Mammary Gland Biol Neoplasia. 2011;16(3):221–33.
31. Linet MS, Slovis TL, Miller DL, Kleinerman R, Lee C, Rajaraman P, et al. Cancer risks associated with external radiation from diagnostic imaging procedures. CA Cancer J Clin. 2012;62:75–100.
32. Adams MJ, Dozier A, Shore RE, Lipshultz SE, Schwartz RG, Constine LS, et al. Breast cancer risk 55+ years after irradiation for an enlarged thymus and its implications for early childhood medical irradiation today. Epidemiol Biomark Prev. 2010;19(1):48–58.
33. Elkin EB, Klem ML, Gonzales AM, Ishill NM, Hodgson D, Ng AK, et al. Characteristics and outcomes of breast cancer in women with and without a history of radiation for Hodgkin's lymphoma: a multi-institutional, matched cohort study. J Clin Oncol. 2011;29:2466–73.
34. Travis LB, Hill D, Dpres GM, Gospodarowicz M, van Leeuwen FE, Holowaty E, et al. Cumulative absolute breast cancer risk for young women treated for Hodgkin lymphoma. J Natl Cancer Inst. 2005;97:1428–37.
35. Bernstein L, Patel AV, Ursin G, Sullivan-Halley J, Press MF, Deapen D, et al. Lifetime recreational exercise activity and breast cancer risk among black women and white women. J Natl Cancer Inst. 2005;97:1671–9.
36. Dallal CM, Sullivan-Halley J, Ross RK, Wang Y, Deapen D, Horn-Ross PL, et al. Long-term recreational physical activity and risk of invasive and in situ breast cancer. The California Teachers Study. Arch Intern Med. 2007;167:408–15.
37. Chlebowski RT, Pettinger M, Stefanick ML, Howard BV, Mossavar-Rahmani Y, McTiernan A. Insulin, physical activity, and caloric intake in postmenopausal women: breast cancer implications. J Clin Oncol. 2004;22:4507–13.
38. McTiernan A, Tworoger SS, Ulrich CM, Yasui Y, Irwin ML, Rajan KB, et al. Effect of exercise on serum estrogens in postmenopausal women: a 12-month randomized clinical trial. Cancer Res. 2004;64:2923–8.
39. Zhu K, Caulfield J, Hunter S, Roland CL, Payne-Wilds K, Texter L. Body mass index and breast cancer risk in African American women. Ann Epidemiol. 2005;15:123–8.
40. Ziegler RG, Hoover RN, Nomura AMY, West DW, Wu AH, Pike MC, et al. Relative weight, weight change, height, and breast cancer risk in Asian-American women. J Natl Cancer Inst. 1966;88:650–60.
41. Hursting SD, DiGiovanni J, Dannenberg AJ, Azrad M, LeRoith D, Demark-Wahnefried W, et al. Obesity, energy balance, and cancer: new opportunities for prevention. Cancer Prev Res. 2012;5(11):1260–72.
42. Terry MB, Zhang FF, Kabat G, Britton JA, Teitelbaum SL, Neugut AI, et al. Lifetime alcohol intake and breast cancer risk. Ann Epidemiol. 2006;16:230–40.
43. Zhang SM, Lee IM, Manson JE, Cook NR, Willett WC, Buring JE. Alcohol consumption and breast cancer risk in the Women's Health Study. Am J Epidemiol. 2007;165:667–76.
44. Collaborative Group on Hormonal Factors in Breast Cancer. Alcohol, tobacco and breast cancer-collaborative reanalysis of individual data from 53 epidemiological studies, including 58,515 women with breast cancer and 95,067 women without the disease. Br J Cancer. 2002;87:1234–45.
45. Deandrea S, Talamini R, Foschi R, Montella M, Dal Maso L, Falcini F, et al. Alcohol and breast cancer risk defined by estrogen and progesterone receptor status in a case-control study. Cancer Epidemiol Biomarkers Prev. 2008;17(8):2025–8.
46. Horn-Ross PL, Canchola AJ, Bernstein L, Clarke CA, Lacey JV, Neuhausen SL, et al. Alcohol consumption and breast cancer risk among postmenopausal women following the cessation of hormone therapy use: the California Teachers Study. Cancer Epidemiol Biomarkers Prev. 2012;21(11):2006–13.
47. Li CI, Chlebowski RT, Freiberg M, Johnson KC, Kuller L, Lane D, et al. Alcohol consumption and risk of postmenopausal breast cancer by subtype: the Women's Health Initiative Observational Study. JNCI. 2010;102(18):1422–31.
48. Brooks PJ, Zakhari S. Moderate alcohol consumption and breast cancer in women: from epidemiology to mechanisms and interventions. Alcohol Clin Exp Res. 2013;1:23–30.
49. Venkitaraman AR. Cancer susceptibility and the functions of BRCA1 and BRCA2. Cell. 2002;108(2):171–82.
50. King MC, Marks JH, Mandell JB, New York Breast Cancer Study Group. Breast and ovarian cancer risks due to inherited mutations in BRCA1 and BRCA2. Science. 2003;302(5645):643–66.
51. Antoniou A, Pharoah PD, Narod S, Risch HA, Eyfjord JE, Hopper JL, et al. Average risks of breast and ovarian cancer associated with *BRCA1* or *BRCA2* mutations detected in case series unselected for family history: a combined analysis of 22 studies. Am J Hum Genet. 2003;72(5):1117–30.
52. Chen S, Parmigiani G. Meta-analysis of *BRCA1* and *BRCA2* penetrance. J Clin Oncol. 2007;25:1329–33.
53. Graeser MK, Engel C, Rhiem K, Gadzicki D, Bick U, Kast K, et al. Contralateral breast cancer risk in BRCA1 and BRCA2 mutation carriers. J Clin Oncol. 2009;27:5887–92.
54. Lakhani SR, Van de Vijver MJ, Jacquemier J, Anderson TU, Osin PP, McGuffog L, et al. The pathology of familial breast cancer: predictive value of immunohistochemical markers estrogen receptor, progesterone receptor, HER-2, and p53 in patients with mutations in BRCA1 and BRCA2. J Clin Oncol. 2002;20(9):2310–8.
55. Lee E, McKean-Cowdin R, Ma H, Spicer DV, Van Den Berg D, Bernstein L, et al. Characteristics of triple-negative breast cancer in patients with a BRCA1 mutation: results from a population-based study of young women. J Clin Oncol. 2011;29(33):4373–80.

56. Mavaddat N, Barrowdale D, Andrulis IL, Domchek SM, Ecceles D, Nevanlina H, et al. Pathology of breast and ovarian cancers among BRCA1 and BRCA2 mutation carriers: results from the Consortium of Investigators of Modifiers of BRCA1/2 (CIMBA). Cancer Epidemiol Biomarkers Prev. 2012;21(1):134–47.
57. Gonzales-Angulo AM, Timms KM, Liu S, Chen H, Litton JK, Potter J, et al. Incidence and outcome of BRCA mutations in unselected patients with triple receptor-negative breast cancer. Clin Cancer Res. 2011;17(5):1082–9.
58. Chrompret A, Abel A, Stoppa-Lyonnet D, Brugieres L, Pages S, Feunteun J, Bonaiti-Pellie C. Sensitivity and predictive value of criteria for p53 germline mutation screening. J Med Genet. 2001;38:43–7.
59. Hisada MM, Garger JE, Fung CY, Fraumeni Jr JF, Li FP. Multiple primary cancers in families with Li-Fraumeni syndrome. J Natl Cancer Inst. 1998;90(8):606–11.
60. Gonzalez KD, Noltner KA, Buzin CH, Gu D, Wen-Fong CY, Nguyen VQ, et al. Beyond Li Fraumeni syndrome: clinical characteristics of families with p53 mutations. J Clin Oncol. 2009;27(8):1250–6.
61. Pilarski R. Cowden syndrome: a critical review of the clinical literature. J Genet Couns. 2009;18(1):13–27.
62. Jeghers H, McKusick VA, Katz KH. Generalized intestinal polyposis and melanin spots of the oral mucosa, lips and digits: a syndrome of diagnostic significance. N Engl J Med. 1949;241(25):993–1005.
63. National Cancer Institute. PDQ® genetics of breast and ovarian cancer. Bethesda: National Cancer Institute. 24 May 2013. Available at: http://cancer.gov/cancertopics/pdq/genetics/breast-and-ovarian/HealthProfessional
64. Hearle N, Schumacher V, Menko FH, Olschwang S, Boardman LA, Gille JJ, et al. Frequency and spectrum of cancers in the Peutz-Jeghers syndrome. Clin Cancer Res. 2006;12(10):3209–15.
65. Lim W, Hearle N, Shah B, Murday V, Hodgson SV, Lucassen A, et al. Further observations on LKB1/STK11 status and cancer risk in Peutz-Jeghers syndrome. Br J Cancer. 2003;89:308–13.
66. Young RH. Sex cord-stromal tumors of the ovary and testis: their similarities and differences with consideration of selected problems. Mod Pathol. 2005;18 Suppl 2:S81–98.
67. Aretz S, Stienen D, Uhlhaas S, et al. High proportion of large genomic STKI11 deletions in Peutz-Jehers syndrome. Hum Mutat. 2005;26(6):513–9.
68. Pharoah PD, Guilford P, Caldas C. Incidence of gastric cancer and breast cancer in CDH1 (E-cadherin) mutation carriers from hereditary diffuse gastric cancer families. Gastroenterology. 2001;121:1348–53.
69. Fitzgerald RC, Hardwick R, Huntsman D, Carneiro F, Guilford P, International Gastric Cancer Linkage Consortium. Hereditary diffuse gastric cancer: updated consensus guidelines for clinical management and directions for future research. J Med Genet. 2010;47:436–44.
70. McColl KE. Cancer of the gastric cardia. Best Pract Res Clin Gastroenterol. 2006;20:687–96.
71. National Society of Genetic Counselors' Definition Task Force, Resta R, Biesecker BB, Bennett RL, Blum S, Hahn SE, et al. A new definition of genetic counseling: National Society of Genetic Counselors' Task Force report. J Genet Couns. 2006;15(2):77–83.
72. Riley BD, Culver JO, Skrzynia C, Senter LA, Peters JA, Costalas JW, et al. Essential elements of genetic cancer risk assessment, counseling, and testing: updated recommendations of the National Society of Genetic Counselors. J Genet Couns. 2012;21(2):151–61.
73. Berliner JL, Fay AM, Cummings SA, Burnett B, Tillmanns T. NSGC practice guideline: risk assessment and genetic counseling for hereditary breast and ovarian cancer. J Genet Couns. 2013;2:155–63.
74. Bennett RL, French KS, Resta RG, Doyle DL. Standardized human pedigree nomenclature: update and assessment of the recommendations of the National Society of Genetic Counselors. J Genet Couns. 2008;17(5):424–33.
75. National Comprehensive Cancer Network. NCCN clinical practice guidelines in oncology, genetic/familial high risk assessment: breast and ovarian (version 1.2013). 2013. Available from: http://www.nccn.org/professionals/physician_gls/pdf/genetics_screening.pdf
76. Weitzel JN, Lagos VI, Cullinane CA, Gambol PJ, Culver JO, Blazer KR, et al. Limited family structure and BRCA gene mutation status in single cases of breast cancer. JAMA. 2007;297(23):2587–95.
77. Mai PL, Garceau AO, Graubard BI, Dunn M, McNeel TS, Gonsalves L, et al. Confirmation of family cancer history reported in a population-based survey. J Natl Cancer Inst. 2011;103(10):788–97.
78. Sijmons RH, Boonstra AE, Reefhuis J, Hordijk-Hos JM, de Walle HE, Oosterwijk JC, et al. Accuracy of family history of cancer: clinical genetic implications. Eur J Hum Genet. 2000;8(3):181–6.
79. Schneider KA. Counseling about cancer: strategies for genetic counseling. 3rd ed. Hoboken: Wiley-Blackwell; 2012.
80. Lipkus IM. Numeric, verbal, and visual formats of conveying health risks: suggested best practices and future recommendations. Med Dec Making. 2007;27(5):696–713.
81. Gail MH, Brinton LA, Byar DP, Corle DK, Green SB, Schairer C, et al. Projecting individualized probabilities of developing breast cancer for white females who are being examined annually. J Natl Cancer Inst. 1989;81(24):1879–86.
82. Costantino JP, Gail MH, Pee D, Anderson S, Redmond S, Benichou J, et al. Validation studies for models projecting the risk of invasive and total breast cancer incidence. J Natl Cancer Inst. 1999;91(18):1541–8.
83. Hoskins KF, Stopfer JE, Calzone KA, Merajver SD, Rebbeck TR, Garber JE, et al. Assessment and counseling for women with a family history of breast cancer. A guide for clinicians. JAMA. 1995;273(7):577–85.
84. National Cancer Institute. Breast cancer risk assessment tool. http://www.cancer.gov/bcrisktool/

85. Antoniou AC, Cunningham AP, Peto J, Evans DG, Lalloo F, Narod SA, et al. The BOADICEA model of genetic susceptibility to breast and ovarian cancers: updates and extensions. Br J Cancer. 2008;98(9):1457–66.
86. Couch FJ, DeShano ML, Blackwood MA, Calzone K, Stopfer J, Campeau L, et al. BRCA1 mutations in women attending clinics that evaluate the risk of breast cancer. N Engl J Med. 1997;336(20):1409–15.
87. Frank TS. Hereditary risk of breast and ovarian carcinoma: the role of the oncologist. Oncologist. 1998;3(6):403–12.
88. Lindor NM, Johnson KJ, Harvey H, Shane Pankratz V, Domchek SM, Hunt K, et al. Predicting BRCA1 and BRCA2 gene mutation carriers: comparison of PENN II model to previous study. Fam Cancer. 2010;9(4):495–502.
89. Parmigiani G, Berry D, Aguilar O. Determining carrier probabilities for breast cancer-susceptibility genes BRCA1 and BRCA2. Am J Hum Genet. 1998;62(1):145–58.
90. Tyrer J, Duffy SW, Cuzick J. A breast cancer prediction model incorporating familial and personal risk factors. Stat Med. 2004;23(7):1111–30.
91. Amir E, Freedman OC, Seruga B, Evans DG. Assessing women at high risk of breast cancer: a review of risk assessment models. J Natl Cancer Inst. 2010;102(10):680–91.
92. Culver J, Lowstuter K, Bowling L. Assessing breast cancer risk and BRCA1/2 carrier probability [review]. Breast Dis. 2006–2007;27:5–20.
93. American Society of Clinical Oncology. Policy statement update: genetic and genomic testing for cancer susceptibility. J Clin Oncol. 2010;28(5):893–901.
94. National Comprehensive Cancer Network. NCCN clinical practice guidelines in oncology, breast cancer screening and diagnosis (version 1.2013). 2013. Available from: http://www.nccn.org/professionals/physician_gls/pdf/breast-screening.pdf
95. United States Preventive Services Task Force (USPSTF). Genetic risk assessment and BRCA mutation testing for breast and ovarian cancer susceptibility: recommendation statement. Ann Intern Med. 2005;143(5):355–61.
96. Menon U, Harper J, Sharma A, Fraser L, Burnell M, ElMasry K, et al. Views of BRCA gene mutation carriers on preimplantation genetic diagnosis as a reproductive option for hereditary breast and ovarian cancer. Hum Reprod. 2007;22(6):1573–7.
97. Quinn G, Vadaparampil S, Wilson C, King L, Choi J, Miree C, et al. Attitudes of high-risk women toward preimplantation genetic diagnosis. Fertil Steril. 2009;91(6):2361–8.
98. Domchek SM, Gaudet MM, Stopfer JE, Fleischaut MH, Powers J, Kauff N, et al. Breast cancer risks in individuals testing negative for a known family mutation in BRCA1 or BRCA2. Breast Cancer Res Treat. 2010;119(2):409–14.
99. Culver J, Brinkerhoff C, Clague J, Yang K, Singh K, Sand S, et al. Variants of uncertain significance in BRCA testing: evaluation of surgical decisions, risk perception, and cancer distress. J Clin Genet. 2013. doi:10.1111/cge.12097.
100. Murray ML, Cerrato F, Bennett RL, Jarvik GP. Follow-up of carriers of BRCA1 and BRCA2 variants of unknown significance: variant reclassification and surgical decisions. Genet Med. 2011;13(12):998–1005.
101. Brierley KL, Campfield D, Ducaine W, Dohany L, Donenberg T, Shannon K, et al. Errors in delivery of cancer genetics services: implications for practice. Conn Med. 2010;7:413–23.
102. Centers for Disease Control and Prevention. Good laboratory practices for molecular genetic testing for heritable diseases and conditions. MMWR. 2009;58(RR-6):9.
103. Schwartz MD, Peshkin BN, Hughes C, Main D, Isaacs C, Lerman C. Impact of BRCA1/BRCA2 mutation testing on psychologic distress in a clinic-based sample. J Clin Oncol. 2002;20(2):514–20.
104. Hamann HA, Somers TJ, Smith AW, Inslicht SS, Baum A. Posttraumatic stress associated with cancer history and BRCA1/2 genetic testing. Psychosom Med. 2005;67(5):766–72.
105. van Roosmale MS, Stalmeier PF, Verhoef LC, Hoekstra-Weebers JE, Oosterwijk JC, Hoogerbrugge N, et al. Impact of BRCA1/2 testing and disclosure of a positive test result on women affected and unaffected with breast or ovarian cancer. Am J Med Genet. 2004;124A(4):346–55.
106. Tambor E, Bernhardt B, Chase G, Faden R, Geller G, Hofman K, et al. Offering cystic fibrosis carrier screening to an HMO population: factors associated with utilization. Am J Hum Genet. 1994;55:626–37.
107. Evers-Kiebooms, van den Berghe H. Impact of genetic counseling: a review of published follow-up studies. Clin Genet. 1979;15:465–74.
108. Lord SJ, Wei W, Craft P, Cawson JN, Morris I, Walleser S, et al. A systematic review of the effectiveness of magnetic resonance imaging (MRI) as an addition to mammography and ultrasound in screening young women at high risk of breast cancer. Eur J Cancer. 2007;43(13):1905–17.
109. Saslow D, Boetes C, Burke W, Harms S, Leach MO, Lehman CD, American Cancer Society Breast Cancer Advisory Group, et al. American Cancer Society guidelines for breast screening with MRI as an adjunct to mammography. Cancer J Clin. 2007;57(2):75–89.
110. Fisher B, Costantino JP, Wickerham DL, Redmond CK, Kavanah M, Cronin WM, et al. Tamoxifen for prevention of breast cancer: report of the National Surgical Adjuvant Breast and Bowel Project P-1 Study. J Natl Cancer Inst. 1998;90(18):1371–88.
111. Vogel VG, Costantino JP, Wickerham DL, Cronin WM, Cecchini RS, Atkins JN, et al. Effects of tamoxifen vs raloxifene on the risk of developing

invasive breast cancer and other disease outcomes: the NSABP Study of Tamoxifen and Raloxifene (STAR) P-2 trial. JAMA. 2006;295(23):2727–51.
112. Iodice S, Barile M, Rotmensz N, Feroce I, Bonanni B, Radice P, et al. Oral contraceptive use and breast or ovarian cancer risk in BRCA1/2 carriers: a meta-analysis. Eur J Cancer. 2010;46(12):2275–84.
113. Rebbeck TR, Friebel T, Lynch HT, Neuhausen SL, van't Veer L, Garber JE, et al. Bilateral prophylactic mastectomy reduces breast cancer risk in BRCA1 and BRCA2 mutation carriers: the PROSE Study Group. J Clin Oncol. 2004;22:1055–62.
114. Rebbeck TR, Kauff ND, Domchek SM. Meta-analysis of risk reduction estimates associated with risk-reducing salpingo-oophorectomy in BRCA1 and BRCA2 carriers. J Natl Cancer Inst. 2009;101:80–7.
115. Evans DGR, Clayton R, Donnai P, Shenton A, Lalloo F. Risk-reducing surgery for ovarian cancer: outcomes in 300 surgeries suggest a low peritoneal primary risk. Eur J Cancer. 2009;17:1381–5.
116. Reitsma W, de Bock GH, Oosterwijk JC, Bart J, Hollema H, Mourits MJE. Support of the fallopian tube hypothesis' in a prospective series of risk-reducing salpingo-oophorectomy specimens. Eur J Cancer. 2013;49:132–41.
117. Medeiros F, Muto MG, Lee Y, Elvin JA, Callahan MJ, Feltmate C, et al. The tubal fimbria is a preferred site for early adenocarcinoma in women with familial ovarian cancer syndrome. Am J Surg Pathol. 2006;30(2):230–6.
118. Greene MH, Mai PL, Schwartz PE. Does bilateral salpingectomy with ovarian retention warrant consideration as a temporary bridge to risk-reducing bilateral oophorectomy in BRCA1/2 mutation carriers? Am J Obstet Gynecol. 2011;204(1):19, e1–6.
119. Domchek SM, Friebel TM, Singer CF, Evans DG, Lynch HT, Isaacs C, et al. Association of risk-reducing surgery in BRCA1 or BRCA2 mutation carriers with cancer risk and mortality. JAMA. 2010;304(9):967–75.
120. Ursin G, Henderson BE, Halle RW, Pike MC, Zhou N, Diep A, et al. Does oral contraceptive use increase the risk of breast cancer in women with BRCA1/BRCA2 mutations more than in other women? Cancer Res. 1997;57(17):1678–81.

10 Lobular Neoplasia: Atypical Lobular Hyperplasia and Lobular Carcinoma In Situ

Miraj G. Shah-Khan and James W. Jakub

Lobular Neoplasia

Introduction

Lobular neoplasia (LN) refers to the spectrum of benign epithelial proliferation including atypical lobular hyperplasia (ALH) and lobular carcinoma in situ (LCIS) [1]. It is usually an incidental finding noted at the time of needle or excisional biopsy and lacks distinctive features on imaging or physical exam.

Lobular neoplasia confers an increased rate of development of invasive carcinoma of about 1–2 % absolute risk per year, which is cumulative over the lifetime of the patient [1–3]. Page et al. determined the risk incurred by women with ALH was lower than that of LCIS, approximately a four- to five-fold relative risk. In comparison, patients with LCIS have an eight- to ten-fold relative risk for the development of breast cancer compared to the general population [4, 5]. Over 50 % of patients diagnosed with LCIS show multiple foci in the ipsilateral breast and approximately 30 % in the contralateral breast [6–8].

Although some studies have demonstrated an increased risk of developing an ipsilateral cancer in patients with LN [4, 9–11], the majority of studies, including data from the Surveillance, Epidemiology, End Results (SEER) Registry, demonstrate a comparable risk in both breasts [2, 12–15] (Table 10.1). Though the majority of cancers that develop are ductal in origin, the SEER data also demonstrated that in patients with LN, 23.1 % of invasive cancers that developed were of lobular histology, as compared to 6.5 % of all invasive breast cancers encountered in the general population [13].

Epidemiology

Since there are no specific physical or imaging findings for LN, it is most commonly noted as an occult lesion in surgical specimens or breast biopsies performed for other indications. This makes clarifying the actual overall incidence somewhat problematic. The prevalence of LN, in an otherwise benign breast biopsy, is approximately 0.02–3.8 % [1, 20–23]. Due to the fact that LN is an incidental finding, the actual prevalence of the disease may be much higher.

LCIS is most commonly diagnosed in women in the fifth decade of life, a decade earlier than those diagnosed with DCIS [1, 18]. The majority of women are premenopausal. Based on SEER data, the age-adjusted incidence of LN increased fourfold from 1978 to 1998 (from 0.9 to 3.2/100,000 person-yrs) [24]. Women between

M.G. Shah-Khan, MD (✉)
Division of Surgical Oncology, Medical College of Wisconsin, 9200 W Wisconsin Ave, Milwaukee, WI 53226, USA
e-mail: mshahkhan@mcw.edu

J.W. Jakub, MD
Department of Surgery, Mayo Clinic, 200 First Street S. W, Rochester, MN 55905, USA
e-mail: jakub.james@mayo.edu

A.I. Riker (ed.), *Breast Disease: Comprehensive Management*,
DOI 10.1007/978-1-4939-1145-5_10,

Table 10.1 Development of malignancy in patients with lobular neoplasia

Study, year (Ref.)	*N*	No. cancers (%)	Mean follow-up (years)	Ipsilateral cancer (%)	Contralateral cancer (%)	Lobular histology (%)
Hutter, 1969 [12]	40	15 (33)	4–27	59	41	NR
Haagensen, 1971 [16]	22	9 (40)	9.5	55	44	NR
Wheeler, 1974 [17]	25	4 (16)	17.5	25	75	25
Andersen, 1977 [2]	44	13 (27.7)	15.9	50	50	NR
Haagensen, 1978 [1]	211	35 (16.5)	14	49	51	54
Rosen, 1978 [14]	84	29 (34)	24	60	50	33
Page, 1985 [4]	126	16 (12.7)	17.5	69	31	19
Page, 2003 [18]	161	25 (16)	16	68	20	NR
Chuba, 2005 [13]	4,853	350 (7.2)	10	46	54	23
Li, 2006 [15]	4,490	282 (6.2)	5.5	58	42	49
Hwang, 2008 [19]	148	4 (2.7)	4.1	75	25	0

the ages of 50 and 59 experienced the greatest absolute increase in incidence over the study period. This increase is likely due to the higher use of screening mammography and increased frequency of breast biopsies for mammographic abnormalities [5, 24].

Histology

Lobular neoplasia is used to describe a spectrum of benign proliferation which encompasses LCIS and ALH. Histologically, LCIS is typically characterized by the proliferation of monotonous, discohesive cells, which fill the acini and cause significant distension [25, 26]. Pagetoid spread, in which the neoplastic cells extend along adjacent ducts and in between intact overlying epithelium and underlying basement membrane, may also be present [8, 27]. In ALH, the cells are cytologically similar to LCIS but with minimal distention of the acini (Fig. 10.1).

The above is a description of classic LCIS and is also referred to as type A cells. Type B cells are a well-recognized subtype of LCIS, with mild to moderately larger nuclei showing some increase in pleomorphism [27]. The entity described as pleomorphic LCIS (PLCIS) has cells with more marked pleomorphism and distinctly larger, eccentrically placed nuclei with nucleoli and eosinophilic cytoplasm. The cells of PLCIS often have central necrosis and calcification within granules [27, 29]. These lesions are often difficult to differentiate from DCIS, with staining for E-cadherin often helpful in differentiating PLCIS from DCIS.

E-cadherin is a transmembrane glycoprotein responsible for calcium-dependent cell-to-cell adhesion [30]. This protein is usually absent in lobular neoplasms such as LCIS but present in disease of ductal origin, such as DCIS. Lack of E-cadherin staining supports a diagnosis of LN. Lobular neoplasia consistently demonstrates estrogen and progesterone receptor positivity. However, Her2/neu receptor expression is variable and may be overexpressed in the PLCIS variant [8].

Although criteria exist for differentiating ALH from LCIS, the distinction can be fairly subjective, with significant intraobserver variability among pathologists when distinguishing between these entities. Rosai et al. [31] reported on a series of 17 cases that were evaluated by 5 expert breast pathologists. These lesions included ten ductal and seven lobular lesions, and the pathologists were asked to diagnose these lesions as typical hyperplasia, atypical hyperplasia, or carcinoma in situ. The 5 pathologists were not in unanimous agreement on a diagnosis for any of the 17 lesions. There were only three lesions in which four of the five pathologists agreed upon the diagnosis.

It has been suggested that lobular neoplasia should possibly be renamed "lobular intraepithelial neoplasia (LIN)" and further subdivided into three grades based upon morphology and an increased risk for the development of invasive

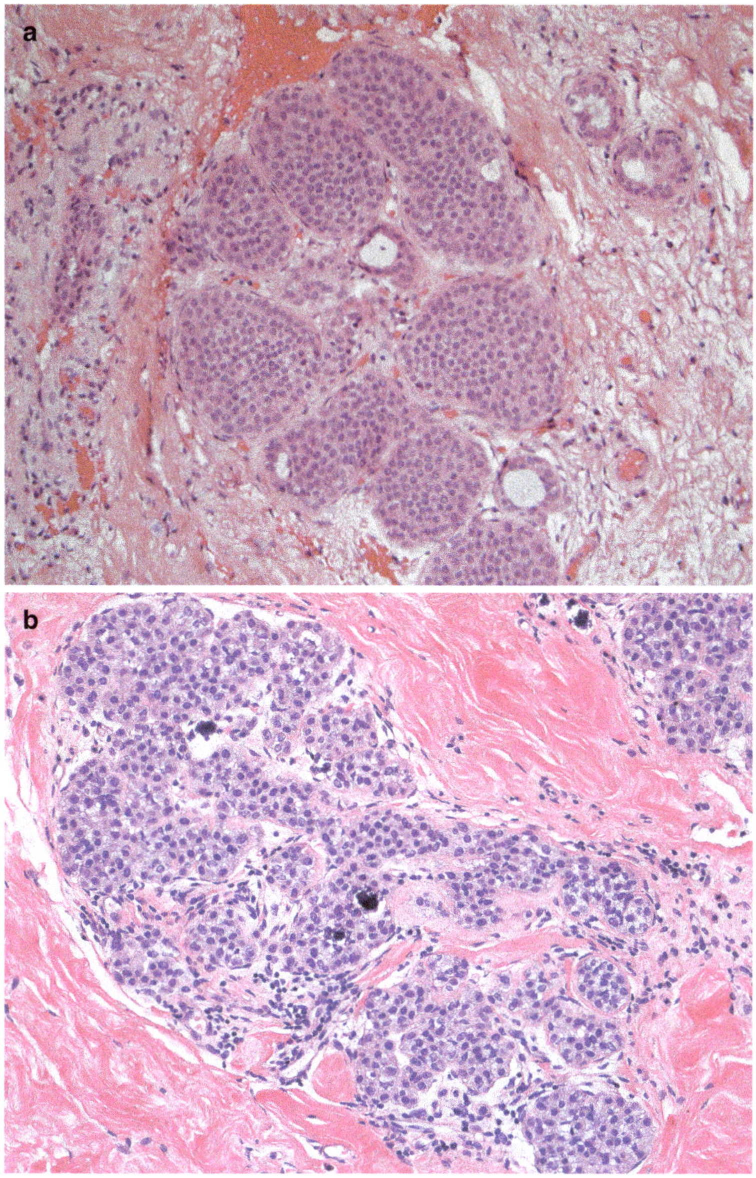

Fig. 10.1 Histopathologic appearance of lobular neoplasia (Reprinted with permission [28]). (**a**) *Lobular carcinoma in situ*. Note that the acini within the lobular unit are filled and show significant distension by the neoplastic proliferation. (**b**) *Atypical lobular hyperplasia*. Cytologically similar to LCIS, with dyshesive and uniform cells, but minimal distension of the acini

cancer (LIN 1, 2, and 3). PLCIS would be described as LIN3 [32]. This modified and new classification system has yet to gain traction, possibly due to the risk of further confusing both clinicians and patients with LN. Also labelling LCIS a "cancer" may have unintended consequences, such as overtreatment. Moving forward, we should consider reserving the word *cancer* for "lesions with a reasonable likelihood of lethal progression if left untreated" as spelled out in a recent JAMA editorial [33].

Lobular Neoplasia Found at Core-Needle Biopsy

The current version of the NCCN treatment guidelines clearly outlines a treatment algorithm for the management of LCIS [34]. The recommendations state that when LCIS is found within the surgical specimen, no additional surgical intervention is necessary. However, when LCIS is encountered on needle biopsy, surgical excision should be performed to rule out a coexisting

Table 10.2 Upstage rate of lobular neoplasia on core-needle biopsy

	ALH		LCIS	
	Malignancies found on surgical excision	% Upgrade	Malignancies found on surgical excision	% Upgrade
Yeh, 2003 [35]	1/12	8	0/3	0
Foster, 2004 [36]	2/14	14	4/12	33
Elsheikh, 2005 [37]	5/20	25	4/13	31
Margenthaler, 2006 [38]	3/19	16	4/16	20
Brem, 2008 [39]	21/97	22	17/67	25
Cangiarella, 2008 [40]	1/18	6	2/20	10
Londero, 2008 [41]	1/8	12	12/20	60
Hwang, 2008 [19]	1/48	2	9/39	23
Rendi, 2012 [42]	2/48	4.1	1/20	5
Shah-Khan, 2012 [28]	1/81	1.5	1/20	5
Murray, 2013 [43]	2/29	6.8	0/42	0

DCIS or possibly an invasive cancer. Many reports have been published to determine the actual rate of lesion upstaging with both LCIS and ALH, varying widely from 0 to 60 % [19, 28, 35–43] (Table 10.2).

There are several possible reasons for such a wide variation in the percentage, such as the majority of the studies being retrospective in nature, often with a small number of patients. One limitation of many of these institutional reviews is the basic methodology, specifically focusing only upon the group that underwent surgical excision. By conducting a retrospective review of all cases that had LN on a preoperative needle biopsy that underwent surgical excision, the entire group of LN at the same institution that did *not* undergo an operation is not included in the analysis. This, of course, will affect the overall incidence of lesion upstaging. This will translate into an inherent selection bias toward the lesions that are excised versus those observed, with subsequent upstaging rates that are falsely elevated.

The other major design flaw of many reviews is that they do not account for radiographic and pathologic concordance, without eliminating those core biopsies that contain other high-risk lesions. Many core-needle biopsy specimens contain heterogenous samples, including other high-risk lesions such as atypical ductal hyperplasia, which is known to have a much higher upstage rate.

In the series by Londero et al. [41], complete excision of LN found on core-needle biopsy was advised, yet only one case of ALH was upstaged at surgical excision. This single mass lesion contained calcifications and the core-needle biopsy revealed ALH. Of the 12 upstaged cases of LCIS, 2 were pleomorphic calcifications extending over a 2-cm area and 6 were hypoechoic nodules [41]. In a recent prospective study of 85 consecutive core-needle biopsies for LN, 80 underwent excisional biopsy and carcinoma was identified in 3 % of concordant cases versus 38 % of discordant cases [43]. The importance of radiographic and pathologic concordance in allowing for an individualized approach to care of this disease cannot be overstated.

When considering whether to excise LN that is encountered on the original core-needle biopsy, it is reasonable to evaluate these situations on a case-by-case basis. The following situations are commonly encountered:

Scenario #1: ALH with No Other High-Risk Lesion, with Radiologic and Pathologic Concordance

Case 1

Forty-five-year-old female with a screening mammogram showing an area of suspicious microcalcifications measuring 5 mm in diameter reported as BIRADS category 4 – a suspicious abnormality.

Table 10.3 Pure ALH with concordance and no other high-risk lesions

Study	Number of cases ALH	Total upstage	Upstage concordant only	Comments
Hwang [19]	48	1/48 (2 %)		1 mass lesion upstaged to DCIS
Shah-Khan [28]	81	1/81 (1.5 %)	0/73 (0 %)	1 *discordant* case upstaged to DCIS
Rendi [42]	48	2/48 (4.1 %)	1/48 (2.1 %)	1 of 2 lesions upstaged was a mass lesion noted to be *discordant*
Murray [43]	72	5/80 (6 %)	2/72 (3 %)	1 upgrade was a 2-mm DCIS, 1 was a 2-mm IDC 3/8 *discordant* lesions (38 %) upstaged
Nagi [44]	35	0/35 (0 %)	0 %	

Stereotactic core-needle biopsy with an 11-gauge needle and a total of ten core samples reveal ALH. On further analysis of the final pathology, there are fibrocystic changes only, with some associated calcium in the benign fibrocystic ducts. There is a single focus of ALH. A clip is in good position and it appears on post-biopsy mammogram that all of the microcalcifications were removed.

Our recommendation for this patient would be for continued observation and a discussion of chemopreventive strategies, such as tamoxifen.

Concordance is achieved when the pathologic findings provide a sufficient explanation for the radiologic appearance. These lesions can generally be observed. It is recommended that the issue of concordance be carefully reviewed and that the surgeon, radiologist, and pathologist are in agreement with these findings. When evaluating the literature carefully, lesions of pure ALH that have demonstrated documented radiologic–pathologic concordance consistently have a low rate of upstaging to a malignancy (Table 10.3).

The data we have collected from the Mayo Clinic addresses the upstage rate of pure LN [28]. We performed a retrospective review evaluating all patients that underwent core-needle biopsy between 1993 and 2010. We excluded any core biopsy that contained an associated high-risk lesion such as PLCIS, ADH, radial scar, papilloma, flat epithelial atypia (FEA), ipsilateral invasive carcinoma, or DCIS. The final analysis included 184 cases, with 74 % of the core biopsies performed for suspicious microcalcifications, 21 % for a solid mass or nodule, and 5 % for an area deemed suspicious by breast MRI. We identified 147 (80 %) patients with ALH and 37 (20 %) with LCIS. Of these, 81 (55 %) of the ALH cases and 20 (54 %) of LCIS cases underwent definitive operative removal of the lesions.

Table 10.4 Mayo Clinic data

	ALH (%)	LCIS (%)	*p*-value
Upstaged at excision	1/81 (1.5)	1/20 (0)	0.36
Concordant cases only	0/73 (0)	1/18 (5.6)	0.2
Developed ipsilateral cancer	2/112 (1.8)	3/26 (11.5)	0.04
Developed contralateral cancer	3/112 (2.7)	1/26 (3.8)	0.57

The rate of upstage upon surgical excision for ALH was 1.5 % (1/81) and 5 % (1/20) for LCIS. The single ALH case that was upstaged had a *discordant* biopsy result and was upgraded to DCIS. Of the ALH lesions that had no other associated high-risk features and pathologic–radiographic concordance on needle biopsy, none were upstaged at the time of excisional biopsy (Table 10.4). These upstage rates are very low and consistent with other studies evaluating the upstage rates of pure LN that have undergone meticulous review of the pathologic–radiographic concordance [19, 42–44]. Similar findings were recently published from a prospective series by Murray et al. [43].

Our series is somewhat unique in that it included the entire cohort of LN lesions, including those that were observed and did not undergo excisional biopsy. Follow-up data was available for 65 cases that were merely observed without surgical excision, with a mean follow-up period of 53 months. In patients with ALH, 1/51 (2 %) developed an ipsilateral cancer and for those with LCIS, 3/14 (21.4 %) developed an ipsilateral cancer. This ipsilateral breast event rate is high; however, it is worth noting that all patients with LCIS that developed a subsequent ipsilateral malignancy did so in a different quadrant than the initial biopsy, suggesting excisional surgical biopsy would not have influenced the future events. This is also a relatively small cohort, as the majority of patients with LCIS in our series did go onto excisional biopsy, thus caution is advised in making conclusions based on this subset of 14 patients. With regard to the contralateral breast, 2.7 % of patients with ALH and 3.8 % with LCIS developed a contralateral malignancy during the follow-up period.

All of the subsequent cancers that developed were invasive ductal carcinoma in origin. Although these rates appear to be much lower than the expected rate of development of malignancy in such patients with LN, the lifetime incidence for the development of ipsilateral or contralateral or malignancy was 21 % (31/145) for those with ALH and 29 % (10/35) for those with LCIS. These lesions are associated with an increased risk of future breast cancer and these patients should be under surveillance and strongly consider chemoprevention. This is discussed in more detail below.

Hwang et al. reported on a series of 48 patients with pure ALH, of which the upstage rate was 2 % [19]. Of note, the upgraded lesion was a biopsy performed for a mass lesion. This report also provided follow-up data for patients that did not undergo excision following a diagnosis of LN. The mean follow-up period was 49 months for 148 cases of LN without subsequent excision and demonstrated a 2 % incidence of subsequent ipsilateral carcinomas, including one case within a different site than the original biopsy identifying LN.

Brem et al. reported on a multi-institution series of LN [39], analyzing 67 LCIS and 97 ALH cases that underwent complete excision. The upgrade rate reported was substantial, 25 % for those with LCIS and 22 % (21/97) for those with ALH. However, of the 164 lesions excised, 74 (45 %) were noted to have radiologic–pathologic discordance. A major limitation of this study lies in the fact that there were several institutions included and no retrospective pathology overview, resulting in potential variability in the interpretation of LN. Rendi et al. reported on 68 patients with pure LN [42]. Two cases (4.1 %) of ALH were upstaged, with one being a mass lesion that was noted to be discordant. Thus, the true upstage rate of pure, concordant ALH in this series is likely closer to 2 %.

Extent of disease is also an important factor to be evaluated. Esserman et al. demonstrated that the extent of lobular neoplasia in a core biopsy specimen may predict whether or not excision is required [45]. They distinguished diffuse lobular neoplasia (>1 lobule per core affected) from focal lobular neoplasia (less than or equal to 1 lobule per core) and found that upgrades to malignancy were more likely to be associated with diffuse LN. Although the number of patients included was small (35 patients), these findings would support that in patients with simply a focus of LN, observation can be considered.

Scenario #2: ALH on Core-Needle Biopsy in the Presence of a Higher-Risk Lesion

Case 2

A 52-year-old female undergoes a screening mammogram that reveals a 1.5-cm diameter area of suspicious microcalcifications (BIRADS 4). A stereotactic biopsy with a 14-gauge core needle and four core samples reveals ALH and ADH with the microcalcifications associated with the atypical ducts. Post-biopsy mammogram reveals the clip in good position with many microcalcifications remaining.

Our recommendation would be for an excisional biopsy to obtain an adequate sample for final pathologic analysis to rule out an underlying occult malignancy. This is a conservative surgical excision. In general, this is a diagnostic procedure, and we are attempting to obtain an adequate representative sample to assure there is no upstaging. The rationale for excision in this case is twofold; the calcifications in question have not been adequately sampled, and a definitive diagnosis must be obtained due to the presence of a higher-risk lesion. As covered in another chapter, excisional biopsy is standard for ADH and results in approximately a 10–20 % upstage [46]. *At the time of this publication, core-needle biopsy alone for ADH has not been able to stratify a low enough risk group that an occult cancer can be excluded. The management of such cases should be directed toward removal of the highest-risk lesion. The higher-risk lesion would trump the ALH and standard of care for the ADH would be followed.*

The disadvantage of a more aggressive wire localized lumpectomy stems from the fact that lobular neoplasia is a risk factor for the development of breast cancer. This risk occurs in all quadrants and is bilateral; thus a more aggressive surgery, short of a bilateral mastectomy, does not prevent the potential development of a future malignancy. We are not prepared at the time of excisional biopsy to proceed to definitive mastectomy, reconstruction, or axillary staging if the lesion is upstaged. In the rare case where there is extensive calcifications throughout a large area or scattered throughout the breast and follow-up imaging may be inadequate, deciding what is an adequate sampling and observing can be unsettling and mastectomy may be an option. This should be the exception, not the rule.

The Role for Chemoprevention

Excisional biopsy reveals post-biopsy changes with a residual focus of ADH. The specimen radiograph revealed the clip and the residual calcifications.

In addition to future surveillance, it is recommended that patients with findings of atypia be counseled regarding their appropriateness for chemoprevention.

Prospective, randomized trials have been conducted to evaluate the effect of chemoprevention in reducing the development of breast cancer in patients at high-risk, including those with LCIS. The NSABP-01, known as the breast cancer prevention trial (BCPT), randomized 13,388 high-risk women to the selective estrogen receptor modulator (SERM), tamoxifen, versus placebo [47, 48]. Patients were determined to be at high risk if they were older than 60, had LCIS or atypical hyperplasia, or had a 5-year risk of developing breast cancer calculated as >1.66 % utilizing the Gail risk model.

The study was unblinded after a median 54.6 months of follow-up due to a significant difference noted in the development of breast cancer in the treatment arm. Tamoxifen treatment reduced the incidence of breast cancer by 49 %, with the subgroup analysis revealing that women with a history of LCIS experienced a similar relative reduction in overall risk. There were 829 women included in the study who had a history of LCIS, with an overall 56 % relative risk reduction in these women. The average annual hazard rate for invasive cancer fell from 12.99 to 5.69 per 1,000 women.

Concerns over the untoward side effects of tamoxifen in postmenopausal women prompted the evaluation of alternatives for chemoprevention. The NSABP P-2 trial, the Study of Tamoxifen and Raloxifene (STAR), compared the two drugs in the prevention of breast cancer in high-risk, postmenopausal women [49, 50]. At a median follow-up of 3.9 years, similar rates of reduction for invasive cancer were reported in both groups, concluding that raloxifene is as effective as tamoxifen in decreasing the risk of invasive breast cancer. Of the 19,747 women included in the study, there were 1,998 with an identified history of LCIS. When comparing subgroups, it is notable that women with LCIS had the highest risk of developing cancer, with 9.6–9.8 cases per 1,000 women. An equal number of invasive cancers occurred in each treatment group in patients with LCIS.

The recent MAP.3 trial was conducted to determine the effectiveness of the aromatase inhibitor, exemestane, for chemoprevention in postmenopausal women at high risk for the development of breast cancer [51]. Patients who took exemestane experienced a 65 % reduction in the relative incidence of invasive breast cancers, from 0.55 to 0.19 %. Subgroup analysis evaluated women with a history of LCIS, ALH, or ADH as a group, showing that although exemestane was found to be superior to placebo, its specific chemopreventive benefit specifically in patients with LN could not be fully determined.

In the data obtained from the Mayo Clinic cohort, of the patients diagnosed with LN that were eligible for chemoprevention, 25 % (30/120) accepted initiation of therapy [28]. There were no patients that started chemoprevention that subsequently developed a malignancy (0/30) during follow-up. However, 10 % of those who did not initiate chemoprevention developed a future breast cancer during a mean follow-up period of 50.3 months. Although no conclusions can be drawn from this due to the small number of patients and limited follow-up, there is substantial evidence that the risk-reducing benefits of this approach is superior to observation alone.

Tchou et al. reported on their data demonstrating a similarly low acceptance rate of chemoprevention [52]. They identified 219 patients treated between 1998 and 2002, with 60 % offered chemoprevention with tamoxifen and 41 % accepting therapy. A total of 30 women were at risk due to LCIS, with 53 % accepting chemoprevention. Lastly, Port et al. reported that among 43 high-risk women offered tamoxifen at MSKCC, 41 declined due to their perception that the personal risks outweighed the benefit of tamoxifen therapy [53].

In an LCIS high-risk surveillance program, 163 women on chemoprevention versus 835 women who did not choose chemoprevention were evaluated. After a median follow-up of 84 months, 6/163 (3.6 %) of those taking chemoprevention developed breast cancer versus 121/835 (14.4 %) patients not on chemoprevention [54]. Although the significance of these findings are limited by the retrospective nature of this study, it does support the benefit of chemoprevention in patients with LN that has been established by the prospective, randomized trials described above.

Prophylactic Mastectomy

In general, we offer close surveillance with or without chemoprevention as the primary strategy for patients diagnosed with LN. Bilateral risk-reducing mastectomy has been shown to offer a 90 % relative risk reduction [55] and is an option for prevention. Although bilateral mastectomy was readily recommended for women with LN in the distant past, we believe this approach is overly aggressive for the majority of patients. A minority of women with LN currently elect risk-reducing surgery. In the Mayo Clinic series, bilateral prophylactic mastectomy was performed in 10 of our 172 patients with LN, which is similar to the 5.6 % of patients undergoing the same operation reported by Memorial Sloan Kettering [56].

In general, women diagnosed with unilateral cancer are choosing bilateral mastectomies with increased frequency [57]. A study evaluating data from the National Cancer Data Base demonstrated the use of contralateral prophylactic mastectomy (CPM) increased from 0.4 to 4.7 % between 1998 and 2007. The increased use was observed to be more associated with patient-related factors rather than stage or biologic characteristics of the tumor [58]. This shift in the operative decision-making is multifactorial, not least of which includes improved reconstructive options. One single institution study compared patients undergoing unilateral mastectomy and CPM [59]. Patients undergoing CPM were more likely to undergo immediate breast reconstruction than those undergoing unilateral mastectomy. Numerous institutional reviews have evaluated this trend of increased CPM, and little consistency exists among studies with respect to factors associated with use of CPM that have statistical significance [58–60]. There is agreement, however, that the use of CPM in patients with unilateral cancer does not improve overall, disease-free, or distant disease-free survival [58–61]. Patients that do consider prophylactic mastectomy should be counseled regarding risks of surgery, limitations of risk reduction, as well as consideration of a possible alteration in body image or sexual health. In general we remain supportive of breast-conserving surgery or a unilateral mastectomy for a cancer diagnosis synchronous with an ipsilateral or contralateral LCIS diagnosis, but certainly some women choose a contralateral risk-reducing mastectomy. LCIS found at the time of definitive breast surgery, including lumpectomy, for DCIS or invasive cancer, should not change the treatment recommendations from lumpectomy to mastectomy, or from a unilateral procedure to a bilateral procedure.

Scenario #3: LCIS on Core-Needle Biopsy

Case 3

A 65-year-old female is found to have a 1-cm well-circumscribed, solid mass on routine screening mammography. An ultrasound-guided core biopsy reveals a fibroadenoma and a focus of LCIS in the surrounding breast tissue. Surgical removal reveals a 1-cm benign fibroadenoma with LCIS in the neighboring background breast parenchyma that extends to a single margin. The patient asks about a unilateral mastectomy.

We would not recommend re-excision or further surgical intervention. A conservative excision to assure the area is adequately sampled is the goal. In general this is considered a marker of high risk surveillance for early detection and a systemic, rather than local, approach to risk reduction should be the mindset. Discussion regarding the risks and benefits of chemoprevention would be held. We would treat both breasts similarly and in general would advise observation. We do perform bilateral, risk-reducing mastectomies with reconstruction for patients with LCIS, but this indication comprises, by far, the minority of cases performed at our institution. We would discuss the woman's future risk for the development of breast cancer. The probability is approximately 1.5 %/year, based on series with long-term follow-up [62, 63]. *Factors such as family history, age at diagnosis of LN, parity, and other factors leading to increased unopposed estrogen exposure certainly affect a woman's overall risk. Risk calculators such as the Gail, IBIS, or the extended Claus model are often used to quantify a woman's risk for the development of breast cancer. It is important to note that these risk models are very reliable for population studies, but less reliable for individual risk assessment; each has limitations and may over (or under) estimate a woman's risk, thus used in combination may offer a more valid estimation* [64]. *Future risk predictions will likely become tissue based. These will allow more individual risk estimates, as opposed to population-based modeling that currently exists.*

The NCCN guidelines recommend that if LCIS is encountered on core biopsy, surgical excision should be performed to rule out the presence of an associated malignancy [34]. The wide range of upstage rates in the literature reflects the lack of consistency among factors that may predict upstaging of these lesions.

The relative risk for the development of a future malignancy in patients with LCIS is about eight- to ten-fold relative risk compared to the general female population [5]. This translates into an approximately a 1.5 %/per year absolute risk [62]. Haagensen and colleagues reviewed 210 breast biopsies containing LCIS, and after a mean follow-up of 14 years, 16.7 % developed carcinoma with an equivalent risk for either breast [1]. Andersen et al. evaluated 52 patients with LCIS with a mean follow-up period of 15 years, with 20 % developing an ipsilateral carcinoma and 17.3 % developing a contralateral carcinoma [2].

Although the equivalent risk with respect to laterality has been well established, some series have demonstrated an increased risk in the ipsilateral breast. The Nashville Breast Cancer Study retrospectively evaluated 252 women with LN (both LCIS and ALH) [9]. Fifty patients developed invasive breast cancer, with 68 % found in the ipsilateral breast and 24 % in the contralateral breast. The Danish Breast Cancer Cooperative Group collected follow-up data for 100 women who underwent excision for LCIS [10, 65]. This study had a follow-up of 19 years, with 18 malignancies developing, of which 16 were in the ipsilateral breast.

Studies looking at the molecular profiling of LN in specimens coexisting with invasive lobular carcinoma have demonstrated shared genetic alterations, including the loss or downregulation of E-cadherin expression; loss of chromosomal material from 16p, 17p, and 22q; and gain of material on 1q and 6q [30, 66–68]. Due to these shared genetic alterations as well as the greater proportion of invasive lobular cancer than in the general population, it has been suggested that LN may serve as a precursor lesion, rather than simply a risk factor. Work is underway with respect to identifying the alterations in genetic content that may make some LCIS lesions act as precursors to invasive lobular cancer [66]. Patients should be referred for a discussion of chemoprevention, as discussed above.

Pleomorphic LCIS on Core Biopsy

The entity described as pleomorphic LCIS (PLCIS) is a variant of LCIS. Histologically, PLCIS has cells with greater pleomorphism, larger nuclei with distinct nucleoli, and often with central necrosis and calcification within granules, complicating the distinction from DCIS [27, 30]. Staining for E-cadherin can help differentiate PLCIS from DCIS. A higher Ki-67 proliferation index and higher percentage of p53 protein positivity has been demonstrated more so in PLCIS compared to classic LCIS lesions, suggesting a more aggressive behavior of this entity [29]. PLCIS has also been described in association with the fairly aggressive pattern of pleomorphic invasive lobular carcinoma [69, 70]. It is recommended that when PLCIS is encountered on core-needle biopsy, excision with negative margins should be undertaken.

Surgical Considerations

Managing LN Found on Core-Needle Biopsy

When evaluating a patient with LN, the main clinical question faced by the surgeon is typically whether an excisional biopsy is warranted. Pleomorphic LCIS should always undergo excisional biopsy and we are more aggressive with this specific entity in regard to obtaining clear histologic margins. Until more data is available, in general LCIS that is identified on a core biopsy should trigger a conservative surgical excisional biopsy to assure a representative pathologic sample. We do not mandate clear histologic margins.

In regard to ALH, we have adopted a more individualized approach. When we face this decision in the clinic, there are a number of factors to consider:

1. Is there *radiographic–pathologic concordance*? This can sometimes appear confusing because it is generally accepted that LN is radiographically occult and merely an incidental finding on core-needle biopsy. Some have argued that by definition, the biopsy results showing LN are *always* considered to be discordant. From our perspective, a few examples may help highlight our thought process.
   - A biopsy is performed for microcalcifications and pathology reveals fibrocystic disease or sclerosing adenosis with associated calcifications. An incidental focus of ALH is identified in the neighboring breast parenchyma. We would consider this concordant.
   - A solid mass that appears consistent with a fibroadenoma on ultrasound undergoes a core biopsy revealing a fibroadenoma with an incidental focus of ALH. We would consider this concordant.

   In these examples the ALH is truly incidental. It is essentially a bystander in the path to the targeted lesion. The radiographic findings are completely explained and consistent with the histologic findings and thus considered concordant.
2. The next question that we ask is, "Was a representative sample obtained by core-needle biopsy?" This takes into account concordance and *extent of disease*. When the extent of radiographic findings is small and an adequate sample was obtained, we are generally more comfortable with observation. Similarly, when there is a minimal amount of ALH on pathological findings, we are less concerned. Descriptions of a "single focus" or "minute focus" in the pathology report are often helpful when appropriate. A few examples may best highlight the point.
   - A single mammographic focus of 4 mm of microcalcifications is completely removed with a core biopsy. Pathology reveals calcifications in benign acini with a small focus of ALH. In this case, we are comfortable that the lesion has been adequately sampled and an excisional biopsy is not needed.
   - If there is a much larger area, such as a 3-cm area of suspicious calcifications with core biopsy revealing extensive ALH, or a

spiculated mass with core biopsy revealing benign breast parenchyma with a small focus of ALH, clearly the lesion of concern has not been adequately sampled. In these cases, ALH is an unrelated finding and the radiographic suspicious finding has not been adequately explained; further tissue is needed, either by repeat core or most commonly excisional biopsy, to determine the etiology.

3. The *size of the biopsy*. This is also related to the above points. A large gauge needle, such as a 9- or 11-gauge biopsy needle with several passes, such as 8–12, with the lesion completely excised is reassuring.
4. No other *high-risk lesions*. If the biopsy reveals ADH or obvious DCIS on the final pathology, appropriate surgery should be discussed with the patient. The highest-risk lesion will always have the priority in terms of adequate removal with excision.

Surgical Pathology

1. When an excisional biopsy is advised following the diagnosis ALH or LCIS by core-needle biopsy, it must be kept in mind that the surgical procedure is diagnostic and not a therapeutic procedure. The goal is to obtain a representative sample in order to obtain a pathologic diagnosis and further rule out a malignancy. As a result, a conservative surgical biopsy is appropriate.
2. *Negative margins* for all atypias are not always a necessity. If a lumpectomy is performed for DCIS or invasive ductal cancer, with the pathology revealing ALH or LCIS at a margin, re-excision is not required [71]. However, this does not apply to the pleomorphic variant of LCIS. Furthermore, in the setting of infiltrating lobular carcinoma arising in a background of extensive LCIS, one may be more concerned about LCIS at the margins. It is institution and individual pathologist dependent whether LN at a margin is even reported. The current standard is not to re-excise margins for ALH or LCIS. There is some data that local recurrence may be higher [72, 73], but this is neither the current consensus nor standard practice and conflicting data exist [74]. There is also some emerging data regarding some classic LCIS lesions serving as a precursor lesion, but this is not well defined. As a rule we do not chase margins for atypia or classic LCIS. It also needs to be kept in mind that clinically the event rate for developing a breast cancer following a diagnosis of LCIS is about 1–1.5 % per year with observation alone [62]. Even if LN at a margin adds a slight increased risk of local recurrence, following a lumpectomy patients with malignancy are treated with radiation and systemic therapy (hormone therapy and/or chemotherapy). Thus, the benefit of trying to clear all LN is likely minimal at best and could compromise cosmesis and increase the mastectomy rate with no established clinical benefit to date.
3. LCIS is a risk marker for cancer, but is considered less important in a patient who is diagnosed with breast cancer. LCIS found at the time of definitive breast surgery, including lumpectomy, for DCIS or invasive cancer, should not change the treatment recommendations from lumpectomy to mastectomy, or from a unilateral procedure to a bilateral procedure.

Summary

- Lobular neoplasia comprises both ALH and LCIS and imparts an increased risk for the development of breast cancer. This risk is conferred bilaterally and the majority of breast cancers that develop are ductal in origin.
- The risk of developing invasive cancer remains steady over time and translates to about a 1–1.5 % per annum risk.
- There is little relationship between the site of breast biopsy demonstrating lobular neoplasia and the future site of breast cancer (if one is to develop).
- As a result of the above, the only logical operation would be a bilateral risk-reducing

mastectomy. At our institution, we consider this to be overly aggressive for the vast majority of patients with this disease, and observation (close surveillance, chemoprevention) is the standard.

- When LN is found on surgical excision, no further operative intervention is required; however, a discussion must be held regarding further follow-up and chemoprevention.
- When ALH is identified on core-needle biopsy, excision is advised if:
  - The LN coexists with another high-risk lesion such as ADH.
  - Discordance exists between clinical, radiologic, and pathologic findings.
  - Biopsy is performed for a mass lesion or architectural distortion and a benign explanation is not obtained.
  - Biopsy performed for microcalcifications and no calcifications are obtained.
  - The LN shows mixed histologic features or a mixed E-cadherin staining pattern.
  - Pleomorphic LCIS is present.

Tips

1. Do not accept LN as a definitive diagnosis. The pathologist should specify ALH or LCIS. In general, LN is not an adequate diagnosis by itself and must be further specified as to the type of LN.
2. If there is a large hematoma after core biopsy, allow 3–8 weeks for it to resolve before excisional biopsy to improve cosmesis. There is little risk in waiting and a much smaller volume of breast tissue can be excised once the hematoma has resolved.
3. If observation is the approach following an excisional biopsy for LN, with no further upstaging, then a discussion should be held with the patient in regard to the role of chemoprevention.
4. Lobular neoplasia alone should not explain a mass lesion seen on imaging and is clearly discordant if there is no other pathologic explanation to account for a suspicious mass on imaging.

References

1. Haagensen CD, Lane N, Lattes R, et al. Lobular neoplasia (so-called lobular carcinoma *in situ*) of the breast. Cancer. 1978;42:737–69.
2. Andersen JA. Lobular carcinoma *in situ* of the breast. An approach to rational treatment. Cancer. 1977;39:2597–602.
3. Bauer TL, Pandelidis SM, Rhoads Jr JE. Five-year survival of 100 women with carcinoma of the breast diagnosed by screening mammography and needle-localization biopsy. J Am Coll Surg. 1994;178:427–30.
4. Page DL, Dupont WD, Rogers LW, Rados MS. Atypical hyperplastic lesions of the female breast. A long-term follow-up study. Cancer. 1985;55(11):2698–708.
5. Oppong BA, King TA. Recommendations for women with lobular carcinoma in situ (LCIS). Oncology (Williston Park). 2011;25(11):1051–6, 1058.
6. Urban JA. Bilaterality of cancer of the breast. Biopsy of the opposite breast. Cancer. 1967;20:1867–70.
7. Rosen PP, Senie R, Schottenfeld D, et al. Noninvasive breast carcinoma: frequency of unsuspected invasion and implications for treatment. Ann Surg. 1979;189(3):377–82.
8. Simpson PT, Reis-Filho JS, Lakhani S. Lobular carcinoma in situ: biology and pathology, diseases of the breast. Philadelphia: Lippincott Williams and Wilkins; 2004.
9. Page DL, Schuyler PA, Dupont WD, et al. Atypical lobular hyperplasia as a unilateral predictor of breast cancer risk: a retrospective cohort study. Lancet. 2003;361:125–9.
10. Ottesen GL, Graversen HP, Blichert-Toft M, et al. Lobular carcinoma *in situ* of the female breast. Short-term results of a prospective nationwide study. The Danish Breast Cancer Cooperative Group. Am J Surg Pathol. 1993;17:14–21.
11. Marshall LM, Hunter DJ, Connolly JL, et al. Risk of breast cancer associated with atypical hyperplasia of lobular and ductal types. Cancer Epidemiol Biomarkers Prev. 1997;6:297–301.
12. Hutter RV, Foote Jr FW. Lobular carcinoma in situ. Long term follow-up. Cancer. 1969;24(5):1081–5.
13. Chuba PJ, Hamre MR, Yap J, et al. Bilateral risk for subsequent breast cancer after lobular carcinoma-in-situ: analysis of surveillance, epidemiology, and end results data. J Clin Oncol. 2005;23:5534–41.
14. Rosen PP, Kosloff C, Lieberman PH, et al. Lobular carcinoma *in situ* of the breast. Detailed analysis of 99 patients with average follow-up of 24 years. Am J Surg Pathol. 1978;2:225–51.
15. Li CI, Malone KE, Saltzman BS, et al. Risk of invasive breast carcinoma among women diagnosed with ductal carcinoma *in situ* and lobular carcinoma *in situ*, 1988–2001. Cancer. 2006;106:2104–12.
16. Haagensen CD. Diseases of the breast. 2nd ed. Philadelphia: WB Saunders; 1971. p. 503–27.
17. Wheeler JE, Enterline HT, Roseman JM, et al. Lobular carcinoma in situ of the breast. Long-term follow up. Cancer. 1974;34(3):554–63.

18. Page DL, Kidd Jr TE, Dupont WD, et al. Lobular neoplasia of the breast: higher risk for subsequent invasive cancer predicted by more extensive disease. Hum Pathol. 1991;22:1232–9.
19. Hwang H, Barke LD, Mendelson EB, Susnik B. Atypical lobular hyperplasia and classic lobular carcinoma in situ in core biopsy specimens: routine excision is not necessary. Mod Pathol. 2008;21(10):1208–16.
20. Liberman L, Sama M, Susnik B, et al. Lobular carcinoma in situ at percutaneous breast biopsy: surgical biopsy findings. AJR Am J Roentgenol. 1999;173:291–9.
21. Berg WA, Mrose HE, Ioffe OB. Atypical lobular hyperplasia or lobular carcinoma in situ at core-needle breast biopsy. Radiology. 2001;218:503–9.
22. Hussain M, Cunnick GH. Management of lobular carcinoma in-situ and atypical lobular hyperplasia of the breast—a review. Eur J Surg Oncol. 2011;37:279–89.
23. Philpotts LE, Shaheen NA, Jain KS, et al. Uncommon high-risk lesions of the breast diagnosed at stereotactic core-needle biopsy: clinical importance. Radiology. 2000;216:831–7.
24. Li CI, Anderson BO, Daling JR, Moe RE. Changing incidence of lobular carcinoma in situ of the breast. Breast Cancer Res Treat. 2002;75(3):259–68.
25. Foote FW, Stewart SF. Lobular carcinoma *in situ*: a rare form of mammary cancer. Am J Pathol. 1941;17(4):491–96.
26. Page DL, Anderson TJ, Rogers LW. Carcinoma *in situ* (CIS). Diagnostic histopathology of the breast. New York: Churchill Livingstone; 1987.
27. Simpson PT, Gale T, Fulford LG, et al. The diagnosis and management of pre-invasive breast disease: pathology of atypical lobular hyperplasia and lobular carcinoma in situ. Breast Cancer Res. 2003;5:258–62.
28. Shah-Khan MG, Geiger XJ, Reynolds C, et al. Long-term follow-up of lobular neoplasia (atypical lobular hyperplasia/lobular carcinoma in situ) diagnosed on core needle biopsy. Ann Surg Oncol. 2012;19(10):3131–8.
29. Sneige N, Wang J, Baker BA, et al. Clinical, histopathologic, and biologic features of pleomorphic lobular (ductal-lobular) carcinoma *in situ* of the breast: a report of 24 cases. Mod Pathol. 2002;15:1044–50.
30. Jacobs TW, Pliss N, Kouria G, et al. Carcinomas *in situ* of the breast with indeterminate features: role of E-cadherin staining in categorization. Am J Surg Pathol. 2001;25:229–36.
31. Rosai J. Borderline epithelial lesions of the breast. Am J Surg Pathol. 1991;15(3):209–21.
32. Tavassoli FA. Pathology of the breast. 2nd ed. Norwalk: Appleton and Lange; 1999.
33. Esserman LJ, Thompson Jr IM, Reid B. Overdiagnosis and overtreatment in cancer: an opportunity for improvement. JAMA. 2013;310(8):797–8.
34. Referenced with permission from The NCCN Clinical Practice Guidelines in Oncology (NCCN Guidelines®) for Breast Cancer V.1.2013. © National Comprehensive Cancer Network, Inc 2013. All rights reserved. Accessed January 1, 2013. To view the most recent and complete version of the guideline, go online to www.nccn.org. National Comprehensive Cancer Network®, NCCN®, NCCN GUIDELINES®, and all other NCCN Content are trademarks owned by the National Comprehensive Cancer Network, Inc.
35. Yeh IT, Dimitrov D, Otto P, et al. Pathologic review of atypical hyperplasia identified by image-guided breast needle core biopsy. Correlation with excision specimen. Arch Pathol Lab Med. 2003;127:49–54.
36. Foster MC, Helvie MA, Gregory NE, et al. Lobular carcinoma in situ or atypical lobular hyperplasia at core-needle biopsy: is excisional biopsy necessary? Radiology. 2004;231:813–9.
37. Elsheikh TM, Silverman JF. Follow-up surgical excision is indicated when breast core needle biopsies show atypical lobular hyperplasia or lobular carcinoma in situ: a correlative study of 33 patients with review of the literature. Am J Surg Pathol. 2005;29(4):534–43.
38. Margenthaler JA, Duke D, Monsees BS, et al. Correlation between core biopsy and excisional biopsy in breast high-risk lesions. Am J Surg. 2006;192:534–7.
39. Brem RF, Lechner MC, Jackman RJ, et al. Lobular neoplasia at percutaneous breast biopsy: variables associated with carcinoma at surgical excision. AJR Am J Roentgenol. 2008;190:637–41.
40. Cangiarella J, Guth A, Axelrod D, et al. Is surgical excision necessary for the management of atypical lobular hyperplasia and lobular carcinoma in situ diagnosed on core needle biopsy? A report of 38 cases and review of the literature. Arch Pathol Lab Med. 2008;132:979–83.
41. Londero V, Zuiani C, Linda A, et al. Lobular neoplasia: core needle breast biopsy underestimation of malignancy in relation to radiologic and pathologic features. Breast. 2008;17:623–30.
42. Rendi MH, Dintzis SM, Lehman CD, et al. Lobular in-situ neoplasia on breast core needle biopsy: imaging indication and pathologic extent can identify which patients require excisional biopsy. Ann Surg Oncol. 2012;19:914–21.
43. Murray MP, Luedtke C, Liberman L, et al. Classic lobular carcinoma in situ and atypical lobular hyperplasia at percutaneous breast core biopsy: outcomes of prospective excision. Cancer. 2013;119(5):1073–9.
44. Nagi CS, O'Donnell JE, Tismenetsky M, et al. Lobular neoplasia on core needle biopsy does not require excision. Cancer. 2008;112:2152–8.
45. Esserman LE, Lamea L, Tanev S, et al. Should the extent of lobular neoplasia on core biopsy influence the decision for excision? Breast J. 2007;13:55–61.
46. Degnim AC, King TA. Surgical management of high-risk breast lesions. Surg Clin North Am. 2013;93(2):329–40.
47. Fisher B, Costantino JP, Wickerham DL, et al. Tamoxifen for the prevention of breast cancer: current status of the National Surgical Adjuvant Breast and Bowel Project P-1 study. J Natl Cancer Inst. 2005;97:1652.
48. Fisher B, Costantino JP, Wickerham DL, et al. Tamoxifen for the prevention of breast cancer:

report of the National Surgical Adjuvant Breast and Bowel Project P-1 study. J Natl Cancer Inst. 1998;90:1371–88.
49. Cummings SR, Eckert S, Krueger KA, et al. The effect of raloxifene on risk of breast cancer in postmenopausal women: results from the MORE randomized trial. Multiple outcomes of raloxifene evaluation. JAMA. 1999;281:2189–97.
50. Vogel VG, Costantino JP, Wickerham DL, et al. Effects of tamoxifen vs raloxifene on the risk of developing invasive breast cancer and other disease outcomes: the NSABP Study of Tamoxifen and Raloxifene (STAR) P-2 trial. JAMA. 2006;295:2727–41.
51. Goss PE, Ingle JN, Ales-Martinez J, et al. Exemestane for breast-cancer prevention in postmenopausal women. N Engl J Med. 2011;364:2381–91.
52. Tchou J, Hou N, Rademaker A, et al. Acceptance of tamoxifen chemoprevention by physicians and women at risk. Cancer. 2004;100(9):1800–6.
53. Port ER, Montgomery LL, Heerdt AS, Borgen PI. Patient reluctance toward tamoxifen use for breast cancer primary prevention. Ann Surg Oncol. 2001;8(7):580–5.
54. Oskar S, Muhsen S, Sung J, et al. Chemoprevention among women with lobular carcinoma in situ. Ann Surg Oncol. 2011;18:S59.
55. Hartmann LC, Schaid DJ, Woods JE, et al. Efficacy of bilateral prophylactic mastectomy in women with a family history of breast cancer. N Engl J Med. 1999;340:77–84.
56. Muhsen S, Junqueira MJ, Park A, et al. Patient characteristics associated with the decision to undergo bilateral prophylactic mastectomy for lobular carcinoma in situ. J Clin Oncol. 2011;29 (S27, A148).
57. Katipamula R, Degnim AC, Hoskin T, et al. Trends in mastectomy rates at the Mayo Clinic Rochester: effect of surgical year and preoperative magnetic resonance imaging. J Clin Oncol. 2009;27(25):4082–8.
58. Yao K, Stewart AK, Winchester DJ, Winchester DP. Trends in contralateral prophylactic mastectomy for unilateral cancer: a report from the National Cancer Data Base, 1998–2007. Ann Surg Oncol. 2010;17(10):2554–62.
59. Chung A, Huynh K, Lawrence C, Sim MS, Giuliano A. Comparison of patient characteristics and outcomes of contralateral prophylactic mastectomy and unilateral total mastectomy in breast cancer patients. Ann Surg Oncol. 2012;19(8):2600–6.
60. Arrington AK, Jarosek SL, Virnig BA, Habermann EB, Tuttle TM. Patient and surgeon characteristics associated with increased use of contralateral prophylactic mastectomy in patients with breast cancer. Ann Surg Oncol. 2009;16(10):2697–704.
61. Lostumbo L, Carbine NE, Wallace J. Prophylactic mastectomy for the prevention of breast cancer. Cochrane Database Syst Rev. 2010;11:CD002748.
62. Bodian CA, Perzin KH, Lattes R. Lobular neoplasia. Long term risk of breast cancer and relation to other factors. Cancer. 1996;78(5):1024–34.
63. Fisher ER, Land SR, Fisher B, et al. Pathologic findings from the National Surgical Adjuvant Breast and Bowel Project: twelve-year observations concerning lobular carcinoma in situ. Cancer. 2004;100:238–44.
64. Pankratz VS, Hartmann LC, Degnim AC, et al. Assessment of the accuracy of the Gail model in women with atypical hyperplasia. J Clin Oncol. 2008;26(33):5374–9.
65. Ottesen GL, Graversen HP, Blichert-Toft M, et al. Carcinoma in situ of the female breast. 10 year follow-up results of a prospective nationwide study. Breast Cancer Res Treat. 2000;62(3):197–210.
66. De Leeuw WJ, Berx G, Vos CB, et al. Simultaneous loss of E-cadherin and catenins in invasive lobular breast cancer and lobular carcinoma in situ. J Pathol. 1997;183:404–11.
67. Hwang ES, Nyante SJ, Yi Chen Y, et al. Clonality of lobular carcinoma in situ and synchronous invasive lobular carcinoma. Cancer. 2004;100:2562–72.
68. Lakhani SR, Collins N, Sloane JP, Stratton MR. Loss of heterozygosity in lobular carcinoma in situ of the breast. Clin Mol Pathol. 1995;48:M74–8.
69. Bentz JS, Yassa N, Clayton F. Pleomorphic lobular carcinoma of the breast: clinicopathologic features of 12 cases. Mod Pathol. 1998;11(9):814–22.
70. Downs-Kelly E, Bell D, Perkins GH, et al. Clinical implications of margin involvement by pleomorphic lobular carcinoma in situ. Arch Pathol Lab Med. 2011;135(6):737–43.
71. Ciocca RM, Li T, Freedman GM, Morrow M. Presence of lobular carcinoma in situ does not increase local recurrence in patients treated with breast-conserving therapy. Ann Surg Oncol. 2008;15(8):2263–71.
72. Apple SK, Matin M, Olsen EP, Moatamed NA. Significance of lobular intraepithelial neoplasia at margins of breast conservation specimens: a report of 38 cases and literature review. Diagn Pathol. 2010;5:54.
73. Jolly S, Kestin LL, Goldstein NS, Vicini FA. The impact of lobular carcinoma in situ in association with invasive breast cancer on the rate of local recurrence in patients with early-stage breast cancer treated with breast-conserving surgery. Int J Radiat Oncol Biol Phys. 2006;66(2):365–71.
74. Li S, Liu J, Yang Y, et al. Impact of atypical hyperplasia at margins of breast-conserving surgery on the recurrence of breast cancer. J Cancer Res Clin Oncol. 2014;140(4):599–605.

11 Current Management of Ductal Carcinoma In Situ (DCIS)

Adam I. Riker, Barbara L. Krueger, and Jami Walloch

Introduction

Ductal carcinoma in situ (DCIS) is the earliest described form of breast cancer, and despite tremendous research into this enigmatic disease process, that continues to puzzle researchers and clinicians around the world. Some clinicians clearly think that we are overtreating DCIS, from the initial screening stages through the surgical management. Although we all recognize the seemingly innocuous natural history of DCIS, we all know of patients that have initially presented with DCIS whom have ultimately died from their disease. Given this, until we are capable of developing better prognostic features that can definitively determine those that will (and will not) go on to develop progressive invasive disease, we are obligated to treat all patients with DCIS (all grades) who present with this noninvasive form of breast cancer.

Epidemiology and Statistics

Ductal carcinoma in situ (DCIS, intraductal carcinoma) is a noninvasive form of breast cancer, represented by a spectrum of various grades ranging from low-grade through high-grade DCIS with comedo necrosis and those with microinvasion (DCISM). Histologically, DCIS is characterized by proliferating malignant epithelial cells that are bounded by the basement membrane of the breast ducts (Fig. 11.1). It is still unclear whether DCIS is considered to be a direct precursor to invasive breast cancer (IBC), with evidence suggesting that it is rather an intermediary between normal breast tissue and IBC.

However, the natural course or history of untreated DCIS is really unknown, partially due to current surgical therapy that often removes the majority of the disease [1–3]. Additionally, the overall percentage of "nonprogressing" DCIS is unclear. There are some model estimates of the incidence of DCIS that will progress into IBC if left untreated as high as 100–270 per 100,000 [3, 4]. This model further estimates that women can survive >30 years with nonprogressing DCIS, while the average time interval for progressive DCIS to become IBC is 3 months, with the IBC remaining subclinical for about 2.5–3 years.

A.I. Riker, MD, FACS (✉)
Advocate Center for Breast Health, Advocate Cancer Institute, Advocate Christ Medical Center, 4400 West 95th Street, Suite 107 POB 408, Oak Lawn, IL 60453, USA
e-mail: adam.riker@advocatehealth.com, ariker1234@gmail.com

B.L. Krueger, MD, FACS
Breast Cancer Program, Advocate Cancer Institute, Advocate Christ Medical Center, 4400 West 95th Street, Oak Lawn, IL 60453, USA
e-mail: barbara.krueger@advocatehealth.com, bkrueger333@comcast.net

J. Walloch, MD
Department of Pathology, Advocate Cancer Institute, Advocate Christ Medical Center, 4400 West 95th Street, Suite 107 POB 408, Oak Lawn, IL 60453, USA

A.I. Riker (ed.), *Breast Disease: Comprehensive Management*,
DOI 10.1007/978-1-4939-1145-5_11, © Springer Science+Business Media New York 2015

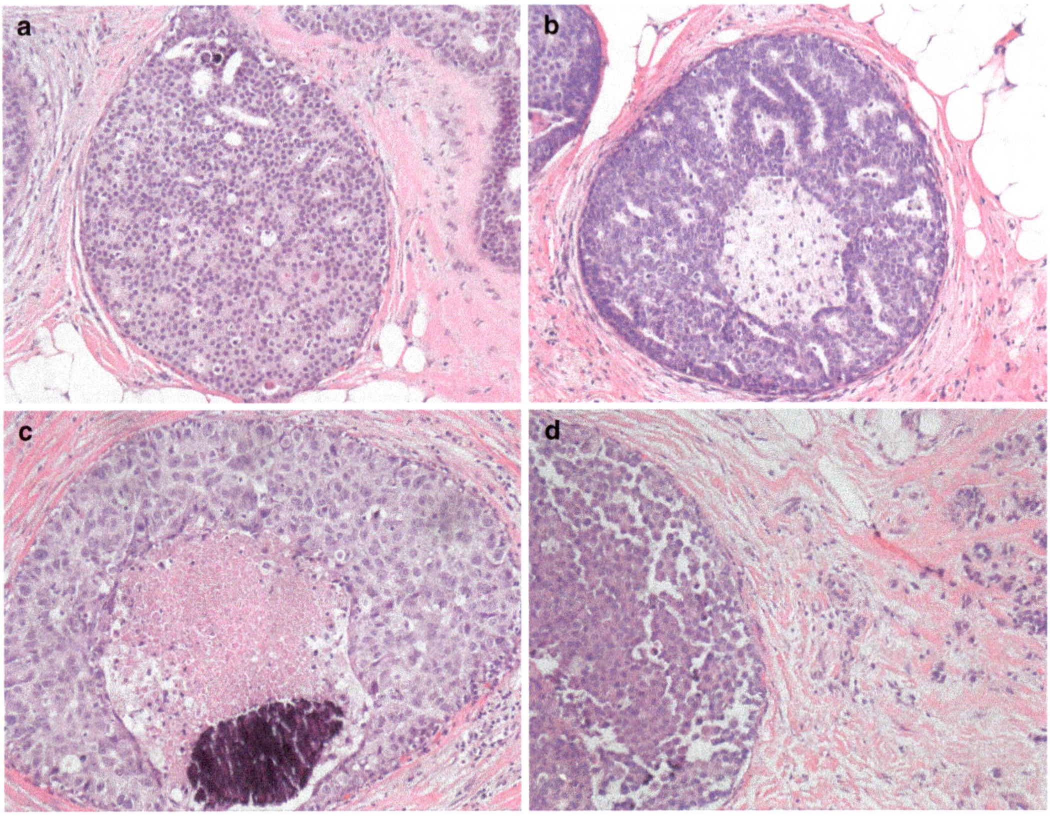

Fig. 11.1 (**a**) Low-grade ductal carcinoma in situ (grade 1): low-grade monomorphic nuclei, inconspicuous nucleoli, diffuse chromatin, cells maintain polarity around gland-like spaces, no comedo necrosis. (**b**) Intermediate-grade ductal carcinoma in situ (grade 2): low- to intermediate-grade nuclei with mild size variation, occasional nucleoli, diffuse to coarse chromatin, polarity loss around gland-like spaces, may have comedo necrosis. (**c**) High-grade ductal carcinoma in situ (grade 3): high-grade pleomorphic nuclei, prominent nucleoli, coarse to clumped chromatin, usually solid with no nuclear polarity, comedo necrosis common. (**d**) Ductal carcinoma in situ with microinvasion: this is an example of ductal carcinoma in situ, grade 2, with microinvasion (pT1mi: ≤1 mm invasion) into the adjacent stroma

The incidence of DCIS has been increasing at a rapid rate since the 1970s, coinciding with the adoption of screening and diagnostic mammography as the key driver for this increase. Over 80 % of all DCIS is diagnosed initially by mammography, accounting for 17–34 % of all mammographically detected breast neoplasms [5, 6]. According to the Surveillance, Epidemiology, and End Results (SEER) program from 1975 to 2008, in situ disease (DCIS and LCIS) accounted for ~15 % of all new breast cancer diagnoses in the United States [7]. Thus, DCIS will account for about 22 % of all newly diagnosed breast cancers or 63,300 cases of DCIS for 2012 [8].

Although it is recognized that DCIS is likely an intermediary to the development of IBC, the risk of death from DCIS remains quite low. Utilizing the SEER database, the 10-year risk of death for DCIS that was diagnosed between the years 1984 and 1989 is 1.9 % [9]. This low rate is consistent with other studies examining the long-term outcomes of DCIS, consistently reported as <2 % at 10 years from diagnosis [10–12]. Although the risk of death from DCIS remains low, the risk of a local recurrence is estimated to be between 2.4 and 15 % at 5 years and 10–24 % at 10 years [13]. Achieving local control is clearly the preferred method of achieving both long-term survival and preventing a local recurrence.

There is also a correlation between tumor grade and patient outcomes, consistently showing that a higher tumor grade (grade 3) is associated with a higher risk of local recurrence with DCIS and IBC compared to intermediate-grade (grade 2) or low-grade (grade 1) DCIS [13, 14]. Other factors associated with a higher risk of local recurrence are cellular architecture (comedo necrosis), the presence of microinvasion, multifocality, and possibly the lack of calcification. One possible tool available is the Van Nuys Index, developed to predict the chances of a local recurrence based upon four different predictors [15]. This predictive model is scored from 4 to 12, based upon tumor size, width of the negative margin, pathologic classification, and patient age, with each predictor scored from 1 to 3. Several studies have revealed a consistent correlation between the Van Nuys risk category and patient outcomes, showing that women within the highest risk category (Van Nuys score of 10–12) have a 224 % greater odds of mortality than women in the 4–6 risk category [16].

There are several demographic risk factors for the development of DCIS, and with few exceptions, with the same factors associated with the development of IBC. The incidence of DCIS is strongly related to age, with DCIS extremely uncommon in women younger than 40 years old. In fact, the incidence is only 2.5 per 100,000 for women ages 30–34, with a steady increase in incidence as the age increases, peaking at 96.7 per 100,000 women aged 65–69 [17, 18]. However, it should be noted that no matter what the age group, IBC is more common than DCIS. Other demographic risk factors associated with an increased likelihood of developing DCIS are race, urban versus rural living, lower educational level, and higher socioeconomic status. In terms of race, the incidence is highest for Caucasian women, followed second by African-American and Asian-Pacific Islanders.

Of note, caution should be taken when the younger patient, <40 years old, who present with DCIS, as they often present with some unique characteristics, such as a palpable mass, nipple discharge, or even breast pain. A recent study by Alvarado et al. shows that younger (<40 years old) patients with DCIS more often have multicentric disease, present with one or more clinical findings, and opt for, or require, mastectomy with immediate reconstruction [19]. Furthermore, the point is made that such patients should only be offered conservative surgery with an understanding that adjuvant radiotherapy will be delivered to the remaining breast.

Several reproductive factors have been shown to have a fairly weak association with an increased development of DCIS, such as late menopause (after 55 years of age), oral contraceptive use, and parity (age of first live birth <30 years of age) [20].

There does not appear to be any definitive evidence that the use of HRT is associated with an increased risk of DCIS. Biologic factors, such as density of the breast tissue, have also been examined. One study showed that premenopausal women with heterogeneous or extreme breast density had the highest risk of developing DCIS than women with scattered density [21]. Other studies have associated a strong family history of IBC or those with obesity, BRCA 1/2 mutational carriers, or a strong family history (high familial risk) with an increased odds for developing DCIS [22, 23]. Lastly, there is ample evidence that point to a protective effect from both tamoxifen and raloxifene for breast cancer prevention, with tamoxifen being more effective for preventing DCIS.

Initial Assessment

The initial assessment of the patient with DCIS begins with a thorough evaluation of all radiographic studies. This usually begins with a screening mammogram, with the vast majority of identified DCIS associated with a new area of microcalcifications when compared to previous films. The usual characteristics of suspicious or malignant-appearing calcifications are typically present, such as pleomorphic, grouped, linear, branching, irregular-shaped, and dystrophic calcifications. Comparative calcifications of a benign nature are generally larger, more rounded, and uniform in density, such as the "popcorn calcifications" associated with a fibroadenoma. Occasionally, DCIS may present initially as a palpable mass in about 10–15 % of all cases, also associated with a significantly higher potential for occult invasion, multicentricity, and locoregional recurrence [24, 25]. Several studies suggest that if left untreated, DCIS has the capacity to progress to invasive breast cancer in 30–50 % of all cases of DCIS [26, 27].

For DCIS, what is identified on the mammogram is often an underestimation of the entire extent of disease, as the DCIS is commonly found to extend along the ducts and may involve a large portion of the breast with multiple foci. Furthermore, even with the latest diagnostic imaging techniques, such as breast MRI, it is still difficult to accurately ascertain the true extent of DCIS. The Agency for Healthcare Research and Quality (AHRQ) as part of the US Department of Health and Human Services has thoroughly examined the utility of the increasing use of breast MRI and its impact upon treatment and outcomes for patients with DCIS [28]. The authors concluded that breast MRI consistently results in changes in treatment, primarily due to a differential ability for it to detect multicentric and contralateral disease, as well as accurately estimate the size of the tumor.

In our practice, we have incorporated breast MRI as an additional tool that often provides supplemental information, in addition to other studies, that is important to discuss with patients in determining the most appropriate operative intervention. It is not uncommon to obtain a breast MRI for patients with a 1.5 cm diameter area of grade 2/3 microcalcifications identified on mammography to ultimately have a much wider diameter area found on breast MRI. Additionally, contralateral abnormalities are often identified, with many found to be biopsy-proven high-risk lesions or even invasive cancer. Of course, this will greatly change the subsequent discussion with our patients, outlining the findings in detail and how this will impact the ultimate operative approach.

We should also point out the significance of additional areas identified on MRI that are deemed suspicious and requiring further intervention. Such areas may further require a biopsy or even a 6-month follow-up study with ultrasound or repeat MRI. Many patients at this point simply "throw in the towel," not wanting to delay their treatment any further with possible further diagnostic testing and biopsy. Most will opt for definitive and expeditious treatment of their cancer with mastectomy. Lastly, once the latter decision is made, many patients will further wish to discuss the risks, advantages, and disadvantages of contralateral prophylactic mastectomy for maximal risk reduction and, secondly, for improved symmetry and cosmetic outcome associated with bilateral breast reconstruction. Of importance, many patients will often strongly express their desire to obtain some semblance of "peace of mind," not wanting to have to worry about developing breast cancer in the contralateral breast in the future. Although it is well established that patients will overestimate their risk, many will still opt for contralateral mastectomy for this reason.

Surgical Management

The surgical management of DCIS is dependent upon a number of factors. One important factor that will ultimately determine the most appropriate surgical approach is the overall size (diameter) of the DCIS. Both mammogram and ultrasound can be very useful in determining the overall size of the area and whether it is multifocal or multicentric. If either is still indeterminate, breast MRI may be beneficial as an adjunct to further assessing the area in question. Once the area has been determined to be unifocal, a discussion about breast conservation can be pursued with the patient.

Once the final pathology has been reviewed, it is important to discuss whether the DCIS is pure low grade, intermediate grade, or high grade, with or without microinvasion (DCISM). We generally divide our operative approach based upon the overall grade of the DCIS, with low-grade DCIS having the smallest chance of spreading to the adjacent draining nodal basin (usually

<2 %). Thus, for patients with pure low-grade DCIS, we do not recommend sentinel lymph node mapping as part of breast conservation. However, we spend some time discussing the importance of adjuvant hormonal and radiation therapy.

Achieving local control is the key to good overall patient outcome and preventing local recurrence. Positive surgical margins (tumor at ink) are consistently shown to be associated with increased DCIS and invasive breast cancer recurrence [29–31]. In our practice, we plan our operative approach with attempting to remove the specimen with 10-mm margins of normal-appearing surrounding breast tissue. Upon removal of the lumpectomy specimen, we orient the specimen (short superior stitch at 12 o'clock and a long lateral stitch at 3 or 9 o'clock) followed by an intraoperative specimen radiograph in order to confirm that the previously placed core biopsy clip has been removed and is within the central portion of the lumpectomy specimen.

Additionally, we then send over the lumpectomy specimen for margin analysis, which involves the pathologist. The pathologist will first gross the specimen followed by inking of all of the surgical margins and subsequent serial gross sectional analysis of the tumor itself and biopsy cavity. A gross measurement is then made in order to assess the closest margin to the tumor, and if less than 2 mm by gross measurement, we will re-excise this margin intraoperatively.

We then await the final pathology based upon any re-excision margins that have been removed. It is uncommon that a return to the operating room is required due to a positive margin, occurring in <5 % of all cases of lumpectomy for DCIS. If the final margins are found to be <2 mm and assuming there is further tissue to be removed with re-excision, we will offer the patient a re-excision of margins in order to achieve negative margins. If there are multiple margins involved with DCIS, we will recommend a completion mastectomy in order to clear extensive, multifocal DCIS. If the deep margin is <2 mm or focally involved and the pectoralis fascia has been previously removed, then we do not recommend a return to the operating room. We will send this patient for radiation therapy with a likely boost to this area.

For patients identified with having either intermediate-grade DCIS, high-grade DCIS, or DCISM, we recommend concomitant sentinel lymph node mapping of the draining ipsilateral nodal basin. The likelihood of identifying SLN positivity in the intermediate- to high-grade group (without microinvasion) is between 5 and 10 % and those with microinvasion between 10 and 16 % [32, 33]. Even so, such positive findings in the SLN in any of these groups are likely to be either micrometastatic disease or isolated tumor cells (ITC's), with little, if any, overall impact on ultimate survival or outcome [32, 33]. However, there remains uncertainty in the preoperative setting as to the accurate identification of pure low-grade DCIS, often found to be upstaged to either intermediate- or high-grade DCIS, DCISM, or even invasive breast cancer. Thus, we discuss the nuances of performing SLNB in all of our patients with DCIS, clearly outlining the above findings and coming to a consensus with the patient about performing SLNB in the setting of DCIS.

There are other situations where SLNB may be justified in patients with DCIS, such as those with high-risk factors for harboring occult invasion. Preoperative factors for harboring occult invasion are older patient age, diagnosis by core needle biopsy, large-diameter DCIS, comedo-type necrosis, high-grade (grade 3) DCIS, a palpable mass, and tumor visible by ultrasound [32, 33]. For those patients that present with a palpable mass, which can be seen in 10–20 % of all cases of DCIS, it is very likely that there will be adjacent areas of invasive cancer found in about 25–35 % of all cases.

Therefore, we would strongly recommend SLNB as part of BCT. The last reason to perform SLN mapping are for those patients with DCIS who are undergoing a mastectomy. Recently, Shah et al. examined the SEER database to identify those patients with DCIS (all grades) between the years 2000 and 2008 (total of 20,177) who also underwent a SLNB as part of the operation [34]. They found that 51 % of all patients did not undergo a SLNB as part of the mastectomy procedure, with various reasons for this low percentage of patients being offered SLNB.

There is ongoing debate as to the benefit of performing a SLNB in patients with DCIS when compared to those with invasive breast cancer. Recent results from the ACOSOG Z10011 trial have examined the role of SLNB in patients with IBC (not DCIS). They conclude that there is no difference in either disease-free or overall survival in those patients with invasive breast cancer who have limited disease within the SLN and subsequently undergo a completion axillary lymph node dissection [35]. Clearly, the role of performing a SLNB in patients with DCIS can be questioned in many cases, with much of the decision based upon the grade of the DCIS, the presence of microinvasion, and the level of suspicion for concomitant areas of unrecognized invasive disease.

Adjuvant Therapy for DCIS

Based upon the current literature, it is clear that patients who have undergone operative removal with BCS (lumpectomy) for their DCIS should follow with adjuvant radiation therapy. Whole breast radiation therapy following BCS is associated with a significant reduction of local DCIS recurrence, with little, if any, impact upon improving overall survival. Both prospective and retrospective studies have demonstrated excellent long-term outcomes at 10 and 15 years after BCT with radiation. There have been four prospective, randomized trials that have extensively examined the utility of adding radiation therapy after lumpectomy, with all showing that the addition of radiation therapy after lumpectomy reduces the risk of local recurrence by about 50 % and for a subset of invasive local recurrence [10, 31, 36–40]. Thus, it is clear that radiation therapy after lumpectomy is an important adjuvant treatment option for patients undergoing BCT with lumpectomy.

However, it is much less certain as to a defined subset of patients that may not benefit from adjuvant radiation therapy. It is likely that not all patients with DCIS require radiation therapy after BCT, but there is a lack of evidence supporting its omission in suspected low-risk patients. To date, there has yet to be a definitive trial that has been able to identify such a group of patients who do not benefit from adjuvant radiation therapy as part of BCT for patients with DCIS. Some studies suggest that if one is able to obtain a >10 mm or greater surgical margin on the lumpectomy specimen, then it may be possible to eliminate the need for adjuvant radiation therapy [41–43].

Current areas of controversy:

1. *Do we overdiagnose and potentially overtreat DCIS?* It is quite likely that we are overdiagnosing and overtreating a fair proportion of patients who present with early findings based upon screening mammography. Recently, the independent UK Panel on Breast Cancer Screening addressed this very question, on whether breast cancer screening does more harm than good [44]. They provide the best available data for the UK setting, based upon a meta-analysis of 11 randomized trials examining the role of breast cancer screening and observational studies of the relative risk of breast cancer mortality for women invited to screening compared to controls. The panel concludes that there is about a 20 % relative risk reduction for those who undergo regular screening mammography, with a best estimate of overdiagnosis in the range of 11–19 %. This translates into about 1 % being overdiagnosed in the next 20 years for >300,000 women aged 50–52 who are invited in the United Kingdom to be screened every year.

   To the contrary, Wallis et al. report that incidence of DCIS rose rapidly since the inception of the National Health Service Breast Screening Programme (NHSBSP) in 1988 [45]. Many consider this rapid increase a representation of both overdiagnosis and overtreatment, with Wallis et al. reporting on the long-term follow-up of 700 noninvasive breast cancers (DCIS) over the first 10-year screening period (1988–1999). After a median follow-up of 183 months (range of 133–259 months), 102/700 (14.6 %) patients were identified with a first local recurrence, with

49/102 (48 %) being invasive breast cancer. The median time to the first noninvasive recurrence was 15 months and 60 months for invasive cancer. Additionally, they show that high-grade DCIS initially is associated with a much shorter interval to local recurrence with invasive recurrence (76 months) compared to those with low-/intermediate-grade DCIS (131 months). Thus, even with short-term follow-up, there will be a significant number of missed events, especially with invasive breast cancer as the first local recurrence.

Bleyer et al. utilized the SEER data to examine the trends from 1976 to 2008 for the incidence of early-stage breast cancer (DCIS and localized disease) and late-stage breast cancer (regional and distant disease) among women >40 years old [46]. They report that as a direct result of screening mammography, the number of cases of early-stage breast cancer that are detected each year has doubled, from 112 to 234 cases per 100,000 women in the United States. They further estimate that breast cancer was overdiagnosed (i.e., tumors are found by mammography that would *not* have led to clinically apparent disease) in 1.3 million women in the past 30 years. In 2008, they estimate that breast cancer was overdiagnosed in >70,000 women, accounting for 31 % of all breast cancers diagnosed that year. This study is supported by several other studies that examine this issue of overdiagnosis of not just DCIS but of invasive breast cancer [47]. Although these studies raise serious questions about the value of screening mammography to our respective societies, it is a much more complicated task to distill down the ever-increasing data in order to discuss the treatment decisions to be made with our patients.

2. *Is there a sequential progression of cellular and molecular events that occurs with high-risk lesions and DCIS becoming invasive breast cancer? Is it possible to differentiate and/or distinguish between DCIS that will progress on to become invasive breast cancer versus DCIS that will remain indolent and unlikely to harm the patient over an extended period of time?* DCIS is a neoplastic proliferation of cells within the ductal/lobular units of the breast that have not penetrated the myoepithelial basement membrane interface. The assumption is that all DCIS will eventually and inevitably progress to invasive breast cancer, with data to the contrary showing that up to 50 % of all cases of DCIS will in fact NOT progress on to invasive breast cancer in a woman's lifetime [39, 48]. The future challenge is to be able to identify those patients with DCIS that will go on to develop invasive breast cancer from those that will not. This will allow for the proper selection of patients who should undergo further therapy for their DCIS from those that can be safely followed without further intervention with surgery.

Bijker et al. examined 775 cases of DCIS as part of a randomized trial of BCT, with or without adjuvant radiotherapy, showing that there was a recurrence in 125 patients (16.1 %) at a median follow-up of 5.4 years [49]. Of the 125 cases of recurrence, 65 were DCIS and 60 were IBC, with the risk of developing a recurrence with IBC independent of whether the initial DCIS was low or high grade. To the contrary, intermediate- and high-grade DCIS was associated with a significantly higher risk of recurrent DCIS compared to low-grade DCIS, with the outcome for recurrent invasive disease differing significantly between the initial grade of the DCIS. The risk of distant metastasis and death was found to be significantly higher in recurrences secondary to high-grade DCIS.

Although DCIS as a whole is associated with an overall excellent outcome, even low-grade DCIS has the potential to progress into IBC. Betsill et al. followed ten patients with a mean follow-up of 21.6 years who were diagnosed with pure low-grade DCIS and treated with biopsy only, finding that 7/10 (70 %) developed IBC at an average interval of 9.7 years (range of 7–30 years) [50]. Saunders et al. provide further evidence for true disease progression of DCIS, as opposed to de novo development of disease, by following 28 women with small, low-grade DCIS treated again with biopsy only [48]. Of the 28 women followed for over 30 years time, 11/28 (39.3 %) developed IBC, with 7/11 (64 %) developing IBC within 10 years of their original biopsy.

In all cases, the IBC developed in the same quadrant of the breast where the original biopsy had been taken from previously, with 5/11 patients ultimately dying of metastatic breast cancer. Further support of this concept comes from recent data from King et al., who demonstrate that low-grade DCIS has a significant likelihood of recurring as high-grade IBC, indicating that grade alone is insufficient to predict the risk of breast cancer mortality [51]. Thus, it is clear that the highest risk for the development of recurrent IBC rests with high-grade DCIS; one should not underestimate the potential risk of recurrence for lower grades of DCIS as well.

3. *How does the increasing use of breast MRI impact patients with DCIS?*

   MRI of the breast has been shown to have a high sensitivity for the detection of invasive breast cancer, with a range of about 89–99 % [52, 53]. However, recent studies on the utility of preoperative breast MRI for the detection of DCIS are variable, with a sensitivity of 73–100 % [54–58]. A study by Kropcho et al. examined the role of preoperative breast MRI in the surgical treatment of DCIS, further evaluating the accuracy of MRI as compared to the final pathologic assessment and overall size of the DCIS [5]. They found that despite a high correlation between the size of the DCIS as assessed by MRI and histopathologic size, MRI appears to overestimate or underestimate the tumor size in over 70 % of the cases. They further conclude that there is a very low level of overall true accuracy in assessing the size of the DCIS, additionally finding that MRI did not favorably impact the surgeon's ability to achieve margins and may therefore not be of value to this end in patients with DCIS [5].

   Recently, Pilewskie et al. examined the effect of MRI on the management of DCIS of the breast in terms of preoperative surgical planning [59]. They divided a group of 352 patients with DCIS into two groups, those that underwent a preoperative MRI and those that did not, comparing the rates of additional biopsies, alterations in surgical management, reoperation rates, and the size of the DCIS as assessed by mammography, MRI, and final pathology. They found a remarkably higher rate of additional biopsies in the preoperative MRI group (38 % versus 7 % in the no-MRI group), with 18 % undergoing >2 additional biopsies compared to just 2 % in the no-MRI group.

   There did not seem to be a significant difference in assessing the size of the DCIS between MRI and mammography. Importantly, in women who underwent preoperative MRI, a higher fraction underwent a mastectomy as the first operation compared to those undergoing conventional imaging (34.6 % versus 27 %), but this was not found to be statistically significant. This must be weighed against the potential benefits of finding a contralateral breast cancer in about 3.2 % of cases, along with the downside of multiple additional biopsies that may yield a false positive on final pathologic analysis.

4. *What is the proper definition of positive surgical margins in the face of randomized controlled trials that clearly show that RT after BCS does not remove the negative prognostic impact of positive margins? Should patients with "close" margins undergo re-excision?* As stated above, it is our practice to take a patient back to the operating room if a final pathology margin on the lumpectomy specimen is positive (tumor at/on ink) or less than 2 mm. We may deviate from this practice for select situations, such as an older patient with a close (<1 mm), but not positive margin. Other situations may include a positive deep margin along the pectoralis muscle where there is clearly nothing further to re-excise. There is currently much controversy as whether "bigger is better," meaning a wider margin for DCIS translating into improved outcomes.

   Wang et al. recently performed a meta-analysis of 21 studies involving >7,500 patients with DCIS treated over a 25-year period [60]. They suggest that a wider margin of >10 mm should be considered a "priority" for all patients with DCIS, regardless of the patient receiving a full course of adjuvant radiation therapy. Furthermore, they show that a margin width of >10 mm was associated with a decreased risk of local recurrence compared to 2 mm or greater margins. However, this observational study has several faults associated with the interpretation of the data, as pointed out in an editorial by Morrow et al. [61]. As of 2012, it is still unclear what a negative surgical margin is, with many different margins accepted by surgeons worldwide, from no tumor cells identified at the inked margin, 1-mm, 2-mm, 4-mm to 10 mm margins. As such, there is currently no compelling evidence that a wider margin is any better than a smaller margin, with a 1–2 mm accepted as a safe, negative margin in most cases.

References

1. Ernster VL, Barclay J, Kerlikowske K, et al. Mortality among women with DCIS of the breast in the population-based surveillance, epidemiology and end-results program. Arch Intern Med. 2000;160(7):953–8.
2. Fisher ER, Land SR, Saad RS, et al. Pathologic variables predictive of breast cancer events in patients with DCIS. Am J Clin Pathol. 2007;128(1):86–91.
3. Yen MF, Tabar L, Vitak B, et al. Quantifying the potential problem of overdiagnosis of DCIS in breast cancer screening. Eur J Cancer. 2003;39(12):1746–54.
4. Duffy SW, Agbaje O, Tabar L, et al. Over-diagnosis and over-treatment of breast cancer: estimates of overdiagnosis from two trials of mammographic screening for breast cancer. Breast Cancer Res. 2005;7(6):258–65.
5. Ernster VL, Ballard-Barbash R, Barlow WE, et al. Detection of DCIS in women undergoing screening mammography. JNCI. 2002;94(20):1546–54.
6. May DS, Lee NC, Richardson LC, et al. Mammography and breast cancer detection by race and Hispanic ethnicity: results from a national program (United States). Cancer Causes Control. 2000;11(8):695–705.
7. Howlader N, Noone A, Krapcho M, et al., editors. SEER Cancer Statistics Review, 1975–2008. Bethesda: National Cancer Institute. http://seer.cancer.gov/csr/1975–2008/.
8. CA Cancer J Clin. 2012 Jan-Feb; 62(1):10–29. doi: 10.3322/caac.20138. PMID: 22237781.
9. Horner M, Rice L, Krapcho M, et al. SEER Cancer Statistics Review, 1975–2006. Bethesda: National Cancer Institute; 2009.
10. Fisher ER, Dignam J, Tan-Chiu, et al. Pathologic findings from the NSABP 8-year follow-up of protocol B-17: intraductal carcinoma. Cancer. 1999;86(3):429–38.
11. Smith BD, Haffty BG, Buchholz TA, et al. Effectiveness of radiation therapy in older women with DCIS. J Natl Cancer Inst. 2006;98(18):1302–10.
12. Solin LJ, Fourquet A, Vicini FA, et al. Long-term outcome after breast conservation treatment with radiation for mammographically detected DCIS of the breast. Cancer. 2005;103(6):1137–46.
13. Solin LJ. The impact of adding radiation treatment after breast conservation surgery for ductal carcinoma in situ of the breast. J Natl Cancer Inst Monogr. 2010;41:187–92.
14. Li CI, Malone KE, Saltzman BS, et al. Risk of invasive breast carcinoma among women diagnosed with DCIS and LCIS, 1998–2001. Cancer. 2006;106(10):2104–12.
15. Silverstein MJ. The University of Southern California/Van Nuys prognostic index for DCIS of the breast. Am J Surg. 2003;186(4):337–43.
16. Di Saverio S, Catena F, Santini D, et al. 259 patients with DCIS of the breast applying the USC/Van Nuys prognostic index: a retrospective review with long-term follow-up. Breast Cancer Res Treat. 2008;109(3):405–16.
17. Coburn NG, Chung MA, Fulton J, et al. Decreased breast cancer tumor size, stage and mortality in Rhode Island: an example of a well-screened population. Cancer Control. 2004;11(4):222–30.
18. Li CI, Daling JR, Malone KE. Age-specific incidence rates of in situ breast carcinoma by histologic type, 1980–2001. Cancer Epidemiol Biomarkers Prev. 2005;14(4):1008–11.
19. Alvarado R, Lari SA, Roses RE, et al. Biology, treatment and outcome in very young and older women with DCIS. Ann Surg Oncol. 2012. doi:10.1245/s10434-012-2413-4. Published online: 24 May 2012.
20. Claus EB, Stowe M, Carter D. Breast carcinoma in situ: risk factors and screening patterns. J Natl Cancer Inst. 2001;93(23):1811–7.
21. MacKenzie TA, Titus-Ernstoff L, Vacek PM, et al. Breast density in relation to risk of DCIS of the breast in women undergoing screening mammography. Cancer Causes Control. 2007;18(9):939–45.
22. Kerlikowske K, Barclay J, Grady D, et al. Comparison of risk factors for DCIS and invasive breast cancer. J Natl Cancer Inst. 1997;89(1):76–82.
23. Brekelmans CT, Seynaeve C, Bartels CC, et al. Effectiveness of breast cancer surveillance in BRCA ½ gene mutation carriers and women with high familial risk. J Clin Oncol. 2001;19(4):924–30.
24. van Deurzen CHM, Hobbelink MGG, van Hillegersberg R, et al. Is there an indication for sentinel node biopsy in patients with DCIS of the breast? A review. Eur J Cancer. 2007;43(6):993–1001.

25. Kurniawan ED, Rose A, Mou A, et al. Risk factors for invasive breast cancer when core needle biopsy shows DCIS. Arch Surg. 2010;145(11):1098–104.
26. Erbas B, Provenzano E, Armes J, et al. The natural history of DCIS of the breast: a review. Breast Cancer Res Treat. 2006;97(2):135–44.
27. Sanders ME, Schuyler PA, Dupont WD, et al. The natural history of low-grade DCIS of the breast in women treated by biopsy only revealed over 30 years of long-term follow-up. Cancer. 2005;103(12):2481–4.
28. Minnesota Evidence-based Practice Center, Minneapolis, Minnesota. Diagnosis and management of ductal carcinoma in situ (DCIS). Evidence Report and Technology Assessment, No. 185, AHRQ Publication No. 09-E018, Sept 2009.
29. MacDonald HR, Silverstein MJ, Mabry H, et al. Local control in DCIS treated by excision alone: incremental benefit of larger margins. Am J Surg. 2005;190(4):521–5.
30. Kerlikowske K, Molinaro A, Cha I, et al. Characteristics associated with recurrence among women with DCIS treated by lumpectomy. J Natl Cancer Inst. 2003;95(22):1692–702.
31. Bijker N, Meijnen P, Peterse JL, et al. Breast conserving treatment with or without radiotherapy in DCIS: 10-year results of EORTC randomized phase 3 trial 10853-A study by the EORTC Breast Cancer Cooperative Group and the EORTC Radiotherapy Group. J Clin Oncol. 2006;24(21):3381–7.
32. Meretoja TJ, Heikkila PS, Salmenkivi K, et al. Outcome of patients with DCIS and sentinel node biopsy. Ann Surg Oncol. 2012;19:2345–51.
33. Lyons JM, Stempel M, Van Zee KJ, et al. Axillary node staging for microinvasive breast cancer: is it justified? Ann Surg Oncol. 2012;19:3416–21.
34. Shah DR, Canter RJ, Khatri VP, et al. Utilization of sentinel lymph node biopsy in patients with DCIS undergoing mastectomy. Ann Surg Oncol. 2012. doi:10.1245/s10434-012-2539-4.
35. Giuliano AE, Hunt KK, Ballman KV, et al. Axillary dissection vs. no axillary dissection in women with invasive breast cancer and sentinel node metastasis. JAMA. 2011;305(6):569–75.
36. Fisher B, Dignam J, Wolmark N, et al. Lumpectomy and radiation therapy for the treatment of intraductal breast cancer: findings from NSABP B-17. J Clin Oncol. 1998;16(2):441–52.
37. Fisher B, Land S, Mamounas E, Dignam ER, et al. Prevention of invasive breast cancer in women with DCIS: an update of the NSABP. Semin Oncol. 2001;28(4):400–18.
38. Wapnir I, Dignam J, Julian TB, et al. Long-term outcomes after invasive breast tumor recurrence (IBTR) in women with DCIS in NSABP B-17 and B-24. J Clin Oncol. 2007;25(suppl):7s.
39. Bijker N, Peterse JL, Duchateau L, et al. Risk factors for recurrence and metastasis after breast conserving therapy for DCIS: analysis of EORTC 10853. J Clin Oncol. 2001;19(8):2263–71.
40. Holmberg L, Garmo H, Granstrand B, et al. Absolute risk reductions for local recurrence after postoperative radiotherapy after sector resection for DCIS of the breast. J Clin Oncol. 2008;26(8):1247–52.
41. Silverstein MJ, Lagios MD, Groshen S, et al. The influence of margin width on local control of DCIS of the breast. NEJM. 1999;340(19):1455–61.
42. Rudloff U, Brogi E, Reiner AS, et al. The influence of margin width and volume of disease near margin on benefit of radiation therapy for women with DCIS treated with breast-conserving surgery. Ann Surg. 2010;251(4):583–91.
43. Independent UK Panel on Breast Cancer Screening. The benefit and harms of breast cancer screening: an independent review. Lancet. 2012;380(9855):1778–86.
44. Wallis MG, Clemets K, Kearins O, et al. The effect of DCIS grade on rate, type and time to recurrence after 15 years of follow-up of screen-detected DCIS. Br J Cancer. 2012;106(10):1611–7.
45. Bleyer A, Welch HG. Effect of three decades of screening mammography on breast-cancer incidence. N Engl J Med. 2012;367(21):1998–2005.
46. Kalager M, Adami HO, Bretthauer M, et al. Overdiagnosis of invasive breast cancer due to mammography screening: results from the Norwegian screening program. Ann Intern Med. 2012;156:491–9.
47. Saunders ME, Schuyler PA, Dupont WD, et al. The natural history of low grade DCIS of the breast in women treated by biopsy only revealed over 30 years of long-term follow-up. Cancer. 2005;103:2481–4.
48. Collins LC, Tamimi RM, Baer HJ, et al. Outcome of patients with DCIS untreated after diagnostic biopsy. Results from the Nurses' Health Study. Cancer. 2005;103:1778–84.
49. Betsill WLJ, Rosen PP, Lieberman PH, et al. Intraductal carcinoma. Long-term follow-up after treatment by biopsy alone. J Am Med Assoc. 1978;239:1863–7.
50. King TA, Sakr RA, Muhsen S, et al. Is there a low-grade precursor pathway in breast cancer? Ann Surg Oncol. 2012;19:1115–21.
51. Lehman CD, Gatsonis C, Kuhl CK, et al. MRI evaluation of the contralateral breast in women with recently diagnosed breast cancer. N Engl J Med. 2007;356:1295–303.
52. Kriege M, Brekelmans CT, Boetes C, et al. Efficacy of MRI and mammography for breast cancer screening in women with a familial or genetic predisposition. N Engl J Med. 2004;351:427–37.
53. Schouten van der Velden AP, Boetes C, Bult P, et al. The value of MRI imaging in diagnosis and size assessment of in situ and small invasive breast carcinoma. Am J Surg. 2006;192:172–8.
54. Santamaria G, Velasco M, Farrus B, et al. Preoperative MRI of pure intraductal breast carcinoma-A valuable adjunct to mammography in assessing cancer extent. Breast. 2008;17:186–94.

55. Kuhl CK, Schrading S, Bieling HB, et al. MRI for diagnosis of pure DCIS: a prospective observational study. Lancet. 2007;370:485–92.
56. Fadare O, Clement NF, Ghofrani M. High and intermediate grade DCIS of the breast: a comparison of pathologic features in core biopsies and excisions and an evaluation of core biopsy features that may predict a close or positive margin in the excision. Diagn Pathol. 2009;4:26.
57. Allen LR, Lago-Toro CE, Hughes JH, et al. Is there a role for MRI in the pre-operative assessment of patients with DCIS? Ann Surg Oncol. 2010;17:2395–400.
58. Kropcho LC, Steen ST, Chung AP, et al. Preoperative breast MRI in the surgical treatment of DCIS. Breast J. 2012;18(2):151–6.
59. Pilewskie M, Kennedy C, Shappell C, et al. Effect of MRI on the management of DCIS of the breast. Ann Surg Oncol. 2012. doi:10.1245/s10434-012-2771. Published online 07 Dec 2012.
60. Wang SY, Chu H, Shamliyan T, et al. Network meta-analysis of margin threshold for women with DCIS. J Natl Cancer Inst. 2012;104(7):507–16.
61. Morrow M, Katz SJ. Margins in DCIS: is bigger really better? Editorials. J Natl Cancer Inst. 2012;104(7):494–5.

Management of Axilla in Invasive Breast Cancer

12

Paulomi Shroff and Philip Israel

Introduction

A large proportion of primary breast cancers will first metastasize to the regional lymphatic nodal basin prior to the patient developing distant metastases. The majority of lymph node metastases from the breast are to the ipsilateral axillary nodal basin, including both central and medial breast cancers, which may also metastasize to the internal mammary lymph nodes. It is surmised that approximately 75 % of the breast lymphatic flow drains directly into the axillary lymph nodes, with about 20 % draining into both axillary and internal mammary lymph nodes. Only 5 % of breast lymphatic drainage is predominantly to the internal mammary nodes [1]. Hence management of the axilla is important for both accurate staging and locoregional control of breast cancer. It is important to note, however, that 30 % of node-negative patients will eventually relapse with distant metastatic disease [2].

Historical Perspective

Prior to the 1990s, all women with invasive breast cancer underwent an axillary dissection, otherwise known as complete axillary lymph node dissection (CALND), as a standard part of their surgical treatment. The landmark NSABP-04 study, which compared patients with mastectomy alone to mastectomy and axillary dissection, revealed no difference in the overall survival in the two groups and a less than expected axillary recurrence rate in the non-axillary dissection arm [3]. This paved the way for sentinel lymph node biopsy (SLNB) in breast cancer. The 1990s saw the advent of axillary sentinel lymph node biopsy in the staging of breast cancer patients that was subsequently substantiated and validated in the NSABP-32 [4]. This further led to questioning whether patients with positive sentinel nodes need to subsequently undergo a completion axillary dissection addresses with the ACOSOG Z00011 clinical trial (macrometastases) [5] and the ISBCG 23-01 trials (micrometastases) [6]. As expected, both of these studies have resulted in a true paradigm shift in our current surgical management of the axilla.

P. Shroff, MD (✉) • P. Israel, MD
Department of Surgery, The Breast Center,
702 Canton Road, Marietta, GA 30060, USA
e-mail: paulomishroff@yahoo.com

Anatomy

Lymphatics in the breast exist in a perilobular and periductal plexus. These and the subareolar plexus of dermal lymphatics drain into the axillary lymph nodes. They first drain into the level 1 axillary lymph nodes, which lie lateral to the pectoralis minor muscle insertion. Thereafter, they drain into the level 2 (deep to pectoralis minor) and level 3 (medial to pectoralis minor) lymph nodes. As the lymphatics arborize extensively, there may be drainage to more than one sentinel lymph node [2] (Figs. 12.1 and 12.2).

A.I. Riker (ed.), *Breast Disease: Comprehensive Management*,
DOI 10.1007/978-1-4939-1145-5_12, © Springer Science+Business Media New York 2015

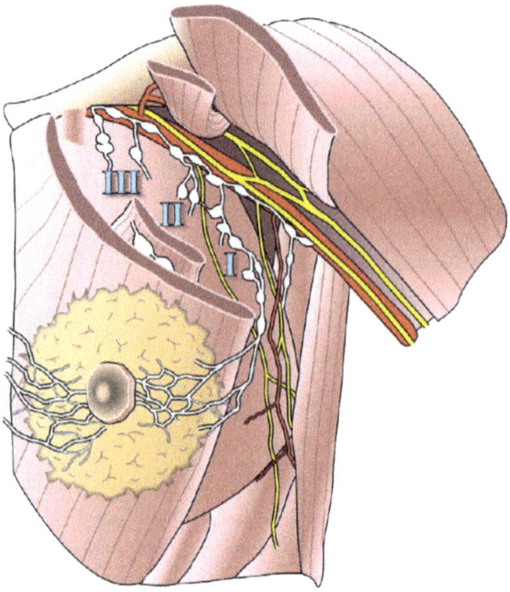

Fig. 12.1 Anatomy of lymphatic flow of the breast (Reproduced with permission from: Benson et al. [2])

Significance of Axillary Evaluation

Evaluation of the axilla is vital for the proper management of invasive breast cancer. It is necessary to adequately stage the breast cancer and for local control of disease metastasis to the axillary lymph nodes. The extent of lymph node involvement guides the need for and type of chemotherapy used. It also guides the extent of the radiation fields that may be necessary to control disease in the axilla [2] (Fig. 12.3).

Preoperative Evaluation of Axilla

Clinical Examination

A critical component of staging is the clinical examination. The axilla is best evaluated clinically in an upright position, with the patient's arm resting by her side. The axilla is then evaluated for any palpable, hard nodes. If identified, it is important to assess if these nodes are matted together, a critical aspect of nodal staging, based solely upon the clinical examination alone.

Ultrasound of the Axilla

Ultrasound of the axilla is an important adjunct in patients with breast cancer, especially in patients with palpable axillary lymphadenopathy. Ultrasound appearance of a normal lymph node reflects its normal anatomy, being transversely oval and hypoechoic, with a central hyperechoic hilum. A pathologic lymph node on ultrasound has an abnormal shape and architecture. It is more rounded with the ratio of the longitudinal to transverse axis being less than two. The cortex is thicker than the hilum, and in some nodes, the hilum may not be visualized at all. This may be preoperatively evaluated further by fine-needle aspiration (FNA) cytology [7] or ultrasound-guided core needle biopsy [8]. Specificity of both modalities approaches 100 %, with sensitivities of FNA and core needle biopsy noted to be 36–42 %, respectively, in the abovementioned studies in cohorts of patients with invasive breast cancer and nonpalpable axillary lymph nodes. Once proven to contain metastatic cancer, it obviates the need for sentinel lymph node biopsy in those patients (Fig. 12.4).

Surgery of the Axilla

Sentinel Lymph Node Biopsy (SLNB)

Indications

The indications for SLNB in breast cancer patients are well established [9] (Table 12.1).

Technique

The technique involves the use of technetium-99m sulfur colloid (99m-Tc). This is injected intradermally in the upper outer quadrant of the areola, about 1–4 h prior to surgery. Intraoperatively, 1–3 cc of 1 % isosulfan blue may additionally be injected subcutaneously, if necessary. A transverse axillary skin crease incision is marked over the site of the maximum frequency of radioactive dye uptake. After incising the skin, subcutaneous tissue, and axillary fascia, afferent blue lymphatics are indentified and followed to the draining lymph node. Alternately, any radioactive lymph

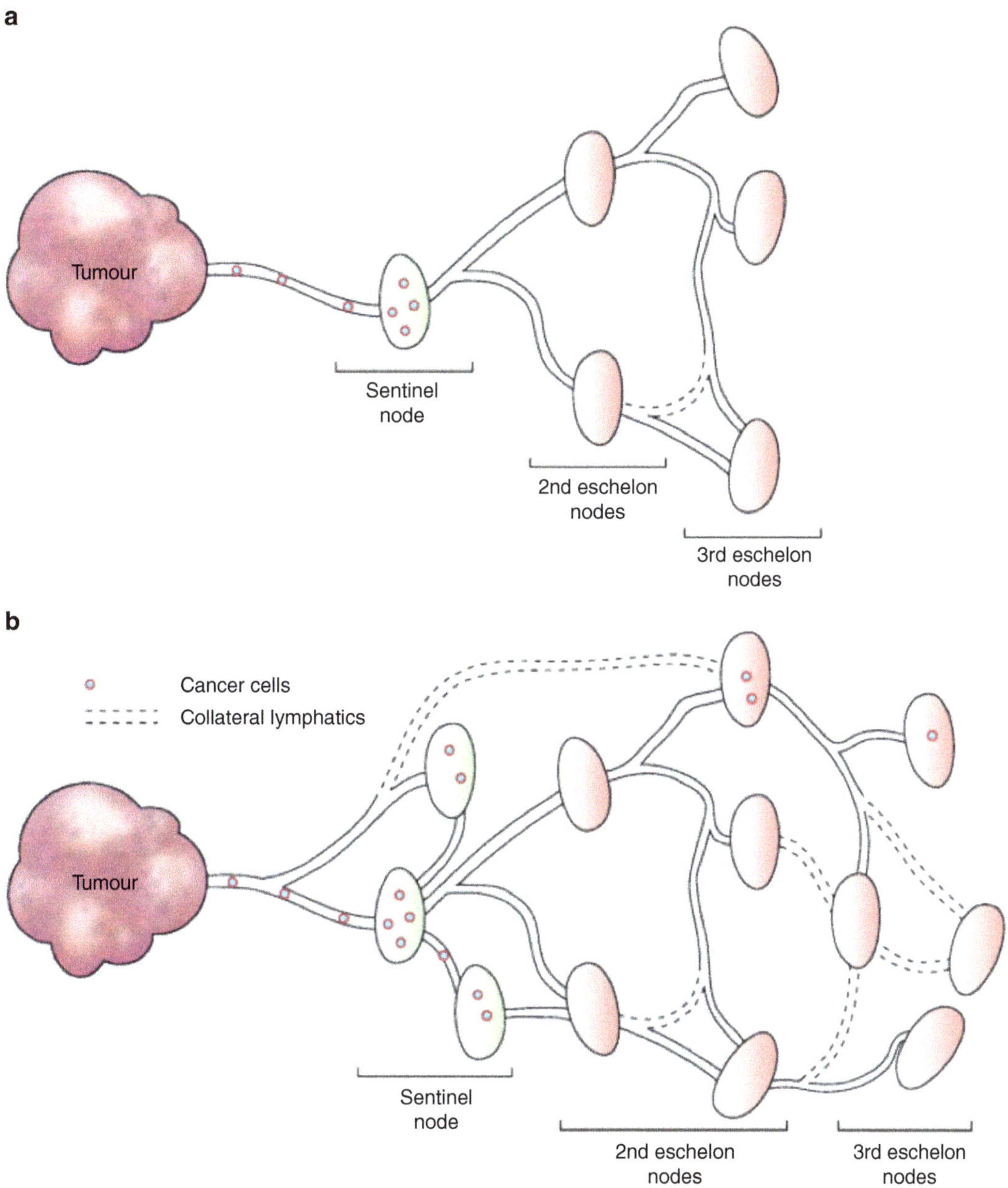

Fig. 12.2 (**a**) Patterns of lymphatic drainage from a primary tumor. (**b**) Note the arborization of lymphatics may result in more than one sentinel lymph node (Reproduced with permission from: Benson et al. [2])

node identified is also considered an SLN and removed. This dual technique for sentinel lymph node identification is considered more sensitive than the use of a single agent. Any suspicious palpable lymph node may also be considered to be a sentinel lymph node and thus removed.

Intraoperative Evaluation SLNs: Sentinel lymph nodes are often sent for intraoperative evaluation. This is done by frozen section analysis of a few sections of the lymph node or by touch preparation of the bivalved lymph node. Of note, the sensitivity is fairly good, although

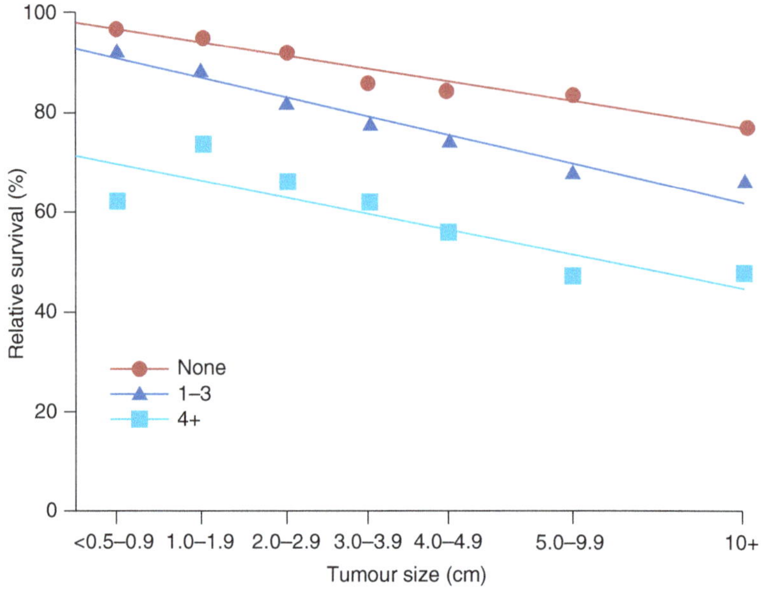

Fig. 12.3 Relative rates of 5-year survival in relation to tumor size and number of positive regional lymph nodes (SEER database 1977–1982) (Reproduced with permission from: Benson et al. [2])

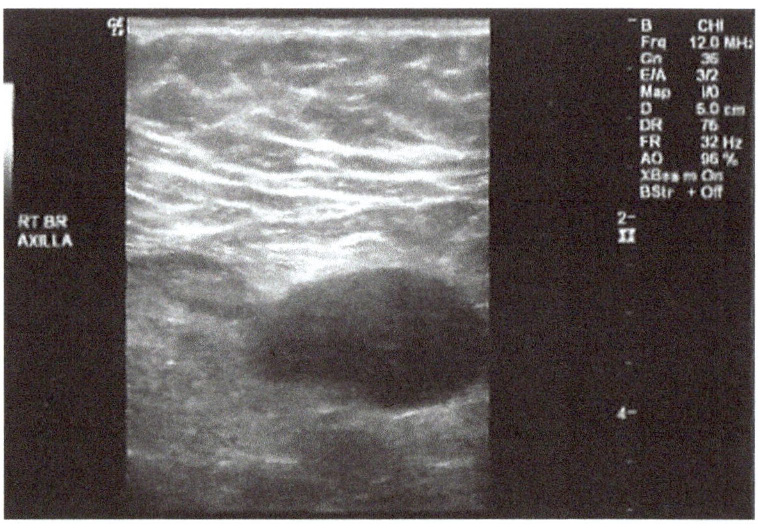

Fig. 12.4 Normal architecture axillary lymph node (*left*) adjacent to abnormal architecture, enlarged lymph node (*right*)

micrometastases and metastases from invasive lobular carcinomas may sometimes be missed.

Other methods less commonly used are rapid cytokeratin immunostain of frozen section of the sentinel lymph node [10] and reverse transcriptase polymerase chain reaction (RT-PCR) on a portion of the sentinel lymph node [11]. These methods are of increasing sensitivity, but the more complex methods have time constraints and utilize more tissue, which may be unavailable for final pathology.

There is about a 10 % incidence of non-sentinel lymph node metastases [12]; however, the Z0011 trial would question the clinical significance of the same [5].

Completion Axillary Lymph Node Dissection (CALND)

This involves removal of levels 1 and 2 axillary lymph nodes. It is indicated for those patients with

Table 12.1 Indications for sentinel lymph node biopsy

Clinical scenarios	Indication of sentinel node biopsy
T1 or T2 tumors	Established
Older age	Established
Obesity	Established
Before preoperative systemic therapy	Established
Male breast cancer	Established
DCIS with mastectomy	Established
Internal mammary chain	Established but controversial
DCIS without mastectomy	Controversial, except for DCIS with suspected or proven microinvasion
Pregnancy	Controversial
Suspicious, palpable axillary nodes	Controversial
T3 or T4 tumors	Controversial
Multicentric or multifocal tumors	Controversial
Prior diagnostic or excisional breast biopsy	Controversial
Prior axillary surgery	Controversial
Prior non-oncologic breast surgery	Controversial
After preoperative systemic therapy	Controversial
Inflammatory breast cancer	Not recommended

Courtesy of Vidal-Siccart S, Olmos R [9]

grossly enlarged axillary lymph nodes proven to contain metastatic disease preoperatively. Also patients with sentinel lymph nodes, with intraoperative confirmation of metastatic lymph node involvement, will warrant CALND. Lastly, CALND is recommended for those patients who have confirmed nodal disease prior to undergoing neoadjuvant chemotherapy.

A transverse axillary skin crease incision is made over the low axilla. The skin, subcutaneous tissue, and axillary fascia are incised. The lateral border of the pectoralis minor muscle is identified and followed superiorly up to the axillary vein. The inferior border of the axillary vein is freed by ligating the tributaries to the vein. The level 2 lymph nodes that lie between the axillary vein and the undersurface of the pectoralis minor muscle are dissected free and brought into the low axilla, to be removed along with level 1 lymph nodes. Thereafter, the long thoracic nerve to the serratus anterior muscle is identified and preserved along the chest wall. The subscapular vessels along with the thoracodorsal nerve to the latissimus anterior muscle are identified and preserved. The tissue between the two nerves and the inferior border of the axillary vein is then delivered out as axillary content, with everything sent to pathology for final diagnosis. Lastly, palpation of the level 3 area is necessary in order to confirm that there are no hard, palpable, suspicious lymph nodes. If present, they must be removed as there is a high likelihood of metastatic disease.

Complications of axillary dissection may range from numbness of the upper, inner aspect of the arm from injury to the intercostobrachial nerve, chronic lymphedema, and nerve or major vessel injury.

Lymphedema: Lymphedema following the operative treatment of breast cancer can be defined as the persistent swelling of the ipsilateral upper extremity.

The overall incidence of lymphedema is about 26 % [13]. It varies based upon treatment modalities—with a <1 % incidence of chronic lymphedema with sentinel lymph node biopsy (SLNB) alone, 9.1 % with axillary sampling combined with radiation therapy, 7.4 % with CALND alone, 8.3 % with axillary radiation alone, and 38.3 % in patients who undergo CALND followed by adjuvant axillary radiation [14]. As the number of lymph nodes removed increases as well as the overall extent of the axillary fields of radiation increases, so does the risk increase for the development of chronic lymphedema [15].

Lymphedema may be measured either subjectively or objectively. Objectively it is defined as an increase in arm volume by 200 ml or an increase in forearm circumference by 2 cm (measured 10 cm inferior to lateral epicondyle) [13].

The treatment of lymphedema includes both prevention and treatment, with prevention focused upon meticulous skin care, skin safety, and prompt attention and treatment of skin infections. Various treatment options include manual lymphatic drainage, compression garments, and pneumatic compression (Fig. 12.5).

AJCC 7 Node Staging for Breast Cancer

Regional lymph nodes (N)

Clinical Classification

•*NX*: Regional lymph nodes cannot be assessed (e.g., previously removed)

•*N0*: No regional lymph node metastasis

•*N1*: Metastasis to movable ipsilateral axillary lymph node(s)

•*N2*: Metastasis to ipsilateral axillary lymph node(s) fixed or matted, or in clinically detected* ipsilateral internal mammary nodes in the absence of clinically evident lymph node metastasis
•*N2a*: Metastasis in ipsilateral axillary lymph nodes fixed to one another (matted) or to other structures
•*N2b*: Metastasis only in clinically detected* ipsilateral internal mammary nodes and in the absence of clinically evident axillary lymph node metastasis

•*N3*: Metastasis in ipsilateral infraclavicular lymph node(s) with or withoutaxillary lymph node Involvement, or in clinically detected* ipsilateral internal mammary lymph node(s) and in the presence of clinically evident axillary lymph node metastasis; or, metastasis in ipsilateral supraclavicular lymph node(s) with or without axillary or internal mammary lymph node involvement
•*N3a*: Metastasis in ipsilateral infraclavicular lymph node(s)
•*N3b*: Metastasis in ipsilateral internal mammary lymph node(s) and axillary lymph node(s)
•*N3c*: Metastasis in ipsilateral supraclavicular lymph node(s)

* Note: "Clinically detected"is defined as detected by imaging studies (excluding lymphoscintigraphy) or by clinical examination and having characteristics highly suspicious for malignancy or a presumed pathologic macrometastasisbased on fine needle aspiration biopsy with cytologic examination. Confirmation of clinically detected metastatic disease by fine needle aspiration without excision is designated with an (f) suffix, for example, cN3a (f). Excisionbiopsy of a lymph node or biopsy of a sentinel lymph node, in the absence of anassignment of a pT, is classified as a clinical N, for example cN1. Information regarding the confirmation of nodal stats will be designated in site-specific factors as clinical, fine needle aspiration, core biopsy or sentinel lymph node biopsy. Pathologic classification(pN) is used for excisionor sentinel lymph node biopsy only in conjunction with a pathologic T assignment.

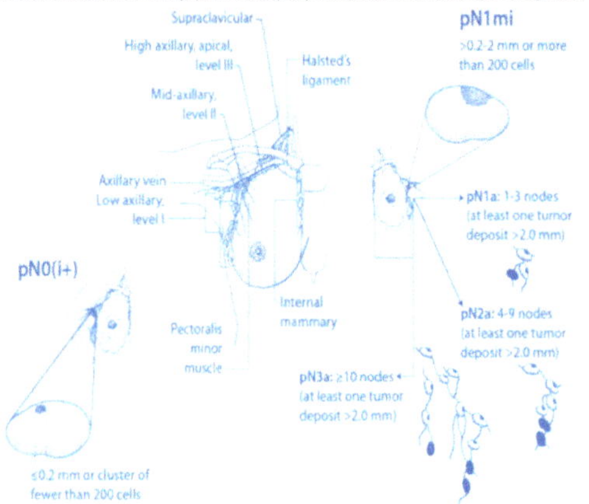

Pathologic classification (pN)*

•*pNX*: Regional lymph nodes cannot be assessed (e.g., notremoved for pathologic study or Previously removed)

•*pN0*: No regional lymph node metastasis histologically.
(Note: Isolated Tumor Cells (ITC) are defined as single tumor cells or small cell clusters not larger than 0.2 mmor a cluster of fewer than 200 cells on a single histologic cross-section. ITCs may be detected by routine histology orby immunohistochemical (IHC) methods. Nodescontaining ITCs are excluded from total positive nodes counted for purposes of N classification, but should be included in total number of nodes evaluated.)
•*pN0(i-)*: No regional lymph node metastasis histologically, negative IHC
•*pN0(i+)*: Malignant cells in regional lymph node(s), no greater than 0.2 mm (detected by H&E or by IHC)
•*pN0(mol-)*: No regional lymph node metastasis histologically, and negative molecular findings (RT-PCR)**
•*pN0(mol+)*: Positive molecular findings (RT-PCR)**, but no regional lymph node metastases detected by histology or IHC.

•*pN1*: Micrometastases or Metastasis in one to three axillary lymph nodes, and/or in internal mammary nodes with metastaticdisease detected by SLN biopsy but not clinically detected***
•*pN1mi*: Micrometastasis (larger than 0.2 mmand more than 200 cells, but none larger than 2.0 mm)
•*pN1a*: Metastasis in one to three axillary lymph no des, at least 1 metastasis larger than 2.0 mm.
•pN1b: Metastasis in internal mammary nodes with micrometastasis or macrometastasis detected by SLN biopsy, but not clinically detected***
•*pN1c*: Metastasis in one to three axillary lymph nodes and in internal mammary lymph nodes with micrometastasis or macrometastasisdetectedby SLN biopsy but not clinically detected***

•*pN2*: Metastasis in four to nine axillary lymph nodes, or in clinically detected**** internal mammary lymph nodes in the absenceof axillary lymph node metastasis.
•*pN2a*: Metastasis in four to nine axillary lymph nodes (at least one tumor deposit larger than 2.0 mm)
•*pN2b*: Metastasis in clinically detected**** internal mammary lymph nodes in the absenceof axillary lymph node metastasis

•*pN3*: Metastasis in ten or more axillary lymph nodes, or in infraclavicular (Level III axillary) lymph nodes, or inclinically detected**** ipsilateral internal mammary lymph node(s) in the presence of one or more positivelevel I and II axillary lymph node(s); or, in more than three axillary lymph nodes and in the internal mammary lymph node(s) with micrometastasis or macrometastasis detected by sentinel lymph node biopsy, but not clinically detected ***, or in ipsilateral supradavicular lymph nodes.
•*pN3a*: Metastasis in ten or more axillary lymph nodes (at least one tumor deposit larger than 2.0 mm); or, metastasis to the infraclavicular(level III axillary) lymph nodes
•*pN3b*: Metastasis in clinically detected**** ipsilateral internal mammary lymph nodes in the presence of one or more positive axillary lymph node(s); or, in more than three axillary lymph nodes and in internal mammary lymphnodes with micrometastasis or macrometastasis detected by sentinel lymph node biopsy but not clinically detected***
•*pN3c*: Metastasis in ipsilateral supraclavicular lymph nodes

* Note: Classification is based on axillary lymph node dissection with or without sentinel lymph node (SLN) dissection. Classification based solely on SLN dissection without subsequent axillary lymph node dissection is designated (sn) for sentinel node, e.g., pN0(I+) (sn).
**Note: RT-PCR: reverse transcriptase-polymerase chain reaction.
***Note: "Not clinically detected" is defined as not detected by imaging studies (excluding lymphoscintigraphy) or by clinical examination and having characteristics highly suspicious for malignancy or a presumed pathologic macrometastsis based on fine needle aspiration biopsy with cytologic examination.
****Note: "Clinically detected" is defined as detected byimaging studies (excluding lymphoscintigraphy) or by clinical examination.

Fig. 12.5 AJCC 7 breast cancer staging (Reprinted with permission, Springer, 2013 [16])

Recent Trends in Axillary Surgery for Invasive Breast Cancer

As the understanding of the biology of breast cancer has shifted from a Halstedian model with an orderly anatomical progression of cancer to a systemic Fischerian model, so has the management of the axilla. Prior to the advent of sentinel lymph node biopsy, all breast cancer patients underwent a CALND as part of their treatment. However, the adoption of sentinel lymph node biopsy, and its subsequent validation, by studies such as the NSABP-32 [4], led to a paradigm shift to lesser axillary surgery. The results of the American College of Surgeons Oncology Group (ACOSOG) Z0011 trial [6] went a step further. This multicenter study randomized T1 and T2 lumpectomy patients with one to two positive sentinel lymph nodes to completion axillary dissection versus no completion axillary dissection, followed by standard whole breast radiation and adjuvant systemic therapy. There was noted to be no significant difference in overall survival, as might be expected. However, there was also no difference in the rates of axillary recurrence. This has led to an appropriate decreased utilization of axillary dissection in selected patients [17]. The American Society of Breast Surgeons (ASBS) has posted a position statement on management of the axilla in patients with invasive breast cancer which references the potentially practice-changing results of the Z0011 trial [18].

The After Mapping of the Axilla: Radiotherapy or Surgery? (AMAROS) phase III study performed by the European Organization for Research and Treatment of Cancer (EORTC) published its preliminary data [19]. This trial randomizes patients with 5–30 mm invasive breast cancers (clinically negative nodes), with a positive sentinel lymph node, to axillary dissection versus axillary radiotherapy. The absence of knowledge of extent of axillary involvement in the non-axillary dissection group did not appear to have any major impact on the determination of adjuvant therapy, per the early results of the trial. Further results of the trial are awaited.

The International Breast Cancer Study Group (IBCSG) trial 23-01 randomizes clinically node-negative T1 and T2 invasive breast cancer patients with micrometastases in sentinel lymph nodes to axillary dissection versus no axillary dissection. While the final results are awaited, the 4-year data reveals very low rates of recurrence in both groups [6].

There is much more work ahead to be done, such as identifying the ideal patient that may not need an axillary dissection after a positive sentinel node and the extent of radiation needed to the axilla for comparable outcomes. The present trend to avoid axillary dissection in appropriately selected patients is admirable. It is essential, however, that we recognize that it may be unwise to trade one set of complications for another and that the advantages of doing less surgery on the axilla are not offset by excessive radiation damage to the axilla. Further studies in this regard are warranted.

Another intriguing study is the American College of Surgeons Surgical Oncology Group (ACOSOG) Z1071 trial. This multicenter study enrolled women with clinical T 0–4, N1–2, M0 in receiving neoadjuvant chemotherapy and thereafter undergoing SLNB and CALND. The overall sensitivity of the SLNB was 84 %, with a false-negative rate of 12.8 %. This puts forth the possibility that some patients with clinical N1–2 disease may avoid an axillary dissection after neoadjuvant chemotherapy, but further work is needed to identify appropriate patient selection for the same [20].

Axillary Management in Special Situations

Sentinel Lymph Node Biopsy (SLNB) and Neoadjuvant Chemotherapy

This remains a controversial topic, with options of performing an SLNB in clinically node-negative patients prior to commencing neoadjuvant chemotherapy versus after the completion of chemotherapy. The proponents of SLNB biopsy prior to chemotherapy maintain that axillary staging is needed to direct the use of anthracyclines in neoadjuvant chemotherapy and radiation. Those in favor of SLNB after neoadjuvant chemotherapy maintain that clinically node-negative patients can safely undergo a single-stage procedure with axillary staging at the time of definitive breast surgery following the completion of neoadjuvant chemotherapy. This may avoid the need for axillary dissection in low-volume axillary disease that may have been cleared by neoadjuvant chemotherapy [21].

The incidence of non-sentinel lymph node metastases, for those completing neoadjuvant chemotherapy in the NSABP 27 trial, was 11 %, not significantly different from the results of the NSABP-32 trial. This would support the validity of performing SLNB after the completion of neoadjuvant chemotherapy [22].

The authors usually perform sentinel lymph node biopsy after neoadjuvant chemotherapy except when the multidisciplinary opinion is that preneoadjuvant sentinel lymph nodes status will significantly change the nature of chemotherapy or adjuvant radiation therapy, or there is a discrepancy in the clinical examination and imaging.

Ductal Carcinoma In Situ (DCIS)

As a routine, patients undergoing surgery for DCIS do not need axillary staging. However, if the patient is undergoing a mastectomy for DCIS, a sentinel lymph node biopsy is warranted. There is a 20 % chance of upgrade of diagnosis to invasive carcinoma, on final pathology [1]. After a mastectomy, the ability to identify a sentinel lymph node is greatly diminished, were there to be an upgrade of diagnosis.

A biopsy suggesting high-grade DCIS, microinvasion, or a mass on mammography predicts a higher risk of invasive carcinoma being found on final pathology. Hence sentinel lymph node biopsy may be selectively utilized in these situations [23].

Micrometastases

These are defined as lymph node metastases that are 0.2–2.0 mm in diameter. These are often not identified intraoperatively. They are classified as N1 (mic) in the TNM classification [16]. Presently, the trend is not to perform a completion axillary dissection in this situation. This is supported by the aforementioned 4-year results of the International Breast Cancer Study Group (IBCSG) trial 23-01, but final results are awaited.

Isolated Tumor Cells (ITC)

These are sentinel lymph node metastases that are <0.2 mm in diameter. They are most often identified only on immunohistochemistry. This is sometimes performed on sentinel lymph nodes, especially for patients with invasive lobular carcinoma. The TNM classification of these is N0 (ihc+), and the ITC metastases have been shown to not be considered clinically significant [24].

Other Breast Malignancies: Lymphoma, Sarcoma, and Malignant Phyllodes

Although uncommon, lymphoma, especially B-cell lymphoma, may present either as a breast lesion or with axillary lymphadenopathy. The role of surgery is limited to diagnosis, either in the form of a core needle biopsy or an excisional biopsy. Fine-needle aspiration cytology is inadequate to definitively diagnose lymphoma. Further management of the lymphoma is with chemotherapy and/or radiation.

In patients diagnosed with sarcoma of the breast or malignant phyllodes tumors, there is no role for performing SLNB of the axilla, as the natural course of spread is not lymphatic, rather hematogenous. However, were there to be clinically enlarged lymph nodes in this situation, there may be a role for surgical removal of the same.

Patients with Previous Ipsilateral Axillary Surgery

Axillary staging is possible in patients with previous axillary surgery. A thorough preoperative evaluation of the patient is essential. A preoperative axillary ultrasound may visualize an abnormal lymph node and an ultrasound-guided fine-needle aspiration of the same may be performed. Clinically node-negative patients, with previous axillary surgery, should have an axillary sentinel lymph node biopsy attempted. Cox et al. had a successful identification rate of the SLN in 89 % of the cases. A CALND may be considered in patients in whom an SLN is not identified, provided there is enough residual axillary tissue in the levels 1 and 2 locations and that the operation can be performed safely. Alternately close observation of the axilla alone may be sufficient, provided there are no enlarged, clinically suspicious lymph nodes palpable [25].

Elderly Patients with Invasive Breast Cancer

Older patients with invasive breast cancer comprise of a heterogeneous group, with varying levels of comorbidity and life expectancy. The surgical management of the axilla in these patients with invasive breast cancer is to be tailored to the individual. Clinically node-positive patients are to be treated with a standard axillary operation, such as a CALND. Controversy remains as to the management of the axilla in the elderly patient with a clinically node-negative axilla.

The recommendation of the International Society of Geriatric Oncology (SIOG) and the European Society of Breast Cancer Specialists (EUSOMA) remains to perform SLNB and CALND in patients with positive lymph nodes [26]. However, there is data to suggest that these patients may not warrant a CALND if they had less than 3 involved lymph nodes with no extranodal extension based upon the results of the ACOSOG Z0011 trial.

The International Breast Cancer study group (IBCSG) trial 10-93 randomized patients older than 60 years, with clinically negative nodes, in whom postoperative tamoxifen was indicated, to axillary clearance versus no axillary surgery. The preliminary results have suggested no significant change in disease-free or overall survival between the two groups, with improved early quality of life in the non-axillary surgery group [27].

SLN Biopsy After Previous Mastectomy

Although less successful, sentinel lymph node biopsy is certainly feasible after mastectomy. It is helpful to inject the Tc99m sulfur colloid into the upper portion of the chest wall. The success rate reported by Karam et al. for SLN biopsy following a mastectomy was 65 % [28].

Male Breast Cancer

Sentinel lymph node biopsy is indicated in men with breast cancer and clinically negative lymph nodes. Men are more likely to have positive sentinel lymph nodes, and in those with positive sentinel lymph nodes, the probability of having non-sentinel lymph node metastases is higher [29].

Pregnant Women with Breast Cancer

Blue dye is thought to be unsafe for the fetus in pregnant women with breast cancer. Studies have found the radiation dose to the uterus from the Tc99m sulfur colloid to be safe. In the second and third trimesters, when organogenesis is considered to be complete, there is still considerable controversy in the use of the radiolabeled dye for sentinel lymph node biopsy. It may be used on an individualized basis, but if it were to be performed, it should be injected on the same day as surgery to reduce the exposure time to the fetus [29].

As evidenced above, there are multiple different approaches to the axillary management of invasive breast cancer. Hence, we created a somewhat oversimplified flow chart for the same (Table 12.2):

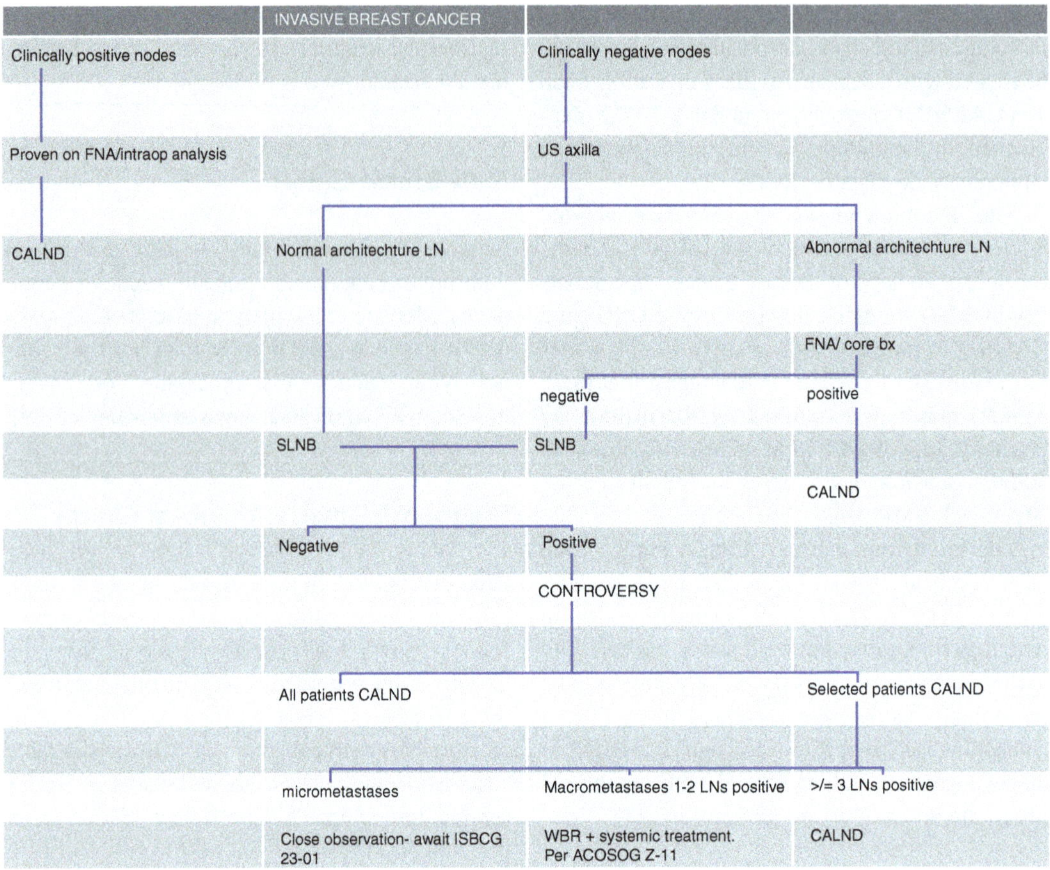

Table 12.2 Approach to axillary management of patient with invasive breast cancer

References

1. Townsend: Sabiston Textbook of surgery. 19th ed. Saunders, 2012.
2. Benson JR. Querci della Rovere G and the Axilla Management Consensus Group. Management of the axilla in women with breast cancer. Lancet Oncol. 2007;8:331–48.
3. Fischer B, Montague F, Redmond C, et al. Ten year results of a randomized trial comparing radical mastectomy and total mastectomy with or without radiation. N Engl J Med. 1985;312:674–81.
4. Krag D, Anderson S, Julian T, et al. Sentinel-lymph-node resection compared with conventional axillary-lymph-node dissection in clinically node-negative patients with breast cancer: overall survival findings from NSABP B-32 randomised phase 3 trial. Lancet Oncol. 2010;11:927–31. Cancer Research: December 15, 2012; Volume 72, Issue 24, Supplement 3.
5. Giuliano A, Hunt K, Ballman K, et al. Axillary dissection vs no axillary dissection in women with invasive breast cancer and sentinel node metastasis. A randomized clinical trial. J Am Med Assn. 2011;305(6):569–75.
6. S3-1. Update of International Breast Cancer Study Group Trial 23-01 to compare axillary dissection versus no axillary dissection in patients with clinically node negative breast cancer and micrometastases in the sentinel node. Galimberti V, Cole BF, Zurrida S, et al. International Breast Cancer Study Group Trial 23-01 Investigators. Abstract presented at San Antonio Breast conference 2011.
7. De Kanter A, Van Eijck C, Van Geel A, et al. Multicenter study of ultrasonographically guided axillary node biopsy in patients with breast cancer. Br J of Surg. 1999;86:1459–62.
8. Damera A, Evans A, Cornford E, et al. Diagnosis of axillary nodal metastases by ultrasound-guided core biopsy in primary operable breast cancer. Br J of Cancer. 2003;89:1310–3.

9. Vidal-Sicart S, Olmos R. Sentinel node mapping for breast cancer: current situation. J Oncol. 2012;2012:361341.
10. Krishnamurthy S, Meric-Bernstam F, Lucci A, et al. A prospective study comparing touch imprint cytology, frozen section analysis and rapid cytokeratin immunostain for intraoperative evaluation of axillary sentinel lymph nodes in breast cancer. Cancer Apr. 2009;115:1555–62.
11. Veys I, Derbecq V, Majjaj S, et al. Eighteen months clinical experience with the Gene search breast lymph node assay. Am J of Surg. 2009;198:203–9.
12. Krag D, Anderson S, Julian T, et al. Technical outcomes of sentinel-lymph-node resection and conventional axillary-lymph-node dissection in patients with clinically node-negative breast cancer: results from the NSABP B-32 randomised phase III trial. Lancet Oncol. 2007;8:881–8.
13. Erickson V, Pearson M, Ganz P, et al. Arm edema in breast cancer patients. J Natl Cancer Inst. 2001; 93:96–111.
14. Kissin M, della Rovere G Q, Easton D, Westbury G. Risk of lymphoedema following the treatment of breast cancer. Br J Surg. 1986;73:580–4.
15. Shah C, Wilkinson J, Baschnagel A, et al. Factors associated with the development of breast cancer-related lymphedema after whole breast irradiation. Int J Radiat Oncol Biol Phys. 2012;83(4):1095–100.
16. American Joint Commission on Cancer, 7th ed. Springer, 2009.
17. Massimino K, Hessman C, Ellis M, et al. Impact of American College of Surgeons Oncology Group Z0011 and National surgical Adjuvant Breast and Bowel Project B-32 trial results on surgeon practice in the Pacific Northwest. Am J of Surg. 2012;203:618–22.
18. Position statement on management of the axilla in patients with invasive breast cancer. The American Society of Breast Surgeons. 2011.
19. Straver M, Meijnen P, van Tienhoven G, et al. Role of axillary clearance after a tumor-positive sentinel node in the administration of adjuvant therapy in early breast cancer. J Clin Oncol. 2010;28:731–7.
20. Boughey JC, Suman VJ, Mittendorf EA, et al. Sentinel lymph node surgery after neoadjuvant chemotherapy in patients with node-positive breast cancer: The ACOSOG Z1071 (alliance) clinical trial. JAMA. 2013;310(14):1455–1461. doi: 10.1001/jama.2013.278932.
21. Sabel MS. Sentinel lymph node biopsy before or after neoadjuvant chemotherapy: pros and cons. Surg Oncol Clin N Am. 2010;19(3):519–38.
22. Mamounas E, Brown A, Anderson S, et al. Sentinel node biopsy after neoadjuvant chemotherapy in breast cancer: results from National Surgical Adjuvant Breast and Bowel Project Protocol B-27. J Clin Oncol. 2005;23:2694–702.
23. Wilke C, White L, et al. An update of sentinel lymph node mapping in patients with ductal carcinoma in situ. Am J Surg. 2005;190:563–6.
24. Hulvat M, Hansen N, Jeruss J. Multidisciplinary care for patients with breast cancer. Surg Clin N Am. 2009;89:133–76.
25. Cox C, Furman B, Kiluk J, et al. Use of reoperative sentinel lymph node biopsy in breast cancer patients. J Am Coll Surg. 2008;207:57–61.
26. Biganzoli L, Wildiers H, Oakman C, et al. Management of elderly patients with breast cancer: updated recommendations of the International Society of Geriatric Oncology (SIOG) and European Society of Breast Cancer Specialists (EUSOMA). Lancet Oncol. 2012;13:e148–60.
27. Galimberti V, Cole B, Viale V, et al. Axillary dissection Vs no axillary dissection in patients with sentinel lymph node micrometastases (IBCSG 23-01): a phase 3 randomised controlled trial. Lancet Oncol. 2013;14:297–305.
28. Karam A, Stempel M, Cody H, Port E. Reoperative sentinel lymph node biopsy after previous mastectomy. J Am Coll Surg. 2008;207:543–8.
29. Ansari B, Boughey J. Sentinel lymph node surgery in uncommon clinical circumstances. Surg Oncol Clin N Am. 2010;19:539–53.

Breast-Conserving Therapy for Breast Cancer

13

Charles E. Cox, Adela Fernandez, Evan Tummel, Richard Betzold, Wei Wei Zhang, Vanessa Prowler, John Chipko, Michelle Jung, Michelle Vice, and Steven C. Shivers

History of Lumpectomy

Essential to the surgical treatment of breast cancer is an understanding of the two critical objectives that have not varied in the last 50 years: (1) local control and (2) accurate staging. While survival may be improved with early detection, its accomplishment is only secured by providing excellent local control of the disease. Every surgeon understands that some cases, though detected early and treated effectively, will go on to metastasize in spite of excellent local control. This substantiates the claim that the disease is systemic in some cases at its earliest development. Therefore, a surgeon's skill and function in the treatment of the disease should be measured by the outcomes of local control and accuracy of staging.

William S. Halsted's description of the radical mastectomy was the great advance at the turn of the last century and remains the mainstay of surgical management for those uncommon cases today of locally advanced breast cancer. The advent of mammography and improved technology has increased the detection rates of very early breast cancer in many instances. Patient advocacy, through the committed efforts of patient advocates such as Rose Kushner, has also greatly helped with advancing breast cancer research funding and the development of a national screening program. Dr. Bernard Fisher, a surgeon, and his brother Dr. Edwin Fisher, a pathologist at the University of Pittsburgh, postulated that breast cancer at these earlier stages could be treated with the combination of local excision to negative margins and the addition of radiation therapy.

To prove this hypothesis, the National Surgical Adjuvant Breast and Bowel Project (NSABP) B-04 trial began in 1971. The trial compared women undergoing radical mastectomies to those obtaining total mastectomies, with and without radiation therapy. In 1977, the first results were published, which showed no difference in treatment failure or survival and, after 25 years, no difference in long-term outcomes [1, 2]. In 1976, the NSABP B-06 trial, which compared mastectomy to lumpectomy, showed that removing a small portion of the breast along with axillary lymph nodes and radiation therapy was just as

C.E. Cox, MD (✉) • M. Jung, BS • M. Vice, BS
S.C. Shivers, PhD
Department of Surgery, USF Breast Health Program, University of South Florida Morsani College of Medicine, 3000 Medical Park Drive, MDC 25, Tampa, FL 33613, USA
e-mail: coxce@hotmail.com; mjung4@mail.usf.edu; mvice1@health.usf.edu; sshivers@health.usf.edu

A. Fernandez, MD • E. Tummel, MD • W.W. Zhang, MD
V. Prowler, MD • J. Chipko, MD
Department of Surgery, Tampa General Hospital, University of South Florida Morsani College of Medicine, 2 Tampa General Circle, 7th Floor, Tampa, FL 33606, USA
e-mail: afernand@health.usf.edu; etummel@gmail.com; wzhang325@gmail.com; vprowler@health.usf.edu; jchipko@health.usf.edu

R. Betzold, MD
Department of Surgery, University of Arkansas for Medical Sciences, Little Rock, AR, 72212, USA
e-mail: rdbetzold@uams.edu

A.I. Riker (ed.), *Breast Disease: Comprehensive Management*,
DOI 10.1007/978-1-4939-1145-5_13, © Springer Science+Business Media New York 2015

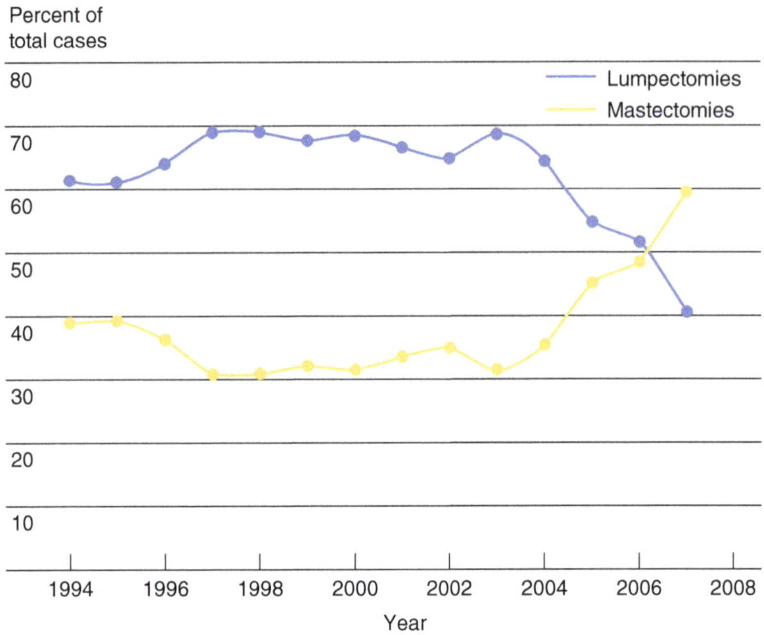

Fig. 13.1 Lumpectomy versus mastectomy (From McGuire et al. [5])

effective as mastectomy. After 20 years of follow-up of the B-06 trial, no significant difference has been found in overall or disease-free survival between those that underwent total mastectomy and lumpectomy [1–3]. Based on the NSABP B-06 trial, breast conservation therapy decreases local recurrences from 39 to 14 % [4].

Lumpectomy, also known as wide local excision or partial mastectomy, combined with sentinel node biopsy and radiation therapy, comprises the package described as "breast conservation therapy" (BCT). Up until 2003, BCT has been the primary treatment option for breast cancer treatment for nearly 60–70 % of all cases treated at major breast cancer treatment centers. A recent decline has been noted in several major programs and a trend back toward mastectomy has occurred (Fig. 13.1). These have been shown to be due primarily to patient-driven decision making and are not physician-driven outcomes [5–7].

Keystone Trials

Over the past 50 years, patient education, screening, and early detection with advancements in mammography, ultrasound, magnetic resonance imaging (MRI), breast-specific gamma imaging (BSGI), and positron emission mammography (PEM) have continued to shape the management of breast cancer. It is the summation of several early studies that have culminated in identifying the equivalency of mastectomy and BCT. For instance, rates of survival of those undergoing a mastectomy in comparison to lumpectomy with radiation achieved no significant differences in outcome. Defined predictors of local recurrence after BCT have led to modifications in surgical and radiation techniques to reduce local recurrence.

NSABP B-06

The National Surgical Adjuvant Breast and Bowel Project (NSABP) Protocol B-06, a federally sponsored clinical trial, raised several aspects of comparisons between surgical options, use of radiation, and systemic therapy. In a step further, it compared the efficacy of chemotherapy in patients with positive axillary nodes after surgical treatment, as well as determining the clinical significance of microscopic multicentricity. The study took place between 1976 and 1984, with a total of 1,851 patients with tumors up to 4 cm in diameter and clinically negative lymph nodes, T1 or T2, N0 or N1, M0. Patients were randomly assigned to a total mastectomy, lumpectomy alone, or lumpectomy with postoperative radiation of the breast. All patients with histologically positive axillary nodes received chemotherapy.

Based on this study, rates of ipsilateral breast cancer recurrence after lumpectomy, with or without breast radiation, were compared. At 20 years follow-up, local recurrence rate in women treated with lumpectomy and radiation was 14.3 % versus those treated with lumpectomy alone with a recurrence rate of 39.2 %. For patients with positive nodes who received chemotherapy, the local recurrence rate was 44.2 % for lumpectomy alone, as opposed to 8.8 % for lumpectomy and radiation therapy. The study concluded that lumpectomy, paired with radiation therapy, and adjuvant chemotherapy in women with positive nodes, was appropriate in patients with tumors equal to or less than 4 cm, placing them at stage I or II disease, provided that the resected margins are free of tumor [2].

EORTC

At about the same time, a similar study compared the overall survival between those patients that underwent a modified radical mastectomy (MRM) and breast conservation therapy (BCT) with radiation. The results would similarly echo those found in the NSABP B-06 trial. The European Organization for Research and Treatment of Cancer Trial 10801 took place between 1980 and 1986, in eight centers in the UK, Netherlands, Belgium, and South Africa. It randomized 868 women to MRM and BCT with radiation. The size of tumors was up to 5 cm, though 80 % of women had tumors larger than 2 cm, and patients with axillary node-negative or axillary node-positive disease were included.

At 20 year follow-up, there was no difference in survival between MRM and BCT with radiation [8]. The overall survival was 44.5 % in MRM group and 39.1 % in the BCT group. There was no difference in time to distant metastases or overall survival by age. The study concluded that as a standard of care, patients with early-stage breast cancer can be offered BCT with radiation as an alternative to MRM.

Danish Breast Center Cooperative Group

From 1983 to March 1989, the Danish Breast Cancer Cooperative Group (DBCG) conducted a randomized trial comparing breast conservation to mastectomy in patients with invasive breast cancer. From a total of 1,153 women, 905 were placed on either mastectomy or breast conservation. The remaining 248 were not randomized. Those placed in the breast conservation arm obtained radiotherapy afterward. Tumor diameter was more than 2 cm in over 50 % of cases. Patients were excluded based on the following criteria: sarcoma of the breast or carcinoma in situ, fixation of the tumor to the muscles, evidence of metastatic disease, history of other malignancies, signs of multicentricity by palpation or mammography, and concerns in cosmesis, such as a large tumor in a small breast. In this trial, patients had the choice of changing arms in terms of the proposed operation. Hence, 33 patients randomly assigned to a mastectomy chose breast conservation, while 55 chose a mastectomy over breast conservation. Regardless of tumor size and palpable nodes, all patients underwent an axillary dissection. The dissection consisted of removal of at least all level I lymph nodes.

The median follow-up was 40 months for all patients. For the purpose of consistency, both patient and tumor characteristics were similar in both breast conservation and mastectomy group. Overall survival in the breast conservation group was 79 %, compared to that of the mastectomy group of 82 %. The recurrence-free survival at 6 years was similar in both groups, 70 % versus 66 % [9].

Milan National Tumor Institute Trial

Under the guidance of the National Cancer Institute in Milan, between the years of 1973 and 1980, this trial enrolled 701 women with breast cancer up to 2 cm in size for the primary tumor and clinically negative nodes. These patients would undergo either a radical mastectomy or quadrantectomy with axillary dissection and postoperative radiation to the ipsilateral residual breast tissue. Chemotherapy was reserved for patients with pathologically positive nodes. Of the 701 patients, 349 had a mastectomy and 352 a quadrantectomy. Factors such as age, size and site of primary tumor, and axillary metastases were similar in both groups.

At a 20 year follow-up, no differences between the two groups were found in overall or disease-free survival [10]. Interestingly, the contralateral breast cancer rates were similar. These findings contraindicated the previous thought that radiation increased the incidence of contralateral breast cancer. Based on this trial, patients with a breast cancer lesion less than 2 cm in size have the option of either a mastectomy or quadrantectomy, without concern for decrease in survival.

The Institute Gustave-Roussy Trial

The trial randomized 179 women with breast cancer into modified radical mastectomy versus lumpectomy. Eighty eight patients had lumpectomy and radiotherapy, while 91 patients underwent mastectomy. Axillary dissection was performed in all patients regardless of the lack of palpable axillary lymph node. At a 15-year follow-up, no differences were observed between the two surgical groups in risk for death, metastases, contralateral breast cancer, or locoregional recurrence [9].

Patient Selection for Lumpectomy

As the advent of mammography and early detection improved, the average tumor sizes of the 1970s and 1980s fell to 2.5 cm, allowing the majority of women to undergo BCT. BCT is indicated in women with a T1 (<2 cm) tumor, T2 that is ≤5 cm, N0, N1 (ipsilateral moveable axillary nodes), and M0 (no metastasis) tumors, which correlates to clinically stages I and II breast cancer. An important consideration as to which patients are candidates for BCT is practicality and cosmesis. The tumor to breast volume as well as location of the tumor, such as central or lower inner quadrant, may require nipple-areola complex removal or result in significant deformity of the breast and preclude standard approaches to BCT. Newer techniques of oncoplastic surgery described by Clough and Silverstein may allow for the accommodation of BCT in otherwise compromising locations. Nearly all BCT has been done on unifocal lesions with multicentric lesions being a contraindication for BCT [4]. Certain cases of closely approximated or "kissing lesions" have been successfully treated with BCT. More extensive areas when completely excised with oncoplastic techniques can result in excellent outcomes with BCT.

To be eligible for breast-conserving therapy, three conditions must be met. One must be able to obtain negative surgical margins, patient is able to undergo adjuvant radiation therapy, and the result must be cosmetically acceptable. Positive margins, due to lobular invasive or ductal in situ disease, require excision to negativity and are amenable to BCT, as long as they meet the aforementioned criteria [4].

Contraindications of lumpectomy are multicentric disease, persistently positive margins, early pregnancy, diffuse microcalcifications on preoperative mammogram, or prior history of breast radiation. Early pregnancy is a contraindication since whole breast radiation is contraindicated during pregnancy. However, breast cancer detected during pregnancy in the second or third trimester may be able to be treated with lumpectomy and sentinel node biopsy after which chemotherapy can be administered followed by radiation following delivery.

With the advent of accelerated partial breast irradiation (APBI) and intraoperative radiation therapy (IORT), some patients may be offered shielded breast irradiation during the second or third trimester of pregnancy. Multicentric disease is defined as two or more primary tumors in separate quadrants of the same breast and is a contraindication to BCT. However, some patients with out-of-field recurrences are now being offered APBI or

IORT to those new areas of disease. Relative contraindications include whole breast radiation to a very large breast, lobular carcinoma in situ (LCIS), active connective tissue disease (such as systemic lupus erythematosus, scleroderma or radiosensitivity due to inherited ataxia telangiectasia), and a tumor larger than 5 cm in a patient with small breasts (due to a poor cosmetic result) [4].

Surgical Principles: Techniques in Breast Lumpectomy

BCT is routinely performed for malignant breast diseases. Particularly for malignant processes, there are myriad of surgical techniques and complementary therapies being performed. All of these techniques have similar efficacy rates, and selection should be a patient-centered decision.

Needle-Localized Lumpectomy

Preoperative image-guided needle localization of breast masses has been performed since the 1960s [11–13]. After being refined to include a hook wire to prevent needle migration, the technique quickly became the standard of care in excising breast masses [12]. Mammography, ultrasonography, and magnetic resonance imaging are all used to guide needle placement. After placement, standard lumpectomy incisions are used to gain a rectangular or cylindrical block of tissue around the wire. Needle localization is a time-tested method, but effective excision depends both on the precision of radiological placement and surgical technique. Unfortunately, it does add another step in the procedure, which could lead to patient discomfort and inconvenience [13]. Nonetheless, it is arguably the most popular technique among surgeons.

Palpable Mass Excision

Excision of a palpable mass is indicated for those masses that are not visualized on mammography or for those with features that portend malignancy. Incisions should be made to facilitate excision while maintaining a good cosmetic result.

Hematoma Ultrasound-Guided Lumpectomy

Ultrasonography can be utilized to directly visualize lesions and post-biopsy hematomas. The hematoma ultrasound-guided lumpectomy was described in 2001 and has become widely performed [14]. After routine biopsy of breast lesions, a hematoma forms that is sometimes palpable and most of the time is easily visualized under ultrasound guidance. Intraoperative ultrasound is used to localize the lesion, which guides incision placement. The ultrasound can then be used to ensure proper margin-free excision, and ex vivo ultrasonography ensures that the lesion is removed. Hematomas do resorb with time, so operative scheduling should be close to the biopsy date (within 6 weeks). This technique obviates the need for needle localization in many patients, but if lesions are not visualized with sonography, needle localization should be performed [14, 15].

Radioisotope (Seed) Localization Lumpectomy

Tc^{99m} radioisotope sulfur colloid is used to identify draining lymph nodes of the primary tumor. It follows that if a different radioisotope could be inserted into target lesions, excision could be similarly guided by gamma counts. This has been performed and widely published since the early 2000s [16]. Radiological or ultrasound placement of radioactive I^{125} seeds can be used to localize the malignant lesion, and any of the gamma detection probes set on the I^{125} setting can detect the seed even in the presence of the Tc^{99m} which has been injected for lymphatic mapping of sentinel nodes. A gamma counter is used to guide both the incision and the extent of excision. This technique does require a preoperative radiological implantation, but improvements in margin negativity have cemented the use of this procedure in the breast surgeon's armamentarium [17].

Cryoablation-Assisted Lumpectomy

Cryoablation can be used in conjunction with intraoperative ultrasound to guide lumpectomy. Essentially, the lesion is visualized under ultrasound guidance and a cryoablation of the area is performed, followed by an ultrasound-guided lumpectomy of the area that was ablated. Margin negativity is acceptable using this technique for lesions less than 18 mm [18]. Larger lesions are more difficult to adequately ablate, and the ablation process makes postoperative pathological analysis more difficult [19]. To further analyze the ability of cryoablation to eradicate intraductal carcinoma, the Cryoablation Trial Z0172 is in clinical Phase II trials at present.

Lumpectomy with Radiofrequency Ablation

Intraoperative radiofrequency ablation of the lumpectomy bed was examined in the early part of year 2000. Performance of this technique requires some specialized equipment and surgical precision, but the consistent 1 cm margin of ablation confirmed on post-ablation cavity wall biopsy could prevent re-excision rates for specimen margin positivity. After lumpectomy, RFA probe is secured in the lumpectomy bed with a purse-string suture. Care is taken to keep the probe from causing skin burns, and Doppler ultrasonography can be used to manipulate the probe to prevent this [20]. It is possible that this could be definitive breast conservation therapy for some patients with favorable lesions, but this requires more evaluation [21].

Lumpectomy with Brachytherapy

Some patients with favorable tumors can avoid whole breast radiation therapy and undergo accelerated partial breast irradiation (APBI) [22] (see Table 13.1). This entails 1 week of radiation therapy that is often delivered through exteriorized catheters placed into or through the lumpectomy cavity. Surgeons can assist with partial breast irradiation by placing brachytherapy catheters through externalized catheters placed into or through the lumpectomy cavity devices into the lumpectomy cavity either intraoperatively or in the office after lumpectomy. The catheter can be cumbersome for some patients, but given that the total radiation time is 1 week, it is widely tolerated [23]. Techniques of multiple polyethylene catheters placed in an array through and through the breast tissue traversing the lumpectomy cavity were first implemented over 30 years ago. Subsequent balloon catheter devices (MammoSite, ClearPath) were developed as well as bundled and strutted device with multiple polyethylene catheters (SAVI) device. Treatment programs of 34 Gy delivered in 10×3.4 Gy fractions twice daily have been employed (see Table 13.2).

Lumpectomy with Intraoperative Radiation Therapy

Intraoperative radiation therapy is a development in the spectrum of breast conservation therapy. This collaboration between breast surgeons and radiation oncologists begins by localizing and removing the tumor. Next, the radiation device (Intrabeam, Xoft) is placed within the lumpectomy cavity and secured the radiation is delivered to the tumor and peritumoral tissues in a single fraction of 20 Gy. Proper therapy can be completed even in noncompliant patients given the one stage lumpectomy and radiation [25]. While intraoperative cost is higher, this eliminates the long-term radiation therapy costs and ensures patient compliance with therapy [26]. The recent results of the TARGIT trial demonstrate excellent short-term results with single 20 Gy doses of IORT.

Margin Assessment

Obtaining adequate margins is of the utmost importance in breast-conserving surgery. Excision of the lesion in its entirety with adequate margins is vital to minimizing the risk of a local tumor recurrence. However, overzealous

Table 13.1 Professional medical society consensus guidelines for patient selection for APBI

	ABS[a]	ASBS[b]	ACRO[c]	ASTRO[d]		
				Suitable	Cautionary	Unsuitable
Age	≥50	≥45	≥45	≥60	50–59	<50
Diagnosis	Unifocal, invasive ductal carcinoma	Invasive ductal carcinoma or DCIS	Invasive ductal carcinoma or DCIS	Invasive ductal or other favorable subtypes (i.e., mucinous, tubular, colloid)	Pure DCIS ≤3 cm EIC ≤3 cm	–
Tumor size (cm)	≤3	≤3	≤3	≤2	2.1–3.0	>3
Surgical margins	Negative microscopic margins of excision	Negative microscopic margins of excision	Negative microscopic margins of excision	Negative by at least 2 mm	Close (<2 mm)	Positive
Nodal status	NØ	NØ	NØ	NØ (i–, i+)	–	Positive

There continues to be growing interest in the use of accelerated partial breast irradiation. To provide additional direction for patients and physicians regarding the use of APBI, consensus guidelines have been issued by the major physician professional societies

[a]Breast Brachytherapy Task Group, American Brachytherapy Society (ABS), February 2007

[b]Consensus statement for accelerated partial breast irradiation. American Society of Breast Surgeons (ASBS), October 7, 2008

[c]American College of Radiation Oncology (ACRO) Statement on Partial Breast Irradiation, September 2008

[d]American Society for Radiation Oncology (ASTRO) Consensus Statement on Partial Breast Irradiation, July 2009

Table 13.2 APBI data review

Institution	# of cases	Median F/U (months)	Local recurrence (%)	Cosmesis good/ excellent (%)
ASBS MammoSite Registry	1,440	60.5	1.8	90
Virginia Commonwealth University	483	24	1.2	91
National Institute of Oncology, Hungary Phase III Trial[a]	APBI 127 WBI 131	66	APBI 4.7 WBI 3.4	APBI 81 WBI 62
William Beaumont Hospital	199	71	1.6	92
Ochsner Clinic	164	65	3	75
RTOG 95–17	99	51	4	Not reported
Mass General Hospital	48	84	2	68
National Institute of Oncology, Hungary Phase I/II Trial	45	80	6.7	84
MammoSite FDA Trial	43	66	0	83
Tufts/Brown	33	84	6.1	88
Total	2,681	65	APBI 3.1 WBI 2.8	84

Adapted from Polgar et al. [24]

Not only does brachytherapy allow for a dramatic change in the treatment schedule from several weeks to just 5 days, it also is associated with fewer radiation-related toxicities and an improved cosmetic outcome. This chart summarizes a multitude of clinical trials evaluating the efficacy of brachytherapy

[a]Conclusion: Partial breast irradiation using interstitial HDR implants or EB to deliver radiation to the tumor bed alone for a selected group of early-stage breast cancer patients produces 5-year results similar to those achieved with conventional WBI. Significantly better cosmetic outcome can be achieved with carefully designed HDR multi-catheter implants compared with the outcome after WBI

resection may lead to a less than desirable cosmetic outcome. Although there is no clear consensus as to what constitutes a negative margin, many authors define a positive margin as tumor at the inked margin and a close margin as tumor less than 2 mm from the inked margin. Definition for an adequate margin in the breast literature ranges from no tumor at ink to 10 mm.

It is important to ensure a negative margin at the time of the initial resection. Although re-excision is possible and often performed for positive margins, this adds patient discomfort, cost and further anesthesia, and surgical risk. Currently re-excision rates for positive margin status vary greatly in the literature. A recent multi-institutional study of 2,206 women undergoing partial mastectomy found an overall re-excision rate of 22.9 %, with 9.4 % of patients requiring re-excision of two or more re-excisions with 8.5 % of patients ultimately requiring a total mastectomy. The study found that younger women (age <35), thinner women (BMI <18.5), and those with initial margins of less than 1 mm are more likely to require a re-excision.

A study by Morrow et al. analyzing the SEER data from several institutions nationwide demonstrated a stunning 40 % re-excision rate. DCIS, lobular carcinoma, and lymphovascular invasion also had higher re-excision rates. Obtaining a negative margin is important because margin status affects the rate of local and overall recurrence. Local recurrence rates with negative margins found in the literature vary between 2 and 13 % and increase to 6–31 % if the margins are positive. However, it is important to remember that negative margins do not guarantee total eradication of disease but that the residual tumor burden is low enough to be treated with chemoradiation. Thus, factors such as intrinsic tumor biology and clinical stage play an important role in the risk of overall recurrence.

Margin assessment is especially difficult in clinically non-palpable lesions or lesions with poorly defined borders. Various techniques have been used to assess specimen margins to ensure adequate resection including optical assessment, intraoperative frozen section, and imprint cytology. Ensuring an adequate margin begins with preoperative imaging. Standard imaging such as mammography, ultrasound, and MRI should be used to determine the size, location, and character of the tumor. Ultrasound- or mammography-guided needle localization or clip placement near non-palpable tumors is helpful in identifying suspicious regions. However, this technique does not define the borders of the lesion in a three-dimensional setting and thus does not ensure a negative margin. After careful surgical dissection, the specimen should be orientated and marked carefully as to ensure facile re-excision if necessary. A gross visual inspection of the specimen is always necessary to assess macroscopic disease. In addition, a number of surgeons use a variety of techniques to ensure adequate margins intraoperatively. Portable radiography systems, such as the Faxitron® and Kubtec® (XPERT 40) systems, allow for immediate radiographic analysis of specimen margins following needle-localized excisions. The images can be sent immediately to radiology for further evaluation.

Although wire-guided localization has traditionally been viewed as the standard of care for localizing non-palpable breast lesions in breast-conserving therapy. Various new technologies have been introduced to augment and even substitute its role in localization and margin assessment. Intraoperative specimen mammography provides an immediate image of the entire excised specimen. This allows radiographic visualization of suspicious areas and allows the surgeon to excise additional margins at the time of lumpectomy, thus decreasing the rate of re-operative surgery. In Bathla et al.'s study of the utility of Faxitron mammographically guided intraoperative re-excision, 84.3 % of patients who underwent primary lumpectomy using this method had histologically clear margins at initial excision versus national rates of 55–68 % [27]. A total of 17.6 % of excisions had positive margins despite the use of 2D Faxitron imaging. The sensitivity and specificity of intraoperative margin assessment via 2D Faxitron imaging for patient with primary breast cancer quoted in this study were 58.5 and 91.8 %, respectively, with a positive predictive value of 82.7 % and negative predictive value of 76.7 %. Thus, although intraoperative specimen mammography improves the rate of negative margins at initial excision, it does not always predict negative histological margin. It should be used carefully in conjunction with the already established assessment tools available to ensure a negative margin.

Intraoperative ultrasonography can also be used to aid margin assessment. Ultrasound localization can be used alone for non-palpable lesions or used as an adjunct to the standard needle localization procedure. Although some studies have shown a superior negative margin rate for ultrasound-guided excision versus needle localization, this technique is only useful for lesions clearly visualized by the ultrasound and is often not useful in DCIS where lesions are diagnosed as calcifications on mammography.

Various other techniques have been used in an attempt to optimize margin negativity. Cryoprobe-assisted location (CAL) is one such method which uses liquid nitrogen or argon to freeze the lesion using an ultrasound-guided cryoprobe, transforming the non-palpable lesion to a solid palpable mass easily viewed by ultrasound. This technique was shown to have similar positive margin rates compared to needle-wire localization lumpectomy while excising a smaller specimen. CAL also showed a benefit in ease of lumpectomy, surgical cosmesis, and procedure time. However, the freezing process associated with this procedure alters the tumor morphology and interferes with pathological analysis of the specimen including tumor grade, distinguishing between in situ and invasive components, assessment of mitoses and lymphovascular invasion, and expression of hormone receptors.

Radio-guided localization (RGL) has emerged as a novel method for localization of non-palpable breast lesions with the promise of improved margin clearance. This technology uses a radioactive tracer placement into the occult breast mass in order to aid with excision. Radio-guided occult lesion localization (ROLL) and radio-guided seed localization (RSL) are two approaches to this technology that has become increasingly popular. ROLL involves injecting (99m)Tc-labeled particles of human serum albumin (7–10 MBq) into the lesion under stereotactic mammographic or ultrasonic guidance then carrying out breast-conserving surgery with the aid of a handheld gamma-detecting probe. After excision, the specimen may be examined by either ultrasonography or mammography to verify complete lesion prior to histological evaluation.

RSL is utilized in a similar fashion but uses an implantable ^{125}I encapsulated titanium seed as the radioactive guide. The seed used in RSL has the added advantage of being easily visible on both mammography and ultrasound. The radioactive seed used in RSL has a relatively long half-life (60 days) compared to that of the Tc-labeled albumin used in ROLL (6 h), so it does not need to be performed on the day of surgery. Furthermore, RSL does not use the same radiotracer (^{99m}Tc) as SLN mapping and causes less confusion when performing both procedures than ROLL. Recent data has shown at least equivalent outcomes between radio-guided localization and wire localization in terms of margin status. It shows promise as a useful tool in the future of breast conservation surgery.

Although the various technologies mentioned above have facilitated complete excision of breast lesions, definitive margin assessment is through pathological analysis. Some surgeons utilize frozen section in an attempt to confirm negative margins at the time of the operation. Frozen section is fairly accurate, with sensitivity and specificity quoted in the literature at approximately 90 and 100 %, respectively [28, 29]. However, this technique can be costly, time consuming, and labor intensive, and its use is often limited by these factors.

Intraoperative touch prep or imprint cytology offers a quicker and easier alternative to intraoperative frozen section. Using this method, each surface of the specimen is touched to a glass slide then stained and air dried. The slides are then screened to look for malignant epithelial cells, with the premise that malignant cells stick to the slide while benign cells do not. Therefore, a negative margin will show no epithelial cells or rare benign epithelial or non-epithelial cells, while a positive margin will show atypical or malignant epithelial cells. This method is useful in determining positive margins but does not indicate when margins are close. Current data shows that imprint cytology demonstrates sensitivities of 80–100 %, specificities of 83–100 %, and diagnostic accuracies of 73–100 %. In addition, the efficacy of intraoperative imprint cytology has been well established in a large series of 1,713 patients published by Weinberg et al. [30].

The study showed that imprint cytology provided an accurate evaluation of lumpectomy margins and was associated with an overall decrease in overall 5-year local recurrence from 8.8 to 2.8 % compared to frozen section.

Recurrence After Lumpectomy

Recurrence after breast-conserving therapy must be broken down into local (occurring in the conserved ipsilateral breast), regional (occurring in the ipsilateral axillary, supraclavicular, infraclavicular, or internal mammary lymph nodes), and distant (outside of the ipsilateral breast and lymph nodes). BCT has been shown to be equivalent compared to MRM in terms of disease-free and overall survival. The overall recurrence rates have been found to be 0.5–2 % per year. Two large randomized studies, the Milan trial and NSABP trial, demonstrated these findings with short- and long-term follow-up for patients with stages 0, I, and II disease. The NSABP B-06 trial evaluated the effectiveness of lumpectomy with and without radiation versus modified radical mastectomy in patients with tumors $\leq$4 cm. The recurrence rate at 5 years for lumpectomy with radiation was 7.7 % [31]. By 8 years after treatment, this was up to 10 % [32]. However, the patients treated with lumpectomy alone (no radiation) had a recurrence rate of nearly 40 %. Patients who had positive nodes and were treated with chemotherapy, radiation, and lumpectomy had a local recurrence rate of only 6 %. Twenty-year follow-up data of this trial has found a hazard ratio for death of 1.05 (lumpectomy without radiation compared to mastectomy) and 0.97 (lumpectomy with radiation compared to mastectomy) [3].

Despite the risk of death being nearly equal, the risk of local recurrence was significantly higher in the lumpectomy without radiation group (39.2 %) compared to the lumpectomy with radiation (14.3 %) and the mastectomy (10.2 %). Over 73 % of the recurrences in the lumpectomy without radiation group occurred within the first 5 years, while 40 % of those undergoing lumpectomy plus radiation had a recurrence within the same time span. The 20-year follow-up data for the Milan trial [10] differs from the NSABP trial suggesting a higher incidence of local recurrence in the breast conservation group (8.8 % $\pm$3.2) compared to the mastectomy group (2.3 % $\pm$0.8). Despite the difference in recurrence rates, both treatment options showed comparable overall survival as well as risk of death from breast cancer (26.1 % vs. 24.3 %, respectively). These results were later confirmed in a large meta-analysis of nearly 42,000 patients [33].

Imprint cytology has shown to decrease the risk of recurrence in patients undergoing breast conservation therapy. In a study published in 2004 [30], recurrences after BCT performed at an outside institution using frozen and permanent sections to determine margins were compared to those performed at the Moffitt Cancer Center where imprint cytology was used to determine margins. The results were dramatic, with imprint cytology reducing the recurrence rate from 8.8 to 2.8 % for all types of breast cancer. The breakdown for each type of cancer can be seen in Table 13.3.

While BCT certainly has advantages to the patient compared to a traditional MRM, there are a number of risk factors that have to be considered prior to surgery that can increase the risk of recurrence in patients undergoing BCT. The most common risk factors debated among the literature are large tumor size, multiple tumors, axillary lymph node involvement, young age, high nuclear grade, hormone receptor status, lack of radiation, and margin status. Of these risk factors, achieving a clear surgical margin is the only factor that can be controlled by the surgeon. Some studies suggest that it is not the width of the negative margin, but the mere status of having a negative margin. It is common practice of many surgeons to perform a re-excision if the cancer is within 2 mm of the margin when examined by the pathologist. Age less than 40 years has been shown to increase the risk of recurrence by 1.8 % while being ER negative increases it by 1.5 % [34]. Their study also confirms what has been shown in many other studies that adjuvant radiation therapy after lumpectomy significantly decreases the chance of recurrence (HR 0.39). Of note, other groups feel the age that worsens prognosis is less than 35 years old [35].

Table 13.3 BCT recurrence rates without and with imprint cytology (IC)

Recurrence	OSH without IC	Moffitt with IC	*P* value
Overall	8.8 %	2.8 %	<0.0001
DCIS	8.8 %	4.0 %	0.105
IDC	9.5 %	2.7 %	<0.0001
ILC	5.1 %	1.5 %	0.166
Mixed	0	2.9 %	0.558

Adapted from Weinberg et al. [30]
DCIS ductal carcinoma in situ, *IDC* invasive ductal carcinoma, *ILC* invasive lobular carcinoma, *Mixed* mixed ductal and lobular carcinoma

Treatment of recurrence after BCT depends on the initial operation and location of recurrence. For local recurrence, patients who undergo BCT with radiation should return to the OR for a total mastectomy with repeat sentinel node biopsy. If follow-up has demonstrated regional or local and regional recurrence in the axilla, the patient should be evaluated for possible resection and then be evaluated for chest wall, supraclavicular, infraclavicular, and axillary radiation. If the regional recurrence is in the supraclavicular or internal mammary nodes, surgical resection may be indicated and the patient should receive localized radiation therapy. When recurrent disease is systemic, then no surgical intervention is warranted and the patient should be evaluated for chemotherapy.

Oncoplastic Reductions

As BCT became an acceptable option for many women instead of a mastectomy, the concept of oncoplastic breast surgery evolved from its early attempts to preserve breast tissue. Over time, BCT has been regarded as a minimalist approach, with the assurance that the cancerous lesion is excised in its entirety. Oncoplastic surgery provides a range of possibilities to allow a more "cosmetic" result. A range of applications stem from breast reduction, skin and nipple sparing, and autologous reconstruction. It combines oncologic principles with plastic surgery techniques, requiring vision of symmetry and aesthetics and understanding of breast anatomy and contour.

For those women with large breasts and breast tumor, the volume of breast tissue allows for tumor resection and reduction mammoplasty. After the tumor has been excised with sufficient tissue to ensure negative margins, large breasts allow for a better aesthetic result. Papp et al. [36] observed an overall improved aesthetic outcome with patients in the immediate mammoplasty group compared to those with delayed reconstruction. Indications for bilateral reduction mammoplasty are large, pendulous breasts, tumor location to allow for negative margins, tumor located in lower quadrants, significant area of redundant skin remaining after tumor resection, and tumor location in area where a poor aesthetic result is likely (for instance, underneath the nipple) [37].

The option to provide a bilateral reduction mammoplasty at the same time of the oncologic resection does increase the overall surgical time. In certain patients with multiple comorbidities, a lengthened anesthetic state may not be suitable. Radiation therapy for certain patients after their reconstruction causes some degree of fibrosis and retraction of tissue [38]. Furthermore, postoperative complications in terms of wound healing can pose a delay in adjuvant therapy. Poor healing can lead to wound dehiscence, fat necrosis, flap necrosis, nipple-areola complex necrosis, wound infection, hematoma, and seroma [39]. A conservative approach to wound dehiscence consists of local debridement and revision if necessary. However, flap necrosis and nipple-areola complex necrosis are due to poor vascularity to area and tension in flap. These complications can be prevented by preservation of perforator vessels and beveling of the flap.

The key concepts to a reduction mammoplasty are to preserve adequate vascular supply to the nipple-areola complex as well as to the remaining breast parenchyma. The Wise pattern, also referred to as the "keyhole" approach, creates the classic inverted T- or anchor-shaped incision. The first line marker is from the suprasternal notch advancing inferiorly as it intersects with a midclavicular line at a point where the current nipple exists. The distance between the midline and new nipple should be approximately 9–10 cm, and the lines from the suprasternal notch and the new nipples on both sides should form a right triangle [40]. The tumor location is marked and a keyhole marks the excision area to include the area of breast to be removed. A pedicle width is chosen, approximately 8–10 cm, based on the tumor location. The inferior- or superior-based pedicle should be within 1.5 cm from the areola. After the tumor is resected, an incision is created along the markings and de-epithelization is performed to create the pedicle. Thickness of the pedicle is between 4 and 8 cm at the base and 3–5 cm at the nipple-areola complex. Flaps are created and the parenchymal tissue is excised, followed by transposition of the pedicle and the flaps aligned and approximated to these new margins of skin [41].

Similarly to the Wise pattern for reduction mammoplasty, a vertical pattern offers similar results. Once the tumor is excised, the breast is pushed medially and laterally against a vertical line. The medial and lateral incision lines delineate the areas of resection. The inferior margin of the excision is 4 cm superior to the inframammary fold. A pedicle 8–10 cm in width with a 1.5 cm margin around the areola is designed. The dermal pedicle is de-epithelialized, parenchymal tissue is excised, and the dermal pedicle is transposed, advancing and closing the skin flaps as performed with the Wise pattern [42].

As to oncologic and adjuvant treatment benefits, for instance, radiation, immediate mammoplasty reduction allows for an overall better tissue composition. In patients with large, pendulous breasts, clinical series note increased complications after radiation, in comparison to smaller breasts [43]. The increased fat content in large breasts, the fatty tissue, results in more fibrosis after radiation therapy. Increased skin retraction and asymmetry is noted in this group of patients, preventing a better cosmetic result.

From an oncologic perspective, the ability to resect and remove further tissue allows for a greater possibility of negative margins. In patients with oncologic mammoplasty reduction, the core of the tumor and substantial excision of surrounding tissue permits a negative resection margin [44]. The reduction allows a larger mean volume of breast tissue, potentially reducing the incidence of margin involvement. One drawback of these oncoplastic approaches is the fact that once the excision has occurred and the breast tissues are rearranged, the margins that remain positive can be nearly impossible to accurately locate and re-excise. The solution to this dilemma has been solved in the authors' experience by placing a Cavity Evaluation Device (CED) into the lumpectomy cavity at the time of primary excision. It is then embedded into the breast, bringing the fill valve just under the skin at a position that would make subsequent catheter-based APBI an appropriate treatment in this population of patients. If indeed the margins remain positive on final pathology, it is relatively easy to go back through the prior incisions to the balloon cavity and re-resect the appropriate margin(s). Again, you must await final pathology, finally exchanging the CED for an APBI treatment catheter.

This method provides a number of advantages: accurate excision of the tumor-bearing area with wide margins, accurate identification of the lumpectomy site for subsequent radiation therapy, accurate identification of margins in the event of a pathologically positive margin, the ability to accurately find and re-excise the margin, and ultimately the ability to apply APBI treatment options. The latter is associated with less breast deformity and shrinkage to a group of patients that have undergone plastic reductive procedures for improved cosmesis that can be greatly altered by the long-term consequences of whole breast irradiation. For those patients with the criteria necessary for whole breast irradiation, the placement of the CED and subsequent APBI for tumor bed boost dosing enhances the accuracy and effectiveness of that treatment. In women with large, pendulous breasts, oncoplastic reduction provides the ability to fully excise the existing tumor without leaving a significant defect from its resection, while remodeling the surrounding breast tissue to provide an aesthetic as well as functional outcome.

Controversial Topics in Breast Conservation Therapy

Breast conservation therapy has an equivalent efficacy when compared with mastectomy for early-stage breast cancers. As surgical techniques and medical treatments advance, more patients are becoming candidates for BCT which is obscuring the boundaries between lumpectomy and mastectomy.

Breast Conservation for Large Tumors

Lumpectomy and radiation had traditionally been offered for tumors less than 20 mm in size. NSABP B-06 included patients with up to 40 mm tumors, and subsequent series of patients with larger tumors have been published. Dongen et al. published a series in 2000 with inclusion criteria up to 50 mm in size [8]. Their series had nearly 900 patients and a 13.4-year median follow-up. With regard to overall survival and distant disease, there was no difference between the BCT and mastectomy groups. However, local recurrence in this series was higher in the BCT group (20 %) than in the group who had mastectomy (12 %). Even for T3/T4 cancers, BCT outcomes were found to be acceptable when compared with mastectomy. In one series with 196 patients, overall survival, breast cancer-related survival, and local recurrence-free survival were equivalent between BCT and mastectomy [45].

Much like large tumors, centrally located tumors have traditionally been treated with mastectomy because the oncoplastic result has previously been in question. A head to head comparison of BCT for central tumors with BCT for tumors on the breast periphery involving 1,485 patients showed no difference in 5-year overall, local, or distant recurrence-free survival between the groups [46]. Furthermore, oncoplastic techniques have improved the cosmesis after these operations. One subset of patients where lumpectomy has shown to be feasible for large tumors includes those women with breast hypertrophy/macromastia. One series used partial mastectomy with immediate reduction mammoplasty to treat tumors 0.05–8.9 cm large. There was no difference in recurrence or complication rate attributable to tumor size [37]. Advances in neoadjuvant therapy and oncoplastic techniques are being explored, and these will continue to allow for broadened indications for BCT, even in the setting of locally advanced disease.

Lumpectomy After Neoadjuvant Therapy

As with other malignancies, neoadjuvant therapy is being utilized to downstage tumors in breast cancer with a couple of goals in mind. The first goal is to offer more patients breast conservation therapy as neoadjuvant therapy pushes tumor size into nationally acceptable parameters. The other is to use response to predict patient outcomes. Large series have been completed, and these have shown that BCT with neoadjuvant therapy has resulted in acceptable rates of recurrence. In a series of 340 patients at MD Anderson Cancer Center, neoadjuvant therapy was used prior to BCT, with 96 % of these patients with initial stage II or stage III disease. BCT after neoadjuvant therapy in their study produced acceptable rates of local recurrence and ipsilateral breast recurrence, but they did notice a subset of patients for whom BCT was less effective in controlling disease. These were patients with nodal involvement at diagnosis, multifocal disease pattern, lymphovascular invasion, and large residual tumor. Consequently, they developed a prognostic index to predict successful BCT after neoadjuvant therapy [47].

A 325-patient study out of Vienna analyzed use of neoadjuvant therapy and BCT in patients with lobular carcinoma [48]. There was no difference in local recurrence in those patients with ductal versus lobular carcinoma. Fifty-three month follow-up showed no difference in local recurrence between those lobular carcinoma patients who had mastectomy and BCT. Furthermore, neoadjuvant therapy made BCT an option in 45 % of patients originally scheduled for mastectomy. Likewise, others have seen neoadjuvant therapy enable BCT in nearly 50 % of patients, while also delineating how response to therapy does impact overall survival [49]. Five-year survival was 100 % for those who achieved a complete response, while partial and nonresponders had 74 and 48 % 5-year survival, respectively. The general trend has been for more widespread use of neoadjuvant therapy. This has been predicated upon the fact that it has allowed more patients to undergo BCT, in addition to enabling assessment of tumor response to therapy as an important prognostic tool for survival.

References

1. Fischer JE. Fischer's mastery of surgery. 6th ed. Philadelphia: Wolters Kluwer Health/Lippincott Williams & Wilkins; 2012.
2. Wickerham DL, Costantino JP, Mamounas EP, Julian TB. The landmark surgical trials of the national surgical adjuvant breast and bowel project. World J Surg. 2006;30(7):1138–46. doi:10.1007/s00268-005-0552-5.
3. Fisher B, Anderson S, Bryant J, Margolese RG, Deutsch M, Fisher ER, Jeong JH, Wolmark N. Twenty-year follow-up of a randomized trial comparing total mastectomy, lumpectomy, and lumpectomy plus irradiation for the treatment of invasive breast cancer. N Engl J Med. 2002;347(16):1233–41. doi:10.1056/NEJMoa022152.
4. Sabiston DC, Townsend CM. Sabiston textbook of surgery: the biological basis of modern surgical practice. 19th ed. Philadelphia: Elsevier/Saunders; 2012.
5. McGuire KP, Santillan AA, Kaur P, Meade T, Parbhoo J, Mathias M, Shamehdi C, Davis M, Ramos D, Cox CE. Are mastectomies on the rise? A 13-year trend analysis of the selection of mastectomy versus breast conservation therapy in 5865 patients. Ann Surg Oncol. 2009;16(10):2682–90. doi:10.1245/s10434-009-0635-x.
6. Balch CM, Jacobs LK. Mastectomies on the rise for breast cancer: "the tide is changing". Ann Surg Oncol. 2009;16(10):2669–72. doi:10.1245/s10434-009-0634-y.
7. Katipamula R, Degnim AC, Hoskin T, Boughey JC, Loprinzi C, Grant CS, Brandt KR, Pruthi S, Chute CG, Olson JE, Couch FJ, Ingle JN, Goetz MP. Trends in mastectomy rates at the Mayo Clinic Rochester: effect of surgical year and preoperative magnetic resonance imaging. J Clin Oncol. 2009;27(25):4082–8. doi:10.1200/JCO.2008.19.4225.
8. van Dongen JA, Voogd AC, Fentiman IS, Legrand C, Sylvester RJ, Tong D, van der Schueren E, Helle PA, van Zijl K, Bartelink H. Long-term results of a randomized trial comparing breast-conserving therapy with mastectomy: European Organization for Research and Treatment of Cancer 10801 trial. J Natl Cancer Inst. 2000;92(14):1143–50.
9. Blichert-Toft M, Rose C, Andersen JA, Overgaard M, Axelsson CK, Andersen KW, Mouridsen HT. Danish randomized trial comparing breast conservation therapy with mastectomy: six years of life-table analysis. Danish Breast Cancer Cooperative Group. Journal of the National Cancer Institute Monographs. 1992;11:19–25.
10. Veronesi U, Cascinelli N, Mariani L, Greco M, Saccozzi R, Luini A, Aguilar M, Marubini E. Twenty-year follow-up of a randomized study comparing breast-conserving surgery with radical mastectomy for early breast cancer. N Engl J Med. 2002;347(16):1227–32. doi:10.1056/NEJMoa020989.
11. Hall FM, Frank HA. Preoperative localization of nonpalpable breast lesions. AJR Am J Roentgenol. 1979;132(1):101–5. doi:10.2214/ajr.132.1.101.
12. Hall FM, Kopans DB, Sadowsky NL, Homer MJ. Development of wire localization for occult breast lesions: Boston remembrances. Radiology. 2013;268(3):622–7. doi:10.1148/radiol.13121943.
13. Ernst MF, Avenarius JK, Schuur KH, Roukema JA. Wire localization of non-palpable breast lesions: out of date? Breast. 2002;11(5):408–13. doi:10.1054/brst.2002.0444.
14. Thompson M, Henry-Tillman R, Margulies A, Thostenson J, Bryant-Smith G, Fincher R, Korourian S, Klimberg VS. Hematoma-directed ultrasound-guided (HUG) breast lumpectomy. Ann Surg Oncol. 2007;14(1):148–56. doi:10.1245/s10434-006-9076-y.
15. Arentz C, Baxter K, Boneti C, Henry-Tillman R, Westbrook K, Korourian S, Klimberg VS. Ten-year experience with hematoma-directed ultrasound-guided (HUG) breast lumpectomy. Ann Surg Oncol. 2010;17 Suppl 3:378–83. doi:10.1245/s10434-010-1230-x.
16. Cox CE, Furman B, Stowell N, Ebert M, Clark J, Dupont E, Shons A, Berman C, Beauchamp J, Gardner M, Hersch M, Venugopal P, Szabunio M, Cressman J, Diaz N, Vrcel V, Fairclough R. Radioactive seed localization breast biopsy and lumpectomy: can specimen radiographs be eliminated? Ann Surg Oncol. 2003;10(9):1039–47.
17. Gray RJ, Pockaj BA, Karstaedt PJ, Roarke MC. Radioactive seed localization of nonpalpable breast lesions is better than wire localization. Am J Surg. 2004;188(4):377–80. doi:10.1016/j.amjsurg.2004.06.023.
18. Sabel MS, Kaufman CS, Whitworth P, Chang H, Stocks LH, Simmons R, Schultz M. Cryoablation of early-stage breast cancer: work-in-progress report of a multi-institutional trial. Ann Surg Oncol. 2004;11(5):542–9. doi:10.1245/ASO.2004.08.003.
19. Bland KL, Gass J, Klimberg VS. Radiofrequency, cryoablation, and other modalities for breast cancer ablation. Surg Clin North Am. 2007;87(2):539–50. doi:10.1016/j.suc.2007.02.003, xii.
20. Klimberg VS, Kepple J, Shafirstein G, Adkins L, Henry-Tillman R, Youssef E, Brito J, Talley L, Korourian S. eRFA: excision followed by RFA-a new technique to improve local control in breast cancer. Ann Surg Oncol. 2006;13(11):1422–33. doi:10.1245/s10434-006-9151-4.
21. Wilson M, Korourian S, Boneti C, Adkins L, Badgwell B, Lee J, Suzanne Klimberg V. Long-term results of excision followed by radiofrequency ablation as the sole means of local therapy for breast cancer. Ann Surg Oncol. 2012;19(10):3192–8. doi:10.1245/s10434-012-2476-2.
22. NSABP B-39, RTOG 0413. A Randomized Phase III Study of conventional whole breast irradiation versus partial breast irradiation for women with stage 0, I, or II breast cancer. Clinical advances in hematology & oncology. H&O. 2006;4(10):719–21.

23. Benitez PR, Keisch ME, Vicini F, Stolier A, Scroggins T, Walker A, White J, Hedberg P, Hebert M, Arthur D, Zannis V, Quiet C, Streeter O, Silverstein M. Five-year results: the initial clinical trial of MammoSite balloon brachytherapy for partial breast irradiation in early-stage breast cancer. Am J Surg. 2007;194(4):456–62. doi:10.1016/j.amjsurg.2007.06.010.
24. Polgar C, Fodor J, Major T, Nemeth G, Lovey K, Orosz Z, Sulyok Z, Takacsi-Nagy Z, Kasler M. Breast-conserving treatment with partial or whole breast irradiation for low-risk invasive breast carcinoma–5-year results of a randomized trial. Int J Radiat Oncol Biol Phys. 2007;69(3):694–702. doi:10.1016/j.ijrobp.2007.04.022.
25. Vaidya JS, Joseph DJ, Tobias JS, Bulsara M, Wenz F, Saunders C, Alvarado M, Flyger HL, Massarut S, Eiermann W, Keshtgar M, Dewar J, Kraus-Tiefenbacher U, Sutterlin M, Esserman L, Holtveg HM, Roncadin M, Pigorsch S, Metaxas M, Falzon M, Matthews A, Corica T, Williams NR, Baum M. Targeted intraoperative radiotherapy versus whole breast radiotherapy for breast cancer (TARGIT-A trial): an international, prospective, randomised, non-inferiority phase 3 trial. Lancet. 2010;376(9735):91–102. doi:10.1016/S0140-6736(10)60837-9.
26. Veronesi U, Orecchia R, Luini A, Galimberti V, Zurrida S, Intra M, Veronesi P, Arnone P, Leonardi MC, Ciocca M, Lazzari R, Caldarella P, Rotmensz N, Sangalli C, Sances D, Maisonneuve P. Intraoperative radiotherapy during breast conserving surgery: a study on 1,822 cases treated with electrons. Breast Cancer Res Treat. 2010;124(1):141–51. doi:10.1007/s10549-010-1115-5.
27. Bathla L, Harris A, Davey M, Sharma P, Silva E. High resolution intra-operative two-dimensional specimen mammography and its impact on second operation for re-excision of positive margins at final pathology after breast conservation surgery. Am J Surg. 2011;202(4):387–94. doi:10.1016/j.amjsurg.2010.09.031.
28. Olson TP, Harter J, Munoz A, Mahvi DM, Breslin T. Frozen section analysis for intraoperative margin assessment during breast-conserving surgery results in low rates of re-excision and local recurrence. Ann Surg Oncol. 2007;14(10):2953–60. doi:10.1245/s10434-007-9437-1.
29. Weber WP, Engelberger S, Viehl CT, Zanetti-Dallenbach R, Kuster S, Dirnhofer S, Wruk D, Oertli D, Marti WR. Accuracy of frozen section analysis versus specimen radiography during breast-conserving surgery for nonpalpable lesions. World J Surg. 2008;32(12):2599–606. doi:10.1007/s00268-008-9757-8.
30. Weinberg E, Cox C, Dupont E, White L, Ebert M, Greenberg H, Diaz N, Vercel V, Centeno B, Cantor A, Nicosia S. Local recurrence in lumpectomy patients after imprint cytology margin evaluation. Am J Surg. 2004;188(4):349–54. doi:10.1016/j.amjsurg.2004.06.024.
31. Fisher B, Bauer M, Margolese R, Poisson R, Pilch Y, Redmond C, Fisher E, Wolmark N, Deutsch M, Montague E, et al. Five-year results of a randomized clinical trial comparing total mastectomy and segmental mastectomy with or without radiation in the treatment of breast cancer. N Engl J Med. 1985;312(11):665–73. doi:10.1056/NEJM198503143121101.
32. Fisher B, Redmond C, Poisson R, Margolese R, Wolmark N, Wickerham L, Fisher E, Deutsch M, Caplan R, Pilch Y, et al. Eight-year results of a randomized clinical trial comparing total mastectomy and lumpectomy with or without irradiation in the treatment of breast cancer. N Engl J Med. 1989;320(13):822–8. doi:10.1056/NEJM198903303201302.
33. Group EBCTC. Effects of radiotherapy and surgery in early breast cancer. An overview of the randomized trials. N Engl J Med. 1995;333(22):1444–55. doi:10.1056/NEJM199511303332202.
34. Miles RC, Gullerud RE, Lohse CM, Jakub JW, Degnim AC, Boughey JC. Local recurrence after breast-conserving surgery: multivariable analysis of risk factors and the impact of young age. Ann Surg Oncol. 2012;19(4):1153–9. doi:10.1245/s10434-011-2084-6.
35. Matthews RH, McNeese MD, Montague ED, Oswald MJ. Prognostic implications of age in breast cancer patients treated with tumorectomy and irradiation or with mastectomy. Int J Radiat Oncol Biol Phys. 1988;14(4):659–63.
36. Papp C, Wechselberger G, Schoeller T. Autologous breast reconstruction after breast-conserving cancer surgery. Plast Reconstr Surg. 1998;102(6):1932–6; discussion 1937–8.
37. Chang E, Johnson N, Webber B, Booth J, Rahhal D, Gannett D, Johnson W, Franzini D, Zegzula H. Bilateral reduction mammoplasty in combination with lumpectomy for treatment of breast cancer in patients with macromastia. Am J Surg. 2004;187(5):647–50. doi:10.1016/j.amjsurg.2004.01.002; discussion 650–1.
38. Gray JR, McCormick B, Cox L, Yahalom J. Primary breast irradiation in large-breasted or heavy women: analysis of cosmetic outcome. Int J Radiat Oncol Biol Phys. 1991;21(2):347–54.
39. Brierley JD, Paterson IC, Lallemand RC, Rostom AY. The influence of breast size on late radiation reaction following excision and radiotherapy for early breast cancer. Clin Oncol. 1991;3(1):6–9.
40. Yang JD, Lee JW, Kim WW, Jung JH, Park HY. Oncoplastic surgical techniques for personalized breast conserving surgery in breast cancer patient with small to moderate sized breast. J Breast Cancer. 2011;14(4):253–61. doi:10.4048/jbc.2011.14.4.253.
41. Berry MG, Fitoussi AD, Curnier A, Couturaud B, Salmon RJ. Oncoplastic breast surgery: a review and systematic approach. J Plast Reconstr Aesthet Surg. 2010;63(8):1233–43. doi:10.1016/j.bjps.2009.05.006.
42. Smith ML, Evans GR, Gurlek A, Bouvet M, Singletary SE, Ames FC, Janjan N, McNeese MD. Reduction mammaplasty: its role in breast conservation surgery

for early-stage breast cancer. Ann Plast Surg. 1998;41(3):234–9.
43. Losken A, Elwood ET, Styblo TM, Bostwick 3rd J. The role of reduction mammaplasty in reconstructing partial mastectomy defects. Plast Reconstr Surg. 2002;109(3):968–75; discussion 976–7.
44. Kaur N, Petit JY, Rietjens M, Maffini F, Luini A, Gatti G, Rey PC, Urban C, De Lorenzi F. Comparative study of surgical margins in oncoplastic surgery and quadrantectomy in breast cancer. Ann Surg Oncol. 2005;12(7):539–45. doi:10.1245/ASO.2005.12.046.
45. Fitzal F, Riedl O, Wutzl L, Draxler W, Rudas M, Pluschnig U, Handl-Zeller L, Dubsky P, Bachleitner-Hofmann T, Steger G, Jakesz R, Gnant M. Breast-conserving surgery for T3/T4 breast cancer: an analysis of 196 patients. Breast Cancer Res Treat. 2007;103(1):45–52. doi:10.1007/s10549-006-9325-6.
46. Fitzal F, Mittlboeck M, Trischler H, Krois W, Nehrer G, Deutinger M, Jakesz R, Gnant M. Breast-conserving therapy for centrally located breast cancer. Ann Surg. 2008;247(3):470–6. doi:10.1097/SLA.0b013e31815b6991.
47. Akay CL, Meric-Bernstam F, Hunt KK, Grubbs EG, Bedrosian I, Tucker SL, Kuerer HM, Hoffman KE, Babiera GV, Strom EA, Buchholz TA, Mittendorf EA. Evaluation of the MD Anderson Prognostic Index for local-regional recurrence after breast conserving therapy in patients receiving neoadjuvant chemotherapy. Ann Surg Oncol. 2012;19(3):901–7. doi:10.1245/s10434-011-2006-7.
48. Fitzal F, Mittlboeck M, Steger G, Bartsch R, Rudas M, Dubsky P, Riedl O, Jakesz R, Gnant M. Neoadjuvant chemotherapy increases the rate of breast conservation in lobular-type breast cancer patients. Ann Surg Oncol. 2012;19(2):519–26. doi:10.1245/s10434-011-1879-9.
49. Spanheimer PM, Carr JC, Thomas A, Sugg SL, Scott-Conner CE, Liao J, Weigel RJ. The response to neoadjuvant chemotherapy predicts clinical outcome and increases breast conservation in advanced breast cancer. Am J Surg. 2013;206(1):2–7. doi:10.1016/j.amjsurg.2012.10.025.

Mastectomy for Invasive Breast Cancer

14

Tracy-Ann Moo and Rache M. Simmons

Abbreviations

DCIS Ductal carcinoma in situ
NAC Nipple-areola complex

Introduction

The mastectomy procedure has evolved considerably since the era of the radical mastectomy. In the late 1800s, Halsted and Mayer described the radical mastectomy in individual reports on the treatment of breast cancer. The radical mastectomy involved removal of the breast and pectoral muscles in conjunction with an axillary and infraclavicular lymph node dissection [1, 2]. At a time when no effective adjuvant treatment existed, this en bloc resection provided the best rates of local control. The obvious drawbacks to such a radical procedure included chronic lymphedema, as well as neurologic deficits related to transection of the long thoracic and thoracodorsal nerves, which was routinely performed at the time.

By the mid-1900s, the modified radical mastectomy, which spared the pectoral muscles, began to gain widespread support as a less morbid procedure that could achieve results equivalent to the radical mastectomy [3–6]. The modified radical mastectomy would in subsequent decades be replaced by the total or simple mastectomy, which eliminated the axillary lymph node dissection. However, around the same time, other groups advocated for a more extensive resection as a means of achieving greater local control, the extended radical mastectomy [7, 8]. The extended radical mastectomy was a more morbid procedure removing not only the infraclavicular and axillary lymph nodes but also the supraclavicular and parasternal lymph nodes.

To address this growing dichotomy in surgical treatment options, the first randomized trials in breast cancer treatment were conceived. These trials examined the debated approaches to local control. As early as 1951, the Danish trial began to enroll patients diagnosed with breast cancer to either simple mastectomy followed by radiation or extended radical mastectomy [9]. In multiple reports from this, as well as other randomized controlled trials, it became evident that there was no difference in survival between the two groups. In the United States, the modified radical mastectomy had replaced the radical mastectomy as the standard therapy for breast cancer by the 1980s [10].

T.-A. Moo, MD (✉)
Department of Breast Surgery, Memorial Sloan Kettering Cancer Center, Evelyn H Lauder Breast Center, 300 East 66th street, 8th floor, New York, NY 10065, USA
e-mail: trm9012@med.cornell.edu

R.M. Simmons, MD, FACD
Department of Surgery, New York Presbyterian Hospital, 425 East 61st street, 10th floor, New York, NY 10065, USA
e-mail: rms2002@med.cornell.edu

A.I. Riker (ed.), *Breast Disease: Comprehensive Management*,
DOI 10.1007/978-1-4939-1145-5_14, © Springer Science+Business Media New York 2015

In the decades that followed, debate centered on the treatment of breast cancer with breast conservation (lumpectomy and radiation) vs. mastectomy. Subsequent randomized controlled trials demonstrated equivalence of the two approaches and have resulted in more women now being treated with breast-conserving surgery [11–14]. However, there are still instances in which mastectomy remains the procedure of choice. The choice of mastectomy technique largely depends on the indication, tumor characteristics, and plans for reconstruction. Currently, several mastectomy techniques can be used including the simple mastectomy, skin-sparing mastectomy, and the nipple-areola-sparing mastectomy.

Indications for Mastectomy

- Presence of contraindications to breast-conserving surgery
  - Multicentric disease
  - Previous chest radiation
- Inability to achieve cosmetically acceptable result with lumpectomy
- Patient preference
- Risk reduction of second ipsilateral or contralateral breast cancer
- Inflammatory breast cancer

Although most women will be candidates for breast-conserving surgery, mastectomy is at times the more appropriate procedure. These situations vary from the presence of an absolute contraindication to breast conservation to patient preference.

Scenario 1

> A patient presents following a workup demonstrating a 1 cm mass within the upper outer quadrant of the right breast, with an additional area of microcalcifications within the right lower inner quadrant. Core needle biopsy of both suspicious areas demonstrates invasive ductal carcinoma in the upper outer quadrant and ductal carcinoma in situ (DCIS) in the lower inner quadrant.

This patient has multicentric disease, for which the current recommended treatment is mastectomy. There is some retrospective evidence demonstrating equivalent outcomes with breast-conserving surgery in select cases of multicentric disease [15–17]. However, there are no prospective, randomized trials that have addressed this issue and so for now the standard remains mastectomy.

Scenario 2

> A 36-year-old female with a past medical history of mantle radiation as a teenager for Hodgkin's lymphoma presents with a new diagnosis of left breast cancer...

Prior chest wall radiation may be a contraindication to breast-conserving surgery depending on the dose and radiation field. In these cases, details on prior radiation exposure are very important in determining the optimal surgical options of either breast conservation or mastectomy.

Scenario 3

> A 54-year-old woman with scleroderma presents with a diagnosis of breast cancer...

Patients with active collagen vascular disease such as systemic lupus erythematosus or scleroderma may not be candidates for radiation therapy (therefore not candidates for breast conservation therapy) secondary to poor wound healing and subsequent complications.

Scenario 4

> A 29-year-old woman at 14 weeks gestation presents with right breast invasive ductal carcinoma...

As radiation therapy cannot be given to patients during pregnancy, breast conservation may not be a feasible option during early pregnancy. This depends on the stage of gestation and whether or not radiation therapy can be timely administered after delivery in relation to chemotherapy, if indicated. Some women will simply prefer to have a mastectomy as definitive treatment during pregnancy.

Scenario 5

> A 39-year-old female with a BRCA gene mutation is recently diagnosed with a right invasive ductal carcinoma and presents to your office desiring bilateral mastectomies…

Mastectomy may be a better option for the patient who is found to have a BRCA gene mutation, as they are certainly at a very high risk of a new primary and contralateral breast cancer. Increasingly common is the election of bilateral mastectomies in this population.

Scenario 6

> A 65-year-old woman presents with inflammatory breast cancer…

The treatment of inflammatory breast cancer mandates a mastectomy. This occurs after the completion of neoadjuvant chemotherapy, with a modified radical mastectomy being the procedure of choice in this scenario.

Mastectomy Techniques

There are several techniques by which a mastectomy can be performed. The procedure involves the removal of the entire breast parenchyma with varying degrees of skin, with or without removal of the nipple-areola complex. The choice of technique depends largely on the size of the breast and whether or not immediate reconstruction is planned. Incision choice is often dictated by the technique as well as the size and shape of the breast and to some extent surgeon and patient preference. The choice of incision also depends on the existence of previous biopsy or lumpectomy incisions and whether or not the tumor is adherent to the skin. In all techniques, the limits of resection are the clavicle superiorly, the lateral border of the sternum medially, the inframammary crease inferiorly, and the anterior border of the latissimus dorsi laterally.

Simple Mastectomy (Non-Skin-Sparing)

The simple mastectomy is well suited for those patients who will not have immediate reconstruction. In this type of mastectomy, most of the skin is removed. On completion, the incision is expected to lie flat against the chest wall without leaving excess amounts of tissue at the medial and lateral limits of the incision. This allows proper positioning of prosthesis and limits potential discomfort resulting from redundant skin.

The simple mastectomy removes all the breast parenchyma with the nipple-areola complex and the skin, leaving just enough skin to close the wound without undo tension. The most commonly used incision is the Stewart elliptical incision, which extends medially from the sternum to the latissimus laterally and will encompass most tumors located central and laterally. Depending on the position of the tumor, the Stewart incision can also be placed obliquely as in the modified Stewart or Orr incision (Fig. 14.1). These oblique incisions can be placed with the medial aspect

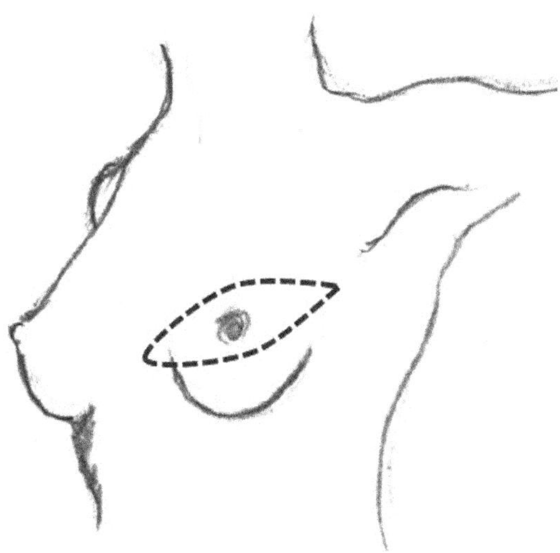

Fig. 14.1 Oblique elliptical incision for simple mastectomy

directed cephalad to encompass tumors in the upper inner quadrant and lower outer quadrant of the breast. They can also be positioned so that the medial aspect is pointing caudad to encompass tumors located in the lower inner quadrant or upper outer quadrant. The incision should encompass any previous lumpectomy scars and any area of the skin that is adherent to the tumor.

An incision is made through the dermis and the skin is elevated using penetrating skin hooks. A dissection plane is developed in the avascular plane between the breast parenchyma and the subcutaneous tissue ensuring preservation of the subcutaneous vasculature. The dissection proceeds utilizing electrocautery as necessary or with a scissors or knife depending on surgeon preference. The mastectomy skin flaps are then created, allowing removal of all breast parenchyma while leaving a layer of subcutaneous fat. Acceptable flap thickness varies by patient and amount of subcutaneous fat present. Skin flaps should not be so thin as to compromise blood supply and lead to skin necrosis. However, creating flaps that are too thick will leave behind breast tissue that may lead to an increased risk of tumor recurrence.

Once the skin flaps have been dissected superiorly to the clavicle, inferiorly to the inframammary fold, medially to the sternal border, and laterally to the latissimus dorsi, the breast is removed from the pectoralis major muscle. Elevation of the breast from the pectoralis major is usually performed with electrocautery. The superior margin of the breast is grasped and retracted caudad, while the pectoralis fascia is removed with the breast leaving the underlying pectoralis major muscle intact. At times when the tumor is abutting or invading the pectoralis muscle, this area of muscle can be removed with the specimen. Perforating vessels should be controlled with electrocautery, clips, or ties. As the dissection progresses inferolaterally, care is taken to preserve the fascia of the serratus muscle. Toward the axillary tail, the lateral mammary branches entering the breast are ligated and divided. The breast is divided at the axilla, which is recognized by visualization of the clavipectoral fascia.

Skin-Sparing Mastectomy

The skin-sparing mastectomy as described by Toth and Lappert [18] achieves removal of all breast parenchyma with the nipple-areola complex and minimal skin excision (figure 14.2). This technique is well suited for patients who are having immediate tissue or implant reconstruction.

Nipple-Areola-Complex-Sparing Mastectomy

First described in the 1960s by Freeman [19] as the subcutaneous mastectomy, the nipple-areola-complex (NAC)-sparing mastectomy was intended to achieve an improved cosmetic result by preserving the NAC. This procedure was initially performed selectively at very few institutions, as there were concerns for oncologic outcomes as well as appropriate selection criteria. In women undergoing prophylactic mastectomy, nipple-areola-sparing mastectomy is well accepted as a safe procedure. There remains controversy regarding its use in women with invasive cancer. However, an increasing body of evidence supports nipple-areola-sparing mastectomy in select patients. This includes women who have small (<3.5 cm), peripherally located tumors that are >2 cm from the nipple, a negative axilla and have not been treated with neoadjuvant chemotherapy [20–23]. Frozen sections are routinely sent in patients with invasive cancer or DCIS to confirm a negative nipple margin before proceeding with nipple-areola-sparing mastectomy. In our experience, the overall rate of nipple involvement was 10.6 % [24].

There are several incisions that can be used for the NAC-sparing mastectomy, including the inframammary fold, various lateral incisions, vertical incision, and an incision that incorporates a reduction mastectomy (Fig. 14.3). The choice of incision is largely predetermined by the size of the breast as well as the extent of ptosis. A well-placed incision facilitates removal of all breast parenchyma within the boundaries of a traditional mastectomy. In women who present with

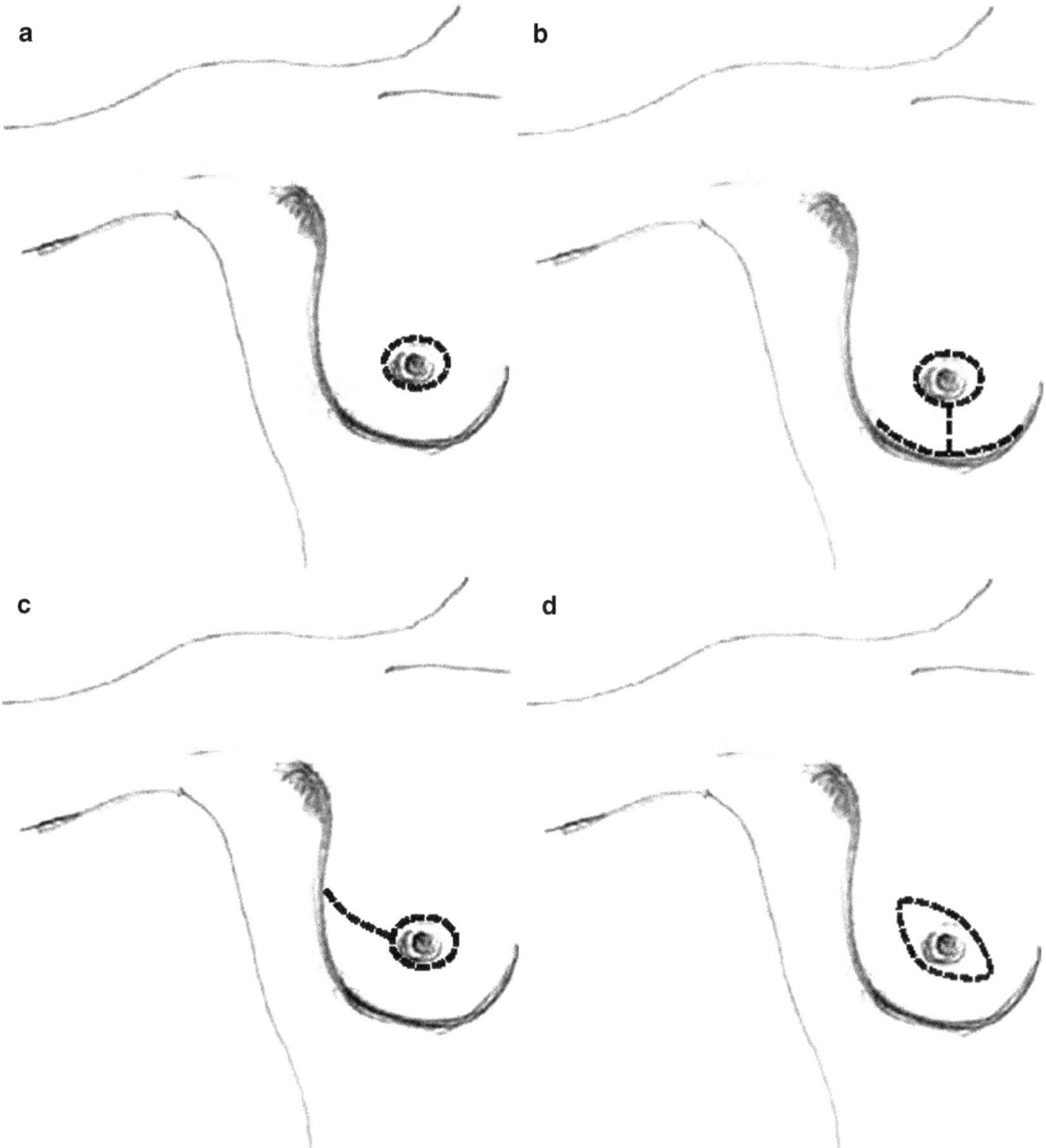

Fig. 14.2 Skin-sparing mastectomy incisions: (**a**) peri-areolar, (**b**) reduction, (**c**) tennis racquet, (**d**) modified ellipse

small, non-ptotic breasts, this can be done through an inframammary incision. However, in the larger ptotic breast, a variation of the lateral or vertical incision is better suited for performing an oncologically safe procedure with survival of the breast skin.

Once the skin incision has been made, flaps are raised in the usual fashion. The creation of skin flaps for the nipple-areola-sparing mastectomy is often more challenging than with the simple mastectomy or skin-sparing mastectomy. The use of a knife, scissors, or electrocautery depends on surgeon preference. As progress is made along the flap, a lighted retractor may be useful to ensure adequate retraction and flap thickness. The nipple is dissected from the underlying duct tissue sharply; this may be done with or without nipple tumescence. We have found that insertion of a 2-0 silk stitch through the nipple allows the assistant to elevate the nipple,

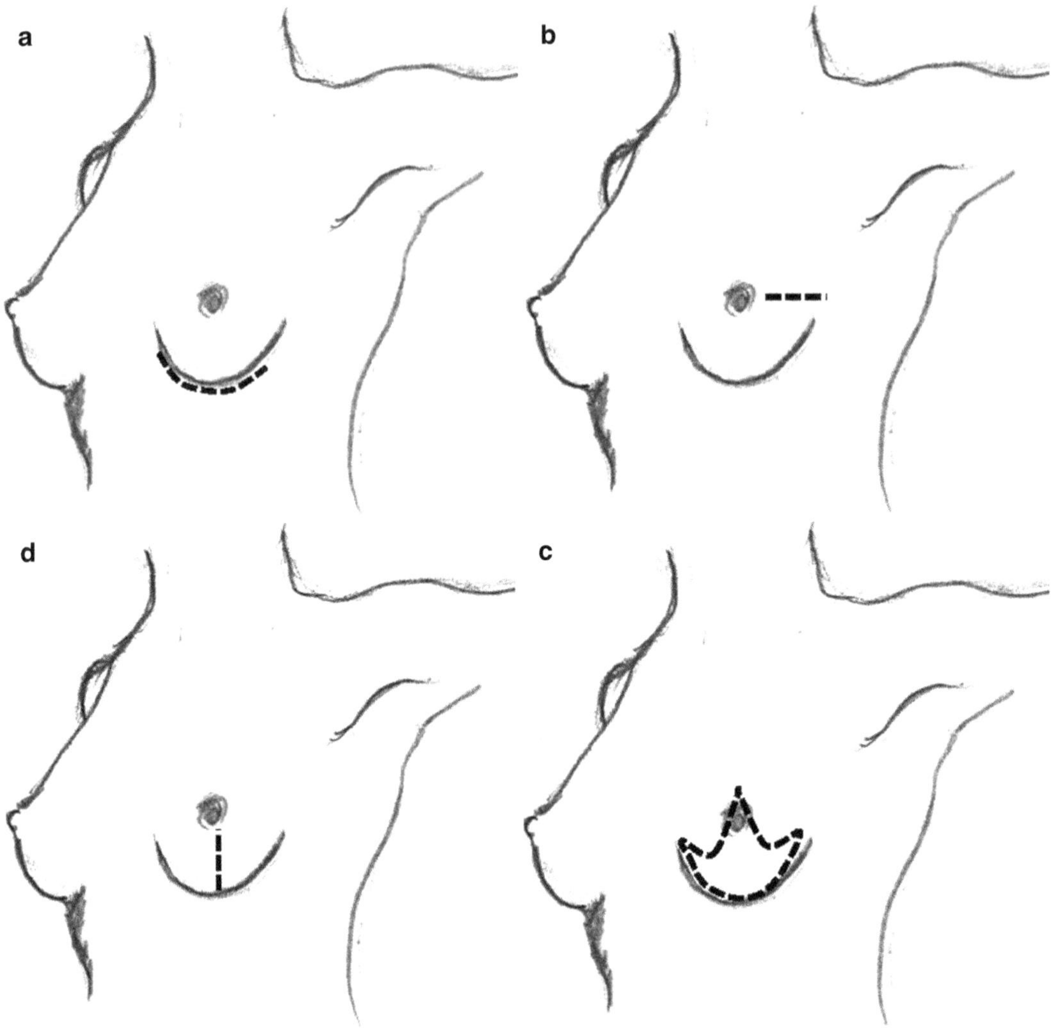

Fig. 14.3 Nipple-areola-complex-sparing incisions: (**a**) inframammary, (**b**) lateral, (**c**) vertical, (**d**) reduction

which facilitates dissection of the underlying ductal tissue.

Once the ductal tissue is removed, the nipple is inverted and an additional nipple margin is taken and sent for frozen section. After the skin flaps have been created, removal of the breast from the chest wall including the pectoral fascia with the specimen must be accomplished. Often this dissection is most easily done by beginning at the lateral aspect of the breast and proceeding medially and inferiorly until the breast is completely removed up to the sternum. The breast can then be delivered through the incision and reflected cranially to facilitate dissection of the superior aspect away from the chest wall. If the mastectomy has been performed through an inframammary incision, then separation of the breast parenchyma beginning at the inframammary crease and progressing superiorly toward the clavicle is more feasible.

Management of the Axilla

The mastectomy procedure (non-skin-sparing, skin-sparing, or nipple-areola-sparing) can be combined with either a sentinel lymph node biopsy for staging of the axilla or a formal axillary lymph node dissection.

The mastectomy incision may also provide access to the axilla for dissection or sentinel lymph node biopsy. In those instances where the incision does not allow axillary access, a small counterincision in the axilla can be made or a lateral extension can be added to the primary incision. In cases where there is a preexisting incision on the breast, the mastectomy incision is designed to incorporate the previous incision. If it is not possible to include the previous incision, the area can be excised separately as long as this can be done without compromising the blood supply to the intervening skin bridge.

In the case of a patient with a positive axilla, a modified radical mastectomy is performed which combines a simple mastectomy, skin-sparing mastectomy, or nipple-areola-sparing mastectomy in an en bloc resection with the axillary lymph node dissection.

Complications

Complications of mastectomy include early and late events. In the early postoperative period, one must be vigilant for ongoing bleeding and hematoma formation, a complication reported in less than 5 % of patients [25]. The use of closed suction drainage will often allow early detection of ongoing bleeding, and a firm swelling on the chest wall usually indicates subsequent hematoma formation. This is often accompanied by complaints of increased pain from the patient. In these situations, the patient should be evaluated by the surgeon and a decision made whether to attempt compression or immediate evacuation. Flap ischemia or necrosis may also be seen in the early postoperative period and are often managed with watchful waiting and delayed debridement of nonviable tissue. Large areas of skin loss requiring debridement may necessitate split-thickness skin grafts or rotational flaps for coverage.

Late complications include infection and seroma formation. Manifestations of infections include superficial cellulitis, wound drainage, and skin breakdown. This may be treated with a combination of antibiotics, aspiration, or debridement. Particularly in the presence of a foreign body (tissue expander or implant), careful attention must be paid to the expedient administration of intravenous antibiotics. Infectious complications are generally handed in conjunction with the plastic surgeon when an expander or implant is present. Seroma formation is the most common complication after mastectomy, reported in 10–30 % of patients [26, 27]. While small fluid collections without evidence of infection may be observed, larger symptomatic seromas require aspiration and sometimes placement of a drainage catheter.

Nipple-sparing mastectomy has particular considerations. The presence of occult metastasis detected on permanent pathology should be treated with resection of the nipple. Partial or complete nipple necrosis may also occur, requiring debridement of the nipple.

Considerations for the Plastic Surgeon

Currently, the treatment of breast cancer with mastectomy includes the proper screening and selection of patients for breast reconstructive surgery. While some patients will decline reconstruction for various reasons, most will meet a plastic surgeon in advance of their operation in order to better understand their options for reconstruction. Once the decision to proceed with mastectomy has been made, the patient should be referred to plastic and reconstructive surgery for consultation. Communication between the breast surgeon and plastic surgeon is important for optimal surgical planning. Decisions on mastectomy technique as well as incision are often made with the input of the patient, breast surgeon, and plastic surgeon.

References

1. Halsted WS. I. The results of operations for the cure of cancer of the breast performed at the Johns Hopkins hospital from June, 1889, to January, 1894. Ann Surg. 1894;20(5):497–555.

2. Meyer W. An improved method for the radical operation for carcinoma of the breast. Breast Med Rec. 1894;46:746.
3. Patey DH. A review of 146 cases of carcinoma of the breast operated on between 1930 and 1943. Br J Cancer. 1967;21(2):260–9. PubMed PMID: 6028079. Pubmed Central PMCID: 2008130. Epub 1967/06/01. eng.
4. Mc WR. The value of simple mastectomy and radiotherapy in the treatment of cancer of the breast. Br J Radiol. 1948;21(252):599–610. PubMed PMID: 18099752.
5. Grace E. Simple mastectomy in cancer of the breast. Am J Surg. 1937;35:512.
6. Madden JL, Kandalaft S, Bourque RA. Modified radical mastectomy. Ann Surg. 1972;175(5):624–34. PubMed PMID: 4555029. Pubmed Central PMCID: 1355229.
7. Urban JA. Radical mastectomy with en bloc in continuity resection of the internal mammary lymph node chain. Am J Roentgenol Radium Ther Nucl Med. 1957;77(3):431–7. PubMed PMID: 13403036.
8. Dahl-Iversen E, Tobiassen T. Radical mastectomy with parasternal and supraclavicular dissection for mammary carcinoma. Ann Surg. 1963;157:170–3. PubMed PMID: 14024626.
9. Johansen H, Kaae S, Jensen MB, Mouridsen HT. Extended radical mastectomy versus simple mastectomy followed by radiotherapy in primary breast cancer. A fifty-year follow-up to the copenhagen breast cancer randomised study. Acta Oncol. 2008;47(4):633–8. PubMed PMID: 18465331.
10. Moxley 3rd JH, Allegra JC, Henney J, Muggia F. Treatment of primary breast cancer. Summary of the National Institutes of health consensus development conference. JAMA. 1980;244(8):797–800. PubMed PMID: 6893059. Epub 1980/08/22. eng.
11. Simone NL, Dan T, Shih J, Smith SL, Sciuto L, Lita E, et al. Twenty-five year results of the national cancer institute randomized breast conservation trial. Breast Cancer Res Treat. 2012;132(1):197–203. PubMed PMID: 22113254. Epub 2011/11/25. eng.
12. Fisher B, Jeong JH, Anderson S, Bryant J, Fisher ER, Wolmark N. Twenty-five-year follow-up of a randomized trial comparing radical mastectomy, total mastectomy, and total mastectomy followed by irradiation. N Engl J Med. 2002;347(8):567–75. PubMed PMID: 12192016. Epub 2002/08/23. eng.
13. Showalter SL, Grover S, Sharma S, Lin L, Czerniecki BJ. Factors influencing surgical and adjuvant therapy in stage I breast cancer: a SEER 18 database analysis. Ann Surg Oncol. 2013;20(4):1287–94. PubMed PMID: 23135311.
14. Veronesi U, Cascinelli N, Mariani L, Greco M, Saccozzi R, Luini A, et al. Twenty-year follow-up of a randomized study comparing breast-conserving surgery with radical mastectomy for early breast cancer. N Engl J Med. 2002;347(16):1227–32. PubMed PMID: 12393819. Epub 2002/10/24. eng.
15. Gentilini O, Botteri E, Rotmensz N, Da Lima L, Caliskan M, Garcia-Etienne CA, et al. Conservative surgery in patients with multifocal/multicentric breast cancer. Breast Cancer Res Treat. 2009;113(3):577–83. PubMed PMID: 18330695. Epub 2008/03/12. eng.
16. Lim W, Park EH, Choi SL, Seo JY, Kim HJ, Chang MA, et al. Breast conserving surgery for multifocal breast cancer. Ann Surg. 2009;249(1):87–90. PubMed PMID: 19106681. Epub 2008/12/25. eng.
17. Bauman L, Barth RJ, Rosenkranz KM. Breast conservation in women with multifocal-multicentric breast cancer: is it feasible? Ann Surg Oncol. 2010;17 Suppl 3:325–9. PubMed PMID: 20853054. Epub 2010/10/01. eng.
18. Toth BA, Lappert P. Modified skin incisions for mastectomy: the need for plastic surgical input in preoperative planning. Plast Reconstr Surg. 1991;87(6):1048–53. PubMed PMID: 1852020. Epub 1991/06/01. eng.
19. Freeman BS. Subcutaneous mastectomy for benign breast lesions with immediate or delayed prosthetic replacement. Plast Reconstr Surg Transplant Bull. 1962;30:676–82. PubMed PMID: 13959443. Epub 1962/12/01. eng.
20. Laronga C, Kemp B, Johnston D, Robb GL, Singletary SE. The incidence of occult nipple-areola complex involvement in breast cancer patients receiving a skin-sparing mastectomy. Ann Surg Oncol. 1999;6(6):609–13. PubMed PMID: 10493632. Epub 1999/09/24. eng.
21. de Alcantara FP, Capko D, Barry JM, Morrow M, Pusic A, Sacchini VS. Nipple-sparing mastectomy for breast cancer and risk-reducing surgery: the memorial sloan-kettering cancer center experience. Ann Surg Oncol. 2011;18(11):3117–22. PubMed PMID: 21847697. Epub 2011/08/19. eng.
22. Crowe Jr JP, Kim JA, Yetman R, Banbury J, Patrick RJ, Baynes D. Nipple-sparing mastectomy: technique and results of 54 procedures. Arch Surg. 2004; 139(2):148–50. PubMed PMID: 14769571. Epub 2004/02/11. eng.
23. Babiera G, Simmons R. Nipple-areolar complex-sparing mastectomy: feasibility, patient selection, and technique. Ann Surg Oncol. 2010;17 Suppl 3:245–8. PubMed PMID: 20853041. Epub 2010/10/01. eng.
24. Simmons RM, Brennan M, Christos P, King V, Osborne M. Analysis of nipple/areolar involvement with mastectomy: can the areola be preserved? Ann Surg Oncol. 2002;9(2):165–8. PubMed PMID: 11888874. Epub 2002/03/13. eng.
25. Winther Lietzen L, Cronin-Fenton D, Garne JP, Kroman N, Silliman R, Lash TL. Predictors of re-operation due to post-surgical bleeding in breast cancer patients: a Danish population-based cohort study. Eur J Surg Oncol. 2012;38(5):407–12. PubMed PMID: 22429495. Epub 2012/03/21. eng.
26. Agrawal A, Ayantunde AA, Cheung KL. Concepts of seroma formation and prevention in breast cancer surgery. ANZ J Surg. 2006;76(12):1088–95.
27. Budd DC, Cochran RC, Sturtz DL, Fouty Jr WJ. Surgical morbidity after mastectomy operations. Am J Surg. 1978;135(2):218–20. PubMed PMID: 626296. Epub 1978/02/01. eng.

15 Inflammatory Breast Cancer

Ricardo Hugo Alvarez, Shaheenah Dawood, and Massimo Cristofanilli

Introduction

Inflammatory breast cancer (IBC) is the most aggressive form of primary breast cancer, with the optimal treatment methods remaining a challenge, primarily due to the early onset of metastasis and rapid tumor progression. In the United States, the incidence is low, reported as 1–6 % of all breast cancers [1]. Data from the Surveillance, Epidemiology, and End Results Program (SEER) revealed that IBC incidence rates between 1988–1990 and 1997–1999 increased from 2 to 2.5 (per 100,000 women-years) ($p<0.001$), whereas those with locally advanced breast cancer (LABC) declined (2.5–2.0; $p=0.0025$) [2]. Improvement in systemic treatment and locoregional managements with surgery and radiation are a crucial part of the curative treatment program of IBC, and several studies have shown the improvement in locoregional control and overall survival when patients are treated with chemotherapy [3, 4]. However, despite the use of multidisciplinary treatment for the IBC, the 5-year survival remains at approximately 30–40 % [5, 6], with no significant change in the overall prognosis over the past 30 years [7].

IBC is a unique entity, characterized by more aggressive clinical features and worse prognosis compared with non-IBC LABC. IBC must be considered a distinct epidemiologic entity within LABC and should be a prolific field for the exploration of innovative systemic treatment. Here, we will review the most current information regarding clinical aspect, molecular targets, and multimodality treatment for IBC.

R.H. Alvarez, MD, MSc (✉)
The Morgan Welch Inflammatory Breast Cancer Research and Clinic Department of Breast Medical Oncology, The University of Texas MD Anderson Cancer Center, 1515 Holcombe Blvd, Unit #1354, Houston, TX 77030, USA
e-mail: ralvarez@mdanderson.org

S. Dawood, MRCP, MPH
Department of Medical Oncology, Department of Health and Medical Services, Dubai Hospital, 8179, Dubai, United Arab Emirates
e-mail: shaheenah_d@yahoo.com

M. Cristofanilli, MD
Breast Cancer Center, Jefferson Medical College, Thomas Jefferson University-Kimmel Cancer Center, 1025 Walnut St, Suite 700, Philadelphia, PA 19107, USA
e-mail: massimo.cristofanilli@jefferson.edu

Definition

Sir Charles Bell is credited with publishing the first description of IBC in 1814 [8]. Subsequently, Klotz [9] in 1869 and Volkmann in 1875 described "mastitis carcinomatosa," a variant of carcinoma of the breast characterized by its clinical virulence, leading to a rapid progression of the disease. A modern description of the clinical features of IBC was introduced by Lee and Tannenbaum in 1924 [10]. This disease has been known by many different names over the last two centuries, including mastitis carcinomatosa, acute mammary carcinoma, acute brawny cancer,

A.I. Riker (ed.), *Breast Disease: Comprehensive Management*,
DOI 10.1007/978-1-4939-1145-5_15, © Springer Science+Business Media New York 2015

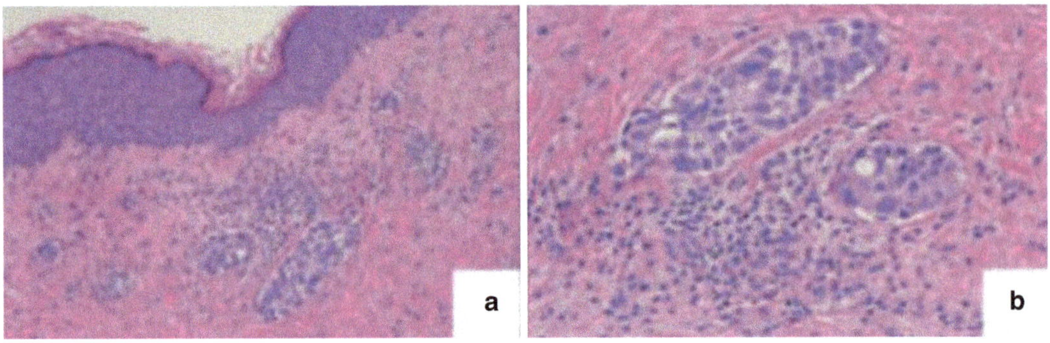

Fig. 15.1 (**a**) Punch biopsy of the skin demonstrates small-, medium-, and large-sized lymphovascular tumor emboli and the superficial dermis from a patient with clinical manifestation of IBC. (**b**) The tumor cells forming the emboli demonstrate high nuclear grade. Note the presence of a mild lymphoplamacytic infiltration in between the emboli

acute scirrhous carcinoma, lymphocytoma of the breast, acute encephaloid cancer, acute cancer of the breast, acute mammary carcinomatosis, and lactation cancer [11].

A key clinical difference compared to non-IBC is that the initial diagnosis of non-IBC is suspected by the presence of mass on imaging studies, whereas the diagnosis of IBC is based upon clinical features of the overlying skin of the breast and rapid evolution. By definition, the clinical features of IBC result in skin changes that arise in a period of less than 6 months, further characterized by discoloration of the skin (ranging from red to purple), extension of the involved area of at least one third of the breast, thickening or fine dimpling (peau d' orange) of the skin, and edema or warmth to touch with palpable ridge at the margin of the induration [12]. The American Joint Committee defined IBC as a clinicopathologic entity characterized by diffuse erythema and edema (peau d'orange) of the breast with or without an underlying palpable mass. However, the term IBC has been used to clinically describe a neglected non-IBC LABC. Both entities have a poor overall prognosis, with several factors blurring the lines of distinction between IBC and LABC.

Pathology Characteristics

The original histopathologic description of IBC was published first by Bryant in 1887 [13]. Initially, this author hypothesized that the clinical findings (erythema, warmth, diffuse enlargement and swelling, pain and tenderness, and edema) were caused by the tumor invasion to the dermal lymph channels. Subsequently, the recognition of the importance of dermal lymphatic invasion (DLI) was considered a "pathologic proof" of IBC. The presence of DLI might be responsible for the lymphatic obstruction causing the marked swelling of the breast with inflammatory signs.

However, DLI is not pathognomonic of IBC, and the presence of tumor embolization of the dermal lymphatic vessels may arise from any breast cancer histopathology. IBC is often misdiagnosed, and the differentiation between primary and secondary IBC is not often made. Taylor and Meltzer categorized patient with IBC as having primary or secondary IBC. Primary IBC is used to describe the "de novo" development of IBC in a previously normal breast. Secondary IBC describes the development of inflammatory skin changes that mimic IBC in either a breast that already has cancer or on the chest wall following mastectomy for a non-IBC. Although the presence of DLI frequently correlates with the clinical findings typical of IBC, the diagnosis of IBC is made on clinical grounds and does not require the pathologic finding of dermal lymphatic invasion [14] (Fig. 15.1a, b).

Epidemiology and Risk Factors

A large population-based study describing the demographic and tumor characteristics of 3,626 women with IBC diagnosis during 1994–1998 demonstrated that the majority of the cases were between 40 and 59 years old [15]. This study also revealed that the incidence of IBC was 1.3 per 100,000 for all races combined. African American women had the highest relative risk (1.6) and Asian and Pacific Islanders women had the lowest (0.7). A large analysis from SEER population-based cancer registry described a marked epidemiologic difference between IBC and LABC [2]. The presence of young age at diagnosis, high nuclear grade, and absence of estrogen receptor (ER)-positive are suggestive of IBC rather than LABC. In a multivariate analysis after adjusting for race, age, tumor size, axillary lymph node status, histologic grade, and ER expression, the risk of death from IBC was nearly twice that compared to LABC [2]. A recent study analyzing the California Cancer Registry of 2,014 IBC patients found that despite an association with stage, HER2-positive status was not an independent adverse prognostic factor for survival among IBC patient cases [16]. These differences in prognostic factor profiles and age-specific incidence patterns support the hypothesis that IBC and LABC are distinct biologic entities.

The number of cases of IBC in Western countries is low; however, they are increasing in overall incidence. There appears to be a striking geographic pattern, with a higher incidence in North African countries (Maghreb) especially Morocco, Algeria, Tunisia, and Egypt, with the incidence of IBC reported to be 10–15 % [17]. However, in these countries, there is some uncertainty about the completeness of case registration and strict definitions used for IBC detection. There are very limited published data on the risk factors for developing IBC. A report from SEER that contains the largest population-based sample of IBC in the United States was published in 1999 [18]. During the period 1975–1981, IBC patients were younger at diagnosis than non-IBC patients. African American women tended to be younger than white women, and the 3-year survival rate for patients with IBC was far lower (34 %) than that for patients with other types of carcinoma (90 %). A second report from SEER demonstrated that between 1975–1977 and 1990–1992, the overall age-adjusted incidence of IBC doubled, increasing among white women from 0.3 to 0.7 cases per 100,000 person-years and among African Americans from 0.6 to 1.1 [1]. Patients with IBC are affected at an early age. Among white women, the mean age at diagnosis for IBC patients (mean = 57 years) was significantly younger than that for other breast carcinoma (62 years, $p = 0.0001$). Among African Americans, IBC were significantly younger (mean = 52 years) than other breast carcinoma patients (mean = 57 years, $p = 0.0003$) [1].

High body mass index (BMI) has been associated with a lower risk of premenopausal breast cancer [19, 20], however, a higher risk of postmenopausal breast cancer [21]. This observation suggests that reproductive hormones and factors related to the body size may partially contribute to the overall risk of developing breast cancer. A single institution report evaluated the BMI as a risk factor for IBC. In this study, a comparison of 68 IBC patients, 143 non-IBC cases, and 134 non-breast cancer cases suggested that IBC patients have an earlier age at menarche and a greater BMI [1]. IBC patients were younger at menarche and at the time of their first live birth than non-IBC and non-breast cancer patients.

The proportion of premenopausal IBC patients was higher than the proportion of premenopausal women in the comparison groups, although differences were not statistically significant. There were no differences in height, but IBC patients were heavier (77.6 kg) than non-IBC (70.0 kg) and non-breast cancer patients (68.0 kg). After adjusting for other factors, women in the highest BMI percentile (BMI >26.65 kg/m^2) relative to the lowest percentile (BMI <22.27) had significantly increased IBC risk (IBC vs. non-IBC, odds ratio [OR] = 2.45, 95 % CI, 1.05–5.73; IBC vs. non-breast cancer, OR = 4.52, 95 % CI = 1.85–11.04). This association was not significantly modified by menopausal status and was independent of age at menarche, family history of breast cancer, gravidity, smoking status, and alcohol use.

In 1936, Bittner and collaborators [22] described the involvement of the mouse mammary tumor virus (MMTV) in mouse mammary carcinogenesis. Subsequently, the sequences of MMTV-like were described in breast cancer samples but absent in normal tissues in multiple reports. More recently, Pogo and collaborators [23] found that retroviral sequences of the

MMTV were present in 40 % of the sporadic breast cancer contrasting with 71 % of IBC in American women. Similar incidence has been found in IBC cancers from Tunisia. Because these conditions represent highly invasive malignancies, it is concluded that HMTV is sometimes associated with a particularly malignant phenotype.

Molecular Insights of IBC

The classical description of IBC attributes to the obstruction of lymphatic vessels the clinical aspect of inflammation. However, the mechanism of "inflammatory" symptoms may be related to a local release of multiple tumor-derived inflammatory cytokines. Besides established and key angiogenic factors like VEGF, chemokines, a superfamily of cytokine-like proteins that bind to seven transmembrane-spanning G protein-coupled receptors, have been associated with angiogenesis under homeostatic conditions. Chemokine receptors, CXCR4 and CCR7, are highly expressed in human breast cancer cells, and metastases. Their respective ligands CXCL12/SDF-1α and CCL21/6Ckine exhibit peak levels of expression in organs representing the first destination of breast cancer metastasis [24].

IBC is characterized by the expression of multiple chemokine receptors, with Cabliogu et al. [24] reporting on IBC patients found to exhibit high levels of expression of CXCR4, EFGR, and HER2-neu amplification. Increased expression of cytoplasmic CXCR4 in almost 50 % of the IBC samples compared with only 5 % expression of T1-tumors lymph node negative, and 11 % of T1-tumors lymph node positive, appears to be at least partially responsible for the metastatic process [25]. EGFR overexpression was detected in 30 % of IBC patients by immunohistochemical staining [24], and it was associated with a higher increase of recurrence and significantly worse 5-year overall survival rate compared to EGFR-negative IBC. Interestingly, co-expression of CXCR4 and growth factor receptors, particularly HER2-neu and EGFR in breast cancer, has been associated with poor outcome. Increased expression of HER2-neu and EGFR in IBC compared with non-IBC appears to be more specific to the IBC phenotype [25].

Experimental models have recently led to the identification of genes involved in IBC, such as *ARHC*, coding for the RhoC GTPase, and *WISP3*, coding for S-glutathione-related protein [26]. In human studies, comparing patients with IBC with stage-matched, non-IBC tumor samples identifies two important genetic characteristics of IBC: loss of WISP3 and overexpression of RhoGTPase [27]. *WISP3* is a tumor suppressor gene that produces proteins that are biologically important, such as with cell proliferation, migration, wound healing, angiogenesis, and carcinogenesis [28]. Expression of *WISP3* was lost in 80 % of the IBC samples versus only 20 % of the stage-matched, non-IBC tumors [29]. In preclinical models, using the IBC cell line SUM149, restoring WISP3 gene expression decreased tumor cell growth, invasiveness, and angiogenic potential [30]. RhoC GTPase is a member of the *Ras* superfamily of small GTP-binding proteins and contributes to the metastatic characteristics of IBC by upregulation of angiogenic factors (VEGF and bFGF) promoting cell motility and invasion [31, 32]. In a comparative study of human tumor samples with stage-matched, non-IBC samples, RhoC was overexpressed in 90 % of the IBC tumors versus 38 % of the non-IBC tumors [27].

Cadherins are integral membrane glycoproteins that mediate calcium-dependent cell-cell adhesion and being responsible of the intercellular signaling trafficking. Loss of E-cadherin expression has been related to a wide spectrum of human cancers, especially prostate and breast. Alterations in the cadherin complexes are directly implicated in tumorigenesis and cancer progression [33]. E-cadherin was found overexpressed in IBC, and strong expression was observed in lymphovascular tumor emboli from IBC [34]. Preclinical data using antibodies against E-cadherin caused dissolution of pulmonary lymphovascular emboli in an IBC xenograft model [35]. The biological role of E-cadherin is not completely known. On the basis of these results, we could hypothesize that the loss of E-cadherin occurs in the early phase of IBC as a transient effect to induce epithelial-to-mesenchymal transition and allow metastasis and that, by the time of diagnosis of IBC, tumor cells have reinstated expression of E-cadherin [29].

It has been validated through many studies that in vitro and in vivo tumor models of IBC have a high expression of proangiogenic and prolymphangiogenic molecules. One of the pioneering studies showed an increased mRNA expression of VEGF-C, VEGF-D, KDR, Flt-4, Ang-1, Tie-1, Tie-2, cyclooxygenease-2, fibroblast growth factor-2 (FGF-2), Prox-2, and LYVE-1 in 16 IBC compared with 20 non-IBC specimens. These factors support the rapid growth of tumor cells under hypoxic conditions and also promote a venue for dissemination. In addition to the classic angiogenic pathways associated with endothelial migration, proliferation, and organization to form new vessels, driven primarily by VEGF and its receptors, IBC tumors exhibit vasculogenesis, which is the de novo formation of vessel-like structures that allow the flow of oxygen and nutrients in the absence of endothelial cells.

The ability of tumor cells to form tubelike structures is defined as vasculogenic mimicry. Evaluation of molecules and pathways that are known to regulate vasculogenesis and lymphangiogenesis represents a very exciting area of drug development and the clinical studies with these new molecules providing new opportunities for understanding the spectrum of angiogenesis that is crucial to the distinct molecular signature of IBC. The anaplastic lymphoma kinase (*ALK*) gene belongs to the insulin receptor superfamily and encodes a receptor tyrosine kinase that is normally expressed only in select neuronal cell types [36]. Aberrant ALK activity results from point mutations, amplifications, chromosomal translocations, or other types of gene rearrangements involving the ALK gene.

Mutations in the ALK gene have been associated with several cancers and chromosomal translocations linking ALK to their fusion partners in anaplastic large cell lymphoma (ALCL), inflammatory myofibroblastic tumors, and neuroblastoma [37]. Recently, a novel gene fusion involving ALK and echinoderm microtubule-associated protein-like 4 (EML4) was discovered in non-small cell lung cancer (NSCLC), and treatment with ALK inhibitors in vitro has been reported to lead to cell cycle arrest and apoptosis. A recent preliminary report revealed evidence for amplification (three- to sevenfold) of the ALK receptor in 13/15 IBC patients and 66 % amplification by FISH in IBC cell lines [38]. A phase I, multicenter study of LDK378 in patients with genetic abnormalities in ALK is currently ongoing (NCT01283516).

Histone deacetylase (HDACs) cooperate with histone acetyltransferases (HATs) to regulate the acetylation status of nuclear histones, transcription factors, and other cellular proteins to regulate a variety of cellular processes including cell division and gene expression and cell death [39]. HDAC inhibitors are also currently being evaluated for their therapeutic potential in breast cancer.

Clinical Characteristics

Patients with IBC typically present with a sudden onset of increase in size of the breast, firmness, tenderness, and redness of the skin overlying the breast. In a seminal publication by Haagensen et al. [13], they described the clinical presentation and associated symptoms of IBC including a breast mass (57 %), redness of the skin (57 %), breast enlargement (48 %), pain in the breast or nipple (29 %), breast tenderness (16 %), generalized breast hardness (16 %), nipple retraction (13 %), edema of the skin (13 %), axillary mass (9 %), and warmness of the skin (8 %). In this analysis, the median duration of these symptoms before the diagnosis of IBC was 2.5 months, compared with 5 months for non-IBCs (Fig. 15.2a, b). Several breast diseases may mimic IBC and this might result in a delay of diagnosis. The two most common are infectious mastitis and breast abscess, both of which can be associated with lactation, skin erythema and redness, fever, and leukocytosis. Ductal ectasia can also mimic IBC, characterized by localized inflammation and enlarged breast that responds quickly to supportive measures.

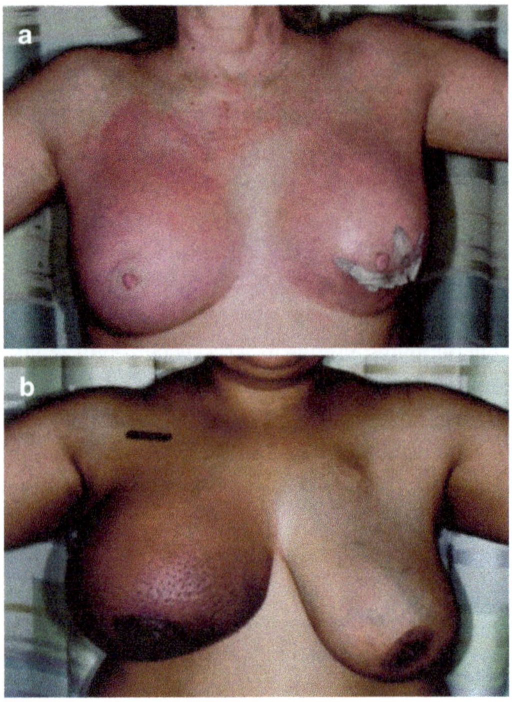

Fig. 15.2 There are variations in clinical presentation of IBC. Patient (**a**) presented with synchronous bilateral erythema. Patient (**b**) is an IBC patient with increased breast size, peau d'orange, and minimal erythema on background of darker skin

Imaging Studies

Evaluation of the patient with IBC involves a diagnostic mammogram, which is almost always abnormal [40]. The most common mammographic characteristics of IBC consist in skin thickening and diffusely increased density in 92 and 81 % of patients, respectively [41]. The authors defined a focal asymmetric density as asymmetry of tissue density, but completely lacking borders and the conspicuity of a true mass. In the same series, axillary lymphadenopathy was seen in 58 % of patients. A series including 22 patients with IBC from Memorial Sloan-Kettering Cancer Center found that 95 % of patients had a breast mass or malignant-appearing calcifications identified on mammography [42]. In a comparative study of PET/CT, magnetic resonance imaging (MRI), mammography, and sonography of 80 patients with IBC, mammography resulted in the least sensitive imaging method for diagnosing multifocal and multicentric disease [43].

Ultrasonography can be very helpful in the evaluation of regional nodal status. The most common findings with sonography are skin thickening, increased vascularity in the axillary lymphadenopathies, and architectural distortion. In a recent study from MD Anderson Cancer Center, regional axillary nodal disease was diagnosed in 93 % of IBC patients with this modality [43]. This percentage of axillary nodal involvement is highest compared with previous reported series where axillary adenopathy was found in 22–56 % (mean 28 %) [2, 11, 18].

The role of MRI in IBC is currently being investigated, with Chow et al. [44] reporting that the affected breast with IBC was most frequently found to have an infiltrative mass represented by a "reticular/dendritic pattern" of enhancement. Yang et al. [43] also reported that MRI revealed a primary breast lesion in 100 % of the cases, compared with 96 % with combined positron emission tomography and computed tomography (PET/CT), 95 % with ultrasonography, and 80 % with mammography. In this study, the most frequent MRI findings were multiple masses with irregular margins and heterogeneous internal enhancement associated with a washout or plateau kinetic curve in 97 % of patients.

PET/CT is an emerging imaging method that is widely gaining clinical acceptance because of its ability to co-register both anatomic and functional information on one image [45]. PET/CT has the advantage of identifying the local extent of metabolically active carcinomas, as well as lymph node and distant metastases, all in one procedure. A single PET study of seven patients with IBC demonstrated diffusely increased or intense foci of increased uptake in enlarged breast with increased skin uptake [46]. A recent retrospective review from MD Anderson Cancer Center in patients with IBC suggest that MRI would be the preferred initial imaging modality for IBC, and PET/CT would be an excellent companion for the detection of distant metastasis [43].

Multimodality Treatment

More than 70 % of patients with IBC have clinically localized disease without distant metastasis at their initial presentation [15]. A potentially curative, combined modality treatment approach should be offered to this group of patients, demonstrating a very good rate of locoregional control (84 %), with a lower distant metastasis-free survival rate of 47 % and an overall 5-year survival rate of 51 % [47]. In this study of 192 patients treated for IBC at the University of Texas MD Anderson Cancer Center with trimodality therapy including neoadjuvant chemotherapy, mastectomy, and postmastectomy radiation, most often delivered in a dose-dense twice-daily fraction to 66 Gy, revealed a 5-year actuarial locoregional control, distant metastasis-free survival, and overall survival of 84, 47, and 51 %, respectively.

The variable with the strongest relationship with locoregional control was the response to neoadjuvant chemotherapy. The 5-year locoregional control rate was 95 % for the 42 patients with a complete response, 86 % in the 111 patients experiencing a partial response, and 51 % in the 30 patients with less than a partial response ($p=0.0001$). Univariate factors significantly associated with locoregional control were response to neoadjuvant chemotherapy, surgical margin status, number of involved lymph nodes, and the use of taxanes. Increasing the total chest wall dose of postmastectomy radiation from 60 to 66 Gy significantly improved locoregional control for patients who experienced less than a partial response to chemotherapy; patients with positive, close, or unknown margins; and patients less than 45 years of age.

Surgical Management

The poor outcome of surgery as the only therapeutic modality was recognized in the 1920s, and observed again in 1950s, resulting in radiotherapy becoming the primary therapeutic treatment modality for the management of IBC until the 1970s [10, 48]. In the 1950s, Hagensen and collaborators [49] reported on 29 patients with IBC treated with radical mastectomy. The mean survival was only 19 months, and no patients were alive at 5 years. Subsequent studies demonstrated that local recurrence, in spite of the combination of chemotherapy, surgery, and radiation, occurred in 25–40 % of the cases.

Modified radical mastectomy has replaced the radical mastectomy as the operative treatment of choice for patients with IBC. However, breast conservation therapy has been used in highly selected patients who achieve a favorable response to neoadjuvant chemotherapy. If residual disease is present within the breast, high radiation dosage (>70 Gy) is required to achieve disease control which may cause substantial tissue damage. Chevalier and collaborators [50] reported a 61 % local failure rate in patients who achieved a complete response to PST and were treated with conservative treatment. Arthur et al. [51] reported slightly higher local control rates among 15 patients who achieved a clinical complete response who were not treated with surgery (87 % at 3 years). However, the follow-up was only 24 months.

Systemic Treatment

Primary Systemic Chemotherapy

The last four decades has seen an evolution in the prognostic outcome of IBC, transforming it from a disease that was once considered uniformly fatal with fewer than 5 % of women surviving past 5 years to rates approaching 40 % [52]. The key component to this transformation was the recognition of the vital importance of a combined modality approach to management, involving from the onset all disciplines of breast cancer management including medical, surgical, and radiation oncology. The recognition of the importance of starting systemic treatment upfront stemmed from the important clinical observation that IBC was, for the most part, not optimally resectable at initial presentation [10]. Furthermore, the disease was often poorly controlled with locoregional modalities alone [53]. The introduction of primary systemic chemotherapy incorporated several advantages: downstaging of the tumor, operability after chemotherapy, in vivo assessment of response to chemotherapy, earlier treatment of subclinical distant micrometastases, and the possibility of obtaining a pathologic complete response. The latter has been shown to be associated with a superior prognostic outcome [54].

Table 15.1 Selected studies of primary systemic chemotherapy for inflammatory breast cancer patients

Author/year of publication	No. of patients	Regimen of chemotherapy	Clinical response rate	5-year overall survival
Ueno et al. 1997 [52]	178	Anthracycline based	71 %	40 %
Cristofanilli et al. 2001 [56]	240	FAC vs. FAC + Pac	74 % vs. 82 %	NA
Harris et al. 2003 [57]	54	CMF or CAF	52 %	56 %
Low et al. 2004 [58]	46	CAF-M	57 %	26.7 % (10 years)
Baldini et al. 2004 [55]	68	CEF or CAF	73.6 %	44 %
Veyret et al. 2006 [59]	120	FEC-HD	91.1 %	41.2 % (10 years)

Abbreviations: *OS* overall survival, *CMF* cyclophosphamide, methotrexate, 5-fluoruracil, *CAF* cyclophosphamide, doxorubicin, f-fluorouracil, *Pac* paclitaxel, *CEF* cyclophosphamide, epirubicin, 5-fluorouracil, *CAF-M* cyclophosphamide, adriamycin, 5-fluorouracil, methotrexate, *HD* high dose, *N/A* not available

Due to the fact that IBC is a rare disease coupled with the fact that it is actively excluded from large clinical trials due to its known associated poor prognostic outcome, most of the available data on systemic management are derived from retrospective studies and small clinical trials. One of the largest series comes from the University of Texas MD Anderson Cancer Center [52] reported on the 20-year experience of a cohort of 178 women with IBC treated on four prospective clinical trials receiving a doxorubicin-based preoperative chemotherapy-based regimen followed by radiation therapy with or without mastectomy. The authors reported 5- and 10-year survival rates of 40 and 33 %, respectively, with 28 % of patients reported to be alive beyond 15 years.

Furthermore, the authors reported 15-year survival rates of 44, 31, and 7 % among patients achieving a clinical complete response, partial response, and less than partial response, respectively, demonstrating the prognostic importance of response to primary systemic therapy. In a more recent review, Baldini et al. [55] reported on a smaller cohort of 68 women with IBC treated with an anthracycline-based regimen (CAF or FEC) followed by surgery, adjuvant chemotherapy, and radiotherapy. Similar to the series from the MD Anderson Cancer Center, the authors reported 5- and 10-year survival rates of 44 and 32 %, respectively. Based on these results and others, an anthracycline-based preoperative chemotherapeutic-based regimen should be considered the current standard of care, as the survival results reported are indeed far superior to those reported historically.

The efficacy of taxanes incorporated into the preoperative anthracycline regimen of patients with IBC has also been explored. In a retrospective study, Cristofanilli and colleagues [56] reported on the results of a comparison of women with IBC who had either been treated with preoperative FAC to those who were treated with preoperative FAC followed by paclitaxel, receiving it either every 3 weeks or weekly. The authors reported a pathological complete response rate of 25 % among the cohort who had received paclitaxel, compared to 10 % among those who did not, with the difference being statistically significant ($p=0.012$). Additionally, the authors reported higher median overall and progression-free survival rates among the group of women who received FAC followed by paclitaxel. Table 15.1 summarizes selected studies of primary systemic chemotherapy for IBC.

Targeted Therapy

The introduction of the humanized monoclonal antibody, trastuzumab, has revolutionized the management of women with breast tumors that overexpress HER2 positively, impacting survival in both early- and advanced-stage breast cancers [56, 60, 61]. Furthermore, the incorporation of trastuzumab into preoperative regimens has been shown to increase pathological complete response rates [62]. With a high incidence of HER2 overexpression in IBC [63], the efficacy of trastuzumab among these women has been explored. Several small prospective studies have explored the incorporation of trastuzumab into the preoperative systemic chemotherapy regimen among women with IBC [64–66]. These studies have reported pathological complete response rates ranging from 17 to 40 %. More recently, Gianni et al. [67] reported on a phase III, randomized clinical trial that included 327 women with HER2-positive locally advanced breast cancer, 27 % of whom had IBC. The objective of the study was to evaluate the efficacy of the addition of trastuzumab to an anthracycline- and taxane-based preoperative regimen. The authors reported that the addition of trastuzumab increased the 3-year event-free survival from 53.3 to 70.1 % ($p=0.0007$).

Lapatinib, a reversible inhibitor of ErbB1 and HER2 [68], has also been investigated in the treatment of women with HER2-positive IBC. Kaufman et al. [69] recently reported on a cohort of 126 women with relapsed or refractory HER2-positive IBC who were treated with single-agent lapatinib (1,500 mg once daily) in a nonrandomized, prospective phase II study. The authors reported 39 % of patients achieving a partial response with a median progression-free survival of 14.6 weeks overall. Cristofanilli et al. [70] recently reported on a cohort of 21 women with newly diagnosed IBC who were treated prospectively with single-agent lapatinib for 14 days followed by a combination of lapatinib and paclitaxel for 12 weeks. Preliminary results of the study showed a good tolerance to the regimen and a clinical response rate of approximately 80 %. The regimen is currently being investigated in larger cohort prospectively (Table 15.2).

Table 15.2 Selected studies of anti-HER2-based primary systemic chemotherapy for inflammatory breast cancer

Author/year of publication	No. of patients	Chemotherapy regimen	pCR
Van Pelt et al. 2003 [71]	22 LABC (9 IBC)	Doc + Tz	40 %
Burstein et al. 2003 [66]	40 (6 IBC)	Pac + Tz	18 %
Hurley et al. 2006 [64]	48 (4 IBC)	Doc + cDDP + Tz	17 %
Cristofanilli et al. 2006 [70]	21 IBC	Pac + Lap	95 % had cRR
Dawood et al. 2007 [72]	40 (4 IBC)	FEC + Pac + Tz	55 %
Limentani et al. 2007 [65]	31 LABC (9 IBC)	Doc + VNR + Tz	39 %
Gianni et al. 2008 [67]	327 LABC (88 IBC)	A/Doc + Pac + CMF + Tz	39 %
Kaufman et al. 2009 [69]	126 IBC relapsed to Tz	Lap	39 % had PR

Abbreviations: *LABC* locally advanced breast cancer, *IBC* inflammatory breast cancer, *pCR* pathologic complete response, *Doc* docetaxel, *Tz* trastuzumab, *Pac* paclitaxel, *cDDP* cisplatin, *FEC* 5-fluorouracil, epirubicin, cyclophosphamide, *VNR* vinorelbine, *A* adriamycin, *CMF* cyclophosphamide, methotrexate, 5-fluorouracil, *Lap* lapatinib, *PR* partial response, *cRR* clinical response rate

A combination of lapatinib with pazopanib, an inhibitor of VEGFR1, VEGFR2, and VEGFR3 and PDGF α/β molecule, was also investigated in a phase II study in patients with trastuzumab-refractory IBC patients (GW-786034; GlaxoSmithKline, London, UK) [73]. A multicenter, phase II study evaluated lapatinib, pazopanib, and its combination in patients with HER2-positive IBC. In cohort 1, 76 patients were randomized 1:1 to receive either lapatinib plus placebo or lapatinib plus pazopanib. This cohort was closed due to an adverse side effect of high-grade diarrhea. In cohort 2, additional 88 patients were randomized in a 5:5:2 ratio to receive daily monotherapy with lapatinib 1,500 mg, lapatinib 1,000 mg plus pazopanib 400 mg, or monotherapy pazopanib 800 mg, respectively. The primary endpoint was ORR, and the secondary endpoint was the duration of response and progression-free survival and safety. The lapatinib-pazopanib combination was associated with numerically higher ORR, but no increase in PFS compared with lapatinib alone. The combination also had increased toxicity resulting in more dose reductions, modifications, and treatment delays.

A preliminary report by Alvarez and collaborators [74] from a prospective phase II study of lapatinib in combination with paclitaxel followed by FEC (5-fluorouracyl, epirubicin, and cyclophosphamide) was discontinued prematurely

Table 15.3 Selected studies of targeted therapy as primary systemic chemotherapy for inflammatory breast cancer

Author/year of publication	No. of patients	Chemotherapy regimen	pCR	Comments
Wedam et al. 2006 [75]	21 LABC (19 IBC)	Bev + A/Doc + Bev	NA	↑ pVEGF 66 %, ↑median apoptosis 128.9 %, no changes in MVD or VEGF A expression
Overmoyer et al. 2007 [76]	18 IBC	SU5416 + Dox	NA	4/18 (22 %) patients developed reversible CHF signs
Sparano et al. 2009 [77]	44 LABC (12 IBC)	DD AC + Tipifarnib	25 %	2/12 IBC patients achieved pCR. Neutropenia G3 50 %

Abbreviations: *LABC* locally advanced breast cancer, *IBC* inflammatory breast cancer, *pCR* pathologic complete response, *Bev* bevacizumab, *Doc* docetaxel, *A* adriamycin, *Pac* paclitaxel, *CBDA* carboplatin, *CHF* congestive heart failure, *Dox* doxorubicin

because of a lack of efficacy and associated high toxicity. Fifteen patients were included in this study in chemo-naïve HER2-positive IBC patients, and the primary endpoint was a complete pathologic response (pCR). Ten out of 15 patients had a modified radical mastectomy and 1 out of 10 (10 %) achieved a pCR. In terms of toxicity, more than half of the patients developed grade 3 diarrhea. The study was closed per protocol boundaries.

Novel Therapies for the Treatment of IBC

Several novel agents, including antiangiogenic agents and Ras pathway inhibitors, are currently being investigated for the treatment of IBC (Table 15.3). Angiogenesis plays an essential role in breast cancer development, invasion, and metastasis [78, 79]. VEGF plays a multifactorial role where it has autocrine pro-survival effects on tumor cells protecting them from stresses such as hypoxia, chemotherapy, and radiotherapy. Bevacizumab, a recombinant humanized monoclonal antibody of VEGF, was evaluated in a pilot study in 21 patients with LABC, 19 of them with IBC [75]. One cycle of bevacizumab was administered, followed by 6 cycles of bevacizumab plus doxorubicin and docetaxel, every 3 weeks. Fourteen out of 21 patients had a clinical partial response, but there were no complete responses observed. The overall response rate was 67 %. The median decrease of pVEGF-R2 was observed in 66.7 % of the samples analyzed, and the median apoptosis was increased 128.9 % in patients. The Ras superfamily of GTPases acts as crucial regulatory switches coordinating a variety of biologic functions. Based on promising preclinical and phase I studies of farnesyl transferase inhibitors, several are being examined in combination with chemotherapy for patients with IBC [80, 81]. Sparano et al. [77] published results from a phase II trial in a group of 44 patients with LABC, including 12 patients with IBC. Eleven out 44 patients obtained a pCR (25 %) after primary systemic therapy with dose-dense AC and tipifarnib, a farnesyl transferase inhibitor. Two out of 12 patients with IBC achieved pCR, with the most common toxicity being grade 3 neutropenia (50 % of patients).

High-Dose Chemotherapy

In an attempt to further improve upon the survival outcomes, several investigators have explored the use of high-dose chemotherapy supported by autologous stem support with promising results. In the PEGASE 02 trial, 90 patients with IBC received high-dose chemotherapy, followed by preoperative anthracycline-based chemotherapy. The authors reported an encouraging 3-year survival rate of 70 % [19]. Cheng and colleagues [82] reported on a cohort of 177 women with breast cancer, 10 % of whom had IBC and received high-dose chemotherapy. The authors reported a 5-year overall survival rate of 36 %.

The results of these studies are certainly encouraging; however, they remain investigational and should only be offered to patients within the context of a clinical trial.

Conclusions

A multidisciplinary approach targeting both local and systemic disease and the incorporation of anthracyclines and taxanes has resulted in survival outcomes far superior to those reported historically for this aggressive disease. However, despite the significant progress made, survival outcomes still remain poor for patients with IBC, with most patients eventually dying from this aggressive disease. IBC is an important model for clinical investigation of targeted therapies, and currently the receptor tyrosine kinase and angiogenesis pathways have been validated in clinical trials as important targets. Further extensive work is still required to determine if the novel molecular targeted therapies in combination with standard chemotherapy can improve the outcomes of patients with IBC.

References

1. Chang S, et al. Inflammatory breast carcinoma incidence and survival: the surveillance, epidemiology, and end results program of the National Cancer Institute, 1975–1992. Cancer. 1998;82(12):2366–72.
2. Hance KW, et al. Trends in inflammatory breast carcinoma incidence and survival: the surveillance, epidemiology, and end results program at the National Cancer Institute. J Natl Cancer Inst. 2005;97(13):966–75.
3. Liao Z, et al. Locoregional irradiation for inflammatory breast cancer: effectiveness of dose escalation in decreasing recurrence. Int J Radiat Oncol Biol Phys. 2000;47(5):1191–200.
4. Liauw SL, et al. Inflammatory breast carcinoma: outcomes with trimodality therapy for nonmetastatic disease. Cancer. 2004;100(5):920–8.
5. Cristofanilli M, et al. Inflammatory breast cancer (IBC) and patterns of recurrence: understanding the biology of a unique disease. Cancer. 2007;110(7):1436–44.
6. Fields JN, et al. Inflammatory carcinoma of the breast: treatment results on 107 patients. Int J Radiat Oncol Biol Phys. 1989;17(2):249–55.
7. Gonzalez-Angulo AM, et al. Trends for inflammatory breast cancer: is survival improving? Oncologist. 2007;12(8):904–12.
8. Bell C. A system of operative surgery, vol. 2. Hartford: Hale and Homse; 1814. p. 136.
9. Lee B. and Tannenbaum E. Inflammatory carcinoma of the breast. Surg Gynecol Obstet. 1924;39:580–95.
10. Lee B, et al. Manganese acts centrally to activate reproductive hormone secretion and pubertal development in male rats. Reprod Toxicol. 2006;22(4):580–5.
11. Jaiyesimi IA, Buzdar AU, Hortobagyi G. Inflammatory breast cancer: a review. J Clin Oncol. 1992;10(6):1014–24.
12. Haagensen CD. Inflammatory carcinoma. In: Disease of the Breast. Philadelphia, PA. W.B. Saunders, 1956.
13. Bryant T. Disease of the breast. London: Cassell & Co Ltd.; 1887.
14. Dawood S, Ueno NT, Cristofanilli M. The medical treatment of inflammatory breast cancer. Semin Oncol. 2008;35(1):64–71.
15. Wingo PA, et al. Population-based statistics for women diagnosed with inflammatory breast cancer (United States). Cancer Causes Control. 2004;15(3):321–8.
16. Zell JA, et al. Prognostic impact of human epidermal growth factor-like receptor 2 and hormone receptor status in inflammatory breast cancer (IBC): analysis of 2,014 IBC patient cases from the California Cancer Registry. Breast Cancer Res. 2009;11(1):R9.
17. Mourali N, et al. Epidemiologic features of rapidly progressing breast cancer in Tunisia. Cancer. 1980; 46(12):2741–6.
18. Levine PH, et al. Inflammatory breast cancer: the experience of the surveillance, epidemiology, and end results (SEER) program. J Natl Cancer Inst. 1985; 74(2):291–7.
19. Willett W, et al. Cigarette smoking, relative weight, and menopause. Am J Epidemiol. 1983;117(6):651–8.
20. Swanson CA, et al. Body size and breast cancer risk assessed in women participating in the Breast Cancer Detection Demonstration Project. Am J Epidemiol. 1989;130(6):1133–41.
21. Ballard-Barbash R, et al. Association of change in body mass with breast cancer. Cancer Res. 1990;50(7):2152–5.
22. Bittner JJ. Some possible effects of nursing on the mammary gland tumor incidence in mice. Science. 1936;84(2172):162.
23. Pogo BG, Holland JF, Levine PH. Human mammary tumor virus in inflammatory breast cancer. Cancer. 2010;116(11 Suppl):2741–4.
24. Muller A, et al. Involvement of chemokine receptors in breast cancer metastasis. Nature. 2001;410(6824):50–6.
25. Bieche I, et al. Molecular profiling of inflammatory breast cancer: identification of a poor-prognosis gene expression signature. Clin Cancer Res. 2004;10(20):6789–95.
26. Kleer CG, van Golen KL, Merajver SD. Molecular biology of breast cancer metastasis. Inflammatory breast cancer: clinical syndrome and molecular determinants. Breast Cancer Res. 2000;2(6):423–9.
27. van Golen KL, et al. A novel putative low-affinity insulin-like growth factor-binding protein, LIBC (lost in inflammatory breast cancer), and RhoC GTPase

correlate with the inflammatory breast cancer phenotype. Clin Cancer Res. 1999;5(9):2511–9.
28. Davies SR, et al. Differential expression and prognostic implications of the CCN family members WISP-1, WISP-2, and WISP-3 in human breast cancer. Ann Surg Oncol. 2007;14(6):1909–18.
29. Yamauchi H, et al. Molecular targets for treatment of inflammatory breast cancer. Nat Rev Clin Oncol. 2009;6(7):387–94.
30. Kleer CG, et al. WISP3 is a novel tumor suppressor gene of inflammatory breast cancer. Oncogene. 2002; 21(20):3172–80.
31. van Golen KL, et al. RhoC GTPase, a novel transforming oncogene for human mammary epithelial cells that partially recapitulates the inflammatory breast cancer phenotype. Cancer Res. 2000;60(20):5832–8.
32. van Golen KL, et al. RhoC GTPase overexpression modulates induction of angiogenic factors in breast cells. Neoplasia. 2000;2(5):418–25.
33. Van Aken E, et al. Defective E-cadherin/catenin complexes in human cancer. Virchows Arch. 2001;439(6): 725–51.
34. Colpaert CG, et al. Inflammatory breast cancer shows angiogenesis with high endothelial proliferation rate and strong E-cadherin expression. Br J Cancer. 2003; 88(5):718–25.
35. Tomlinson JS, Alpaugh ML, Barsky SH. An intact overexpressed E-cadherin/alpha, beta-catenin axis characterizes the lymphovascular emboli of inflammatory breast carcinoma. Cancer Res. 2001;61(13):5231–41.
36. Morris SW, et al. ALK, the chromosome 2 gene locus altered by the t(2;5) in non-Hodgkin's lymphoma, encodes a novel neural receptor tyrosine kinase that is highly related to leukocyte tyrosine kinase (LTK). Oncogene. 1997;14(18):2175–88.
37. Pulford K, Morris SW, Turturro F. Anaplastic lymphoma kinase proteins in growth control and cancer. J Cell Physiol. 2004;199(3):330–58.
38. Robertson FM, PE, Chu K, et al. Amplification of Anaplastic Lymphoma Kinase (ALK) as a common genetic alteration in inflammatory breast cancer. In: 2011 CTRC-AACR San Antonio Breast Cancer Symposium; 2011.
39. Lane AA, Chabner BA. Histone deacetylase inhibitors in cancer therapy. J Clin Oncol. 2009;27(32):5459–68.
40. Tardivon AA, et al. Mammographic patterns of inflammatory breast carcinoma: a retrospective study of 92 cases. Eur J Radiol. 1997;24(2):124–30.
41. Kushwaha AC, et al. Primary inflammatory carcinoma of the breast: retrospective review of mammographic findings. AJR Am J Roentgenol. 2000;174(2):535–8.
42. Dershaw DD, et al. Inflammatory breast carcinoma: mammographic findings. Radiology. 1994;190(3):831–4.
43. Yang WT, et al. Inflammatory breast cancer: PET/CT, MRI, mammography, and sonography findings. Breast Cancer Res Treat. 2008;109(3):417–26.
44. Chow CK. Imaging in inflammatory breast carcinoma. Breast Dis. 2005;22:45–54.
45. Fueger BJ, et al. Performance of 2-deoxy-2-[F-18] fluoro-D-glucose positron emission tomography and integrated PET/CT in restaged breast cancer patients. Mol Imaging Biol. 2005;7(5):369–76.
46. Baslaim MM, et al. 18-Fluorodeoxyglucose-positron emission tomography in inflammatory breast cancer. World J Surg. 2003;27(10):1099–104.
47. Bristol IJ, et al. Locoregional treatment outcomes after multimodality management of inflammatory breast cancer. Int J Radiat Oncol Biol Phys. 2008; 72(2):474–84.
48. Chris SM. Inflammatory carcinoma of the breast; a report of 20 cases and a review of the literature. Br J Surg. 1950;38(150):163–74.
49. Haagensen CD, Stout AP. Carcinoma of the breast. III. Results of treatment, 1935–1942. Ann Surg. 1951;134(2):151–72.
50. Chevalier BS, et al. Design, activity, and structure of a highly specific artificial endonuclease. Mol Cell. 2002;10(4):895–905.
51. Arthur DW, et al. Accelerated superfractionated radiotherapy for inflammatory breast carcinoma: complete response predicts outcome and allows for breast conservation. Int J Radiat Oncol Biol Phys. 1999;44(2):289–96.
52. Ueno NT, et al. Combined-modality treatment of inflammatory breast carcinoma: twenty years of experience at M. D. Anderson Cancer Center. Cancer Chemother Pharmacol. 1997;40(4):321–9.
53. Atkins HL, Horrigan WD. Treatment of locally advanced carcinoma of the breast with roentgen therapy and simple mastectomy. Am J Roentgenol Radium Ther Nucl Med. 1961;85:860–4.
54. Kuerer HM, et al. Clinical course of breast cancer patients with complete pathologic primary tumor and axillary lymph node response to doxorubicin-based neoadjuvant chemotherapy. J Clin Oncol. 1999;17(2): 460–9.
55. Baldini E, et al. Long-term results of combined-modality therapy for inflammatory breast carcinoma. Clin Breast Cancer. 2004;5(5):358–63.
56. Cristofanilli M, et al. Paclitaxel improves the prognosis in estrogen receptor negative inflammatory breast cancer: the M. D. Anderson Cancer Center experience. Clin Breast Cancer. 2004;4(6): 415–9.
57. Harris EE, et al. Ten-year outcome after combined modality therapy for inflammatory breast cancer. Int J Radiat Oncol Biol Phys. 2003;55(5):1200–8.
58. Low JA, et al. Long-term follow-up for locally advanced and inflammatory breast cancer patients treated with multimodality therapy. J Clin Oncol. 2004;22(20):4067–74.
59. Veyret C, et al. Inflammatory breast cancer outcome with epirubicin-based induction and maintenance chemotherapy: ten-year results from the French Adjuvant Study Group GETIS 02 Trial. Cancer. 2006;107(11):2535–44.

60. Piccart-Gebhart MJ, et al. Trastuzumab after adjuvant chemotherapy in HER2-positive breast cancer. N Engl J Med. 2005;353(16):1659–72.
61. Slamon DJ, et al. Use of chemotherapy plus a monoclonal antibody against HER2 for metastatic breast cancer that overexpresses HER2. N Engl J Med. 2001;344(11):783–92.
62. Buzdar AU, et al. Significantly higher pathologic complete remission rate after neoadjuvant therapy with trastuzumab, paclitaxel, and epirubicin chemotherapy: results of a randomized trial in human epidermal growth factor receptor 2-positive operable breast cancer. J Clin Oncol. 2005;23(16):3676–85.
63. Parton M, et al. High incidence of HER-2 positivity in inflammatory breast cancer. Breast. 2004;13(2):97–103.
64. Hurley J, et al. Docetaxel, cisplatin, and trastuzumab as primary systemic therapy for human epidermal growth factor receptor 2-positive locally advanced breast cancer. J Clin Oncol. 2006;24(12):1831–8.
65. Limentani SA, et al. Phase II study of neoadjuvant docetaxel, vinorelbine, and trastuzumab followed by surgery and adjuvant doxorubicin plus cyclophosphamide in women with human epidermal growth factor receptor 2-overexpressing locally advanced breast cancer. J Clin Oncol. 2007;25(10):1232–8.
66. Burstein HJ, et al. Preoperative therapy with trastuzumab and paclitaxel followed by sequential adjuvant doxorubicin/cyclophosphamide for HER2 overexpressing stage II or III breast cancer: a pilot study. J Clin Oncol. 2003;21(1):46–53.
67. Gianni L, et al. Neoadjuvant trastuzumab in patients with HER2-positive locally advanced breast cancer: primary efficacy analysis of the NOAH trial. In: San Antonio Breast Cancer Symposium. San Antonio: Breast Cancer Res Treat; 2008.
68. Xia W, et al. Anti-tumor activity of GW572016: a dual tyrosine kinase inhibitor blocks EGF activation of EGFR/erbB2 and downstream Erk1/2 and AKT pathways. Oncogene. 2002;21(41):6255–63.
69. Kaufman B, et al. Lapatinib monotherapy in patients with HER2-overexpressing relapsed or refractory inflammatory breast cancer: final results and survival of the expanded HER2+ cohort in EGF103009, a phase II study. Lancet Oncol. 2009;10(6):581–8.
70. Cristofanilli M, et al. A phase II combination study of lapatinib and paclitaxel as a neoadjuvant therapy in patients with newly diagnosed inflammatory breast cancer (IBC). In: San Antonio Breast Cancer Symposium. San Antonio: Breast Cancer Res Treat; 2006.
71. Van Pelt AE, et al. Neoadjuvant trastuzumab and docetaxel in breast cancer: preliminary results. Clin Breast Cancer. 2003;4(5):348–53.
72. Dawood S, et al. Efficacy and safety of neoadjuvant trastuzumab combined with paclitaxel and epirubicin. Cancer. 2007;110(6):1195–200.
73. Cristofanilli M, et al. A randomized phase II study of lapatinib + pazopanib versus lapatinib in patients with HER2+ inflammatory breast cancer. Breast Cancer Res Treat. 2013;137(2):471–82.
74. Alvarez RH, et al. Limited efficacy and significant toxicities of lapatinib (Lap) plus chemotherapy as neoadjuvant therapy (NAC) for HER2-positive inflammatory breast cancer (IBC) patients (Pts). ASCO Meet Abstr. 2012; 30 15 suppl:594.
75. Wedam SB, et al. Antiangiogenic and antitumor effects of bevacizumab in patients with inflammatory and locally advanced breast cancer. J Clin Oncol. 2006;24(5):769–77.
76. Overmoyer B, et al. Inflammatory breast cancer as a model disease to study tumor angiogenesis: results of a phase IB trial of combination SU5416 and doxorubicin. Clin Cancer Res. 2007;13(19):5862–8.
77. Sparano JA, et al. Phase II trial of tipifarnib plus neoadjuvant doxorubicin-cyclophosphamide in patients with clinical stage IIB-IIIC breast cancer. Clin Cancer Res. 2009;15(8):2942–8.
78. Gasparini G. Prognostic value of vascular endothelial growth factor in breast cancer. Oncologist. 2000;5 Suppl 1:37–44.
79. Folkman J. What is the evidence that tumors are angiogenesis dependent? J Natl Cancer Inst. 1990; 82(1):4–6.
80. Johnston SR, et al. Phase II study of the efficacy and tolerability of two dosing regimens of the farnesyl transferase inhibitor, R115777, in advanced breast cancer. J Clin Oncol. 2003;21(13):2492–9.
81. NCI. Phase Ib/II neoadjuvant study of tipifarnib, docetaxel, and capecitabine in patients with locally advanced or metastatic solid tumors or stage IIIA or IIIB breast cancer 8/11/2006 [cited 2003 9/24/2006; Clinical Trials].
82. Cheng YC, et al. The use of high-dose cyclophosphamide, carmustine, and thiotepa plus autologous hematopoietic stem cell transplantation as consolidation therapy for high-risk primary breast cancer after primary surgery or neoadjuvant chemotherapy. Biol Blood Marrow Transplant. 2004;10(11): 794–804.

16 Operative Management of Metastatic Breast Cancer

Hannah W. Hazard

Introduction

Worldwide, breast cancer is the second most common malignancy in women. The World Health Organization estimates 1.67 million new cases of breast cancer and 521,818 deaths from the disease in 2012 [1]. The worldwide incidence of breast cancer is increasing as life expectancy lengthens and as non-western societies adopt the lifestyle practices of western society [2]. In the United States, the American Cancer Society estimates 234,580 new breast cancers will be diagnosed and 40,030 deaths will occur in 2013. For women, a new diagnosis of breast cancer in 2013 will represent 29 % of all malignancies diagnosed [3]. Despite the increase in incidence, breast cancer-related mortality has shown a steady decline over the last decade [4]. The decline in mortality can primarily be attributed to two factors: the first is a better understanding of and adherence to screening guidelines, and the second is the advances made in the systemic treatment of breast cancer patients.

The most important predictor of survival is the stage of disease at the time of diagnosis. The American Joint Commission on Cancer (AJCC) staging of breast cancer includes the size of the tumor at diagnosis (in centimeters), how many lymph nodes are involved, and if there is metastatic spread. Staging for breast cancer ranges from Stage 0 when the diagnosis is ductal carcinoma in situ to Stage 4 when there is disease distant from the breast or regional lymph nodes. Survival estimates from the National Cancer Institute (NCI) illustrate the need to diagnose the disease in the earlier stages, if possible, as the 5-year overall survival for localized breast cancer is 98.4 %. Patients diagnosed with early-stage disease comprise approximately 60 % of the entire patient population. As the tumor spreads to the locoregional lymph nodes, the relative 5-year survival drops to 83.9 %. While the metastatic population represents only 5 % of newly diagnosed cancers, the 5-year overall survival drops dramatically to only 23.8 % [5]. By diagnosing women at an earlier stage, the disease can be treated with a curative intent. Once the patient is diagnosed with metastatic disease, treatment is designed to contain the disease and can no longer be considered as having a curative intent.

Metastatic spread of breast cancer is generally classified by the end organ affected. Solid organ metastases to the liver and lung have a better outcome when compared to those with brain metastasis, while those with bony metastasis seem to have the longest survival. The standard treatment of metastatic (Stage 4) breast cancer is palliative, with systemic treatment as the mainstay of therapy. In this situation, the primary breast cancer is most often left intact as the patient undergoes

H.W. Hazard, MD, FACS
Department of Surgery, Health Sciences Center – South, West Virginia University School of Medicine, 1 Medical Center Drive, 9238, Morgantown, WV 26506, USA
e-mail: hhazard@hsc.wvu.edu

A.I. Riker (ed.), *Breast Disease: Comprehensive Management*,
DOI 10.1007/978-1-4939-1145-5_16,

their systemic therapy. This principle is derived from the traditional belief that metastatic disease burden is the greatest predictor of survival, while the complete operative removal of the primary breast cancer seemingly has no impact upon overall survival.

The development of treatment algorithms for patients with metastatic disease has always focused upon the systemic treatment of breast cancer, reserving an operative approach with removal of the primary lesion only for palliation of uncontrolled or rapidly growing disease. Recently, several investigators have questioned the dogma of this approach, instead asking whether resection of the primary lesion (breast cancer and other tumor histologies) in the presence of known metastatic disease may be beneficial to the patient, possibly improving their overall survival. For example, the resection of a primary renal cell carcinoma improves the overall survival when compared to leaving the primary cancer intact and treating solely with chemotherapy [6]. Additionally, it is well known that maximal tumor debulking of ovarian cancer improves, though marginally, survival for women with metastatic ovarian cancer. The stem cell theory is well established in malignancies such as leukemia and has been postulated to have implications in metastatic breast cancer. In the normal setting, this is a line of cells that are self-renewing and are best exemplified by the hematopoietic system. Hematopoietic stem cells must continue to renew and differentiate to maintain hemostasis. There is now a rapidly growing body of work indicating the presence of cancer stem cells (csc) with the first clear delineation of their existence in leukemia cells [7]. Further work in solid tumor cells has been able to reproduce similar results. Of greatest interest is the potential for metastatic cancer stem cells. These cells seem to have unique properties allowing for honing on metastatic sites as well as resistance to chemotherapy and radiation therapy [8]. More specific to the metastatic spread of breast cancer, Al-Hajj et al. demonstrated the presence of a unique cell line in heterogeneous breast cancer in nonobese diabetic/severe combined immunodeficiency mice with a higher propensity to be tumorigenic. CD44 and CD24 are adhesion molecules, and in the work by Al-Hajj, CD44+/CD24− cell lines were tumorigenic; a similar pattern found in normal stem cells [9]. The source of such cancer stem cells is still not well understood. The following questions remain: Are the csc derived from the primary tumor or from the metastatic deposit? Is it the primary lesion or the metastasis seeding and reseeding metastatic lesions? Can removing the primary tumor not only reduce the disease burden but also the source of the cancer stem cells and thereby improve overall survival?

On these principles, Khan et al. have challenged the traditional secondary role of surgery in the newly diagnosed metastatic breast cancer patient. Analysis of the National Cancer Data Base (NCDB) from 1990 to 1993 indicated approximately 57 % of metastatic breast cancer patients received either a partial mastectomy or a total mastectomy. Despite their diagnosis of metastatic disease, those who did have negative surgical margins had an improvement in their 3-year survival [10]. In this chapter, we will analyze the role of resecting the primary breast cancer and the distant metastatic sites, by reviewing the recent literature for trends in the overall outcome of Stage 4 patients.

Resection of the Primary Breast Tumor

The inclusion of surgical intervention in the treatment plan of patients with metastatic breast cancer remains somewhat controversial, with several investigators questioning the utility of an operative approach in a traditionally palliative treatment plan. The 2002 paper by Khan et al. examined the NCDB database from 1990 to 1993, finding a total of 16,023 Stage 4 breast cancer patients with 9,162 undergoing either a partial or a total mastectomy as part of their treatment. This represented 57.2 % of the patient population. The median age was 62.5 years, and of the 9,162 undergoing operative intervention, 3,513 (38 %) had a partial mastectomy and 5,649 had a total mastectomy. The 3-year observed survival rate for the entire group of Stage 4 patients was 24.9 % with a mean survival duration of 19 months. Once restricted to patients having either a partial mastectomy or a total mastectomy, the mean survival duration increased to 26.9 months and 31.9 months, respectively. Similar increases in the 3-year observed survival were also noted with 17.3 % (no surgical intervention), 27.7 % (partial mastectomy), and 31.8 % (total mastectomy). Using the nonsurgical group as a reference, the hazard ratio (HR) of death was 0.88 in the partial mastectomy cohort and 0.74 in those undergoing a total mastectomy. One of the criticisms of this study, and others to follow, is the retrospective nature of the data. The authors admit there is no way to control for the biases that lead to the resection of the primary tumor [6].

In 2006, Rapiti et al. published a similar study using the Geneva Cancer Registry, examining a total of 300 metastatic breast cancer patients from 1977 to 1996. In this cohort, 127 of the 300 (42 %) women had surgical intervention, 40 patients had a partial mastectomy, and 87 patients had a total mastectomy. Negative margins were accomplished in 61 (48 %) patients, and margin status was unknown in 26 % of the population. They found that excision of the intact primary breast cancer in the face of known metastatic disease imparted an impressive 40 % risk reduction in death due to breast cancer. The 5-year breast cancer-specific survival was 27 % when negative margins were achieved and 16 % and 12 % when the margins were either positive or unknown, respectively. Those women who underwent a surgical resection, but had positive margins on the final pathology, did not have a significant difference in survival when compared to those without surgical intervention. The adjusted HR for the four groups of patients were 1.0 for the nonintervention group, 0.6 for the group with negative margins, 1.3 for positive margins, and 1.1 for the margin-unknown cohort of patients. In comparing the characteristics of the two patient cohorts, the surgical intervention group tended to be younger, treated in the private (vs. public) sector of their healthcare system, and had lower T- and N-stages (as defined by the AJCC standard staging practices for breast cancer) at initial diagnosis.

Additionally, in the Rapiti et al. analysis, 61 % of the patients who had resection had only one site of metastasis, while 41 % of the patients who did not have an operation had one metastatic site of disease. A smaller proportion of the operative group had visceral metastasis (43 %) as compared to the inoperative group (58 %). Thus, the authors conclude that the complete resection of the primary tumor improves the long-term survival in women with metastatic breast cancer [11]. When interpreting these results, it is important to recognize the role of selection bias in the sample. The younger age and less distant disease burden at the time of surgical intervention may have contributed to the differences in the improved overall survival in those undergoing operative intervention compared to those who did not.

Finally, in 2007, Gnerlich et al. looked at the data from the Surveillance, Epidemiology, and End Results (SEER) program. The SEER program began collecting data in 1973, initially collecting just a series of small datasets. It has now become the largest inclusive dataset in the United States, comprised of over 22 population-based cancer registries and encompassing approximately 28 % of the entire US population [12]. Gnerlich and colleagues analyzed data from SEER datasets between 1988 and 2003, identifying 9,734 patients with Stage 4 breast cancer. Definitive operative intervention to remove the primary breast cancer in the face of known metastatic disease occurred in 47 % (4,578) of the women. Simple mastectomy was performed on 2,485 (54.3 %) patients, and 7,844 (40.3 %) had a partial mastectomy.

As in the study by Rapiti and colleagues, the women who had surgery were younger (age 62 vs. 66 $p<0.001$) with smaller tumors that were grade 3 and estrogen receptor (ER) and progesterone receptor (PR) positive. The authors also noted that if the patients were Caucasian, married, or diagnosed earlier in the study period, they were more likely to have surgery compared to others. To control for such confounders, they developed six multivariate Cox regression models that were applied to the dataset. Utilizing the most conservative estimates of the relationship between surgery and survival, the data indicates that women who underwent an operation had a 37 % reduced risk of dying during the study period [13].

In addition to the large population-based studies, several smaller single-institutional, retrospective studies have indicated a survival benefit with extirpation of the primary breast tumor in the setting of metastatic disease. A study by Babiera et al. looked at 224 patients treated at the University of Texas M.D. Anderson Cancer Center. They found that 82 (37 %) of the women with Stage 4 breast cancer underwent an operation (48 % had a partial mastectomy, 52 % had a total mastectomy). Twenty-nine of the 82 had an excisional biopsy, 41 had definitive treatment, and only seven had an operation for palliation of their symptoms. Again, it was found that women who were treated operatively tended to be younger in age, have a lower N-stage, have only a single site of metastatic disease, have liver metastases, have amplification of the Her-2/neu receptor, and have neoadjuvant chemotherapy. Only 14 (17 %) of the patients who underwent operative intervention had multiple metastatic sites, whereas 40 of the 142 (28 %) of the non-operative group had multiple metastatic sites. With a median follow-up time of 32 months, the study demonstrated a trend toward an overall survival benefit to surgical resection of the primary tumor. The authors were able to demonstrate a statistically significant difference in metastatic progression-free survival for those in the surgical group with an HR of 0.54 ($p=0.0007$). There was a trend toward an overall survival benefit on univariant analysis that did not reach statistical significance [14].

With the growing amount of data demonstrating a possible overall and progression-free survival benefit with resection of the primary tumor in the face of metastatic disease, Rao et al. analyzed patients treated at the University of Texas Southwestern Medical Center with metastatic breast cancer. They identified a study population of 75 patients and further classified them based upon the time to surgical resection from the time of their original diagnosis. They were divided into three groups: surgical resection at 0–2.9 months, 3–8.9 months, and at 9 months or more after diagnosis. During the time of the study period, from 1997 to 2002, most of the patients had an excisional biopsy to diagnose their disease (37 of 75 patients) resulting in a higher rate of incomplete resection due to the higher positive margin rate in this cohort. Forty-one underwent an operation with a curative intent and seven for palliation. The authors reported that those patients who had an operation ≥3 months after diagnosis had a better metastatic progression-free survival compared to those who were operated on within the first 3 months of their diagnosis but were not able to demonstrate a difference in overall survival. On univariant analysis, the size of the tumor, method of diagnosis, number of distant metastatic sites, and type of axillary surgery were all associated with an improvement in overall and progression-free survival. However, on multivariant analysis, only the patient's race (Caucasian), fewer metastatic sites, and negative margins had better metastatic progression-free survival.

It was noted by the authors that most of the patients in the first group (surgery prior to 3 months from diagnosis) had an operation for purely diagnostic purposes and less for curative intent and, as expected, had a much higher rate of positive surgical margins. Additionally, they noted that those undergoing surgery at 3 months or greater had likely finished a chemotherapy regimen as their first-line treatment. Therefore, these patients were more likely to have had a response to systemic treatment, thereby highlighting the inherent selection biases of the retrospective study. The study authors recommend patients who have metastatic disease at the time of diagnosis to undergo systemic therapy as a first-line treatment followed by a surgical intervention, with the goal of obtaining negative margins as these patients had an improvement in the metastatic progression-free survival without an impact on overall survival [15].

It is important to understand that breast cancer represents a markedly heterogeneous group of tumors, highly variable in both genotypic and phenotypic expressions. Such heterogeneity is highly variable between any two patients, and as such, differences seen in overall survival may be impacted by any number of factors. Extensive research has been performed in order to classify various breast cancers based upon their molecular classification, finding four major breast cancer subtypes: luminal A, luminal B, Her-2/neu positive, and basal-like. Luminal A breast cancers are strongly ER and/or PR positive and Her-2/neu negative with a low Ki67 and have the best overall survival. Luminal B cancers are ER and/or PR positive and Her-2/neu positive with a high Ki67 and comprise about 20 % of the tumors diagnosed. The so-called basal-like cancers are negative for all three markers, ER, PR, and Her-2/neu, and, as such, have the worst overall survival. The final subtype is ER/PR negative and Her-2/neu positive [16]. The most common of the subtypes are the luminal breast cancers (A and B), comprising approximately two-thirds of all breast cancers. Breast cancers with the ER-/PR-negative and Her-2/neu pattern are the second most common at approximately 20% of the population. The least common, basal-like, comprises only 10–15 % of the patient population, but these numbers vary with ethnicity. Basal-like breast cancers are more common in the Hispanic and Black patient population (16 % and 24 %, respectively) as compared to White patients (11.5 %) [17]. Acknowledging the impact of these subtypes of survival, Blanchard et al. investigated the role of the molecular classification of breast cancer and their influences upon the overall survival and metastatic progression-free survival compared to historical data.

The authors identified 16,401 patients in the database of the University of Texas Health Science Center at San Antonio who had hormone receptor assays performed. Of those patients, 807 had Stage 4 metastatic breast cancer at presentation, and in contrast to the previously discussed papers, the women receiving surgery in the study tended to be older, with an average age of 63.3 years as compared to 57.1 years in the non-operative group. The patients in the study were more likely to be ER positive and PR negative and have T2 tumors at presentation, and the most common site of distant metastases was the bone. A total of 242 patients (61.3 %) underwent an operation with the majority of the patients undergoing a modified radical mastectomy.

In univariant analysis, significant improvement in overall survival was noted if the patients were ER positive, PR positive, or both ER and PR positive. ER-positive patients who underwent surgical intervention had a significantly improved overall survival as compared to those who did not have surgery (27.1 months vs. 16.8 months, $p<0.0001$), and this was maintained in patients with ER-negative disease. On multivariate analysis, controlling for ER/PR, age, race, visceral metastases, number of metastatic sites, and histology, the surgical removal of the intact primary breast cancer in the face of metastatic disease remained an independent factor associated with improved overall survival. The authors also found that ER/PR receptor status and the total number of distant metastatic sites were independent factors; ER-/PR-positive patients and those with less metastatic sites had better overall survival. Using multivariate models, surgical intervention demonstrated an overall HR of 0.71. In subset analysis, the HR improved to 0.606 if the tumor was ER positive, but when patients had more than one metastatic site, the HR was 1.268. The group also looked at the survival differences based on site of metastases and found survival to be worse if the patient had visceral metastases or more than one site of metastatic disease [18].

Using the clinical database from the Dana-Farber Cancer Institute, Brigham and Women's Hospital, and Massachusetts General Hospital, Bafford et al. examined 147 patients diagnosed with synchronous primary and metastatic breast cancer, of which 41 % underwent removal of the primary lesion. Interestingly, by examining the timing of their diagnosis as either preoperative or postoperative, they found that only 25/147 (17 %) patients were diagnosed with metastatic disease prior to their surgical intervention. There was no statistically significant difference in age, but patients receiving surgery were more likely to receive adjuvant radiation therapy and have fewer sites of distant disease. The authors further adjusted for ER and Her-2/neu receptor status, age, total number and location of metastases, and the various regimens of systemic therapy, finding that surgery was still a predictor of improved survival. The median overall survival, unadjusted, was 3.52 years in the surgical group versus 2.36 years in the nonsurgical group. Perhaps more important was the subset analysis of survival between those diagnosed before and after surgical intervention. For those patients who were diagnosed with metastatic disease prior to surgery, the overall survival was not impacted by surgical resection, and these patients had overall survival comparable to those who did not have surgical intervention at 2.4 years and 2.36 years, respectively [19].

In the Netherlands, Rashaan et al. accessed the database of two Dutch hospitals and identified 171 patients diagnosed with metastatic breast cancer between 1989 and 2009. Thirty-five percent of these patients had surgical intervention (59 of 171 patients) of whom 35 % (21 of 59 patients) were undiagnosed with metastatic disease at the time of their surgical intervention. The patients who had extirpation of their primary tumor were younger and had a lower T-stage, lower-grade tumors, and less comorbid conditions. In univariant analysis, there was an association between surgery and survival; however, this finding was not significant when examined by multivariate analysis.

The authors identified that patients who were younger at presentation and had an overall favorable health profile were operated on more frequently as a result, thus translating into a survival benefit with removal of the primary tumor. While a small patient population, and contrary to the aforementioned study by Bafford et al., they did not identify differences in outcomes between those who were operated on pre- and post-identification of metastatic disease. The authors again acknowledge the selection bias inherent in the retrospective nature of the study and recognize the need for a prospective randomized control trial to help reduce these confounders [20].

In a much larger study, Nguyen et al. identified 733 women with newly diagnosed metastatic breast cancer in the British Columbia Cancer Agency (years 1996–2005). They analyzed tumor characteristics, overall survival, and locoregional progression-free survival and compared locoregional treatment to those who had no local treatment. Fifty-two percent (378 of 733) had locoregional intervention defined as surgery alone (67 %), radiation alone (22 %), or a combination of the two (11 %). Those who were less than 50 years of age and had better performance status, tumors <5 cm, and low nodal disease burden had a higher rate of locoregional intervention. Additionally, patients who had less than five metastatic lesions and/or were asymptomatic from their metastatic disease were also more likely to have locoregional treatment.

Eighty percent of those who underwent local intervention were diagnosed with metastatic disease prior to their intervention, and 20 % had distant disease diagnosed with 4 months of presentation and diagnosis. The authors found the overall survival rate and the locoregional progression-free survival were better for women who underwent locoregional treatment as compared to those who did not. The 5-year overall survival was 21 % for those who underwent local regional therapy as compared to 14 % in the group who did not ($p<0.001$). Additionally, the local progression-free survival was 72 % in the regional therapy group and 46 % in those that did not ($p<0.001$). Importantly, the type of locoregional therapy did not seem to play a role; it was merely that locoregional therapy had been provided. The improvement in overall survival was maintained upon multivariant analysis, with locoregional therapy associated with an improved overall survival and negative resection margins, receiving chemotherapy and hormonal therapy [21].

In 2008, Hazard et al. published a small, single-institution, retrospective review of 111 women treated at the Lynn Sage Breast Cancer Center at Northwestern University. The authors found that surgery alone did not improve overall survival, but gaining locoregional control of chest wall disease was associated with an improved overall survival. The authors determined the lack of chest wall disease, whether by surgery, radiation, systemic therapy, or any combination thereof, imparted an overall survival benefit to women diagnosed with metastatic disease. Of the 111 women included in the study, 103 had information regarding chest wall disease. Surgery was performed in 42 % of the patients, with successful chest wall control maintained in 82 % of those patients as compared to only 34 % who did not have surgical intervention. The overall hazard ratio associated with chest wall control was highly significant ($p<0.0002$). Thus, the authors conclude that maintaining chest wall control, whether by surgery or not, may play a role in improving overall survival in women diagnosed with metastatic disease at presentation. The reason for this overall survival benefit is not well understood but may be related to the reduction in tumor volume and thus a potential for seeding and reseeding of metastatic sites. Again, the authors called for a randomized control trial to help discern the role locoregional intervention plays in overall survival and progression-free survival in metastatic breast cancer patients [22].

While all the previously referenced studies indicate a marginal benefit of locoregional therapy to the patient with metastatic breast cancer diagnosed at presentation, a study published in 2011 by Dominici et al. contradicts these findings. Using the National Comprehensive Cancer Network (NCCN) Breast Cancer Outcomes Database, they looked at patients who were treated with surgical intervention prior to systemic treatment and compared them to women who received no surgical intervention. They matched the patients based on age, ER status, Her-2/neu status, and number of metastatic sites. A total of 1,048 patients with metastatic disease were identified, but the appropriate data was only available for 551 patients. The authors matched 236 patients without intervention to 54 patients with surgical intervention. They found the survival was similar between the two groups, 3.4 years in the nonsurgical versus 3.5 years in the surgical group [23].

Each of these studies provides a variation on the hypothesis that surgical intervention, or at least locoregional intervention, will help impart an overall survival benefit for patients diagnosed with metastatic breast cancer. While it is easy to attribute all of the survival benefit to the selection bias inherent in retrospective studies, this may be underestimating the role primary tumor resection has on distant disease control. As our knowledge of cancer stem cells and other mechanisms of tumorigenesis improves, it is possible that reducing local disease burden with complete surgical resection, in and of itself, may play a key role in an improved overall survival. With a 5-year survival rate of less than 25 %, it behooves us to continue to strive to find ways of improving this relatively dismal prognosis. To this end, there is now one randomized controlled trial in the United States whose sole aim is to identify the possible role that surgery or locoregional treatment may play in improving the outcome in Stage 4 patients. The Eastern Cooperative Oncology Group (ECOG) 2108 study is a randomized phase III trial examining the value of early local therapy for the intact primary tumor in patients with metastatic breast cancer. All women enrolled in the trial will undergo induction systemic treatment after the diagnosis of metastatic disease is made. Patients may be enrolled either at the time of diagnosis or up to week 30 of systemic treatment. Systemic therapy is up to the provider, but the patient must have completed 16 weeks of therapy. Those who respond to treatment with either stable or decreased metastatic disease burden defined as (1) no new sites of disease, (2) no enlargement of existing disease ≥20 %, and (3) no deterioration of symptoms will be randomized into one of two arms.

In the first arm, patients will not undergo any surgical intervention and continue their systemic treatment. In the second arm, the patient will undergo surgical resection of the primary tumor and then continue with further systemic therapy at the discretion of the provider and as needed for palliation of local progression. The intervention arm will be the definitive treatment of the primary breast cancer with either lumpectomy or mastectomy with concomitant axillary nodal staging and followed by radiation therapy if necessary [24]. However, due to the small population of patients who fit the eligibility criteria, we are unlikely to know the answer in short order. In the meantime, it appears that there is enough data to consider the curative resection of the primary tumor when the overall metastatic disease burden is minimal and/or locoregional control of chest wall disease can be achieved.

Liver Metastasis

One of the most common solid organ metastatic sites for breast cancer is the liver. This is often in combination with disseminated disease to other locations such as to the bone, lung, and brain. However, approximately 5 % of Stage 4 breast cancer patients will have isolated metastasis to the liver [25]. Originally, the morbidity and mortality associated with partial liver resections made the risks of surgery outweigh the potential benefit of improved overall survival. However, the advent of several new surgical devices and techniques has considerably shifted this ratio to a more favorable outcome for those undergoing a resection of isolated liver metastases. Taking a cue from the role of partial hepatectomy for metastatic colon cancer and its associated improvement in overall survival, many groups in the United States, Europe, and Asia have assessed the possible benefits of similar, aggressive, operative intervention for patients with breast cancer liver metastases.

In 2000, investigators at Duke University retrospectively evaluated 17 patients accrued over a 10-year period. There were 33 patients eligible for curative resection; however, 16/33 (48 %) were found to be unresectable at the time of the operation. Of the remaining 17 patients, 10 received neoadjuvant chemotherapy. Twelve (71 %) had a single metastatic liver lesion, and five patients had two lesions. The median size of the liver metastasis was 2.5 cm with none larger than 5 cm. There was one death in the immediate postoperative period. The median survival of the remaining 16 patients was 27 months, with a 5-year actuarial survival rate of 22 % and a 5-year disease-free survival of 17 %. Local recurrences were high, with 12/16 (75 %) developing recurrent disease at a median time to recurrence of any type was 7 months [26].

A second group at the Institut Curie also published data in 2000 regarding their experiences with liver resection for patients with breast cancer metastases. Pocard et al. identified 52 patients who underwent surgery between 1988 and 1997. Forty-six (88.5 %) had chemotherapy or endocrine therapy prior to surgical intervention (3–24 cycles) with the mean interval from diagnosis to surgery of 11 months. Solitary liver metastasis were present in 36 (69.2 %) of the patients. Eight-six percent had an operation for curative intent. With a median follow-up of 23 months, the overall survival after surgery was 86 % at 12 months, 79 % at 24 months, and 49 % at 36 months. Survival was dependent on the length of time from the diagnosis of the primary breast cancer to the diagnosis of metastatic disease. The overall survival at 36 months was 45 % for those patients who were diagnosed with metastases within 48 months of the original tumor and 82 % if the patient's diagnosis of breast cancer was >48 months ($p=0.023$) [27]. The authors acknowledge the highly selective patient population but postulate the potential for a greater role in partial liver resections in this small, highly selective subset of patients.

Around the same time, Yoshimoto et al. published a study of 25 patients with liver metastasis who underwent surgery with a curative. This retrospective study of women treated from 1985 to 1998 included those with both liver and extrahepatic metastases. Fourteen patients (56 %) had a solitary metastasis, 11 patients had multiple lesions, and 8 had extrahepatic disease. Of the 25 patients, recurrence occurred in 18 (72 %); the liver was the sole site of recurrence in 12 (67 %) patients. The 2-year and 5-year cumulative survival rates were 71 % and 27 %, respectively, and the median duration of survival was 34.3 months. In this study, overall survival was not impacted by the number or size of the metastatic lesions, the interval between diagnoses, or the presence of extrahepatic metastases [28].

Vlastos et al. published a single institution's experience with aggressive management of breast cancer liver metastases at the University of Texas M.D. Anderson Cancer Center. A total of 31 patients treated between 1991 and 2002 were retrospectively evaluated. These patients had liver-only disease and the median size of the lesions was 2.9 cm. Twenty of the patients (65 %) had a solitary lesion and the vast majority of them had chemotherapy prior to surgical intervention. The median survival was 63 months and the overall 2-year and 5-year survival rates were 86 % and 61 %, respectively. The disease-free survival was 39 % and 31 % at 2 years and 5 years, respectively. The median time to recurrence was 13 months and only four patients (13 %) had recurrences in the liver [29]. Again, this is a highly selective patient population but with a median survival of 63 months; it substantially exceeds the range of survival reported in the literature for those not undergoing surgical intervention.

Two different studies have looked at the extent of resection and its impact, if any, on survival. The first, published in 2006 by Adam et al., is a single institution, retrospective study of 85 patients with a median age of 47. Twenty-seven (32 %) had evidence of extrahepatic metastases, 32 had a solitary lesion in the liver, and 26 had greater than 3 metastases. On final pathology, 65 % of the patients had negative margins (R0 resection). Eighteen percent of patients had microscopic disease evident at the margins of resection (R1), and 17 % had macroscopic disease (R2) at the resection margin. Thirty-two patients (38 %) were alive at a median follow-up of 38 months. The median survival was 32 months and the median disease-free survival was 20 months. The 5-year overall survival was 37 % and the 5-year disease-free survival was 21 %. Only an R2 resection was found to be a predictor of poor prognosis [30].

Van Walsum et al. also evaluated the degree of resection relative to survival. In their series of 32 patients, the median diameter of the lesions was 2.5 cm, all patients had previously undergone resection of their primary breast tumor, and the median age was 50 years. With a median follow-up time of 26 months (range 0–188), the 5-year overall survival and disease-free survival were 37 % and 19 %, respectively. The median overall survival was 55 months and the median time to recurrence was 11 months. All but three patients (91 %) had R0 sections of the metastatic lesions. The overall survival and the median survival were not significantly different; however, there were three patients with microscopic disease at the resection margin (R1). The authors indicated having a solitary lesion was associated with an improved overall survival of 68 % as opposed to those with multiple lesions with 37 % [31].

As this impacts survival, the receptor status of the primary tumor and its correlation to the metastatic lesion have become a point of interest. Liu et al. published an interesting study comparing the receptor status of the primary tumor to the receptor status of the metastatic lesion(s) in the liver. In a population of 58 patients diagnosed with metastatic breast cancer to the liver, 12 had a simultaneous diagnosis of the primary and the metastatic lesion, and 46 had a diagnosis of liver metastases remote to the diagnosis and treatment of the primary tumor. Of those diagnosed with Stage 4 at presentation, the ER status did not change between the primary tumor and the metastases. However, in four cases, PR status changed and in one patient the Her-2/neu status changed. By contrast, there was a significant variation in receptor status when the diagnosis of Stage 4 disease was made remote to the diagnosis of the primary tumor. ER status was different between the tumors in 14 of 46 (30.4 %) patients, PR changed in 25 patients (54.3 %), and Her-2/neu was altered in 5 of 46 (11 %) patients [32]. Thus, the clinician should not assume the receptor status of the primary tumor and the metastatic site are the same, and therefore it is important to assess for the ER, PR, and Her-2/neu status of the metastatic lesion as the systemic therapy may need to be adjusted to the new receptor patterns.

Martinez et al. from the John Wayne Cancer Institute evaluated the impact of the ER status on overall survival. Their retrospective study evaluated 20 patients meeting criteria out of a pool of 1,147 patients treated at their institution between 1995 and 2004. They demonstrated the overall survival was better if the ER was positive but did not identify a correlation with PR status. The median survival was 32 months, and the 2-year and 5-year survival rates of the entire cohort were 61 % and 33 %, respectively. However, if the patient was ER positive on the primary tumor, the survival was 3.52 years in comparison to 1.5 years if the primary was ER negative. Similarly, if the ER was positive on the liver metastasis, the survival was 3.14 years as compared to 0.77 years when the ER was negative. Additionally, patients with two or more metastases or who were less than 50 years of age had worse overall survival [33].

Finally, Abbot et al. evaluated the ER status and the response to chemotherapy as a predictor of improved survival in patients. Patients treated between 1997 and 2010 were identified and 86 patients met study criteria. With a median follow-up of 62 months, the median disease-free survival was 14.2 months and the median actuarial overall survival was 57 months. In this patient population, 27 patients had synchronous liver metastases, 90 % had an R0 resection, and 62 % had a solitary liver metastasis. The vast majority (86 %) of the patient's liver lesions were less than 5 cm, and 65 of the 86 (76 %) patients had neoadjuvant chemotherapy or antiestrogen therapy. If the patient had an ER-positive tumor, the median disease-free survival was 19.8 months as compared to ER-negative tumors in which disease-free survival was 7.8 months ($p=0.031$). The median overall survival for ER-positive tumors was 76.8 months and 61.8 months for PR-positive tumors. If the patient's tumor was ER and PR negative, the median overall survival was 28.3 months. However, the authors found the most significant predictor of survival advantage with liver resection was radiographic evidence of response to preoperative chemotherapy or antiestrogen therapy [34].

Thus, studies would indicate patients with a prolonged interval between diagnosis of the primary lesion and liver metastasis, solitary liver lesion, older age, ER-positive tumors, and radiographic evidence of response to neoadjuvant systemic therapy may benefit the most from an evaluation for and potentially curative surgical resection of liver metastases.

Lung Metastasis

The lung is the second most common solid organ to which breast cancer will metastasize. However, the role of surgical resection is somewhat controversial. During the initial evaluation of a pulmonary nodule in a patient with a prior diagnosis of breast cancer, it is important to delineate benign versus malignant etiology. If the lesion returns as malignant, it is important to then differentiate a primary lung cancer from metastatic breast cancer. Historically, the aggressive surgical treatment of pulmonary metastases was isolated to a select few academic centers, and the patients chosen for intervention had to have had a long disease-free interval. As with liver metastasectomy, the resection of breast cancer lung metastasis with curative intent was fostered by the development of supportive data derived from another malignancy, in this case, osteosarcoma.

Data from the Mayo Clinic in Rochester, Minnesota, indicated an improved 5-year overall survival from 17 % to 32 % when pulmonary metastases were resected in patients with metastatic osteosarcoma [35]. Most pulmonary metastases are asymptomatic, especially when there is limited disease in the thoracic cavity. Thus, the experience with metastasectomy is confined to a very small, highly selective, subpopulation derived from the larger pool of Stage 4 patients. As with liver metastases, the role of surgical intervention is gaining greater prominence as the morbidity and mortality of chest surgery continue to decline.

The initial experience at the University of Texas M.D. Anderson Cancer Center was published in 1992. The authors reported on 44 eligible patients accumulated from 1981 to 1990. All patients had thoracic metastasis and prior treatment of their primary tumor. Seven patients were excluded, three for benign disease and four for incomplete resection (due to hilar or nodal disease), for a total of 37 patients. The median age was 55 years, there were no deaths, most patients had either preoperative or postoperative systemic therapy, and the vast majority (27 patients) had a single lesion. The median survival for complete resection (R0) was 47 months ± 5.5 months, and the actuarial 5-year survival was 49.5 %. The authors noted the disease-free interval was a significant predictor in this population. If greater than 12 months had elapsed from the diagnosis of the primary tumor, the median survival was 82 months, and the 5-year survival was 57 %. By comparison, if the diagnosis of the primary was less than 12 months prior, the median survival was 15 months, and the 5-year survival was 0 %. Two additional factors assessed by the authors were the role of the ER status and the number of pulmonary metastasis. Twenty-seven patients had a single pulmonary lesion, and ten patients had two or more lesions. The median survival was 82 months for the group with an isolated lesion and 24 months for multiple lesions; the 5-year survival was 59 % in the former group and only 36 % in the latter. This difference did not reach statistical significance ($p=0.229$). Similarly, those with ER-positive disease had a trend toward a survival advantage, but with only a total of 29 patients with known ER status, statistical significance was not achieved ($p=0.98$) [36].

McDonald et al. published their single-institution experience of 60 patients with a median age of 58 years. Solitary metastasis was identified in 31 patients, and 40 of the 60 patients had an R0 resection. Of the 39 survivors, 32 patients eventually had a recurrence of their disease. The median disease-free interval was 1.6 years. The overall 5-year survival was 37.8 %, and the survival was not influenced by the age of the patient, the type of breast cancer, the original stage, the tumor-free interval, the estrogen receptor status, and the type of pulmonary resection. Only the number of metastasis approached clinical significance, with the low number of patients in each category making statistical significance difficult to achieve [37].

Friedel et al. assessed the benefit of lung metastasectomy using the International Registry of Lung Metastases. There were 467 patients in the database of whom 84 % had a complete resection of their pulmonary metastatic burden. The overall 5-, 10-, and 15-year survival was 38, 22, and 20 %, respectively. With further analysis, the authors noted that disease-free interval was a significant predictor of overall survival. For patients whose primary tumor was diagnosed greater than or equal to 36 months prior to lung resection, the 5-, 10-, and 15-year survival was 45, 26, and 21 %, respectively ($p=0.0001$). Single metastasis was not a significant predictor of survival. The authors analyzed a subset of patients who had (1) R0 resection, (2) prolonged disease-free interval, and (3) a single lung metastasis. This highly selected population did not have a significant survival benefit [38].

Several subsequent single-institutional studies have been published with conflicting results. The first, by Tanaka et al., was published in 2005. Fifty-two breast cancer patients, diagnosed between 1992 and 2001, underwent surgical treatment of pulmonary nodules. All patients had prior surgical resection of the primary tumor and the mean age was 55.8 years. Of the 52 patients, 39 (75 %) had breast cancer metastasis, six had primary lung cancer, and seven had benign lesions on final pathology. Complete resection was accomplished in 33 of the 39 patients (84.6 %), and multiple nodules/lesions were present in 24 patients. None of the patients had extrathoracic disease. The median overall survival was 32 months and the 5-year survival was 30.8 %. The number of metastases, the disease-free interval, and the presence of unilateral versus bilateral disease did not influence survival. Interestingly, the patients with pulmonary nodules from metastatic disease had a disease-free interval of 66 months as compared to 272 months when the nodule was due to a new primary lung cancer [39].

Contradictory to these findings, Rena et al. found that disease-free interval positively influenced overall survival rates. In this retrospective study of 79 patients, the mean age was 63 and none of the patients had extrathoracic disease. All of the patients had previously undergone curative resection of the primary tumor. Of the 79 patients, 27 (34 %) had metastatic breast cancer, 38 had primary pulmonary malignancy, and 14 had benign pathology. Again, the average disease-free interval was much longer when the pathology of the lung lesion was a primary lung cancer. The patients were stratified to disease-free intervals of <36 or >36 months. The 5-year and 10-year survival rates were 38 % and 23 % when the diagnosis was made greater than 36 months from the primary tumor. This is significantly longer than if the diagnosis was made prior to 36 months, 21 % and 9 % ($p=0.014$) [40].

Finally, one study showed a significant difference in survival based on the receptor status of the primary and the metastatic tumor. Welter et al. retrospectively evaluated 47 patients treated between 1998 and 2007. The mean age was 56.2 years, and the median disease-free interval from the primary diagnosis was 3.66 years. Complete resection was accomplished in 27 of 47 (57 %) patients. Residual microscopic and macroscopic disease at the margins of resection was identified on final pathology in 6 and 14 patients, respectively. The authors noted that 11 of 39 (28 %) patients had a change in the ER status and 4 of 16 patients had a change in Her-2/neu status. The overall survival and 5-year survival rates for the entire cohort were 32 months and 36 %, respectively. If the patient was ER positive, the 5-year survival rate was 76 % as compared to 12 % when the patient had ER-negative disease ($p=0.002$). The authors did not find a correlation with the age of the patient, the number of metastases, original tumor stage, completeness of resection (R0 vs. R1/R2), or the presence of nodal involvement [41].

Thus, the approach to the patient diagnosed with new pulmonary nodules or documented pulmonary metastasis is complex. Nichols et al. suggest assessing five key factors that are, in part, supported by the data presented above. The author advocates evaluating for (1) control of the primary tumor, (2) the number of metastatic lesions in the lung, (3) the presence or absence of extrathoracic metastases, (4) whether or not the patient can physiologically tolerate the resection, and finally (5) the disease-free interval [42]. These factors can help the clinician decide whether or not a patient should be referred for an evaluation with the intent of resecting pulmonary metastases.

Brain Metastasis

Breast cancer is the second most common malignancy to metastasize to the brain, while non-small cell lung cancer is the most common. The incidence of brain metastasis may be increasing as patients live longer as a result of improvements in both local and systemic therapies. At the time a diagnosis of metastatic breast cancer to the brain is made, the average survival is between 11 and 14 months, and this is significantly impacted by the number of metastatic lesions. To understand this poor prognosis, it is important to discuss some of the factors making treatment of brain metastasis difficult. Unique to the central nervous system (CNS) is the blood-brain barrier. This system of tightly woven endothelial cells functions as an effective defense mechanism. It protects the CNS from exposure to the highly variable composition of the blood as well as the brain from infection and other pathogens. The endothelial cells form tight junctions and are without the standard transendothelial pathways that allow for movement of substances from the blood vessel into the brain. While this is an excellent protective measure, it is detrimental in the setting of metastatic lesions. The relative difficulty of effectively getting therapeutic agents such as chemotherapy across the barrier to treat the malignancy within the CNS parenchyma makes systemic treatment of these lesions problematic.

In an autopsy study published in 1983, Tsukada et al. found 309 of 1,044 (30 %) patients with breast cancer had CNS disease. Of those 309 patients, 193 (62 %) had parenchymal involvement (as compared to leptomeningeal) resulting in a calculated overall incidence of approximately 19 %. The authors point out that only 31 % of the 309 patients were clinically diagnosed with CNS disease prior to their death [43]. Quigley et al. published a retrospective review of 88 patients who presented with a new diagnosis of brain metastasis at a single institution. They found that 68 % had multiple lesions and 17 % had a solitary lesion and the factors negatively impacting survival were the presence of leptomeningeal disease and triple-negative status (ER/PR and Her-2/neu negative). The median survival of the patients in each of these latter two groups was 3.1 months [44].

One key factor in determining both overall survival and treatment in this group of patients is the number and location of the lesions detected. The majority of metastatic lesions are confined to the cerebral cortex with the remaining metastatic deposits located in the cerebellum and the brain stem. Local treatment, depending on the location of the lesion, can result in significant physical and cognitive impairments. Thus, the locoregional approach to the single metastatic deposit is different than that of diffuse lesions within the brain. Broadly speaking, surgical treatment of the brain metastasis can be subclassified into true microsurgical resection and stereotactic radiofrequency surgery (SRS). While not a true surgical technique, SRS can effectively target the lesion and the surrounding parenchyma.

There are very few studies dedicated to the treatment of breast-only metastatic disease to the brain. However, several randomized studies have been published regarding the treatment of brain metastasis. In 1990 Patchell et al. published a randomized study comparing surgical resection and radiation therapy of a single metastatic deposit to radiation therapy alone. There were 25 patients in the radiation and surgery arm; however, only 2 of the 25 were breast cancer metastases. This arm had an overall length of survival of 40 weeks, and the patients maintained good functional indices until week 38. By contrast, the radiation alone arm had 23 patients (one breast cancer patient) with an overall length of survival of 15 weeks, and the patients maintained good functional status until week 8. The recurrence rate was 20 % in the combined treatment arm as compared to 52 % in the radiation alone arm [45].

While the patient population was predominantly non-breast cancer patients, the study set the stage for further work published in 1998 by the same group where a comparison of radiation plus surgery to surgical resection alone was reported. In this randomized, multicenter trial of 95 patients, 49 (51.5 %) patients were randomized to radiation and surgery, and 46 patients were randomized to surgery alone. Again, all patients had a single metastatic deposit. The recurrence rate was 18 % for the combined therapy group and 70 % for the surgery alone group; there was no difference in overall survival. Of the patients in this cohort, only nine patients had a primary breast malignancy [46]. Both of these studies seem to indicate that combination therapy is a better means of reducing risk of brain recurrences and, in at least one study, potentially improving overall survival.

More recently, focus has turned to the role of surgery and radiation in the treatment of more than one metastatic site in the brain. Rades et al. published in *Cancer* in 2007 a series of 201 patients who had one to two brain metastases and were treated with combined therapy. The arms were (1) surgery plus whole breast radiation (99 patients) and (2) surgery, whole brain radiation with a boost dose to the tumor bed (102 patients). The 1-year overall survival for the arm treated with surgery and whole brain radiation was 41 % as compared to 66 % in the cohort of patients who received an additional boost dose ($p<0.001$). Of this 201 patient cohort, breast cancer was the primary malignancy in 43 (21 %) patients. On multivariant analysis, the use of the boost dose, complete surgical resection, and the interval between tumor diagnosis and whole breast radiation therapy (12 m) were associated with improved overall survival. There was no difference in survival based on the tumor type [47].

The same authors also investigated the role of a boost dose to the metastatic site in patients who presented with a single metastatic site. This study had 105 patients in the surgery plus whole breast radiation and 90 patients who underwent the same regimen but with an added boost of radiation to the metastatic bed. Of these 195 patients, 34 were breast cancer patients (17 %). They found that the local control rates were much better for the group who had an additional boost dose at 1 year (67 % vs. 38 %), 2 years (51 % vs. 20 %), and 3 years (33 % vs. 9 %) as compared to those patients who did not receive a boost dose ($p=0.002$). However, despite the improved local control, the addition of the boost dose did not impart an overall survival benefit. The overall survival at 1 year for the boost group was 60 % and 52 % for the non-boost group; the 2-year survival was 40 % versus 25 %, and the 3-year survival was 26 % versus 19 %. The authors concluded that the addition of a boost dose should be considered in most patients as local control is important in controlling the neurologic complications of CNS metastasis, but they do caution this should be confirmed by a randomized control trial [48].

In 2012, the Cochrane Collaboration published updated recommendations for the treatment of newly diagnosed multiple brain metastases from various primary cancers. The group searched MEDLINE, EMBASE, and the Cochrane Central Register of Controlled Trials (CENTRAL) for randomized control trials comparing whole brain radiation therapy to other treatment therapies in adults. To the original review published in 2006, the authors added nine additional articles and 1,420 patients for a total of 39 articles reviewed and 10,835 patients. Based on the updated data, the authors conclude (1) the standard dose-fractionation plans are equally as effective as others and (2) the use of boost to the metastatic site in combination with whole brain radiation therapy improves local control but does not affect overall survival in patients with multiple brain metastases. Finally, it appears those who are treated with radiosurgery alone have better neurocognitive outcomes than those treated with whole brain radiation and radiosurgery, but caution this is based on one randomized control trial [49].

In conclusion, the recommendations for treatment of a patient diagnosed with metastatic breast cancer to the brain depend upon the number of lesions present at the time of diagnosis. If you extrapolate the data from studies looking at brain metastasis from all sources, the use of microsurgical resection and/or radiosurgical resection of a solitary lesion seems to impart a survival advantage especially if complete resection is obtained and supplemental radiotherapy is used. However, in the setting of multiple metastases, the use of radiation therapy, whole brain with boost or with radiosurgery, does not seem to impart an overall survival benefit but it does appear to improve local control. Therefore, a patient may have better neurocognitive outcomes as compared to a treated patient who does not undergo any local treatment. Thus, the use of surgical resection and/or radiation therapy should be considered in patients who present with brain metastasis in an attempt to at least control local disease and possibly improve survival in the patient with a solitary metastatic deposit.

Conclusion

Surgical treatment of the metastatic breast cancer patient is difficult as the indications for intervention are, at best, unclear. The majority of the published data supports an aggressive operative treatment approach of the intact primary tumor. This data is all retrospective and with that comes the inherent bias toward survival benefit. The metastatic patient who responds well to systemic therapy is far more likely to be offered surgical intervention than the metastatic patient who has progressive disease despite systemic therapy. The women from the latter group are, by and large, not present in the published studies discussed in the beginning of this chapter. Despite the relative ambiguity at this time, it seems reasonable to offer surgical resection of an intact primary breast tumor when there is demonstrated response to systemic therapy. This is especially true with low volume of disease burden or even more so in the setting of complete radiographic response. When contemplating resecting the primary tumor in the metastatic setting, a detailed discussion of the patient's surgical options should also include the basis for the recommendation that comes from data with an inherent selection bias. Patients should be cautioned that the data supporting these recommendations comes from retrospective trials and a definitive answer as the role surgery plans in overall survival is forthcoming, but it will take many years for maturation of the data.

The recommendations for, or against, resection of solid organ metastasis are even more difficult to make. The focus of a clinician's assessment should include the time interval from diagnosis of the primary tumor, the ability to perform a resection with curative intent, and the patient's ability to tolerate the intervention. With the increasing complex systemic therapy, many argue that the survival advantages seen in some studies regarding liver and lung resection may be confounded by the systemic treatment of the disease and that the biology of the tumor itself and not the surgical resection is a greater predictor of the patient's overall survival.

Until randomized controlled trials are initiated and completed, our information is predominantly limited to retrospective reviews of an exceedingly small patient population. At this time, national guidelines are not possible. The treatment of the metastatic patient is truly individualized and must honor the goals and desires of the patient.

References

1. GLOBOCAN. Estimated Cancer Incidence, Mortality and Prevalence Worldwide in 2012.
2. World Health Organization. Breast cancer: prevention and control. http://www.who.int. Accessed 21 Dec 2012.
3. Siegel R, Naishadham D, Jemal A. SEER stat fact sheets: breast cancer. Cancer statistics, 2013. CA: Cancer J Clin. 2013;63:11–30.
4. American Cancer Society. Cancer facts and figures, 2012. http://www.cancer.org. Accessed 21 Dec 2012.
5. National Cancer Institute. SEER Stat Fact Sheets: Breast Cancer. www.cancer.gov. Accessed 21 Dec 2012.
6. Flanigan RC, Salmon SE, Blumenstein BA, et al. Nephrectomy followed by interferon alfa-2b compared with interferon alfa-2wb alone for metastatic renal-cell cancer. NEJM. 2001;345:1655–9.
7. Bonnet D, Dick JE. Human acute myeloid leukemia is organized as a hierarchy that originates from a primitive hematopoietic cell. Nat Med. 1997;3(7):730–7.
8. Li F, Tiede B, Massague J, et al. Beyond tumorigenesis: cancer stem cells in metastasis. Cell Res. 2007;17:3–14.
9. Al-Hajj M, Wicha MS, Benito-Hernandez AB, et al. Prospective identification of tumorigenic breast cancer cells. Proc Natl Acad Sci U S A. 2003;100(7):3983–8.
10. Khan SA, Stewart AK, Morrow M. Does aggressive local therapy improve survival in metastatic breast cancer? Surgery. 2002;132(4):620–7.
11. Rapiti E, Verkooijen HM, Blastos G, et al. Complete excision of primary breast tumor improves survival of patients with metastatic breast cancer at diagnosis. J Clin Oncol. 2006;24(18):2743–9.
12. National Cancer Institute. Surveillance, Epidemiology, and End Results (SEER). http://www.seer.cancer.gov/. Accessed 24 Dec 2012.
13. Gnerlich J, Jeffe DB, Deshpande AD, et al. Surgical removal of the primary tumor increases overall survival in patients with metastatic breast cancer: analysis of the 1988–2003 SEER data. Ann Surg Oncol. 2007;14(8):2187–94.
14. Babiera GV, Rao R, Fen L, et al. Effect of primary tumor extirpation in breast cancer patients who present with stage IV disease and an intact primary tumor. Ann Surg Oncol. 2006;13(6):776–82.
15. Rao R, Fen L, Kuerer HM, et al. Timing of surgical intervention for the intact primary in stage IV breast cancer patients. Ann Surg Oncol. 2008;15(6):1696–702.
16. Sorlie T, Perou CM, Tibshirani R, et al. Gene expression patterns of breast carcinomas distinguish tumor subclasses with clinical implications. Proc Natl Acad Sci U S A. 2011;98(19):10869–74.
17. Kuran A, Fish K, Shema SJ, et al. Lifetime risks of specific breast cancer subtypes among women in four racial/ethnic groups. Breast Cancer Res. 2010;12:R99.
18. Blanchard DK, Shetty PB, Hilsenbeck SG, Elledge RM. Association of surgery with improved survival in stage IV breast cancer patients. Ann Surg. 2008;247(5):732–8.
19. Bafford AC, Burstein HJ, Barkley CR, et al. Breast surgery in stage IV breast cancer: impact of staging and patient selection on overall survival. Breast Cancer Res Treat. 2009;115:7–12.
20. Rashan ZM, Bastiaannet E, Portielje JEA, et al. Surgery in metastatic breast cancer: patients with a favorable profile seem to have the most benefit from surgery. Eur J Surg Oncol. 2012;38:52–6.
21. Nguyen DHA, Truong PT, Alexander C, et al. Can locoregional treatment of the primary tumor improve outcomes for women with stage IV breast cancer at diagnosis? Int J Radiat Oncol. 2012;84(1):39–45.
22. Hazard HW, Gorla SR, Scholtens D, et al. Surgical resection of the primary tumor, chest wall control, and survival in women with metastatic breast cancer. Cancer. 2008;113(8):2011–9.
23. Dominici L, Najita J, Hughes M, et al. Surgery of the primary tumor does not improve survival in stage IV breast cancer. Breast Cancer Res Treat. 2011;129:459–65.
24. Eastern Oncology Cooperative Group. Physician and patient education materials for E2108. http://www.ecog.org/general/E2108info.html. Accessed 28 Dec 2012.
25. Al H, Royle GT. Taylor I. Breast liver metastases – incidence, diagnosis and outcome. J R Soc Med. 1991;84(12):714–6.
26. Selzner M, Morse M, James J, et al. Liver metastases from breast cancer: long-term survival after curative resection. Surgery. 2000;127:383–9.
27. Pocard M, Pouillart P, Asselain B, et al. Hepatic resection in metastatic breast cancer: results and prognostic factors. Eur J Surg Oncol. 2000;26:155–9.
28. Yoshimoto M, Tada T, Saito M, et al. Surgical treatment of hepatic metastases for breast cancer. Breast Cancer Res. 2000;59(2):177–84.
29. Vlastos G, Smith DL, Singletary SE, et al. Long-term survival after an aggressive surgical approach in patients with breast cancer hepatic metastases. Ann Surg Oncol. 2004;11(9):869–74.

30. Adam R, Aloia T, Krissat J, et al. Is liver resection justified for patients with hepatic metastases from breast cancer? Ann Surg Oncol. 2006;244(6): 897–907.
31. Van Walsum GAM, de Ridder JAM, Verhoef C, et al. Resection of liver metastases in patients with breast cancer: survival and prognostic factors. Eur J Surg Oncol. 2012;38:910–7.
32. Liu J, Deng H, Jia W, et al. Comparison of ER/PR and HER2 statuses in primary and paired liver metastatic sites of breast cancer in patients with or without treatment. J Cancer Res Clin Oncol. 2012;138:837–42.
33. Martinez SR, Young SE, Giuliano AE, et al. The utility of estrogen receptors, progesterone receptors, and Her-2/neu status to predict survival in patients undergoing hepatic resection for breast cancer metastases. Am J Surg. 2006;191:281–3.
34. Abbott ED, Brouquet A, Mittendorg EA, et al. Resection of liver metastases from breast cancer: Estrogen receptor status and response to chemotherapy before metastasectomy define outcome. Surgery. 2012;151:710–6.
35. Rashid OM, Takabe K. The evolution of the role of surgery in the management of breast cancer lung metastasis. J Thorac Dis. 2012;4(4):420–4.
36. Lanza LA, Nataragan G, Roth JA, et al. Long-term survival after resection of pulmonary metastases from carcinoma of the breast. Ann Thorac Surg. 1992; 54:244–8.
37. McDonald ML, Deschamps C, Illstrup DM, et al. Pulmonary resection for metastatic breast cancer. Ann Thorac Surg. 1994;58:1599–602.
38. Friedel G, Pastorino U, Ginsberg RJ, et al. Results of lung metastasectomy from breast cancer: prognostic criteria on the basis of 467 cases of the International Registry of Lung Metastases. Eur J Cardiothorac Surg. 2002;22:335–44.
39. Tanaka F, Li M, Hanaoka N. Surgery for pulmonary nodules in breast cancer patients. Ann Thorac Surg. 2005;79:1711–5.
40. Rena O, Papalia E, Ruffini E, et al. The role of surgery in the management of solitary pulmonary nodule in breast cancer patients. Eur J Surg Oncol. 2007;33: 546–60.
41. Welter S, Jacobs J, Krbek T, et al. Pulmonary metastases of breast cancer. When is resection indicated? Eur J Cardiothorac Surg. 2008;34(6):1228–34.
42. Nichols FC. Pulmonary metastasectomy. Thorac Surg Clin. 2012;22:91–9. vii.
43. Tsukada Y, Fouad A, Pickren JW, et al. Central nervous system metastasis from breast carcinoma. Autopsy study. Cancer. 1983;52(12):2349–54.
44. Quigley MR, Fukui O, Chew B, et al. The shifting landscape of metastatic breast cancer to the CNS. Neurosurg Rev. 2013;36(3):377–82.
45. Patchell RA, Tibbs PA, Walsh JW, et al. A randomized trial of surgery in the treatment of single metastases to the brain. N Engl J Med. 1990;322:494–500.
46. Patchell R, Tibbs PA, Regine WF, et al. Post-operative radiation therapy in the treatment of single metastases to the brain. JAMA. 1998;280(17):1485–9.
47. Rades D, Pluemer A, Beninga T, et al. A boost in addition to whole brain radiotherapy improves patient outcome after resection of 1–2 brain metastases in recursive partitioning analysis class 1 and 2 patients. Cancer. 2007;110(7):1551–9.
48. Rades D, Kueter JD, Gliemroth J, et al. Resection plus whole-brain irradiation versus resection plus whole-brain irradiation plus boost for the treatment of single brain metastasis. Strahlenther Onkol. 2012;188:143–7.
49. Tsao MN, Lloyd N, Wong RKS, et al. Whole brain radiotherapy for the treatment of newly diagnosed multiple brain metastases (Review). The Cochrane Collaboration. http://www.thecochranelibrary.com.

A History of Breast Reconstruction Following Mastectomy

17

Charles Dupin, James Mayo, and M'liss Hogan

Why Reconstruct the Breast?

The human breast has great significance in Western culture. It is associated with femininity and sexual attraction. The breast is a symbol of nurturing and is highly prized by fashion designers who tailor their clothing to flatter the breasts.

Loss of the breast destroys the patient's self-image and makes her feel deformed and less feminine. Her feeling that she is sexually attractive is severely impacted, even to a loving partner. Her ability to conceal the deformity impacts her ability to dress and to engage in with the normal activities of life. Many times patients may delay therapy or refuse to undergo procedures for fear of mutilation. This is very common and frequently results in untoward outcomes in patients who have had previous breast augmentation procedures.

One of the goals in breast reconstruction is to mitigate the patient's psychological fear of losing her breast [1–3]. The more physical goals of breast reconstruction include providing a mound that is aesthetically acceptable, both in clothing and without. The breasts should be symmetrical in unilateral mastectomy. The mound should be soft and pliable. If the opposite breast is aesthetically deficient (macromastia or ptosis), it should be modified to match the reconstructed breast. A nipple/areola reconstruction should also be provided.

The relatively recent development of skin-sparing mastectomy has allowed for preservation of the skin envelope and inframammary fold, both of which improve cosmesis in a reconstructed breast. The reconstructive surgeon must, however, work within the confines of the remaining tissue. If there is a sizable excision of the breast skin (or excess skin in the case of larger breasts), scarring will be visible on the final result. The shape and symmetry of the breast is considered more important than visible scars. A team approach with the oncologic surgeon and reconstructive surgeon is necessary to provide optimal outcomes in breast reconstruction.

The possibility of reconstruction gives the patient faced with mastectomy hope that some of the physical and emotional impact of undergoing a mastectomy can be avoided. The diagnosis of breast cancer has both an immediate and long-lasting impact upon the patient. Having a plan to deal with the tumor is very beneficial to patients struggling with their diagnosis. It is helpful for surgeons to understand the history of breast reconstruction because it is an essential part of the comprehensive approach to treatment.

The Women's Health and Cancer Rights Act of 1998 ensures that insurers pay for reconstruction following mastectomy. It was assumed that with the passage of legislation, doors would open and reconstruction would become widely available to all women diagnosed with breast cancer. Population-based studies have demonstrated

C. Dupin, MD (✉) • J. Mayo, MD • M. Hogan, MD
Division of Plastic Surgery, Department of Surgery, Louisiana State University Health Sciences Center, 1542 Tulane Avenue, New Orleans, LA 70112, USA
e-mail: cldupinmd@gmail.com; jameslmayo@gmail.com; mhoga1@lsuhsc.edu

A.I. Riker (ed.), *Breast Disease: Comprehensive Management*,
DOI 10.1007/978-1-4939-1145-5_17,

a significant increase in breast reconstruction following mastectomy. The rate of reconstruction remains below what many surgeons expected in view of the availability of reconstruction. A longitudinal study taken from the nationwide inpatient sample database analyzed immediate reconstruction following mastectomy (1998–2008). In 1998, immediate reconstruction was noted to be 20.8 % with an increase in levels in 2008 to 37.8 % [4].

Reasons for the relatively low reconstruction rates seem to be multifold. First, lack of awareness of breast reconstructive options on both the patient's and physician's part may play a role in low rates of reconstruction. Alderman et al. determined that a large proportion of general surgeons still do not refer breast cancer patients to plastic surgery at the time of surgical decision making. This greatly impacts the number of breast reconstruction recipients [5]. In a survey for the year 2008 of the American Society of Plastic Surgeons (ASPS), Alderman et al. demonstrated factors associated with low- and high-volume breast reconstruction practices among plastic surgeons in the United States. Poor professional reimbursement for breast reconstruction and lack of resident coverage were identified as significant factors associated with low volume [6]. Socioeconomic factors have also been implicated in low reconstruction rates in some populations [4].

Challenges to Reconstruction

The treatment of breast cancer was dominated by William Halstead at the turn of the century. He performed the first radical mastectomy in 1882 and published the procedure in 1889. His approach of radical surgery went unchallenged for over 60 years. He further advised against attempts to reconstruct the breast for fear of jeopardizing local control of the disease [7]. Despite Halstead's tenets, attempts were made to reconstruct the breast as early as 1895, when Czerny reported a case of breast reconstruction [8]. In 1906, Tanzini et al. described the use of a latissimus flap for breast reconstruction [9]. Despite these early attempts, several issues arose which

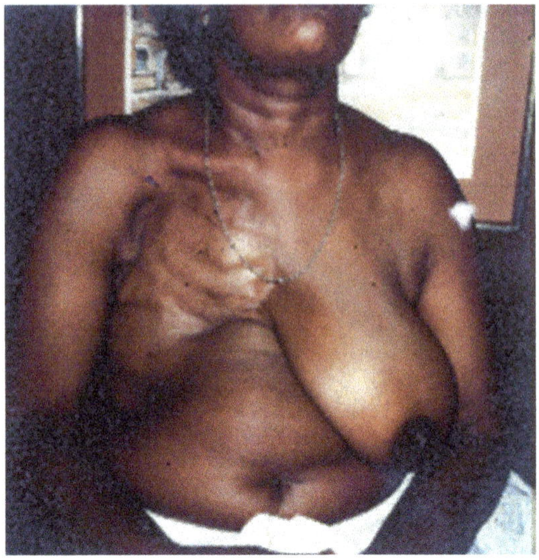

Fig. 17.1 Radical mastectomy defect

made breast reconstruction more difficult to perform. The first was the attitude of the surgeon that reconstruction would somehow jeopardize either local control or possibly overall survival. The second was the massive defects resulting from the standard Halstead radical mastectomy that was performed during this era, which made closure of such large defects quite challenging (Fig. 17.1).

It was not until the late 1960s that strong evidence became available to prove that a less deforming operation was able to deliver similar rates of survival and local recurrence [10].

The third driving force that affected the change to a less deforming operation was the more frequent diagnosis of less advanced disease that did not require radical surgery. Shortly thereafter, evidence was presented that even less aggressive surgery (lumpectomy) followed by radiation therapy offered similar survival rates to mastectomy. Although conserving the breast, radiation therapy was necessary to provide comparable outcomes. In the United States, this external beam radiation was administered at 6,000 gray, although in Europe the dose was normally 4,500 gray. The number of patients in the United States who choose breast conservation (lumpectomy, followed by radiation therapy) has recently declined. This is in part due to many patients not wanting to undergo adjuvant radiation therapy

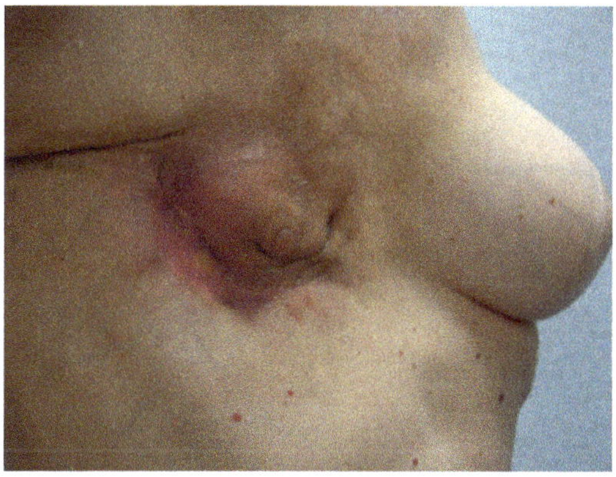

Fig. 17.2 Unusual severe case of radiation mastitis following lumpectomy and radiation therapy

after lumpectomy, partly due to the time commitment required and partly due to the adverse side effects associated with radiation therapy to the breast. The use of radiation therapy, which in the United States is normally given as 4500 gray with a "boost" of 1500 gray, has produced unfortunate radiation induced deformities in the residual breast (Fig. 17.2).

The concept of a skin-sparing mastectomy originated with Freeman in 1962. He suggested a modification of the traditional mastectomy before an implant-based breast reconstruction for benign disease [11]. The skin-sparing mastectomy as a cancer procedure was further described by Toth and Lappert in 1991 [12]. They described preoperative planning of mastectomy incisions to maximize skin preservation and to facilitate breast reconstruction. These modifications in tissue removal have made reconstruction much simpler to achieve. Along with the abandoning of the radical mastectomy in favor of the skin-sparing modified radical mastectomy, other devices were introduced to assist in reconstructing the breast mound.

An important milestone was the development of the silicone breast implant by Cronin (originally for breast augmentation) [13]. The concept of providing a breast mound substitute without a donor site was immediately attractive and popular with patients. Breast augmentation with silicone implants provided far superior results than previous materials, and it seemed possible to use the implants within the mastectomy defect. Unfortunately, postmastectomy reconstruction and augmentation are two very different surgical situations. In the augmentation patient, there is normally ample soft tissue coverage and supple skin. In the mastectomy patient, thinner flaps are the rule and the breast tissue is absent. This results in a lack of adequate soft tissue coverage over the implant, sometimes resulting in significant postoperative complications. These problems included a high rate of capsule contracture, exposure of the implant, deformity from skin rippling over the implant, frequent revision operations, and displaced implants.

The concept of tissue expansion developed by Radovan was an important step. The use of expanders could "recruit" additional soft tissues (skin, fat, and muscle) that attempt to make up for the deficiencies following mastectomy. In fact, the most common use of tissue expanders currently is in breast reconstruction [14]. An effort to improve the soft tissue envelope led to developing procedures that provide "total muscle" coverage of the implants using the serratus as well as the pectoralis muscle. The use of tissue expanders and the use of flaps were utilized to improve the soft tissue envelope. Although these efforts reduced the deformity from skin irregularities and exposure of the implant, the problems with capsule contracture and long-term failure of the reconstruction continued.

Acellular dermal matrix is a biologically altered product that is harvested from cadaveric donors and then processed to remove the cells. It has become popular as an adjunct to soft tissue coverage over the lower third of implants and expanders in cases of immediate breast reconstruction. These materials require no donor site and act as a dermal brassiere to help cover and support the implants. All of these efforts have improved the results of non-autologous reconstruction, still the most common procedure for breast reconstruction undertaken in the United States. Unfortunately, there is still a relatively high failure rate, both short and long term. The FDA post-approval CORE studies of breast implants describe, "between 20–40 % of augmentation patients and 40–70 % of reconstruction patients had re-operations during the first 8–10 years after they received their implants. Although routine replacement is not necessary, many women will need additional surgery to modify, remove, or replace their implants." Additionally, 17 % of patients in whom implants were used for reconstruction had their implants removed without replacement [15].

Reconstruction with the Patient's Own Tissue

Because of the problems with implant reconstruction, there has always been interest in using the patient's own tissue to recreate the breast mound. As early as the turn of the century, the latissimus muscle was described for reconstruction. It was not until Carl Hartrampf popularized the transverse rectus abdominis muscle (TRAM) flap in the 1970s that a procedure was devised to use the patulous abdomen (a very favorable donor site) to replace the missing breast [16]. This procedure was truly revolutionary for its time, with the original case experiences reported by Hartrampf found to be very favorable. It was, however, based on very selective patient criteria, excluding those with a history of smoking, diabetes, obesity, macromastia, and hypertension. Nonetheless, the procedure eventually was being performed more commonly, with less rigorous selection.

When the patient selection was not as rigorous, problems with necrosis of the flap and abdominal wall donor site problems (hernia, bulges, etc.) became evident. There were a number of issues that contributed to these problems. First, the procedure harvested the entire rectus muscle and most of the pre-rectus fascia (Fig. 17.3).

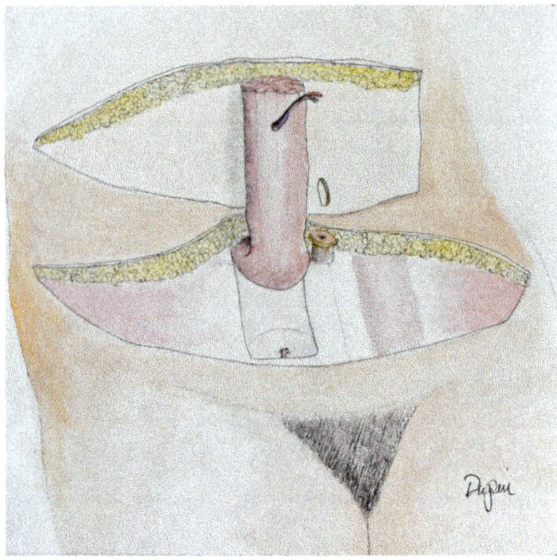

Fig. 17.3 The rotational TRAM flap

This tended to result in functional abdominal wall weakness, more severe for bilateral procedures. The second issue was the circulation to the fat and skin. The primary circulation to the lower abdomen arises from the deep inferior epigastric artery (DIEA). The TRAM flap circulation relied on the deep superior epigastric artery, a continuation of the internal mammary artery. Frequently, the connection of the two vessels around the umbilicus can be tenuous, and without its primary blood supply, ischemia of the flap was a considerable risk. Additionally, in order to move the pedicle flap into the breast defect, a large tunnel had to be created to move the flap (Fig. 17.4). This further impacted the circulation to the upper abdomen.

Several techniques were proposed to try to improve the reliability, including delay of the flaps and using both rectus muscles.

As a result of these issues, attention was turned to the free transfer of tissue. This procedure would utilize the primary blood supply (DIEA), using the lower abdominal tissue as a free transfer, rather than as a pedicle flap. The free TRAM flap was first reported by Holmstrom in 1979 [17] (Fig. 17.5). This procedure also did not require extensive undermining of the upper abdominal as was necessary in the TRAM flap to pass the flap from the abdomen to the chest.

This procedure increased the reliability of the transfer, especially in patients with risk factors such as smoking and obesity. The problem with hernia and bulges in the abdominal wall did not significantly change from the TRAM flap, as the amount of muscle and fascia removed was the same (Fig. 17.6). Lejour and Dome reported a series of patients from whom abdominal flaps were harvested and found significant persistent weakness of the abdominal wall [18].

Due to the significant weakening of the abdominal wall, efforts were made to reduce the amount of muscle and fascia harvested. The muscle-sparing

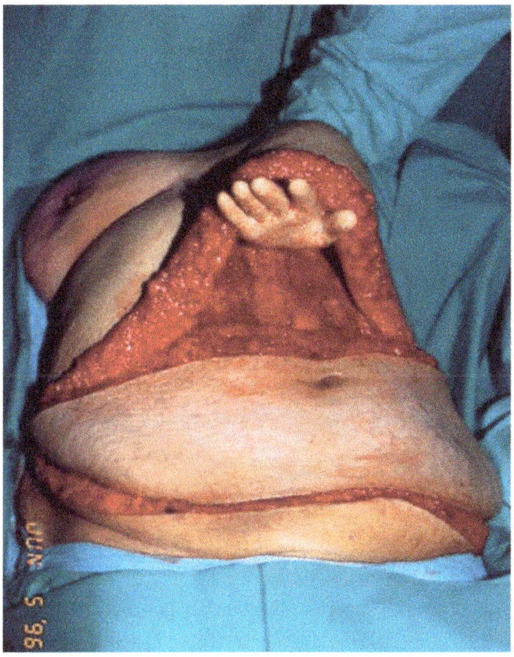

Fig. 17.4 Extensive tunnel required to transfer rotational TRAM flap

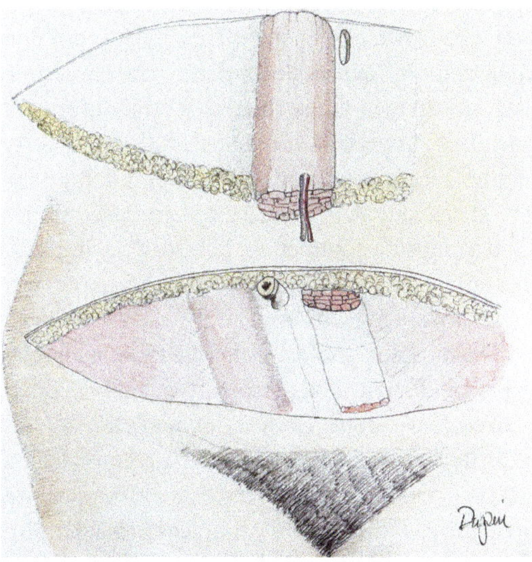

Fig. 17.5 The free TRAM flap

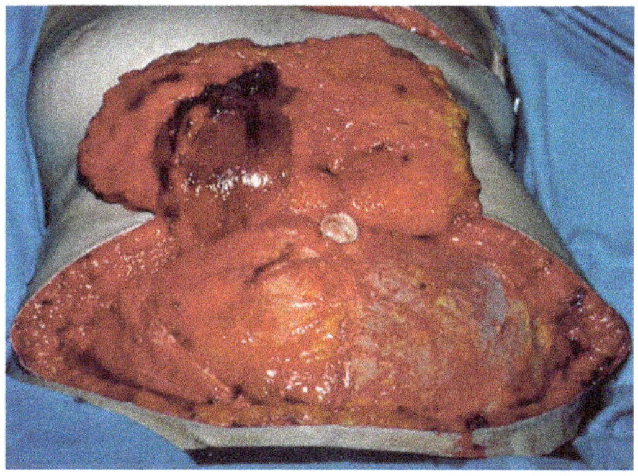

Fig. 17.6 Defect in fascia and muscle in free TRAM

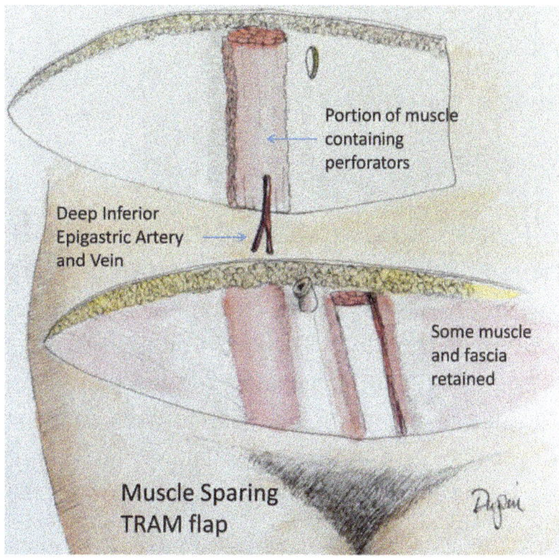

Fig. 17.7 The muscle-sparing TRAM flap

TRAM flap was developed that did not remove all of the muscle or fascia (Fig. 17.7). This procedure retains that which is medial or lateral to the perforators arising from the DIEA.

Unfortunately the bulge/hernia rate between the two procedures was found to be about the same. To address this, the use of plastic mesh was advised to reduce the bulge/hernia rate for these procedures. Although the rate of hernia/bulge is improved by mesh, there are attendant problems with its use and there does not appear to be any improvement in the muscle function [19, 20].

In an effort to reduce abdominal wall complications, procedures to harvest the skin and fat without the rectus muscle or fascia were developed. The most common is the deep inferior epigastric artery perforator (DIEP) flap. This free flap is based on vessels that emerge from the deep inferior epigastric artery, enter and pass through the muscle and fascia, and provide blood supply to the overlying skin (perforating vessels) (Fig. 17.8).

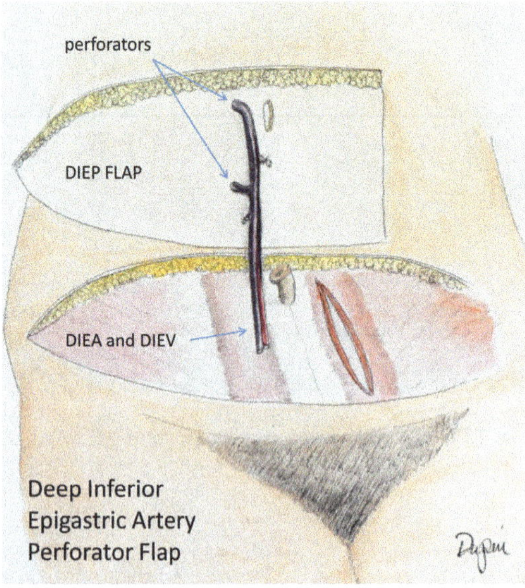

Fig. 17.8 The DIEP flap

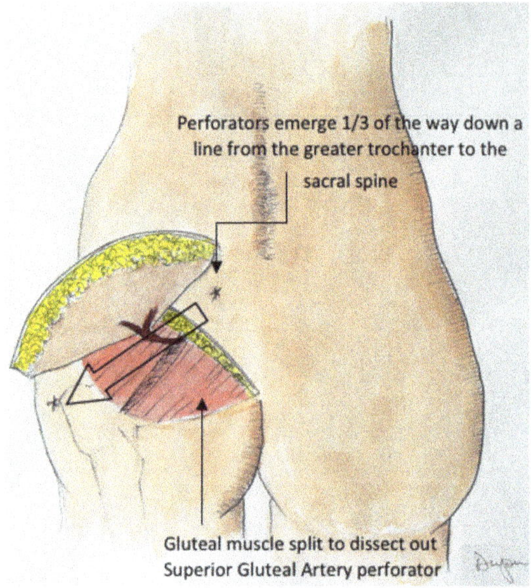

Fig. 17.9 The superior gluteal artery perforator flap

First described by Allen and Blondeel [21, 22], the use of the DIEP flap has increased dramatically as a reconstructive option for autologous breast reconstruction. The very low rate of hernia or bulges without the need for mesh repair was a tremendous improvement, despite the somewhat longer operative time. Even bilateral DIEP flaps can be repaired primarily with no tension on the fascia [23].

Once the perforator concept was described, other sources of tissue for reconstruction were rapidly developed based on the concept of "perforator flaps." These include flaps from the buttocks, thighs, and other areas where there is sufficient fat and skin to harvest. The buttock flaps include those based on perforators arising from the superficial gluteal artery (S-GAP) [24] (Fig. 17.9) and the inferior gluteal artery (I-GAP) [25].

The thigh flaps include the anterolateral thigh flap [26], the gracilis myocutaneous flap [27], and, more recently, a flap based on the second perforating branch of the profunda femoris (Fig. 17.10) [28].

These flaps are typically used in patients when the DIEP flap cannot be used. Patients with a previous abdominoplasty, for example, cannot have the DIEP flap transferred, as all of the perforators to the lower abdomen have been destroyed.

Current Choices

Therefore, two distinct approaches to reconstruction are currently used. The most common approach is expander/implant reconstruction. The advantages are a relatively straightforward operative procedure, a reduced initial morbidity and hospitalization, and the lack of a donor site. The disadvantages include implant-based issues such as capsule contracture, failure of the implant, multiple procedures, and lack of adequate soft tissue coverage (see above).

The most favorable patients are those with relatively small, non-ptotic breasts, especially in bilateral reconstructions. The least favorable are patients with large ptotic breasts, delayed reconstruction patients, and patients who have undergone, or will undergo, radiation therapy. Implant/expander procedures are also less satisfactory in obese patients and patients with macromastia or severe ptosis. The rate of complications, while initially low, also tends to increase over time. Revision procedures have a higher complication rate than the original procedure. Nonetheless, the majority of these procedures are successful and have a high level of patient satisfaction [29].

The second approach to breast reconstruction is autologous in nature, utilizing the patient's own

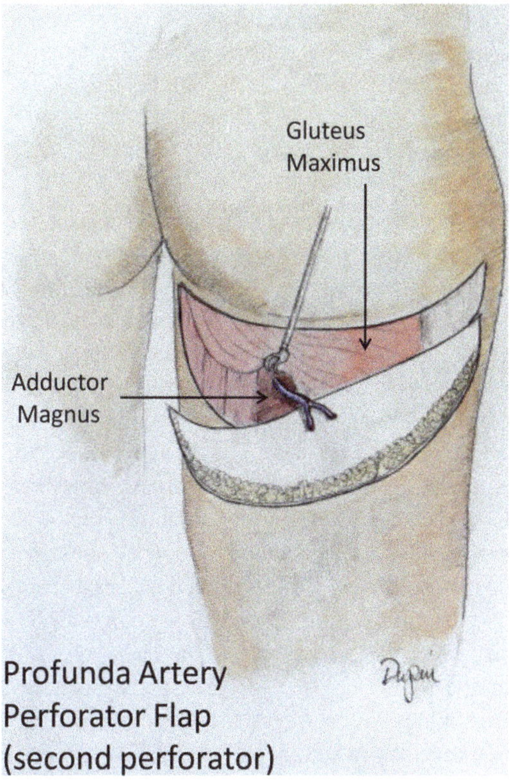

Fig. 17.10 The profunda artery perforator flap

tissue. The advantages are as follows: permanence, lack of implant problems, ease of reshaping the breast mound, and (for most patients) a tight, flat postoperative abdomen. The disadvantages are higher early complication rate (including the loss of the flap), donor site problems, longer initial operative time, and scars in the donor site area. The rate of total flap loss in microsurgical breast reconstruction is 5 % or less in most series. Patient satisfaction with the procedure and overall cosmetic outcome is quite high [30].

The optimal candidates are patients with delayed reconstruction (especially with radiation changes), patients with poor quality chest wall soft tissues, patients with macromastia or ptosis, and patients with bilateral reconstruction. Patients with extensive disease may require chest wall reconstruction and benefit from free transfers. Poor candidates are patients who cannot withstand anesthesia risks of long surgery, hypercoagulable patients, morbidly obese patients, and smokers.

Other factors that have tended to increase the rate of breast reconstruction include patient demand for mastectomy instead of conservative breast treatment and the discovery of genetic predisposition (BRCA1 and BRCA2) for breast cancer. Despite the original optimism for breast conservation surgery, a significant number of patients continue to select mastectomy as their desired surgical option, with a growing number further opting to undergoing prophylactic mastectomy of the contralateral breast with immediate reconstruction. Although the data is clear that the statistical chance of survival is based upon the original cancer, many patients will still fear a recurrence, no matter how small or insignificant the risk.

The discovery of genetic factors [BRCA gene mutations] responsible for the development of breast cancer has resulted in a new population of patients that requires therapy. Many of these patients, especially those who have seen close family members struggling with breast cancer, opt for bilateral mastectomy, additionally wanting immediate reconstruction.

Immediate Versus Delayed Breast Reconstruction

In the subset of breast cancer patients who require or choose mastectomy, the discussion with the patient focuses upon whether to proceed immediately with reconstruction or to wait a period of time for a delayed procedure. There are sound oncologic reasons for delaying reconstruction in some patients. Patients who will require radiation therapy are more likely to have a much better outcome with delayed reconstruction, especially when autologous reconstruction is performed. A full course of chest wall radiation can result in significant and sometimes unpredictable changes within the radiated flap, including fat necrosis, scarring, and loss of tissue volume. The aesthetic outcomes are far better with delayed reconstruction in these patients. Patients treated with expanders and implants have a significantly higher complication rate for all complications when radiation therapy is used.

Immediate reconstruction provides several benefits. The preservation of the breast skin envelope around the reconstructed breast produces a more aesthetically pleasing result and reduces the visible scar. Immediate reconstruction also avoids the emotional distress of awakening without a breast mound. Immediate reconstruction was noted by Rozen to have a positive effect on anxiety, depression, self-image, and emotional as well as sexual function [31]. There is no evidence that forcing the patient to wait and live with her defect improves patient acceptance.

There have been numerous studies examining the safety of immediate breast reconstruction, with no apparent increase in the rates of local or distant recurrences noted in this group of patients. There was also no significant delay in the timeliness of delivering adjuvant chemotherapy. Furthermore, the detection of a local recurrence in the immediate reconstruction patients is not impaired. However, the rates of postoperative complications with respect to radiation are increased. This will be discussed further below [32].

Prophylactic Mastectomy and Breast Reconstruction

Gurunluoglu et al. demonstrated that around 16 % of all breast reconstructions were performed after prophylactic mastectomy. Prophylactic mastectomy has a demonstrated cancer risk reduction of up to 90 %. It appears that more women are electing to have a bilateral mastectomy in the setting of unilateral breast cancer to reduce their risk of developing breast cancer in the other breast. Many reasons are given, such as a strong family history, fear of developing breast cancer, having had chemotherapy or knowing someone who has struggled with chemotherapy, or positive genetic testing results for the BRCA1 or BRCA2 mutations [33]. Spear et al. notes that in regard to prophylactic mastectomy with breast reconstruction, surgical results vary from center to center and are even surgeon specific. He hypothesizes, "the best prophylaxis and best cosmetic results from prophylactic mastectomy and reconstruction will come from centers that become most skilled at these operations" [34]. Patients undergoing prophylactic mastectomy who do not have invasive cancer should have treatment directed by a team approach. In these patients the aesthetic result is more critical, and the decision on mastectomy incision and skin- and nipple-sparing issues should be carefully addressed.

Oncoplastic Surgery

The practice of partial mastectomy and radiation for the treatment of select breast tumors has become more common over the past decade. With 25 years of follow-up data, reports have shown equivalent disease-free and overall survival when comparing partial mastectomy and radiation to total mastectomy alone [35–37]. The 2008 National Cancer Database reported the national rate of breast conservation therapy to be 64 % [38]. As breast conservation therapy for the treatment of breast cancer has increased, the aesthetic outcomes of these procedures have come under scrutiny. Partial mastectomy can refer to a size of breast tissue resection as small as a lumpectomy up to a full quadrantectomy. Depending on the size of the breast, these resections can have a significant impact on the postoperative breast shape and volume.

The option to allow a woman to keep her breast is attractive, if the result does not leave a significant deformity. However, poor aesthetic outcomes have been reported in 25–30 % of cases [39]. As a result, oncoplastic surgical techniques have developed with an overall goal for "a complete surgical resection of disease, prevention of tumor recurrence, and preservation of a natural and cosmetically acceptable breast" [40]. One benefit of oncoplastic surgery is the ability to resect a wider tissue margin without compromising aesthetic outcomes [41]. Though not affecting overall survival, a wider surgical margin has been shown to significantly decrease recurrence rate [42]. Additionally, for women with macromastia, an oncoplastic reduction prior to radiation therapy may allow for easier radiation planning, with an ultimate decrease in long-term radiation fibrosis [43, 44]. If a reduction is not performed prior to radiation and a patient has significant deformity with radiation treatment, a postradiation reduction can be quite difficult.

Numerous articles have outlined techniques and algorithms aimed at providing the best surgical approach to various breast tumors [39, 45–50].

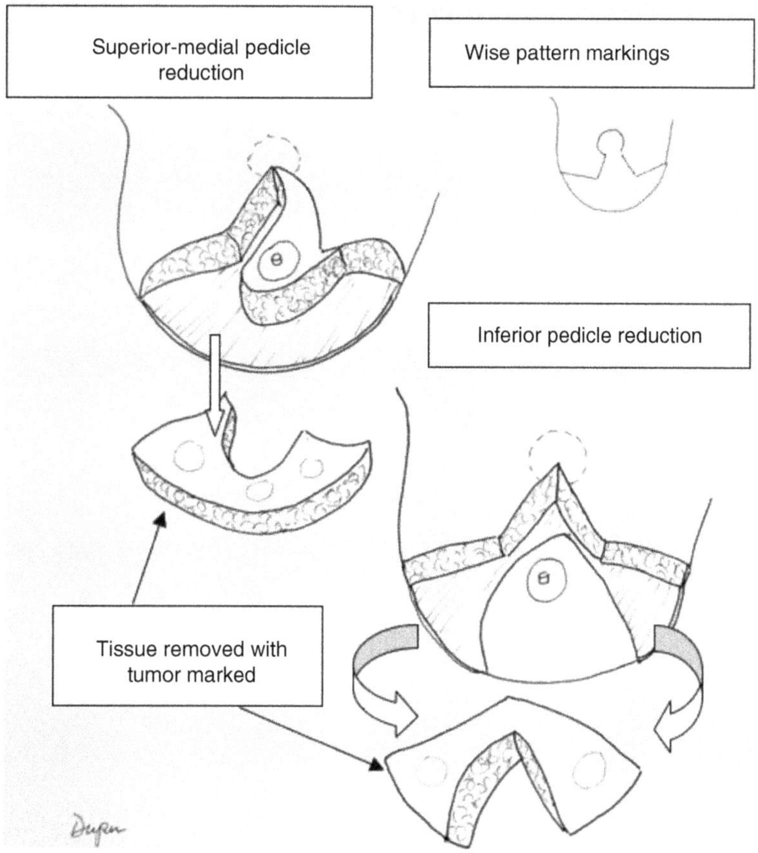

Fig. 17.11 Reduction techniques that can be used to remove localized breast tumor

As Kronowitz outlines in his algorithm, an A or B cup breast is often best treated either by a mastectomy and reconstruction or by filling the defect with a local or regional flap [45]. Those patients with a C cup or larger breasts, once evaluated for tumor location and ptosis, will undergo tissue remodeling or an oncologic reduction. These patients will require whole breast radiation. Whole versus partial breast radiation has been a further trend since the Z0011 trial as patients with favorable tumors and a positive sentinel node can forego an axillary dissection if undergoing whole breast radiation therapy [51].

If a patient has a C cup breast without ptosis, a tissue rearrangement approach can assist in filling a partial mastectomy defect. This involves mobilizing the entire skin envelope from the breast, then redraping the tissue over a breast mound remolded with local breast or subcutaneous tissue. Preserving the breast tissue perforators from the base of the breast is essential for ensuring tissue viability. Other options for those with minimal ptosis involve various mastopexy-type resections. A donut mastopexy can be performed by excising a ring of skin surrounding the nipple and then resecting the tumor and closing with a purse-string stitch. Another possibility for a superior tumor in either a central or medial position is performing the resection with a batwing-shaped skin excision. These two options allow for smaller scars with a minor lifting procedure [48].

For those patients with large breasts and ptosis, the best breast conservation surgical intervention is an oncoplastic reduction. For reasons described above, the best timing of this surgery is at the time of tumor resection. A symmetry procedure on the opposite breast can then be completed after radiation therapy. In our practice, a Wise pattern resection is predominantly performed. The reduction technique utilizes a superiorly based pedicle for inferior tumors and an inferiorly based pedicle for superior tumors (Fig. 17.11).

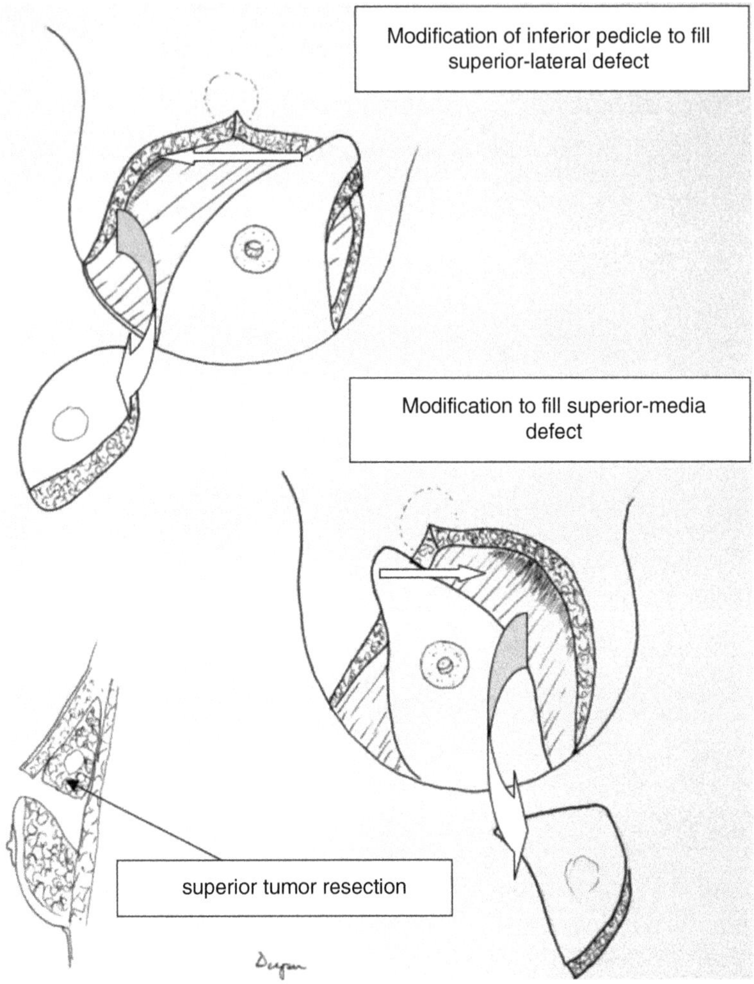

Fig. 17.12 Modifications of standard technique to repair nipple areola defects

The pedicles can be tailored to assist in replacing the volume lost with the resection, depending on tumor location. Often, a limb of tissue that would have been resected in a standard reduction mammoplasty is retained to rotate into the defect created by the tumor resection. Kronowitz reports using an inframedial pedicle for superior and infralateral tumors [45]. He purports that the additional medial tissue adds both volume and additional blood supply. If the tumor is located in a central and inferior location, a vertical reduction mammoplasty can be performed with a superior pedicle. Clough describes rotating the Wise pattern toward the tumor to resect the skin with the tumor [39] (Fig. 17.12).

Regardless of the technique, the principles remain consistent, that is, to maintain an oncologic resection while utilizing local tissue to remold a breast mound with an appropriate skin pocket. Oncoplastic surgery will continue to evolve as breast conservation therapy persists and grows. With a sound understanding of breast anatomy and effective planning/communication with the oncologic surgeon, favorable outcomes from both an oncologic and aesthetic standpoint can be attained (Table 17.1).

In summary, during the senior author's 35-year career, the field of breast reconstruction has had an amazing development. In 1976, in which the author began training,

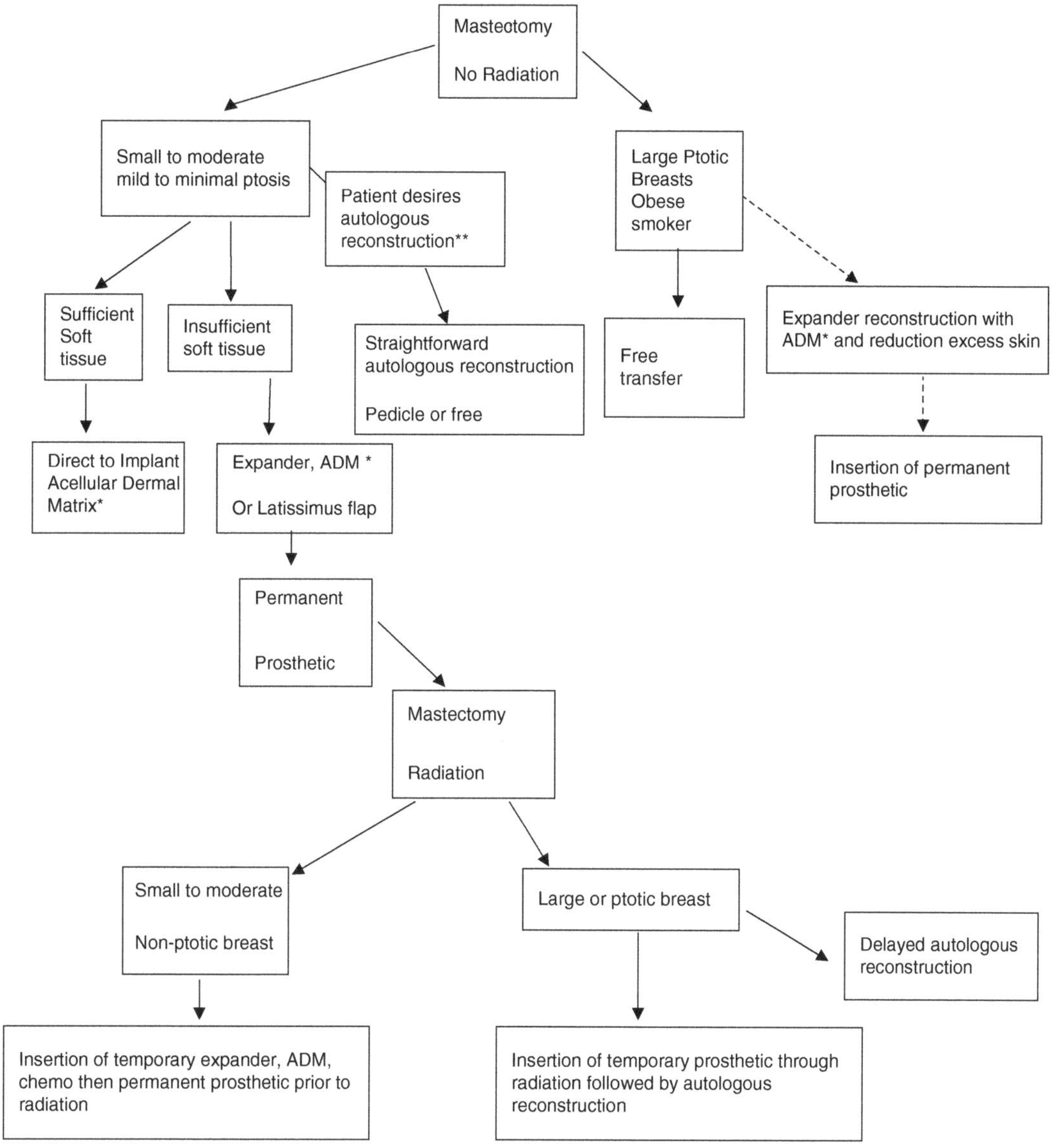

Table 17.1 Our algorithm for breast reconstruction

there was virtually no breast reconstruction performed. Techniques were not available and patient's deformities were severe and complicated. Today, we have good reliable options for reconstruction with a high rate of patient satisfaction.

It has been the privilege of plastic surgeons to help these patients feel whole again after mastectomy.

References

1. Dean C, Chetty U, Forrest AP. Effects of immediate breast reconstruction on psychosocial morbidity after mastectomy. Lancet. 1983;320:459–62.
2. Schain WS. Breast reconstruction: update of psychosocial and pragmatic concerns. Cancer. 1991;68:1170–5.
3. Cederna PS, Yates WR, Chang P, Cram AE, Ricciardelli EJ. Post mastectomy reconstruction:

comparative analysis of the psychosocial, functional, and cosmetic effects of transverse rectus abdominis musculocutaneous versus breast implant reconstruction. Ann Plast Surg. 1995;35:458–68.
4. Wilkins EG, Alderman AK. Breast reconstruction practices in North America: current trends and future priorities. Semin Plast Surg. 2004;18(2):149–55.
5. Alderman AK, Hawley ST, Waljee J, et al. Correlates of referral practices of general surgeons to plastic surgeons for mastectomy reconstruction. Cancer. 2007; 109:1715.
6. Alderman AK, Atisha D, Streu R, et al. Patterns and correlates of postmastectomy breast reconstruction by U. S. Plastic surgeons: results from a national survey. Plast Reconstr Surg. 2011;127:1796.
7. Halsted WS. The results of radical operations for the cure of cancer of the breast. Ann Surg. 1907;46:1.
8. Czerny V. Plastischer Ersatz der Brustdrusse durch ein Lipom. Drei Plastiche Operationen. Verh Dtsch Ges Chir. 1895;24:216.
9. Tansini I. Sopra il mio nuovo processo di amputazione della mammella. Gazz Med Ital. 1906;57:141.
10. Papatestas AE, Lesnick GJ. Treatment of carcinoma of the breast by modified radical mastectomy. Surg Gynecol Obstet. 1975;140(1):22–6.
11. Freeman BS. Subcutaneous mastectomy for benign breast lesions with immediate or delayed prosthetic replacement. Plast Reconstr Surg. 1962;30:676.
12. Toth BA, Lappert P. Modified skin incisions for mastectomy: the need for plastic surgical input in preoperative planning. Plast Reconstr Surg. 1991; 87:1048.
13. Cronin TD, Gerow FJ. Augmentation mammaplasty: a new "natural feel" prosthesis. In: Broadbent TR, editor. Transactions of the Third International Congress of Plastic and Reconstructive Surgery, Oct 13–18, 1963, Amsterdam, The Netherlands, Excerpta Medica Foundation, pp. 41–49.
14. Radovan C. Breast reconstruction after mastectomy using the temporary expander. Plast Reconstr Surg. 1982;69:195.
15. FDA update on the safety of silicone gel-filled breast implants. Center for Devices and Radiological Health U.S. Food and Drug Administration. Accessed Jun 2011.
16. Hartrampf CR, Scheflan M, Black PW. Breast reconstruction with a transverse abdominal island flap. Plast Reconstr Surg. 1982;69:216.
17. Holmstrom H. The free abdominoplasty flap and its use in breast reconstruction. An experimental study and clinical case report. Scand J Plast Reconstr Surg. 1979;13:423.
18. Lejour M, Dome M. Abdominal wall function after rectus abdominis transfer. Plast Reconstr Surg. 1991;87:1054.
19. Zienowicz RJ, May Jr JW. Hernia prevention and aesthetic contouring of the abdomen following TRAM flap breast reconstruction by the use of polypropylene mesh. Plast Reconstr Surg. 1995;96:1346.
20. Shestak KC, Fedele GM, Restifo RJ. Treatment of difficult TRAM flap hernias using intraperitoneal synthetic mesh application. Plast Reconstr Surg. 2001;107:55.
21. Blondeel PN, Vanderstraeten GG, Monstrey SJ, et al. The donor site morbidity of free DIEP flaps and free TRAM flaps for breast reconstruction. Br J Plast Surg. 1997;50:322.
22. Allen RJ, Treece P. Deep inferior epigastric perforator flap for breast reconstruction. Ann Plast Surg. 1994;32:32.
23. Gill P, Hunt J, Guerra A, et al. A 10-year retrospective review of 758 DIEP flaps for breast reconstruction. Plast Reconstr Surg. 2004;113:1153.
24. Guerra A, Metzinger S, Bidros R, et al. Breast reconstruction with gluteal artery perforator (GAP) flaps: a critical analysis of 142 cases. Ann Plast Surg. 2004; 52:118.
25. Robert J, Allen RJ, Levine JL, Granzow JW. The in-the-crease inferior Gluteal artery perforator flap for breast reconstruction. Plast Reconstr Surg. 2006;118(2):333–9.
26. Wei FC, Suominen S, Cheng M, Celik N, Lai Y. Anterolateral thigh flap for postmastectomy breast reconstruction. Plast Reconstr Surg. 2002;110(1):82–8.
27. Fansa H, Schirmer S, Warnecke IC, Cervelli A, Frerichs O. The transverse myocutaneous gracilis muscle flap: a fast and reliable method for breast reconstruction. Plast Reconstr Surg. 2008;122(5): 1326–33.
28. Allen RJ, Haddock NT, Ahn CY, Sadeghi A. Breast reconstruction with the Profunda artery perforator flap. Plast Reconstr Surg. 2012;129(1):16e–23.
29. Macadam SA, Ho AL, Cook Jr EF, Lennox PA, Pusic AL. Patient satisfaction and health-related quality of life following breast reconstruction: patient-reported outcomes among saline and silicone implant recipients. Plast Reconstr Surg. 2010;125(3):761–71.
30. Alderman AK, Wilkins EG, Lowery JC, Myra K, Davis JA. Determinants of patient satisfaction in postmastectomy breast reconstruction. Plast Reconstr Surg. 2000;106(4):769–76.
31. Rozen WM, Ashton MW, Taylor GI. Defining the role for autologous breast reconstruction after mastectomy: social and oncologic implications. Clin Breast Cancer. 2008;8(2):134–42.
32. Taylor CW, Horgan K, Dodwell D. Oncological aspects of breast reconstruction. Breast. 2005;14(2): 118–30.
33. Gurunluoglu R, Gurunluoglu A, Williams SA, Tebockhorst S. Current trends in breast reconstruction. Ann Plast Surg. 2011;70(1):103–10.
34. Spear SL, Mary Ella C, Karl S. Prophylactic mastectomy: indications, options, and reconstructive alternatives. Plast Reconstr Surg. 2005;115(3):891–909.
35. Fisher B, Anderson S, Bryant J, et al. Twenty-year follow-up a randomized trial comparing total mastectomy, lumpectomy, and lumpectomy plus irradiation for the treatment of invasive breast cancer. N Engl J Med. 2002;347:1233–41.

36. Veronesi U, Cascinelli N, Mariani L, et al. Twenty-year follow-up of a randomized study comparing breast conserving surgery with radical mastectomy for early breast cancer. N Engl J Med. 2002;347: 1227–32.
37. Fisher B, Jeong JH, Anderson S, et al. Twenty-five year follow-up of a randomized trial comparing radical mastectomy, total mastectomy, and total mastectomy followed by irradiation. N Engl J Med. 2002; 347:567–75.
38. Nelson MC, Norton HJ, Greene FL. Breast conservation therapy versus mastectomy in the community-based setting: can this rate be used as a benchmark for cancer care? Surg Oncol Clin N Am. 2011;20:427–37.
39. Clough KB, Cuminet J, Fitoussi A, et al. Cosmetic sequelae after conservative treatment for breast cancer: classification and results of surgical treatment. Ann Plast Surg. 1998;41:471–81.
40. Losken A, Elwood ET, Styblo TM, et al. The role of reduction mammaplasty in reconstructing partial mastectomy defects. Plast Reconstr Surg. 2002;109: 968–75.
41. Kaur N, Petit JY, Rietjens M, et al. Comparative study of surgical margins in oncoplastic surgery and quadrantectomy in breast cancer. Ann Surg Oncol. 2005;12:539–45.
42. Veronesi U, Volterrani F, Luini A, et al. Quadrantectomy versus lumpectomy for small size breast cancer. Eur J Cancer. 1990;26:671–3.
43. Smith ML, Evans GR, Gurlek A, et al. Reduction mammaplasty: its role in breast conservation surgery for early-stage breast cancer. Ann Plast Surg. 1998;41:234–9.
44. Brierly JD, Paterson IC, Lallemand RC, et al. The influence of breast size on late radiation reaction following excision and radiotherapy for early breast cancer. Clin Oncol (R Coll Radiol). 1991;3:6–9.
45. Kronowitz SJ, Kuerer HM, Buchholz TA. A management algorithm and practical oncoplastic surgical techniques for repairing partial mastectomy defects. Plast Reconstr Surg. 2008;122:1631–47.
46. Kronowitz SJ, Hunt KK, Kuerer HM. Practical guidelines for repair of partial mastectomy defects using the breast reduction technique in patients undergoing breast conservation therapy. Plast Reconstr Surg. 2007;120:1755–68.
47. Berry MG, Fitoussi AD, Curnier A, et al. Oncoplastic breast surgery: a review and systemic approach. J Plast Reconstr Aesthet Surg. 2010;63:1233–43.
48. Anderson B, Masetti R, Silverstein M. Oncoplastic approaches to partial mastectomy: an overview of volume-displacement techniques. Lancet Oncol. 2005;6:145–57.
49. Gainer SM, Lucci A. Oncoplastics: techniques for reconstruction of partial breast defects based on tumor location. J Surg Oncol. 2011;103:341–7.
50. Masetti R, Di Leone A, Franceshini G, et al. Oncoplastic techniques in the conservative surgical treatment of breast cancer: an overview. Breast. 2006;12:174–80.
51. Giuliano AE, McCall L, Beitsch P, et al. Locoregional recurrence after sentinel lymph node dissection with or without axillary dissection in patients with sentinel lymph node metastases: the American College of Surgeons Oncology Group Z0011 randomized trial. Ann Surg. 2010;252:426–32.

18 Breast Reconstruction with Expanders and Implants

Charles Dupin, M'liss Hogan, Haiqiao Jiao, and M. Whitten Wise

Non-autologous breast reconstruction remains the predominant type of reconstruction in the United States today. In 2011, the American Society of Plastic Surgeons reported in their yearly statistical analysis that up to 75 % of their breast reconstructions were implant based [1].

Autologous reconstruction was the mainstay from 1998 to 2001, until in 2002, implant reconstruction became the most common form of breast reconstruction. In 2008, data showed that expander/implant reconstruction outnumbered autologous nearly 2:1 [2, 3].

There are a number of patient choice reasons for this shift in reconstructive options: (1) the decreased time for recovery, (2) an apparent reduction in operative time and hospitalization (when compared to autologous procedures), and (3) the lack of additional donor site. Many patients find these to be appealing advantages. There is also an institutional and individual surgeon bias. Autologous reconstruction is more arduous, technically difficult, for the surgeon, with longer operative time, more risk of early complications in the breast, and the possibility of donor site complications that will require further treatment. Physician reimbursement rates also play a role in the type of reconstructions being performed.

C. Dupin, MD (✉) • M. Hogan, MD
M.W. Wise, MD
Division of Plastic Surgery, Department of Surgery, Louisiana State University Health Sciences Center, 1542 Tulane Avenue, New Orleans, LA 70112, USA
e-mail: cldupinmd@gmail.com; mhoga1@lsuhsc.edu; mwhitwise@gmail.com

H. Jiao, MD
Department of Surgery, Louisiana State University Health Sciences Center, 1542 Tulane Avenue, New Orleans, LA 70124, USA
e-mail: jiao@lsuhsc.edu

Immediate Breast Reconstruction with Expanders and Implants

The surgeon should be certain that the patient has realistic expectations of the likely outcome from reconstruction and the patient must understand the risks of implant/expander reconstruction. Breast reconstruction is not the same operation as augmentation mammoplasty, and patients should not expect the same outcome. The frequent request to "be larger" should be tempered, and the significantly increased rates of complications with larger prosthetics should be discussed. The implant chosen should have a base diameter that is similar to the native breast. Cohesive silicone gel implants are used in order to minimize rippling of the overlying mastectomy skin and to provide a more natural appearance and feel.

Patients with large and/or ptotic breasts must be counseled about the complications of skin reduction at the time of mastectomy. Nonetheless, the breast must be reduced to avoid reconstruction of an aesthetically undesirable breast. The excess skin resected will remove questionably viable skin. Mastectomy flaps are thinner and

A.I. Riker (ed.), *Breast Disease: Comprehensive Management*,
DOI 10.1007/978-1-4939-1145-5_18, © Springer Science+Business Media New York 2015

have more tenuous blood supply than those associated with reduction mammoplasty. It is important to avoid standard reduction mammoplasty patterns when attempting implant breast reconstruction. Mastectomy flaps created are fragile and have an unreliable blood supply. These patients are better served with a transverse incision for the mastectomy approach. Additionally, the loss of the mastectomy skin flap in the face of an implant is far more problematic than necrosis in reduction mammoplasty because of the underlying implant.

Some patients are candidates for replacing the excised tissue with an implant at the time of mastectomy (direct-to-implant reconstruction). In some cases, the reconstruction may be accomplished in a single stage. Ideal patients for the single-stage direct-to-implant technique are women with smaller breasts and no ptosis. Patients of this type are good candidates for mastectomy via inframammary fold incision. Surgeons must be willing to perform the mastectomy through this incision, and plastic surgeons must be willing to accept the somewhat restricted access for mound reconstruction. Nonetheless, the results from a nipple-sparing mastectomy performed through the inframammary incision clearly provide a superior aesthetic result. Either implant or autologous reconstruction can be undertaken via this approach.

Patients who require excision of the nipple-aureola complex or resection of excess skin may also be candidates for reconstruction initially with an implant, if the skin is adequate in size and viability.

Some patients, however, have complicating issues that make "direct-to-implant" reconstruction technically challenging. Patients who have had a substantial skin/nipple resection may require skin expansion because the remaining skin may be insufficient to cover the required implant. Patients with large ptotic breasts or women with obesity and a small, thin pectoralis muscle or questionably robust mastectomy skin will do better with a staged (expander) reconstruction. In both cases, the soft tissue deficiency should be addressed by using an expander rather than a permanent implant at the time of mastectomy. Expanders are devices that are made with a silicone shell and a valve that is used to add saline percutaneously to increase the volume. Expanders must be replaced with permanent implants when the volume is appropriate.

Appropriate tissue expanders or implants should be available. The diameter of the expander should fit within the base diameter of the breast to be removed. Both tissue expanders and implants are produced in a number of shapes and sizes. Anatomic tissue expanders aid in greater lower pole expansion, giving the appearance of a natural breast. Most tissue expanders incorporate a valve that can be identified externally with a magnet. In the office setting, a needle is used to access the port for adding volume.

Reconstructive surgeons should be present for preoperative markings on patients undergoing mastectomy. At this time, the skin incisions can be marked. Excessive removal of mastectomy skin will limit the volume of fill at the time of mastectomy. The oncologic and plastic surgeons should arrive at a consensus about the amount of skin to be removed. Landmarks such as the inframammary fold, the limits of breast excision, and previous biopsy sites in the skin to be excised are marked. The oncologic surgeon, taking care not to devitalize the skin envelope of the breast, performs the mastectomy. Every attempt should be made by the oncologic surgeon to respect the boundaries of the breast. Preserving the inframammary fold and the lateral borders of the breast will improve the subsequent stages of reconstruction. The "Wise" pattern markings, used in reduction, are risky because the mastectomy skin flap viability is much more tenuous than the thick flaps found in reduction mammoplasty. Transverse incisions, which preserve blood supply to the lower flaps, are safer. The primary goal of the oncologic surgeon is to ensure that the cancer is removed with the necessary and appropriate margins, with a collaborative effort and discussion with the plastic surgeon to optimize patient outcome.

Mastectomy skin flaps alone are not enough to provide adequate soft tissue coverage of the implant or tissue expander. Thin flaps have a significant risk of skin flap necrosis, extrusion of implant, visible folds, or rippling of the implant. In order to address the soft tissue deficiency, the pectoralis major muscle is raised from the chest wall to cover the superior two-thirds of the implant/expander. Dissection is taken superiorly to the second rib. Medial attachments of the pectoralis major to the sternum are kept intact to prevent symmastia. All lateral and costal attachments are raised. A tissue expander is then placed in the pocket. At this time the tissue expander should be partially filled to the tolerance of the mastectomy flaps and pectoralis major. If the space around the expander is not partially filled, there is increased risk of seroma. In most patients, the upper two-thirds of the device will be covered by the muscle. This leaves a deficiency in the coverage of the lower portion of the device that needs to be addressed. The choices are either to raise the serratus muscle to attempt to cover the lower pole, which is technically difficult, or to cover the lower pole with a free dermal graft or acellular dermal matrix.

Today, the majority of US reconstructive surgeons who perform expander-based reconstruction use some type of acellular dermal matrix (ADM) to cover and support the inferior pole of tissue expander and eventual implant [3–5]. ADM is an allograft of human dermis. Cellular components of the dermis are removed which render the graft nonimmunogenic. The ADM forms a brassiere extending along the inframammary fold to the lateral edge of the pectoralis at the anterior axillary fold. The dermal side of the ADM should face the mastectomy flap in order to allow vascular ingrowth. The matrix is sutured medially and inferiorly to the chest wall at the level of the IMF. Once lateral to the IMF, the matrix is sutured to the chest wall itself. The ADM is then attached to the chest wall, along the lateral margin of the breast pocket (Fig. 18.1). Prior to completing the closure, the expander is placed and the ADM is then sutured into place superiorly at the lower edge of the previously elevated pectoralis major muscle. The ADM allows for better pocket control, reduces stress on the mastectomy skin flaps, and allows greater initial tissue expansion. This can decrease the total number of expansions needed. Reports have shown an improved stability of the IMF, as well as a protection of inferior pole of the expander. Suction drains are placed in the subpectoral and skin pocket. A drain may also be placed in the axilla if an axillary dissection has been performed.

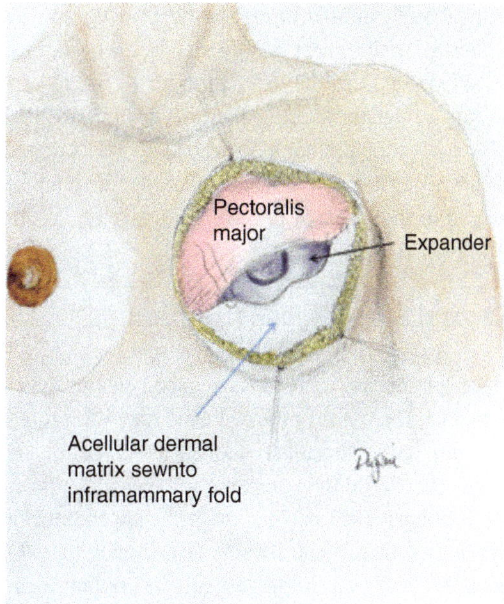

Fig. 18.1 Expander reconstruction with acellular dermal matrix

Postoperative Course

The postoperative course of non-autologous reconstruction patients is straightforward. It consists of an overnight stay in the hospital with drain-care teaching. Drains are removed 1–2 weeks postoperatively when output falls to <30 cc/day. It is extremely important to treat the drains as one would treat a central line, with meticulous site care. Infection arising from the drains is a serious problem and may well cause cellulitis, periprosthetic infection, or loss of the implant.

After healing of incisions (2–3 weeks), tissue expansion may begin. The magnetic port finder is used to locate the valve. The amount to sterile saline injected is surgeon dependent; amounts from 50 to 120 cc can be injected. Patient comfort often dictates the amount of saline injected at one time. Care must be taken to avoid overexpansion at a single setting, which can lead to skin flap necrosis. Expansions can occur weekly and last from 3 to 6 months, until the desired volume is achieved. In the unilateral setting, the contralateral breast size guides the expansion need. Some surgeons advocate overexpansion of up to 110–120 % over the patient's desired size. This creates a natural ptotic result when a smaller implant is placed in the larger skin envelope.

Second Stage Reconstruction

Once appropriate volume is reached in the tissue expander, the patient returns to the operating room for implant placement. Cohesive silicone gel implants are used for a more natural feel and appearance. Cohesive gel also decreases the appearance of rippling of the reconstructed breast. During the past decade, continuing improvements in implant technology has made a tremendous improvement in outcomes. If the patient has had a shaped expander, a matching implant should be used. Preoperatively, with the patient standing, landmarks of the breast are marked. The capsule is assessed; areas in need of capsulorrhaphy or capsulotomy are appropriately marked. The base diameter is again confirmed. Several sizes of previously chosen implants should be available. The un-inflated tissue expander can add as much as 100 cc to the total volume needed. This needs to be taken into consideration when deciding upon the final volume of the implant, and not just the amount of fill.

A portion of the previous skin incision is opened. If the mastectomy was previously performed through a transverse incision and the breast has good contour and projection, another option is to utilize an inframammary incision along the lateral aspect of the breast rather than reoperating through a central transverse scar. This avoids flattening of the anterior breast with the additional surgery through the old scar. Occasionally, a Z-plasty must be performed to further release the central scar. Dissection is taken through the subcutaneous tissue to the pectoralis muscle. The muscle is split with the electrocautery and capsule is incised. Capsulorrhaphy or capsulotomy is performed as needed. Once hemostasis is achieved, the appropriately sized implant is placed in the pocket. The wound is then closed in multiple layers paying special attention to avoid piercing the newly placed implant. At this stage, patients may elect to undergo a symmetry procedure on contralateral breast. This can include reduction, mastopexy or augmentation, depending upon the patient's need. This is performed as an outpatient procedure performed without need for drains. A soft bra is worn for several weeks. Nipple reconstruction is usually performed up to 2–3 months following implant placement and will be discussed later in the chapter on revision surgery.

Variations of Implant-Based Reconstructions

Delayed Reconstruction with Implants

When reconstruction is delayed, the challenges of using implants and expanders are much greater compared to immediate reconstruction. This is especially true when there has been a long period of time between the mastectomy and reconstruction. The skin is deficient and usually adherent to the underlying pectoralis. Frequently the inframammary fold is distorted or lost and providing adequate soft tissue becomes a challenge. This insufficient, thin, and scarred skin is very difficult to expand with an expander alone. Patients having delayed reconstruction are most effectively treated with an autologous reconstruction rather than implant based reconstruction. If implant based reconstruction is to be accomplished the deficiency can be remied. The deficiency can be remedied by adding tissue to the mastectomy site, in the form of regional flaps. The latissimus dorsi muscle transfer is the most common transfer (Fig. 18.2). Even with the improved soft tissue envelope, an expander may have to be used to provide space for an eventual prosthesis.

Direct-to-Implant Breast Reconstruction

The use of ADM has renewed interest in an old method of implant-based reconstruction. In the past, when implants were placed beneath thin mastectomy flaps without adequate soft tissue coverage, complications were common and the aesthetic results were suboptimal. With the scaffolding

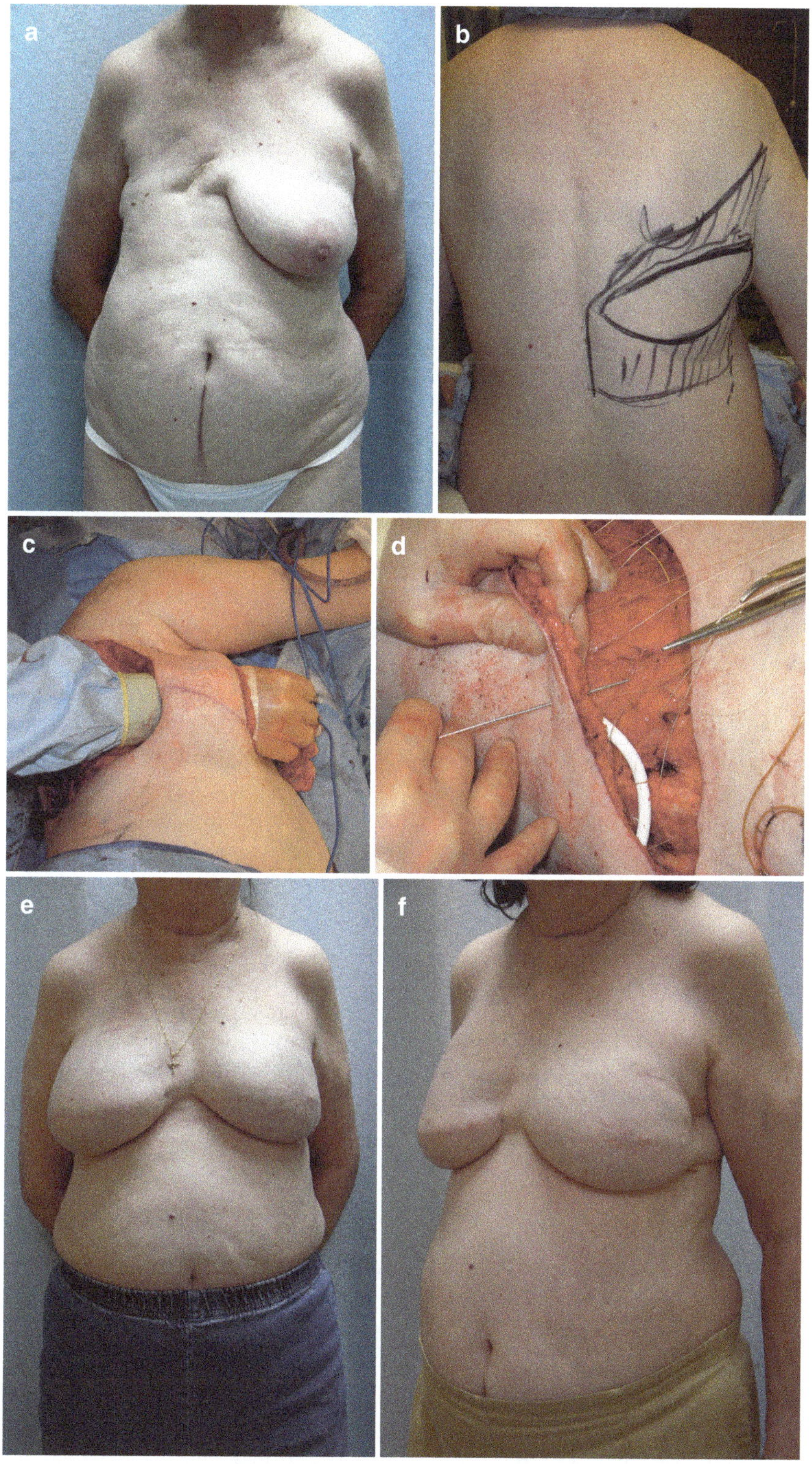

Fig. 18.2 Delayed reconstruction with latissimus dorsi myocutaneous flap and expander. (**a**) Preoperative view showing shortage of soft tissue. (**b**) Preoperative markings for latissimus myocutaneous flap. (**c**) Intraoperative view of tunnel through which the flap is passed. (**d**) Sewing the acellular dermal matrix to the lateral chest wall to shape pocket for expander. (**e, f**) Three postoperative result (Patient had opposite side mastectomy and implant reconstruction)

created by utilizing ADM, immediate implant-based reconstruction is now a feasible option.

This reconstruction may be done as a single-stage procedure. The ideal candidate for the single-stage direct-to-implant technique is a patient with a medium or small breast size, grade 0–1 ptosis, and good skin quality. A nipple-sparing mastectomy and the absence of skin resection make this procedure possible. The ideal incision in patients with small, well-shaped breasts is the inframammary incision. The ADM is placed the same as was previously discussed in the tissue expander section. Instead of an expander, the final implant is placed. The wounds are closed over two drains and kept in place for 7–14 days [5].

Patients who have resection of the nipple-aureola complex and skin, but who have mastectomy flaps which are adequate, in both size and vitality, may also be reconstructed with a direct-to-implant technique. They will require a secondary procedure to reconstruct the nipple.

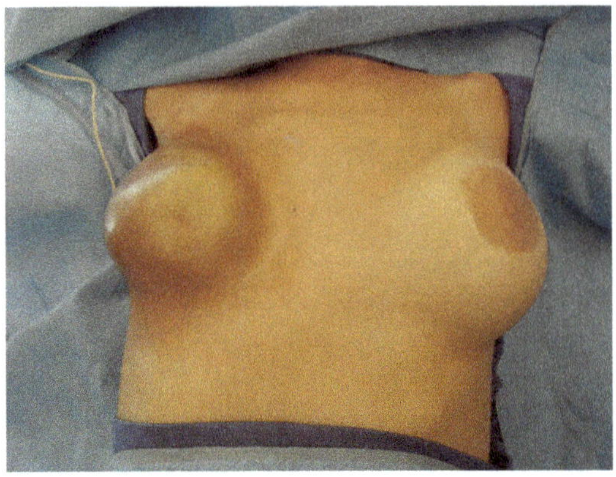

Fig. 18.3 Severe capsule contracture in implant reconstruction following radiation therapy

The Effect of Radiation on Breast Reconstruction

Current recommendations for postmastectomy radiation are in T3 or T4 tumors, tumors involving the skin, and tumors with three or more positive lymph nodes or one lymph node with extracapsular invasion. There is much debate about the timing of reconstruction with respect to the initiation of radiation. In the delayed setting, implant-based reconstruction is often difficult. Radiated skin is fibrosed and fixated to the chest wall, making tissue expansion difficult and compromising the aesthetic quality of the reconstructed breast (Fig. 18.3). In this group of patients, problems with wound healing may occur, as well as higher rates of capsular contracture [6, 7]. Patients who have had postmastectomy radiation and still desire implant reconstruction may benefit from the use of a latissimus dorsi (LD) flap. The patient will have a large skin deficit, which will be hard to expand. The benefits of this flap are multiple. The fibrosed postradiation skin may be removed and replaced by the healthy skin paddle that the LD flap provides. Additionally, the bulky latissimus muscle provides for an optimal adjunct for implant coverage. It is the author's practice to offer the patient with a previously radiated chest the option of autologous reconstruction, which provides optimal skin coverage and produces a more aesthetically acceptable breast in this type of patient. The author also feels strongly that chest wall radiation following flap reconstruction can cause fibrosis and loss of volume in the flap. We make every effort to avoid immediate reconstruction in patients who will have radiation therapy planned, whether with autologous or non-autologous procedures.

The choice is made to proceed with implant/expander reconstruction despite the inherent problems of wound healing and high rates of capsule contracture, and some protocol must be found to reduce complications. The key to successful implant-based reconstruction in the immediate reconstruction patient who faces radiation therapy is to maintain the natural breast skin envelope during radiation. Two published series have addressed these issues.

MD Anderson employs the "delayed immediate" reconstruction tactic for use in this setting. The patient undergoes placement of a completely filled tissue expander at the time of the mastectomy. Once the pathology is finalized and it is confirmed that the patient will not require radiation, immediate reconstruction may then be performed. If radiation will be needed, the tissue

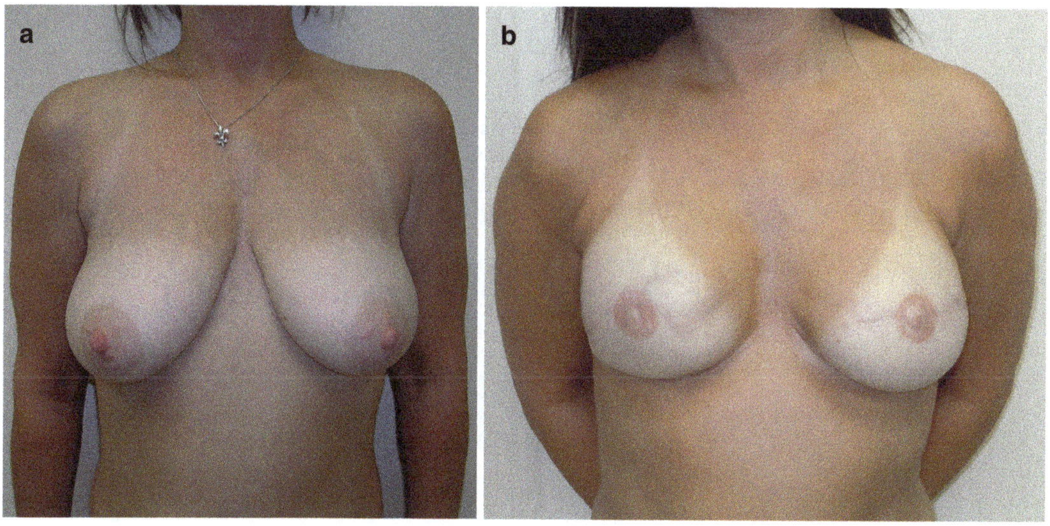

Fig. 18.4 (**a**, **b**) Patient with grade two ptosis following two-stage implant reconstruction with ADM

expander is deflated. Once radiation is complete, tissue expansion may commence, followed by definitive reconstruction [8, 9].

Memorial Sloan Kettering uses a different protocol. The treatment algorithm begins as a modified radical mastectomy with immediate placement of tissue expanders that are not fully expanded. At approximately 5 weeks postoperatively, chemotherapy is initiated with concurrent expander inflation. Four weeks following the completion of chemotherapy, patients undergo exchange of the tissue expanders for permanent implants. Postmastectomy radiation is usually initiated about 1 month following implant placement [10]. Their reported incidence of postradiation complications is more favorable than that reported by the MD Anderson series. Additionally, radiation delivery is more easily achieved with implants rather than expanders.

Kronowitz states "despite advances in reconstructive devices and materials, post-mastectomy radiation therapy still appears to have an adverse impact on outcomes of implant-based breast reconstruction." In a review of the literature, he notes that most postmastectomy radiation therapy tissue expander reconstructions had a significant amount of unplanned or major corrective surgery. Approximately one-third of patients develop Baker grade III or IV capsular contracture, characterized by pain and distortion. Despite the complications and additional surgery, the majority of patients who undergo implant-based reconstruction and postmastectomy radiation therapy ultimately keep the implant-based reconstruction (Figs. 18.4 and 18.5) [11]. There is some evidence that acellular dermal matrix may have protective effects to avoid complications, this topic is being researched extensively.

Complications Specific to Non-autologous Reconstruction

Mastectomy flap necrosis is always a threat in implant-based breast reconstruction. Flap necrosis can be minor with mild skin sloughing, which may be treated with local wound care. More severe necrosis can lead to implant exposure or extrusion. If this occurs, the implant will likely require removal, and other reconstruction options will need to be explored. This is why soft tissue coverage of implant or expander is crucial with implant-based reconstruction (Fig. 18.6).

Postoperative seroma appears to occur more frequently with ADM use when compared with total muscle coverage. Possible causes include the following: (1) tissue preservatives, (2) fat

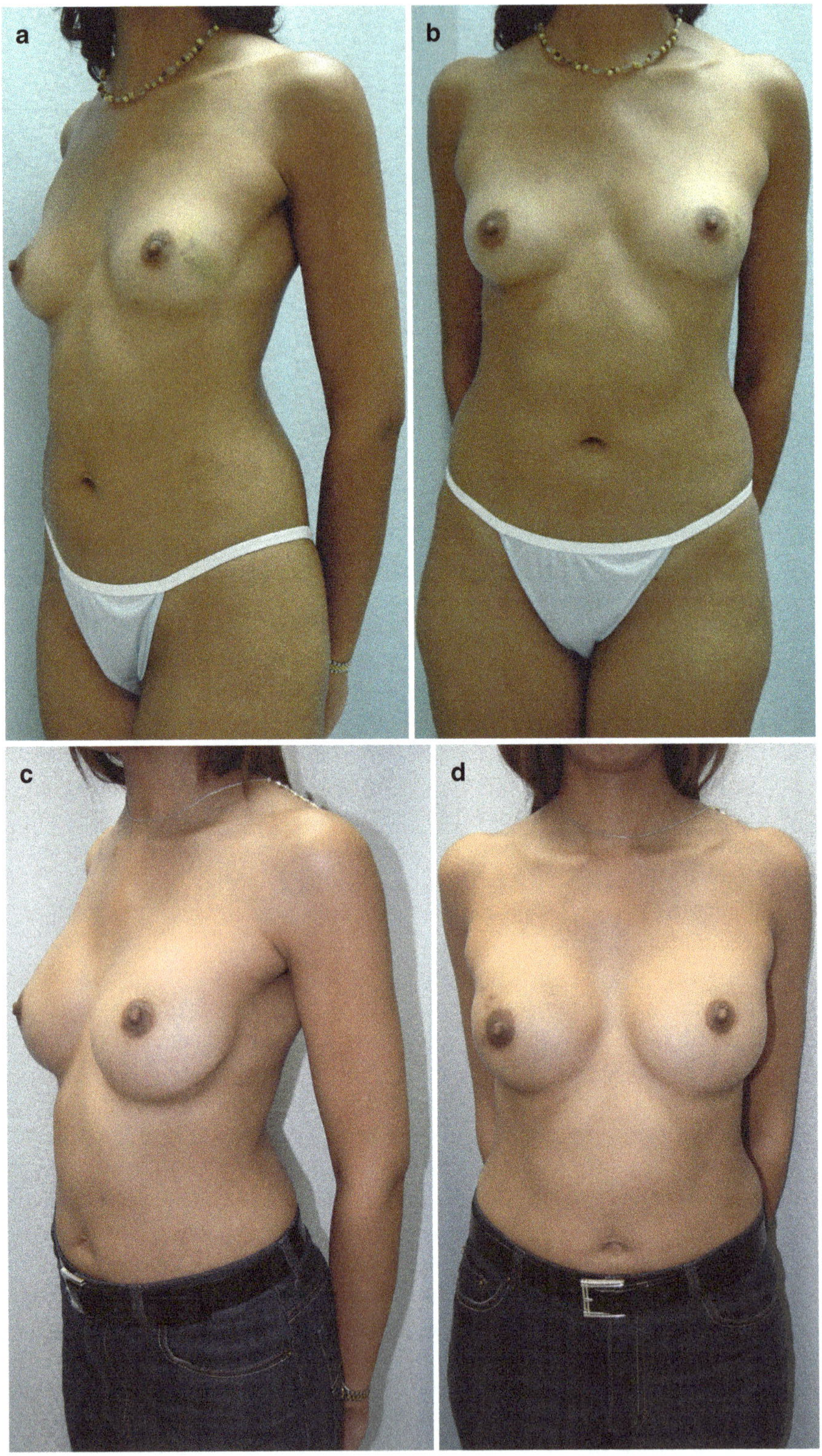

Fig. 18.5 (**a**, **b**) Preoperative and (**c**, **d**) postoperative of patient with BRAC-1 who had nipple-sparing mastectomy and direct-to-implant reconstruction

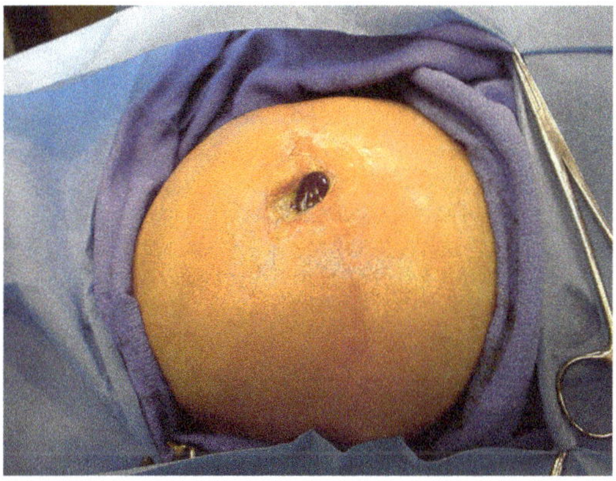

Fig. 18.6 Exposed implant following mastectomy flap necrosis

and other operative debris, (3) stymied revascularization, and (4) axillary surgery. Each is associated with a higher seroma rate [12–18]. Seroma rates have been reduced with newer ADMs or by the use of vicryl mesh in place of ADM. Various strategies to prevent the development of a seroma have been advocated., Examples include intraoperative washes of the breast pocket, quilting sutures to minimize dead space, fenestration of the graft to allow passage of sub-graft fluid, multiple prolonged drains and providing volume to reduce dead space. If the ADM does not adhere to the overlying mastectomy flap, it will behave as a foreign body, complicating the seroma. Once the seroma has established itself, the key intervention is to evacuate via washout or percutaneous drains and prevent secondary infection [19].

Implant infection incidence is noted to develop in ~0.2–7 % of patients [20]. Simple cellulitis around the incision does not warrant immediate operative exploration. A trial of oral antibiotics is a reasonable option. However, in the presence of infected fluid around the implant, drainage with implant removal may be necessary. Patients who are symptomatic (fever, malaise, fluid around the implant) have a periprosthetic infection that cannot be controlled with antibiotics alone. An attempt may be made to salvage the reconstruction by removal of the infected implant, irrigation with antibiotics and replacement with a new implant.

Implant exposure is another complication that occurs in non-autologous reconstruction. Operative debridement, irrigation, and closure may be attempted if implant exposure is threatened and if the soft tissue can be approximated without tension. In more severe cases of implant exposure, local or distant flaps with implant exchange may be necessary in order to salvage the reconstruction (Fig. 18.4).

Complication rates following expander/implant reconstruction vary greatly. Cordeiro and McCarthy reviewed a 12-year, single surgeon's experience with 1,522 expander/implant reconstructions in 1,221 patients. The incidence of complications after tissue expander insertion was 8.5 %, significantly higher than after the exchange procedure, 2.7 %. Complications were increased with a history of preoperative chest wall irradiation [21]. Capsular contraction is a potential serious complication in non-autologous reconstruction. It occurs when the tissue interface with the implant undergoes contraction. The cause is not clearly defined. In the mastectomy patient, without overlying breast tissue, capsule contracture is more clinically evident. Capsular contracture was classified by Baker into four classes with respect to cosmetic breast augmentation. Sear et.al revised this classification after prosthetic breast reconstruction into five classes. Class III has a moderately firm reconstructed breast with a readily detected implant, but the results may still be acceptable. Class IV contracture produces patient symptoms and/or compromises aesthetic result requiring surgical intervention [22]. Surgical intervention could include a capsulotomy or a capsulectomy. Implant exchange at that time is warranted as well. If capsular contracture recurs, autologous reconstruction may need to be offered as an alternative.

Implant and autologous breast reconstruction techniques have different long-term complications, with the aging process also affecting the aesthetic appearance of the reconstructed breast [23–26]. Clough et al. performed a prospective, single-center cohort study evaluating aesthetic outcomes in patients with TRAM versus expander/implant reconstructions over an 8-year time period. The number of patients satisfied with implant reconstruction diminished from

86 % at post-reconstructive year 2 to 54 % at post-reconstructive year 5. However, the number of patients satisfied with TRAM reconstruction was 96 % at year 2 and remained at 94 % at year 5 [24–26]. A study by Hu et al. has yielded similar results, but from the patient's perspective, 82 % of patients 5 years or less post surgery were satisfied with the size of their implant. However, this rate dropped to only 42 % satisfaction among those more than 8 years after surgery [27].

Autologous tissue reconstruction provides a more stable aesthetic outcome. Implants will likely fail during the patient's life and will require replacement. Additionally surveillance of implants with MRI, as advised by the Food and Drug Administration, is a long-term issue, which increases the cost of this type of reconstruction. Implants do not become naturally ptotic with age and are prone to capsular contracture, which can lead to distortion of the breast mound. Additionally, implants do not change in size as a patient gains or loses weight over time. This is an important issue for women to consider, since most women do not remain the same size throughout their lifetime. With changing implant technology and use of ADM in implant-based breast reconstruction, long-term prospective studies must be designed to establish the outcomes of implant-based breast reconstruction.

References

1. American Society of Plastic surgeons. Department of public relations 444 east Algonquin road, Arlington Heights Illinois. Available at www.plasticsurgery.org/documents/media/2011-r.
2. Albornoz CR, Bach RB, Meharar BJ. A paradigm shift in U.S. breast reconstruction: increasing implant rates. Plast Reconstr Surg. 2013;131(1):15–23.
3. Dean C, Chetty U, Forrest AP. Effects of immediate breast reconstruction on psychosocial morbidity after mastectomy. Lancet. 1983;320:459–62.
4. Gurunluoglu R, Gurunluoglu A, Williams SA, Tebockhorst S. Current trends in breast reconstruction. Ann Plast Surg. 2011;70(1):103–10.
5. Breuing KH, Colwell AS. Inferolateral AlloDerm hammock for implant coverage in breast reconstruction. Ann Plast Surg. 2007;59(3):250–5.
6. Salzberg CA. Focus on technique: one-stage implant-based breast reconstruction. Plast Reconstr Surg. 2012;130(5):95s–103. 2nd ser.
7. Spear SL, Carter ME, Schwarz K. Prophylactic mastectomy: indications, options, and reconstructive alternatives. Plast Reconstr Surg. 2005;115(3):891–909.
8. Chalfoun C, Lane K. Adjuvant therapy and breast reconstruction. In: Hall-Findlay E, Evans G, editors. Aesthetic and reconstructive surgery of the breast. Saunders/Elsevier, Edenburgh; 2010. p. 11–9.
9. Kronowitz SJ, Kuerer HM. Advances in surgical decision making for breast reconstruction. Cancer. 2006; 107(5):893–907.
10. Kronowitz SJ, Robb GI. Breast reconstruction with postmastectomy radiation therapy: current issues. Plast Reconstr Surg. 2004;114(4):950–60.
11. Ho A, Cordeiro P, Disa J. Long-term outcomes in breast cancer patients undergoing immediate 2-stage expander/implant reconstruction and postmastectomy radiation. Cancer. 2012;118:2552–9.
12. Kronowitz SJ. Current status of implant-based breast reconstruction in patients receiving postmastectomy radiation therapy. Plast Reconstr Surg. 2012;130.4:513e–24.
13. Kim JYS, Davila AA, Persing S, et al. A meta-analysis of human acellular dermis and submuscular tissue expander breast reconstruction. Plast Reconstr Surg. 2012;129:28–41.
14. Sbitany H, Serletti JM. Acellular dermis-assisted prosthetic breast reconstruction: a systematic and critical review of efficacy and associated morbidity. Plast Reconstr Surg. 2011;128:1162–9.
15. Chun YS, Verma K, Rosen H, et al. Implant-based breast reconstruction using acellular dermal matrix and the risk of post-operative complications. Plast Reconstr Surg. 2010;125:429–36.
16. Antony AK, McCarthy CM, Cordeiro PG, et al. Acellular human dermis implantation in 153 immediate two-stage tissue expander breast reconstructions: determining the incidence and significant predictors of complications. Plast Reconstr Surg. 2010;125:1606–14.
17. Hoppe IC, Yueh JH, Wei CH, Ahuja NK, Patel PP, Datiashvili RO. Complications following expander/implant breast reconstruction utilizing acellular dermal matrix: a systematic review and meta-analysis. Eplasty. 2011;11:417–28.
18. Spear SL, Parikh PM, Peisin E, Menon NG. Acellular dermis assisted breast reconstruction. Aesth Plast Surg. 2008;32:418–25.
19. Kim JYS. Focus on technique: two-stage implant-based breast reconstruction. Plast Reconstr Surg. 2012;130(5):104s–15. 2nd ser.
20. Spear SL, Howard MA, Boehmler JH, Ducic I, Low M, Abbruzzesse MR. The infected or exposed breast implant: management and treatment strategies. Plast Reconstr Surg. 2004;113(6):1634–44.
21. Cordeiro PG, McCarthy CM. A single surgeon's 12-year experience with tissue expander/implant breast reconstruction: Part 1. A prospective analysis of early complications. Plast Reconstr Surg. 2006; 118:825.
22. Spear SL, Baker JL. Classification of capsular contracture after prosthetic breast reconstruction. Plast Reconstr Surg. 1995;96(5):1119–23.

23. Alderman AK, Kuhn LE, Lowery JC, et al. Does patient satisfaction with breast reconstruction change over time? Two year results of the Michigan Breast Reconstruction Outcomes Study. J Am Coll Surg. 2007;204:7–12.
24. Clough KB, O'Donoghue JM, Fitoussi AD, et al. Prospective evaluation of late cosmetic results following breast reconstruction: I. Implant reconstruction. Plast Reconstr Surg. 2001;107:1702–9.
25. Spear SL, Onyewu C. Staged breast reconstruction with saline-filled implants in the irradiated breast: recent trends and therapeutic implications. Plast Reconstr Surg. 2000;105:930–42.
26. Clough KB, O'Donoghue JM, Fitoussi AD, et al. Prospective evaluation of late cosmetic results following breast reconstruction: II. TRAM flap reconstruction. Plast Reconstr Surg Plast Reconstr Surg. 2001;107: 1710–6.
27. Hu ES, et al. Patient-reported aesthetic satisfaction with breast reconstruction during the long-term survivorship period. Plast Reconstr Surg. 2009;124(1): 1–8.

Autologous Breast Reconstruction 19

M. Whitten Wise, Hugo St.Hilaire, Ali Sadeghi,
M'liss Hogan, and Charles Dupin

The advance in autogenous breast reconstruction has been phenomenal in the past 25 years. Some patients do not like the idea of an implant or the negative consequences that can accompany implant reconstruction. Many patients are poor candidates for implant reconstruction because of either their body habitus or the lack of an appropriate soft tissue envelope. Additionally the soft tissue envelope may be scarred and tight following external beam radiation therapy, which also increases the risk of capsule contracture and implant reconstruction failure. Until 2002, the most common type of breast reconstruction was autologous tissue transfer. However, since 1998, the use of non-autologous reconstruction has, for a number of reasons, eclipsed autologous reconstruction by nearly 2:1 [1]. Nonetheless, autologous reconstruction continues to be an essential form of reconstruction. There are two types of autologous reconstruction flaps: pedicle flaps and free tissue transfer.

M.W. Wise, MD • H. St.Hilaire, MD, DDS (✉)
A. Sadeghi, MD • M. Hogan, MD • C. Dupin, MD
Division of Plastic Surgery, Department of Surgery, Louisiana State University Health Sciences Center, 1542 Tulane Avenue, New Orleans, LA 70112, USA
e-mail: mwhitwise@gmail.com; hugost1@gmail.com; alsadeghi@gmail.com; mhoga1@lsuhsc.edu; cldupinmd@gmail.com

Pedicle Flap Reconstruction

Latissimus Dorsi Breast Reconstruction

The latissimus dorsi (LD) myocutaneous flap is considered by many to be the "workhorse" flap in breast reconstructive surgery. The thoracodorsal system offers a reliable blood supply that makes reconstructive outcomes predictable. Its use in breast reconstruction can be traced back to the late 1890s to Iginio Tansini [2]. In the late 1970s and early 1980s, its use in breast surgery became more widespread, with the LD flap utilized in immediate and delayed reconstruction. The main disadvantage of the LD is the lack of volume it offers. Often times, it is used in conjunction with a tissue expander or an implant, effectively creating a hybrid reconstruction.

Anatomy of the Latissimus Dorsi

The LD is a broad muscle that originates on the spinous process of T7–L5, the thoracolumbar fascia, the iliac crest, and the inferior angle of the scapula. It inserts on the floor of the intertubercular groove of the humerus. Blood supply to the LD flap is via the thoracodorsal artery, which is the terminal branch of the subscapular artery. The neurovascular pedicle consists of the artery, two veins, and the thoracodorsal nerve. The neurovascular bundle can be identified at the undersurface of the LD, approximately 10–12 cm below the axillary artery and 2–3 cm medial from the lateral border. A serratus branch can be given off

A.I. Riker (ed.), *Breast Disease: Comprehensive Management*,
DOI 10.1007/978-1-4939-1145-5_19, © Springer Science+Business Media New York 2015

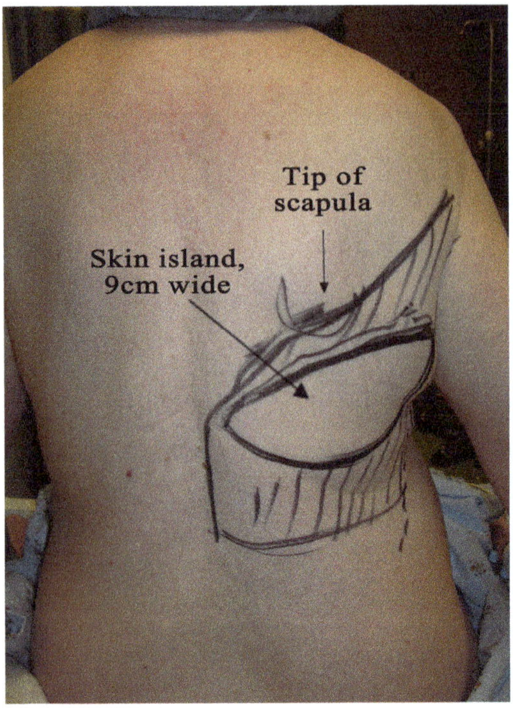

Fig. 19.1 Preoperative markings for a latissimus flap

of the thoracodorsal artery immediately prior to its entry into the LD.

Preoperative Evaluation

The latissimus dorsi muscle borders are marked. If the patient has had a previous axillary lymphadenectomy, the thoracodorsal vessels may have been injured. The innervation of the muscle should be examined. If the muscle contracts, it is likely that the vessels are intact. It is possible to raise the flap based on the serratus branch if the thoracodorsal vessels were previously damaged.

The midline, tip of the scapula, and posterior iliac crest are reliable landmarks that help delineate the LD borders. Commonly, a skin paddle is used. The surgeon should fashion a template of the defect and translate it to the back (Fig. 19.1). Care must be taken to ensure primary closure of the donor site. A skin paddle of less than 10 cm should close with acceptable tension. The arc of rotation of the flap needs to be evaluated to ensure adequate transposition to the chest wall [3].

Procedure

In cases of immediate reconstruction, after the mastectomy is complete, the reconstructive surgeon must ensure that the thoracodorsal vasculature is unharmed. While dissecting within the axillary pocket, the anterior border of the LD muscle can be defined. An anterior axillary tunnel is made for the rotation of the flap into the mastectomy defect. The mastectomy flaps are then temporarily closed with staples and covered with an occlusive dressing. In unilateral reconstruction, the patient is then placed in the lateral decubitus position. If bilateral reconstruction is being performed, the patient is placed in the prone position.

If a skin paddle is being included, the skin island should be incised. The plane of dissection is taken below Scarpa's fascia, leaving the layer of deep fat overlying the muscle as added bulk to the flap. The superior aspect of the muscle is identified at the level of the inferior border of the scapula, and the anterior margin is separated from the serratus anterior. The muscle is then raised cephalad and toward the midline. The midline attachments are then dissected. The plane in the inferior portion of the LD is less defined than the other parts of the muscle, and electrocautery is used to dissect it. The flap is then raised in the areola tissue below the muscle superiorly toward the axilla.

Once the pedicle is identified, care is taken not to injure the vessels. It is not always necessary to completely dissect the pedicle, as its arc of rotation should be adequate to rotate into the mastectomy defect even if the serratus branch is intact. The insertion of the LD at the bicipital groove of the humerus is taken down to allow for an increased arc of rotation. Great care is taken to avoid traction on the pedicle. The thoracodorsal nerve is then isolated and divided. The muscle is then freely rotated into the pocket through the previously dissected tunnel in the axilla and into the mastectomy defect (Fig. 19.2).

The donor site is closed in layers. Quilting sutures are used along with two closed suction drains. This helps to prevent postoperative seroma formation. Once the wound is closed, the patient is again placed in supine position.

The subcutaneous tunnel is made high in the axilla to help recreate the anterior axillary fold.

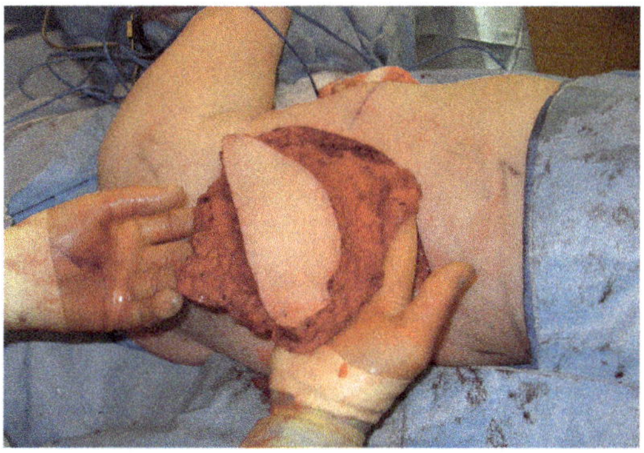

Fig. 19.2 Skin island on the isolated latissimus muscle

In the case of a small breast mound, or delayed reconstruction, the flap is inset over the pectoralis major muscle. The skin paddle is then shaped, and if the entire paddle is being used, the flap can be approximated to the edges of the mastectomy flaps. Drains are placed under the flap and in the axilla. If only part of the skin paddle is being used, it is de-epithelized and inset appropriately.

In the setting of alloplastic reconstruction, the LD flap can be an alternative to the acellular dermal matrix to cover the infralateral pole of the tissue expander. The pectoralis muscle is raised and the LD is then inset at the inframammary fold. The tissue expander is then placed, with the LD flap secured to the lateral chest wall to maintain the lateral border of the breast and to keep the implant from migrating laterally (Fig. 19.3).

Postoperative Course

Postoperative care usually consists of an overnight stay in the hospital. The ipsilateral arm is elevated on several pillows to prevent undue pressure on the vascular pedicle. The skin paddle is monitored for temperature and color to ensure vascular patency. The patient will go home with drains and keep a record of the output.

Complications of Latissimus Dorsi Reconstruction

Seroma formation at the LD donor site is the most common complication following LD breast reconstruction. Closing the LD donor site with quilting sutures helps close the dead space left by the dissection. Closed suction drains are

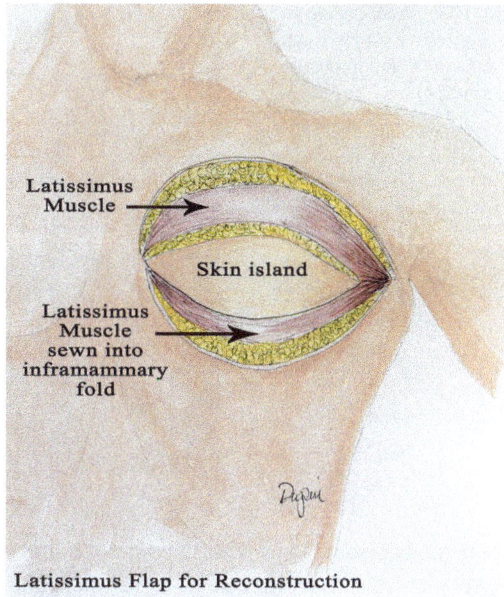

Fig. 19.3 Latissimus flap

imperative, with the drains kept in place for 1–2 weeks, or longer, if output is persistently elevated. Some surgeons also advocate the use of a fibrin sealant within the donor site to help seal the raw edges of the dead space. Only small retrospective studies have addressed the use of fibrin sealants, but most have noted a decrease in postoperative seroma formation as well as a shorter duration of drain usage when compared to the quilting suture groups alone [4] (Fig. 19.4).

Transverse Rectus Abdominis Flap

Since its introduction in the early 1980s by Hartrampf, Schleflan, and Black, the pedicle transverse rectus abdominis muscle (TRAM) has been the most commonly used form of autologous breast reconstruction. It uses the excess lower abdominal tissue that would otherwise be discarded in an abdominoplasty procedure. The use of the abdominal tissue is appealing because it is soft and moldable and therefore can be shaped to the form of a native breast. The appeal of the pedicle TRAM to surgeons is its proven reliability, predictable blood supply, and ease of harvest. However, patient

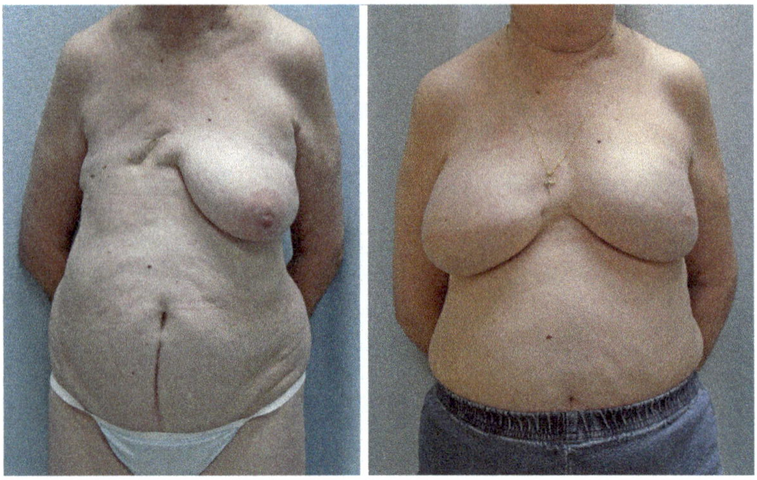

Fig. 19.4 Preoperative and postoperative prophylactic mastectomy and implant reconstruction

selection is critical to providing good outcomes. Associated comorbidities such as obesity, diabetes, and hypertension all dramatically increase the risk of complications [4–8].

Anatomy of the Pedicle TRAM Flap

The pedicle TRAM flap is based upon the deep superior epigastric artery (a continuation of the internal mammary artery). Above the level of the umbilicus, the vessels coalesce with the deep inferior epigastric artery. There may be a significant reduction in caliber around and above the umbilicus, which impacts reliability. This anatomical variation has promoted recommendations for delay of the flap and even consideration for using both rectus muscles for transporting the flap. The deep inferior epigastric artery is a branch of the internal iliac artery and is the dominant arterial blood supply to the rectus abdominis muscle and its overlying skin. In the pedicle TRAM technique, the dominant blood supply (deep inferior epigastric artery) is ligated to allow for rotation into the mastectomy site. The valves of the deep superior epigastric veins will inhibit flow until congestion renders them incompetent [9].

The available skin is considered in four vascular zones. Numbered in order of decreasing blood supply, zone I overlays the muscle to be transposed. Zone II lies lateral to zone I and usually has a reliable blood supply stemming from zone I. Zone III is adjacent to zone I but across the midline. The viability of this zone must be

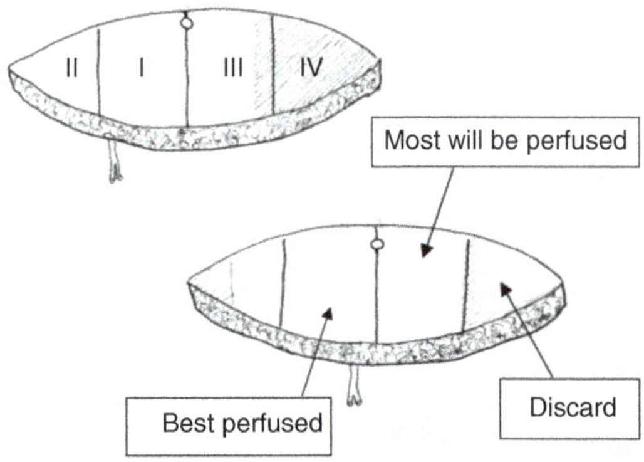

Fig. 19.5 Zones of perfusion for DIEP flap

explored, and portions of this zone should not be incorporated into the flap if there is any question of viability. Zone IV (the portion of the flap most remote from the vessels) is discarded in the unilateral pedicle TRAM as its perfusion is unreliable (Fig. 19.5). In bilateral procedures, each hemi-abdomen consists of zone I and zone II [10]. Basically, tissue remote to the entry of the vessels into the flap will be increasingly poorly perfused as they become further away.

In the case of a subcostal incision due to previous cholecystectomy, the right superior deep epigastric vessel and rectus muscle are usually compromised. Therefore, pedicle TRAM should not be raised from that side. The contralateral hemi-abdomen, however, can be considered for a pedicle TRAM transposition. Vertical midline scars do not preclude the use of the pedicle

TRAM method, but tissue across the midline should not be used. A lower abdominal or Pfannenstiel incision or previous appendectomy incision do not interfere with elevation of a pedicle TRAM reconstruction [11].

Preoperative Approach and Procedure

With the patient standing, the inframammary folds are marked. The midline is also delineated. The upper abdominal marking is a transverse line 1–2 cm above the umbilicus. The lower abdominal marking is a suprapubic curvilinear incision that extends to the anterior superior iliac spine bilaterally. In the immediate setting, the mastectomy may proceed concomitantly with the TRAM dissection. The superior edge of the flap island is incised first, beveling cephalad until abdominal wall fascia is reached. The dissection is continued toward the costal margins. The medial and lateral edges of the rectus muscle are then identified. At the level of the costal margins, the anterior rectus sheath is incised on both sides of the rectus muscle down to the level of the skin island, leaving the anterior rectus sheath attached to the muscle and making the muscle dissection less difficult.

Next, the inferior border of the flap is incised down to the level of the abdominal wall fascia. The side contralateral to the rectus muscle supplying the flap is elevated first. The external oblique and rectus fascia are left intact, and large perforating vessels are ligated. The umbilicus is sharply incised to its base and separated from the flap. Attention is now directed to the ipsilateral side of the flap. Dissection proceeds until the lateral border of the rectus fascia is encountered. At this point, bipolar cautery is used to incise the rectus fascia, taking care not to injure perforating vessels. The same is done to the medial side of the rectus muscle. The medial and lateral rectus sheath incisions are extended caudally to the inferior border of the flap, where the two incisions merge. The inferior aspect of the rectus muscle is incised, and the deep inferior epigastric vascular bundle is identified and ligated. Using blunt dissection, the flap can be elevated caudally toward the costal margins (Fig. 19.6). In the area of inscriptions, the muscle can be quite thin and care must be taken not to damage the muscle and its accompanying vessels.

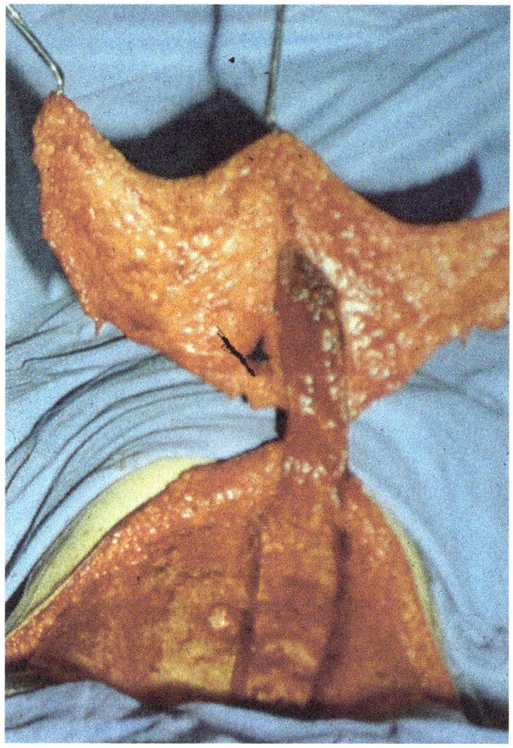

Fig. 19.6 TRAM flap

At the level of the costal margin, a tunnel is made at the medial aspect of the IMF to allow for passage of the skin island. This tunnel must be wide enough to easily pass the skin island into place without undue traction (Fig. 19.7).

Attention is then directed to the mastectomy site, and the tunnel is completed while staying within the same plane as the dissected flap. The vascular pedicle is then identified near the level of the costal margins. Lateral attachments near the pedicle are carefully excised in order to prevent tension of the pedicle when rotated into the mastectomy site. Prior to flap rotation, the inadequately perfused part of the flap from zone IV and part of zone III will need to be excised. The flap is then rotated into the mastectomy site via the previously dissected tunnel. Care is taken to avoid any undue tension on the vascular pedicle. The flap is then temporarily stapled in the mastectomy wound.

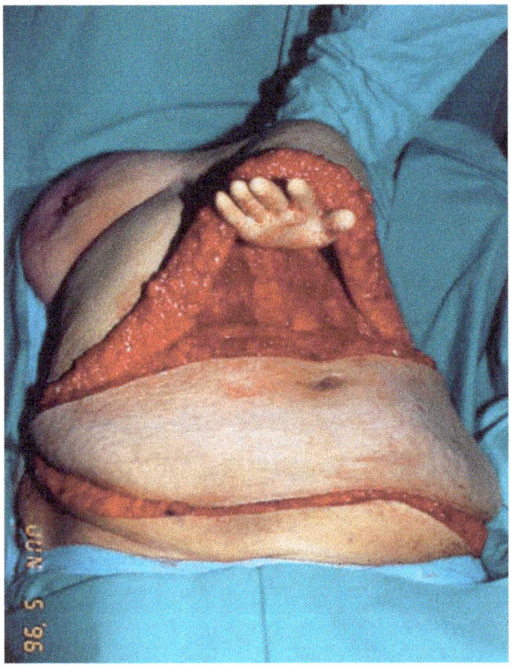

Fig. 19.7 Extensive tunnel required to transfer rotational TRAM flap

A sound abdominal wall closure is essential in order to prevent bulging or hernia formation. The rectus fascia is closed primarily, with the superior aspect of the rectus fascia left open to prevent compression of the vascular pedicle. Once the fascia is closed, most surgeons place a mesh overlay to prevent bulge or hernia formation, a well-known complication of the pedicle TRAM. The OR table is then put into a flexed position to aid in abdominal skin closure. Scarpa's fascia is approximated with a series of simple, interrupted absorbable sutures with placement of two suction drains. The umbilicus is repositioned in the midline and delivered through a new opening. Both the abdominal incision and the umbilicus are closed with a running subcuticular suture.

The flap is then inspected to assure adequate perfusion. It may need to be repositioned if it appears congested or compromised. Areas to be buried under mastectomy flaps are marked and de-epithelized. The flap is tacked down to the chest wall, being mindful of the borders of the breast. The skin paddle is sutured to the mastectomy flap. This allows for flap monitoring in the early postoperative period.

Bilateral Pedicled TRAM Flaps

The procedure is similar to the unilateral pedicle TRAM. The difference is in the size of the abdominal fascial defect that cannot be primarily closed. Therefore, mesh prosthesis is fashioned to the size of the fascial defect, and starting at the level of the umbilicus, the mesh is inserted. The two sutures on the opposite sides of the umbilicus set the tension of the abdominal wall repair. This is continued superiorly and inferiorly. The mesh is trimmed if necessary, and a running suture reinforces the repair of the fascial defect. The umbilicus is delivered through a hole in the mesh, and abdominal closure is completed over drains [12].

Postoperative Care

The patient is admitted to a unit capable of monitoring flaps. Temperature and color are monitored, and the surgeon is notified of any changes. The patient is encouraged to ambulate as early as postoperative day 1 and is discharged when tolerating a regular diet and when pain is controlled with oral pain medications. Patient is taught proper drain care prior to discharge.

Risk Factors in Pedicle TRAM Procedures

Smoking and obesity have been associated with deleterious outcomes following pedicle TRAM flap reconstruction. Wound healing problems, flap infections, and partial and total flap loss are greatly increased in these subsets of patients. Spear et al. reported that active smokers are at a high risk of complications with a statistically significant increase in various flap complications and infection. It was further noted that former smokers were also at increased risk of flap complications and delayed wound healing [4]. Obesity has long been considered a relative contraindication for TRAM flap reconstruction. Kroll and Netscher found that complications after pedicle TRAM flap reconstruction increased proportionally to the degree of obesity [5]. Paige et al. found obesity to be associated with an increase incidence of postoperative fat necrosis, partial flap loss, and infection. Complication rates of 31–41 % have been reported with the pedicle TRAM flap reconstruction in obese patients, with an 8–21 % incidence of partial flap loss [6]. With the introduction of the free TRAM flap, which greatly increase flap perfusion, complication rates have improved in both smokers and obese patients [6–8].

Microvascular Breast Reconstruction

Along with the development of microsurgical techniques, and in order to improve outcomes in autogenous breast reconstruction, the free TRAM (F-TRAM) flap was developed. Microsurgical transfer allows the use of the dominant deep inferior epigastric artery as the vascular pedicle to the lower abdominal flap. The more vigorous blood supply provided by the deep inferior epigastric artery decreases the incidence of fat necrosis and wound healing complications. In order to minimize donor site morbidity, the F-TRAM evolved to the muscle-sparing TRAM (MS-TRAM). The latter minimizes the amount of muscle and abdominal fascia violation, significantly reducing the incidence of hernia and bulges. The ultimate muscle-sparring TRAM is the deep inferior epigastric artery perforator flap where the perforating artery and veins are dissected through the muscle and fascia.

Anatomy of the Abdominal Wall

It is imperative to understand the anatomy of the abdominal wall in order to appreciate the fundamental difference between these procedures. The blood supply to the F-TRAM, MS-TRAM, and DIEP flap is via the deep inferior epigastric artery, a branch of the internal iliac artery. At the level of the arcuate line, the deep inferior epigastric artery often splits into a lateral and medial row after entering the rectus muscle. Occasionally there is only one vessel identified, with perforating vessels traversing the anterior rectus sheath and entering the overlying abdominal fat and skin.

Moon and Taylor described the vascular anatomy of the abdomen [10]. The primary blood supply is derived from the deep inferior epigastric artery. While there is flow across the midline to the contralateral abdominal skin and fat, it is variable. When performing unilateral reconstructions, about half of the contralateral skin and fat (zones III and IV shown above) is reliably perfused, with the remainder of the tissue discarded. In the case of bilateral breast reconstruction, the abdomen is divided in the midline so there is no concern with contralateral perfusion.

The Free Flaps Harvested from the Abdominal Donor Site

The four procedures that utilize the abdominal donor site are the free TRAM (F-TRAM), the muscle-sparing TRAM (MS-TRAM), the superficial inferior epigastric artery (SIEA), and the deep inferior epigastric artery perforator (DIEP) flap. Due to many aspects of three of the flaps being similar, only the dissection of each flap will be discussed separately.

Preoperative Evaluation and Markings

Preoperative evaluation of the abdominal wall is crucial when choosing to proceed with any abdominal tissue transfer. Close attention must be made to previous abdominal surgeries and the resulting scars. Scars in the upper abdomen increase the risk of necrosis of the abdominal donor site tissue. Scars from appendectomies and vertical midline incisions will likely jeopardize perfusion across the scar [13, 14]. Examination of the skin with an 8 MHz Doppler will give an indication of the location of the perforators. Preoperative CT angiogram is a useful adjunct that can aid in preoperative planning. Perforator size can be documented, as can their location [15, 16].

Once the dominant perforator is identified in supine position, the remaining markings are performed in the standing position. The superior edge of the flap is a transverse line typically above the umbilicus. Approximately one third of the dominant perforators are above the umbilicus [17]. It should be noted that the critical mark is the *level of the cranial (superior) incision line* and the dominant perforator needs to be included within the design of the flap.

The inferior edge is based on the superior marking. It is marked at a distance below the superior incision that will provide enough flap volume for the reconstruction. This may be just above the pubis or higher and extends laterally to the anterior superior iliac spine. Care should be taken to avoid making the height of the flap excessive, as this will make primary closure difficult and may result in wound healing complications. Depending upon the size of the patient, the presence of a panniculus, the size of the breast to be reconstructed, and the volume needed, the height of the flap varies from 12 to 16 cm.

In the case of immediate reconstruction, the breast skin to be excised is marked, including previous biopsy sites. The inframammary folds are marked and should be used by the oncologic surgeons as the inferior limit of dissection.

Positioning

The patient is placed in the supine position. Bilateral sequential compression devices are used and a Foley catheter is placed. In immediate reconstruction, the arm is prepped and placed out but will be tucked during the microvascular portion of the procedure. The mastectomy can occur concomitantly with raising of the flap. In delayed reconstruction, two teams are useful as while one team is dissecting the flaps, the other team dissects the recipient vessels.

Common Aspects of the Procedures

All three procedures are similar in the early dissection. The procedure begins by incising the inferior incision as marked. Frequently, there is a large (4–5 mm) vein approximately halfway between the ASIS and the midline. It is very superficial and should be carefully dissected inferiorly for a moderate distance. This vein can be used to drain the flap if there are problems with the venae comitantes of the deep inferior epigastric artery.

As the dissection proceeds deep to Scarpa's fascia, another set of vessels are encountered. These are the superficial inferior epigastric vessels (SIEA and SIEV) that frequently emerge from the femoral artery, as a branch of the lateral femoral circumflex vessels. If this system is large (3–4 mm), it is possible to transfer the flap without dissecting the rectus muscle at all. A flap transferred on the SIEA vessels is termed an SIEA flap. Unfortunately, the vessels are usually too small to perfuse the flap and the muscular dissection must proceed.

The superior incision is made. As noted above, it should be made at least 1–2 cm above any periumbilical dominant perforator. This incision should be beveled superiorly away from the flap. A periumbilical incision is then made, and the umbilicus dissected down to the abdominal wall, leaving some soft tissue to perfuse it.

In unilateral reconstructions, the flap is dissected from lateral to medial. The dissection is rapid until the lateral rectus sheath is visualized. In order to approach the medial rectus sheath, the opposite flap will have to be raised to the midline. It is important to be sure that the flap chosen has adequate perforators on the initial side, as elevation to the midline will obviously destroy the contralateral perforators. In bilateral reconstructions, the medial rectus sheath can be approached from the midline incision as well.

If a F-TRAM is to be harvested, the fascia is incised cephalad to the skin island. Incisions are then made in the fascia on either side until the level of the lower edge of the skin island is reached. The fascia can then be opened in the midline for the caudal dissection. Next, the muscle is elevated with blunt dissection from cranial to caudal, until the deep inferior epigastric vessels are seen entering the muscle. The deep inferior epigastric vessels are then dissected to their origin. Muscular side branches are ligated using clips. The surgeon and assistant must take great care at this time to ensure no undue tension is placed on the pedicle. Once adequate pedicle length is dissected, the vessels are marked in situ with a marking pen to prevent twisting or kinking of the pedicle (Fig. 19.8). The MS-TRAM attempts to save muscle and, more importantly, fascia. The dissection is extended over the rectus fascia until the lateral row of perforators is identified. Fascia that is lateral to these perforators can be preserved. The same technique can be done on the medial side, preserving some fascia (Fig. 19.9). The muscle is split at the same level, leaving some on either side. The rest of the dissection is similar to the F-TRAM flap. If the patient is found to have dominant perforators on either row, additional fascia/muscle can be preserved by ligating the nondominant perforator row and increasing the amount of fascia and muscle spared. It should be cautioned, however, that these perforators may have long intramuscular courses and run in a transverse fashion before connecting with the deep inferior epigastric vessels. Leaving only a small cuff of muscle may injure the intramuscular vasculature (Fig. 19.9).

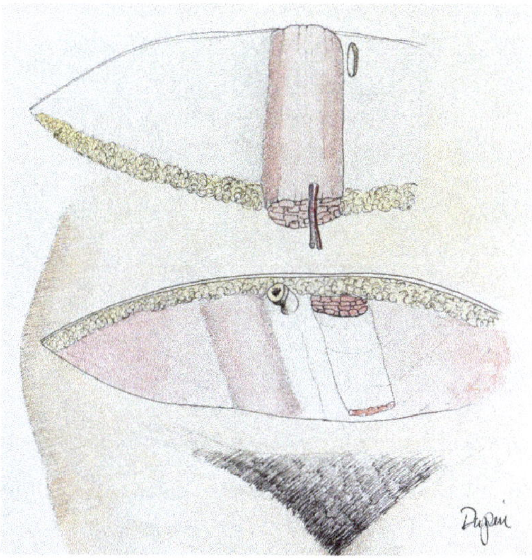

Fig. 19.8 The free TRAM flap

Deep Inferior Epigastric Artery Perforator Flap and Superficial Inferior Epigastric Artery Flap

Preoperative Planning

The success of the DIEP flap is dependent upon harvesting adequate perforators. Therefore, it is important to be certain of their size and location. Preoperatively, our patients undergo a CT angiogram of the abdominal wall. The CTA allows visualization of the dominant perforators. It demonstrates the location and also the intramuscular course of the perforating vessels. Dominant perforators are >2.5 mm in diameter at the level of the fascia. Occasionally, the ipsilateral flap is chosen if it contains dominant perforators. Flaps

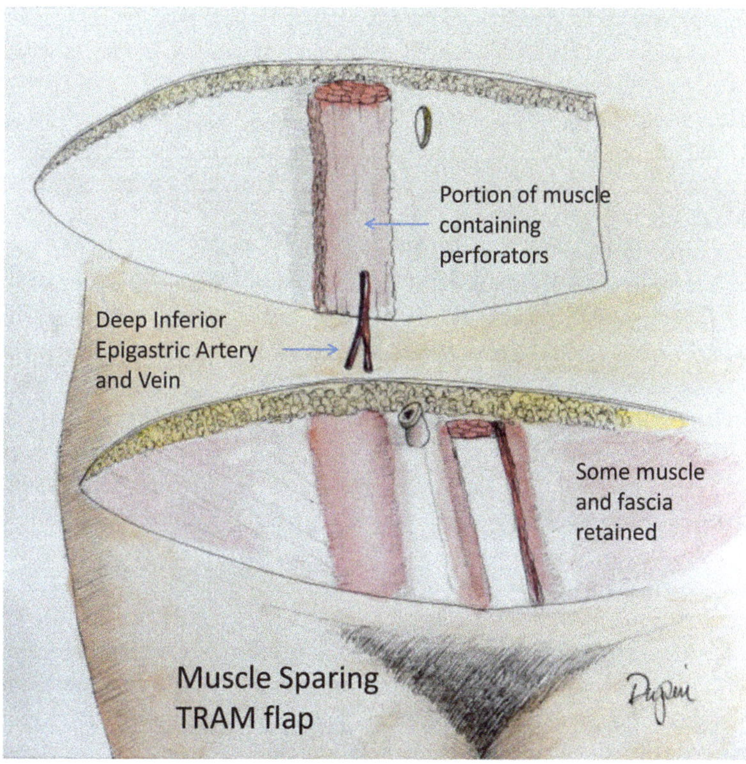

Fig. 19.9 The muscle-sparing TRAM flap

harvested with only small perforators, even multiple, will not be as well perfused as those harvested with dominant perforators. Occasionally, the CTA fails to identify any dominant perforators. Those patients may be more reliably converted to a MS-TRAM flap to ensure adequate circulation. The CTA also gives an estimate of the caliber of the dominant perforating vessel. Furthermore, it guides the best location of the DIEP flap designs. Saad et al. noted that nearly one third of dominant perforators were located superior and within 2 cm of the umbilicus. We move the flap design superiorly to encompass the dominant perforator [17].

In the preoperative holding area, the patient is marked with the assistance of the oncologic surgeon. Landmarks such as at the IMF and the midline are marked, and previous biopsy sites are marked for excision as well. The abdominal wall is then marked. Using a Doppler, abdominal perforating vessels are marked. The upper abdominal incision is designed to incorporate the dominant perforator. At least half of the time, it is 1–2 cm above the umbilicus. Once the level of the upper incision is decided upon, the lower incision is marked. The lower abdominal incision is marked in the suprapubic region and extends in a curved fashion to the ASIS bilaterally. Care is taken to avoid excess width of the flap. Incisional wound in very small, thin, or nulliparous patients may be closed with only a 12 cm-wide flap; those in patients with a large panniculus can be closed with a 16 cm-wide flap (Fig. 19.10).

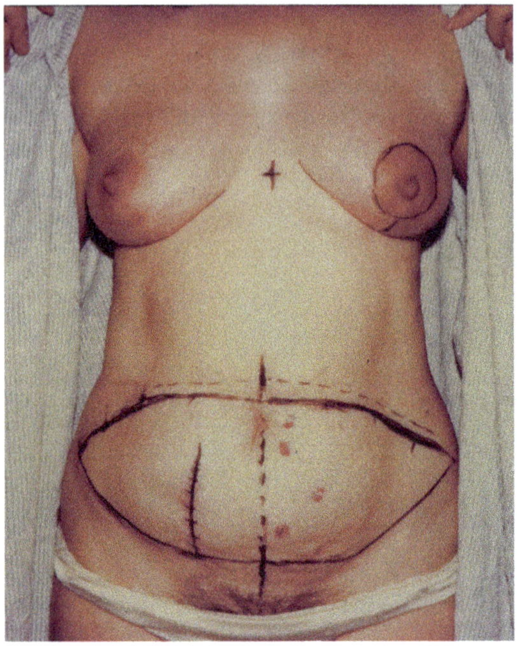

Fig. 19.10 Preoperative markings contralateral DIEP flap for left mastectomy

The patient is then taken to the operating room. Sequential compression devices and Foley catheter are placed. The patient also receives preoperative antibiotics which are re-dosed appropriately throughout the procedure.

Operative Procedure

In immediate breast reconstruction, the oncologic surgeon undertakes the mastectomy at the same time as the plastic surgeon dissects the DIEP flap. The lower abdominal incision is made first and the superficial epigastric system is explored at this time. The superficial inferior epigastric vein (SIEV) is approximately 4–5 cm lateral from the midline. If it is large in size, it should be dissected inferiorly, ligated, and preserved. Very large superficial veins may indicate that they, rather than the venae comitantes, are the primary drainage for the flap. The superficial inferior epigastric artery (SIEA) is located about 2–3 cm lateral to the SIEV but deep to Scarpa's fascia. It is identified and examined. Occasionally the superficial system is very large (>2.5 mm in diameter). If this situation is found, it is possible to harvest the flap based on the superficial system as previously described.

A very large superficial system may also indicate that the perforators are very small. In such cases, it may be safer to harvest the flap utilizing the superficial system. This should be seen on the CTA as well. If the SIEA is large, the dissection proceeds in an inferior (caudal) direction until the SIEA is found emerging from the femoral artery. It may (48 %) join the superficial circumflex vessels before joining the femoral vessel. This is a more favorable situation as harvesting the superficial circumflex artery allows a much greater caliber vessel (2 mm) than the SIEA

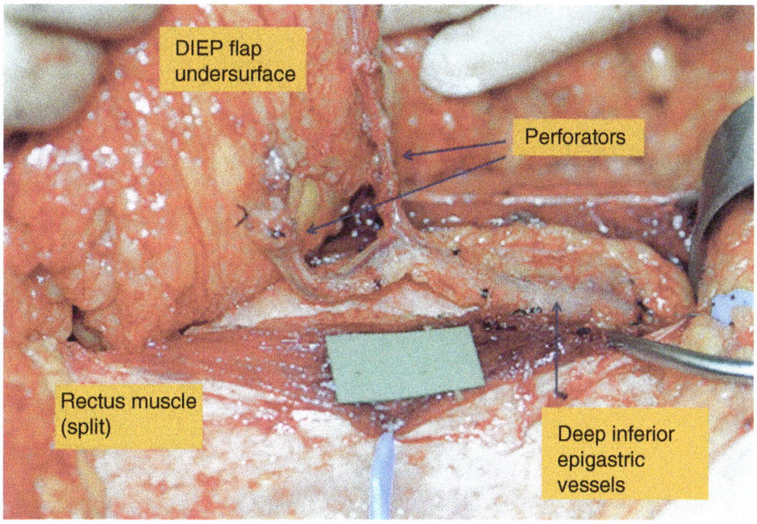

Fig. 19.11 DIEP flap dissections showing perforating vessels

alone. The small size of the SIEA makes for a mismatch with the internal mammary artery (IMA), and anastomosis may be easier with a perforating branch of the IMA, rather than the IMA itself. The donor site of the SIEA flap is prone to postoperative development of a seroma, but the rectus muscle and fascia are not dissected.

If the decision is made to proceed with the DIEP flap, the superior skin incision is made and beveled superiorly to allow for more tissue inclusion in the flap and aid in abdominal wall closure. The umbilicus is dissected down to the abdominal wall. Laterally, the skin and fat is elevated from the abdomen using electrocautery. Near the lateral edge of the rectus sheath, bipolar dissection takes place and perforating vessels are preserved. If the patient is undergoing a bilateral procedure, or if a small amount of tissue needed in the reconstruction, a midline abdominal incision is made. Dissection is then taken medially to explore the medial row perforators. The periumbilical perforators can usually be visualized by dissecting caudally from the upper incision, without taking the lateral perforators.

The perforators are then evaluated. The ideal perforator is 2.5 mm or greater in diameter and should have vigorous pulsations. The accompanying vein should be a larger caliber vessel, to allow for venous outflow of the flap. The most common problem causing pedicle inadequacy is, in our experience, the venous outflow tract, not the inflow arterial tract. If the vessels are small or moderate in size, two or more perforators should be included in the flap. Including the dominant perforator is critical, however. A number of small perforators cannot carry the volume of a single large perforator. In the mid-1850s, a French physicist named Poiseuille determined that the flow of a liquid was proportional to the fourth power of the radius of the tube. Thus, a single 2-mm vessel will carry four times as much blood as two 1-mm vessels.

Once the best perforator is selected, it is dissected circumferentially. The rectus fascia is then incised longitudinally toward the next lower perforator. It is important to carefully open the sheath because there may be a subfascial course of the vessel that could be easily injured in this dissection. The most tedious portion of the dissection is the intramuscular course (Fig. 19.11). Great care must be taken to protect the pedicle; patients should be paralyzed to prevent muscular contraction. Small intramuscular branches are clipped using hemoclips or bipolar cautery. At this time it is important to avoid any undue tension on the flap or the perforating vessels. The assistant must be very involved and go to great lengths not to place tension on the pedicle while he retracts as it is being dissected.

The pedicle is dissected toward its origin near the iliac vessels. If bilateral flaps are to be

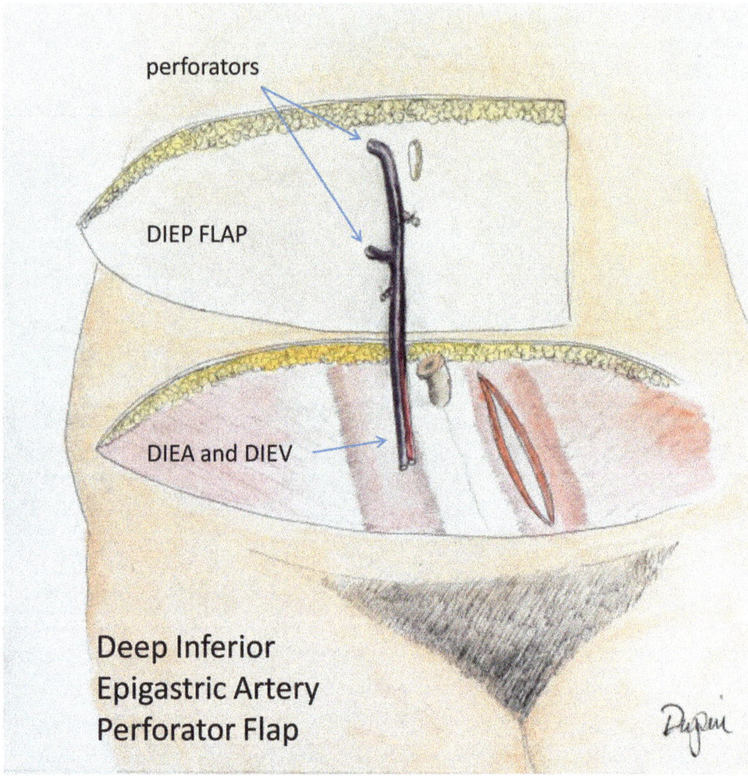

Fig. 19.12 The DIEP flap

harvested, the other side may be dissected at this time. Flaps are kept intact until mastectomy and recipient vessels are dissected, and the microvascular portion of the case is ready to commence (Fig. 19.12).

Recipient Vessels

Internal Mammary Recipient Vessels

Dissection of internal mammary vessels is undertaken between the second and third rib. Access below the third rib, especially on the left, may have inadequate veins [18]. Meticulous dissection is imperative. The pectoralis muscle is incised parallel to the muscle fibers and the interspace is exposed. Bipolar cautery is then used to remove the intercostal muscles. Branches to the intercostal muscle are ligated with micro clips, instead of electrocautery. This is important to prevent damage to the underlying vasculature. The third rib costal cartilage may need to be removed in order to fully expose the length needed to perform the anastomosis. The cartilage is scored, and an elevator is used to raise the perichondrium. The cartilage is removed using a rongeur, and bipolar cautery is used to excise the remaining perichondrium (Fig. 19.13). At this point, with vessels exposed, dissection is stopped. Finer dissection can be undertaken when the microscope is moved into position.

Thoracodorsal Artery

Currently, most free flap breast reconstructions are anastomosed to the internal mammary vessels. The internal mammary vessels permit more centralization of the breast mound and allow for easy operative access by the surgeon and assistant. In the delayed or previously radiated axilla, most surgeons elect to use the IMA for microvascular anastomosis.

On rare occasions, it may be necessary to use the subscapular system as the recipient vessels.

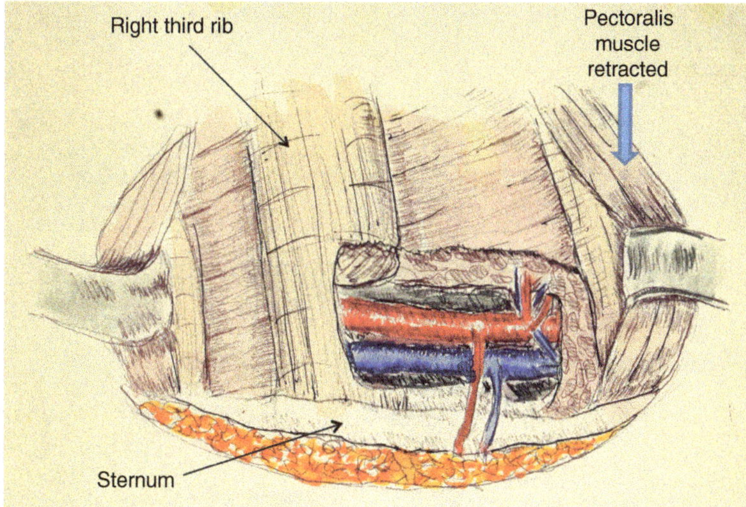

Fig. 19.13 The internal mammary artery

In immediate reconstruction with axilla exploration, the thoracodorsal vessels are easily exposed. With skin-sparing mastectomies, a separate axillary incision may be necessary to expose the thoracodorsal vessels. The thoracodorsal vessels can be identified in a plane deep to the axillary fat. Once identified, they are ligated just proximal to the serratus anterior branch. This allows for the thoracodorsal vessels to be delivered into the surgical field.

Microanastomosis

Once the recipient vessels are exposed, attention is again directed to the donor site. Using a retractor, the deep inferior epigastric vessels are dissected down to their origin near the external iliac vessels. Prior to ligation, the vessels are marked along their axis using a marking pen. This helps to orient the pedicle after transfer to help reduce the chance of twisting. The artery and vein(s) are ligated using hemoclips. The flap is weighed and then positioned on the chest in preparation for microvascular anastomosis.

The flap is temporarily secured with sutures onto the chest wall. Once the flap is in position, the microscope is brought into the field. The donor vein is carefully separated from the artery. It is helpful to mark the internal mammary vein (IMV) to be sure that it does not twist. The IMV is clamped proximally with a microsurgery clamp, and it is clipped distally and cut. A coupler sizer is then used to measure the diameter of the veins. An appropriately sized venous coupler is then used for the venous anastomosis. The surgeon must take great care to ensure the vein is not twisted and that there is no tension on the vein which can lead to avulsion. The IMA is then clamped proximally and ligated distally. A double approximating clamp is then used to position the flap and recipient arteries. A background is placed into the field. Simple interrupted 9-0 nylon is used for the arterial anastomosis, but a running suture can also be used. The temporary clips are removed. Any significant leaks are repaired using 9-0 nylon. There should be pulsatile flow in the pedicle after the clamps are released (Fig. 19.14). An internal venous Doppler is then placed on the donor vein and connected to the monitor box.

Once it is noted that good flow has been established through the flap, insetting may begin. The audible venous Doppler signal helps to ensure that the flap continues to be well perfused while the insetting takes place. The signal should resemble "waves at the beach" and should vary with respiration. Momentary clamping of the vein should result in immediate loss of the audible signal. If, during the insetting process, the signal is lost, the flap must be removed and the vessels must be visualized and rearranged so

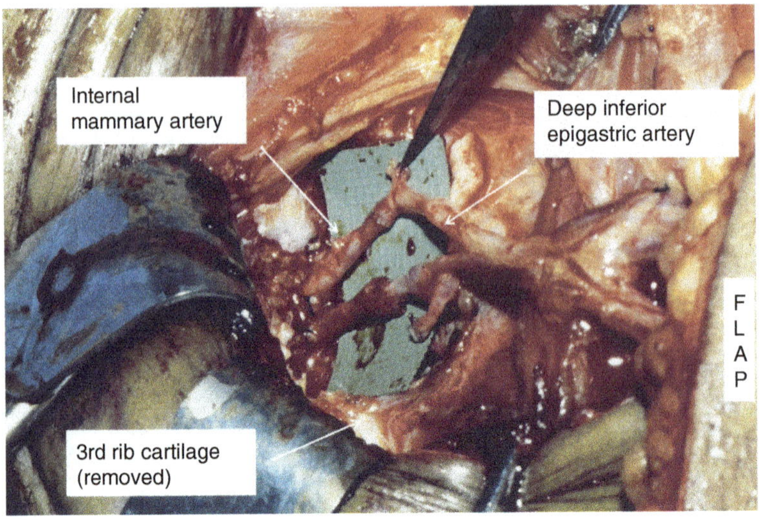

Fig. 19.14 Internal mammary to DIEP flap anastomosis

that they are not twisted, kinked, or compressed. The flap is tacked down using Vicryl sutures at the level of the IMF. The flap is then internalized within the mastectomy skin flaps.

At this point, the skin of the flap is marked. The skin not included in the external skin paddle is de-epithelized. It is critical to be certain that the mastectomy flaps are well perfused before de-epithelializing the flap. If there is questionable viability, the abdominal skin can be retained beneath the flap for a short period of time prior to the final removal of either the abdominal skin or the overlying mastectomy skin. This will avoid the need for a skin graft to replace nonviable mastectomy skin. The use of the intraoperative angiogram using indocyanine green helps to make the decision about the viability of the mastectomy skin. Skin that is not viable should be removed. Layered closure is performed. Using a handheld Doppler, the location of arterial and venous signals is marked on the skin paddle with a 5-0 Prolene suture so that it can be easily found in the postoperative period.

The patient is then placed in a flexed position for the abdominal wall closure. In a unilateral MS-TRAM procedure, the fascia is approximated using PDS suture in a running fashion. The contralateral abdominal wall may need to be plicated to centralize the umbilicus. In bilateral MS-TRAM or unilateral F-TRAM reconstruction, soft mesh is recommended to repair the fascial defect in order to prevent hernia or bulging. There is no need for mesh in the DIEP patients, including bilateral DIEP flaps.

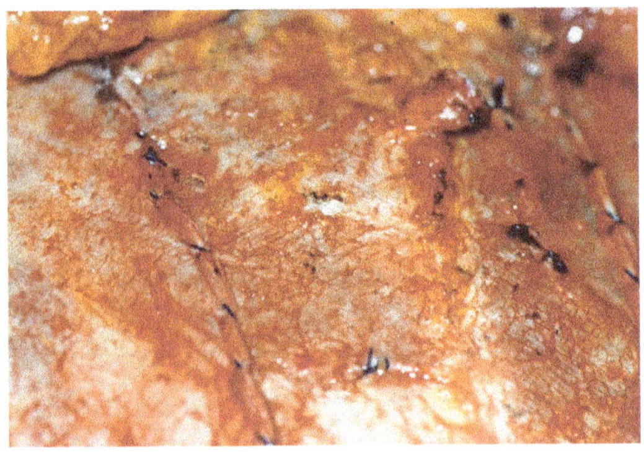

Fig. 19.15 Bilateral DIEP flap harvest, closure is tension-free with no muscle or fascia missing

The abdominal wall is undermined superiorly to the level of the xiphoid process in the midline. Lateral dissection is performed as needed. Significant perforators from the lateral row are preserved if possible. Perforators inferior to a subcostal scar should be preserved to avoid necrosis. Diastasis of the rectus is plicated if necessary. Closure even in bilateral flap harvest is straightforward and without tension (Fig. 19.15). Two suction drains are placed. Vicryl (0) sutures are used to close Scarpa's fascia in a simple interrupted fashion. The umbilicus is marked in the midline; an ellipse of skin is excised. The

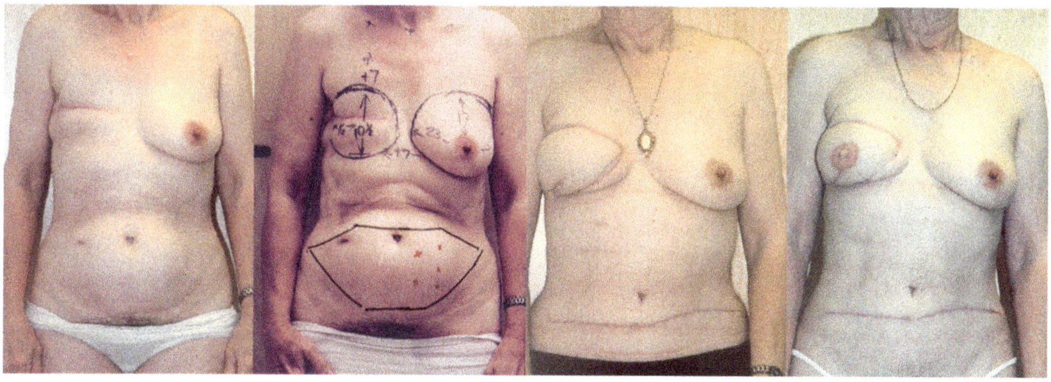

Fig. 19.16 Delayed unilateral DIEP flap: preoperative, planning, postoperative, after nipple

umbilicus is delivered through the wound and sutured into place. The abdominal skin wound is closed using 2/0 barbed suture in the deep dermal layer. The abdominal wound is dressed with surgical adhesive and an occlusive dressing; the patient is placed in a girdle. The breast wound edges are also dressed with surgical adhesive and left open for close observation.

Postoperative Course

The patient is sent to the ICU for frequent postoperative flap checks. It is important to be sure that the ICU nurse is oriented to the signals when the patient reaches the ICU. The ICU nurse records color, temperature, external arterial Doppler sounds, and internal venous Doppler sounds. These observations should be every 15 min for 4 h, then hourly. Any changes are immediately reported to the surgeon. Vascular inflow is verified by external arterial Doppler signals. Venous outflow is followed by both the internal Doppler signal and flap color. It is also possible to hear venous signals with the external Doppler. The patient remains in the 30° beach chair position. Sequential compression devices continue until ambulating, and DVT prophylaxis is started in the morning to prevent venous thromboembolism. On the first postoperative day, the Foley catheter is removed and the patient is allowed to ambulate. The patient must wear a support bra at all times when out of bed. The patient is discharged on the fourth postoperative day. They must be able to tolerate a general diet and able to ambulate without difficulty, and their pain must be controlled with oral pain medications.

The DIEP flap has become an integral part of autologous breast reconstruction. It utilizes a highly desirable donor site (patulous abdomen) and has a high degree of reliability with excellent aesthetic outcomes (Figs. 19.16 and 19.17).

Complications Associated with Free Flap

Overall, complete or partial flap loss rates following free flap breast reconstruction range from 1.5 to 5 %, with published postoperative vascular complications running on the order of 0.6–0.8 % for arterial thrombosis and 1.5–2.3 % for venous thrombosis [19–23]. Flap success in microsurgery is greatly dependent on the surgeon's technical skills and experience. There are three basic principles to successful microvascular reconstruction. First, during the dissection of the flap, care must be taken to avoid damaging the vessels. Second, the recipient vessels must be carefully dissected. Third, the microvascular anastomosis must be atraumatic, and the vessels must not be kinked or twisted. Marking the vessels in situ can help alleviate this complication. If these three steps are accomplished, a good outcome will likely result. The most common early complication is hematoma. Hematomas are manifest by swelling, pain, congestion, and excessive oozing

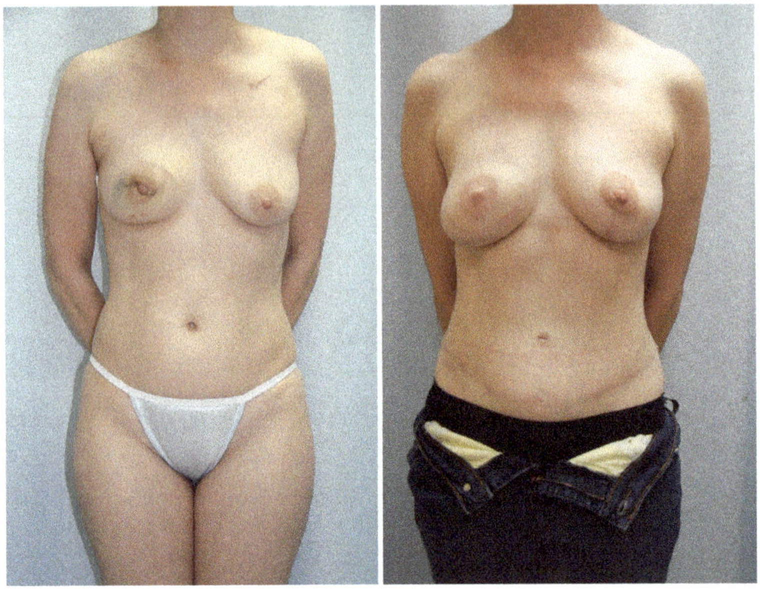

Fig. 19.17 Unilateral immediate reconstruction with DIEP flap

around the flap. Unfortunately, hematomas may compromise venous outflow and should be dealt with promptly.

Catastrophic complications most commonly occur in the first 12–24 h postoperatively. The majority of these compromised free flaps can be salvaged, but only if the complication is recognized in a timely fashion and prompt surgical intervention is made. For instance, Kroll et al. examined the timing of free flap vascular complications and found that 80 % of thrombosis occurred within the first 2 postoperative days. A number of authors have suggested a 2-day postoperative window as the "golden period" for potential salvage of free flaps compromised by pedicle thrombosis [19–25]. The largest series examining techniques in free flap salvage concluded that successful salvage was more likely to occur in the early postoperative period, within hours of diagnosis [26]. It is important to have a very low threshold for bringing a patient back to the operating room. With any suspected compromise, the flap should be explored [27].

The abdominal donor site also has possible complications. The most common is seroma formation. Seromas are far more common in obese patients. Prevention of seromas includes the use of quilting sutures between Scarpa's fascia and the abdominal wall and the use of suction drains. A prolonged seroma can lead to cellulitis and wound breakdown. Skin necrosis can also occur. This is far more common in smokers and obese patients. If extensive, the necrotic tissue will require debridement and the use of negative pressure (VAC) treatment. Virtually all heal with this protocol, but scar revision may need to be undertaken once the tissue softens.

Another frequent problem with autologous reconstruction is fat necrosis. This problem presents within the first weeks after surgery as a firm area within the flap. The extent may be difficult to define. It involves about 20 % of flaps, and the exact cause has not been determined. If small in area, it may be removed when the flap is revised. Partial excision, however, may lead to long-term drainage and is not advised. Concerns about recurrence can be alleviated by a small biopsy with closure.

When the flap has healed well, a second operative procedure is performed as an outpatient. This may include a nipple areolar reconstruction, revising abdominal dog ears and performing surgery on the opposite breast for symmetry, if indicated. Finally, patients are encouraged to undergo tattoo pigmentation for color matching to the contralateral nipple.

Other Perforator Flaps

Following the introduction of the perforator flap concept with the DIEP flap, a sizable number of other perforator flaps have been described, utilizing other perforating vessels. These include flaps harvested from the superior and inferior gluteal arteries (S-GAP and I-GAP), the profunda femoris artery (PAP), and the vessel perfusing the gracilis muscle. It is theoretically possible to develop perforator-based flaps wherever the donor site is not objectionable, and there is enough fat and skin to accomplish the reconstruction.

Gluteal Artery Perforator Flaps

The abdominal wall has become the gold standard in autologous breast reconstruction. The tissue is soft and pliable and can be easily shaped into a natural appearing ptotic breast. However, in patients who are thin and have undergone prior abdominoplasty or prior breast reconstruction with the abdominal flap, alternative donor sites for free tissue transfer are available.

Fujino et al. was the first to report the free transfer of gluteal tissue in 1975 [28]. It was originally described as a musculocutaneous flap, which resulted in a bulky flap with a short vascular pedicle. Vein grafts were needed for microvascular anastomosis. In the early 1990s, perforator flaps became of great interest for use in breast reconstruction. Allen and Tucker proposed an alternative to the gluteal musculocutaneous flap. They described the gluteal fascio-cutaneous perforator flap in which the gluteus maximus muscle is preserved and the pedicle length is adequate to perform microsurgical anastomosis without vein grafting [29].

The choice between S-GAP flaps and I-GAP flaps depends on the distribution of fat, the patient-desired scar position, and the location of sizeable perforators in the patient's gluteal area. Gluteal artery perforator flaps are considered an alternative when abdominal tissue is not available due to previous abdominoplasty, abdominal surgery, or extensive scarring. The procedure is technically demanding and more time consuming, since simultaneous teamwork cannot be accomplished with the patient in the prone position. However, in cases where abdominal tissue is not available, the gluteal fascio-cutaneous free flap provides adequate volume and projection that can mimic the contralateral breast.

Anatomy

The superior and inferior gluteal arteries (SGA and IGA) arise from the external iliac artery and pass through the sciatic foramen. Both vessels supply the gluteus maximus muscle. The SGA runs superior to the piriformis muscle and gives off several branches to the gluteus maximus muscle. Through the muscle, perforators supply the superior and lateral aspect of the buttock.

The inferior gluteal artery runs inferior to the piriformis muscle and proximal to coccygeus muscle. When exiting the sciatic foramen, the IGA runs with the internal pudendal vessels, pudendal nerve, sciatic nerve, and posterior cutaneous nerve of the thigh. The IGA penetrates the inframedial aspect of the gluteus maximus muscle and courses with the posterior cutaneous nerve of the thigh before penetrating the subcutaneous tissue of the buttock. The perforators of the IGA can be found in the middle third of the gluteal region, just above the gluteal crease [30–32] (Fig. 19.18).

Preoperative Imaging

CTA or MRA of the gluteal region has become a useful adjunct in GAP flaps. It aids in identifying the largest perforators with the least tortuous course through the gluteus maximus muscle. Rozen et al. noted regularly abundant S-GAP and I-GAP identifiable within the gluteal region. While many are diminutive in size, the identification of suitable perforators with CTA aids the operative planning for gluteal flap harvest [33].

S-GAP Flap Preoperative Marking

The marking take place in the preoperative holding area with the patient in the lateral decubitus position or prone position. The posterior superior iliac spine is marked along with the greater

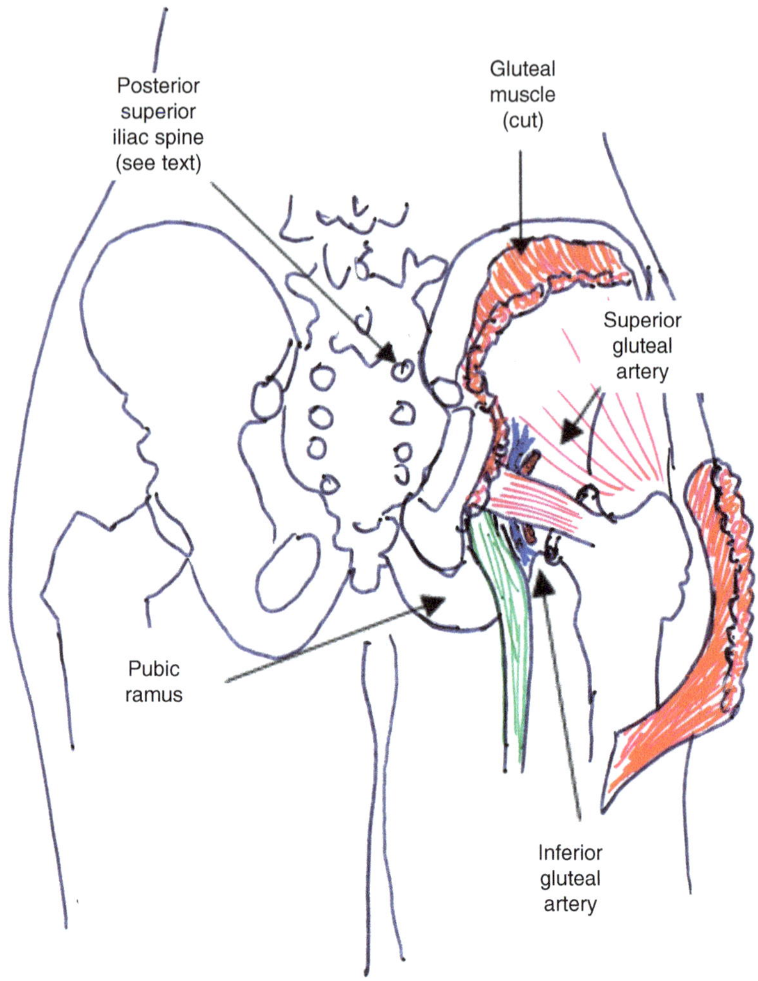

Fig. 19.18 Anatomical location of SGA and IGA

trochanter of the femur. The SGA perforators are found along this line in the medial one third [34, 35]. An elliptical skin paddle is designed to encompass the perforators. A donor site width of 6–8 cm can be closed primarily with minimal tension.

Procedure

The patient is placed in supine position. If immediate reconstruction is taking place, the oncologic surgeon completes the mastectomy and the IMA recipient vessels are dissected. In the delayed setting, the previous mastectomy incision is excised and skin flaps are raised. The IMA vessels are then prepared for microvascular anastomosis. The wounds are temporarily closed with staples and an occlusive dressing. The patient is then rotated to the prone position, paying attention not to place undue tension on the mastectomy skin flaps.

Incisions are made along the previously marked markings on the buttocks. A beveling technique can be employed to incorporate more subcutaneous tissue, adding bulk to the flap. Excessive beveling will result in a depressed scar. Dissection is then taken down to the subfascial plane. Unlike the DIEP flap, this dissection is performed in the subfascial plane. The flap is dissected from lateral to medial, preserving larger perforators along the way. The largest perforator(s) is preserved. Many times, however, the perforators will not join prior to arriving at the sacral fascia, and the flap is based on a single perforator.

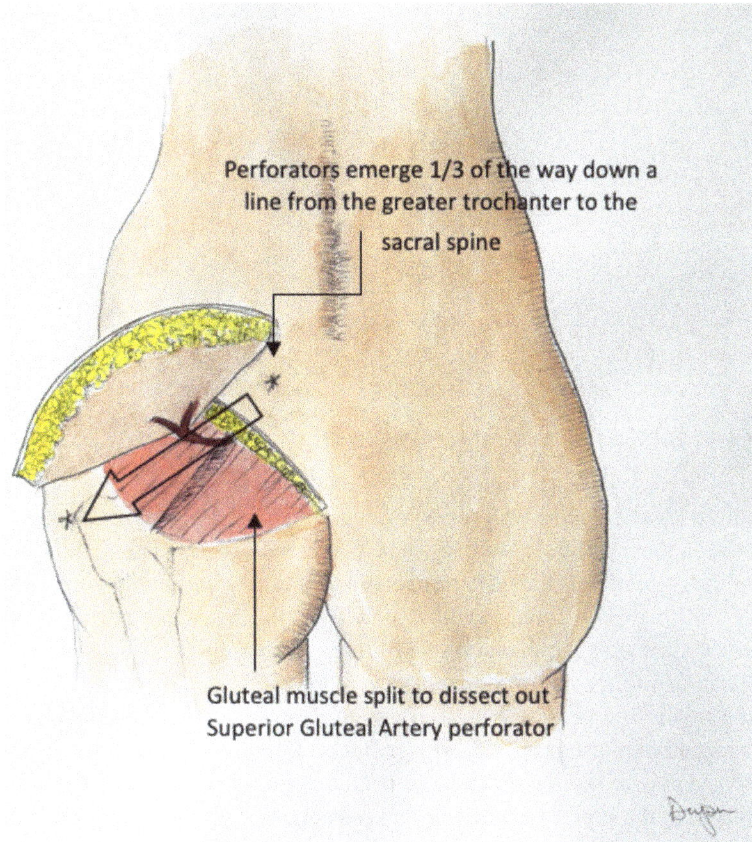

Fig. 19.19 The S-GAP flap

At the level of the perforator, the muscle is split along its fibers, and a self-retaining retractor is used to expose the vessels. The perforator is traced down to its origin near the piriformis muscle. Any side branches are ligated using hemoclips, taking care to achieve hemostasis. The vessels pass under the sacral fascia, and there are a number of large veins and arterial branches which require tedious dissection until the perforator joins the superior gluteal artery. Dissection ends when an acceptable artery diameter is reached (2 mm). A longer pedicle may be dissected by using a more lateral perforator. In this portion of the procedure, the assistant must be very careful to avoid tension or stretching of the pedicle. The pedicle is then ligated and the flap placed in a moist lap while the donor site is closed. The superior and inferior aspects of the donor site are undermined. The wound is closed in layers over a drain. Sterile dressings are applied and the patient is turned over into the supine position (Fig. 19.19).

Preoperative Marking: I-GAP Flap

The patient is marked in the supine position. The posterior superior iliac spine and ischial tuberosity are identified. The IGA perforators can be found half way between these points, just above the gluteal crease. An ellipse encompasses the perforators, and the inferior incision is made in the gluteal crease to hide the scar [30].

Procedure

Incisions are made along the markings and beveled out conservatively to include the subcutaneous tissue in the periphery. The flap is then elevated from lateral to medial in the subfascial plane, taking care to preserve perforating vessels. Near the ischial tuberosity, it is important to preserve adipose tissue. This helps minimize donor site morbidity. Once the dominant perforator is chosen, the gluteus muscle is split along its fibers. The IGA tends to have a more torturous

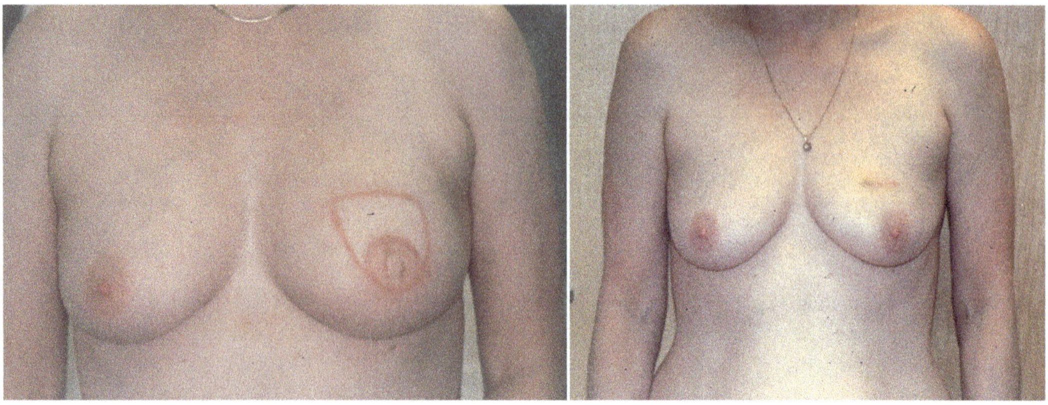

Fig. 19.20 Unilateral S-Gap, post-op and pre-op

intramuscular course than the SGA, making dissection more difficult. Adding to the complexity of the dissection is the posterior cutaneous nerve of the thigh, which runs with the IGA at this level. Care must be taken to avoid injury to the nerve and to prevent postoperative numbness of the thigh. The pedicle is ligated and the flap is wrapped in moist gauze. The donor site is closed in layers over suction drains. The patient is then placed in the supine position for flap anastomosis and inset.

Microvascular

The S-GAP or I-GAP flap is loosely approximated to the chest being careful not to twist the pedicle. The veins are prepared and sized. A venous coupler is used for this anastomosis. The artery is sutured using 9-0 nylon in an interrupted or running fashion. Once flow has been established, an internal venous Doppler is placed for monitoring in the postoperative period.

The flap is then inset, suturing the inferior portion of the flap at the level of the IMA. Areas of the flap that will be covered by the mastectomy skin are de-epithelized. The flap skin paddle is closed in layers with the mastectomy skin. An arterial signal is found using the handheld Doppler, and this site is marked with a stitch so that it can easily be found for monitoring.

Postoperative Care

The patient is monitored for the first 24 h in the ICU setting with the same protocol as the DIEP flap (see above). On postoperative day 1, the Foley is removed and the patient is encouraged to ambulate. The patient is discharged when they are ambulating and tolerating a diet and pain is under control with oral analgesics.

I-GAP vs. S-GAP

The I-GAP flap has several advantages over the S-GAP flap. The inferior gluteal region has more tissue readily available, and the scar is hidden in the crease of the buttock, which is more aesthetically pleasing. The S-GAP flap is technically easier to dissect, but the scar may lead to a contour deformity in the buttock. Both flaps require a skilled surgeon who is cognizant of the unique anatomy of the gluteal region. In the appropriately selected patient, the GAP flaps can achieve a natural appearing breast with adequate projection (Figs. 19.20 and 19.21).

Profunda Femoris Artery Perforator Flap

In 1983, Baek et al. described the skin territory supplied by the third perforator of the profunda femoris artery [36]. Since then, the application of this flap had primarily been explored as a source of tissue for local advancement and lower extremity reconstruction. In 2001, Angrigiani et al. described posterior thigh flaps based on the profunda femoris artery [37]. It was not until 2012 that descriptions for the profunda femoris

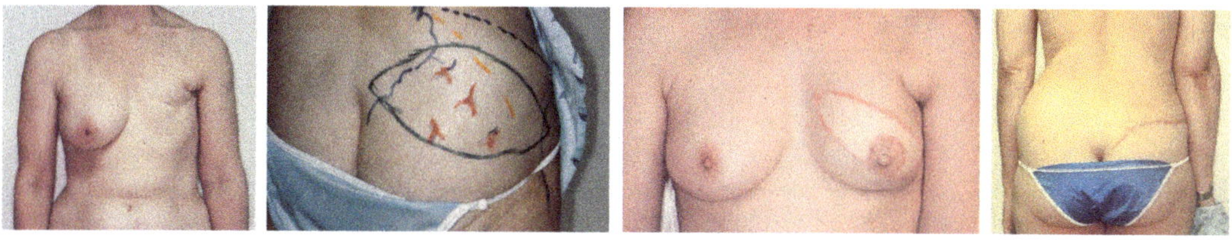

Fig. 19.21 Delayed reconstruction with S-GAP flap

artery perforator (PAP) flap were used in autologous breast reconstruction [38].

Though the DIEP flap for breast reconstruction remains our number one choice for autologous breast reconstruction, the abdomen as a donor site may be excluded by previous surgery or lack of soft tissue. In these cases, we utilize the profunda artery perforator flap as a second option. The PAP flap offers a mean tissue weight of 385 g, is easily harvested with the patient in the supine position, and provides an acceptable donor site scar.

Anatomy

The posterior thigh is bordered medially by the adductor muscle, laterally by the iliotibial tract, superiorly by the gluteal fold, and inferiorly by the popliteal fossa. The profunda femoris branches from the femoral artery at approximately the level of the lesser trochanter. Immediately after branching, the internal (medial) and external (lateral) circumflex arteries branch off toward the posterior and anterior aspects, respectively. The profunda femoris artery then dives deep, to supply flow to the posterior thigh. There are three main perforators that branch off. The first supplies the adductor magnus and gracilis, and the second and third perforators supply the semimembranosus, the biceps femoris, and the vastus lateralis. There are both medial and lateral perforators. More commonly, the medial perforators are dominant and tend to be located posterior to the gracilis muscle [38].

From a study of cadavers, several estimations of the arteries were developed: (1) Average distance inferior to the gluteal crease was 3.5 cm (1–5 cm). (2) Average distance from the midline was 6.2 cm (3–12 cm). (3) The average pedicle length was 10.6 cm. (4) Diameters of the artery and vein averaged 2.3 mm and 2.8 mm. (5) The flaps averaged 28 × 8 cm. (6) Average weight was 206 g (100–260 g). Per computed tomography angiograms of the same 20 thighs, measurements were taken from the gluteal crease and midline to the perforator. The average distance caudal from the gluteal crease was 4.4 cm (1.1–7.2 cm), and the average distance lateral from the midline was 5.1 cm (2.5–9 cm) [39].

Perioperative Imaging

Preoperative imaging is essential to identify the profunda perforator coursing through the adductor magnus muscle. CTA or MRI of the pelvis and thigh with contrast is especially important if the procedure is to be done in supine position because there is no "rescue" flap if the PAP flap cannot be harvested. This will be discussed in more detail below.

Marking

The patient is marked the day before surgery in a standing position after identifying the perforator with a Doppler probe. The transverse ellipse is drawn such that the medial marking lies at the adductor longus, the superior border travels 1 cm below the gluteal crease, the inferior marking is 7–8 cm below this, and the posterior marking is just at the edge of the gluteal crease. The transverse width averages 27 cm. The location of the flap should be on the median posterior thigh so that the scar neither extends into the visible medial nor lateral thigh.

Procedure

This procedure has been successful in both a prone and supine approach. We greatly favor the supine approach. Each will be described with its respective advantages and disadvantages.

Supine: The patient is placed in a modified dorsal recumbent, or "frog leg," position. An

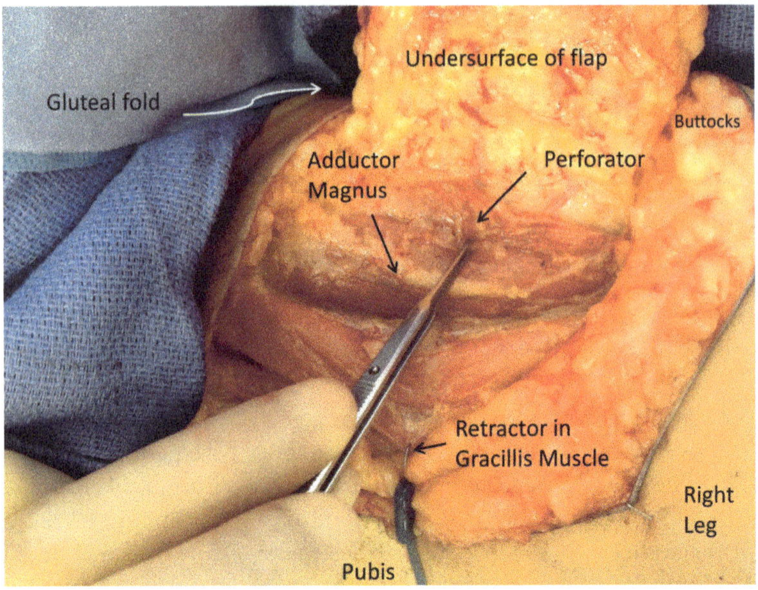

Fig. 19.22 Perforating vessel (second perforator off of profunda) emerging through adductor magnus (patient in supine/frog leg position)

elliptical incision is made and dissection is taken to the level of the supra-fascial plane. Dissection proceeds in an anterior or a medial to posterior or lateral fashion, and the gracilis muscle is identified. The fascia is entered over the gracilis muscle, and the perforator is identified, entering the flap from its emergence from the adductor muscle. The pedicle, which averages 10 cm in length, is dissected through the adductor magnus to its origin at the profunda artery. The wound is closed in multiple layers over a drain with emphasis placed on suturing the inferior subcutaneous fascia to Colles' fascia superiorly. The flap is inset in a coned fashion. Complications are minimal and include donor site seroma, minor wound dehiscence, and flap fat necrosis rate less than 7 %. The profunda perforator flap to date has proven to be a great option as a second option in free flap autologous breast reconstruction.

The advantage of performing this procedure in the supine position is that there is a shorter operative duration, because there is no need for repositioning and the rapid medial to lateral dissection. The disadvantage is that there is no alternative to the flap if the perforating vessels are not found (Fig. 19.22).

Prone: The prone position approaches the flap from lateral to medial. The dissection occurs in the supra-fascial layer until it nears the previously marked perforators. At that time, dissection is taken to the subfascial level as this facilitates better exposure of the perforators (Fig. 19.23). The advantage of this approach is that it preserves the ability to perform a transverse upper gracilis flap if there are inadequate perforators. The disadvantage is that intraoperative repositioning is required, adding to the total operative time.

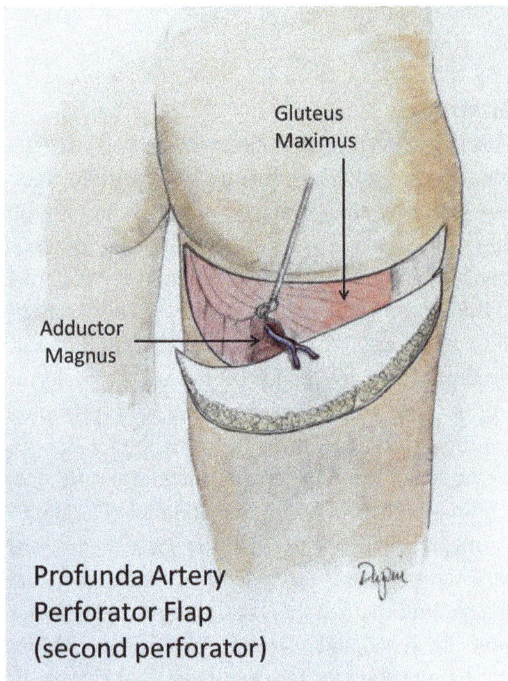

Fig. 19.23 The profunda artery perforator flap

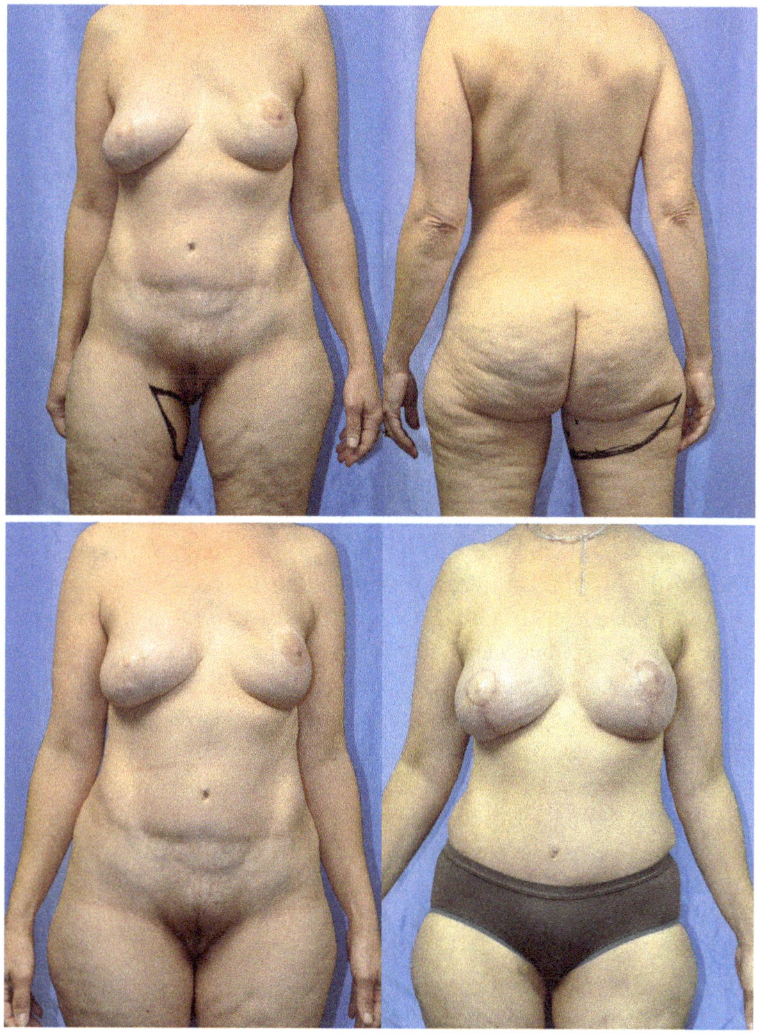

Fig. 19.24 A fifty-five-year-old with history of right breast cancer and right DIEP breast reconstruction developed a new breast cancer in the left breast and underwent a nipple-sparing mastectomy and left PAP flap breast reconstruction. These results are at 6 weeks postoperatively from a second-stage balancing operation

For both approaches, beveling in the lateral thigh can help increase the flap volume, as well as improved postoperative donor site contour. Beveling should not be done in such a way as to lose the contour of the gluteal fold. In the study by Allen et al., the flap size ranged from 235 to 695 g with an average of 385 g. This could be an insufficient volume for women with large breasts that require more tissue for reconstruction.

Postoperative Care

Standard free flap postoperative care should be used to monitor this flap: The patient is admitted to the intensive care unit, and every 15 min vascular checks are performed for the first 4 h and then every 1 h for the next 20 h. Once transferred to a standard bed, the patient is allowed to ambulate but should avoid any strenuous exercise for 4 weeks.

Complications

As noted by Allen et al., there is a potential to accentuate a preoperatively prominent "saddle-bag" if the flap is not beveled to include the subcutaneous soft tissue from the donor site. There is commonly a lowering of the infra-gluteal fold. Another possibility is damage to the posterior femoral cutaneous never during dissection. If the medial pedicle is chosen, dissection in the supra-fascial plane after pedicle identification should avoid injury to the nerve (Figs. 19.24 and 19.25).

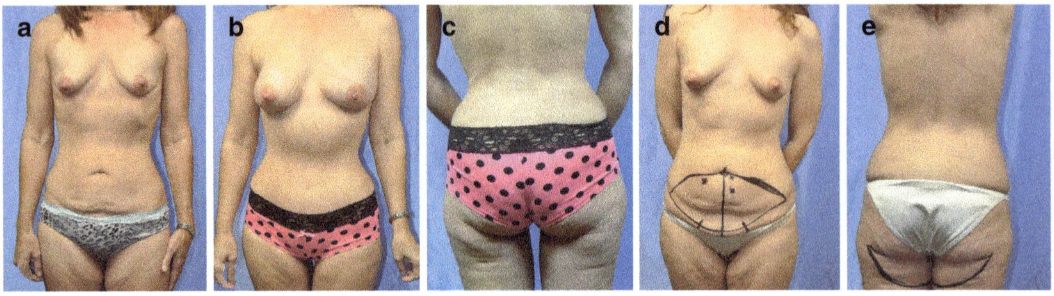

Fig. 19.25 (**a**–**e**) A thirty-five-year-old with strong family history of breast cancer underwent bilateral nipple-sparing mastectomies with bilateral DIEP and PAP stacked flaps for breast reconstruction. These results are at 6 months postoperatively. (**a**) Pre- and (**b**, **c**) postoperative views and (**d**, **e**) preoperative markings

Stacked Perforator Flaps in Bilateral Breast Reconstruction

The DIEP flap for breast reconstruction at times does not offer adequate volume. Our practice has addressed this volume deficiency by providing additional tissue by "stacking" two flaps to reconstruct each breast. Previous reports have described utilizing either two DIEP flaps for a unilateral reconstruction or a DIEP and a superior gluteal artery perforator flap. The addition of the S-GAP necessitated having the patient in both the prone and supine position and offered the firmer, less malleable fat quality of the upper gluteal fat. In an effort to avoid the drawbacks of the S-GAP but provide autologous reconstruction when the abdominal soft tissue volume is not sufficient, we have combined the profunda artery perforator flap with the DIEP flap for bilateral stacked breast reconstruction.

Two experienced microsurgeons harvest all four flaps. They are harvested in a standard fashion with the patient in the supine/frog leg position. The internal mammary vessels are exposed with resection of portions of the superior and inferior ribs within the third intercostal space. The PAP flap is first anastomosed to the antegrade internal mammary vessels, and then the DIEP flap is anastomosed to the retrograde internal mammary vessels. The flap pedicles actually cross as the DIEP is placed superiorly to provide superior pole and medial volume and the PAP is placed in a transverse orientation along the lower pole, providing a pleasing contour. The addition of two free flaps to our bilateral breast reconstructions has not increased our flap loss rate which remains below 1 %, and donor site morbidity is on par with that historically for each individual flap. Stacked flaps are ideal for autologous reconstruction when the abdomen does not provide sufficient volume for reconstruction. Combining the PAP with the DIEP offers superior aesthetics while allowing operative efficiency and no increase in morbidity (Figs. 19.24 and 19.25).

References

1. Albornoz CR, Bach RB, Meharar BJ, et al. A paradigm shift in U.S. breast reconstruction: increasing implant rates. Plast Reconstr Surg. 2013;131(1): 15–23.
2. Maxwell GP. Iginio Tnasini and the origin of the latissimus dorsi musculocutaneous flap. Plast Reconstr Surg. 1980;65:686.
3. Boehmler JH, Butler CE. Latissimus dorsi flap breast reconstruction. In: Hall-Findlay EJ, Evans GRD, editors. Aesthetic and reconstructive surgery of the breast. Edinburgh: Elsevier Limited; 2010. p. 51–60.
4. Spear SL, Ducic I, Cuoco F, Hannan C. The effect of smoking on flap and donor-site complications in pedicled TRAM breast reconstruction. Plast Reconstr Surg. 2005;116(7):1873–80.
5. Kroll SS, Netscher DT. Complications of TRAM flap breast reconstruction in obese patients. Plast Reconstr Surg. 1989;84(6):886–92.
6. Paige KT, Bostwick J, Bried JT, Jones G. A comparison of morbidity from bilateral, unipedicled and unilateral, unipedicled TRAM flap breast reconstructions. Plast Reconstr Surg. 1998;101(7):1819–27. Print.

7. Berrino P, Campora E, Leone S, et al. The transverse rectus abdominis musculocutaneous flap for breast reconstruction in obese patients. Ann Plast Surg. 1991;27:221.
8. Moran SL, Serletti JM. Outcome comparison between free and pedicled TRAM flap breast reconstruction in the obese patient. Plast Reconstr Surg. 2001;108(7): 1954–60. Print.
9. Bailey SH, Oni G, Guevara R, Wong C, Saint-Cyr M. Latissimus dorsi donor-site morbidity: the combination of quilting and fibrin sealant reduce length of drain placement and seroma rate. Ann Plast Surg. 2012;68(6):555–8.
10. Moon H, Taylor I. The vascular anatomy of the rectus abdominis musculocutaneous flaps based on the deep superficial epigastric system. Plast Reconstr Surg. 1988;82:815.
11. Takeishi M, Shaw W, Ahn C, et al. TRAM flaps in patients with previous abdominal scars. Plast Reconstr Surg. 1982;69:216.
12. Weiss PR. TRAM flap breast reconstruction. In: Hall-Findlay EJ, Evans GRD, editors. Aesthetic and reconstructive surgery of the breast. Edinburgh: Elsevier Limited; 2010. p. 61–80.
13. Parrett BM, Caterson SA, Tobia AM, Lee BT. DIEP flaps in women with abdominal scars: are complication rates affected? Plast Reconstr Surg. 2008;121(5): 1527–31.
14. Takeishi M, Shaw WW, Anh CY, Borud LJ. TRAM flaps in patients with abdominal scars. Plast Reconstr Surg. 1997;99(3):713–22.
15. Scott JR, Liu D, Said H, et al. Computed tomographic angiography in planning abdomen-based microsurgical breast reconstruction: a comparison with color duplex ultrasound. Plast Reconstr Surg. 2010;125:446–53.
16. Rozen W, Ashton M, Stella D, et al. The accuracy of computed tomographic angiography for mapping the perforators of the DIEA: a cadaveric study. Plast Reconstr Surg. 2008;122:363–9.
17. Saad A, Rebowe RE, Hogan ME, Wise MW, Hilaire HS, Sadeghi A, Dupin CL. Localization of the dominant deep inferior epigastric artery perforator by computed tomography angiogram: does the standard deep inferior epigastric artery perforator flap design include the dominant perforator? Ann Plast Surg. 2014;72(6): 670–3.
18. Dupin CL, Allen RJ, Glass CA, Bunch R. The internal mammary artery and vein as a recipient site for free-flap breast reconstruction: a report of 110 consecutive cases. Plast Reconstr Surg. 1996;98(4):685–9.
19. Greco III JA, Castaldo ET, Nanney LB, et al. Autologous breast reconstruction: the Vanderbilt experience (1998 to 2005) of independent predictors of displeasing outcomes. J Am Coll Surg. 2008;207:49–56.
20. Mehrara BJ, Santoro TD, Arcilla E, Watson JP, Shaw WW, Da Lio AL. Complications after microvascular breast reconstruction: experience with 1195 flaps. Plast Reconstr Surg. 2006;118:1100–9; discussion 1110–1.
21. Sullivan SR, Fletcher DR, Isom CD, Isik FF. True incidence of all complications following immediate and delayed breast reconstruction. Plast Reconstr Surg. 2008;122:19–28.
22. Selber JC, Kurichi JE, Vega SJ, Sonnad SS, Serletti JM. Risk factors and complications in free TRAM flap breast reconstruction. Ann Plast Surg. 2006;56:492–7.
23. Fosnot J, Jandali S, Low DW, Kovach SJ, Wu LC, Serletti JM. Closer to an understanding of fate: the role of vascular complications in free flap breast reconstruction. Plast Reconstr Surg. 2011;128(4): 835–43.
24. Kroll SS, Schusterman MA, Reece GP, Miller MJ, Evans GR, Robb GL, Baldwin BJ. Timing of pedicle thrombosis and flap loss after free-tissue transfer. Plast Reconstr Surg. 1996;98:1230–3.
25. Khouri RK, Cooley BC, Kunselman AR, Landis JR, Yeramian P, Ingram D, Natarajan N, Benes CO, Wallemark C. A prospective study of microvascular free-flap surgery and outcome. Plast Reconstr Surg. 1998;102:711–21.
26. Chang EI, Mehrara BJ, Festekjian JH, Da Lio AL, Crisera CA. Vascular complications and microvascular free flap salvage: the role of thrombolytic agents. Microsurgery. 2011;31(7):505–9.
27. Bui DT, Cordeiro PG, Hu QY, Disa JJ, Pusic A, Mehrara BJ. Free flap reexploration: indications, treatment, and outcomes in 1193 free flaps. Plast Reconstr Surg. 2007;119:2092–100.
28. Fujino T, Harasina T, Aoyagi F. Reconstruction for aplasia of the breast and pectoral region by microvascular transfer of a free flap from the buttock. Plast Reconstr Surg. 1975;56:178–81.
29. Allen RJ, Tucker Jr C. Superior gluteal artery perforator free flap for breast reconstruction. Plast Reconstr Surg. 1995;95:1207–12.
30. Allen RJ, Levine JL, Granzow JW. The in-the-crease inferior gluteal artery perforator flap for breast reconstruction. Plast Reconstr Surg. 2006;118:333–9.
31. Zenn M, Milard JA. Free inferior gluteal flap harvest with sparing of the posterior femoral cutaneous nerve. J Reconstr Microsurg. 2006;22:509–12.
32. Ahmadzadeh R, Bergeron L, Tang M, Morris SF. The superior and inferior gluteal artery perforator flaps. Plast Reconstr Surg. 2007;120:1551–6.
33. Rozen WM, Ting JWC, Grinsell D, Ashton MW. Superior and inferior gluteal artery perforators: in-vivo anatomical study and planning for breast reconstruction. J Plast Reconstr Aesthet Surg. 2010;64(2): 217–25.
34. Codner MA, Nahai F. The gluteal free flap breast reconstruction: making it work. Clin Plast Surg. 1994;21:289–96.
35. Guerra AB, Metainger SE, Bidros RS, et al. Breast reconstruction with gluteal artery perforator flaps: a critical analysis of 142 cases. Ann Plast Surg. 2004;52:118–25.
36. Baek SM. Two new cutaneous free flaps: the medial and lateral thigh flaps. Plast Reconstr Surg. 1983; 71:354.

37. Angrigiani C, Grilli D, Thorne CH. The adductor flap: a new method for transferring posterior and medial thigh skin. Plast Reconstr Surg. 2001;107:1725–31.
38. Allen RJ, et al. Breast reconstruction with the profunda artery perforator flap. Plast Reconstr Surg. 2012;129(1):16e–23.
39. Saad A, Sadeghi A, Allen RJ. The anatomic basis of the profunda femoris artery perforator flap: a new option for autologous breast reconstruction – a cadaveric and computer tomography angiogram study. J Reconstr Microsurg. 2012;28(6):381–6.

Reconstruction for Locally Advanced and Recurrent Breast Cancer

20

Christopher Sanders and Charles Dupin

Background

Locally advanced breast cancer (LABC) represents a unique problem for both the oncologic therapy and reconstruction of breast cancer patients.

LABC patients may require resection of large amounts of skin and soft tissue and may require resection of the chest wall as well. Reconstructive surgeons may also face challenges with altered healing as a result of radiation and other adjuvant therapies. According to the 2010 American Joint Committee on Cancer (AJCC) and the International Union for Cancer Control (IUCC), the TNM breast cancer staging system for LABC includes advanced primary tumors and/or patients with advanced regional nodal disease. Advanced primary tumors include: (1) tumors >5 cm in greatest dimension (T3); (2) direct extension to the chest wall, involvement of skin with skin nodules, edema, or *peau d'orange*; and (3) inflammatory breast cancer, a distinct entity that will be discussed later in the chapter. Advanced regional nodal disease includes (1) ipsilateral level I and II axillary lymph nodes that are clinically fixed or matted or clinically detected internal mammary lymph nodes in the absence of axillary lymph node metastasis (N2) and (2) ipsilateral level III lymph nodes, ipsilateral internal mammary lymph nodes with axillary lymph node metastasis, or ipsilateral supraclavicular lymph node (N3). These clinical and pathologic findings define LABC as stage III disease.

Inflammatory breast cancer is included in the definition of LABC but represents a unique pathologic entity. Rare and aggressive, the AJCC and IUCC define inflammatory breast cancer as diffuse erythema and edema, with *peau d'orange*, involving one-third or more of the skin of the breast. These skin changes are caused by tumor emboli within the dermal lymphatics. Based on the TNM staging system, inflammatory breast cancer is considered a T4b lesion. Characteristics of inflammatory breast cancer include rapid progression, highly angiogenic and angioinvasive. It is the aggressive involvement of vasculature that accounts for the high metastatic potential that is an intrinsic feature of the tumor (Fig. 20.1).

Epidemiology

LABC represents 5–20 % of all breast cancer in developed countries. While the incidence is decreasing in mammographically screened populations (less than 5 % of those in the United States), LABC cases represent up to 40–50 % of new cases in underdeveloped countries. The incidence also appears to be higher in younger women and African-American and Hispanic women. In contrast, inflammatory breast cancer (IBC) represents 0.5–2 % of cases in the United

C. Sanders, MD (✉) • C. Dupin, MD
Division of Plastic Surgery, Department of Surgery, Louisiana State University Health Sciences Center, 1542 Tulane Avenue, New Orleans, LA 70112, USA
e-mail: csand7@lsuhsc.edu; cldupinmd@gmail.com

A.I. Riker (ed.), *Breast Disease: Comprehensive Management*,
DOI 10.1007/978-1-4939-1145-5_20, © Springer Science+Business Media New York 2015

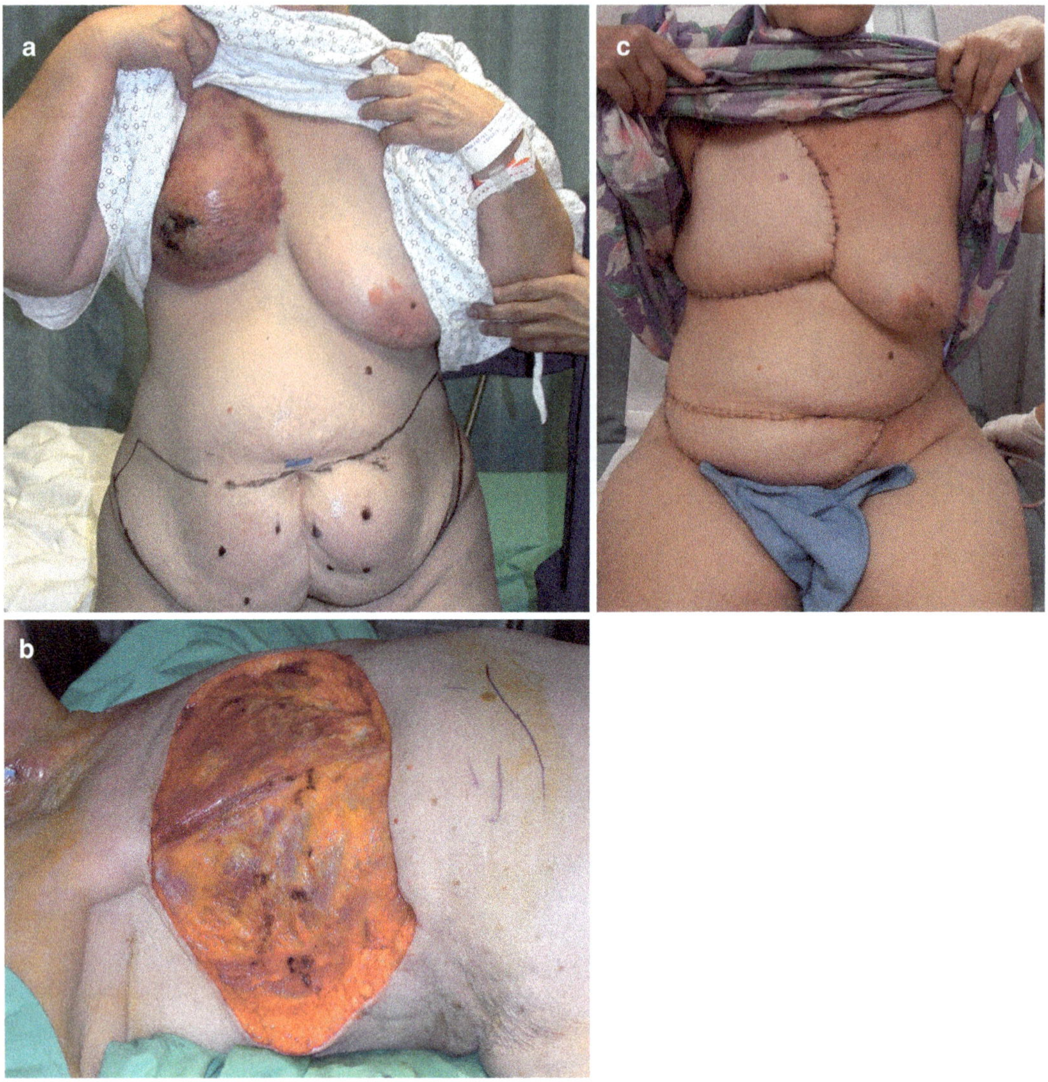

Fig. 20.1 (**a**–**c**) Inflammatory breast cancer of the right breast: chest wall reconstruction with extended DIEP flap 25 × 25 cm; abdominal donor site closed with V-Y advanced DIEP flap from the right side of the abdomen

States. However, it appears to be increasing in incidence, particularly in white women. It is important to note that the incidence of IBC remains higher in African-Americans. It also tends to be diagnosed at an earlier age (median 59 vs. 66) as compared to LABC [1–3].

Treatment

Although the specific treatment options are too in-depth for discussion here, some important aspects of treatment for LABC are useful to keep in mind. In general, the treatment of LABC utilizes multimodality therapy that includes systemic chemotherapy, either in the neoadjuvant or adjuvant setting, and locoregional therapy with radiation. As radiation therapy is the standard in the multimodal treatment of LABC and IBC, special attention must be given to its physiologic side effects on the breast. The mechanism of injury may involve vaso-occlusive processes as well as chromosomal alterations in fibroblasts that result in dysfunctional collagen formation [4, 5].

These physiologic aberrations result in markedly increased complication rates after radiation treatment in patients treated primarily with mastectomy. One study cites an institutional complication rate (including wound infections, dehiscence, and necrosis) in up to 50 % of mastectomy patients and 30–87 % of chest wall reconstruction patients previously treated with postoperative radiation [6–9].

The reconstructive surgeon must be prepared to excise much of the irradiated tissue, which can result in a much larger defect than anticipated. Local tissue may often be inadequate because of radiation damage and microsurgical efforts may be complicated by alterations in the wound bed, as well as recipient vessels. As a result, donor tissue must be well outside of the irradiated fields to ensure the greatest potential for flap survival.

Chest Wall Reconstruction

Patients with LABC without evidence of distant metastasis can undergo operative treatment with curative intent. The goals of chest wall reconstruction in LABC patients are to alleviate symptoms, to enhance quality of life, and to cover vital structures. Several options are available for chest wall reconstruction, with multiple factors to consider before any particular case. Some of these factors are the patient's desire, outcome, and willingness to undergo multiple (often lengthy) procedures and extended hospital stays. Physiologic factors that impact operative strategy include size, composition of the defect, quality of donor and recipient tissues, and the effects of radiation as described above.

Skin Grafting

Although much discussion has been given to the "reconstructive ladder" and after primary closure, the next "simplest" option for chest wall reconstruction is placement of a split-thickness skin graft (STSG). The STSG is only an option, however, when the defect is limited to the skin and subcutaneous tissue. When skin grafts are applied to irradiated tissue, they may not "take" as skin grafts rely on recipient beds for their blood supply. Skin grafting is also the least aesthetically acceptable option of all options for chest wall reconstruction, but it remains a valuable adjunct for coverage of muscle flaps employed in larger defects. The muscle flap that has not been irradiated is an acceptable recipient site for STSG.

Flaps

Local Flaps

Local flaps can be employed for the coverage of smaller defects of the chest wall. The limitation of local flaps is the dependence on the quality of the surrounding tissue. Local flaps are often excluded from use because of the effects of radiation, the size of flap available, and their limited utility in chest wall reconstruction for LABC.

Regional Flaps

As previously stated, LABC typically requires extensive resection of tissue and causes large defects. Myocutaneous flaps are the most commonly employed approach, since these flaps provide enough bulk and coverage for large defects of the chest wall.

Latissimus Dorsi Flap

The latissimus dorsi flap is one of the most commonly used flaps for chest wall reconstruction for LABC. A class V muscle flap with a dominant pedicle (the thoracodorsal artery and vein) and a secondary blood supply (the posterior intercostal perforators), the latissimus flap was first described by Tansini in 1897 for chest wall reconstruction. Over the years, multiple revisions and improvements in harvesting techniques have led the latissimus flap to become one of the most versatile flaps in all of plastic surgery.

The latissimus dorsi flap has several benefits. The dissection is rapid, relatively straightforward, and safe. The muscle has a long pedicle that facilitates local transfer as a pedicle-based flap or as a microvascular free tissue transfer. A skin island can be oriented in virtually any direction, and its proximity to the chest makes it ideal for breast reconstruction. Disadvantages of the flap are few, but not insignificant. The width of the traditional elliptical skin island cannot exceed 9–10 cm or the donor site cannot be closed primarily. For large defects, a skin graft will be needed to cover the exposed portions of the muscle. A modification of the traditional skin pattern by Micali and Carramaschi described below allows for a larger skin island.

Many of the disadvantages are related to donor site morbidity. Seroma formation after latissimus dorsi harvest has been reported to have an incidence of anywhere between 4 % and 80 % of patients [10]. Dynamic testing has shown that there is a decrease in strength in the affected extremity after latissimus dorsi muscle transfer [11]. That effect appears to be greater in women than in men [12]. While this decrease in strength has not been shown to affect normal daily activities, special consideration must be given to patients with increased reliance on shoulder girdle strength, such as those who are walker dependent. While radiation to the axilla or previous axillary dissection is not a contraindication to latissimus dorsi flap utilization, one must keep in mind that the vascular supply may be compromised in irradiated fields or disrupted by axillary dissection.

A modification of the latissimus dorsi flap has been described by Micali and Carramaschi [13]. They describe what they refer to as an extended V-Y musculocutaneous flap; the primary benefits include decrease in the morbidity of the donor site and ability to close the donor site primarily. The skin island of this flap is a large triangle, with its base along the chest wall defect (in the case of mastectomy, the posterior-lateral resection edge). The apex of the flap is at the midline of the back, and the flap is situated over musculocutaneous perforators that emerge from the underlying latissimus dorsi muscle.

The large triangular skin flap is incised circumferentially down to the underlying latissimus flap. The skin of the back is then elevated above the latissimus muscle until the entire muscle outer surface is exposed. The muscle is then harvested in the normal manner, based on the thoracodorsal circulation. Once freed from its origin and insertion, the flap will easily move into the chest defect, carrying the large skin island (as much as 22 cm in width and 42 cm in length). The donor site is closed as a V-Y [10]. Fierreira, Mendoca, et al. reported a series of 25 patients with excellent outcomes [14] (Figs. 20.2 and 20.3).

Rectus Abdominis Flaps

Rectus abdominis flaps have been a mainstay of reconstructive surgery for nearly 50 years. Like the latissimus dorsi flap, the rectus abdominis flap has the benefit of relative ease of elevation, reliable vascular pedicle (arising from the superior and deep inferior epigastric arteries), and a large amount of tissue available for harvest. The collateral circulation between these vessels allows the rectus to be oriented in a variety of configurations.

The vertically oriented rectus abdominis muscle myocutaneous (VRAM) flap can be used in reconstruction after resection of LABC. However, because of the VRAM's limited vertically oriented skin paddle, the transverse rectus abdominis (TRAM) flap is much more commonly employed for breast cancer reconstruction. The TRAM flap is one of the most common tools in the reconstructive surgeon's repertoire, owing to larger tissue and skin paddle available and an aesthetically appealing donor site scar. TRAM flaps may be designed as pedicle-based flaps or free tissue transfer. Free TRAM flaps have the benefit of being versatile in terms of position. Multiple vessels may be exposed during chest wall resection and can be used for recipient vessels for free tissue transfer.

Utility of the TRAM flap may be limited in patients who smoke, have diabetes, and have had previous abdominal surgery or in patients where the dominant pedicle (internal mammary artery)

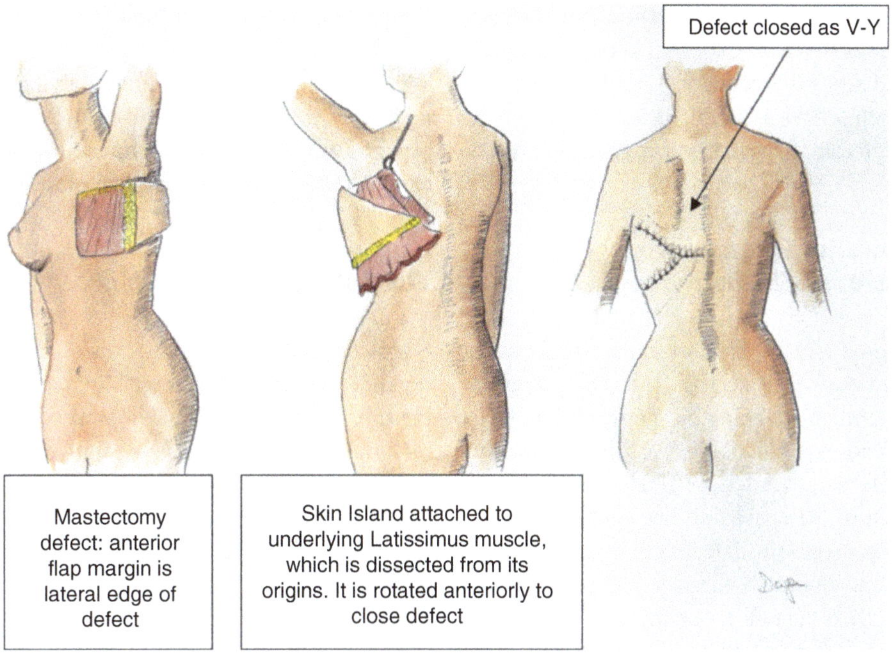

Fig. 20.2 The latissimus musculocutaneous V-Y rotational flap

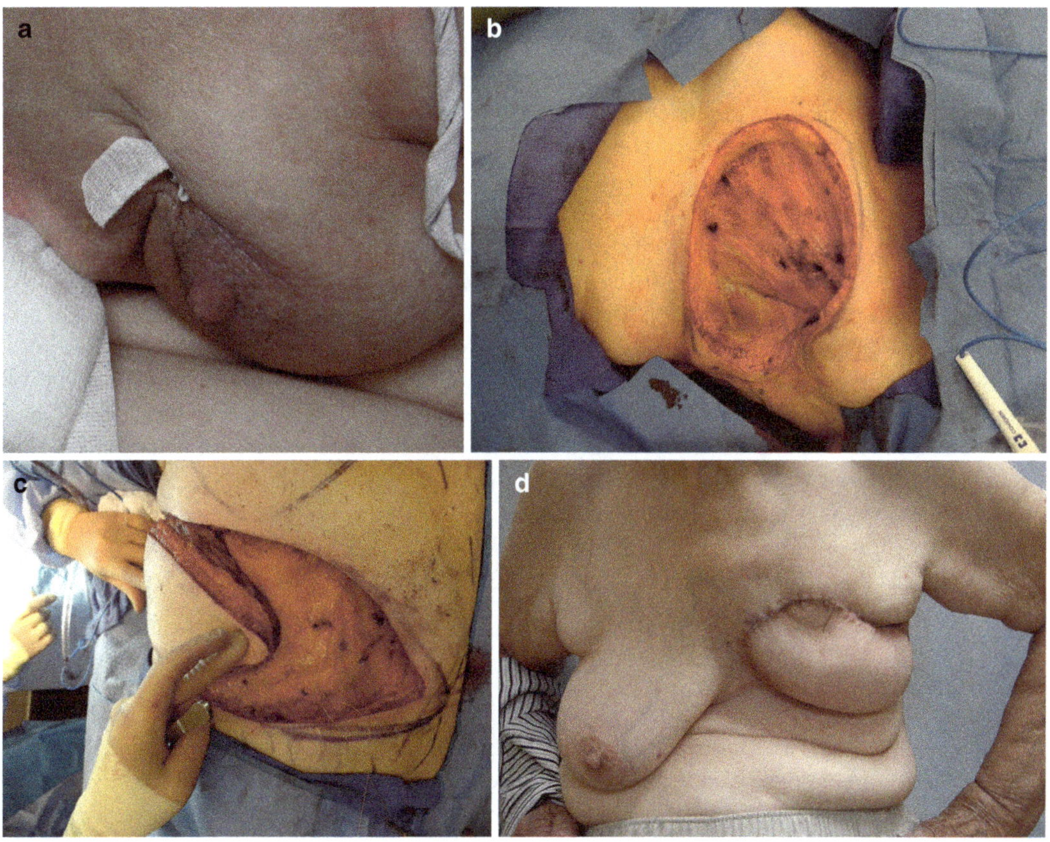

Fig. 20.3 Mastectomy patient with large wound closed with V-Y latissimus myocutaneous flap. (**a**) Locally advanced breast cancer with involved skin (**b**) defect after resection (**c**) latissimus advanced with overlying skin in V-Y fashion (**d**) final result

is compromised by tumor excision. Another disadvantage is the morbidity associated with muscle harvested from the abdominal wall and increase risk of hernia. This morbidity is decreased with the use of perforator flaps that will be discussed below.

Deep Inferior Epigastric Artery Perforator (DIEP) Flap

While some authors have raised concerns about reported rates of fat necrosis, the DIEP flap has become the most common flap in our breast reconstruction practice. It is used in both patients with early stage and LABC. In cases where a large area of the chest wall has been resected or a large mastectomy defect is present, we have been able to employ both sides of the lower abdomen as DIEP flaps to cover the area. While this necessitates two microvascular anastomoses, it can provide coverage for very large areas of the chest wall. Drawbacks of the DIEP relate mostly to the need for microsurgical skill. As previously described, the donor site morbidity in TRAM flaps is decreased by the DIEP flap that does not harvest muscle or fascia from the abdominal wall.

Omental flaps have been used in chest wall reconstruction for decades. While both the right and left gastroepiploic arteries may be used as a pedicle, the right gastroepiploic typically affords a greater arch of rotation. The use of the right gastroepiploic artery allows approximately 5–10 cm of additional rotation. While the omentum is easy to harvest and can cover large areas, the use of the flap requires a laparotomy. Obvious concern includes hernia formation as well as difficult fixation to chest wall, retraction, and instability of an overlying skin graft. These concerns have led to the use of omentum as a form of salvage flap when others have failed.

Negative Pressure Therapy

Clinical indications and applications for negative pressure therapy have grown exponentially since its introduction in the 1990s. Negative pressure therapy can be used as both a bridge to and replacement for flap transfer in selected patients. Wounds treated by negative pressure therapy typically require a longer time to heal, however, this remains useful in patients who are not otherwise candidates for extensive surgical procedures.

The Full-Thickness Defect

Stabilization and reconstruction of the rib cage remain a controversial topic. Reconstruction of the rib cage has an end goal of preserving respiratory function. Typically, resection of one or two ribs does not adversely affect respiration. However, more extensive resection generally requires stabilization by application of prosthetic mesh and tissue coverage. Resection of the sternum and multiple ribs can result in paradoxical chest wall abnormalities and respiratory compromise. Rigid chest wall stabilization is desirable, and studies have shown that fixation with rib plating systems, synthetic mesh, or methylmethacrylate has improved outcomes in terms of ventilator dependency (Fig. 20.4). It is of paramount importance that adequate soft tissue coverage is available to prevent potentially lethal infectious complications, especially in cases where mediastinal structures are exposed. While pectoralis flaps have been the "workhorse" flap for cases of sternal dehiscence and mediastinitis, these flaps are likely compromised in LABC from either primary excision or radiation injury. As such, latissimus dorsi flaps or rectus abdominis-based flaps are good options because they provide bulk and can compensate for the loss of ribs by stabilizing the chest wall.

Controversies

Timing

Since the days of Halstead, timing of breast reconstruction has been a controversial topic. Over the years, consensus on timing of reconstruction has shifted from "never" to a focus on immediate breast

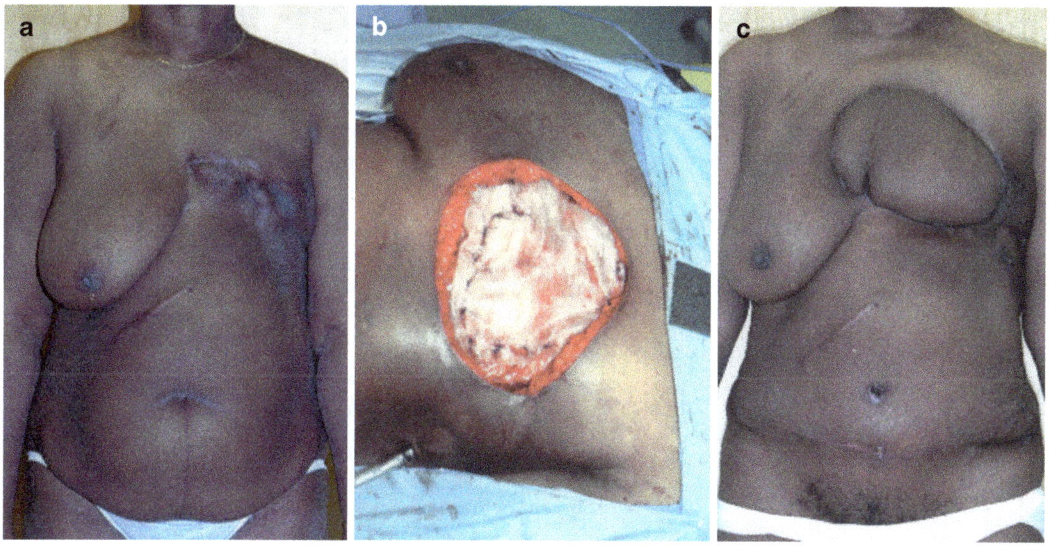

Fig. 20.4 Recurrent breast cancer with chest wall resection covered with DIEP flap. (**a**) Recurrent breast cancer involving the chest wall, (**b**) chest wall reconstruction with Marlex mesh, and (**c**) DIEP flap to cover mesh

reconstruction. Immediate breast reconstruction has multiple advantages: (1) relative technical ease, (2) improved cosmesis, (3) lower overall cost, (4) decreased recovery times, (5) improved coping, (6) improved quality of life, and (7) improved body image for patients. Multiple studies have shown that immediate reconstruction is safe and effective in patients with early-stage cancer, but immediate reconstruction in LABC remains somewhat controversial.

Concerns about immediate reconstruction in LABC result from the fact that LABC carries a high risk of recurrence. As was the case with Halstead, many surgeons fear that immediate reconstruction may lead to a delay in diagnosis of recurrence and a theoretical potential for an increased incidence of local recurrence in the reconstructed breast. Other factors that raise concern over immediate reconstruction include delays in adjuvant therapy caused by wound complications and the ability of the reconstructed breast to withstand postoperative irradiation. It should also be understood that the reason for reconstruction may not be reconstruction of the breast, but rather stable reconstruction of the chest so that radiation can be administered. The goals may be limited in the aesthetic sense but important in the therapeutic sense.

Crisera et al. acknowledge that, in the past, most studies assessing the feasibility of immediate reconstruction in LABC were small and did not assess the long-term complication rates. In 2011, they published a retrospective review to evaluate the safety and efficacy of microvascular autogenous immediate breast reconstruction in women with LABC. They evaluated 766 patients with clinical stage IIB or greater breast cancer that were followed over the course of 10 years, evaluating the rates of early and late complications, local recurrence, and delays in adjuvant therapy. They also employed a rating scale to assess the cosmetic outcome following radiation [15]. They concluded that immediate reconstruction in patients with LABC is safe and well tolerated.

The authors based this conclusion on the results of their study, which demonstrated that their complication rates were not statistically different than those treated with mastectomy alone and were similar to those patients with early-stage breast cancer. They also state that their rates of microvascular complications, flap loss, length of hospital stay, and need for blood transfusions are also comparable to published data on early-stage breast cancer. Additionally, they reported delays in postoperative chemotherapy in 4.7 % of patients. This was comparable to rates reported after mastectomy without reconstruction in women with advanced stage breast cancer, with a maximal delay of only 3 weeks.

Others found no differences in local or distant recurrence rates when chemotherapy was initiated less than or greater than 10 weeks postoperatively, making a delay of 3 weeks oncologically insignificant [16]. In terms of local recurrence, incidence was not greater than other published data, and those that did develop recurrence did so in areas that were not obstructed by the reconstruction and did not have a delay in diagnosis. While radiation can have negative effects on a microsurgically reconstructed breast in terms of distortion and shrinkage, the authors found that these changes were relatively minor and could be easily corrected by outpatient procedures. While it seems further investigation is certainly warranted, based on the current literature, immediate reconstruction for LABC is safe and effective.

Conclusions

The treatment of LABC is continuously evolving. LABC still carries a relatively low 5-year survival rate when compared to those patients with early-stage breast cancer. Improvements in chemotherapy, targeted therapeutics, and radiation therapy will continue to increase the overall survival rates as well as improve quality of life. As breast cancer is an extremely complex disease, so is the treatment of these patients. Although the ultimate goal is the long-term survival of these patients, one cannot understate the importance of breast reconstruction or stable chest wall coverage to the overall quality of life. As such, there are a myriad of options for breast reconstruction available to the surgeon in the treatment of these patients, and while no one option can be, or should be, a catch all, it is important for the surgeon to be familiar with the options available to both surgeon and patient.

References

1. Hance KW, Anderson WF, Devesa SS, et al. Trends in inflammatory breast carcinoma incidence and survival: the surveillance, epidemiology, and end results program at the National Cancer Institute. J Natl Cancer Inst. 2005;97:966.
2. Anderson WF, Schairer C, Chen BE, et al. Epidemiology of inflammatory breast cancer (IBC). Breast Dis. 2005–2006;22:9.
3. Tai P, Yu E, Shiels R, et al. Short- and long-term cause-specific survival of patients with inflammatory breast cancer. BMC Cancer. 2005;5:137.
4. Rudolph R, Vande BJ, Schneider JA, et al. Slowed growth of cultured fibroblasts from human radiation wounds. Plast Reconstr Surg. 1988;82:669–77.
5. Hopewell JW, Calvo W, Jaenke R, et al. Microvasculature and radiation damage. Recent Results Cancer Res. 1993;130:1–166.
6. Chuang VP. Radiation-induced arthritis. Semin Roentgenol. 1994;29:64–9.
7. Williams KJ, Carlson GW, Bostwick III J, et al. The effects of radiation treatment after TRAM flap breast reconstruction. Plast Reconstr Surg. 1997;100:1153–60.
8. Tran NV, Chang DW, Gupta A, et al. Comparison of immediate and delayed free TRAM flap breast reconstruction in patients receiving postmastectomy radiation therapy. Plast Reconstr Surg. 2001;108:78–82.
9. Beahm E, Chang DW. Chest wall reconstruction and advanced disease. Semin Plast Surg. 2004;18:117–29.
10. Delay E, Gounot N, Bouillot A, et al. Autologous latissimus breast reconstruction: a 3-year clinical experience with 100 patients. Plast Reconstr Surg. 1998;102:1461–78.
11. Lin CH, Wei FC, Levin LS, Chen MC. Donor-site morbidity comparison between endoscopically assisted and traditional harvest of free latissimus dorsi muscle flap. Plast Reconstr Surg. 1999;104:1070–7.
12. Fraulin FO, Louie G, Zorrilla L, Tilley W. Functional evaluation of the shoulder following latissimus dorsi muscle transfer. Ann Plast Surg. 1995;35:349–53.
13. Micali E, Carramaschi FR. Extended V-Y latissimus dorsi musculocutaneous flap for anterior chest wall reconstruction. Plast Reconstr Surg. 2001;107(6): 1382–90.
14. Munhoz AM, Montag E, Arruda E, Okada A, Brasil JA, Gemperli R, Filassi JR, Ferreira MC. Immediate local advanced breast cancer and chest wall reconstruction: surgical planning and reconstruction strategies with extended V-Y latissimus dorsi myocutaneous flap. Plast Reconstr Surg. 2011;127(6):2186–97.
15. Crisera CA, Chang EI, Da Lio AL, Festekjian JH, Mehrara BJ. Immediate free flap reconstruction for advanced- stage breast cancer: is it safe? Plast Reconstr Surg. 2011;128(1):32–41.
16. Buzdar AU, Smith TL, Powell KC, Blumenschein GR, Gehan EA. Effect of timing of initiation of adjuvant chemotherapy on disease-free survival in breast cancer. Breast Cancer Res Treat. 1982;2:163–9.

Revision Breast Reconstruction and General Complications

21

M'liss Hogan and Charles Dupin

Breast Reconstruction Revision

Breast reconstruction is rarely completed with a single operative procedure. With the exception of direct to implant reconstruction in nipple-sparing mastectomy, additional procedures are required for the best cosmetic outcomes.

Autologous reconstructions also are completed in two stages. In the first stage (if the contralateral breast is aesthetically acceptable), the flap is used to create a match for the opposite breast mound. A contralateral ptotic or macromastic breast should not be replicated. It is either reduced or lifted at the time of the second procedure. It is far easier to balance the final size and nipple position at the second procedure.

Expander-based reconstruction always has a planned second-stage procedure. Expanders are normally implanted at less than optimal volume in order to decrease the stress placed upon the mastectomy flaps. After expansion to the desired volume, the expander is removed and a permanent implant is placed.

M. Hogan, MD (✉) • C. Dupin, MD
Division of Plastic Surgery, Department of Surgery, Louisiana State University Health Sciences Center, 1542 Tulane Avenue, New Orleans, LA 70112, USA
e-mail: mlisshogan@gmail.com; cldupinmd@gmail.com

Fat Grafting in Breast Reconstruction

Contour deformities in autologous and nonautologous reconstruction can be addressed at the second stage. Fat grafting is a promising adjunct in breast reconstruction. Contour deformities and areas deficient in volume can be injected to improve the final appearance of the reconstructed breast. Previous apprehensions with respect to risks of fat necrosis or mammogram changes due to fat grafting can be minimized with proper technique. To date, no measurable increase in breast cancer recurrence rates secondary to fat grafting on long-term follow-up have been noted [1].

Preoperative markings are made with the patient standing. Fat is harvested from the abdomen using tumescent technique; this is done under low pressure (−10 mmHg of suction). Once the fat is aspirated, the fat is allowed to separate from the tumescent fluid. This is accomplished using a centrifuge or gravity. Fat is then placed in 10 cc syringes and injected into previously marked areas. This is done at about 1 cc per pass, and the fat is always injected as the syringe is being withdrawn from the injection site. The fat is dispersed in multiple passes.

In implant-based reconstruction, fat is injected prior to removal of the expander so there is no risk of damage to the permanent implant. Once fat injection is complete, implant exchange proceeds. In autologous reconstruction fat grafting is performed at the time of other procedures whose goal is to achieve symmetry.

A.I. Riker (ed.), *Breast Disease: Comprehensive Management*,
DOI 10.1007/978-1-4939-1145-5_21, © Springer Science+Business Media New York 2015

Nipple Areolar Reconstruction

Nipple/areola reconstruction is generally not done at the time of the mastectomy. The mastectomy flaps that will be the donor tissue used to create the nipple are too unstable at that time. The procedure can be performed at the time of the exchange for a permanent implant as the mastectomy flaps have matured and are stable. The flaps however may be thin and great care must be taken in elevating the flaps that form the nipple (Fig. 21.1). As noted in the chapter on implant based reconstruction (Chap. 18), if at the time of initial reconstruction, the lower edge of the pectoralis muscle was advanced inferiorly to a position below the level of the proposed nipple, there is less risk of implant exposure.

Although the reconstruction of a mound has become much more predictable, the reconstruction of a nipple areola complex has been challenging. This is mostly due to a loss of projection of the nipple over time. There have been many designs for nipple and areola reconstruction. All utilize some form of interposed rotational flaps to create the nipple. These flaps are harvested from the flap skin paddle in autologous reconstruction or the mastectomy skin flaps in implant reconstruction.

The "skate" flap was an early design that incorporated interposed flaps [2]. In 1994, Bostwick et al. reported a nipple reconstruction with the C-V flap [3]. The two flaps are interposed and the donor sites closed primarily. This technique has many variations (Fig. 21.2).

We have proposed a procedure that also uses interposed flaps, but the donor site is closed in a circular fashion, which looks like the edge of the areola. A dermal graft, harvested from the abdominal "dog ear" or acellular dermal matrix, is inserted into the flap to increase projection of the nipple (Figs. 21.3 and 21.4).

Once stable, the nipple and the areola can be tattooed to match the pigment on the other areola. This is typically the last step in the reconstruction (Fig. 21.5).

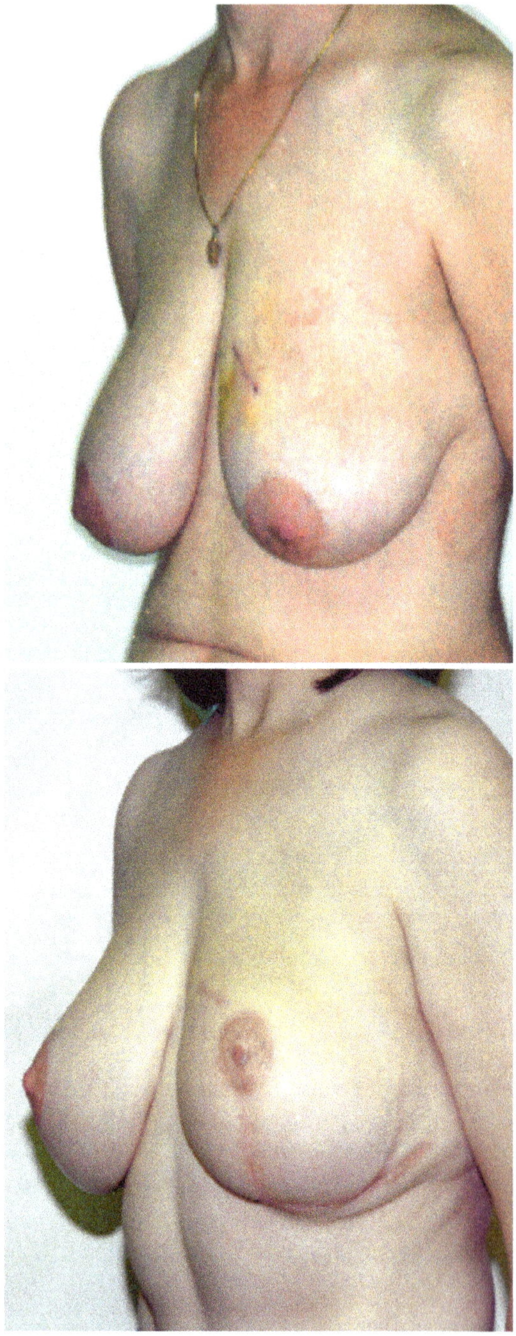

Fig. 21.1 Patient with ptosis and left breast cancer. The left breast was reconstructed with a DIEP flap. A mastopexy was performed on the right to match the more aesthetic reconstructed left breast

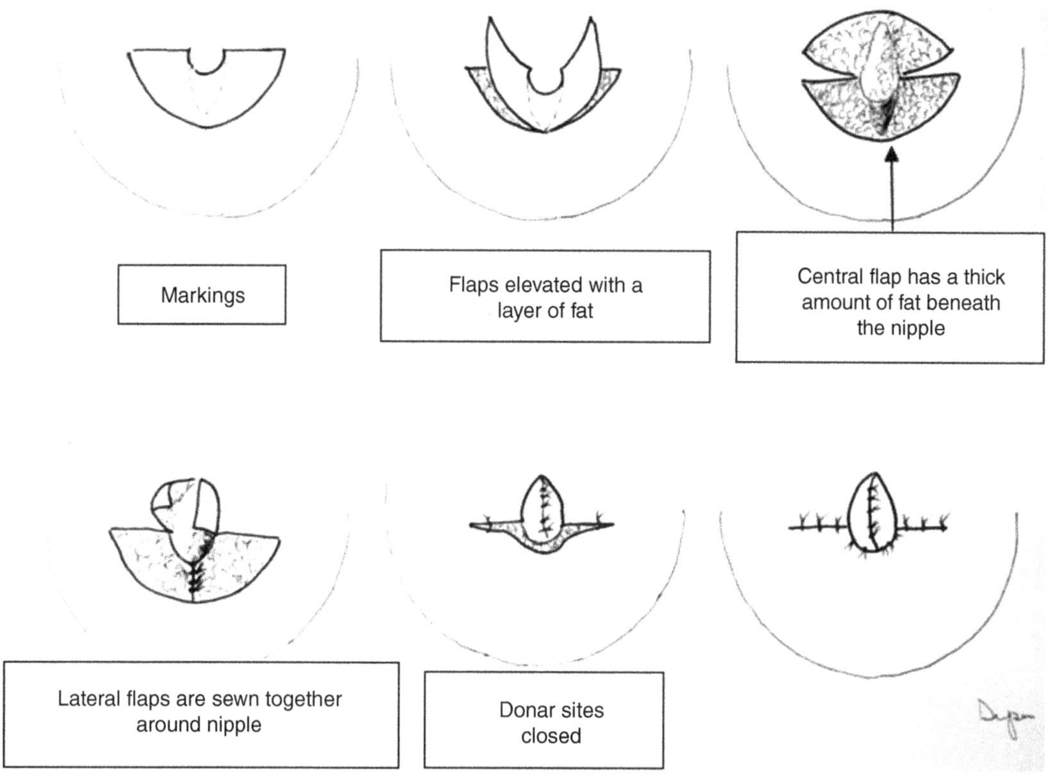

Fig. 21.2 The SKATE flap: note that two flaps of mastectomy or flap skin are interposed to form the nipple skin flaps

Complications in Breast Reconstruction

Fortunately, life-threatening complications are rare and are still most commonly associated with the development of a postoperative pulmonary embolism. Adhering to the recommendations of the American College of Chest Physicians, accounting for thrombosis risk factors and prophylaxis should minimize this potentially lethal complication [4].

Unfortunately, breast cancer patients are frequently in the 41–60 age group (1 point), and many or obese (1 point). They all have malignancy (2 points) and all have major surgery (2 points). Thus, a reconstructive patient who is over the age of 60, obese, and undergoing a flap procedure will start with a score of 6. These patients should have chemoprophylaxis unless contraindicated with low molecular weight heparin as our drug of choice. It requires no monitoring and poses minimal risk of bleeding, even if given preoperatively [4]. We treat our patients with a score of 6 or less for a week postoperatively. Patients with risk factors of 7 or greater require longer prophylaxis.

There is no specific risk of infection that differs from other clean surgical procedures, other than periprosthetic infection in implant reconstructions. These infections can become life threatening and lead to sepsis if not addressed.

Seroma formation is common in the donor sites of autologous tissue. They tend to occur more

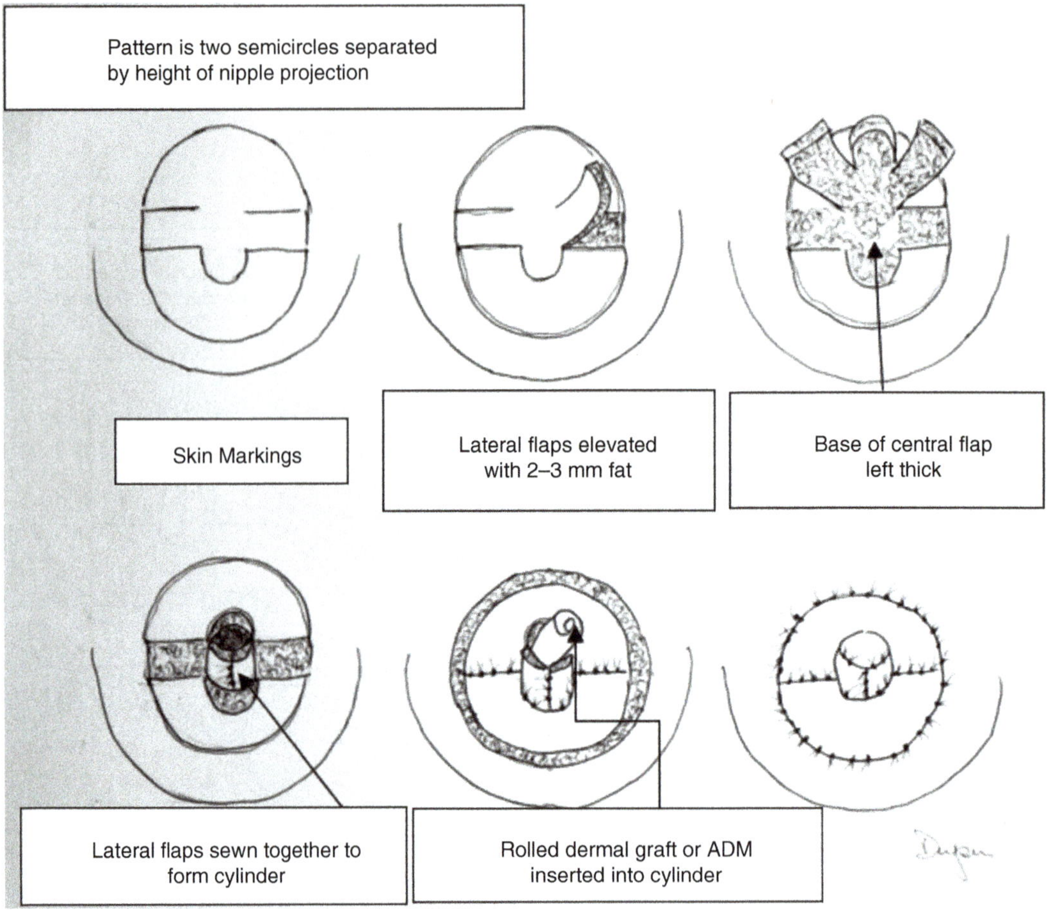

Fig. 21.3 Nipple reconstruction with dermal graft or ADM

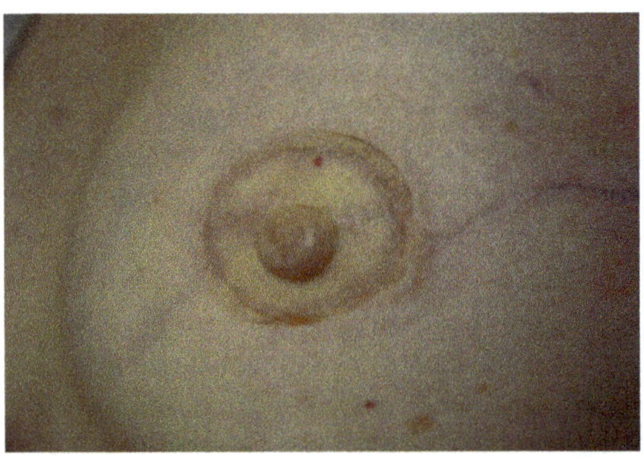

Fig. 21.4 Nipple reconstruction with dermal graft

frequently in obese patients. Seromas should be prevented if possible, with long-term effective drainage and the use of "quilting" sutures, which fix the flap down to the underlying deep fascia. Once a seroma is identified, it is best treated with an ultrasound-placed indwelling pigtail drain, and the area should be compressed. Most are amenable to nonsurgical treatment; occasionally the seroma cavity may require excision and a second set of quilting sutures and drains placed. Seroma problems with expanders or implants are addressed specifically in the chapter on nonautologous reconstruction.

Hematomas are more commonly associated with autologous reconstruction. The more common sources of hematoma are the lateral chest wall when an axillary dissection has been done or from the edges of the flap or de-epithelialized dermis. Care should be taken with hemostasis when trimming or de-epithelializing the flaps. It is important to recognize evolving hematomas

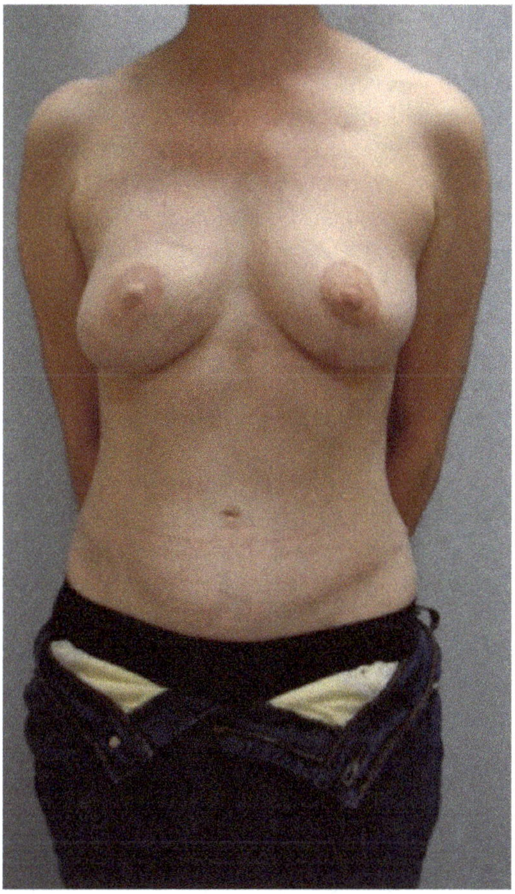

Fig. 21.5 The completed reconstruction, with right DIEP flap, right nipple areola reconstruction, and left mastopexy

when flaps are done, because the pressure from the hematoma may compromise the outflow from the flap. Hematomas should be addressed by promptly returning to the operating room, removal of hematoma, and irrigation. Waiting for a hematoma to resolve spontaneously is risky, because the hematoma will cause thinning of the soft tissues and will likely drain through the wound, allowing ingress of infection.

Problems with mastectomy flap necrosis are associated with cellulitis, wound disruption and exposure of the prosthesis. Patients with macromastia or significant ptosis of the breast frequently require excision of excess skin. This leaves additional wounds and increases the chance of necrosis and infection. Small areas of partial necrosis can be treated with careful wound

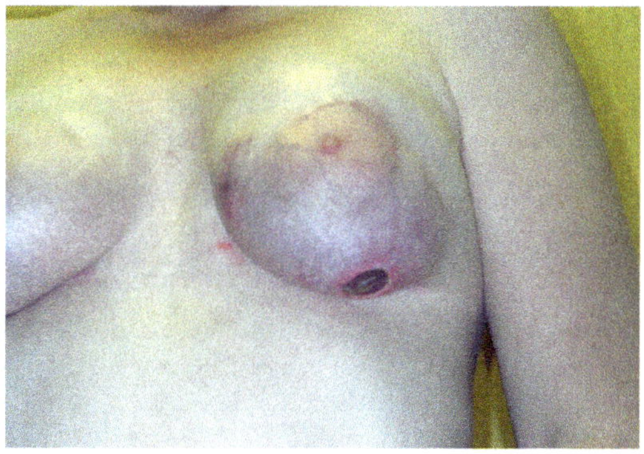

Fig. 21.6 Exposed prosthetic; note poor-quality soft tissue coverage

care and will frequently heal without implant exposure, but larger areas of necrosis are very troublesome. Large amounts of mastectomy flap necrosis may require autologous reconstruction of either the entire mound with another flap or to replace the debrided skin (Fig. 21.6).

Exposed Prosthetic

Cellulitis should be treated aggressively. It is our practice to use intravenous antibiotics with broad-spectrum coverage and try to resolve the cellulitis, to prevent infection involving the prosthetic itself. Swelling in the reconstructed breast, fluid collection around the prosthetic, persistent cellulitis, and drainage are indicators of periprosthetic infection. Patients with periprosthetic infections will frequently have fever and other constitutional symptoms of infection.

There have been reports of salvaging the reconstructive effort with explantation, washing out the wound, replacing the prosthetic, and incorporating antibiotic irrigation for a period of time. Periprosthetic infections require either removal of the prosthesis or some attempt at salvage, including removal of the prosthetic, irrigation of the pocket, and replacement of the prosthetic combined with wound irrigation with antibiotic solution. Prince et al. reported a 75 % salvage rate with early aggressive therapy [5].

Capsule contracture and failure of the implant are the two primary long-term complications of

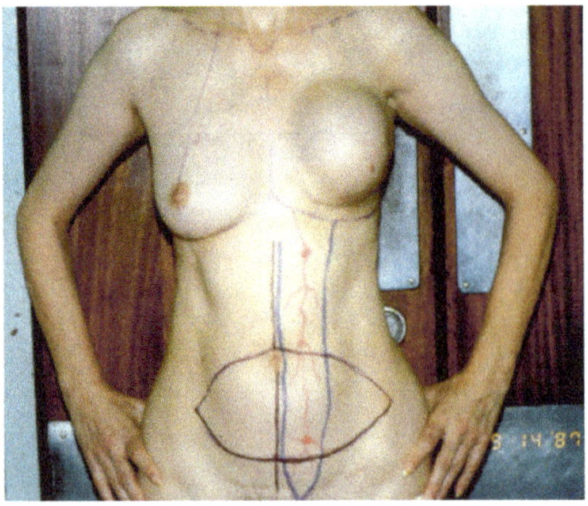

Fig. 21.7 Patient with grade 4 Baker capsule contracture marked for TRAM flap

implant reconstruction. The advent of capsule contracture is a linear risk. The longer the implant is in place, the more likely that contracture will occur. Contracture can distort the breast and be a cause of pain. Most will require revision surgery but the result of surgery for capsule contracture is unpredictable. Its cause is unknown but there is a much higher incidence in patients who have had radiation therapy. Patients that develop series of problems with implants are frequently improved with a change to autologous reconstruction rather than multiple attempts to revise the implant-based reconstruction (Fig. 21.7).

While the life span of a silicone implant is hard to define, it is not a lifetime product. Patients who have implant reconstructions should be told that they will need a replacement at some point in the future, and possibly more than one. If the implant fails and the gel is restricted to the scar capsule, it can be difficult to diagnose. The FDA has developed recommendations for follow-up on silicone implants, which include intermittent MRI surveillance [6].

Complications in Autologous Reconstruction

Autologous reconstruction patients have a different set of problems. Unlike implant-based reconstructions, they have a donor site. They also are at risk of partial or total necrosis of the flap. Flap loss in the rotational abdominal procedures is more likely due to insufficient periumbilical connections between the deep superior epigastric vessels and the deep inferior epigastric vessels. Contributing factors include smoking and obesity. Kroll et al. reported a very high complication rate among smokers [7]. Morbidly obese patients are poor candidates for rotational procedures and are at high risk of severe abdominal complications (necrosis, hernia, and seroma).

In order to reduce the problem of necrosis, multiple variations have been proposed to the standard rotational flap. These include surgical delay of the flap, using both rectus muscles in the pedicle and using a more caudal level for the flap donor site [8–10].

The most common donor site problem is seroma formation. These can be troublesome and lead to cellulitis and loss of skin and fat. Suturing Scarpa's fascia to the abdominal wall (quilting sutures) can reduce the development of a seroma. Drains are left until the output is less than 50 cc per day. If skin necrosis is superficial or minor, local wound care, topical antibiotics, and dressings are used. If the necrosis is full thickness, surgical debridement will be needed to remove all necrotic tissue. As it is not possible to close again at that time, a VAC device is used until the wound is closed. Most of these patients will need eventual scar revision. It is best to debride the wound as soon as significant necrosis is discovered.

Flaps from other areas (buttocks, back, and thigh) also have potential to form seroma. This is especially true of the latissimus dorsi transfers. Quilting suture are again helpful, and long-term drains may be required.

Besides the donor site issues, free transfers have potential for microvascular anastomotic compromise. While the accepted flap survival rate is 95 %, returns to the operating room remain at about 5–10 % [11]. The three causes of microvascular dysfunction are arterial thrombosis, venous thrombosis, and hematoma. A hematoma in the flap/mastectomy wound needs to be promptly treated because pressure from the hematoma can obstruct the venous outflow. Observation in the face of swelling and pain can lead to loss of the flap. Early intervention for hematoma normally does not require revision of the anastomosis.

Arterial thrombosis can occur. It is typically manifested by loss of the external arterial signal in the flap and a pale flap. If the patient has an internal venous Doppler, the signal will be lost as well. Most thrombosis occurs shortly after anastomosis. The problems may be technical issues, flap or recipient arteries that have fragile walls, or hypercoagulability of the patient. Revision of the anastomosis will generally solve the problem unless the patient is hypercoagulable.

Venous thrombosis has become much less common since the advent of the venous anastomotic coupler. It is manifested by dark bleeding from the flap edges, rapid capillary refill and plethoric skin color, swelling, and loss of either skin venous signal or implantable Doppler signal. At the onset, the arterial Doppler signal in the skin is present. It is critical to recognize this condition as early as possible. Continuing outflow problems causes blood to accumulate in the flap and leads to thrombosis in the small vessels in the flap. Revising the anastomosis when there is extensive clotting within the flap will result in pulsatile flow into the flap but no venous return. This is called the "no reflow" phenomenon and is associated with flap loss.

Clotting in the microcirculation of the flap resulting from venous occlusion requires thrombolysis. Either thrombin plasmin activator (TPA) or urokinase may be used. The TPA is injected through a previously ligated arterial branch in the flap pedicle. It may also be injected directly into the artery at the anastomotic end. The venous anastomosis should be uncoupled and outflow must be allowed to drain into the wound, rather than the circulation. If the declotting is successful, the vein is recoupled. If the intra-flap clot cannot be lysed, the flap will be lost even if the anastomosis is successfully revised.

Other than the surgical skills of the operator, the most important factor in a successful outcome is close observation of the flap. Early intervention is the key to successful flap salvage. If the flap is not warm, pink, soft, and with good Doppler signals, it is wise to return to the OR, rather than waiting until intravascular clotting or irreconcilable ischemia occurs. Color and size of the flap, external arterial (and venous) Doppler examination, and internal venous Doppler signals are all helpful.

Muscle flaps without perfusion are likely not salvageable after 4 hours. Fascio-cutaneous flaps are somewhat more resistant, but when the clot is adherent to the intima for prolonged periods, it will be impossible to restore circulation. Communication with the receiving nurses in the close care unit should be routinely done. The surgical team should demonstrate what the sounds are like and where to look for them. If a problem occurs, early return to the operating room is the key to success.

References

1. Seth AK, Hirsch EM, et al. Long-term outcomes following fat grafting in prosthetic breast reconstruction: a comparative analysis. Plast Reconstr Surg. 2005;130(5):984–90.
2. Little III, SW. Nipple-areolar reconstruction. Clin Plast Surg. 1984;11:351–64.
3. Bostwick J. Nipple-areolar reconstruction. Op Tech Plast Reconstr Surg. 1994;1(1):35.
4. Schuunemann HJ, American College of Chest, Guyatt GH, Akl EA, Mark C, Gutterman DD. Physicians antithrombotic, therapy and prevention of thrombosis panel, evidence-based clinical practice guidelines, American college of chest physicians, therapy and prevention of thrombosis, 9th. Chest. 2012;141: 7S–47.
5. Prince MD, Suber JS, Aya-ay ML, Cone Jr JD, Greene JN, Smith Jr DJ, Smith PD. Prosthesis salvage in breast reconstruction patients with periprosthetic infection and exposure. Plast Reconstr Surg. 2012; 129(1):42–8.
6. FDA Update on the safety of silicone gel-filled breast implants. 2011. Screening for rupture. p. 29. www.fda.gov/.../ProductsandMedicalProcedures/ImplantsandProsthetics/BreastImplants/UCM260090.pdf
7. Kroll Stephen S. Necrosis of abdominoplasty and other secondary flaps after TRAM flap breast reconstruction. Plast Reconstr Surg. 1994;94(5):637–43.
8. Codner MA, Bostwick III J, Nahai F, Bried JT, Eaves FF. TRAM flap vascular delay for high-risk breast reconstruction. Plast Reconstr Surg. 1995;96(7):1615–22.
9. Wagner DS, Michelow BJ, Hartrampf Jr CR. Double-pedicle TRAM flap for unilateral breast reconstruction. Plast Reconstr Surg. 1991;88(6):987–97.
10. Spear SL, Ducic I, Cuoco F, Taylor N. Effect of obesity on flap and donor-site complications in pedicled TRAM flap breast reconstruction. Plast Reconstr Surg. 2007;119(3):788–95.
11. Gill P, Hunt J, Guerra A, et al. A 10-year retrospective review of 758 DIEP flaps for breast reconstruction. Plast Reconstr Surg. 2004;113:1153.

22 Molecular Medicine and Personalized Therapy for Breast Cancer Patients

Pamela N. Munster

Historical Perspective

Personalized medicine or targeted therapy in breast cancer has been practiced for well over a century. Even before the recognition of the estrogen receptor as one the most relevant therapeutic targets, Beatson described the benefits of estrogen withdrawal by oophorectomy in 1986 [1]. Other hormonal ablation interventions that were pursued in postmenopausal women included adrenalectomies and hypophysectomies [2, 3].

These non-estrogen-selective surgical interventions were replaced when the first estrogen analogs were synthesized. For several decades, synthetic estrogens were an integral part in the treatment of breast cancer. First described in 1938, diethylstilbestrol (DES) received approval by the US Food and Drug Administration as a synthetic estrogen by the Food and Drug Administration in 1941 [4–6]. However, in the setting of the well-recognized benefits that were observed with estrogen withdrawal using surgical interventions, the noted benefits of synthetic estrogen administration were only poorly understood. Furthermore, routine assessment of estrogen receptor expression was not yet available due to the absence of robust tests that were able to accurately measure it. Hence, albeit approved in 1941, the use of DES for metastatic breast cancer in postmenopausal was not formally recommended until the 1960 council on drugs (*JAMA* 1960) [4–6].

High doses of estrogens remained the nonsurgical treatment of choice until the development of the antiestrogen modulator, tamoxifen. While unsuccessful as a contraceptive, a small, randomized phase II trial demonstrated the efficacy of tamoxifen at two doses in postmenopausal women with advanced breast cancer who had progressed on prior hormonal intervention. Tested against DES, tamoxifen showed sustained activity in patients with breast cancer, comparable to those seen with DES [7–9]. However, tamoxifen was much better tolerated. The successful introduction and recognition of an antiestrogen as a crucial therapeutic target was followed by a 30-year intense focus on selective estrogen receptor modulators (SERMs), selective estrogen receptor downregulators (SERDs), and selective aromatase inhibitors ranging from the treatment of advanced disease to breast cancer prevention. The estrogen receptor remains to be the most important target in breast cancer and is expressed in two-thirds of patients with breast cancer.

In 1987, Slamon and colleagues' seminal discovery of HER2 described the second important target in breast cancer [10, 11]. Expressed in 15–25 % of all breast cancers, overexpression of HER2 has been shown to be an adverse prognostic

P.N. Munster, MD
Division of Hematology and Oncology, Department of Medicine, Helen Diller Family Cancer Center, University of California, San Francisco, 1600 Divisadero St., 1770, San Francisco, CA 94143, USA
e-mail: pmunster@medicine.ucsf.edu

A.I. Riker (ed.), *Breast Disease: Comprehensive Management*,
DOI 10.1007/978-1-4939-1145-5_22, © Springer Science+Business Media New York 2015

indicator with shortened overall survival and notable resistance to hormonal therapy. However, HER2 can be successfully inhibited by several modalities directed to the receptor itself or by interference with its interaction with other HER2 family members such as EGFR (HER1) and HER3. While the development in targeting the ER took almost a century, the approval of the first monoclonal antibody against HER2 was received a decade after Slamon's initial description of its relevance in treating breast cancer [12–18].

Over the last 10 years, several novel agents have been developed, tested, and approved, including VEGF, VEGFR, PI3kinase, mTOR, and PARP inhibitors that have entered clinical testing in early-stage breast cancer.

In addition to the development of individual predictive and prognostic biomarkers, much emphasis has been placed upon the discovery of gene array patterns to define prognostic and predictive factors. There are currently two commercially available assays that are routinely used in clinical practice to determine the need and benefit of adjuvant chemotherapy. The trademarks for these assays are the Oncotype DX and MammaPrint molecular assays [19–24]. A third multigene predictive marker has recently been introduced, evaluating a 50-gene signature, the PAM50 assay. As more targeted therapies are being approved for patients with metastatic disease, a personalized approach to therapy for early-stage breast cancer has taken center stage for such patients.

Molecular Assessment of Therapeutic Targets in Breast Cancer

Select Molecular Targets

The most widely used molecular assessment of therapeutic targets in early-stage breast cancer includes the qualitative and quantitative assessment of the estrogen receptor (ER) and progesterone receptor (PR), human epidermal growth factor 2 (HER2), and the proliferation marker, Ki67. The first three tests are routinely performed tests in local or central laboratories and are based on immunohistochemical assessment of the protein expression of these targets. These tests are the backbone for clinical decision making in breast cancer that assists in guiding systemic therapy and influences local therapy decisions. All three tests should be assessed for each patient with a diagnosis of breast cancer. The Ki67 proliferative index has been evaluated in multiple neoadjuvant and adjuvant studies and has been found to be a strong predictive marker of hormone therapy resistance. However, the testing and scoring of Ki67 has not been standardized uniformly, and hence the test is still only used selectively.

Estrogen and Progesterone Receptors

Both the ER and the PR are strong predictors of outcome and hormonal therapy response. The estrogen receptor is expressed in 70–80 % of women with breast cancer, and tumors are typically tested with immunohistochemistry [25]. However, the benefits of hormone therapy has been recognized and used in breast cancer long before the standardized testing for hormone receptors was introduced. Historically, hormonal therapy was recommended for 5 years after an initial diagnosis of early-stage breast cancer with early studies demonstrating the clear benefits of hormone therapy in both ER-positive and ER-unknown disease. Hormone therapy was beneficial in women of all ages, nodal status, and regardless of chemotherapy use [26–29].

The most commonly used hormonal interventions are antiestrogens or aromatase inhibitors. The aromatase inhibitors are the treatment of choice for postmenopausal woman with early-stage breast cancer due to improved disease-free survival rates compared to tamoxifen and fewer detrimental long-term sequelae such as endometrial cancer or strokes [30–32]. The benefits of aromatase inhibitors over tamoxifen have been shown for all three currently available aromatase inhibitors, either upfront (ATAC), after 2–3 years of tamoxifen (TEAM trial) or after 5 years of tamoxifen (MA17) [33–35]. Aromatase inhibitors are not effective in premenopausal women and tamoxifen remains the drug of choice for women with intact ovaries or those who do not tolerate aromatase inhibitors.

An initial third arm in the Arimidex, Tamoxifen Alone, or in Combination (ATAC) trial evaluating the potential benefit of combining both tamoxifen and anastrozole found no additional benefit from the combination. Data from individual large randomized trials and quinquennial meta-analyses of worldwide collaboration summarizing all large trials suggest that hormonal therapy reduced the risk of breast cancer recurrence by about 50 % and breast cancer mortality by 30 % in patients whose tumors express ER [26–29]. However, strongly confounded by the almost universal use of adjuvant chemotherapy in addition to hormonal therapy, much emphasis has been placed on determining which patients would be adequately treated by hormonal therapy only, without the use of concomitant chemotherapy. Recognizing the importance of the estrogen receptor as a prognostic molecular marker and its successful inhibition in the majority of patients, a vast effort has been focused on predictors of hormone therapy response in ER-positive tumors.

While data in the meta-analysis from the worldwide overview and most large randomized trial clearly suggested a lesser benefit or hormonal interventions in ER-poor tumors or those with ER-negative disease, the role of PR and its impact on outcome and therapy response has been less clear (ref overview, big 98). Several individual studies demonstrated a worse outcome in patients whose tumors do not express PR [36]; however, this has not been found in the meta-analyses [37–40]. PR is a response gene of ER signaling and, therefore, an integral part of ER signaling. Yet using IHC assessment of PR, its role as a prognostic or predictive marker in the adjuvant setting could not clearly be determined [34, 36, 41–44]. Utilizing DNA microarrays, breast cancers have been divided into at least four major subtypes, with the role of PR as predictive markers validated with in-depth molecular classification of tumors that have subdivided ER-positive tumors in those with positive expression of PR and those with absent PR [45–49].

Ki-67

Several neoadjuvant studies have suggested that the pathological response to chemotherapy in ER-positive tumors was low, yet the overall survival and breast cancer-specific outcomes were excellent. These findings suggest that only a small subgroup of patients with ER-positive tumors may truly need and benefit from chemotherapy. Furthermore, disease stabilization is often the predominant clinical response to hormonal therapy in advanced cancer with little to no tumor regression. In the absence of tumor regression, more emphasis has been placed upon finding biological markers such as a change in proliferation to accurately predict outcomes and therapy response.

One of the most promising proliferation markers is Ki67. Based on xenograft models suggesting Ki67 could predict a decrease in proliferation and induction of apoptosis, multiple studies have evaluated Ki67 as a biological endpoint for treatment effects in hormonal therapy. Extensive preclinical and smaller clinical studies have suggested that low expression of Ki-67 is associated with hormonal response, whereas higher levels of Ki67 may point to hormone therapy resistance. Furthermore, two neoadjuvant trials evaluated the baseline expression and a change in Ki67 to predict the response to hormonal therapy after a 2- and 12-week exposure to hormonal therapy.

The P024 trial that compared letrozole and tamoxifen and the IMPACT study (Immediate Preoperative Anastrozole, Tamoxifen, or Combined with Tamoxifen) showed that baseline Ki67 expression, and the degree of Ki67 suppression during treatment, paralleled the risk reduction in the overall recurrence-free survival that was seen in other larger adjuvant trials examining tamoxifen or an aromatase inhibition, such as the ATAC and BIG 98 trials [50, 51]. The integration of Ki67 in a multivariate assessment of posttreatment changes of Ki67 in conjunction with pathological tumor size, pathological node status, and ER status (PEPI score: preoperative endocrine prognostic index) was further found to be highly predictive of the risk of recurrence. Hence, patients with a low PEPI score may be adequately treated with hormonal therapy and do not require chemotherapy [52, 53].

These data have supported the further testing of Ki67 as a predictive marker in shorter presurgical window trials. A 2-week exposure to neoadjuvant hormonal therapy followed by a biopsy of the tumor is currently being studied to determine whether patients would be candidates for endocrine therapy only or whether the high pretreatment levels of Ki67 and the absence of treatment-induced suppression may be used to identify patients' change with a need for adjuvant chemotherapy. The role of KI67 as a predictive marker of endocrine therapy in a short-term trial is currently being studied in a 4,000-patient trial (POETIC trial: PeriOperative Endocrine Therapy for Individualizing Care) [54]. A prospective analysis of the role of Ki67 as a predictive marker is currently ongoing in the ACOSOG Z1031 trial.

The predictive value of Ki67 for therapy response to tamoxifen and letrozole has been further studied in a large randomized adjuvant trial (BIG-98). A retrospective analysis analyzing Ki67 in tumors derived from 2,685 of the 8,010 enrolled patients showed that a high Ki67 expression was associated with worse outcome and patients with high Ki67 expression may derive a higher benefit from an aromatase inhibitor than tamoxifen [55]. As the robustness and the test standardization for Ki67 is evolving, the routine assessment of Ki67 has not been introduced into practice universally.

Human Epidermal Growth Factor 2 (HER2)

Early studies have suggested that the overexpression of HER2 is associated with a high risk of recurrence in early-stage breast cancer and decreased survival. In a seminal discovery in 1987, Slamon et al. described the human epidermal growth factor receptor, HER2, as an oncogene [11, 56]. Typically found as a transmembrane point mutation and oncogenic mutation in virus, the HER2 receptor in breast cancer is found as a gene amplification and overexpression, rather than as mutations [57]. While HER2 is expressed in other tissues, most of the advances in targeting HER2 have focused on breast cancer. Treatment decisions of HER2 targeting are based on the tumor expression of HER2 typically measured by immunohistochemistry, using a grading ranging from 0, +1, +2 to +3. HER2 protein is mostly located to the membrane, and overexpression of the protein has been associated with worse outcome and is a very strong predictor of treatment response to HER2 targeting. However, the protein-based studies faced several challenges with marked differences seen between HER2 protein and gene expression [58–61]. This may be accounted for biologically by transcriptional and posttranslational modification and technically by a less robust protein-based assay. Hence, clinically 0 and +1 protein expression of HER2 are considered HER2 negative. Patients whose tumors express 2+ or 3+ by IHC are considered positive and often further analyzed for gene overamplification with FISH (fluorescent in situ hybridization) analysis. Given the importance of HER2 as a therapeutic target, detailed guidelines on the testing procedures and interpretation of HER testing have been recommended by the American Society of Clinical Oncology and the College of American Pathologists in a joint venture [62–64] (Table 22.1).

Table 22.1 HER2 testing

Test	IHC	Fish
Positive for *HER2*	*HER2* 3+ (defined as uniform intense membrane staining of >30 % of invasive tumor cells)	HER2 amplified (FISH ratio of *HER2* to CEP17 of >2.2 or average *HER2* gene copy number > six signals/nucleus for those test systems without an internal control probe)
Equivocal for *HER2*	IHC 2+	FISH ratio of 1.8–2.2 or average *HER2* gene copy number four to six signals/nucleus for test systems without an internal control probe
Negative for *HER2*	IHC 0–1+	FISH ratio of <1.8 or average *HER2* gene copy number of < four signals/nucleus for test systems without an internal control probe

BRCA Gene Mutations

Many of the basal-like tumors share similarities with tumors from carriers of BRCA mutations. Dysfunction of the BRCA pathway interferes with DNA repair and activation of cell-cycle checkpoints and disturbs chromosomal stability. BRCA1 tumors are predominantly ER negative, a clear link observed between the basal-like phenotype and germline mutation of *BRCA1* gene [65–68]. However, there are many distinct features between BRCA1-positive triple-negative tumors and the basal-like triple-negative tumors [69–75].

Tumors with a BRCA2 gene mutation have a wider range of phenotypes and are more commonly found to be ER positive. With the recent removal of patent protection for BRCA gene mutation testing in June 2013, more information on the genes and their manifestation as a prognostic and predictive factor, as well as a therapeutic target, is expected. The BRCA mutation carriers who develop ovarian cancer as a result seem to have a better survival and overall outcome after receiving chemotherapy compared to those with sporadic ovarian cancer [76, 77]. It is less clear as to the role of BRCA mutational status as a predictor of chemotherapy response in breast cancer. However, the response to PARP inhibitors for both BRCA-related ovarian and breast cancer is much higher than for sporadic tumors [78–83].

VEGF, VEGFR, PI3kinase, mTOR, and PARP

Multiple targets have been studied to match specific therapeutic interventions. Vascular endothelial growth factors (VEGFs) and vascular endothelial growth factor receptors (VEGFRs) have been evaluated in patients treated with agents targeting these ligands and receptors, with no clear association with improved outcomes clearly identified [84–86]. There has been extensive research recently that has focused on defining predictive markers for inhibitors of the phosphoinositol 3 kinase (PI3k) and mammalian target of rapamycin (mTOR) pathways, with many clinical trials examining the patients with tumors that have somatic mutations in PI3KCA [84–90].

Molecular Assessment of Breast Cancer Outcomes and Predictive Patterns by Gene Expression Profiling

Distinguished Breast Cancer Subtypes

Complimentary to the assessment of long-established markers, a large effort has been put forth by many in order to determine whether larger networks of biomarkers and pathways may provide for a better description of a specific resistance phenotype. To this end, gene expression profiling by cDNA expression microarrays has subclassified breast cancer into four distinguished molecular classes based upon similarities in gene expression characteristics [45–49].

Luminal A Subtype

Molecular profiling demonstrated that ER-positive tumors can be categorized into two distinct subtypes based upon the expression of their receptors, with tumors expressing both ER and PR considered luminal A tumors. These tumors are hormone sensitive and should be treated with hormonal therapy. Luminal A tumors are frequently less responsive to treatment with chemotherapy, which is further supported by the low pathological response rates in neoadjuvant studies [91–95]. However, given the very favorable overall survival in these tumors, chemotherapy may not be needed in patients with luminal A tumors.

Luminal B Subtype

ER + tumors with low or absent PR are considered luminal B cancers. Luminal B tumors carry a worse overall prognosis in patients. They also are found to have an aggressive phenotype, high proliferation rates, high-grade features, and resistance to hormonal therapy. The estrogen receptor signaling is often dysregulated with genomic instability, mutations, and epigenetic modification in the ER gene [47, 53, 96].

HER2-Positive Subtype

Tumors in this subtype have overexpression or amplification of HER2 and HER2-related genes on the same amplicon. In HER2-positive, early-stage breast cancer, ER is expressed in about 50 % of the patients. However, even in the setting of maintained expression of ER positivity, the predominant driver of this disease is the HER2 gene. It has been identified as a very strong prognostic and predictive molecular marker, with the specific targeting and inhibition of HER2 seen as one of the most important milestones in the treatment of breast cancer. Furthermore, the efficacy of HER2 targeting is not influenced by the expression or absence of ER. HER2 targeting with trastuzumab, or in combination with other HER2 targeting agents, should be explored in all patients with tumors that express HER2 who otherwise have no contraindications [97–99].

Nonetheless, in tumors that express both, HER2 and ER, therapy should be directed against both targets. In addition to HER2-targeting therapy, current recommendations for hormonal therapy are similar to those for ER-positive, HER2-negative tumors. While early assessment suggested that tamoxifen was less active than aromatase inhibitors in HER2-positive disease, recent studies, such as the TRANS ATAC and PHARE trials, have found similar efficacy for antiestrogens as well as aromatase inhibitors [97–100]. However, the risk of recurrence and breast cancer-related death remains high, suggesting an increase in resistance to hormonal therapy.

Basal-Like Breast Cancers

Basal-like tumors are ER-negative, PR-negative, and HER2-negative tumors, often referred to as triple-negative (TN) tumors. These tumors are genetically unstable and highly altered at the gene level. Although the majority of basal-like tumors have common morphologic features, there are no distinct features to discern prognostic or predictive patterns of therapy. Basal-like and triple-negative tumors tend to have a higher response rate to chemotherapy, but clear predictive markers to which chemotherapy is more likely to increase the disease-free and overall survival remains elusive at present.

Multigene Signature Assays

In addition to the routine assessment of ER, PR, HER2, and Ki67, several multigene signatures are currently being utilized to better predict outcomes and treatment response. The most commonly used tests are MammaPrint and OncotypeDX, which are both cleared for clinical use and have been approved by the Food and Drug Administration (FDA). The assessment and utilization of the recurrence score (RS) with Oncotype DX is endorsed by both ASCO and NCCN treating guidelines to assess the need and potential benefit of chemotherapy in early-stage breast cancer. These tests are typically used for patients with ER-positive tumors that are node-negative and are not recommended for patients with HER2-positive and triple-negative tumors.

The Oncotype DX assay was developed using real-time reverse transcriptase polymerase chain reaction (RT-PCR) for gene expression in paraffin-embedded tumors. This assay examines the expression of 21 genes (16 breast cancer genes and 5 reference genes) to estimate the 10-year distant recurrence risk of breast cancer and the potential benefit of adjuvant chemotherapy and hormonal therapy in patients with estrogen receptor-positive breast cancer [101–106]. This test has been validated from large retrospective studies of women with early-stage, estrogen receptor-positive breast cancer without lymph node involvement, with a subgroup of patients with <4 nodes involved with metastatic disease. This test was originally designed to assign a recurrence score that reflected the 10-year risk of recurrence in women with ER-positive disease with no involved lymph nodes. Patients were treated with either tamoxifen alone or tamoxifen and chemotherapy in two large NSAPBP studies (B14, n-668 and B20, n-651) [105–107]. The results of the tests are strongly influenced by the expression of the estrogen receptor and are negatively impacted by the absence of progesterone expression and a high HER2 expression. The assay may not be clinically as relevant in those patients with HER2 overexpressing and ER-positive tumors.

The assay initially grouped tumors in three groups with low risk (recurrence score 0–18), intermediate risk (recurrence score 18–30), and high risk for recurrence (recurrence score >31). Patients with a recurrence score in the low- and intermediate-risk groups were found to have limited additional benefit from adjuvant chemotherapy compared to tamoxifen alone. A special focus of the prospective studies has been to quantify the benefits of adjuvant chemotherapy in the intermediate-risk group. While initially only evaluated for women with node-negative disease, more recent studies have been expanded for women with 1–3 or >4 lymph nodes involved with metastatic disease. It also shows that they may not benefit from adding chemotherapy to hormonal therapy, as the benefits over adjuvant chemotherapy may not warrant the excess risk in toxicity [104, 108–111].

A retrospective analysis of the recurrence score in the ATAC trial evaluated recurrence scores from 1,231 evaluable patients treated with either tamoxifen or anastrozole. This trial further supported the use of the recurrence score to assess outcomes for distant recurrence in both node-positive ($n=306$) and node-negative patients ($n=872$), showing that the prognostic value for aromatase inhibitors is similar to those found with tamoxifen. The distribution of risk groups was similar in both groups, with the high risk representing 15 % and 17 %, respectively, of the entire group, and 59 % and 52 %, respectively, for those with a low risk based upon their recurrence score. However, the 9-year risk of distant recurrence was considerably higher in node-positive patients compared to node-negative patients, demonstrating both its prognostic and predictive value in each setting. The distant recurrence rates were 4, 12, and 25 % in low, intermediate, and high recurrence score, node-negative patients and 17, 28, and 49 % for node-positive patients. Further studies have suggested that the RS remains to be a very strong predictor for late recurrences and may be used to determine who should receive hormonal therapy beyond 5 years [112].

The impact of the Oncotype DX breast cancer assay on clinical decision making has been quite dramatic. A recent analysis of over 4,000 women revealed that the utilization of this assay altered the recommendations for adjuvant therapy in 33 % of the patients. These studies further suggested that adjuvant chemotherapy was offered in 6 % of low-risk patients, 37 % intermediate, and 83 % with high recurrence score [104, 108–110, 113–117].

Lastly, we await the results of prospective studies, such as the TailorRx and Responder trials, which will further elucidate the value of this test for clinical decision making (Fig. 22.1).

The MammaPrint gene assay utilizes cDNA microarrays obtained from fresh samples of breast cancer (not paraffin-embedded) to subclassify tumors into five subtypes, based upon their distinct gene expression profiles. These include luminal epithelial cell phenotypes (subtypes A and B), a basal epithelial cell type phenotype, a HER2 (+) phenotype, and a group of cancers expressing a "normal-like" gene profile. Based on earlier observations that the ER levels vary considerably between luminal or basal types [46–48], Van't Veer and colleagues designed a 70-gene microarray platform to identify a "poor-prognosis signature" involving genes associated with the cell cycle, tumor invasion, metastasis, and angiogenesis [19, 21, 118]. An initial validation of this gene assay revealed a poor-prognosis signature as well as a good-prognosis signature. Those in the former group had a significantly worse 10-year overall survival rate [19, 21, 118, 119]. While initially developed as primarily a prognostic test, it has been further developed into a test with predictive value in adjuvant and neoadjuvant trials. Retrospective studies have suggested that the patients with a good-prognosis signature are unlikely to have a significant pathological response rate to chemotherapy [119–123].

The PAM50 gene assay test was recently approved in the United States to determine the

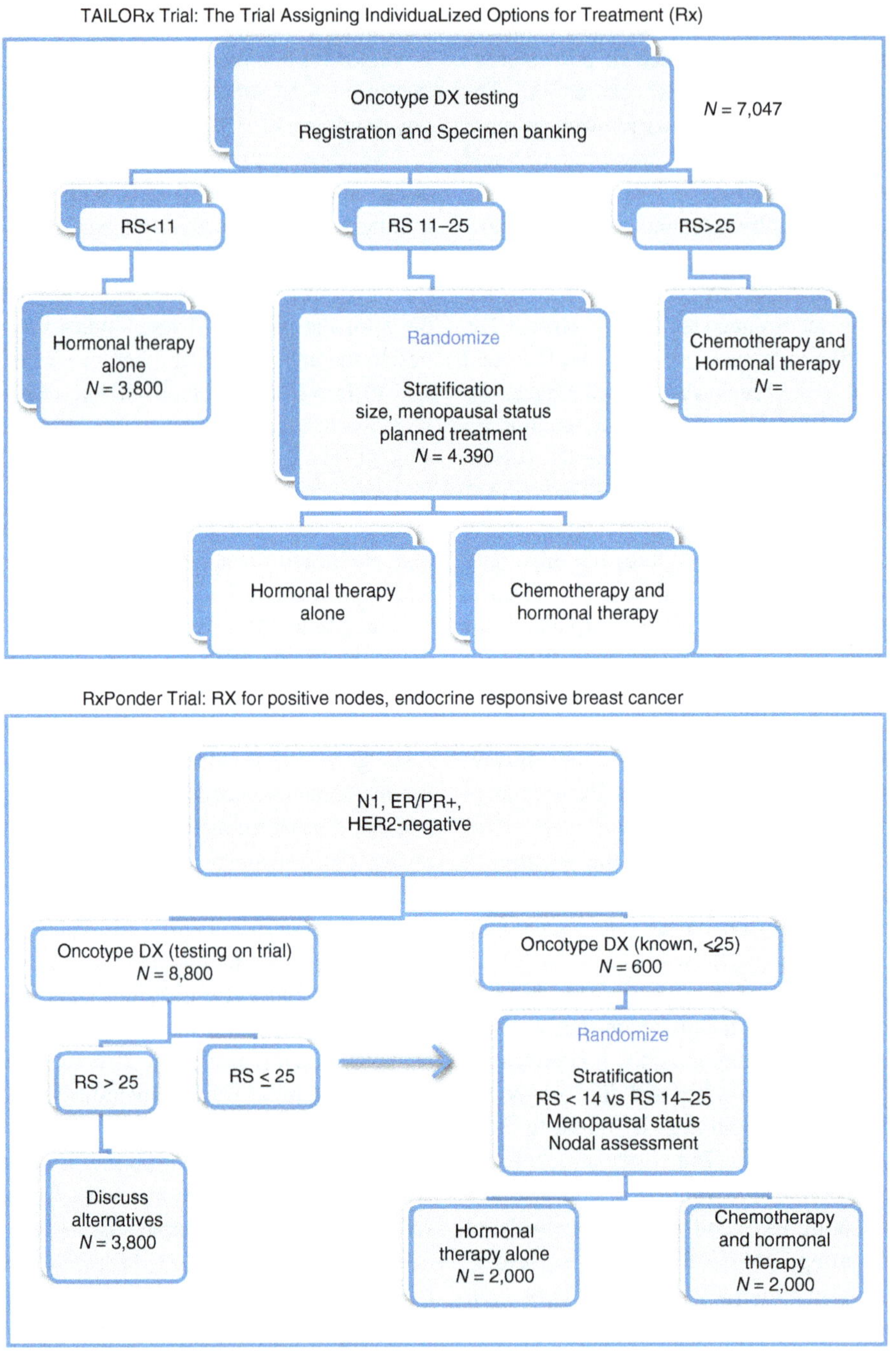

Fig. 22.1 TAILORx Trial: the *T*rial *A*ssigning *I*ndividua*L*ized *O*ptions for Treatment (*Rx*) and RxPonder Trial: RX for positive nodes, endocrine-responsive breast cancer

risk of recurrence (ROR) score for patients with stage I/II, node-negative or stage II, node-positive (1–3 nodes) disease that is hormone receptor positive. A clinical challenge posed by the Oncotype DX assay is the uncertainly on whether to treat patients with an intermediate-risk recurrence score. The PAM50 assay measures the gene profile of 50 genes based on the four basic tumor subtypes (luminal A, luminal B, HER2 enriched, and basal-like) with the goal of defining a better distinction between the intermediate- and high-risk groups.

In two recent studies, tumor samples were obtained from 1,017 women with hormone receptor-positive breast cancer who received either anastrozole or tamoxifen in the TransATAC trial. The recurrence score utilizing the PAM50 (ROR) assay was then compared to the recurrence score for the Oncotype DX assay, showing that the ROR may offer a more definitive discrimination between intermediate- and high-risk groups. They identified more patients that were reclassified as high risk based upon the ROR score compared to the Oncotype DX recurrence score [124–131]. Furthermore, this test may be able to determine a group of patients that benefit from paclitaxel-based chemotherapy [126]. However, further prospective studies will be needed to validate the use of this assay in order to determine its validity and ultimate clinical use in decision making.

Conclusion

The most commonly used prognostic and predictive molecular markers for early-stage breast cancer in clinical practice are ER, PR, and HER-2, as well as Ki67. The latter remains somewhat limited at present, until further studies can assess its validity in clinical practice. Genetic assessments of BRCA mutations are more commonly used to determine the risk for developing primary tumors and to guide the use of novel agents directed against DNA damage. There are three multigene assays that are able to assist clinicians in decision making for their breast cancer patients: the Oncotype DX, MammaPrint, and, more recently, the PAM50 gene assay. Genetic assessments of BRCA mutations are more commonly used to determine the risk for developing primary tumors and to guide the use of novel agents directed against DNA damage repair.

Future Perspective

Over the last two decades, important strides have been made in our attempt to select those patients who are more likely to benefit from therapy from those that will not. Furthermore, gene assays will continue to develop that will better allow us to determine those who need therapy and define those who are less likely to develop metastatic disease. The value of many other genes as predictors of response or as therapeutic targets, as well as the assessment of proteomics and polymorphisms, is undergoing vigorous preclinical and clinical testing and will hopefully emerge as useful tools in the future. Other important predictors may arise from the evaluation of environment modifiers, next-generation sequencing, and molecular bio-imaging. These efforts will be even more important in an area of expensive and often toxic therapy.

References

1. Beatson GT. On the treatment of inoperable cases of carcinomas of the mamma: suggestions for a new method of treatment, with illustrative cases. Lancet. 1896;2:104–7.
2. Dao TL. Estrogen excretion in women with mammary cancer before and after adrenalectomy. Science. 1953;118:21–2.
3. Pearson OH. Hypophysectomy in the treatment of metastatic mammary cancer. CA Cancer J Clin. 1959; 9:159–62.
4. Dodds EC, Goldberg L, et al. Oestrogenic activity of certain synthetic compounds. Nature. 1938;141:247–8.
5. Haddow A, Watkinson JM, et al. Influence of synthetic oestrogens upon advanced malignant disease. BMJ. 1944;2:393–8.
6. Council on Drugs. Androgens and estrogens in the treatment of disseminated mammary carcinoma: retrospective study of nine hundred forty-four patients. JAMA. 1960;172:1271–83.
7. Cole MP, Jones CT, et al. A new anti-oestrogenic agent in late breast cancer. An early clinical appraisal of ICI46474. Br J Cancer. 1971;25:270–5.

8. Ward HW. Anti-oestrogen therapy for breast cancer: a trial of tamoxifen at two dose levels. Br Med J. 1973; 1:13–4.
9. Ingle JN, Ahmann DL, et al. Randomized clinical trial of diethylstilbestrol versus tamoxifen in postmenopausal women with advanced breast cancer. N Engl J Med. 1981;304:16–21.
10. Slamon DJ, Godolphin W, et al. Studies of the HER-2/neu proto-oncogene in human breast and ovarian cancer. Science. 1989;244:707–12.
11. Slamon DJ, Clark GM, et al. Human breast cancer: correlation of relapse and survival with amplification of the HER-2/neu oncogene. Science. 1987;235:177–82.
12. Pegram MD, Lipton A, et al. Phase II study of receptor-enhanced chemosensitivity using recombinant humanized anti-p185HER2/neu monoclonal antibody plus cisplatin in patients with HER2/neu-overexpressing metastatic breast cancer refractory to chemotherapy treatment. J Clin Oncol. 1998;16:2659–71.
13. Cobleigh MA, Vogel CL, et al. Multinational study of the efficacy and safety of humanized anti-HER2 monoclonal antibody in women who have HER2-overexpressing metastatic breast cancer that has progressed after chemotherapy for metastatic disease. J Clin Oncol. 1999;17:2639–48.
14. Pegram MD, Konecny G, et al. The molecular and cellular biology of HER2/neu gene amplification/overexpression and the clinical development of herceptin (trastuzumab) therapy for breast cancer. Cancer Treat Res. 2000;103:57–75.
15. Slamon DJ, Leyland-Jones B, et al. Use of chemotherapy plus a monoclonal antibody against HER2 for metastatic breast cancer that overexpresses HER2. N Engl J Med. 2001;344:783–92.
16. Vogel CL, Cobleigh MA, et al. Efficacy and safety of trastuzumab as a single agent in first-line treatment of HER2-overexpressing metastatic breast cancer. J Clin Oncol. 2002;20:719–26.
17. Pegram MD, Pienkowski T, et al. Results of two open-label, multicenter phase II studies of docetaxel, platinum salts, and trastuzumab in HER2-positive advanced breast cancer. J Natl Cancer Inst. 2004;96: 759–69.
18. Slamon D, Eiermann W, et al. Adjuvant trastuzumab in HER2-positive breast cancer. N Engl J Med. 2011; 365:1273–83.
19. Bueno-de-Mesquita JM, van Harten WH, et al. Use of 70-gene signature to predict prognosis of patients with node-negative breast cancer: a prospective community-based feasibility study (RASTER). Lancet Oncol. 2007;8:1079–87.
20. Modlich O, Bojar H. Can a 70-gene signature provide useful prognostic information in patients with node-negative breast cancer? Nature clinical practice. Oncology. 2007;4:216–7.
21. Weigelt B, Hu Z, et al. Molecular portraits and 70-gene prognosis signature are preserved throughout the metastatic process of breast cancer. Cancer Res. 2005;65:9155–8.
22. Bueno-de-Mesquita JM, Linn SC, et al. Validation of 70-gene prognosis signature in node-negative breast cancer. Breast Cancer Res Treat. 2009;117:483–95.
23. Na KY, Kim KS, et al. The 70-gene prognostic signature for Korean breast cancer patients. J Breast Cancer. 2011;14:33–8.
24. Torrisi R, Garcia-Etienne CA, et al. Potential impact of the 70-gene signature in the choice of adjuvant systemic treatment for ER positive, HER2 negative tumors: a single institution experience. Breast. 2013;22:419–24.
25. Allred DC, Carlson RW. NCCN Task Force Report: estrogen receptor and progesterone receptor testing in breast cancer by immunohistochemistry. J Natl Compr Cancer Netw. 2009;7 Suppl 6:S1–21; quiz S22–3.
26. Effects of chemotherapy and hormonal therapy for early breast cancer on recurrence and 15-year survival: an overview of the randomised trials. Lancet 2005;365:1687–717.
27. Tamoxifen for early breast cancer: an overview of the randomised trials. Early Breast Cancer Trialists' Collaborative Group. Lancet 1998;351:1451–67.
28. Polychemotherapy for early breast cancer: an overview of the randomised trials. Early Breast Cancer Trialists' Collaborative Group. Lancet 1998;352:930–42.
29. Ovarian ablation in early breast cancer: overview of the randomised trials. Early Breast Cancer Trialists' Collaborative Group. Lancet 1996;348:1189–96.
30. van Hezewijk M, Bastiaannet E, et al. Effect of local therapy on locoregional recurrence in postmenopausal women with breast cancer in the Tamoxifen Exemestane Adjuvant Multinational (TEAM) trial. Radiother Oncol. 2013;108:190–6.
31. van Nes JG, Fontein DB, et al. Quality of life in relation to tamoxifen or exemestane treatment in postmenopausal breast cancer patients: a Tamoxifen Exemestane Adjuvant Multinational (TEAM) Trial side study. Breast Cancer Res Treat. 2012;134:267–76.
32. van de Velde CJ, Rea D, et al. Adjuvant tamoxifen and exemestane in early breast cancer (TEAM): a randomised phase 3 trial. Lancet. 2011;377:321–31.
33. Goss PE, Ingle JN, et al. Late extended adjuvant treatment with letrozole improves outcome in women with early-stage breast cancer who complete 5 years of tamoxifen. J Clin Oncol. 2008;26:1948–55.
34. Goss PE, Ingle JN, et al. Randomized trial of letrozole following tamoxifen as extended adjuvant therapy in receptor-positive breast cancer: updated findings from NCIC CTG MA.17. J Natl Cancer Inst. 2005;97:1262–71.
35. Mann BS, Johnson JR, et al. Letrozole in the extended adjuvant treatment of postmenopausal women with history of early-stage breast cancer who have completed 5 years of adjuvant tamoxifen. Clin Cancer Res. 2005;11:5671–7.
36. Viale G, Regan MM, et al. Prognostic and predictive value of centrally reviewed expression of estrogen and progesterone receptors in a randomized trial comparing letrozole and tamoxifen adjuvant therapy for postmenopausal early breast cancer: BIG 1-98. J Clin Oncol. 2007;25:3846–52.

37. Arpino G, Weiss H, et al. Estrogen receptor-positive, progesterone receptor-negative breast cancer: association with growth factor receptor expression and tamoxifen resistance. J Natl Cancer Inst. 2005;97:1254–61.
38. Bardou VJ, Arpino G, et al. Progesterone receptor status significantly improves outcome prediction over estrogen receptor status alone for adjuvant endocrine therapy in two large breast cancer databases. J Clin Oncol. 2003;21:1973–9.
39. Clark GM, Osborne CK, et al. Correlations between estrogen receptor, progesterone receptor, and patient characteristics in human breast cancer. J Clin Oncol. 1984;2:1102–9.
40. Osborne CK, Yochmowitz MG, et al. The value of estrogen and progesterone receptors in the treatment of breast cancer. Cancer. 1980;46:2884–8.
41. Singh L, Wilson AJ, et al. The relationship between histological grade, oestrogen receptor status, events and survival at 8 years in the NATO ('Nolvadex') trial. Br J Cancer. 1988;57:612–4.
42. Baum M, Budzar AU, et al. Anastrozole alone or in combination with tamoxifen versus tamoxifen alone for adjuvant treatment of postmenopausal women with early breast cancer: first results of the ATAC randomised trial. Lancet. 2002;359:2131–9.
43. Regan MM, Neven P, et al. Assessment of letrozole and tamoxifen alone and in sequence for postmenopausal women with steroid hormone receptor-positive breast cancer: the BIG 1-98 randomised clinical trial at 8.1 years median follow-up. Lancet Oncol. 2011;12:1101–8.
44. Coates AS, Keshaviah A, et al. Five years of letrozole compared with tamoxifen as initial adjuvant therapy for postmenopausal women with endocrine-responsive early breast cancer: update of study BIG 1-98. J Clin Oncol. 2007;25:486–92.
45. Kaufmann M, Pusztai L. Use of standard markers and incorporation of molecular markers into breast cancer therapy: consensus recommendations from an International Expert Panel. Cancer. 2011;117:1575–82.
46. Sorlie T. Introducing molecular subtyping of breast cancer into the clinic? J Clin Oncol. 2009;27:1153–4.
47. Sorlie T, Perou CM, et al. Gene expression profiles do not consistently predict the clinical treatment response in locally advanced breast cancer. Mol Cancer Ther. 2006;5:2914–8.
48. Sorlie T, Wang Y, et al. Distinct molecular mechanisms underlying clinically relevant subtypes of breast cancer: gene expression analyses across three different platforms. BMC Genomics. 2006;7:127.
49. Kristensen VN, Sorlie T, et al. Gene expression profiling of breast cancer in relation to estrogen receptor status and estrogen-metabolizing enzymes: clinical implications. Clin Cancer Res. 2005;11:878s–83.
50. Smith IE, Dowsett M, et al. Neoadjuvant treatment of postmenopausal breast cancer with anastrozole, tamoxifen, or both in combination: the Immediate Preoperative Anastrozole, Tamoxifen, or Combined with Tamoxifen (IMPACT) multicenter double-blind randomized trial. J Clin Oncol. 2005;23:5108–16.
51. Dowsett M, Smith IE, et al. Short-term changes in Ki-67 during neoadjuvant treatment of primary breast cancer with anastrozole or tamoxifen alone or combined correlate with recurrence-free survival. Clin Cancer Res. 2005;11:951s–8.
52. Dowsett M, Nielsen TO, et al. Assessment of Ki67 in breast cancer: recommendations from the International Ki67 in Breast Cancer working group. J Natl Cancer Inst. 2011;103:1656–64.
53. Cheang MC, Chia SK, et al. Ki67 index, HER2 status, and prognosis of patients with luminal B breast cancer. J Natl Cancer Inst. 2009;101:736–50.
54. Dowsett M, Smith I, et al. Endocrine therapy, new biologicals, and new study designs for presurgical studies in breast cancer. J Natl Cancer Inst Monogr. 2011;2011:120–3.
55. Viale G, Giobbie-Hurder A, et al. Prognostic and predictive value of centrally reviewed Ki-67 labeling index in postmenopausal women with endocrine-responsive breast cancer: results from Breast International Group Trial 1-98 comparing adjuvant tamoxifen with letrozole. J Clin Oncol. 2008;26:5569–75.
56. Slamon DJ, Clark GM. Amplification of c-erbB-2 and aggressive human breast tumors? Science. 1988;240: 1795–8.
57. Xie Y, Pendergast AM, et al. Dominant-negative mutants of Grb2 induced reversal of the transformed phenotypes caused by the point mutation-activated rat HER-2/Neu. J Biol Chem. 1995;270:30717–24.
58. Xing WR, Gilchrist KW, et al. FISH detection of HER-2/neu oncogene amplification in early onset breast cancer. Breast Cancer Res Treat. 1996;39:203–12.
59. Brien TP, Odze RD, et al. HER-2/neu gene amplification by FISH predicts poor survival in Barrett's esophagus-associated adenocarcinoma. Hum Pathol. 2000;31:35–9.
60. Persons DL, Bui MM, et al. Fluorescence in situ hybridization (FISH) for detection of HER-2/neu amplification in breast cancer: a multicenter portability study. Ann Clin Lab Sci. 2000;30:41–8.
61. Walch A, Bink K, et al. HER-2/neu gene amplification by FISH predicts poor survival in Barrett's esophagus-associated adenocarcinoma. Hum Pathol. 2000;31:1332–4.
62. Wolff AC, Hammond ME, et al. Recommendations for human epidermal growth factor receptor 2 testing in breast cancer: american society of clinical oncology/college of american pathologists clinical practice guideline update. J Clin Oncol. 2013;31:3997–4013.
63. Wolff AC, Hammond ME, et al. Re: predictability of adjuvant trastuzumab benefit in N9831 patients using the ASCO/CAP HER2-positivity criteria. J Natl Cancer Inst. 2012;104:957–8.
64. Hammond ME, Hayes DF, et al. American Society of Clinical Oncology/College of American Pathologists guideline recommendations for immunohistochemical testing of estrogen and progesterone receptors in breast cancer. J Clin Oncol. 2010;28:2784–95.
65. Zakhartseva LM, Gorovenko NG, et al. Breast cancer immunohistochemical features in young women with BRCA 1/2 mutations. Exp Oncol. 2009;31:174–8.

66. Musolino A, Bella MA, et al. BRCA mutations, molecular markers, and clinical variables in early-onset breast cancer: a population-based study. Breast. 2007;16:280–92.
67. Robson M, Gilewski T, et al. BRCA-associated breast cancer in young women. J Clin Oncol. 1998;16:1642–9.
68. Osin P, Gusterson BA, et al. Predicted anti-oestrogen resistance in BRCA-associated familial breast cancers. Eur J Cancer. 1998;34:1683–6.
69. Ersahin C, Chivukula M, et al. Basal-like subtype breast cancers in women older than 40 years of age. Int J Surg Pathol. 2010;18:42–7.
70. Maegawa RO, Tang SC. Triple-negative breast cancer: unique biology and its management. Cancer Invest. 2010;28:878–83.
71. Bal A, Verma S, et al. BRCA1-methylated sporadic breast cancers are BRCA-like in showing a basal phenotype and absence of ER expression. Virchows Arch. 2012;461:305–12.
72. Deb S, Jene N, et al. Genotypic and phenotypic analysis of familial male breast cancer shows under representation of the HER2 and basal subtypes in BRCA-associated carcinomas. BMC Cancer. 2012;12:510.
73. De Summa S, Pinto R, et al. BRCAness: a deeper insight into basal-like breast tumors. Ann Oncol. 2013;24 Suppl 8:viii13–21.
74. Turner NC, Reis-Filho JS, et al. BRCA1 dysfunction in sporadic basal-like breast cancer. Oncogene. 2007;26:2126–32.
75. Turner NC, Reis-Filho JS. Basal-like breast cancer and the BRCA1 phenotype. Oncogene. 2006;25:5846–53.
76. Boyd J, Sonoda Y, et al. Clinicopathologic features of BRCA-linked and sporadic ovarian cancer. JAMA. 2000;283:2260–5.
77. Cass I, Baldwin RL, et al. Improved survival in women with BRCA-associated ovarian carcinoma. Cancer. 2003;97:2187–95.
78. Arun B, Bayraktar S, et al. Response to neoadjuvant systemic therapy for breast cancer in BRCA mutation carriers and noncarriers: a single-institution experience. J Clin Oncol. 2011;29:3739–46.
79. Schott S, Sohn C, et al. Preoperative systemic treatment in BRCA-positive breast cancer patients: case report and review of the literature. Breast Care. 2011; 6:395–8.
80. Alsop K, Fereday S, et al. BRCA mutation frequency and patterns of treatment response in BRCA mutation-positive women with ovarian cancer: a report from the Australian Ovarian Cancer Study Group. J Clin Oncol. 2012;30:2654–63.
81. Gallagher DJ, Cronin AM, et al. Germline BRCA mutation does not prevent response to taxane-based therapy for the treatment of castration-resistant prostate cancer. BJU Int. 2012;109:713–9.
82. Fong PC, Boss DS, et al. Inhibition of poly(ADP-ribose) polymerase in tumors from BRCA mutation carriers. N Engl J Med. 2009;361:123–34.
83. Fong PC, Yap TA, et al. Poly(ADP)-ribose polymerase inhibition: frequent durable responses in BRCA carrier ovarian cancer correlating with platinum-free interval. J Clin Oncol. 2010;28:2512–9.
84. Yavuz S, Paydas S, et al. VEGF-C expression in breast cancer: clinical importance. Adv Ther. 2005; 22:368–80.
85. Bender RJ, Mac Gabhann F. Expression of VEGF and semaphorin genes define subgroups of triple negative breast cancer. PLoS One. 2013;8:e61788.
86. Greb RR, Maier I, et al. Vascular endothelial growth factor A (VEGF-A) mRNA expression levels decrease after menopause in normal breast tissue but not in breast cancer lesions. Br J Cancer. 1999;81:225–31.
87. Loi S, Michiels S, et al. PIK3CA genotype and a PIK3CA mutation-related gene signature and response to everolimus and letrozole in estrogen receptor positive breast cancer. PLoS One. 2013;8:e53292.
88. Weigelt B, Warne PH, et al. PIK3CA mutation, but not PTEN loss of function, determines the sensitivity of breast cancer cells to mTOR inhibitory drugs. Oncogene. 2011;30:3222–33.
89. Cizkova M, Cizeron-Clairac G, et al. Gene expression profiling reveals new aspects of PIK3CA mutation in ERalpha-positive breast cancer: major implication of the Wnt signaling pathway. PLoS One. 2010;5: e15647.
90. Campbell IG, Russell SE, et al. Mutation of the PIK3CA gene in ovarian and breast cancer. Cancer Res. 2004;64:7678–81.
91. Petrelli FandBarni S. Response to neoadjuvant chemotherapy in ductal compared to lobular carcinoma of the breast: a meta-analysis of published trials including 1,764 lobular breast cancer. Breast Cancer Res Treat. 2013;142:227–35.
92. Metzger-Filho O, de Azambuja E. Neoadjuvant chemotherapy and targeted therapies: a promising strategy. J Natl Cancer Inst Monogr. 2011;2011:116–9.
93. Zambetti M, Mansutti M, et al. Pathological complete response rates following different neoadjuvant chemotherapy regimens for operable breast cancer according to ER status, in two parallel, randomized phase II trials with an adaptive study design (ECTO II). Breast Cancer Res Treat. 2012;132:843–51.
94. Huober J, von Minckwitz G, et al. Effect of neoadjuvant anthracycline-taxane-based chemotherapy in different biological breast cancer phenotypes: overall results from the GeparTrio study. Breast Cancer Res Treat. 2010;124:133–40.
95. Chang HR, Glaspy J, et al. Differential response of triple-negative breast cancer to a docetaxel and carboplatin-based neoadjuvant treatment. Cancer. 2010;116: 4227–37.
96. Guiu S, Michiels S, et al. Molecular subclasses of breast cancer: how do we define them? The IMPAKT 2012 Working Group Statement. Ann Oncol. 2012;23: 2997–3006.
97. Goldhirsch A, Gelber RD, et al. 2 years versus 1 year of adjuvant trastuzumab for HER2-positive breast cancer (HERA): an open-label, randomised controlled trial. Lancet. 2013;382:1021–8.

98. Pivot X, Romieu G, et al. 6 months versus 12 months of adjuvant trastuzumab for patients with HER2-positive early breast cancer (PHARE): a randomised phase 3 trial. Lancet Oncol. 2013;14:741–8.
99. Romond EH, Perez EA, et al. Trastuzumab plus adjuvant chemotherapy for operable HER2-positive breast cancer. N Engl J Med. 2005;353:1673–84.
100. Perez EA, Romond EH, et al. Four-year follow-up of trastuzumab plus adjuvant chemotherapy for operable human epidermal growth factor receptor 2-positive breast cancer: joint analysis of data from NCCTG N9831 and NSABP B-31. J Clin Oncol. 2011;29:3366–73.
101. Tang G, Shak S, et al. Comparison of the prognostic and predictive utilities of the 21-gene Recurrence Score assay and Adjuvant! for women with node-negative, ER-positive breast cancer: results from NSABP B-14 and NSABP B-20. Breast Cancer Res Treat. 2011;127:133–42.
102. Albain KS, Paik S, et al. Prediction of adjuvant chemotherapy benefit in endocrine responsive, early breast cancer using multigene assays. Breast. 2009;18 Suppl 3:S141–5.
103. Yothers G, O'Connell MJ, et al. Validation of the 12-gene colon cancer recurrence score in NSABP C-07 as a predictor of recurrence in patients with stage II and III colon cancer treated with fluorouracil and leucovorin (FU/LV) and FU/LV plus oxaliplatin. J Clin Oncol. 2013;31(36):4512–19.
104. Mamounas EP, Tang G, et al. Association between the 21-gene recurrence score assay and risk of locoregional recurrence in node-negative, estrogen receptor-positive breast cancer: results from NSABP B-14 and NSABP B-20. J Clin Oncol. 2010;28:1677–83.
105. Paik S, Tang G, et al. Gene expression and benefit of chemotherapy in women with node-negative, estrogen receptor-positive breast cancer. J Clin Oncol. 2006;24:3726–34.
106. Paik S, Shak S, et al. A multigene assay to predict recurrence of tamoxifen-treated, node-negative breast cancer. N Engl J Med. 2004;351:2817–26.
107. Hornberger J, Cosler LE, et al. Economic analysis of targeting chemotherapy using a 21-gene RT-PCR assay in lymph-node-negative, estrogen-receptor-positive, early-stage breast cancer. Am J Manag Care. 2005;11:313–24.
108. Albain KS, Barlow WE, et al. Prognostic and predictive value of the 21-gene recurrence score assay in postmenopausal women with node-positive, oestrogen-receptor-positive breast cancer on chemotherapy: a retrospective analysis of a randomised trial. Lancet Oncol. 2010;11:55–65.
109. Dowsett M, Cuzick J, et al. Prediction of risk of distant recurrence using the 21-gene recurrence score in node-negative and node-positive postmenopausal patients with breast cancer treated with anastrozole or tamoxifen: a TransATAC study. J Clin Oncol. 2010;28:1829–34.
110. Lo SS, Mumby PB, et al. Prospective multicenter study of the impact of the 21-gene recurrence score assay on medical oncologist and patient adjuvant breast cancer treatment selection. J Clin Oncol. 2010;28:1671–6.
111. Goldstein LJ, Gray R, et al. Prognostic utility of the 21-gene assay in hormone receptor-positive operable breast cancer compared with classical clinicopathologic features. J Clin Oncol. 2008;26:4063–71.
112. Hannouf MB, Xie B, et al. Cost effectiveness of a 21-gene recurrence score assay versus Canadian clinical practice in post-menopausal women with early-stage estrogen or progesterone-receptor-positive, axillary lymph-node positive breast cancer. Pharmacoeconomics. 2013;2:135–47.
113. Eiermann W, Rezai M, et al. The 21-gene recurrence score assay impacts adjuvant therapy recommendations for ER-positive, node-negative and node-positive early breast cancer resulting in a risk-adapted change in chemotherapy use. Ann Oncol. 2013;24:618–24.
114. Hannouf MB, Xie B, et al. Cost-effectiveness of a 21-gene recurrence score assay versus Canadian clinical practice in women with early-stage estrogen- or progesterone-receptor-positive, axillary lymph-node negative breast cancer. BMC Cancer. 2012; 12:447.
115. Reed SD, Dinan MA, et al. Cost-effectiveness of the 21-gene recurrence score assay in the context of multifactorial decision making to guide chemotherapy for early-stage breast cancer. Genet Med. 2013; 15:203–11.
116. Blohmer JU, Rezai M, et al. Using the 21-gene assay to guide adjuvant chemotherapy decision-making in early-stage breast cancer: a cost-effectiveness evaluation in the German setting. J Med Econ. 2013; 16:30–40.
117. Kondo M, Hoshi SL, et al. Economic evaluation of the 21-gene signature (Oncotype DX) in lymph node-negative/positive, hormone receptor-positive early-stage breast cancer based on Japanese validation study (JBCRG-TR03). Breast Cancer Res Treat. 2011;127:739–49.
118. Buyse M, Loi S, et al. Validation and clinical utility of a 70-gene prognostic signature for women with node-negative breast cancer. J Natl Cancer Inst. 2006;98:1183–92.
119. Straver ME, Glas AM, et al. The 70-gene signature as a response predictor for neoadjuvant chemotherapy in breast cancer. Breast Cancer Res Treat. 2010;119:551–8.
120. Hornberger J, Alvarado MD, et al. Clinical validity/utility, change in practice patterns, and economic implications of risk stratifiers to predict outcomes for early-stage breast cancer: a systematic review. J Natl Cancer Inst. 2012;104:1068–79.
121. Retel VP, Joore MA, et al. Cost-effectiveness of the 70-gene signature versus St Gallen guidelines and Adjuvant Online for early breast cancer. Eur J Cancer. 2010;46:1382–91.

122. Knauer M, Mook S, et al. The predictive value of the 70-gene signature for adjuvant chemotherapy in early breast cancer. Breast Cancer Res Treat. 2010; 120:655–61.
123. Mook S, Schmidt MK, et al. The 70-gene prognosis-signature predicts disease outcome in breast cancer patients with 1–3 positive lymph nodes in an independent validation study. Breast Cancer Res Treat. 2009;116:295–302.
124. Hu Y, Bai L, et al. Genetic background may contribute to PAM50 gene expression breast cancer subtype assignments. PLoS One. 2013;8:e72287.
125. Dowsett M, Sestak I, et al. Comparison of PAM50 risk of recurrence score with oncotype DX and IHC4 for predicting risk of distant recurrence after endocrine therapy. J Clin Oncol. 2013;31:2783–90.
126. Martin M, Prat A, et al. PAM50 proliferation score as a predictor of weekly paclitaxel benefit in breast cancer. Breast Cancer Res Treat. 2013;138:457–66.
127. Bastien RR, Rodriguez-Lescure A, et al. PAM50 breast cancer subtyping by RT-qPCR and concordance with standard clinical molecular markers. BMC Med Genomics. 2012;5:44.
128. Prat A, Parker JS, et al. PAM50 assay and the three-gene model for identifying the major and clinically relevant molecular subtypes of breast cancer. Breast Cancer Res Treat. 2012;135: 301–6.
129. Ebbert MT, Bastien RR, et al. Characterization of uncertainty in the classification of multivariate assays: application to PAM50 centroid-based genomic predictors for breast cancer treatment plans. J Clin bioinforma. 2011;1:37.
130. Ellis MJ, Suman VJ, et al. Randomized phase II neoadjuvant comparison between letrozole, anastrozole, and exemestane for postmenopausal women with estrogen receptor-rich stage 2 to 3 breast cancer: clinical and biomarker outcomes and predictive value of the baseline PAM50-based intrinsic subtype – ACOSOG Z103. J Clin Oncol. 2011;29: 2342–9.
131. Nielsen TO, Parker JS, et al. A comparison of PAM50 intrinsic subtyping with immunohistochemistry and clinical prognostic factors in tamoxifen-treated estrogen receptor-positive breast cancer. Clin Cancer Res. 2010;16:5222–32.

23 Adjuvant Chemotherapy in Breast Cancer

Elgene Lim, Shom Goel, and Eric P. Winer

Introduction

The biological rationale for adjuvant systemic therapy is to eradicate micrometastases and therefore improve patient outcomes. Adjuvant combination chemotherapy regimens result in a significant reduction in risk of 5-year recurrence and 15-year mortality rates, with a greater benefit in women <50 years of age [1]. In the clinical setting, the decision to use adjuvant chemotherapy is guided by the clinician's estimation of the patient's prognosis (both her risk of cancer recurrence and overall life expectancy) and assessment of the chemosensitivity of the tumor. Not surprisingly, the use and choice of adjuvant chemotherapy regimen in clinical practice are highly variable. Prognostic determinants of breast cancer recurrence may be broadly divided into the categories of tumor stage (including both tumor size and nodal status) and tumor biology (such as tumor grade, estrogen receptor (ER), progesterone receptor (PR) status, and HER2/neu expression).

It is important to note that the relapse risk for small tumors is relatively small, and it is important to consider the limited benefits in this patient subgroup in the context of the potential risks of toxicities with systemic chemotherapy. Substantial progress has been made in our current understanding of the genes involved in breast cancer, with gene profiling techniques confirming the biological heterogeneity of breast cancer at a molecular level. Researchers have identified at least two intrinsic luminal subtypes (luminal A and luminal B) with distinct gene expression, a basal-like subtype, comprised of primarily triple-negative breast cancer (TNBC, defined as ER negative, PR negative, and HER2/neu negative), and a HER2/neu-positive subtype [2, 3]. Broadly speaking, strongly hormone receptor (HR)-positive tumors are considered less chemosensitive than HR-negative breast cancers [4], with the degree of HR positivity thought to correlate with endocrine therapy responsiveness. As such, the optimal use of adjuvant chemotherapy in HR-positive breast cancer has become quite complex [5]. The identification of the specific subgroup of patients with HR-positive tumors that will benefit the most from adjuvant chemotherapy remains a major challenge to clinicians at present.

Prospective data on the utility on biomarkers to predict chemosensitivity are limited, with the most promising biomarkers likely to be multigene prognostic signatures that are able to capture the multiple biological pathways that determine chemotherapy response. The earlier National Institute of Health (NIH) clinical guidelines on adjuvant therapy have recommended chemotherapy for those patients with tumors >1 cm and in the presence of involved nodes [6]. However, recent advances in our understanding

E. Lim, MBBS, FRACP, PhD (✉)
S. Goel, MBBS, FRACP • E.P. Winer, MD
Division of Women's Cancers, Dana-Farber Cancer Institute, 450 Brookline Ave, Boston, MA 02115, USA
e-mail: elgene_lim@dfci.harvard.edu

A.I. Riker (ed.), *Breast Disease: Comprehensive Management*,
DOI 10.1007/978-1-4939-1145-5_23,

of breast cancer have resulted in several revisions to these guidelines, taking into account the tumor biology of breast cancer.

This chapter will focus on the use of adjuvant chemotherapy primarily in the HER2/neu-negative subtype of breast cancer. HER2-directed therapy will be covered in detail in a separate chapter. The regimens that will be discussed are used in both the ER-positive and triple-negative breast cancer TNBC subtypes and in both preoperative (neoadjuvant) and adjuvant settings. Specifically, the use of biomarkers and multigene tests to identify the subset of patients with HR-positive breast cancer will be discussed in detail. Finally, we will also discuss special considerations for the use of adjuvant chemotherapy in the setting of inflammatory breast cancer, elderly, young, and pregnant patients and will conclude with a discussion on the management of chemotherapy-associated toxicities.

Standard Chemotherapy Regimens

The choice of an adjuvant chemotherapy regimen should take into account the tumor burden and breast cancer subtype, as the absolute reduction in the risk of recurrence and mortality from adjuvant chemotherapy is dependent upon the baseline risk. There are a number of commonly utilized adjuvant chemotherapy regimens in clinical practice today (Table 23.1), with most typically given over 4–8 cycles in total. As many of these regimens have not been compared head to head in clinical trials, there is currently no single uniformly accepted standard adjuvant chemotherapy regimen.

Commonly used regimens for breast cancer are summarized in Table 23.1 *and can broadly be divided into:*

1. Non-anthracycline-containing regimens (i.e., CMF and TC)
2. Anthracycline-containing regimens (i.e., AC, FAC, FEC)
3. Anthracycline- and taxane-containing regimens which incorporate both anthracyclines and taxanes (i.e., AC → T, FEC → taxane and TAC)

The Early Breast Cancer Trialists' Collaborative Group (EBCTCG) has published a large meta-analysis of different polychemotherapy regimens used in over 100,000 women from 123 randomized trials [1]. The most effective adjuvant chemotherapy regimens included both anthracycline and taxanes, but these were also associated with the highest frequency of toxicity. Overall, the addition of adjuvant chemotherapy reduced breast cancer mortality by about one third, and the proportional risk reductions in the trials analyzed were only minimally affected by age, tumor burden (tumor size and nodal status), tumor grade, ER status, or tamoxifen use.

A summary of the key findings are as follows [1]:

- *Standard AC (4 cycles) and standard CMF (6 cycles) are equivalent.*
- *Anthracycline-based regimens such as FAC or FEC, which have a higher cumulative anthracycline dosage than standard AC (4 cycles), are superior to standard oral CMF (6 cycles).*
- *The addition of 4 cycles of a taxane to a fixed anthracycline-based control regimen reduced breast cancer mortality. However, there was no significant difference in outcomes when the extra 4 taxane cycles were counterbalanced with extra cycles of a non-taxane chemotherapy.*

More recently, results from the large phase III randomized National Surgical Adjuvant Breast and Bowel (NSABP) B-38 trial were reported, comparing the three adjuvant chemotherapy regimens, dose-dense AC → T, dose-dense AC → T plus gemcitabine, and TAC, in a large cohort of approximately 5,000 patients (65 % with nodal involvement and 80 % with ER-positive disease) [20]. The 5-year DFS and overall survival (OS) rates were similar in all three groups; however, the incidence of grade 3 or 4 toxicity was the lowest with the AC → T regimen.

Another area of variability is the frequency of administering chemotherapy. Dose-dense chemotherapy typically refers to the administration of chemotherapy over a shorter interval. The best example of this is with AC, which can be administered at the same doses in a standard three-weekly interval or a dose-dense fashion every 2 weeks [9, 11]. With treatment administered every 2 weeks, growth factor support with filgrastim is required. With dose-dense AC regimens, paclitaxel may be given following AC

Table 23.1 Commonly used adjuvant chemotherapy regimens for breast cancer

Regimen	Dose	Cycle duration	No cycles	Notes	Reference
Non-anthracycline containing					
Oral CMF	Cyclophosphamide (100 mg/m^2, PO) d1 to 14 Methotrexate (40 mg/m^2) d1, 8 5-Fluorouracil (500 mg/m^2) d1, 8	q4 weeks	6	*Nonstandard IV* **CMF** (600/60/600 mg/m^2), d1, 8, q4 weeks is occasionally given	[7–9]
TC	Docetaxel (T; 75 mg/m^2) Cyclophosphamide (600 mg/m^2)	q3 weeks	4		[10]
Anthracycline containing					
AC	Doxorubicin (A; 60 mg/m^2)^a Cyclophosphamide (600 mg/m^2)	q3 weeks	4	*Dose-dense* **AC** is given q2 weeks with ^{d}filgrastim support	[9, 11]
FAC	5-Fluorouracil (500 mg/m^2) AC (50/500 mg/m^2)^b	q3 weeks	6		[12, 13]
CAF	Cyclophosphamide (600 mg/m^2) Doxorubicin (A; 30 mg/m^2)^b d1, 8 5-Fluorouracil (500 mg/m^2)	q4 weeks	6	**C** may be given PO at 100 mg/m^2 on d1 to 14 of each cycle	[14]
FEC_{60} (*Canadian*)	5-Fluorouracil (500 mg/m^2) Epirubicin (60 mg/m^2)^c Cyclophosphamide (75 mg/m^2, PO) d1 to14	q4 weeks	6		[15]
FEC_{100}	5-Fluorouracil (500 mg/m^2) Epirubicin (100 mg/m^2)^c Cyclophosphamide (500 mg/m^2)	q3 weeks	6	Filgrastim support should be considered	[16]
Anthracycline and taxane containing					
AC → T	Dose-dense **AC**^{a,d} → Paclitaxel (T; 175 mg/m^2)	q2 weeks	4 → 4		[17]
	AC → Paclitaxel (T; 80 mg/m^2)	q3 weeks → weekly × 12	4 → 12		[18]
FEC_{100} → D	**FEC_{100}** → Docetaxel (T; 75 mg/m^2)	q3 weeks	3 → 3	Filgrastim support should be considered	[16]
FEC_{100} → P	**FEC_{100}** → Paclitaxel (P; 100 mg/m^2)	q3 weeks → weekly × 8	4 → 8		[19]
TAC	Docetaxel (T; 75 mg/m^2) **AC** (50/500 mg/m^2)$^{a, d}$	q3 weeks	6	Filgrastim support should be considered	[12]

All chemotherapy is given intravenously unless otherwise stated. Cumulative doses ^{a}240 mg/m^2, ^{b}>240 mg/m^2, ^{c}>300 mg/m^2, ^{d}Given with filgrastim support

either every 2 weeks for 4 cycles or weekly for 12 weeks (at 175 mg/m^2 and 80 mg/m^2, respectively), and it is unclear at this point if either approach is associated with improved outcomes. A recent meta-analysis of dose-dense chemotherapy for early breast cancer, which included 10 randomized trials involving over 10,000 patients, reported a better DFS and OS with dose-dense regimens, particularly in women with HR-negative breast cancer [21].

Chemotherapy in Different Breast Cancer Subtypes

Endocrine therapy forms the basis of adjuvant therapy in patients with HR-positive breast cancer, and the addition of chemotherapy benefits a subset of these patients. When given for HR-positive breast cancer, adjuvant chemotherapy usually sequenced ahead of, and completed before endocrine therapy. In patients with HER2/

neu-positive tumors, HER2-directed therapy alone has not been tested in large adjuvant trials, and the addition of chemotherapy given concurrently with HER2-directed therapy is considered to be the current standard of care. Finally, for TNBC, there are no targeted therapies recommended for use outside of a clinical trial in the adjuvant setting, and combination chemotherapy remains the standard of care.

Chemotherapy in Hormone Receptor-Positive Breast Cancer

While adjuvant endocrine therapy is the standard of care in patients with tumors that express HRs, the indication for adjuvant chemotherapy in patients with HR-positive disease is undergoing reevaluation. Adjuvant chemotherapy is typically given in sequence with, and prior to, endocrine therapy, as there have been conflicting outcomes with concurrent therapy [22–24]. On average, patients with HR-positive breast cancers derive less benefit from chemotherapy compared to HR-negative tumors [25]. However, there still appears to be a subset of patients with HR-positive tumors that are chemosensitive. The basis for the addition of chemotherapy to adjuvant endocrine therapy is usually guided by the clinician's estimation of prognosis and assessment of the endocrine- and chemosensitivity of the tumor. Patients for whom systemic chemotherapy should be strongly considered include patients with grade 2 or 3 disease, those with high-risk features based upon the gene signature (such as Oncotype DX and MammaPrint), and patients with a higher disease burden. That said, not every patient with node-positive disease has to be treated with chemotherapy, and multigene signatures are particularly useful in guiding the clinicians in regards to the decision to recommend chemotherapy [26].

The EBCTCG overview reported a benefit in terms of 5-year recurrence-free survival with adjuvant sequential chemoendocrine therapy over endocrine therapy alone with hazard ratios of 0.64 and 0.85 in patients with ER-positive tumors aged <50 and >50 years, respectively [27]. The larger impact of chemotherapy in younger patients may be partially explained by the endocrine effect of chemotherapy on ovarian function [6]. Similar long-term DFS benefits with the addition of chemotherapy to adjuvant endocrine therapy were also noted in the phase III randomized NSABP B-20 and Southwest Oncology Group (SWOG) 8814 trials [26, 28]. The identification of predictors of chemosensitivity in HR-positive tumors has been identified as a key challenge.

There is evidence suggesting an inverse relationship between HR expression and chemotherapy benefit in luminal breast cancers. In a study of postmenopausal women with ER-positive and node-positive cancers from the International Breast Cancer Study Group (IBCSG) Trials VII and 12-93, the addition of adjuvant chemotherapy to endocrine therapy improved the DFS (hazard ratio $=0.81$, $p=0.02$, median follow-up of 13 years) [29]. Nonparametric subpopulation treatment effect pattern plot (STEPP) analyses demonstrated that this benefit was limited to the patients whose tumors had low to intermediate levels of estrogen expression. The level of ER appears to predict the response to both endocrine and chemotherapies in opposite directions, but these factors may not entirely overlap. It is likely that there are other biological factors that interact with the ER-signaling pathway to determine chemosensitivity. The assumption that chemosensitivity is inversely related to endocrine sensitivity in ER-positive breast cancer is therefore not clearly defined. Tumors that are endocrine sensitive may also be chemosensitive; conversely, endocrine resistant tumors with poor prognostic factors may not always be chemosensitive.

One biomarker that has been examined in chemosensitive ER-positive tumors is Ki67, a marker of cellular proliferation. In an analysis of 1,521 premenopausal and postmenopausal patients with ER-positive tumors from the IBCSG VIII and IX trials, respectively, a high Ki67 index was found to be associated with poorer DFS, but did not predict an OS benefit with the addition of chemotherapy to endocrine therapy [30]. The adjuvant chemotherapy used in these trials was CMF and did not include anthracyclines and taxanes. In contrast, a high Ki67 index was predictive of both outcome and benefit to adjuvant taxane chemotherapy in ER-positive breast cancers in subset analyses of the PACS 01 and Breast Cancer International Research Group (BCIRG) 001 trials [31, 32]. An important caveat of these findings is that these were unplanned subset analyses. At this point, Ki67 should not be used as a basis of recommendation for adjuvant chemotherapy outside of a clinical trial setting, at least in part because the test is not always reliable.

A major advancement in the identification of biomarkers of chemosensitivity in HR-positive breast cancers has been the development of multigene prognostic signatures. These are typically derived from high-throughput analyses of tumor specimens for gene expression patterns and subsequently validated in patient cohorts from clinical trials. These assays have the potential to identify subsets of patients that would benefit from the addition of adjuvant chemotherapy to endocrine therapy. The 21-gene assay, called the Oncotype DX (Genomic Health, Redwood City, CA, USA), provides a recurrence score (RS) that predicts for risk of 10-year distant recurrence. The RS is derived from a complex algorithm calculated on the gene expressions of a preselected list of 16 genes of biological interest, including genes involved in estrogen signaling, cell proliferation, and HER2/neu signaling and 5 reference genes for normalization purposes [28]. The utility of the RS as a predictor of distant recurrence risk at 10 years was initially assessed in the NSABP B-14 trial, in which patients with ER-positive, node-negative breast cancer were randomized to receive either tamoxifen or placebo. The RS was shown to more accurately predict for distant recurrence than conventional clinicopathologic characteristics in the tamoxifen-treated patients [33].

The utility of the RS to accurately predict 10-year distance recurrences was demonstrated in a retrospective analysis of the NSABP B-20 trial, in which patients with ER-positive, node-negative breast cancer were randomized to either tamoxifen or tamoxifen plus chemotherapy. Patients with a low or intermediate RS (defined as <18, and ≥18 and <31, respectively) were found not to benefit from chemotherapy, while those with a high RS (defined as ≥31) derived a significant benefit from chemotherapy [28]. The absolute difference in the 10-year distant recurrence rates with the addition of chemotherapy in these RS groups was an increase of 1.1 % and 1.8 % and a reduction of 28.6 %, respectively. Similar results were obtained in a retrospective analysis of the SWOG 8814 trial, in which postmenopausal patients with ER-positive, node-positive breast cancer were randomized to receive either tamoxifen or tamoxifen plus anthracycline-based chemotherapy [26]. One of the primary strengths of this assay is that RNA may be extracted from archived formalin-fixed, paraffin-embedded tissue, which is the primary mode of preserving tissue in most pathology departments.

Another multigene signature with prognostic utility is the FDA-approved 70-gene MammaPrint signature (Agendia, Amsterdam, Netherlands). Unlike the Oncotype RS assay where genes are preselected, MammaPrint was developed using an unsupervised hierarchical clustering approach whereby the high-risk gene signature predicted a poor clinical outcome in tumors of all subtypes [34]. A retrospective analysis of pooled patient cohorts with ER-positive, node-negative breast cancer demonstrated that the 70-gene score had prognostic value and predicted improved survival outcomes with the addition of chemotherapy to endocrine therapy only in the subgroup of 70-gene high-risk patients [35].

While both the Oncotype and MammaPrint assays were tested retrospectively, the Oncotype RS was evaluated retrospectively in a prospectively assembled clinical trial. For this reason, there is far greater confidence, at this time, that the Oncotype assay can reliably predict which patients will benefit from chemotherapy, and even more importantly, which ones will not. In addition, unlike the Oncotype assay, MammaPrint is performed on fresh-frozen tissue that may limit its feasibility for routine use. Both of these multigene signatures are currently undergoing prospective validation in large ongoing studies (Oncotype RS, TAILORx and RxPONDER trials; MammaPrint, MINDACT trial), which include over 100,000 patients collectively to definitively address their predictive value for chemosensitivity in ER-positive breast cancer [36, 37].

In considering the benefits of adjuvant chemotherapy in patients with HR-positive tumors, it is important to consider common relapse patterns. Patients with HR-positive tumors are at a continued risk of relapse for many years after initial breast cancer diagnosis [38]. More than half of all recurrences among women treated with adjuvant tamoxifen therapy occur between 6 and 15 years after diagnosis, and the greatest benefit with the addition of chemotherapy in DFS was seen primarily within the first 5 years from diagnosis [27]. The limited benefit from chemotherapy in preventing late relapses is also reflected in the DFS patterns of patients with poor prognosis multigene signatures with both the Oncotype RS and MammaPrint assays [28, 39]. Late recurrences and deaths remain a formidable clinical challenge in HR-positive breast cancer, and chemotherapy is unlikely to be the answer to this problem.

The summary recommendations for adjuvant chemotherapy in hormone receptor-positive breast cancer are as follows:

- *Adjuvant chemotherapy should be strongly considered in the setting of node-positive disease, high-grade tumors, and high-risk gene multigene signatures.*
  - *In regard to the utility of the Oncotype DX Recurrence Score:*
  - *The use of Oncotype for node-positive disease is discouraged in poorer prognosis disease, for example, ≥4 positive nodes, or in the setting of high-grade disease, as chemotherapy should routinely be given in these settings.*
  - *The use of chemotherapy is strongly encouraged in patients with Oncotype RS ≥31.*
  - *In node-positive patients, particularly those with one to three positive nodes, consideration can be given to omitting chemotherapy if the Oncotype RS is low (<18) and there are no other unfavorable features.*
  - *Recommendations for patients with intermediate-risk multigene signatures* (i.e., *Oncotype RS 18-31*) *are an area of controversy and active research, and prospective trials in this population are currently underway* [36, 37].

Chemotherapy in HER2-Positive Breast Cancer

The advent of HER2-directed therapy has revolutionized the management of HER2/neu-positive, early-stage breast cancer. Based on the results of five randomized clinical trials, 12 months of adjuvant trastuzumab is now an integral part of systemic therapy for these patients [40–42]. In all studies, trastuzumab was added to a chemotherapy backbone, and there is currently no data to support the use of adjuvant trastuzumab monotherapy. Evidence-based chemotherapy backbones in this context include AC → T (NSABP B-31, NCCTG N9831), AC → docetaxel (BCIRG 006) and docetaxel + carboplatin (BCIRG 006). Given the increased cardiotoxicity risk upon administering trastuzumab concurrently with an anthracycline in the metastatic setting [43], trastuzumab is omitted during the period of anthracycline chemotherapy.

There remains controversy about the treatment of small HER2/neu-positive cancers. There are limited data on outcomes for patients with small, stage I HER2/neu-positive breast cancers because the seminal adjuvant trastuzumab trials excluded patients with these tumors. Current guidelines from St. Gallen and the European Society for Medical Oncology (ESMO) do not recommend adjuvant trastuzumab and chemotherapy for node-negative HER2/neu-positive tumors that are <1 cm [44]. In contrast, the National Comprehensive Cancer Network (NCCN) treatment guidelines have factored in the indirect evidence obtained from retrospective and subset analyses of trials and recommend consideration be given to the use of trastuzumab-based therapy in T1bN0 tumors, in particular, in the hormone receptor-negative subset [45].

However, there is a wide variation in clinical practice in this subgroup. Recently, interest has developed in using less intensive, and therefore potentially less toxic, partner chemotherapies with adjuvant trastuzumab for low-risk HER2-positive tumors. In a phase II study in women with HER2/neu-positive metastatic breast cancer, weekly paclitaxel and trastuzumab resulted in a 67–81 % response rate, and a 6 % incidence of grade 3 or 4 neutropenia [46]. The Dana-Farber Cancer Institute led a multicenter, phase II, nonrandomized study of weekly paclitaxel plus trastuzumab for 12 weeks, followed by maintenance trastuzumab for a further 9 months in patients with node-negative, HER2/neu-positive tumors that are <3 cm (information available at ClinicalTrials.gov; identifier NCT00542451). This trial has completed accrual of 410 patients, of whom approximately 50 % had tumors <1 cm. If the 3-year DFS is >95 %, the regimen will be deemed worthy of further investigation. The results of this trial were reported at the San Antonio Breast Cancer Conference in 2013. There was a high disease free survival rate of 98.7% at a median follow up of 4 years in the population studied, and there were very few adverse events associated with this regimen [47]. In light of these findings, the combination of paclitaxel and trastuzumab should be considered for patients with stage 1 breast cancer.

The adjuvant therapy of HER2/neu-positive breast cancer will be discussed in detail in a separate chapter. The summary recommendations for systemic adjuvant chemotherapy in HER2/neu-positive breast cancer are as follows:

- *Systemic adjuvant chemotherapy should be given in combination with trastuzumab, especially in tumors >0.5 cm.*
- *Trastuzumab is omitted during the period of anthracycline chemotherapy but can be given concurrently with taxanes.*
- *Consideration of less intensive adjuvant chemotherapy regimens such as paclitaxel plus trastuzumab should be considered for T1N0 HER2/neu-positive breast cancers*

Preoperative Chemotherapy (Neoadjuvant)

Most early systemic chemotherapy trials for operable breast cancer were conducted in the adjuvant setting, with the use of preoperative (neoadjuvant) chemotherapy limited primarily to inflammatory and locally advanced breast cancer. The original rationale for neoadjuvant chemotherapy (NAC) was to render locally advanced tumors operable by shrinking the diameter of these tumors, thereby reducing the extent of surgery required in operable breast cancer. Studies comparing the adjuvant and NAC approaches have found the survival to be equivalent when using identical systemic agents (Table 23.2). These trials also demonstrated that patients who achieved a pathological complete response (pCR) following NAC had improved clinical outcomes compared to patients who did not.

The NAC and adjuvant chemotherapy regimens used clinically are identical. The NAC approach is now increasingly used in smaller, operable TNBC and HER2/neu-positive tumors, although less commonly with HR-positive tumors as they are inherently less chemosensitive [4, 51]. There has also been a trend by many clinicians to evaluate novel therapies in the preoperative setting. A NAC approach allows for the study of the biological impact of systemic therapy on pre- and posttreatment tissue and therefore represents a fertile setting for tissue-intensive correlative research. The goal of biomarker discovery in NAC clinical trials is to identify surrogate end points of clinical outcomes, such as predictive biomarkers of therapeutic response or resistance. The US Food and Drug Administration (FDA) is

Table 23.2 Seminal trials comparing neoadjuvant chemotherapy to adjuvant chemotherapy for early-stage breast cancer

				Neoadjuvant vs. adjuvant therapy			
Trial	Chemotherapy	pCR rate (%)	pCR vs. non-pCR hazard ratio	BCS rates	DFS HR	OS HR	Reference
NSBAP B-18	AC×4	13	OS: 0.32†	68 % vs. 60 %*	0.93	0.99	[48]
EORTC 10902	FEC_{60}×4	3.7	OS: 0.91	35 % vs. 22 %	1.12	1.09	[49]
ECTO	AP×4→CMF×3	20	RFS: 0.43†	65 % vs. 34 %*	1.21	1.10	[50]

BCS breast cancer survival, *DFS* disease-free survival, *OS* overall survival, *pCR* pathological complete response
*$p < 0.05$

considering the possibility of using pCR in the NAC setting as a surrogate end point for clinical benefit and as an indication for accelerated drug approval [52].

Practically, NAC should be managed only in a multidisciplinary team setting, with initial assessments made by the breast surgeon and medical and radiation oncologists. Evaluation of treatment response to NAC could potentially allow the treating team to tailor individual treatment based upon tumor response, particularly if there is the suggestion of disease progression. There have been two trials in which patients were randomized mid-treatment to non-cross-resistant chemotherapy regimens according to their mid-treatment response [53, 54]. In both trials, deviating from the initial course of therapy in clinical nonresponders did not increase either the clinical or pathological response rates or improve survival. For operable breast cancer, in the event of disease progression mid-NAC, we would recommend an immediate reevaluation by the breast surgeon in order to assess the feasibility of surgical resection with mastectomy. Decisions about additional chemotherapy can be deferred until the adjuvant setting. For patients with non-resectable disease, radiation or alternative investigational approaches should be considered [55].

Special Clinical Scenarios

Inflammatory and Locally Advanced Breast Cancer

Inflammatory breast cancer (IBC) represents a unique biological entity characterized by distinct clinical and histopathological features, aggressive behavior, and an exceptionally poor prognosis (median survival with current therapy <4 years) [56]. The current standard of care for management of stage 3B IBC is a multimodality approach consisting of NAC followed by surgery and radiotherapy. Achieving a pCR to NAC is the single most important prognostic factor in IBC [57, 58].

Given the relative rarity of IBC, there have been no specific randomized trials examining the optimal NAC regimen, and moreover patients with IBC have historically been excluded from NAC systemic therapy studies due to their poor prognosis. Single-arm studies and retrospective case series show that anthracycline-based regimens are effective (clinical response rates around 70 %) [57] and that their efficacy is enhanced by the subsequent addition of a taxane as evidenced by increased clinical and pCR rates [59, 60]. As such, regimens included in the "Anthracycline and Taxane" section of Table 23.1 are recommended.

Although outside the scope of this chapter, it is noteworthy that approximately 40 % of IBC are HER2/neu positive, and evidence from randomized phase 3 clinical trials strongly supports the routine addition of trastuzumab to NAC in this setting [61].

Elderly Patients

Although the incidence of breast cancer rises sharply with age, there is a lack of quality data discussing the optimal choices regarding adjuvant chemotherapy in the elderly. This is particularly true for patients with advanced comorbidities and frailty, who are generally excluded from phase 3 clinical trials. For this reason, groups such as the International Society of Geriatric Oncology (SIOG) and European Society of Breast Cancer Specialists (EUSOMA) have developed consensus guidelines specific to the issues facing elderly patients with breast cancer [62]. Compared to their younger counterparts, elderly patients are more likely to present with larger primary tumors and positive lymph nodes [63], at least in part attributable to greater delays in initial diagnosis. Breast cancers in the elderly are also more frequently HR positive [64].

Prescribing adjuvant chemotherapy to elderly patients require several unique considerations. First, elderly patients often suffer comorbid illnesses that provide competing mortality risks. As such, determining the potential overall survival gains from adjuvant chemotherapy for an individual patient is more challenging. Groups such as the Cancer and Leukemia Group B (CALGB) have developed tools for pre-chemotherapy geriatric assessment to help address this problem

[65]. It is also important to note that despite competing risks, >40 % of patients diagnosed with breast cancer after the age of 80 will die from breast cancer [66].

Second, elderly patients may be more susceptible to certain chemotherapy toxicities. Although there is no evidence to support modifying chemotherapy doses because of age, strict monitoring of renal and hepatic function during treatment is essential. Furthermore, routine assessment of left ventricular ejection fraction is recommended for patients scheduled to receive anthracyclines. Thirdly, data suggests that elderly patients are more likely to experience difficulties with medication compliance [63], particularly oral medications such as antiemetics. It is thus critical to ensure that patients with any degree of cognitive impairment clearly understand their drug regimens and are adequately educated and supervised if necessary.

There is little prospectively collected, randomized trial data to suggest a particular adjuvant chemotherapy regimen for elderly patients beyond the general standards of care. In general terms, adjuvant chemotherapy is feasible in patients over 65–70 years of age, but increasing age, reduced functional status, and presence of comorbidities are associated with more frequent dose reductions and/or delays [67]. A landmark CALGB study compared standard chemotherapy regimens (either AC or CMF) to oral capecitabine in patients >65 years of age with early-stage breast cancer [68]. The study was stopped early after an interim analysis suggested that the capecitabine regimen was inferior, resulting in an almost doubled risk of recurrence or death. This study reinforces the efficacy of standard chemotherapy in an elderly population. Nonrandomized data also suggest tolerability of the TC regimen patients >65 years [69], although elderly patients do seem more prone to taxane-induced hematological toxicities [70].

Young Patients

Breast cancer in young patients typically demonstrates a worse prognosis and more aggressive phenotype, characterized by higher-grade disease, more advanced stage at initial presentation, and lower rates of HR positivity. While some studies point toward breast cancer in younger patients as having a unique biology [71, 72], others have illustrated that the poor prognosis in younger patients is more a result of higher frequencies of aggressive breast cancer subtypes [73, 74]. The incidence of germline mutations in genes known to predispose to breast cancer is also increased among women <35 years old with breast cancer, with 10–15 % harboring a *BRCA1* and *BRCA2* germline mutation [75]. Diagnosis of a familial breast cancer syndrome has implications for additional treatment decisions including consideration of prophylactic surgeries (i.e., prophylactic mastectomy and/or prophylactic bilateral salpingo-oophorectomy) that have been shown to improve outcomes for this patient population [76, 77].

While general principles for the selection of cytotoxic and targeted agents are quite similar between younger patients and the general population, specific issues that should be considered in prescribing chemotherapy to younger women include the effect of chemotherapy on their future fertility as well as potential long-term toxicities (i.e., cardiac dysfunction and secondary malignancies), which are more relevant in light of their life expectancy. There are a number of options for fertility preservation including oocyte and embryo cryopreservation. Although outside the scope of the current review, all women of child-bearing potential facing a diagnosis of BC should be educated on the risk of infertility at the earliest opportunity.

An early referral to a reproductive physician is important, as fertility preservation often involves a delay in the start of adjuvant chemotherapy treatment while the oocytes and/or ovarian tissue are harvested [78]. The return of the ovarian function is dependent on the ovarian reserve and age of the patient, and the relative intensity of the chemotherapy regimen. Testing for ovarian reserve involves the measurement of serum anti-Müllerian hormone and inhibin B levels. Recent data from the phase III Prevention of Early Menopause Study (POEMS) comparing chemotherapy versus chemotherapy plus goserelin in premenopausal patients with early stage, hormone receptor-negative breast cancer, demonstrated a lower rate of ovarian failure in the goserelin containing treatment arm (Stratified Odds Ratio = 0.30, p = 0.04, 8 % vs. 22 % in evaluable patients) [79]. The study also reported as a secondary end point, a higher pregnancy attempts (24 % vs. 16 %), successful pregnancy attempts (21 % vs. 11 %) and no increase in the pregnancy associated adverse events with goserelin containing treatment arm. This data suggests that lutenizing hormone releasing hormone analogues may be a potentially useful to prevent premature ovarian failure in premenopausal women receiving chemotherapy. Finally, it is recommended that sexually active women should be prescribed nonhormonal contraception regardless of menstrual status because they may still ovulate and become pregnant.

Pregnant Patients

Pregnancy and an early-stage breast cancer diagnosis can intersect in one of two ways: Either a patient receiving adjuvant chemotherapy may fall pregnant during treatment or a new diagnosis of breast cancer is made in a pregnant patient. Both require intensive management by a multidisciplinary team including surgeons, oncologists, radiation oncologists, obstetricians, and psychologists. The first of these scenarios is rare, and due to the highly teratogenic effects of systemic cytotoxics during the first trimester, all patients receiving adjuvant chemotherapy should be counseled on appropriate use of contraceptive measures during treatment. In this section, we will discuss the second scenario in more detail.

Like all younger women with breast cancer, patients diagnosed during pregnancy are more likely to have a higher-risk disease [80]. As such, a large proportion of these patients will be candidates for systemic adjuvant chemotherapy. There are no data to suggest that concurrent pregnancy per se is an adverse prognostic factor in early-stage breast cancer [81].

As a general principle, adjuvant chemotherapy regimens should be chosen with the goal of recommending a regimen that is as close to the standard care for nonpregnant patients as possible [81]. The critical issue is the timing of therapy. Systemic chemotherapy should not be prescribed during the first trimester (the period of organogenesis) due to the high risk of fetal malformation. Therefore, in patients diagnosed during this time, options include termination of pregnancy followed by systemic chemotherapy or continuation of pregnancy, delaying the onset of chemotherapy till after 14 weeks of gestation. In patients diagnosed during the second trimester (12–28 weeks), surgery can be followed by adjuvant chemotherapy. In both of these situations, it is prudent to suspend adjuvant chemotherapy at about 35 weeks of gestation, allowing for delivery at about 37 weeks and resumption of any remaining chemotherapy after this. In women diagnosed in the final trimester, it is most sensible to allow for delivery at 35–37 weeks before initiating chemotherapy [81].

The adverse consequences of systemic chemotherapy on fetal health and early child development are reported to be minimal. Deferring treatment till after the first trimester abrogates the risk of fetal malformation. There is a lack of long-term data on the consequences of chemotherapy during pregnancy on subsequent child development, but case series suggest no obvious problems with neurodevelopment or risk of second cancers [81]. Only a small fraction of the total delivered anthracyclines, cyclophosphamide, or taxanes crosses the placenta [82, 83], and together with the altered pharmacokinetics of these drugs in pregnancy [84], exposure of the fetus is thought to be limited. Methotrexate (and hence the CMF regimen) is best avoided to avoid its accumulation in third space fluid compartments. There is limited data on the safety of dose-dense chemotherapy regimens in pregnancy.

Chemotherapy Toxicities

Acute Toxicities

Chemotherapy toxicities are listed in Table 23.3 and can be broadly divided into acute and long-

Table 23.3 Common chemotherapy-associated toxicities and recommended management

System	Toxicity	Chemotherapy regimens	Management
General	Fatigue	Majority	
	Weight gain	Majority	
	Vasomotor	Majority	Gabapentin and low dose SSRIs
Ovarian	Amenorrhea and infertility	Majority, especially CMF	Discussion of testing for ovarian reserve, egg and zygote, preservation and GNRH agonist pre-chemotherapy
Gastrointestinal	Nausea and vomiting	Majority, especially anthracyclines	Prophylactic antiemetics
	Anorexia	Majority	
	Mucositis	Majority	Analgesic mouthwash
	Hepatotoxicity	Majority	
Skin	Alopecia	Majority, except CMF	
Hematological	Neutropenia	Majority, especially dose-dense and docetaxel-containing regimens	Prophylactic filgrastim
	Anemia	Majority	Replace serum iron, Vitamin B12 and folate if low
		Specific agents	
Cardiac	Congestive cardiac failure	Anthracyclines	Screening of left ventricular ejection fraction in patients >50 years old or with cardiac risk factors
Secondary malignancy	Acute myeloid leukemia and myelodysplastic syndrome	Anthracyclines	
Neurological	Peripheral neurotoxicity	Taxanes	
Musculoskeletal	Arthralgia and myalgia	Taxanes	Simple analgesics, NSAIDs

Dose reduction and/or delay should be considered standard management for all high-grade toxicities
SSRI selective serotonin reuptake inhibitor

term toxicities. There has been much progress in the management of short-term toxicity, particularly in regard to the prevention and management of nausea and neutropenia. A major development in this area has been the publication of guidelines for the use of effective preventative antiemetic therapies such as dexamethasone, 5-hydroxytryptamine-3 (5-HT3) receptor antagonists (such as ondansetron, granisetron, and palonosetron), and neurokinin 1 (NK1) receptor antagonists (such as aprepitant and fosaprepitant) [85]. Prophylaxis against neutropenia is highly effective. The routine use of prophylactic granulocyte colony-stimulating factors (such as filgrastim and pegfilgrastim) with moderately myelosuppressive chemotherapy regimens, such as dose-dense and docetaxel-containing regimens, markedly reduces the rate of febrile neutropenia, febrile neutropenia-related hospitalizations, and intravenous anti-infective use [86].

Fatigue and weight gain are common general side effects [87] and may be interrelated. Other factors that contribute may include alterations in serum hormonal levels and insulin resistance. Evidence for the health-related benefits of increased physical activity continues to expand [88], and exercise and dietary management is an important aspect of patient care during adjuvant chemotherapy. Another common side effect is decreased ovarian function resulting in menopausal vasomotor symptoms such as hot flashes, mood swings, and decreased ovarian reserve. Selective serotonin reuptake inhibitors (SSRIs) have been used successfully to manage some of the vasomotor symptoms; careful consideration of the use of SSRIs is important in patients on tamoxifen, as some of the SSRIs affect the tamoxifen-metabolizing hepatic enzyme CYP2D6.

Long-Term Toxicities

A comprehensive review of long-term complications of chemotherapy has recently been published by Azim et al. [89]. Cardiac toxicity is especially a concern with anthracycline- and trastuzumab-containing regimens, and the main risk factors are older age, other cardiovascular risk factors, mediastinal radiation, and total dose of anthracyclines received. A number of studies looking at the long-term cardiac toxicity of anthracycline regimens have demonstrated a decrease in cardiac function in up to 11 years of median follow-up, with up to 8 % of anthracycline-treated patients having evidence of systolic dysfunction compared to 2 % in non-anthracycline-treated patients, although the incidence of symptomatic cardiac failure was only in approximately 10 % of this patient subset [90–92]. In a large population study from the Surveillance, Epidemiology, and End Results (SEER) Medicare database of women >65 years of age with early breast cancer, the adjusted hazard ratio of congestive cardiac failure was 1.26 in women aged 66–70 treated with anthracyclines compared to other chemotherapy regimens, but not in women aged 71–80 [93]. There are potential biases at play in evaluating these data sets, and the findings need to be viewed with some caution. It is recommended to restrict the cumulative dose of anthracyclines to no greater than 360 mg/m^2 for doxorubicin and 720 mg/m^2 for epirubicin, and to screen patients >50 years of age or with known cardiovascular risk factors with a baseline left ventricular ejection assessment prior to starting anthracycline and trastuzumab therapy.

Acute myeloid leukemia (AML) and myelodysplastic syndrome are uncommon long-term adverse events associated with anthracycline use. A combined analysis of six adjuvant studies with AC conducted by the NSABP reported a 5-year incidence of AML ranging from 0.3 % to 1.2 % [94]. In clinical practice, the risk of leukemia is likely to be very low if the cumulative doses of anthracyclines and cyclophosphamide are not exceeded [95].

Concluding Statements

Although the basic goals of adjuvant chemotherapy for early-stage breast cancer – eradication of disseminated micrometastases to reduce risk of recurrence – remain the same, there have been significant refinements in the way adjuvant therapy is prescribed in the last three decades. Fundamental to these improvements is our ability to estimate (1) the absolute recurrence risk for tumors of varying stages and biological subtypes and (2) the chemosensitivity of individual tumors.

More so now than ever before, it is realized that certain tumors pose a high risk of distant relapse in spite of a relatively smaller tumor burden (i.e., TNBC, HER2/neu-positive tumors). Patients with such tumors may therefore be good candidates for adjuvant chemotherapy in order to reduce this recurrence risk. Conversely, multigene tools with the capacity to predict relative chemosensitivity now allow for the omission adjuvant chemotherapy in a subset of patients with HR-positive breast cancer (regardless of tumor size and possibly nodal status), sparing unnecessary toxicities.

Moving forward, it is unlikely that we will see a large number of phase III trials comparing different regimens of conventional cytotoxics in the adjuvant setting. The more pressing questions now are clearly as follows: Which patients derive the greatest relative benefit from adjuvant chemotherapy? Which patients derive little or no benefit from adjuvant chemotherapy and can therefore be spared it? With the advent of newer targeted therapies for certain tumors (e.g., HER2/neu-positive cancers), to what extent can biological therapies replace conventional adjuvant chemotherapy or should the two therapies be given together?

As outcomes for patients with early-stage breast cancer continue to improve incrementally, the conduct of phase III clinical trials to evaluate new approaches becomes more challenging. Lower event rates drive the need for higher sample sizes, and it is only through the cooperation of several institutions, often across multiple continents, that we have been able to continue to drive progress. It is difficult to predict the landscape of adjuvant therapy in the next 10–20 years, but research will undoubtedly focus on further tailoring therapy to the individual tumor at hand, taking into account various aspects of histology, biology, and stage.

References

1. Peto R, Davies C, Godwin J, Gray R, Pan HC, Clarke M, et al. Comparisons between different polychemotherapy regimens for early breast cancer: meta-analyses of long-term outcome among 100,000 women in 123 randomised trials. Lancet. 2012;379(9814):432–44.
2. Perou CM, Sorlie T, Eisen MB, van de Rijn M, Jeffrey SS, Rees CA, et al. Molecular portraits of human breast tumours. Nature. 2000;406(6797):747–52.
3. Sorlie T, Perou CM, Tibshirani R, Aas T, Geisler S, Johnsen H, et al. Gene expression patterns of breast carcinomas distinguish tumor subclasses with clinical implications. Proc Natl Acad Sci U S A. 2001;98(19):10869–74.
4. Carey LA, Dees EC, Sawyer L, Gatti L, Moore DT, Collichio F, et al. The triple negative paradox: primary tumor chemosensitivity of breast cancer subtypes. Clin Cancer Res. 2007;13(8):2329–34.
5. Piccart-Gebhart MJ. New developments in hormone receptor-positive disease. Oncologist. 2011;16 Suppl 1:40–50.
6. Sheri A, Dowsett M. Predicting response to cytotoxic drugs–the endocrine part of the story. Breast. 2011;20 Suppl 3:S28–30.
7. Fisher B, Dignam J, Mamounas EP, Costantino JP, Wickerham DL, Redmond C, et al. Sequential methotrexate and fluorouracil for the treatment of node-negative breast cancer patients with estrogen receptor-negative tumors: eight-year results from National Surgical Adjuvant Breast and Bowel Project (NSABP) B-13 and first report of findings from NSABP B-19 comparing methotrexate and fluorouracil with conventional cyclophosphamide, methotrexate, and fluorouracil. J Clin Oncol. 1996; 14(7):1982–92.
8. Tancini G, Bonadonna G, Valagussa P, Marchini S, Veronesi U. Adjuvant CMF in breast cancer: comparative 5-year results of 12 versus 6 cycles. J Clin Oncol. 1983;1(1):2–10.
9. Fisher B, Brown AM, Dimitrov NV, Poisson R, Redmond C, Margolese RG, et al. Two months of doxorubicin-cyclophosphamide with and without interval reinduction therapy compared with 6 months of cyclophosphamide, methotrexate, and fluorouracil in positive-node breast cancer patients with tamoxifen-nonresponsive tumors: results from the National Surgical Adjuvant Breast and Bowel Project B-15. J Clin Oncol. 1990;8(9):1483–96.
10. Jones SE, Savin MA, Holmes FA, O'Shaughnessy JA, Blum JL, Vukelja S, et al. Phase III trial comparing doxorubicin plus cyclophosphamide with docetaxel plus cyclophosphamide as adjuvant therapy for operable breast cancer. J Clin Oncol. 2006;24(34): 5381–7.
11. Shulman LN, Cirrincione CT, Berry DA, Becker HP, Perez EA, O'Regan R, et al. Six cycles of doxorubicin and cyclophosphamide or Paclitaxel are not superior to four cycles as adjuvant chemotherapy for breast cancer in women with zero to three positive axillary nodes: Cancer and Leukemia Group B 40101. J Clin Oncol. 2012;30(33):4071–6.
12. Martin M, Pienkowski T, Mackey J, Pawlicki M, Guastalla JP, Weaver C, et al. Adjuvant docetaxel for node-positive breast cancer. N Engl J Med. 2005; 352(22):2302–13.
13. Martin M, Villar A, Sole-Calvo A, Gonzalez R, Massuti B, Lizon J, et al. Doxorubicin in combination with fluorouracil and cyclophosphamide (i.v. FAC regimen, day 1, 21) versus methotrexate in combination with fluorouracil and cyclophosphamide (i.v. CMF regimen, day 1, 21) as adjuvant chemotherapy for operable breast cancer: a study by the GEICAM group. Ann Oncol. 2003;14(6):833–42.
14. Hutchins LF, Green SJ, Ravdin PM, Lew D, Martino S, Abeloff M, et al. Randomized, controlled trial of cyclophosphamide, methotrexate, and fluorouracil versus cyclophosphamide, doxorubicin, and fluorouracil with and without tamoxifen for high-risk, node-negative breast cancer: treatment results of Intergroup Protocol INT-0102. J Clin Oncol. 2005;23(33): 8313–21.
15. Levine MN, Pritchard KI, Bramwell VH, Shepherd LE, Tu D, Paul N. Randomized trial comparing cyclophosphamide, epirubicin, and fluorouracil with cyclophosphamide, methotrexate, and fluorouracil in premenopausal women with node-positive breast cancer: update of National Cancer Institute of Canada Clinical Trials Group Trial MA5. J Clin Oncol. 2005;23(22):5166–70.
16. Roche H, Fumoleau P, Spielmann M, Canon JL, Delozier T, Serin D, et al. Sequential adjuvant epirubicin-based and docetaxel chemotherapy for node-positive breast cancer patients: the FNCLCC PACS 01 Trial. J Clin Oncol. 2006;24(36):5664–71.
17. Mamounas EP, Bryant J, Lembersky B, Fehrenbacher L, Sedlacek SM, Fisher B, et al. Paclitaxel after doxorubicin plus cyclophosphamide as adjuvant chemotherapy for node-positive breast cancer: results from NSABP B-28. J Clin Oncol. 2005;23(16):3686–96.
18. Sparano JA, Wang M, Martino S, Jones V, Perez EA, Saphner T, et al. Weekly paclitaxel in the adjuvant treatment of breast cancer. N Engl J Med. 2008; 358(16):1663–71.
19. Martin M, Rodriguez-Lescure A, Ruiz A, Alba E, Calvo L, Ruiz-Borrego M, et al. Randomized phase 3 trial of fluorouracil, epirubicin, and cyclophosphamide

alone or followed by Paclitaxel for early breast cancer. J Natl Cancer Inst. 2008;100(11):805–14.
20. Swain SM, Tang G, Geyer CE, Rastogi P, Atkins JN, Donnellan PP, et al. NSABP B-38: definitive analysis of a randomized adjuvant trial comparing dose-dense (DD) AC followed by paclitaxel (P) plus gemcitabine (G) with DD AC followed by P and with docetaxel, doxorubicin, and cyclophosphamide (TAC) in women with operable, node-positive breast cancer. J Clin Oncol. 2012;30(15 s):LBA1000. Abst.
21. Bonilla L, Ben-Aharon I, Vidal L, Gafter-Gvili A, Leibovici L, Stemmer SM. Dose-dense chemotherapy in nonmetastatic breast cancer: a systematic review and meta-analysis of randomized controlled trials. J Natl Cancer Inst. 2010;102(24):1845–54.
22. Hug V, Hortobagyi GN, Drewinko B, Finders M. Tamoxifen-citrate counteracts the antitumor effects of cytotoxic drugs in vitro. J Clin Oncol. 1985;3(12):1672–7.
23. Rivkin SE, Green S, Metch B, Cruz AB, Abeloff MD, Jewell WR, et al. Adjuvant CMFVP versus tamoxifen versus concurrent CMFVP and tamoxifen for post-menopausal, node-positive, and estrogen receptor-positive breast cancer patients: a Southwest Oncology Group study. J Clin Oncol. 1994;12(10):2078–85.
24. Pritchard KI, Paterson AH, Fine S, Paul NA, Zee B, Shepherd LE, et al. Randomized trial of cyclophosphamide, methotrexate, and fluorouracil chemotherapy added to tamoxifen as adjuvant therapy in postmenopausal women with node-positive estrogen and/or progesterone receptor-positive breast cancer: a report of the National Cancer Institute of Canada Clinical Trials Group. Breast Cancer Site Group. J Clin Oncol. 1997;15(6):2302–11.
25. Berry DA, Cirrincione C, Henderson IC, Citron ML, Budman DR, Goldstein LJ, et al. Estrogen-receptor status and outcomes of modern chemotherapy for patients with node-positive breast cancer. JAMA. 2006;295(14):1658–67.
26. Albain KS, Barlow WE, Ravdin PM, Farrar WB, Burton GV, Ketchel SJ, et al. Adjuvant chemotherapy and timing of tamoxifen in postmenopausal patients with endocrine-responsive, node-positive breast cancer: a phase 3, open-label, randomised controlled trial. Lancet. 2009;374(9707):2055–63.
27. EBCTCG. Effects of chemotherapy and hormonal therapy for early breast cancer on recurrence and 15-year survival: an overview of the randomised trials. Lancet. 2005;365(9472):1687–717.
28. Paik S, Tang G, Shak S, Kim C, Baker J, Kim W, et al. Gene expression and benefit of chemotherapy in women with node-negative, estrogen receptor-positive breast cancer. J Clin Oncol. 2006;24(23):3726–34.
29. Pagani O, Gelber S, Simoncini E, Castiglione-Gertsch M, Price KN, Gelber RD, et al. Is adjuvant chemotherapy of benefit for postmenopausal women who receive endocrine treatment for highly endocrine-responsive, node-positive breast cancer? International Breast Cancer Study Group Trials VII and 12-93. Breast Cancer Res Treat. 2009;116(3):491–500.
30. Viale G, Regan MM, Mastropasqua MG, Maffini F, Maiorano E, Colleoni M, et al. Predictive value of tumor Ki-67 expression in two randomized trials of adjuvant chemoendocrine therapy for node-negative breast cancer. J Natl Cancer Inst. 2008;100(3):207–12.
31. Hugh J, Hanson J, Cheang MC, Nielsen TO, Perou CM, Dumontet C, et al. Breast cancer subtypes and response to docetaxel in node-positive breast cancer: use of an immunohistochemical definition in the BCIRG 001 trial. J Clin Oncol. 2009;27(8):1168–76.
32. Penault-Llorca F, Andre F, Sagan C, Lacroix-Triki M, Denoux Y, Verriele V, et al. Ki67 expression and docetaxel efficacy in patients with estrogen receptor-positive breast cancer. J Clin Oncol. 2009;27(17):2809–15.
33. Paik S, Shak S, Tang G, Kim C, Baker J, Cronin M, et al. A multigene assay to predict recurrence of tamoxifen-treated, node-negative breast cancer. N Engl J Med. 2004;351(27):2817–26.
34. van't Veer LJ, Dai H, van de Vijver MJ, He YD, Hart AA, Mao M, et al. Gene expression profiling predicts clinical outcome of breast cancer. Nature. 2002; 415(6871):530–6.
35. Buyse M, Loi S, van't Veer L, Viale G, Delorenzi M, Glas AM, et al. Validation and clinical utility of a 70-gene prognostic signature for women with node-negative breast cancer. J Natl Cancer Inst. 2006; 98(17):1183–92.
36. Sparano JA, Paik S. Development of the 21-gene assay and its application in clinical practice and clinical trials. J Clin Oncol. 2008;26(5):721–8.
37. Cardoso F, Van't Veer L, Rutgers E, Loi S, Mook S, Piccart-Gebhart MJ. Clinical application of the 70-gene profile: the MINDACT trial. J Clin Oncol. 2008;26(5):729–35.
38. Lim E, Metzger-Filho O, Winer EP. The natural history of hormone receptor-positive breast cancer. Oncology (Williston Park). 2012;26(8):688–94. 96.
39. Mook S, Schmidt MK, Viale G, Pruneri G, Eekhout I, Floore A, et al. The 70-gene prognosis-signature predicts disease outcome in breast cancer patients with 1–3 positive lymph nodes in an independent validation study. Breast Cancer Res Treat. 2009;116(2): 295–302.
40. Perez EA, Romond EH, Suman VJ, Jeong JH, Davidson NE, Geyer Jr CE, et al. Four-year follow-up of trastuzumab plus adjuvant chemotherapy for operable human epidermal growth factor receptor 2-positive breast cancer: joint analysis of data from NCCTG N9831 and NSABP B-31. J Clin Oncol. 2011;29(25):3366–73.
41. Gianni L, Dafni U, Gelber RD, Azambuja E, Muehlbauer S, Goldhirsch A, et al. Treatment with trastuzumab for 1 year after adjuvant chemotherapy in patients with HER2-positive early breast cancer: a 4-year follow-up of a randomised controlled trial. Lancet Oncol. 2011;12(3):236–44.
42. Slamon D, Eiermann W, Robert N, Pienkowski T, Martin M, Press M, et al. Adjuvant trastuzumab in HER2-positive breast cancer. N Engl J Med. 2011;365(14):1273–83.

43. Slamon DJ, Leyland-Jones B, Shak S, Fuchs H, Paton V, Bajamonde A, et al. Use of chemotherapy plus a monoclonal antibody against HER2 for metastatic breast cancer that overexpresses HER2. N Engl J Med. 2001;344(11):783–92.
44. Goldhirsch A, Ingle JN, Gelber RD, Coates AS, Thurlimann B, Senn HJ. Thresholds for therapies: highlights of the St Gallen International Expert Consensus on the primary therapy of early breast cancer 2009. Ann Oncol. 2009;20(8):1319–29.
45. National Comprehensive Cancer Network Guidelines for Breast Cancer. http://www.nccn.org/professionals/physician_gls/f_guidelines.asp. Accessed 01 Jan 2013.
46. Seidman AD, Fornier MN, Esteva FJ, Tan L, Kaptain S, Bach A, et al. Weekly trastuzumab and paclitaxel therapy for metastatic breast cancer with analysis of efficacy by HER2 immunophenotype and gene amplification. J Clin Oncol. 2001;19(10):2587–95.
47. Tolaney SM, Barry WT, Dang CT, Yardley DA, Moy B, Marcom PK, et al. Adjuvant paclitaxel and trastuzumab for node-negative HER2+ breast cancer. In Press. N Engl J Med.
48. Rastogi P, Anderson SJ, Bear HD, Geyer CE, Kahlenberg MS, Robidoux A, et al. Preoperative chemotherapy: updates of National Surgical Adjuvant Breast and Bowel Project Protocols B-18 and B-27. J Clin Oncol. 2008;26(5):778–85.
49. van Nes JG, Putter H, Julien JP, Tubiana-Hulin M, van de Vijver M, Bogaerts J, et al. Preoperative chemotherapy is safe in early breast cancer, even after 10 years of follow-up; clinical and translational results from the EORTC trial 10902. Breast Cancer Res Treat. 2009;115(1):101–13.
50. Gianni L, Baselga J, Eiermann W, Porta VG, Semiglazov V, Lluch A, et al. Phase III trial evaluating the addition of paclitaxel to doxorubicin followed by cyclophosphamide, methotrexate, and fluorouracil, as adjuvant or primary systemic therapy: European Cooperative Trial in Operable Breast Cancer. J Clin Oncol. 2009;27(15):2474–81.
51. Rouzier R, Perou CM, Symmans WF, Ibrahim N, Cristofanilli M, Anderson K, et al. Breast cancer molecular subtypes respond differently to preoperative chemotherapy. Clin Cancer Res. 2005;11(16): 5678–85.
52. Prowell TM, Pazdur R. Pathological complete response and accelerated drug approval in early breast cancer. N Engl J Med. 2012;366(26):2438–41.
53. Smith IC, Heys SD, Hutcheon AW, Miller ID, Payne S, Gilbert FJ, et al. Neoadjuvant chemotherapy in breast cancer: significantly enhanced response with docetaxel. J Clin Oncol. 2002;20(6):1456–66.
54. von Minckwitz G, Blohmner JU, Loehr A, et al. Comparison of docetaxel/doxorubicin/cyclophosphamide (TAC) versus vinorelbine/capecitabine (NX) in patients non-responding to cycles of neoadjuvant TAC chemotherapy: first results of the phase III GEPARTRIO-Study by the German Breast Group. Breast Cancer Res Treat. 2005;94(S19):38.
55. Gralow JR, Burstein HJ, Wood W, Hortobagyi GN, Gianni L, von Minckwitz G, et al. Preoperative therapy in invasive breast cancer: pathologic assessment and systemic therapy issues in operable disease. J Clin Oncol. 2008;26(5):814–9.
56. Hance KW, Anderson WF, Devesa SS, Young HA, Levine PH. Trends in inflammatory breast carcinoma incidence and survival: the surveillance, epidemiology, and end results program at the National Cancer Institute. J Natl Cancer Inst. 2005;97(13):966–75.
57. Ueno NT, Buzdar AU, Singletary SE, Ames FC, McNeese MD, Holmes FA, et al. Combined-modality treatment of inflammatory breast carcinoma: twenty years of experience at M. D. Anderson Cancer Center. Cancer Chemother Pharmacol. 1997;40(4):321–9.
58. Robertson FM, Bondy M, Yang W, Yamauchi H, Wiggins S, Kamrudin S, et al. Inflammatory breast cancer: the disease, the biology, the treatment. CA Cancer J Clin. 2010;60(6):351–75.
59. Cristofanilli M, Buzdar AU, Sneige N, Smith T, Wasaff B, Ibrahim N, et al. Paclitaxel in the multimodality treatment for inflammatory breast carcinoma. Cancer. 2001;92(7):1775–82.
60. Cristofanilli M, Gonzalez-Angulo AM, Buzdar AU, Kau SW, Frye DK, Hortobagyi GN. Paclitaxel improves the prognosis in estrogen receptor negative inflammatory breast cancer: the M. D. Anderson Cancer Center experience. Clin Breast Cancer. 2004;4(6):415–9.
61. Gianni L, Eiermann W, Semiglazov V, Manikhas A, Lluch A, Tjulandin S, et al. Neoadjuvant chemotherapy with trastuzumab followed by adjuvant trastuzumab versus neoadjuvant chemotherapy alone, in patients with HER2-positive locally advanced breast cancer (the NOAH trial): a randomised controlled superiority trial with a parallel HER2-negative cohort. Lancet. 2010;375(9712):377–84.
62. Biganzoli L, Wildiers H, Oakman C, Marotti L, Loibl S, Kunkler I, et al. Management of elderly patients with breast cancer: updated recommendations of the International Society of Geriatric Oncology (SIOG) and European Society of Breast Cancer Specialists (EUSOMA). Lancet Oncol. 2012;13(4):e148–60.
63. Wildiers H, Van Calster B, van de Poll-Franse LV, Hendrickx W, Roislien J, Smeets A, et al. Relationship between age and axillary lymph node involvement in women with breast cancer. J Clin Oncol. 2009;27(18): 2931–7.
64. Schonberg MA, Marcantonio ER, Li D, Silliman RA, Ngo L, McCarthy EP. Breast cancer among the oldest old: tumor characteristics, treatment choices, and survival. J Clin Oncol. 2010;28(12):2038–45.
65. Hurria A, Cirrincione CT, Muss HB, Kornblith AB, Barry W, Artz AS, et al. Implementing a geriatric assessment in cooperative group clinical cancer trials: CALGB 360401. J Clin Oncol. 2011;29(10): 1290–6.
66. Rosso S, Gondos A, Zanetti R, Bray F, Zakelj M, Zagar T, et al. Up-to-date estimates of breast cancer survival for the years 2000–2004 in 11 European countries: the role of screening and a comparison with

data from the United States. Eur J Cancer. 2010; 46(18):3351–7.
67. Garg P, Rana F, Gupta R, Buzaianu EM, Guthrie TH. Predictors of toxicity and toxicity profile of adjuvant chemotherapy in elderly breast cancer patients. Breast J. 2009;15(4):404–8.
68. Muss HB, Berry DA, Cirrincione CT, Theodoulou M, Mauer AM, Kornblith AB, et al. Adjuvant chemotherapy in older women with early-stage breast cancer. N Engl J Med. 2009;360(20):2055–65.
69. Jones S, Holmes FA, O'Shaughnessy J, Blum JL, Vukelja SJ, McIntyre KJ, et al. Docetaxel with Cyclophosphamide is associated with an overall survival benefit compared with Doxorubicin and Cyclophosphamide: 7-year follow-up of US Oncology Research Trial 9735. J Clin Oncol. 2009;27(8):1177–83.
70. Loibl S, von Minckwitz G, Harbeck N, Janni W, Elling D, Kaufmann M, et al. Clinical feasibility of (neo)adjuvant taxane-based chemotherapy in older patients: analysis of >4,500 patients from four German randomized breast cancer trials. Breast Cancer Res. 2008;10(5):R77.
71. Bleyer A, Barr R, Hayes-Lattin B, Thomas D, Ellis C, Anderson B. The distinctive biology of cancer in adolescents and young adults. Nat Rev Cancer. 2008;8(4):288–98.
72. Anders CK, Hsu DS, Broadwater G, Acharya CR, Foekens JA, Zhang Y, et al. Young age at diagnosis correlates with worse prognosis and defines a subset of breast cancers with shared patterns of gene expression. J Clin Oncol. 2008;26(20):3324–30.
73. Gabriel CA, Domchek SM. Breast cancer in young women. Breast Cancer Res. 2010;12(5):212.
74. Gnerlich JL, Deshpande AD, Jeffe DB, Sweet A, White N, Margenthaler JA. Elevated breast cancer mortality in women younger than age 40 years compared with older women is attributed to poorer survival in early-stage disease. J Am Coll Surg. 2009; 208(3):341–7.
75. Sørlie T, Perou CM, Tibshirani R, Aas T, Geisler S, Johnsen H, et al. Gene expression patterns of breast carcinomas distinguish tumor subclasses with clinical implications. Proc Natl Acad Sci U S A. 2001;98(19): 10869–74.
76. Tai YC, Domchek S, Parmigiani G, Chen S. Breast cancer risk among male BRCA1 and BRCA2 mutation carriers. J Natl Cancer Inst. 2007;99(23):1811–4.
77. Swerdlow AJ, Schoemaker MJ, Higgins CD, Wright AF, Jacobs PA. Cancer incidence and mortality in men with Klinefelter syndrome: a cohort study. J Natl Cancer Inst. 2005;97(16):1204–10.
78. Lee SJ, Schover LR, Partridge AH, Patrizio P, Wallace WH, Hagerty K, et al. American Society of Clinical Oncology recommendations on fertility preservation in cancer patients. J Clin Oncol. 2006;24(18):2917–31.
79. Moore HCF, Unger JM, Phillips KA, Boyle F, Hitre E, Porter D, et al. Phase III trial of LHRH analog during chemotherapy to reduce ovarian failure in early stage, hormone receptor negative breast cancer: an international Intergroup trial of SWOG, IBCSG, ECOG, and CALGB (Alliance). J Clin Oncol 32:5s, 2014 (suppl, abstr LBA505).
80. Loibl S, Amant F, Kaufmann M, Ring A, Sileny H, Giermek J, et al., editors. Patients with breast cancer during pregnancy – results from a prospective and retrospective registry (GBG-20/BIG02-03). San Antonio Breast Cancer symposium. San Antonio, TX; 2010.
81. Amant F, Loibl S, Neven P, Van Calsteren K. Breast cancer in pregnancy. Lancet. 2012;379(9815):570–9.
82. Calsteren KV, Verbesselt R, Devlieger R, De Catte L, Chai DC, Van Bree R, et al. Transplacental transfer of paclitaxel, docetaxel, carboplatin, and trastuzumab in a baboon model. Int J Gynecol Cancer. 2010;20(9): 1456–64.
83. Van Calsteren K, Verbesselt R, Beijnen J, Devlieger R, De Catte L, Chai DC, et al. Transplacental transfer of anthracyclines, vinblastine, and 4-hydroxy-cyclophosphamide in a baboon model. Gynecol Oncol. 2010;119(3):594–600.
84. Van Calsteren K, Verbesselt R, Ottevanger N, Halaska M, Heyns L, Van Bree R, et al. Pharmacokinetics of chemotherapeutic agents in pregnancy: a preclinical and clinical study. Acta Obstet Gynecol Scand. 2010;89(10):1338–45.
85. Basch E, Prestrud AA, Hesketh PJ, Kris MG, Feyer PC, Somerfield MR, et al. Antiemetics: American Society of Clinical Oncology clinical practice guideline update. J Clin Oncol. 2011;29(31):4189–98.
86. Aapro MS, Bohlius J, Cameron DA, Dal Lago L, Donnelly JP, Kearney N, et al. 2010 update of EORTC guidelines for the use of granulocyte-colony stimulating factor to reduce the incidence of chemotherapy-induced febrile neutropenia in adult patients with lymphoproliferative disorders and solid tumours. Eur J Cancer. 2011;47(1):8–32.
87. Vance V, Mourtzakis M, McCargar L, Hanning R. Weight gain in breast cancer survivors: prevalence, pattern and health consequences. Obes Rev. 2011; 12(4):282–94.
88. Pekmezi DW, Demark-Wahnefried W. Updated evidence in support of diet and exercise interventions in cancer survivors. Acta Oncol. 2011;50(2):167–78.
89. Azim Jr HA, de Azambuja E, Colozza M, Bines J, Piccart MJ. Long-term toxic effects of adjuvant chemotherapy in breast cancer. Ann Oncol. 2011;22(9): 1939–47.
90. Zambetti M, Moliterni A, Materazzo C, Stefanelli M, Cipriani S, Valagussa P, et al. Long-term cardiac sequelae in operable breast cancer patients given adjuvant chemotherapy with or without doxorubicin and breast irradiation. J Clin Oncol. 2001;19(1):37–43.
91. Bonneterre J, Roche H, Kerbrat P, Fumoleau P, Goudier MJ, Fargeot P, et al. Long-term cardiac follow-up in relapse-free patients after six courses of fluorouracil, epirubicin, and cyclophosphamide, with either 50 or 100 mg of epirubicin, as adjuvant therapy

for node-positive breast cancer: French adjuvant study group. J Clin Oncol. 2004;22(15):3070–9.
92. Ganz PA, Hussey MA, Moinpour CM, Unger JM, Hutchins LF, Dakhil SR, et al. Late cardiac effects of adjuvant chemotherapy in breast cancer survivors treated on Southwest Oncology Group protocol s8897. J Clin Oncol. 2008;26(8):1223–30.
93. Pinder MC, Duan Z, Goodwin JS, Hortobagyi GN, Giordano SH. Congestive heart failure in older women treated with adjuvant anthracycline chemotherapy for breast cancer. J Clin Oncol. 2007;25(25):3808–15.
94. Smith RE, Bryant J, DeCillis A, Anderson S. Acute myeloid leukemia and myelodysplastic syndrome after doxorubicin-cyclophosphamide adjuvant therapy for operable breast cancer: the National Surgical Adjuvant Breast and Bowel Project Experience. J Clin Oncol. 2003;21(7):1195–204.
95. Karp JE, Blackford A, Visvanathan K, Rugo HS, Moy B, Goldstein LJ, et al. Myelodysplastic syndrome and/or acute myelogenous leukemia (MDS and/or AML) after a breast cancer diagnosis: the National Comprehensive Cancer Network (NCCN) experience. Cancer Res. 2012;72(24 Supp):98s.

Adjuvant Therapy for Breast Cancer: Hormonal Therapy

24

William J. Gradishar

Introduction

Approximately two-thirds of patients diagnosed with early-stage breast cancer have hormone-sensitive disease (estrogen receptor [ER]-positive and/or progesterone receptor [PR]-positive), and as a result, adjuvant endocrine therapy plays a critical role in reducing the risk of recurrence and improving survival. Data generated from clinical trials over the last 30 years has definitively demonstrated the positive impact of adjuvant endocrine therapy, first with the use of tamoxifen and more recently with the use of aromatase inhibitors either as monotherapy or in sequence with tamoxifen. Many issues need to be understood when considering the optimal approach for adjuvant endocrine therapy in an individual patient, both in terms of optimizing risk reduction and maintaining quality of life. The following discussion will summarize the current state of the art in 2013 and also highlight unresolved research issues of clinical importance.

The rationale for the administration of adjuvant systemic therapy of early-stage breast cancer is to eradicate microscopic metastatic disease that may lead to systemic recurrence. The clinician must decide whether adding systemic chemotherapy and/or endocrine therapy will reduce the odds of recurrence and improve survival. Tools that assist in determining the risk of disease recurrence are related to clinical and biologic features of the tumor (i.e., prognostic factors). With respect to the use of adjuvant endocrine therapy, all patients who have invasive breast cancers expressing the ER and/or the PR are considered potential candidates for treatment with agents such as tamoxifen or an aromatase inhibitor. The best option for an individual patient is based on a variety of factors.

The benefit of adjuvant systemic therapy has been well established through the conduct of randomized clinical trials that compared adjuvant therapy to no adjuvant therapy in patients with early-stage breast cancer. The early clinical trials convincingly showed that disease-free survival (DFS) and overall survival (OS) were improved with systemic treatment. Over the last three decades, numerous clinical trials have been completed to address whether one adjuvant treatment regimen is superior to another in patients with early-stage breast cancer. Early clinical trials were often sized inadequately, not controlled for staging, and accepted a heterogeneous mix of local treatment. Many of these clinical trials were underpowered to address the primary objectives of the study, and as a result, the conclusions of these early trials were undermined.

Modern randomized clinical trials of adjuvant therapy frequently require the accrual of

W.J. Gradishar, MD
Medicine – Division of Hematology/Oncology, Maggie Daley Center for Women's Cancer Care, Robert H. Lurie Comprehensive Cancer Center, Northwestern University Feinberg School of Medicine at Northwestern Memorial Hospital, 676 North St. Clair, Suite 850, Chicago, IL 60611, USA
e-mail: w-gradishar@northwestern.edu

A.I. Riker (ed.), *Breast Disease: Comprehensive Management*,
DOI 10.1007/978-1-4939-1145-5_24, © Springer Science+Business Media New York 2015

thousands of patients in order to address the primary objectives. Equally important in the analysis of data generated by these trials is the requirement for adequate follow-up so that enough events (i.e., recurrences and deaths) have occurred to distinguish differences, if present, between the treatment arms. As an example, the patients followed in a clinical trial conducted in axillary node-negative patients need to be followed for a significantly longer time than a similar trial conducted in patients with higher-risk, axillary node-positive disease. Simply put, the prognosis is worse for patients with axillary node-positive disease, and as a result, one would expect that recurrences would occur with greater frequency and earlier in follow-up than in a population of patients with axillary node-negative disease. Similarly, late recurrences are more common with hormone-sensitive breast cancer compared to early recurrences in those with hormone-insensitive breast cancer.

Tamoxifen

Tamoxifen remains one of the most widely used cancer therapies, even more than three decades following its introduction. The value of tamoxifen was initially established in hormone-sensitive, metastatic breast cancer. Approximately every 5 years since the 1980s, the Early Breast Cancer Trialists' Collaborative Group (EBCTCG), sometimes referred to as the Oxford Overview, undertakes a systematic overview of all randomized trials of adjuvant systemic therapy (chemotherapy and endocrine therapy) in early-stage breast cancer. The advantage of this approach is the ability to pool data from numerous randomized trials creating much more statistical power upon which to ask very relevant clinical questions. Collectively, the large number of patients in these trials results in a greater number of events (recurrences and deaths) compared to any individual trial. With ongoing follow-up of these trials, the meta-analysis methodology has provided important clinical observations, first about the benefits of tamoxifen and more recently regarding the use of aromatase inhibitors (AI). Some of the key findings from the meta-analyses are summarized below [1–5].

1995 Overview

- Huge magnitude of effect of 5 years of tamoxifen compared to no therapy.
- Five years of tamoxifen clearly better than 1 or 2 years of tamoxifen.
- Tamoxifen prevented contralateral breast cancer in women with ER-positive disease.

2000 Overview

- Fifteen-year effects of 5 years of tamoxifen sustained and of significant magnitude
- Door opened to question of 5 years versus longer durations of tamoxifen
- Ovarian suppression/ablation effective but not significantly so when added to chemotherapy

2010 Overview: Tamoxifen

- Five years in ER+ disease
  - ↓ recurrence by 38 %.
  - ↓ breast cancer (BC) death by 30 %.
  - ↓ all deaths by 22 %.
  - ↓ contralateral BC by 40 %.
  - Benefits all women with ER+ disease.
  - Unclear benefits in ER-/PgR+ disease.
  - Benefits women with ER rich tumors most.
  - ↑ endometrial cancer by 2.3-fold.
  - PR does not predict for benefit of adjuvant tamoxifen.
  - For ER-/PgR+ patients, the tumor should be retested, and if doubt remains, tamoxifen therapy is discussed with the patient.
  - Little evidence to prescribe more than 5 years of tamoxifen to postmenopausal women, especially in women with a uterus.

Previously reported information from the NSABP B-14, a randomized, placebo controlled study, demonstrated that patients with ER-positive breast cancer and negative axillary lymph nodes experienced a highly statistically significant improvement in DFS through 5 years of follow-up among tamoxifen-treated women of all ages [6, 7]. The advantage was related to a reduction in the rate of tumor recurrence at local-regional and distant sites in patients who were treated with tamoxifen.

A second objective of the study was to determine whether more than 5 years of tamoxifen administration would provide an advantage greater than that observed in patients where the duration of tamoxifen therapy was limited to 5 years.

Patients who were initially randomized to 5 years of tamoxifen therapy and who were free of disease were re-randomized to either an additional 5 years of tamoxifen therapy or 5 years of placebo. At the time of the final analysis, the data suggested that tamoxifen administration beyond 5 years would offer no additional benefit to patients and may in fact be deleterious. The trial was unblinded and treatment with tamoxifen was discontinued. With follow-up through 7 years after re-randomization, a slight advantage was observed in patients who discontinued tamoxifen relative to those who continued to receive it (DFS: 82 % versus 78 %, $p = .03$ and survival: 94 % versus 91 %, $p = .07$). Based on these findings, limiting the duration of adjuvant tamoxifen to 5 years in patients with ER-positive, node-negative breast cancer was concluded to be optimal at that time (see below).

The Scottish Adjuvant Tamoxifen Trial was initiated in 1978 and was designed to assess the effect of tamoxifen administered to patients postmastectomy (adjuvant arm) versus those who received tamoxifen only after they developed a recurrence (control arm) [6, 7]. A total of 1,323 patients were randomized: 667 to the adjuvant arm and 656 to the control arm. If patients in the adjuvant arm were disease-free after 5 years and agreeable, they were randomly assigned to no further tamoxifen therapy ($n = 169$) or to continue taking it indefinitely until relapse or death ($n = 173$). The initial results of this trial, with a follow-up ranging from 2.5 to 8 years, showed a survival advantage and a reduction in disease recurrence for those patients receiving tamoxifen immediately compared with those receiving delayed tamoxifen therapy. With a median follow-up of 15 years, no additional benefit in terms of total survival, systemic relapse, or death from breast cancer has been observed in those patients receiving tamoxifen beyond 5 years duration [6, 7].

As a result, the standard of care for the duration of adjuvant tamoxifen therapy was established at 5 years. Although strategies for postmenopausal women have evolved to include longer durations of therapy in certain situations (with the addition of an AI), the optimal duration of tamoxifen remained 5 years. Despite the practice-changing data from the NSABP, the duration of tamoxifen has remained an open question to the present time.

Recently, investigators from the Adjuvant Tamoxifen: Longer Against Shorter (ATLAS) trial reported findings of a trial involving 12,894 women with early-stage breast cancer who were treated with 5 years of tamoxifen after which they were randomly allocated (1:1) to stop tamoxifen or continue for another 5 years [8]. All recurrences, second cancers, and deaths were tabulated. This trial did not exclude patients with ER-negative tumors, but the recent report provides results on the 6,846 patients with ER-positive disease.

Among patients with ER-positive disease, those receiving 10 years of therapy experienced statistically fewer recurrences (617 versus 711, $p = 0.002$) and fewer deaths (331 versus 397, $p = 0.01$). Interestingly the effect of longer durations of tamoxifen was not as striking during years 5–9 which may reflect the ongoing carryover effect of tamoxifen administered during the first 5 years. The reductions in adverse breast cancer outcomes appeared to be less striking before, than after, year 10 (recurrence rate ratio [RR] 0.90] during years 5–9 and 0.75 in later years; breast cancer mortality RR 0.97 during years 5–9 and 0.71 in later years).

The cumulative risk of recurrence during years 5–14 was 21.4 % for women allocated to continue versus 25.1 % for controls (5 years); breast cancer mortality during years 5–14 was 12.2 % for women allocated to continue versus 15.0 % for controls (absolute mortality reduction 2·8 %). The cumulative risk of endometrial cancer during years 5–14 was 3.1 % (mortality 0.4 %) for women allocated to continue versus 1.6 % (mortality 0.2 %) for controls (absolute mortality increase 0.2 %) [8].

The ATLAS data, along with the report of a similar trial, Adjuvant Tamoxifen-Treatment

Table 24.1 Adverse events associated with tamoxifen (P-1 trial)

Toxicity	HR
Endometrial cancer	3.28
Pulmonary embolism	2.15
Deep venous thrombosis	1.44
Bone fractures	0.68

Offer More? (aTTom) at the 2013 ASCO meeting [9] and the update of the Oxford Overview Analysis of randomized tamoxifen trials due in the coming year, will bring more clarity to the issue of whether longer durations of tamoxifen beyond 5 years should be recommended. The aTTom trial recruited almost 7,000 patients to 5 versus 10 years of tamoxifen. There was a statistically significant 15 % relative reduction in the odds of recurrence favoring longer durations of tamoxifen, but survival is not statistically different. The optimal duration of tamoxifen is particularly relevant to high-risk premenopausal women where aromatase inhibitors cannot be used. In postmenopausal women, the aromatase inhibitors have supplanted tamoxifen, but whether tamoxifen should be initiated after 5 years of an aromatase inhibitor and whether tamoxifen for 5 years should be followed by an aromatase inhibitor followed by more tamoxifen are all research questions that will have to be considered anew.

Toxicity of Tamoxifen

The side effect profile of tamoxifen is well established. Individual clinical trials, the Oxford Overview, and chemoprevention trials have provided information on the expected adverse events associated with tamoxifen. In the NSABP P-1 trial, which compared tamoxifen to placebo in over 13,000 women with a high risk for developing breast cancer, women who received tamoxifen had increased hot flashes, vaginal discharge, and difficulties in some areas of sexual functioning (Table 24.1). The more serious side effects associated with tamoxifen include endometrial cancer, pulmonary embolism, and deep venous thrombosis; however, the incidence of bone fractures was reduced [10, 11].

In the most recent Oxford Overview Analysis, there was a nonsignificant increase in stroke deaths (3 extra per 1,000 during the first 15 years) balanced by a nonsignificant reduction in cardiac deaths (3 fewer per 1,000 during the first 15 years), with a resulting minimal net effect of tamoxifen on overall cardiovascular mortality. In the recent ATLAS trial evaluating 10 years of tamoxifen therapy, the benefits of longer durations of tamoxifen outweighed the side effects [8]. After 10 years of treatment with tamoxifen, there was an increased risk for endometrial cancer (relative risk [RR], 1.74) and for pulmonary embolism (RR, 1.87). Endometrial cancers occurred in 3.1 % (with mortality of 0.4 %) in the long-duration group and in 1.6 % (with mortality of 0.2 %) of the 5-year group. There were only 18 pulmonary embolism events and there was an equal amount of mortality (0.2 %) in each treatment group. Additionally, there was no increase in the incidence of stroke and a decrease in the incidence of ischemic heart disease in the long-duration group.

Biomarkers for Tamoxifen Efficacy

Endoxifen, one of two active metabolites that mediate tamoxifen's therapeutic effect, is formed through the action of the CYP2D6 enzyme [12–14]. Several polymorphisms of the *CYP2D6* gene that influence the enzyme's activity and, therefore, endoxifen levels have been identified. However, studies designed to uncover the link between patient response to tamoxifen and CYP2D6 enzyme activity (or *CYP2D6* genotype) have yielded inconsistent results, perhaps as a result of limited sample sizes. Regan and colleagues [15] studied 4,861 postmenopausal patients with hormone receptor-positive breast cancer who were randomized to receive tamoxifen, letrozole, or both. Extracted DNA was used to genotype *CYP2D6* and classify each patient as a poor metabolizer (PM), intermediate metabolizer (IM), or extensive metabolizer (EM). No significant association was observed between *CYP2D6* phenotype and disease recurrence in tamoxifen-treated patients. Contrary to an

Table 24.2 Comparison of adverse events: AI and tamoxifen

Adverse event	OR	*P* value	Abs incidence with AI (%)	Abs incidence with tamoxifen (%)
Endometrial CA	0.34	<0.001	0.1	0.5
Cardiovascular	1.30	1.30	4.2	3.4
Hypercholesterolemia	2.36	2.36	–	–
Venous thromboembolism	0.55	<0.001	1.6	2.8

existing hypothesis that high rates of tamoxifen-induced hot flashes are a surrogate for EM phenotype, PM and IM phenotype patients experienced the highest rates of hot flashes.

Rae and colleagues studied 1,203 patients with hormone receptor-positive early-stage breast cancer from the ATAC clinical trial who were available for genotyping of *CYP2D6* and for whom 10 years of follow-up data were available [16]. Patients were classified as a PM, IM, or EM based on *CYP2D6* genotyping. No significant associations were observed between *CYP2D6* genotype and recurrence in tamoxifen-treated patients. These two studies confirm that there is no compelling evidence to support *CYP2D6* testing in patients who are being considered for tamoxifen therapy and the NCCN treatment guidelines do not support their use [17].

Antidepressants (selective serotonin reuptake inhibitor (SSRI)) are commonly prescribed to breast cancer patients for depression and to reduce the effects of hot flashes, but there is evidence that the concurrent use of certain antidepressants can reduce the efficacy of tamoxifen via the CYP2D6 pathway. Although clinicians should not stop antidepressants prescribed for a psychiatric disorder, better choices among the SSRIs may be considered with concurrent use of tamoxifen and the patient should be aware of the potential interaction [18].

Aromatase Inhibitors

The use of AIs has increased dramatically over the last decade with the introduction of new, more selective aromatase inhibitors, such as anastrozole, exemestane, and letrozole. Current guidelines by ASCO [19] and NCCN [17] recommend third-generation AIs as a component of adjuvant therapy in postmenopausal women, either as monotherapy or in a sequential strategy with tamoxifen. The guidelines do not distinguish between the AIs, even though individual trials used a specific agent. There is no compelling evidence that one agent is superior to another either from an efficacy or tolerability standpoint.

This class of agents effectively blocks the extra-ovarian sites of estradiol synthesis, decreasing its serum concentration by more than 90 % in postmenopausal women [20, 21]. In contrast to tamoxifen, the newer AIs lack partial agonist activity and thus appear to avoid a concerning toxicity associated with tamoxifen, that is the highest risk for developing endometrial cancer [22]. There also appears to be a reduced risk of thromboembolic disease associated with the use of the AIs [22]. Because of this lack of estrogen agonist activity, AIs can potentially result in the loss of bone density (Table 24.2) [22]. Unlike tamoxifen, the AIs do not appear to be beneficial in premenopausal women. Even the newer aromatase inhibitors are unable to inhibit ovarian aromatase activity and, as a result, are unable to suppress estrogen synthesis in premenopausal women.

Data is available from several randomized clinical trials in the adjuvant setting that show a superior clinical outcome for postmenopausal patients who receive an AI as a component of their adjuvant therapy program. Trial designs compared (1) an aromatase inhibitor to tamoxifen, each for 5 years, (2) a sequence of tamoxifen with an aromatase inhibitor versus either alone as monotherapy for 5 years duration, or (3) 5 years of tamoxifen followed by no additional therapy or 5 years of an AI. Findings from some of the key pivotal trials are summarized below:

- The Arimidex (anastrozole), Tamoxifen Alone, or in Combination (ATAC) study ($n=9{,}366$) compared tamoxifen versus anastrozole versus tamoxifen plus anastrozole [23, 24]. At 120 months, DFS was significantly improved in the anastrozole group versus the tamoxifen group. Among women with hormone receptor-positive tumors, those randomly assigned to receive treatment with anastrozole had a 4.3 % lower absolute rate of breast cancer recurrence after 10 years, and a 2.6 % lower absolute rate of distant metastasis, than those randomly assigned to receive treatment with tamoxifen. The differences between anastrozole and tamoxifen in time to relapse, contralateral breast cancer, and DFS were greatest in the first 2 years of treatment but were maintained throughout the follow-up period, including the period after treatment was completed. This so-called carryover effect is similar to that observed in tamoxifen-treated patients once therapy is discontinued. OS was not significantly different between the groups.
- The Breast International Group (BIG) 1-98 trial was a randomized, phase 3, double-blind trial of 8, 010 postmenopausal women with hormone receptor-positive, early breast cancer that compared 5 years of tamoxifen or letrozole monotherapy or sequential treatment with 2 years of one of these drugs followed by 3 years of the other [25, 26]. At a median follow-up of 8.7 years from randomization, letrozole monotherapy was significantly better than tamoxifen: DFS HR 0.82, OS HR 0.79, distant relapse-free interval (DRFI) HR 0.79, and breast cancer-free interval (BCFI) HR 0.80. At a median follow-up of 8.0 years from randomization for the comparison of the sequential groups with letrozole monotherapy, there were no statistically significant differences in any of the endpoints for either sequence. The 8-year intention-to-treat estimates for letrozole monotherapy, letrozole followed by tamoxifen, and tamoxifen followed by letrozole were 78.6 %, 77.8 %, and 77.3 % for DFS; 87.5 %, 87.7 %, and 85.9 % for OS; 89.9 %, 88.7 %, and 88.1 % for DRFI; and 86.1 %, 85.3 %, and 84.3 % for BCFI [27]. Sequential treatments involving tamoxifen and letrozole do not improve outcome compared with letrozole monotherapy, but it could be considered for an individual patient based on risk of recurrence and treatment tolerability.
- The Intergroup Exemestane Study ($n=4{,}742$) compared 2–3 years of tamoxifen followed by exemestane to 2–3 years of tamoxifen followed by further tamoxifen, each to a total of 5 years of therapy [28, 29]. After a median follow-up of 55.7 months, the exemestane arm showed significantly improved DFS (HR, 0.76) but showed no significant benefit for overall survival. Time to contralateral breast cancer, time to relapse, and time to distant relapse were also significantly improved in women who switched to exemestane. Overall survival was significantly improved only in a subgroup analysis that excluded patients with estrogen receptor-negative disease (HR, 0.83).
- The Italian Tamoxifen Arimidex (anastrozole) (ITA) trial ($n=426$) compared tamoxifen (20 mg daily) for 2 or more years followed by further tamoxifen or anastrozole (1.0 mg daily) to a total of 5 years of adjuvant hormone therapy [30, 31]. At 64 months follow-up, DFS was significantly improved in women who switched to anastrozole (HR, 0.57). There was no significant difference in OS between therapy arms.
- The Austrian Breast and Colorectal Cancer Study Group (ABCSG)-8 and German Adjuvant Breast Cancer Group Arimidex/Nolvadex (ARNO)-95 trials had arms identical ($n=3{,}224$) to the ITA trial described above [32]. At 28-months median follow-up, a combined analysis showed significantly improved DFS for women who switched to anastrozole (HR, 0.60). Distant metastases-free survival was also significantly longer with anastrozole (HR, 0.61). There was no significant difference in OS. There were significantly more fractures ($p=0.015$) and significantly fewer thromboses ($p=0.034$) in patients treated with anastrozole than in those on tamoxifen.

- A meta-analysis of the ABCSG-8, ARNO-95, and ITA trials, involving 4,006 patients at a median follow-up of 30 months, found improvements in DFS (HR, 0.59; $p<0.0001$), DRFI (HR 0.61, $p=0.002$), and OS (HR, 0.71; $p=0.04$) for women who switched to anastrozole [33]. In absolute terms, there were significantly fewer recurrences (92 events [4.6 %] versus 159 events [8.0 %]) and significantly fewer deaths (66 [3.3 %] versus 90 [4.5 %]) in the group switched to anastrozole versus those remaining on tamoxifen.
- The NCI of Canada study, MA.17, was conducted to determine whether letrozole improves outcome after discontinuation of tamoxifen. Postmenopausal women with hormone receptor-positive breast cancer ($N=5{,}187$) were randomized to letrozole 2.5 mg or placebo once daily for 5 years [34–36]. At a median follow-up of 30 months, letrozole significantly improved DFS ($P<0.001$), the primary end point, compared with placebo (HR for recurrence or contralateral breast cancer 0.58, $P<0.001$). Furthermore, letrozole significantly improved DRFI ($HR=0.60$; 0.84; $P=0.002$) and, in women with node-positive tumors, OS ($HR=0.61$; $P=0.04$). Clinical benefits, including an OS advantage, were also seen in women who crossed over from placebo to letrozole after unblinding, indicating that tumors remain sensitive to hormone therapy despite a prolonged period since discontinuation of tamoxifen. The efficacy and safety of letrozole therapy beyond 5 years is being assessed in a re-randomization study, following the emergence of new data suggesting that clinical benefit correlates with the duration of letrozole. MA.17 showed that letrozole is extremely well tolerated relative to placebo. Letrozole (or an alternative aromatase inhibitor) could be considered for all women completing tamoxifen; results from the post-unblinding analysis suggest that letrozole treatment could also be considered for all disease-free women for periods up to 5 years following completion of adjuvant tamoxifen [34].

Recent reports have also suggested that obese women with early-stage breast cancer, in particular those with body mass index (BMI) ≥ 35 kg/m^2, may have a greater risk of disease recurrence when treated with anastrozole compared to their ideal weight counterparts or those treated with tamoxifen. These findings raise a concern that aromatase inhibition in obese women may be a less effective risk reduction strategy and/or the use of the less potent aromatase inhibitors can adversely impact on clinical outcome [37]. To date, the clinical evidence suggesting that one third-generation aromatase inhibitor is more effective than another has been sparse, but preclinical data and clinical surrogates of clinical activity have shown that letrozole is more potent than anastrozole at suppressing estradiol and estrone sulfate [38]. Whether the differences in estrogen suppression with anastrozole or letrozole actually translate into a different clinical outcome cannot be determined from these data. The ALIQUOT study (Anastrozole vs. Letrozole, an Investigation of Quality of Life and Tolerability) compared the ability of anastrozole and letrozole to suppress estrogen in obese postmenopausal women with early-stage breast cancer. Letrozole appeared to be more effective; however, this small study did not demonstrate a differential effect on clinical outcome. Furthermore, the association between obesity and breast cancer is certainly more complicated than suggesting estradiol alone is the culprit. Increased levels in insulin, inflammatory mediators, and other proteins have been implicated as risk factors for breast cancer and breast cancer recurrence in obese patients [37].

Toxicity of AIs

All of the trials that have included an AI have also reported an increase in musculoskeletal (MS)/joint complaints in patients receiving an AI compared to those receiving tamoxifen alone [23, 24]. As an example, the ATAC trial, which compared 5 years of tamoxifen to 5 years of anastrozole, reported an incidence of MS disorders in 35.6 % of patients versus 29.4 % of patients receiving tamoxifen. Symptoms peaked within 6 months of starting therapy in 29 % of patients receiving anastrozole versus 20 % receiving tamoxifen. Symptoms resolved in 36 % of patients [39]. To gain a "real-world" assessment of the prevalence and severity of AI-induced joint complaints, Crew et al. conducted a 200-patient cross-sectional survey of consecutive postmenopausal patients with early-stage breast cancer who are receiving an AI as part of their adjuvant therapy [40]. Of 200 patients who completed the study, 47 % reported having AI-related joint pain and 44 % complained of AI-related joint stiffness.

In real-life practice, some patients discontinue AI therapy completely due to associated side effects, and as a result, their symptoms are no longer captured in a prospective manner. Though intuitively it is difficult to explain, some patients get relief of these symptoms by simply trying an alternative AI and as such may indicate that they have no joint-related symptoms. The analysis suggests that AI-induced joint complaints are very frequent and better methods of treating symptoms need to be developed. Most patients experiencing these symptoms take oral medications including NSAIDs, pain relievers, and glucosamine as well as exercise with some improvement in their reported joint discomfort.

Although AIs have improved outcome in patients with breast cancer, they can have long-term detrimental effects on bone health [41–44]. AI-induced estrogen depletion has been reported to result in musculoskeletal complications, including bone loss and osteoporotic fractures. Bone loss seen during AI treatment appears to be similar for the three agents within this class of drugs, with the incidence of osteoporosis and fractures approximately 4 % higher for patients receiving an AI compared to tamoxifen in primary adjuvant trials [19].

Ovarian Suppression/Ablation

The role of ovarian suppression/ablation as a component of adjuvant therapy in premenopausal patients has been an area of interest for several decades, but clinical trials of sufficient size and/or rigorous design have been lacking to provide clear evidence of the contribution of this strategy to existing adjuvant endocrine therapy. A meta-analysis of data from 16 studies involving nearly 12,000 women found that ovarian suppression with a luteinizing hormone-releasing hormone (LHRH) agonist, added to tamoxifen, chemotherapy, or both, reduced the risk of recurrence by 12.7 % [45]. Previous studies have looked at the effects of LHRH agonists such as goserelin or *leuprolide* alone or in combination with tamoxifen and other adjuvant therapies or compared to an adjuvant chemotherapy regimen [46, 47].

The results from these trials were inconclusive about the effects of LHRH agonists on TTR, death after recurrence, or OS. The TEXT and SOFT trials are large international randomized trials that have been completed, but not yet reported, that will determine whether chemotherapy adds to the effect of ovarian suppression and whether ovarian suppression adds to other endocrine therapy [48]. Although some guidelines suggest that the addition of ovarian suppression to adjuvant endocrine therapy (i.e., tamoxifen) could be considered, definitive support is lacking until the large randomized trials are reported.

Evidence-Based Approach to Patients

Adjuvant Endocrine Therapy 2013 [17]

- Premenopausal women
  - Tamoxifen (5–10 years) (±ovarian suppression/ablation)
- Postmenopausal women
  - AI × 5 years or tamoxifen (5–10 years) if AI contraindicated, intolerant
  - Tamoxifen (2–3 years), then AI (to complete 5 years or up to 5 more years)
  - AI (2–3 years), then tamoxifen (to complete 5 years if not tolerating AI)
  - Tamoxifen (~5 years), then AI (5 years)
  - Guidelines view AI choices as interchangeable [17]

References

1. Tamoxifen for early breast cancer: an overview of the randomised trials. Early Breast Cancer Trialists' Collaborative Group. Lancet. 1998;351(9114):1451–67.
2. Effects of adjuvant tamoxifen and of cytotoxic therapy on mortality in early breast cancer. An overview of 61 randomized trials among 28,896 women. Early Breast Cancer Trialists' Collaborative Group. N Engl J Med. 1988;319(26):1681–92.
3. Systemic treatment of early breast cancer by hormonal, cytotoxic, or immune therapy. 133 randomised trials involving 31,000 recurrences and 24,000 deaths among 75,000 women. Early Breast Cancer Trialists' Collaborative Group. Lancet. 1992;339(8785):71–85.
4. Dowsett M, et al. Meta-analysis of breast cancer outcomes in adjuvant trials of aromatase inhibitors versus tamoxifen. J Clin Oncol. 2010;28(3):509–18.
5. Early Breast Cancer Trialists' Collaborative Group, et al. Relevance of breast cancer hormone receptors and other factors to the efficacy of adjuvant tamoxifen: patient-level meta-analysis of randomised trials. Lancet. 2011;378(9793):771–84.
6. Stewart HJ, Prescott RJ, Forrest AP. Scottish adjuvant tamoxifen trial: a randomized study updated to 15 years. J Natl Cancer Inst. 2001;93(6):456–62.
7. Stewart HJ, et al. Randomised comparison of 5 years of adjuvant tamoxifen with continuous therapy for operable breast cancer. The Scottish Cancer Trials Breast Group. Br J Cancer. 1996;74(2):297–9.
8. Davies C, et al. Long-term effects of continuing adjuvant tamoxifen to 10 years versus stopping at 5 years after diagnosis of oestrogen receptor-positive breast cancer: ATLAS, a randomised trial. Lancet. 2013;381: 805–16.
9. Earl H, et al. The optimal duration of adjuvant tamoxifen treatment for breast cancer remains uncertain: randomize into aTTom. Clin Oncol. 1997;9(3):141–3.
10. Day R, et al. Health-related quality of life and tamoxifen in breast cancer prevention: a report from the National Surgical Adjuvant Breast and Bowel Project P-1 study. J Clin Oncol. 1999;17(9):2659–69.
11. Fisher B, et al. Tamoxifen for prevention of breast cancer: report of the National Surgical Adjuvant Breast and Bowel Project P-1 study. J Natl Cancer Inst. 1998;90(18):1371–88.
12. Goetz MP. Tamoxifen, endoxifen, and CYP2D6: the rules for evaluating a predictive factor. Oncology (Williston Park). 2009;23(14):1233–4, 1236.
13. Hoskins JM, Carey LA, McLeod HL. CYP2D6 and tamoxifen: DNA matters in breast cancer. Nat Rev Cancer. 2009;9(8):576–86.
14. Rae JM, et al. CYP2D6 genotype and tamoxifen response. Breast Cancer Res. 2005;7(5):E6.
15. Regan MM, et al. CYP2D6 genotype and tamoxifen response in postmenopausal women with endocrine-responsive breast cancer: the breast international group 1-98 trial. J Natl Cancer Inst. 2012;104(6):441–51.
16. Rae JM, et al. CYP2D6 and UGT2B7 genotype and risk of recurrence in tamoxifen-treated breast cancer patients. J Natl Cancer Inst. 2012;104(6):452–60.
17. NCCN.org. NCCN clinical practice guidelines in oncology: breast cancer version 2.2013, 2013.
18. Higgins MJ, et al. Pharmacogenetics of tamoxifen: who should undergo CYP2D6 genetic testing? J Natl Compr Canc Netw. 2009;7(2):203–13.
19. Burstein HJ, et al. American society of clinical oncology clinical practice guideline update on adjuvant endocrine therapy for women with hormone receptor-positive breast cancer. J Oncol Pract. 2010;6(5):243–6.
20. Santen RJ, Harvey HA. Use of aromatase inhibitors in breast carcinoma. Endocr Relat Cancer. 1999;6(1):75–92.
21. Osborne CK. Aromatase inhibitors in relation to other forms of endocrine therapy for breast cancer. Endocr Relat Cancer. 1999;6(2):271–6.
22. Amir E, et al. Toxicity of adjuvant endocrine therapy in postmenopausal breast cancer patients: a systematic review and meta-analysis. J Natl Cancer Inst. 2011;103(17):1299–309.
23. ATAC Trialists' Study Group, et al. Effect of anastrozole and tamoxifen as adjuvant treatment for early-stage breast cancer: 100-month analysis of the ATAC trial. Lancet Oncol. 2008;9(1):45–53.
24. Baum M, et al. Anastrozole alone or in combination with tamoxifen versus tamoxifen alone for adjuvant treatment of postmenopausal women with early breast cancer: first results of the ATAC randomised trial. Lancet. 2002;359(9324):2131–9.
25. BIG 1-98 Collaborative Group, et al. Letrozole therapy alone or in sequence with tamoxifen in women with breast cancer. N Engl J Med. 2009;361(8):766–76.
26. Breast International Group 1-98 Collaborative Group, et al. A comparison of letrozole and tamoxifen in postmenopausal women with early breast cancer. N Engl J Med. 2005;353(26):2747–57.
27. Regan MM, et al. Assessment of letrozole and tamoxifen alone and in sequence for postmenopausal women with steroid hormone receptor-positive breast cancer: the BIG 1-98 randomised clinical trial at 8.1 years median follow-up. Lancet Oncol. 2011;12(12):1101–8.
28. Coombes RC, et al. Survival and safety of exemestane versus tamoxifen after 2–3 years' tamoxifen treatment (Intergroup Exemestane Study): a randomised controlled trial. Lancet. 2007;369(9561):559–70.
29. Coombes RC, et al. A randomized trial of exemestane after two to three years of tamoxifen therapy in postmenopausal women with primary breast cancer. N Engl J Med. 2004;350(11):1081–92.
30. Boccardo F, et al. Switching to anastrozole versus continued tamoxifen treatment of early breast cancer: long term results of the Italian Tamoxifen Anastrozole trial. Eur J Cancer. 2013;49:1546–1554.
31. Boccardo F, et al. Switching to anastrozole versus continued tamoxifen treatment of early breast cancer. Updated results of the Italian Tamoxifen Anastrozole (ITA) trial. Ann Oncol. 2006;17 Suppl 7:vii10–4.

32. Jakesz R, et al. Switching of postmenopausal women with endocrine-responsive early breast cancer to anastrozole after 2 years' adjuvant tamoxifen: combined results of ABCSG trial 8 and ARNO 95 trial. Lancet. 2005;366(9484):455–62.
33. Jonat W, et al. Effectiveness of switching from adjuvant tamoxifen to anastrozole in postmenopausal women with hormone-sensitive early-stage breast cancer: a meta-analysis. Lancet Oncol. 2006;7(12):991–6.
34. Goss PE, et al. Late extended adjuvant treatment with letrozole improves outcome in women with early-stage breast cancer who complete 5 years of tamoxifen. J Clin Oncol. 2008;26(12):1948–55.
35. Goss PE, et al. Randomized trial of letrozole following tamoxifen as extended adjuvant therapy in receptor-positive breast cancer: updated findings from NCIC CTG MA.17. J Natl Cancer Inst. 2005;97(17):1262–71.
36. Goss PE, et al. A randomized trial of letrozole in postmenopausal women after five years of tamoxifen therapy for early-stage breast cancer. N Engl J Med. 2003;349(19):1793–802.
37. Folkerd EJ, et al. Suppression of plasma estrogen levels by letrozole and anastrozole is related to body mass index in patients with breast cancer. J Clin Oncol. 2012;30(24):2977–80.
38. Dixon JM, et al. Letrozole suppresses plasma estradiol and estrone sulphate more completely than anastrozole in postmenopausal women with breast cancer. J Clin Oncol. 2008;26(10):1671–6.
39. Sestak I, et al. Risk factors for joint symptoms in patients enrolled in the ATAC trial: a retrospective, exploratory analysis. Lancet Oncol. 2008;9(9):866–72.
40. Crew KD, et al. Prevalence of joint symptoms in postmenopausal women taking aromatase inhibitors for early-stage breast cancer. J Clin Oncol. 2007;25(25):3877–83.
41. Hadji P. Breast cancer: aromatase inhibitors–bone health assessment is crucial. Natl Rev Clin Oncol. 2012;9(5):254–5.
42. Hadji P. Aromatase inhibitor-associated bone loss in breast cancer patients is distinct from postmenopausal osteoporosis. Crit Rev Oncol Hematol. 2009;69(1):73–82.
43. Hadji P, et al. Practical guidance for the management of aromatase inhibitor-associated bone loss. Ann Oncol. 2008;19(8):1407–16.
44. Clunie GP, et al. Evaluating bone health in women with oestrogen receptor positive breast cancer (ERBC) starting aromatase inhibitors. Eur J Surg Oncol. 2009;35(5):475–80.
45. LHRH-agonists in Early Breast Cancer Overview group, et al. Use of luteinising-hormone-releasing hormone agonists as adjuvant treatment in premenopausal patients with hormone-receptor-positive breast cancer: a meta-analysis of individual patient data from randomised adjuvant trials. Lancet. 2007;369(9574):1711–23.
46. Jonat W. Luteinizing hormone-releasing hormone analogues–the rationale for adjuvant use in premenopausal women with early breast cancer. Br J Cancer. 1998;78 Suppl 4:5–8.
47. Robertson JF, et al. Combined endocrine effects of LHRH agonist (Zoladex) and tamoxifen (Nolvadex) therapy in premenopausal women with breast cancer. Br J Surg. 1989;76(12):1262–5.
48. Love RR. Adjuvant hormonal therapy in premenopausal women with operable breast cancer: not-so-peripheral perspectives. Oncology (Williston Park). 2010;24(4):322–7.

Adjuvant Biologic Agents for Breast Cancer

25

Virginia G. Kaklamani and William J. Gradishar

Introduction

In the year 2013, a total of 234,580 new cases of breast cancer were diagnosed in the USA [1]. Although the incidence of breast cancer is increasing, the 5-year survival rate has continued to improve. This improvement to overall survival (OS) is largely due to new chemotherapeutic and biologic agents. Biologic agents currently in use in early-stage breast cancer mainly target the human epidermal growth factor receptor 2 (HER2). HER2 belongs to the family of epidermal growth factor receptors (EGFRs) and is overexpressed in 20–30 % of all breast cancers [2, 3]. Further, the overexpression of HER2 is a negative prognostic and predictive factor [4, 5]. Patients with HER2+ breast cancers have more aggressive disease, a higher likelihood of lymph node involvement, decreased estrogen receptor (ER) expression, and increased resistance to endocrine therapy, while also found to have an increased responsiveness to anthracycline treatment [6–10]. Initially approved by the Food and Drug Administration (FDA) in 1998 for treatment of HER2+ metastatic breast cancer, trastuzumab has been approved in the adjuvant setting after pivotal trials revealed a statistically significant reduction in the risk of recurrence by nearly 50 % and an improvement of overall survival (OS) by a third [11, 12]. Several other biologic agents are currently under investigation with the goal to improve the long-term survival in women with early-stage breast cancer.

Trastuzumab (Herceptin)

Trastuzumab is a recombinant, humanized IgG monoclonal antibody that targets the extracellular domain of the HER2 receptor [13]. The exact mechanism of action of trastuzumab remains unclear, although several theories have been proposed [14, 15]. Trastuzumab may decrease the concentration of HER2 at the cellular membrane, thus preventing homodimerization and heterodimerization [14]. Trastuzumab also appears to cause arrest of the cell cycle through the inhibition of phosphatidylinositol 3-kinase (PI3K) and mitogen-activated protein kinase (MAPK) cascades by the down-modulation of HER2. In addition, trastuzumab activates phosphatase and tensin homologue (PTEN)

V.G. Kaklamani, MD (✉)
Department of Medicine Hematology/Oncology, Northwestern University, 676 N St Clair st suite 850, Chicago, IL 60611, USA
e-mail: v-kaklamani@northwestern.edu

W.J. Gradishar, MD
Medicine – Division of Hematology/Oncology, Maggie Daley Center For Women's Cancer Care, Robert H. Lurie Comprehensive Cancer Center, Northwestern University Feinberg School of Medicine at Northwestern Memorial Hospital, 676 North St. Clair, Suite 850, Chicago, IL 60611, USA
e-mail: w-gradishar@northwestern.edu

A.I. Riker (ed.), *Breast Disease: Comprehensive Management*,
DOI 10.1007/978-1-4939-1145-5_25, © Springer Science+Business Media New York 2015

phosphatase causing dephosphorylation of Akt resulting in cessation of cell growth [14, 16]. Additionally, trastuzumab has been shown to sensitize HER2-overexpressed breast cancer cell lines to cytotoxic therapy (i.e., taxanes and etoposide) through reducing the levels of Mcl-1, an antiapoptotic protein that promotes cell death [17]. As seen in in vivo studies, trastuzumab may also inhibit angiogenesis [18]. Another mechanism of action is through antibody-dependent cellular cytotoxicity (ADCC) by which the Fc domain of trastuzumab activates natural killer cells to attack and destroy cells expressing HER2 [19].

What Patient Would Be Eligible for Trastuzumab Therapy?

The overexpression of HER2 can be measured by evaluating protein expression via immunohistochemistry (IHC) or gene amplification via fluorescent in situ hybridization (FISH). IHC measures the intensity of staining for HER2 and is classified as 0, 1+, 2+, or 3+. The pivotal clinical trials involving trastuzumab required an IHC score of 3+ to be considered positive. An equivocal IHC score of 2+ requires that FISH be performed on the sample, in which each copy of the *HER2* gene and its centromere 17 (*CEP17*) reference are examined and can be counted in the tissue section. To define HER2 amplification, the presence of at least twice as many *HER2* signals as *CEP17* signals per tumor cell is recommended ($\geq$2.0). These criteria were used in the adjuvant trastuzumab clinical trials [11, 12, 20]. The American Society of Clinical Oncology (ASCO) and the College of American Pathologists (CAP) have published specific guidelines for HER2 positivity [21]. However, recent data suggest that patients with lower levels of HER2 expression may benefit from adjuvant trastuzumab therapy [20]. Although there is no definitive explanation for this discrepancy, future trials are addressing this issue of trastuzumab use in the adjuvant setting for those with lower levels of HER2 expression.

Trastuzumab in Metastatic Breast Cancer (MBC)

Trastuzumab was initially approved for treatment of HER2+ MBC. Trastuzumab has shown single-agent activity in HER2+ MBC with a response rate (RR) of approximately 30 % [22]. However, in combination with chemotherapy, trastuzumab has a higher RR. Based on preclinical data showing synergy of trastuzumab with taxanes and anthracyclines, a randomized trial was conducted comparing anthracycline/cyclophosphamide (AnC) and paclitaxel with or without trastuzumab [23]. A total of 234 patients received chemotherapy alone compared to 235 patients who received chemotherapy plus trastuzumab. Patients who received the combination of chemotherapy plus trastuzumab had a median time to progression (TTP) of 7.4 months compared to 4.6 months for the chemotherapy alone arm ($p<0.001$).

Furthermore, there was an improvement in median OS for those patients receiving chemotherapy plus trastuzumab compared to those receiving chemotherapy alone (25.1 month versus 20.3 months; $p=0.046$). At the completion of therapy, crossover in patients not receiving trastuzumab as initial therapy was allowed. However, it was shown that when comparing "upfront" trastuzumab to crossing over (later initiation), there was an improvement in outcome with the "upfront use" of trastuzumab. Interestingly, 39 patients (27 %) in the AnC plus trastuzumab treatment arm had symptomatic congestive heart failure (CHF) or asymptomatic cardiac dysfunction, whereas in the AC alone arm, 8 % of patients had cardiac dysfunction. Due to the relatively high incidence of cardiotoxicity in the anthracycline-containing arm (AnC plus trastuzumab), the FDA approved the combination of paclitaxel and trastuzumab for use in MBC.

After preclinical studies evaluated the feasibility of combining trastuzumab with chemotherapeutic agents [24, 25], several phase II and III trials using agents such as docetaxel, Navelbine, capecitabine [26–29], or carboplatin and paclitaxel [30, 31] were completed in MBC. All studies demonstrated a significant enhancement in RR when chemotherapy was combined with trastuzumab compared with chemotherapy alone.

Table 25.1 Adjuvant trastuzumab trials

	Number of patients	DFS/RFS HR (95 %CI or p value)	OS	Cardiotoxicity	Comments
NSABP B31/ N9831 [35]	5,548	0.60 (0.53–0.68)	0.63 (0.54–0.73)	4.1 %	The N9831 also included a sequential trastuzumab arm. Data showed that the sequential arm was inferior to the concomitant arm
HERA [37]	5,102	0.76 ($p<0.0001$)	0.76 ($p=0.0005$)	4.1 %	The study also showed that there was no difference between 1 year and 2 years of trastuzumab
BCIRG 006 [12]	3,222	AC-DH: 0.64 ($p<0.001$) DCarboH: 0.75 ($p=0.04$)	AC-DH: 0.63 ($p<0.001$) DCarboH: 0.77 ($p=0.04$)	AC-DH: 2 % DCarboH: 0.4 %	Although the study was not powered to compare the two trastuzumab arms, there was no statistical difference between them
FINher [39]	232	0.42 (0.21–0.83)	0.41 (0.16–1.05)	No decrease	This trial included 12 weeks of trastuzumab therapy
PACS 04 [38]	528	0.86 (0.61–1.22)	0.86 (0.61–1.22)	1.7 %	The only adjuvant trial to not show a significant benefit from 1 year of trastuzumab therapy. This could be attributed to the relatively small number of patients it included
PHARE [40]	3,381	1.28 (1.05–1.56)	NA	NA	This trial showed that 6 months of trastuzumab was not non-inferior to 12 months

Abbreviations: *HERA* Herceptin adjuvant, *BCIRG* Breast Cancer International Research Group, *FINher* Finland Herceptin, *DFS* disease-free survival, *CI* confidence interval, *A* doxorubicin, *C* cyclophosphamide, *D* docetaxel, *H* trastuzumab, *Carbo* carboplatin, *CI* confidence interval, *u/k* unknown

Use of Trastuzumab in Early-Stage Breast Cancer

Trials including trastuzumab in early-stage breast cancer are summarized in Table 25.1 and discussed in detail below.

NSABP B31 and NCCTG 9831 Joint Analysis

Since trastuzumab was effective in improving RR, duration of response, and OS in MBC, large randomized adjuvant trials were initiated [11, 12]. These trials showed that the integration of trastuzumab into adjuvant therapy regimens significantly improved patient outcomes and led to the FDA approval of trastuzumab for HER2+ early-stage breast cancer. The National Surgical Adjuvant Breast and Bowel Project (NSABP)-B31 published a joint analysis with the North Central Cancer Treatment Group (NCCTG) N9831 [11]. These trials were closed prematurely due to the superiority of the trastuzumab arm. The B31 trial enrolled 2,043 node-positive, HER2+ patients with early-stage breast cancer and randomized them to 4 cycles of doxorubicin (A) and cyclophosphamide (C) ($A=60$ mg/m^2 and $C=600$ mg/m^2, q 21 days) followed by paclitaxel ($T=125$ mg/m^2) given every 3 weeks for 4 cycles (Group 1) or the same chemotherapy with weekly trastuzumab ($H=4$ mg/kg loading dose, than 2 mg/kg weekly) for 52 weeks starting with the paclitaxel (Group 2). The protocol was later amended to allow weekly paclitaxel similar to the N9831 trial.

The N9831 trial randomized 3,505 HER2+ (IHC 3+ or HER2 amplified by FISH), axillary node-positive (the protocol was amended at a later point to include high-risk node-negative (tumor size greater than 2 cm ER + or >1 cm if ER-)) patients into three groups: The control group, Group A, received 4 cycles of AC followed by weekly T (80 mg/m^2) for 12 weeks; Group B received 4 cycles of AC followed by 12 weekly doses of T followed by sequential weekly trastuzumab for 52 weeks; and Group C received 4 cycles of AC, followed by 12 weekly doses of T concomitantly with weekly trastuzumab which would be continued for 40 more weeks after completion of paclitaxel. The combined analysis grouped the control groups (Group 1 and Group A from B31 and N9831, respectively) and compared them to Group 2 and Group C from B31 and N9831, respectively. Since there was no group in the B31 trial that evaluated sequential trastuzumab, N9831's Group B was not included in the combined analysis.

Patients in both studies were excluded if they had any history of coronary disease, arrhythmias, cardiomegaly, CHF, or cardiomyopathy or required medications for angina pectoris or valvular heart disease. Furthermore, in order to ascertain any compromise in left ventricular ejection fraction (LVEF), multiple-gated acquisition scanning (MUGA) and echocardiography were obtained (B31 used MUGA scanning only) at treatment initiation and every 3 months until completion of the treatment.

Both trials were terminated early by the independent data-monitoring committee based on the significant benefits trastuzumab added compared to the control arm of chemotherapy. The primary endpoint, DFS, was reached, and at a median follow-up of 2 years, there was a statistically significant reduction in recurrence of 52 % ($p<0.0001$) with an absolute distant recurrence in the trastuzumab-containing arm at 3 and 4 years of 8.8 % and 15.9 %, respectively. The OS was improved by a third (HR, 0.67, $p=0.015$). The absolute survival difference was 2.5 % (94.3 % versus 91.7 %) at 3 years and 4.8 % (91.4 % versus 86.6 %) at 4 years. Interestingly, brain metastases were more commonly seen as a first site of recurrence in the trastuzumab-treated group compared to the control. Possible explanations for the latter observation include delayed failures at local sites compared to distant sites and the limitation that trastuzumab has in crossing the blood-brain barrier [32, 33].

The incidence of symptomatic CHF (New York Heart Association [NYHA] class III or IV) or other cardiac-related deaths at 3 years in the B31 study was 0.8 % in the control group compared to 4.1 % in the trastuzumab-treated group. Additionally, 14 % of trastuzumab-treated patients had to discontinue therapy secondary to asymptomatic decreases in LVEF, whereas 4 % stopped secondary to symptomatic cardiotoxicity [11]. In the N9831 trial, the 3-year cumulative incidence of NYHA class III or class IV CHF was 2.9 % in the trastuzumab-treated group compared to 0 % in the control group. Interestingly, interstitial pneumonitis, albeit rare, occurred more commonly in the trastuzumab-treated group compared with the control. Patients with stage I–IIA breast cancer who required radiation therapy did not have any increase incidence of radiation adverse events when radiation was given concurrently with trastuzumab [11]. The combined analysis revealed the significant benefit in the reduction of recurrence and death.

An unplanned interim analysis revealed that concurrent use of trastuzumab with paclitaxel was more effective than sequential use in both DFS and OS [34].

These two trials were recently updated for a final analysis [35]. At a median follow-up of 8.4 years, DFS was 73.7 % in the trastuzumab arm compared with 62.2 % in the chemotherapy arm (HR, 0.60; $p<0.0001$). The OS was again significantly better in the trastuzumab arm (84.0 % versus 75.2 % respectively; HR, 0.63; $p<0.0001$), with the survival benefit noted to be of similar magnitude in the ER + and the ER– subgroup of patients.

Herceptin Adjuvant (HERA) Trial

Another large, phase III international, multicenter trial, the HERA trial, conducted by the Breast International Group (BIG), sequenced trastuzumab after primary surgery and after a minimum of 4 cycles of adjuvant or neoadjuvant chemotherapy [36]. A total of 5,102 HER2+ patients with early-stage breast cancer were randomized, to receive trastuzumab for 1 or 2 years versus observation alone. If randomized to receive trastuzumab, patients received an initial dose of 8 mg/kg followed by maintenance doses of 6 mg/kg every 3 weeks for either 1 or 2 years. All eligible patients were required to have node-positive disease or, if node negative, a tumor diameter of >1 cm. Cardiac monitoring via MUGA or ECHO was done at baseline and 3, 6, 12, 18, 24, 30, 36, and 60 months after randomization. Trastuzumab was stopped in any patient with LVEF ≤45 % or who developed a 10 % absolute decrease in their baseline LVEF and below 50 %. Trastuzumab was permanently discontinued if the LVEF did not return to above LLN within 3 weeks.

At a median follow-up of 8 years and 734 DFS events, the final analysis was recently presented [37]. This analysis was complicated by the fact that 885 of the 1698 patients assigned to the observation group elected to cross over to trastuzumab after the initial results of the trial were presented. However, in the intention-to-treat analysis, there was a significant risk reduction of 24 % (HR, 0.76; $p<0.0001$) in DFS and an identical reduction in OS (HR, 0.76; $p=0.0005$). The benefit of 1 year of trastuzumab was seen in both HR + and HR– patients.

An analysis comparing both trastuzumab arms did not show any additional benefit with 2 years of trastuzumab compared with 1 year. The DFS in the 2-year arm was 75.8 % compared with 76.0 % in the 1-year arm (HR, 0.99; $p=0.86$). The lack of benefit was seen in both the HR + and HR– subgroups. Similarly there was no benefit in OS (86.4 % in the 2 year arm versus 87.6 % in the 1 year arm; HR, 1.05; $p=0.63$).

The incidence of cardiac toxicity was increased with the use of trastuzumab and was even higher in the 2-year arm. More specifically, the incidence of a significant decrease in the ejection fraction (EF) was 0.9 % in the observation arm, 4.1 % in the 1-year trastuzumab arm, and 7.2 % in the 2-year trastuzumab arm.

The HERA trial evaluated the use of sequential trastuzumab in order to circumvent added cardiotoxicity of combining anthracycline with trastuzumab as well as to determine the optimal duration of trastuzumab therapy. Sequential therapy appears to improve DFS by 24 %. Cardiotoxicity was lower than seen in the joint analysis [11, 36]. There are multiple reasons for the lower incidence of cardiotoxicity including more frequent monitoring, different modalities of monitoring, sequential therapy, as well as fewer patients exposed to anthracycline therapy. The results of the HERA trial clearly confirm the benefit of trastuzumab in patients with HER2+ early-stage breast cancer and demonstrate that durations of trastuzumab beyond 1 year confer no additional clinical benefit.

Breast Cancer International Research Group (BCIRG) 006

The BCIRG initiated a phase III, multicenter trial to evaluate the adjuvant use of trastuzumab concurrently with a non-anthracycline chemotherapy regimen after multiple phase II trials confirmed the feasibility of this approach [12]. The BCIRG 006 is a randomized trial of 3,222 HER2+ patients (FISH only) with axillary lymph node-positive or high-risk lymph node-negative (tumor size >2 cm, ER/PR negative, histologic and/or nuclear grade 2–3, or age <35) breast cancer. The two arms were randomized to adjuvant AC followed by docetaxel (D, 100 mg/m^2 q 21 days for 4 cycles) with or without trastuzumab (H, weekly during chemotherapy and then every 21 days), while the third arm included docetaxel and carboplatin (DCarbo) (D, 75 mg/m^2; Carbo (AUC of 6 every 3 weeks × 6) with H for 1 year). At a median follow-up of 65 months, the DFS was 75 % in the patients receiving AC-D, 84 % in the patient receiving AC-DH (HR, 0.64; $p<0.001$), and 81 % in patients receiving DCarboH (HR, 0.75; $p=0.04$). OS was 87 %, 92 % (HR, 0.63; $p<0.001$), and 91 % (HR, 0.77; $p=0.04$), respectively. Although there was no statistically significant difference between either trastuzumab arms, the study was not powered to detect equivalence between these two regimens.

The BCIRG 006 results were similar to the combined analysis in highlighting the benefit from adjuvant trastuzumab [11], showing that non-anthracycline chemotherapy given concurrently with trastuzumab was effective [12]. The incidence of CHF in the two trastuzumab-containing regimens was higher in the group receiving AC-DH (2.0 %) than in the AC-D group (0.7 %) or the TCH group (0.4 %). The difference in rates of CHF between the two trastuzumab-containing regimens significantly favored DCarboH over AC-D plus trastuzumab ($p<0.001$). There was no significant difference in the incidence of leukemia between arms with six cases seen in the AC-D arm and one each for AC-DH and DCarboH.

PACS-04 Trial

This trial evaluated the role of trastuzumab in women with early-stage, HER2+, lymph node-positive breast cancer [38]. A total of 528 patients were randomized to trastuzumab or observation. This trial had a second randomization to chemotherapy with FEC100 for 6 cycles versus epirubicin (75 mg/m^2) and docetaxel (75 mg/m^2) for 6 cycles. The primary endpoint of the trial was DFS. Trastuzumab started after chemotherapy and radiation therapy. At 47 months of median follow-up, patients on the trastuzumab arm had a nonsignificant 14 % reduction in the risk of relapse (HR, 0.86; $p=0.41$), with no significant difference in OS (HR, 1.27). The incidence of CHF was low (1.7 %) in the trastuzumab arm, and the two regimens overall were well tolerated. Although this is the only reported trial that does not show a benefit from adjuvant trastuzumab, the number of patients included is smaller than the other trials and the sequencing of chemotherapy and trastuzumab may be another plausible explanation for the lack of benefit.

FINher Trial

The FINher (FINl and Herceptin) trial examined whether an abbreviated course of trastuzumab was effective [39]. The FINher trial included patients with early-stage breast cancer (axillary node positive or tumor >2 cm with negative axillary nodes and negative PR). A total of 232 HER2+ patients were randomized to receive either adjuvant docetaxel (100 mg/m^2) every 3 weeks for 3 cycles or vinorelbine on days 1, 8, and 15 of 21-day cycle for 3 cycles with or without concurrent weekly trastuzumab (4 mg/kg loading dose, then 2 mg/kg weekly) for 9 weeks. All patients then received fluorouracil (600 mg/m^2), epirubicin (60 mg/m^2), and cyclophosphamide (600 mg/m^2) (FEC, q 21 days for 18 weeks for 6 cycles after their initial therapy). After a median follow-up of 3 years, HER2+ patients treated with trastuzumab had a significantly improved relapse-free survival (RFS) (HR, 0.42; $p=0.01$) and decreased distant recurrence (HR, 0.29; $p=0.002$) compared to HER2+ patients treated without trastuzumab therapy.

Moreover, a nonsignificant improvement in OS was seen in the trastuzumab-treated arm (HR, 0.41; $p=0.07$). The HR for recurrence in HER2-amplified, trastuzumab-treated patients did not significantly change with the type of chemotherapy, the number of lymph nodes involved, or the center providing the therapy. The HER2+ patients treated with trastuzumab had a similar survival free of distant DFS at 3 years compared with HER2-negative patients (HR, 1.09; 95 % CI 0.52–2.29; $p=0.82$). As expected, HER2+ patients treated without trastuzumab did worse than HER2-negative patients. There was no decline in LVEF in HER2+ patients treated with

9 weeks of trastuzumab. The short course of trastuzumab therapy was effective in this small sample size and raises the possibility that shorter durations of trastuzumab therapy may ultimately prove as effective, and possibly safer, than a standard 1 year regimen.

Protocol of Herceptin Adjuvant with Reduced Exposure (PHARE) Trial

The goal of the PHARE trial was to evaluate the efficacy of 6 months of adjuvant trastuzumab compared with 1 year of therapy [40]. Patients had to have operable, nonmetastatic HER2+ breast cancer and a ≥1 cm tumor and had received at least four cycles of adjuvant chemotherapy for their breast cancer. After the completion of 6 months of adjuvant trastuzumab, eligible patients were randomized to either stop therapy or continue for a total of 1 year. This trial had a non-inferiority design, and a total of 3,381 patients were randomized. In 2010, the trial was suspended after the data-monitoring committee concluded that the 6-month arm had a trend of more DFS events when compared to the 1-year arm. Although this difference was not statistically significant (HR, 1.28; $p=0.29$), there was a trend showing that the 6-month arm was inferior to the 1-year arm. When analyzing patients according to tumor types, there was a significant difference in the ER- patients favoring the 1-year trastuzumab arm (HR, 1.34; $p=0.037$), whereas there was no significant difference in the ER + patients. These results failed to show that 6 months of trastuzumab is non-inferior to 12 months. Other clinical trials are under way, but until further data is available, the results from the PHARE trial viewed in combination with the HERA trial suggest that the optimal duration of therapy with trastuzumab remains at 1 year.

Neoadjuvant Clinical Trials with Trastuzumab

Baselga et al. reported the results of the NeoALTTO trial, conducted by the Breast International Group [41]. This was an open-label, phase 3 trial in which 455 patients with HER2+, early-stage breast cancer (tumors >2 cm) were randomly assigned to oral lapatinib (1500 mg daily), intravenous trastuzumab (standard dose), or a combination of both agents (lapatinib 1000 mg/day plus standard trastuzumab dosing). Lapatinib is an oral, dual HER2 and EGFR tyrosine kinase inhibitor (TKI) which has demonstrated preclinical and clinical activity in HER2+ breast cancer [42–45]. The anti-HER2 therapy was administered alone for the first 6 weeks at which point weekly paclitaxel was added to the assigned anti-HER2 therapy for an additional 12 weeks followed by definitive surgery.

Following surgery, patients received adjuvant therapy along with the same anti-HER2 therapy as assigned preoperatively for a total of 52 weeks of anti-HER2 therapy. The primary endpoint of the study was the pathologic complete response (pCR) rate in the breast. The pCR rate was significantly higher in the group of patients receiving both lapatinib and trastuzumab (51.3 %) versus trastuzumab alone (29.5 %) or lapatinib alone (24.7 %). Additionally, the difference between trastuzumab alone and lapatinib alone was statistically significant, in favor of trastuzumab. Although there was no difference in cardiac events between the treatment arms, the use of lapatinib alone or in combination with trastuzumab was associated with greater frequency of grade 3 diarrhea and liver enzyme abnormalities than those receiving trastuzumab alone. This study suggests that dual HER2 therapy was superior to either anti-HER2 therapy alone, yet trastuzumab was superior to lapatinib as a monotherapy approach.

The GeparQuinto GBG 44, a German Breast Group study, is a phase 3 trial in which 620 patients with HER2+ operable, or locally advanced, breast cancer were randomized to receive neoadjuvant treatment with 4 cycles of epirubicin/cyclophosphamide (EC), every 3 weeks, followed by 4 cycles of docetaxel (T), every 3 weeks, with either concurrent, standard dose, trastuzumab (H) or lapatinib (L) [46]. The primary endpoint of the study was pCR in both the breast and axillary lymph nodes at the time of surgery. The pCR rate for those patients receiving chemotherapy plus H was 30.3 % versus 22.7 % for those receiving chemotherapy plus L (HR, 0.68, $p=0.04$). There was a greater incidence of dyspnea and edema in patients receiving chemotherapy/trastuzumab, while patients receiving chemotherapy/L had a greater incidence of skin rash and diarrhea. A total of 33.1 % of patients receiving chemotherapy/L discontinued treatment due to toxicity compared with 14 % of patients receiving chemotherapy/H.

Another neoadjuvant clinical trial performed by the MD Anderson group incorporated trastuzumab to an epirubicin-based regimen [47]. A total of 64 patients were included in the trial which was conducted in two phases. Patients were randomized to receive 4 cycles of paclitaxel at 225 mg/m^2 as a 24-h infusion at 3-week intervals, followed by 4 cycles of FEC therapy, which consisted of 500 mg/m^2 fluorouracil on days 1 and 4, 500 mg/m^2 i.v. cyclophosphamide on day 1 only, and 75 mg/m^2 epirubicin on day 1 only. Patients randomized to receive trastuzumab received 4 mg/kg trastuzumab i.v. over 90 min on day 1 of the first cycle of paclitaxel. These patients received 2 mg/kg trastuzumab weekly, administered i.v. over 30 min during the 24 weeks of chemotherapy. pCR for patients receiving trastuzumab was 60 % and 26.3 % in the non-trastuzumab group. Cardiac safety data suggested that even though trastuzumab was given concurrently with epirubicin, there was no cardiac dysfunction. This study is relatively small compared with other neoadjuvant and adjuvant clinical trials. However, the efficacy of the trastuzumab arm and apparent lack of cardiac toxicity provide good preliminary data for using this combination in the clinical setting.

Novel Agents

Novel modalities exist to circumvent resistance to trastuzumab by targeting more than one member of the EGFR family, such as lapatinib. As a monotherapy in early clinical studies, lapatinib was found to be both clinically active and well tolerated in heavily pretreated, HER2-amplified patients with advanced breast cancer [48]. The combination of lapatinib (1,250 mg/m^2 daily for 3 weeks) with capecitabine (1,000 mg/m^2/bid on days 1–14 q 3 weeks) is currently approved for use in metastatic HER2+ breast cancer given its superiority to capecitabine alone (1,250 mg/m^2/bid on days 1–14 q 3 weeks) [42]. A neoadjuvant clinical trial conducted in our institution combining lapatinib to *nab*-paclitaxel for four cycles produced a pathologic complete response rate of 17.9 %, showing it to be an active and well-tolerated regimen [49].

In a review of over 2,800 patients exposed to lapatinib, the incidence of symptomatic declines of LVEF was 1.3 %, and in the majority of cases, it was transient and lapatinib was restarted [50]. An interesting finding was the lower incidence of brain metastases as a site of disease progression, possibly due to lapatinib having a better central nervous penetration compared to trastuzumab. The Adjuvant Lapatinib and/or Trastuzumab Treatment Optimisation (ALTTO) trial has currently completed accrual [51]. This trial randomizes patients with HER2+ early-stage breast cancer to one of four treatment arms: (1) trastuzumab, (2) lapatinib, (3) trastuzumab and lapatinib in combination, and (4) trastuzumab followed by lapatinib. Treatment duration for all arms was 1 year. Standard adjuvant chemotherapy was given in all treatment arms. After recommendations for the Independent Data Monitoring Committee, the lapatinib arm was discontinued due to the finding that the lapatinib alone arm was unlikely to meet the pre-specified criteria of demonstrating non-inferiority to trastuzumab alone with respect to DFS. The other arms continue without any changes.

Given its potential lack of cardiac toxicity and benefit in CNS penetration, adjuvant clinical trials are under way comparing its efficacy to trastuzumab as well as evaluating its combination with trastuzumab. In a phase III clinical trial, 3,161 women with HER2+ early-stage breast cancer who had previously received adjuvant chemotherapy, but not trastuzumab, were randomly assigned (1:1) to receive daily lapatinib (1500 mg) or daily placebo for 12 months [52]. After a median follow-up of 47.4 months in the lapatinib group and 48.3 in the placebo group, there was a nonsignificant difference in DFS favoring the lapatinib arm (HR, 0.83; $p=0.053$). Central review of HER2 status showed that only 2,490 (79 %) of the randomized women were HER2+. When the data was analyzed for women with centrally confirmed HER2+ breast cancer, the lapatinib arm had a significant improvement in DFS compared with placebo (HR, 0.82; $p=0.04$).

Another novel agent, pertuzumab (Omnitarg™, Genentech, San Francisco, CA, USA), is a humanized monoclonal antibody directed against heterodimerization of HER2 and HER3 [53]. Known as a dimerization inhibitor, pertuzumab binds to HER2 at a different site than trastuzumab and near the dimerization domain and blocks the ability of the receptor to dimerize with other receptors of the EGFR family. In a large randomized phase III clinical trial in metastatic HER2+ breast cancer, the combination of pertuzumab trastuzumab and docetaxel produced superior results compared with trastuzumab and docetaxel [53]. This leads to the approval of pertuzumab, as a first-line therapy for metastatic HER2+ breast cancer. Phase III clinical trials are under way in early-stage breast cancer combining pertuzumab and trastuzumab in patients with HER2+ breast cancer.

The phase II NeoSphere trial evaluated neoadjuvant trastuzumab/docetaxel, pertuzumab/trastuzumab/docetaxel, pertuzumab/trastuzumab, and docetaxel/pertuzumab in HER2+ stage II or III breast cancer ($N=417$) [54]. The pCR rate was 45.8 % with pertuzumab/trastuzumab/docetaxel, significantly higher than the 29.0 % rate with trastuzumab/docetaxel alone ($p=0.0141$); conversely, the 16.8 % pCR rate with pertuzumab/trastuzumab was significantly lower than that with trastuzumab/docetaxel ($p=0.0198$). Pertuzumab/trastuzumab/docetaxel was associated with a grade ≥3 toxicity profile primarily consisting of neutropenia, febrile neutropenia, leukopenia, and diarrhea (in 45 %, 8 %, 5 %, and 6 % of patients, respectively); with trastuzumab/docetaxel alone these were observed in 57 %, 7 %, 12 %, and 4 %, respectively. Grade ≥3 toxicity with pertuzumab/trastuzumab was limited to neutropenia and drug hypersensitivity (1 % and 2 %, respectively).

Targeting Other Pathways

Angiogenesis Inhibitors

Bevacizumab is a humanized monoclonal antibody that binds VEGF-A and thus is an indirect inhibitor of angiogenesis. Trials in metastatic breast cancer have shown an improvement in progression-free survival (PFS) with the combination of bevacizumab and chemotherapy compared with chemotherapy alone [55, 56]. However, these trials have not shown a benefit in OS. Given the initial enthusiasm behind bevacizumab, several randomized clinical trials were initiated in early-stage breast cancer. Although most of these trials have not matured, a clinical trial in triple-negative breast cancer was recently presented [57]. The Bevacizumab Adjuvant Therapy in Triple-Negative Breast Cancer (BEATRICE) trial randomized patients with triple-negative early-stage breast cancer to 4–8 cycles of chemotherapy with or without bevacizumab. Bevacizumab was administered for a total of 1 year. The primary endpoint was invasive DFS (IDFS) with secondary endpoints of DFS, OS, and safety. A total of 2,591 patients were randomized and with a median follow-up of 32 months; IDFS was similar between the two arms (82.7 % in the non-bevacizumab arm and 83.7 % in the bevacizumab arm; HR, 0.87; $p=0.18$). OS was also similar in the two arms (HR, 0.84; $p=0.23$). There was a small but increased risk of class III and IV heart failure in the bevacizumab arms. The results of this clinical trial show that there is no benefit for the use of bevacizumab in the adjuvant therapy of triple-negative breast cancers.

State of the Art: 2013 Recommendations

- Pathology reports should include HER2 status assessed by IHC and/or FISH.
- Patients with tumors >6 mm, HER2+ (regardless of nodal status) should be considered for anti-HER2-based therapy.
- The standard duration of adjuvant trastuzumab is 1 year.
- Patients with HER2+ breast cancer who are candidates for preoperative systemic therapy should have trastuzumab incorporated into their regimen (Table 25.2).

Table 25.2 Preferred adjuvant and neoadjuvant trastuzumab-containing regimens according to the NCCN guidelines [58]

Regimen	AC→T+H	DCarboH	D+H→FEC	AC→D+H	T+H→CEF+H
Preferred	Yes	Yes			
Adjuvant/neoadjuvant	Both	Both	Both	Both	Neoadjuvant

A doxorubicin, *C* cyclophosphamide, *T* paclitaxel, *H* trastuzumab, *D* docetaxel, *E* epirubicin, *F* 5- fluorouracil

References

1. Siegel R, Naishadham D, Jemal A. Cancer statistics, 2013. CA Cancer J Clin. 2013;63:11–30.
2. Reese DM, Slamon DJ. HER-2/neu signal transduction in human breast and ovarian cancer. Stem Cells. 1997;15:1–8.
3. Slamon DJ, Godolphin W, Jones LA, Holt JA, Wong SG, Keith DE, Levin WJ, Stuart SG, Udove J, Ullrich A. Studies of the HER-2/neu proto-oncogene in human breast and ovarian cancer. Science. 1989;244:707–12.
4. Pegram MD, Pauletti G, Slamon DJ. HER-2/neu as a predictive marker of response to breast cancer therapy. Breast Cancer Res Treat. 1998;52:65–77.
5. Seshadri R, Firgaira FA, Horsfall DJ, McCaul K, Setlur V, Kitchen P. Clinical significance of HER-2/neu oncogene amplification in primary breast cancer. The South Australian Breast Cancer Study Group. J Clin Oncol. 1993;11:1936–42.
6. Carlomagno C, Perrone F, Gallo C, De Laurentiis M, Lauria R, Morabito A, Pettinato G, Panico L, D'Antonio A, Bianco AR, De Placido S. c-erb B2 overexpression decreases the benefit of adjuvant tamoxifen in early-stage breast cancer without axillary lymph node metastases. J Clin Oncol. 1996;14:2702–8.
7. Pietras RJ, Arboleda J, Reese DM, Wongvipat N, Pegram MD, Ramos L, Gorman CM, Parker MG, Sliwkowski MX, Slamon DJ. HER-2 tyrosine kinase pathway targets estrogen receptor and promotes hormone-independent growth in human breast cancer cells. Oncogene. 1995;10:2435–46.
8. Pritchard KI, Shepherd LE, O'Malley FP, Andrulis IL, Tu D, Bramwell VH, Levine MN. HER2 and responsiveness of breast cancer to adjuvant chemotherapy. N Engl J Med. 2006;354:2103–11.
9. Tetu B, Brisson J. Prognostic significance of HER-2/neu oncoprotein expression in node-positive breast cancer. The influence of the pattern of immunostaining and adjuvant therapy. Cancer. 1994;73:2359–65.
10. Tiwari RK, Borgen PI, Wong GY, Cordon-Cardo C, Osborne MP. HER-2/neu amplification and overexpression in primary human breast cancer is associated with early metastasis. Anticancer Res. 1992;12:419–25.
11. Romond EH, Perez EA, Bryant J, Suman VJ, Geyer Jr CE, Davidson NE, Tan-Chiu E, Martino S, Paik S, Kaufman PA, Swain SM, Pisansky TM, Fehrenbacher L, Kutteh LA, Vogel VG, Visscher DW, Yothers G, Jenkins RB, Brown AM, Dakhil SR, Mamounas EP, Lingle WL, Klein PM, Ingle JN, Wolmark N. Trastuzumab plus adjuvant chemotherapy for operable HER2-positive breast cancer. N Engl J Med. 2005;353:1673–84.
12. Slamon D, Eiermann W, Robert N, Pienkowski T, Martin M, Press M, Mackey J, Glaspy J, Chan A, Pawlicki M, Pinter T, Valero V, Liu MC, Sauter G, von Minckwitz G, Visco F, Bee V, Buyse M, Bendahmane B, Tabah-Fisch I, Lindsay MA, Riva A, Crown J. Adjuvant trastuzumab in HER2-positive breast cancer. N Engl J Med. 2011;365:1273–83.
13. Carter P, Presta L, Gorman CM, Ridgway JB, Henner D, Wong WL, Rowland AM, Kotts C, Carver ME, Shepard HM. Humanization of an anti-p185HER2 antibody for human cancer therapy. Proc Natl Acad Sci U S A. 1992;89:4285–9.
14. Albanell J, Codony J, Rovira A, Mellado B, Gascon P. Mechanism of action of anti-HER2 monoclonal antibodies: scientific update on trastuzumab and 2C4. Adv Exp Med Biol. 2003;532:253–68.
15. Nahta R, Esteva FJ. Herceptin: mechanisms of action and resistance. Cancer Lett. 2006;232:123–38.
16. Nagata Y, Lan KH, Zhou X, Tan M, Esteva FJ, Sahin AA, Klos KS, Li P, Monia BP, Nguyen NT, Hortobagyi GN, Hung MC, Yu D. PTEN activation contributes to tumor inhibition by trastuzumab, and loss of PTEN predicts trastuzumab resistance in patients. Cancer Cell. 2004;6:117–27.
17. Henson ES, Hu X, Gibson SB. Herceptin sensitizes ErbB2-overexpressing cells to apoptosis by reducing antiapoptotic Mcl-1 expression. Clin Cancer Res. 2006;12:845–53.
18. Izumi Y, Xu L, di Tomaso E, Fukumura D, Jain RK. Tumour biology: herceptin acts as an anti-angiogenic cocktail. Nature. 2002;416:279–80.
19. Cooley S, Burns LJ, Repka T, Miller JS. Natural killer cell cytotoxicity of breast cancer targets is enhanced by two distinct mechanisms of antibody-dependent cellular cytotoxicity against LFA-3 and HER2/neu. Exp Hematol. 1999;27:1533–41.
20. Perez EA, Press MF, Dueck AC, Jenkins RB, Kim C, Chen B, Villalobos I, Paik S, Buyse M, Wiktor AE, Meyer R, Finnigan M, Zujewski J, Shing M, Stern HM, Lingle WL, Reinholz MM, Slamon DJ. Immunohistochemistry and fluorescence in situ hybridization assessment of HER2 in clinical trials of adjuvant therapy for breast cancer (NCCTG N9831, BCIRG 006, and BCIRG 005). Breast Cancer Res Treat. 2013;138:99–108.
21. Wolff AC, Hammond ME, Schwartz JN, Hagerty KL, Allred DC, Cote RJ, Dowsett M, Fitzgibbons PL, Hanna WM, Langer A, McShane LM, Paik S, Pegram MD, Perez EA, Press MF, Rhodes A, Sturgeon C, Taube SE, Tubbs R, Vance GH, van de Vijver M, Wheeler TM, Hayes DF. American Society of Clinical Oncology/College of American Pathologists guideline

recommendations for human epidermal growth factor receptor 2 testing in breast cancer. J Clin Oncol. 2007;25:118–45.
22. Vogel CL, Cobleigh MA, Tripathy D, Gutheil JC, Harris LN, Fehrenbacher L, Slamon DJ, Murphy M, Novotny WF, Burchmore M, Shak S, Stewart SJ, Press M. Efficacy and safety of trastuzumab as a single agent in first-line treatment of HER2-overexpressing metastatic breast cancer. J Clin Oncol. 2002;20:719–26.
23. Slamon DJ, Leyland-Jones B, Shak S, Fuchs H, Paton V, Bajamonde A, Fleming T, Eiermann W, Wolter J, Pegram M, Baselga J, Norton L. Use of chemotherapy plus a monoclonal antibody against HER2 for metastatic breast cancer that overexpresses HER2. N Engl J Med. 2001;344:783–92.
24. Pegram MD, Lopez A, Konecny G, Slamon DJ. Trastuzumab and chemotherapeutics: drug interactions and synergies. Semin Oncol. 2000;27:21–5.
25. Pegram MD, Konecny GE, O'Callaghan C, Beryt M, Pietras R, Slamon DJ. Rational combinations of trastuzumab with chemotherapeutic drugs used in the treatment of breast cancer. J Natl Cancer Inst. 2004;96:739–49.
26. Esteva FJ, Valero V, Booser D, Guerra LT, Murray JL, Pusztai L, Cristofanilli M, Arun B, Esmaeli B, Fritsche HA, Sneige N, Smith TL, Hortobagyi GN. Phase II study of weekly docetaxel and trastuzumab for patients with HER-2-overexpressing metastatic breast cancer. J Clin Oncol. 2002;20:1800–8.
27. Marty M, Cognetti F, Maraninchi D, Snyder R, Mauriac L, Tubiana-Hulin M, Chan S, Grimes D, Anton A, Lluch A, Kennedy J, O'Byrne K, Conte P, Green M, Ward C, Mayne K, Extra JM. Randomized phase II trial of the efficacy and safety of trastuzumab combined with docetaxel in patients with human epidermal growth factor receptor 2-positive metastatic breast cancer administered as first-line treatment: the M77001 study group. J Clin Oncol. 2005;23:4265–74.
28. Nabholtz JM, Gligorov J. Docetaxel/trastuzumab combination therapy for the treatment of breast cancer. Expert Opin Pharmacother. 2005;6:1555–64.
29. Schaller G, Fuchs I, Gonsch T, Weber J, Kleine-Tebbe A, Klare P, Hindenburg HJ, Lakner V, Hinke A, Bangemann N. Phase II study of capecitabine plus trastuzumab in human epidermal growth factor receptor 2 overexpressing metastatic breast cancer pretreated with anthracyclines or taxanes. J Clin Oncol. 2007;25:3246–50.
30. Perez EA, Suman VJ, Rowland KM, Ingle JN, Salim M, Loprinzi CL, Flynn PJ, Mailliard JA, Kardinal CG, Krook JE, Thrower AR, Visscher DW, Jenkins RB. Two concurrent phase II trials of paclitaxel/carboplatin/trastuzumab (weekly or every-3-week schedule) as first-line therapy in women with HER2-overexpressing metastatic breast cancer: NCCTG study 983252. Clin Breast Cancer. 2005;6:425–32.
31. Robert N, Leyland-Jones B, Asmar L, Belt R, Ilegbodu D, Loesch D, Raju R, Valentine E, Sayre R, Cobleigh M, Albain K, McCullough C, Fuchs L, Slamon D. Randomized phase III study of trastuzumab, paclitaxel, and carboplatin compared with trastuzumab and paclitaxel in women with HER-2-overexpressing metastatic breast cancer. J Clin Oncol. 2006;24:2786–92.
32. Bendell JC, Domchek SM, Burstein HJ, Harris L, Younger J, Kuter I, Bunnell C, Rue M, Gelman R, Winer E. Central nervous system metastases in women who receive trastuzumab-based therapy for metastatic breast carcinoma. Cancer. 2003;97:2972–7.
33. Burstein HJ, Lieberman G, Slamon DJ, Winer EP, Klein P. Isolated central nervous system metastases in patients with HER2-overexpressing advanced breast cancer treated with first-line trastuzumab-based therapy. Ann Oncol. 2005;16:1772–7.
34. Perez EA, Suman VJ, Davidson NE, Gralow JR, Kaufman PA, Visscher DW, Chen B, Ingle JN, Dakhil SR, Zujewski J, Moreno-Aspitia A, Pisansky TM, Jenkins RB. Sequential versus concurrent trastuzumab in adjuvant chemotherapy for breast cancer. J Clin Oncol. 2011;29:4491–7.
35. Romond E, Suman VJ, Jeong J-H, Sledge Jr GW, Geyer CE, Martino S, Rastogi P, Gralow JR, Swain SM, Winer E, Colon-Otero G, Hudis C, Paik S, Davidson NE, Mamounas EP, Zujewski JA, Wolmark N, Perez EA. S5-5 Trastuzumab plus adjuvant chemotherapy for HER2-positive breast cancer: Final planned joint analysis of overall survival (OS) from NSABP B-31 and NCCTG N9831. Cancer Res. 2012;72(24 Suppl):105s.
36. Piccart-Gebhart MJ, Procter M, Leyland-Jones B, Goldhirsch A, Untch M, Smith I, Gianni L, Baselga J, Bell R, Jackisch C, Cameron D, Dowsett M, Barrios CH, Steger G, Huang CS, Andersson M, Inbar M, Lichinitser M, Lang I, Nitz U, Iwata H, Thomssen C, Lohrisch C, Suter TM, Ruschoff J, Suto T, Greatorex V, Ward C, Straehle C, McFadden E, Dolci MS, Gelber RD. Trastuzumab after adjuvant chemotherapy in HER2-positive breast cancer. N Engl J Med. 2005;353:1659–72.
37. Goldhirsch A, Piccart-Gebhart M, Procter M, de Azambuja E, Weber HA, Untch M, Smith I, Gianni L, Jackisch C, Cameron D, Bell R, Dowsett M, Gelber RD, Leyland-Jones B, Baselga J. S5-2. HERA TRIAL: 2 years versus 1 year of trastuzumab after adjuvant chemotherapy in women with HER2-positive early breast cancer at 8 years of median follow up. Cancer Res. 2013;72(24 suppl):103s.
38. Spielmann M, Roche H, Delozier T, Canon JL, Romieu G, Bourgeois H, Extra JM, Serin D, Kerbrat P, Machiels JP, Lortholary A, Orfeuvre H, Campone M, Hardy-Bessard AC, Coudert B, Maerevoet M, Piot G, Kramar A, Martin AL, Penault-Llorca F. Trastuzumab for patients with axillary-node-positive breast cancer: results of the FNCLCC-PACS 04 trial. J Clin Oncol. 2009;27:6129–34.
39. Joensuu H, Kellokumpu-Lehtinen PL, Bono P, Alanko T, Kataja V, Asola R, Utriainen T, Kokko R, Hemminki A, Tarkkanen M, Turpeenniemi-Hujanen T, Jyrkkio S,

Flander M, Helle L, Ingalsuo S, Johansson K, Jaaskelainen AS, Pajunen M, Rauhala M, Kaleva-Kerola J, Salminen T, Leinonen M, Elomaa I, Isola J. Adjuvant docetaxel or vinorelbine with or without trastuzumab for breast cancer. N Engl J Med. 2006; 354:809–20.
40. Pivot X, Romieu G, Bonnefoi H, Pierga J-Y, Kerbrat P, Guastalla J-P, Lortholary A, Espie M, Fumoleau P, Khayat D, Pauporte I, Kramar A. S5-3. PHARE Trial results of subset analysis comparing 6 to 12 months of trastuzumab in adjuvant early breast cancer. Cancer Res. 2013;72(24 suppl):105s.
41. Baselga J, Bradbury I, Eidtmann H, Di Cosimo S, de Azambuja E, Aura C, Gomez H, Dinh P, Fauria K, van Dooren V, Goldhirsch G, Chang TW, Horvath Z, Coccia-Portugal M, Domont J, Tseng LM, Kunz G, Sonz JH, Semiglazov V, Lerzo G, Palacova M, Probachai V, Pusztai L, Untch M, Gelber RD, Piccart-Gebhart M. Lapatinib with trastuzumab for HER2-positive early breast cancer (NeoALTTO): a randomised, open-label, multicentre, phase 3 trial. Lancet. 2012;379:633–40.
42. Geyer CE, Forster J, Lindquist D, Chan S, Romieu CG, Pienkowski T, Jagiello-Gruszfeld A, Crown J, Chan A, Kaufman B, Skarlos D, Campone M, Davidson N, Berger M, Oliva C, Rubin SD, Stein S, Cameron D. Lapatinib plus capecitabine for HER2-positive advanced breast cancer. N Engl J Med. 2006;355: 2733–43.
43. Gomez HL, Doval DC, Chavez MA, Ang PC, Aziz Z, Nag S, Ng C, Franco SX, Chow LW, Arbushites MC, Casey MA, Berger MS, Stein SH, Sledge GW. Efficacy and safety of lapatinib as first-line therapy for ErbB2-amplified locally advanced or metastatic breast cancer. J Clin Oncol. 2008;26:2999–3005.
44. Johnston S, Pippen Jr J, Pivot X, Lichinitser M, Sadeghi S, Dieras V, Gomez HL, Romieu G, Manikhas A, Kennedy MJ, Press MF, Maltzman J, Florance A, O'Rourke L, Oliva C, Stein S, Pegram M. Lapatinib combined with letrozole versus letrozole and placebo as first-line therapy for postmenopausal hormone receptor-positive metastatic breast cancer. J Clin Oncol. 2009;27:5538–46.
45. Zhou Y, Li S, Hu YP, Wang J, Hauser J, Conway AN, Vinci MA, Humphrey L, Zborowska E, Willson JK, Brattain MG. Blockade of EGFR and ErbB2 by the novel dual EGFR and ErbB2 tyrosine kinase inhibitor GW572016 sensitizes human colon carcinoma GEO cells to apoptosis. Cancer Res. 2006;66:404–11.
46. Untch M, Loibl S, Bischoff J, Eidtmann H, Kaufmann M, Blohmer JU, Hilfrich J, Strumberg D, Fasching PA, Kreienberg R, Tesch H, Hanusch C, Gerber B, Rezai M, Jackisch C, Huober J, Kuhn T, Nekljudova V, von Minckwitz G. Lapatinib versus trastuzumab in combination with neoadjuvant anthracycline-taxane-based chemotherapy (GeparQuinto, GBG 44): a randomised phase 3 trial. Lancet Oncol. 2012;13:135–44.
47. Buzdar AU, Valero V, Ibrahim NK, Francis D, Broglio KR, Theriault RL, Pusztai L, Green MC, Singletary SE, Hunt KK, Sahin AA, Esteva F, Symmans WF, Ewer MS, Buchholz TA, Hortobagyi GN. Neoadjuvant therapy with paclitaxel followed by 5-fluorouracil, epirubicin, and cyclophosphamide chemotherapy and concurrent trastuzumab in human epidermal growth factor receptor 2-positive operable breast cancer: an update of the initial randomized study population and data of additional patients treated with the same regimen. Clin Cancer Res. 2007;13:228–33.
48. Burris III HA, Hurwitz HI, Dees EC, Dowlati A, Blackwell KL, O'Neil B, Marcom PK, Ellis MJ, Overmoyer B, Jones SF, Harris JL, Smith DA, Koch KM, Stead A, Mangum S, Spector NL. Phase I safety, pharmacokinetics, and clinical activity study of lapatinib (GW572016), a reversible dual inhibitor of epidermal growth factor receptor tyrosine kinases, in heavily pretreated patients with metastatic carcinomas. J Clin Oncol. 2005;23:5305–13.
49. Kaklamani VG, Siziopikou K, Scholtens D, Lacouture M, Gordon J, Uthe R, Meservey C, Hansen N, Khan SA, Jeruss JS, Bethke K, Cianfrocca M, Rosen S, Von Roenn J, Wayne J, Parimi V, Jovanovic B, Gradishar W. Pilot neoadjuvant trial in HER2 positive breast cancer with combination of nab-paclitaxel and lapatinib. Breast Cancer Res Treat. 2011;132: 833–42.
50. Perez EA, Koehler M, Byrne J, Preston AJ, Rappold E, Ewer MS. Cardiac safety of lapatinib: pooled analysis of 3689 patients enrolled in clinical trials. Mayo Clin Proc. 2008;83:679–86.
51. ALTTO (Adjuvant Lapatinib And/Or Trastuzumab Treatment Optimisation) Study; BIG 2-06/N063D. 2013. http://www.cancer.gov/clinicaltrials/search/view?cdrid=558836&version=healthprofessional.
52. Goss PE, Smith IE, O'Shaughnessy J, Ejlertsen B, Kaufmann M, Boyle F, Buzdar AU, Fumoleau P, Gradishar W, Martin M, Moy B, Piccart-Gebhart M, Pritchard KI, Lindquist D, Chavarri-Guerra Y, Aktan G, Rappold E, Williams LS, Finkelstein DM. Adjuvant lapatinib for women with early-stage HER2-positive breast cancer: a randomised, controlled, phase 3 trial. Lancet Oncol. 2013;14:88–96.
53. Baselga J, Cortes J, Kim SB, Im SA, Hegg R, Im YH, Roman L, Pedrini JL, Pienkowski T, Knott A, Clark E, Benyunes MC, Ross G, Swain SM. Pertuzumab plus trastuzumab plus docetaxel for metastatic breast cancer. N Engl J Med. 2012;366:109–19.
54. Gianni L, Pienkowski T, Im YH, Roman L, Tseng LM, Liu MC, Lluch A, Staroslawska E, Haba-Rodriguez J, Im SA, Pedrini JL, Poirier B, Morandi P, Semiglazov V, Srimuninnimit V, Bianchi G, Szado T, Ratnayake J, Ross G, Valagussa P. Efficacy and safety of neoadjuvant pertuzumab and trastuzumab in women with locally advanced, inflammatory, or early HER2-positive breast cancer (NeoSphere): a randomised multicentre, open-label, phase 2 trial. Lancet Oncol. 2012;13:25–32.
55. Miller K, Wang M, Gralow J, Dickler M, Cobleigh M, Perez EA, Shenkier T, Cella D, Davidson NE. Paclitaxel plus bevacizumab versus paclitaxel alone

for metastatic breast cancer. N Engl J Med. 2007; 357:2666–76.

56. Robert NJ, Dieras V, Glaspy J, Brufsky AM, Bondarenko I, Lipatov ON, Perez EA, Yardley DA, Chan SY, Zhou X, Phan SC, O'Shaughnessy J. RIBBON-1: randomized, double-blind, placebo-controlled, phase III trial of chemotherapy with or without bevacizumab for first-line treatment of human epidermal growth factor receptor 2-negative, locally recurrent or metastatic breast cancer. J Clin Oncol. 2011;29:1252–60.

57. Cameron D, Brown J, Dent R, Jackisch C, Mackey J, Pivot X, Steger G, Suter T, Toi M, Parmar M, Bubuteishvili-Pacaud L, Henschel V, Laeufle R, Bell R. S6-5. Primary results of BEATRICE, a randomized phase III trial evaluating adjuvant bevacizumab-containing therapy in triple-negative breast cancer. Cancer Res. 2013;72(24 Supp):55s.

58. NCCN Clinical practice guidelines in Oncology. NCCN, 2008. http://www.nccn.org/professionals/physician_gls/pdf/breast.pdf.

26 External Beam Radiation Therapy

Paul Crossan

Radiation therapy has been used to treat malignancies for well over 100 years. One of the first examples in the literature comes from Emil Grubbe from Chicago, who treated a woman with breast cancer with X-rays in 1896 [1]. Radiation therapy continues to play an instrumental role in the management of the patient with breast cancer, regardless of the overall stage. When administered in an adjuvant setting, radiation dramatically reduces recurrence rates [2, 3] and does so with an acceptable toxicity profile [4] Most importantly, large meta-analysis has shown that irradiation of the breast in the adjuvant setting prolongs survival [5] The goal of this chapter is to highlight the role of radiation therapy in the management of breast cancer.

Basic Radiation Concepts

The therapeutic basis of radiation requires a basic review of atomic substructure, DNA damage, DNA repair processes, and the biologic principles of malignant cells. In most clinical circumstances, radiation therapy takes the form of either high-energy photon beams (X-rays) or electrons generated in a linear accelerator. To create photons, amplified microwaves are used to accelerate electrons along a waveguide where they collide with a target composed of a high atomic number material thereby generating secondary X-rays. These X-rays are then shaped in the head of the machine and directed according to the previously generated plan toward the target tissue [6]. X-rays are penetrating beams that attenuate according to their interaction with the absorbing material but exit the opposite side. Alternatively, electrons, which are the negatively charged subatomic particles surrounding the atomic nucleus, travel a limited distance through the absorption medium. These beams are typically chosen for more superficial applications where limited dose beyond the target is desired. Other subatomic particles used for therapy including protons and neutrons are beyond the scope of this chapter.

Upon entering the body, X-rays impart their energy primarily to the electrons of the tissue. The energy transferred to the electrons increases their energetic state that generates secondary ions [7]. These ions then interact with the primary target of the cell the DNA. Electron beams directly impart their energy on the target molecules and through secondary ionizing events. Most of the DNA damage is in the form of single-strand breaks, base deletions, and base alterations [8]. These DNA aberrations occur both in the normal and malignant cell, but it is the perturbed state of the malignant cell that creates the therapeutic benefit. As the malignant cell has altered cell cycle kinetics, weakened repair mechanisms, and an altered microenvironment, it is more likely to manifest this DNA damage and die by mitotic crisis.

P. Crossan, MD
Department of Radiation Oncology,
Advocate Christ Hospital Medical Center,
4440 W. 95th street, Oak Lawn, IL 60435, USA
e-mail: pcrossa@gmail.com

A.I. Riker (ed.), *Breast Disease: Comprehensive Management*,
DOI 10.1007/978-1-4939-1145-5_26, © Springer Science+Business Media New York 2015

The DNA damage and repair mechanics are the defining biologic processes that dictate the logistics of radiation therapy treatments. The four Rs repair, re-assortment, repopulation, and reoxygenation are the radiobiology terms used to define the cell's response to radiation injury. These processes help to clarify why different treatment fractionation patterns are chosen. Rapid repair of sublethal radiation damage by cells in a relatively resistant phase of mitosis explains the increase in cell population after a radiation treatment. The surviving cells then progress through the cell cycle in a process described as re-assortment. There is then regrowth of the remaining cells termed repopulation [9]. Reoxygenation of hypoxic cells due to death of adjacent aerated cells increases their sensitivity to subsequent radiation. These processes have implications not only for tumor control but also in how normal tissues respond to therapy and the long-term manifestations and therefore risks of treatment. In general, smaller, more frequent doses of radiation are more effective in rapidly dividing cancers and are more likely to cause increased acute toxicities with fewer long-term toxicities. Larger doses are likely to be more effective in more indolent malignancies but also carry a higher risk of permanent injury to surrounding normal tissues [10]. Therefore, it is the radiation oncologist's responsibility to determine the fractionation pattern most appropriate for the given disease and the patient's expected longevity and goals of therapy. Most fractionation patterns originate from historical standards but have continued to evolve through the results obtained from prospective clinical trials.

Breast Conservation

Prior treatment paradigms concentrated on surgical cures. Large clinical trials in the later part of the twentieth century demonstrated that minimal surgery and radiation are an acceptable alternative to mastectomy. The goal of radiation is to eliminate microscopic residual disease and reduce local recurrence rates within the breast.

Table 26.1 Contraindications to breast conservation

Relative	Absolute
Disproportionate tumor to breast size	Pregnancy
Collagen vascular diseases	Multicentric disease
	Scleroderma
	Prior chest wall radiation therapy

Suitability Criteria for Breast Conservation

Most women are candidates for breast-conserving therapy. Like all treatments; however, there are situations where there are relative and absolute contraindications (Table 26.1).

The primary tumor size in proportion to the breast size: The general concept is breast conservation or organ preservation. The size of disease relative to the size of the breast is an important consideration for the surgeon. In cases where the extent of surgery required to perform an adequate lumpectomy exceeds that where a proportional breast can be retained, then consideration of mastectomy should be entertained. The NSABP-B06 [2] study required that patients have a lumpectomy resulting in clear margins and an acceptable cosmetic result. Selected patients who are unwilling to have a mastectomy may be considered for neoadjuvant therapy in an effort to pursue breast conservation [11].

Prior Thoracic Radiation

Patients who may have had mediastinal radiation due to childhood lymphomas are typically not considered candidates for breast conservation, due to the concern regarding repeat treatment to previously irradiated tissues. However, there are single-institution, retrospective series that describe repeat radiation to the breast in these patients with acceptably low rates of morbidity [12, 13]. There are a handful of case series that describe experiences in patients who have had prior breast-conserving radiation and have gone on to receive partial breast radiation for local recurrences with acceptable morbidity and local control [14, 15].

Pregnancy

The implications of the irradiation of a developing fetus are relatively well described and vary according to the gestational age. Early in pregnancy, exposure to radiation yields an all or nothing outcome where either the embryo is sufficiently altered that it is unable to develop into a fetus or it is completely normal. The greatest implications for injury occur during the period of organogenesis where malformations are most likely. Late in pregnancy, radiation is less likely to cause fetal death but may cause microcephaly, impaired cognition, growth retardation, and potential sterility [16]. It is hard to conceive of a situation where breast radiation therapy would need to be delivered on such an urgent basis where the safety of the fetus would be called into question. Even if breast conservation was preferred, it can usually be delayed until after the birth. Chemotherapy is typically considered safe to deliver during the second trimester and may be used to extend the interval to radiation [17, 18].

Collagen Vascular Diseases

The spectrum of these disorders is broad, and even within each disorder, the penetrance of symptoms can be varied. Each patient's case must be considered independently. Descriptions in the literature of patient's with collagen vascular disease who have received radiation generally describe a particularly increased risk of significant treatment morbidity for patients with active scleroderma. Other diseases such as rheumatoid arthritis or mild lupus are unlikely to bear clinical significance [19] (reference).

Multicentric Disease

Multicentric disease is the description of disease that encompasses more than one quadrant of the breast. The implication is that due to the extent of surgery required to perform adequate lumpectomies in two separate quadrants, the remaining breast is unlikely to retain sufficient tissue to meet the spirit of breast conservation. This is clearly dependent on the patient's breast size and the goals of the patient, particularly one who may consider contralateral breast reduction mammoplasty [20].

Data Supporting Breast Conservation

Ductal Carcinoma In Situ (DCIS)

For patients with ductal carcinoma in situ (DCIS), there is abundant data that supports a role for adjuvant breast radiation therapy. Radiation has been shown to reduce the risk of recurrence not only of noninvasive but also of invasive disease. The four randomized studies looking at adjuvant radiation therapy in noninvasive ductal disease are presented in Table 26.1. All four studies demonstrated a statistically significant reduction in the rate of in-breast recurrences. The NSABP [21], EORTC [22], and Swedish [23] studies had roughly equivalent reduction of both invasive and noninvasive disease, but the UKCCCR [24] study had twice as many noninvasive recurrences as invasive recurrences. The UKCCCR study was a two-by-two randomization between adjuvant radiation therapy and adjuvant tamoxifen therapy. There were too few events in the analysis between the tamoxifen arms to demonstrate a meaningful significance between the groups. Tamoxifen was not routinely used in the other studies (Table 26.2).

Additional prospective studies have also tried to find a subpopulation of low-risk patients that may be observed. A single-arm multicenter study of low-risk DCIS patients in Boston was closed early due to a higher risk of local recurrence. This study that started in 1995 enrolled 153 women who had $\leq$2.5 cm mammographically grade 1 or 2 DCIS with 1 cm surgical margins to observation alone without the use of tamoxifen. By 2002 the stopping rule was reached and the study closed with a recurrence rate of 12 % at 5 years [25]. A larger ECOG registry study conducted on 565 women with low-grade DCIS and 105 with high-grade disease who were treated with surgery alone found a recurrence rate of 6 % for the low-risk group and 15 % for the high-risk group. The median follow-up was 6.2 years, and tamoxifen use in both groups was quite low, only about 10 % of all patients [26]. A prospective randomized study by the RTOG of women with completely resected low-grade disease has been reported in abstract form with a median follow-up of almost 6 1/2 years [27]. Women were either observed or

Table 26.2 DCIS studies

Study	*N*	Years	Follow-up (years)	Whole breast	LRR (%)	OS (%)
NSABP-B17[a,b] [21]	818	1985–1990	15	50 Gy	19.8	92.0
				Lumpectomy	35.0	91.8
EORTC[a,b] [22]	1,010	1986–1996	15	50 Gy	18	90
				Lumpectomy	31	88
Swedish [23]	1,067	1987–1999	8	50 Gy	12.1	91.6
				Lumpectomy	27.1	90.4
UKCCCR[b] [24]	1,701	1990–1998	4.4	50 Gy + Tam	6	93
				50 Gy – Tam	8	98
				Lumpectomy + Tam	18	90
				Lumpectomy – Tam	22	96

[a]Tamoxifen not routine
[b]Boost not standard

treated with adjuvant whole-breast radiation therapy. While not necessary, adjuvant hormone therapy use was much higher (62 %) compared to the previously mentioned single-arm, prospective studies. Five-year recurrence rates in the radiation group were 0.4 % vs. 3.2 % with observation.

Additional follow-up analysis of the prospective, randomized studies has been performed by meta-analysis with the goal of identifying patients at a very low risk of recurrence who may derive little benefit from radiation therapy [28]. In all comparisons, there was a significant improvement in local control with adjuvant radiation therapy. Particularly surprising was that the magnitude of risk reduction was higher in older patients and even in patients with low-grade, small lesions with negative margins, there was an absolute 18 % reduction of breast events. While adjuvant therapy has not demonstrated a reduction in the risk of death due to breast cancer, there is a true reduction in the recurrence of both noninvasive and invasive disease. The EBCTCG meta-analysis of invasive disease found a small improvement in 15-year survival by reducing 5- and 10-year local recurrence rates [5, 29]. While additional follow-up is required to see the long-term outcomes, observation can be considered for highly selected women who consent to adjuvant hormone therapy. Thoughtful consideration must be made regarding expected longevity and the patient's appetite for additional surgery in the event of a recurrence.

Invasive Disease

Breast conservation for invasive disease has evolved significantly over the past 40 years. The studies completed on patients with invasive disease were performed in the late twentieth century, as the pendulum of care was swinging away from the radical Halstedian surgical paradigm. On balance, the data demonstrate that women can preserve their breasts without compromising their longevity. Six major studies performed in randomized fashion are presented in table form (Table 26.3).

All of the studies required routine axillary dissection and adjuvant chemotherapy was indicated for patients with node-positive disease. Adjuvant supraclavicular nodal radiation was included as a routine measure for patients who were found to have nodal disease after mastectomy on the EORTC study and the Danish study that also required chest wall radiation for high-risk patients. Nodal radiation after mastectomy was the subject of a second randomization for node-positive mastectomy patients in the Milan and Gustave-Roussy trials.

Further long-term analysis of the data has resulted in several pooled analyses that have demonstrated improved local control from adjuvant breast radiation that translates to an improvement in overall survival for many patients. A meta-analysis performed by the Early Breast Cancer Trialists' Collaborative Group of 17 randomized studies examined the role of adjuvant radiation therapy after lumpectomy [5]. This

Table 26.3 Breast conservation

Study	*N*	Years	Follow-up (years)	Arms	LRR (%)	OS (%)
NSABP-B06[a,b] [2]	1,851	1976–1984	20	Mastectomy	10.2	47
				Lumpectomy	39.2	46
				Lumpectomy + RT	14.3	46
Milan[a,b] [30]	701	1973–1980	20	Radical Mastectomy	2.3	58.2
				Lumpectomy + RT	8.8	58.3
Danish[a,b] [31]	793[c]	1983–1989	19.6	Mastectomy	21	49.1
				Lumpectomy + RT	13	53.7
Institut Gustave-Roussy[b] [32]	179	1972–1979	15	Mastectomy	18	65
				Lumpectomy + RT	13	72
NCI[a,b] [33]	247	1979–1987	10	Mastectomy	10	75
				Lumpectomy + RT	5	77
EORTC 1081[a,b] [34]	902	1980–1986	10	Mastectomy	12.2	66.1
				Lumpectomy + RT	19.7	65.2

[a]Adjuvant chemo for node-positive disease
[b]Routine axillary node dissection
[c]Analysis of "correctly randomized patients"

Table 26.4 Observation

Study	*N*	Years	Follow-up (years)	Arms	LRR (%)	OS (%)
NSABP-B21 [35]	1,009	1989–1998	8	Whole breast + tamoxifen	2.8	93.4
				Whole breast + placebo	9.3	94
				Tamoxifen	16.5	94
CALGB-9343 [36]	636	1994–1999	12.6	Whole breast + tamoxifen	2	67
				Tamoxifen	10	66
Canadian [37]	769	1992–2000	5.6	Whole breast + tamoxifen	0.6	91
				Tamoxifen	7.7	92
Austrian [38]	869	1996–2004	4.5	Whole breast + Tam/anastrozole	0.4	97.9
				Tam/anastrozole	5.1	94.5

analysis of over 10,000 women demonstrated a consistent, proportional reduction in the rate of local recurrence in women, regardless of their age. An additional important finding was that a reduction in the rate of local recurrence translated to an improved 15-year breast cancer survival advantage that ranged from 3.3 % for node-negative women to 8.5 % for node-positive women.

Not unexpectedly, patient and disease characteristics identify those who derived smaller absolute risk reductions. Several studies have examined the role of adjuvant radiation in favorable risk patients to test the hypothesis if radiation is required for patients who take hormonal therapy. The results suggest that patients of advancing age with a small tumor size, positive receptor status, negative nodal status, and negative resection margins may have a smaller absolute improvement of local control. This data suggests that hormone therapy alone can be considered for highly selected patients who are amenable to close follow-up (Table 26.4).

After Neoadjuvant Chemotherapy

The traditional sequence of care for patients who pursue breast conservation has been the initial surgery followed by adjuvant chemotherapy, if

Table 26.5 Boost studies

Study	N	Follow-up (years)	Whole breast	Boost	LRR
EORTC [41]	5,318	10.8	50 Gy	16 Gy electrons, photons, or brachytherapy	10.2 %
			50 Gy		6.2 % ($p<0.0001$)
Lyon [42]	1,024	3.3	50 Gy (2.5/fx)	10 Gy electrons	4.5 %
			50 Gy (2.5/fx)		3.6 % ($p=0.044$)
Budapest [43]	208	5.3	50 Gy	16 Gy electron or brachytherapy	15.5 %
			50 Gy		6.7 % ($p=0.044$)

needed, followed by radiation therapy. However, neoadjuvant chemotherapy prior to surgery can convert more women who would otherwise require mastectomies to breast-conserving therapy. The NSABP-B18 [39] clinical trial examined the role of neoadjuvant versus adjuvant chemotherapy with 4 cycles of Adriamycin and Cytoxan. Early analysis demonstrated a 12 % increase in the likelihood that a lumpectomy could be performed. There was almost a doubling of the rate of lumpectomy in women with breast cancers greater than 5 cm. Long-term analysis failed to demonstrate a survival advantage between the two arms, although there was a nonsignificant increased risk of ipsilateral breast recurrence for women who were treated preoperatively at 10.7 % vs. 7.6 %. The B-27 [40] trial demonstrated an increased possibility of pCR with the addition of Taxol-based chemotherapy to about 25 % of patients. Radiation therapy was routinely employed in patients who underwent lumpectomy. Radiation remains routine care for lumpectomy patients who have received neoadjuvant chemotherapy as a part of their treatment. Care must be taken when a woman is converted to a breast conservation candidate that the entire preoperative tumor extent has been marked prior to chemotherapy and subsequently excised to avoid the possibility of multifocal residual disease left in the breast.

Boost in Breast Conservation

A boost is a commonly utilized technique in radiation oncology. The concept is that while a larger area may receive a prophylactic dose of radiation therapy, the surgical bed or area of initial gross disease will require a higher dose. This is due to a greater disease burden or to compensate for reduced therapeutic efficacy due to lower oxygen concentrations as a result of the surgical changes. For invasive disease of the breast, the concept of a boost has been most rigorously studied in the conservation setting. A Danish study randomized over 5,000 patients who had undergone a lumpectomy and breast-conserving radiation therapy to either no further therapy or a boost via one of three different techniques. The study demonstrated that there was an improvement in local control with the use of the boost. Other studies have corroborated these results although with shorter follow-ups. On analysis, all studies have found a higher degree of absolute benefit for younger women. All found an increased rate of physician-reported adverse cosmetic changes; however, patient perception of cosmetic outcome was largely satisfactory in groups treated with and without boost (Table 26.5).

The role of a boost in DCIS remains an unanswered question. There are at least two published retrospective series that have demonstrated some improvement in local control [44, 45]. There are two ongoing prospective, the French BONBIS and the Trans Tasmanian 07.01 trial, randomized studies that will provide some guidance on this topic. A boost should be considered for younger women and those with negative prognostic features such as necrosis and higher grade.

Surgical Margins and Breast-Conserving Therapy

Margins of resection at the time of lumpectomy are frequently a topic of discussion between surgeons and radiation oncologists at tumor boards.

Unfortunately, the data regarding the significance of a close (<1 mm) or positive margin (tumor on the inked margin) is mixed, and mainly derived from secondary analysis of prospective studies or retrospective series. It is the heterogeneity of the enrollment criteria of prospective series and the inconsistency of margin assessment that further compound the complexity of these evaluations. A review of the literature by Singletary highlighted the variability in reporting of margin status of surgical results and that there was great variability of recurrence rates reported for a given margin [46]. There is strong evidence that true positive margins result in higher recurrence rates and positive margins for invasive disease should prompt the surgeon to consider additional surgery to clear the margin.

A recent meta-analysis of over 14,000 patients found a strong connection between the risk of local recurrence and margin status (positive vs. negative) [47]. This showed a nonsignificant trend in reduced rates of local recurrence with decreasing negative margin depth. However, the trend was completely lost with the addition of a boost or hormonal therapy. While it may reduce the significance of a close margin, the ability for radiation to correct for positive margins is questionable. A retrospective analysis of patients treated at Thomas Jefferson by DiBiase [48] found that despite higher doses of adjuvant radiation therapy in patients with positive margins, there was still a significantly lower rate of local control at 5 and 10 years. Therefore, while the ideal depth of margin is unclear, positive margins at lumpectomy significantly compromise local control and may not be accounted for with additional radiation.

Accelerated Partial Breast Radiation (ABPI)

With the evolution of the surgical paradigm away from large Halstedian surgeries to breast-preserving lumpectomies and radiation, the next logical question in radiation therapy was whether whole-breast radiation therapy was indicated. Indeed, analyses of patients who failed in the breast, either after lumpectomy alone or after radiation therapy, has demonstrated that the most frequent site of failure is in the same quadrant as the initial lumpectomy [49, 50]. Distant failure in the breast is an uncommon event. Several small single-institution studies demonstrated favorable local control in patients treated with radiation therapy limited to the lumpectomy cavity and surrounding area. However, many of the brachytherapy techniques described in these studies were beyond the scope of many practices and did not gain wide acceptance [51].

With the advent of a series of FDA-approved devices in the late twentieth century, this technique was relatively simple to bring to a wide scope of practices. With the rapid adoption of this technique, a randomized study was commissioned by several groups to examine the effectiveness of this treatment compared to whole-breast radiation therapy. The American Society of Breast Surgeons [52] and the American Brachytherapy Society [53] both have put forth position statements regarding the appropriate candidates and use of accelerated partial breast radiation. The American Society of Radiation Oncology (ASTRO) has a well-developed consensus statement [54] that subdivides patients into appropriate, cautionary, and inappropriate candidates for APBI. Further details of accelerated breast radiation are the subject of a separate chapter.

Explanation of Radiation Planning and Techniques

From a historical standard, whole-breast radiation therapy, as employed in the previously reviewed NSABP studies, consists of what is commonly referred to as tangent radiation therapy. Patients are positioned in a supine position usually at a 10–15° incline. The ipsilateral arm to the affected breast or both arms are extended above the head and supported in an immobilization device. Devices that accomplish all of these positions are often referred to as breast boards. After the patient has been placed in a satisfactory position, wires may be placed on the skin to mark the surface anatomy of the medial, lateral, superior, and inferior aspects of the breast tissue with a margin. The lumpectomy scar is also marked if a boost is anticipated. Once patient setup is complete, a set of images is taken to construct the fields that will be used to treat the patient.

The process of field construction has changed substantially over the past two decades. Traditionally, radiation fields were set either clinically or with the use of a conventional simulator. A conventional simulator is a kilovoltage X-machine setup to replicate the patient position during treatment. Treatment fields were constructed by using single-plane fluoroscopic guidance to adjust the gantry angle to create a beam coming at the breast from a lateral orientation so that a profile of the breast was created with as little lung in the field as possible while still covering the breast. Skin wires placed at the medial and lateral aspects of the breast could be aligned on fluoroscopy to establish appropriate entry and exit points of the beam. Once found to be acceptable, this field was often mirrored with a field from the medial direction.

Simple blocks or collimation and wedges were used to further minimize the dose to the lung and to homogenize the dose across the breast, respectively. The drawback of this planning technique was in the limited data available to moderate the dose and therefore avoid "hot" and "cold" spots within the breast tissue or adjacent normal tissues. The current standard of care is CT-based 3D conformal treatment planning. After the patient positioning is completed, a noncontrast CT scan is performed from the upper neck through the upper abdomen. These images are imported into a treatment planning computer system where the CT images are then reconstructed into a 3D model. The physician and physics staff then contour or identify in three dimensions the tissue to be irradiated and the adjacent normal structures to be shielded. By using a beam's eye view, the beam can be constructed to conform to the target and shield the normal structures and tissues. Using a mathematical algorithm that models the dose, the physician and physics staff can review the fields and make adjustments to the energy and shape and otherwise modulate the field to better conform the dose to meet the ideal treatment constraints.

Radiation therapy plans are evaluated by reviewing isodose lines which are essentially topographical lines representing different doses of radiation, a dose volume histogram and the parameters of each field used for treatment. While the desired doses and target may change from patient to patient, the usual goal is for a homogeneous distribution of the prescription dose of radiation across the target with minimization of hot and cold spots (keeping the dose within 15 % of the prescribed dose). The other aspect of plan evaluation is the review of doses delivered to the normal organs in the vicinity of the target. With the evolution of radiation therapy into 3D-based planning, more accurate dose thresholds have been generated for normal organs. Organs of particular concern when planning breast radiation include the lung, heart (for left-sided disease), brachial plexus, and spinal cord. Upon acceptance of a plan, a variety of quality assurance procedures are performed by the physician and physics staff in order to assure accurate and safe delivery of the radiation.

Fractionation Schemes

Traditionally, radiation therapy has been delivered with prescribed doses of 1.8–2.0 Gy per treatment delivered on a daily basis, 5 days a week over the course of 5–7 weeks. These radiation schedules or fractionation patterns were born out of the previously described trials that laid the groundwork for breast-conserving surgery and radiation. However, alternative whole-breast fractionation patterns have been evaluated in clinical trials resulting in similar outcomes. Hypofractionated radiation therapy condenses the time frame over which the course of therapy and is given typically at a higher dose per fraction. Treatments may still be given daily, but higher doses (>5 Gy) are often given less often. Recent prospective studies have looked at condensing treatment into fewer weeks of therapy (Table 26.6).

Each series has long-term follow-up allowing for reasonable conclusions regarding the value of hypofractionation. A study from Canada has the most mature data, and compared a traditional 25-fraction course of radiation therapy to a 16-fraction course. On the whole the groups performed

Table 26.6 Hypofractionation

Study	N	Years	Follow-up (years)	Radiation	LR (%)	OS (%)
Whelan et al. [55]	1,234	1993–1996	10	50 Gy in 25 Fx	6.7	84.4
				42.5 Gy in 16 Fx	6.2	84.6
START A [56, 57]	2,236	1998–2002	9.3	50 Gy in 25 Fx	7.4	82.6
				41.6 Gy in 13	6.3	82.9
				39 Gy in 13	8.8	81.8
START B [57, 58]	2,215	1999–2001	9.9	50 Gy in 25 Fx	5.5	82.6
				40 Gy in 15 Fx	4.3	85.7

comparably, but there was a significantly higher local recurrence rate for patients with high-grade disease treated with the hypofractionated regimen (15.6 %) compared to those treated with conventional fractionation (4.7 %). The two UK START studies were performed with even more hypofractionated regimens that also demonstrated equivalent local control rates. Follow-up on these studies is at 10 years and provides mature data to support this treatment regimen. Another UK study was performed comparing 50 Gy in 25 fractions to two regimens of five, once weekly radiation, with doses of either 5.7 or 6 Gy. The primary endpoint was cosmesis, finding that the 6 Gy fraction arm was inferior to the conventional and 5.7 Gy fraction arm. The study was not powered to evaluate differences in local control, but failure rates were essentially equivalent [59].

The decision to treat with a particular schedule is multifactorial. Most of the women enrolled on the hypofractionation studies were postmenopausal, over the age of 50, and had early-stage disease that did not require regional nodal radiation. Systemic therapy use was somewhat limited on these studies and may underestimate the impact of combination therapy on cosmesis. ASTRO (American Society of Radiation Oncology) has published guidelines [60] for whole-breast hypofractionated radiation therapy based largely on the results of the abovementioned studies.

Boost Techniques

As discussed above, boost radiation can be utilized to treat the lumpectomy bed after whole-breast radiation in order to improve local control at that site. The technical means of delivering the boost are varied. Commonly, a boost is delivered via an en face electron beam. Different than X-ray or photon radiation as described above, electrons are subatomic particles that directly interact with the target atoms as opposed to imparting energy to the native electrons or nuclei. Due to their small mass relative to their negative charge, the path they take is highly influenced by the tissue through which they pass. As a result, the electrons deposit most of their energy within a few centimeters of the skin surface with no exit dose. Depth of beam penetration and surface dose both increase with increasing electron energies. An easy rule to remember is that 80 % of the prescribed dose is delivered to a depth that is one-third the maximum energy of the electron beam. The electron beam is preferred in patients with a lumpectomy bed close to the skin surface as it can usually encompass the target with one beam and limit the dose to the underlying lung and chest wall.

For deep-seated targets, a combination of photon fields is typically preferred, as one beam will very rarely obtain the desired homogeneous dose distribution over the target. The boost volume is often created from the treatment planning CT where the lumpectomy cavity is frequently evident on the scan. However, this can be more challenging for patients with dense breasts or who may have had a long interval since their surgery. Therefore, surgical clips placed at the periphery of the lumpectomy bed at the time of surgery can frequently be helpful to direct the radiation oncologist. Brachytherapy options are available in addition to the external beam techniques. A conventional interstitial low-dose-rate brachytherapy technique was an option in the original

Table 26.7 Postmastectomy radiation therapy

Study	*N*	Years	Follow-up (years)	Radiation	LRR	OS
British Columbia [66]	318	1979–1986	20	37.5 Gy in 16 fx to the chest wall and IMs	18 % chemo	37 %
				35 Gy in 16 fx to the supraclav and axilla	7 % chemo + RT	47 %
Danish 82b [67] (Premenopausal)	1,708	1982–1989	9.5	50 Gy in 25 or 48 Gy in 22 to chest wall and regional nodes (including IM)	32 % chemo	45 %
					9 % chemo + RT	54 %
Danish 82c [3] (Postmenopausal)	1,460	1982–1990	9.9	50 Gy in 25 or 48 Gy in 22 to chest wall and regional nodes (including IM)	35 % tam alone	36 %
					8 % tam + RT	45 %

Danish boost study [41]. Patients may also have a boost delivered by the now more commonly used brachytherapy catheters [61]. In the same way, intraoperative radiation therapy may be used to treat the lumpectomy cavity at the time of surgery as a boost if not appropriate as a sole modality [62]. Accelerated partial breast and intraoperative radiation therapy techniques and indications are discussed in more detail in their respective chapters.

Postmastectomy Radiation Therapy

Breast radiation therapy has been demonstrated to improve local control for women who desire breast preservation. In early-stage disease, women can choose between breast-conserving surgery and radiation therapy or a mastectomy with equivalent overall survival rates. Women who are not conservation candidates or who choose to have mastectomies may also benefit from adjuvant radiation therapy. Radiation therapy to the chest wall after mastectomy is generally agreed to provide a benefit in local regional control for women with more advanced primary disease and node-positive disease [63]. Several randomized studies and meta-analyses indicate a survival advantage for women in the higher-risk categories. The NCCN [64] and the ACR appropriateness criteria [65] indicate that radiation therapy should be offered or strongly considered for women with cancers that have these high-risk characteristics on final pathology. We would advocate that women with high-risk features should be evaluated by a radiation oncologist to review the risks and benefits that treatment may confer. Discussion is particularly important in the more nuanced settings of mastectomies for women with intermediate risk factors, after neoadjuvant therapy and when breast reconstruction is desired.

Node-Positive and Locally Advanced Disease

The role of radiation therapy in the postmastectomy setting for node-positive and locally advanced disease has been extensively studied. There are three completed randomized studies that have examined the role of radiation therapy after mastectomy in this setting (Table 26.7).

In total, these studies demonstrated a statistical improvement in local regional control and overall survival compared to mastectomy and systemic therapy alone. Of note, only the British Columbia study enrolled women with node-positive disease alone, the Danish studies enrolled women with locally advanced disease as well. The Danish studies have been subject of many subset analyses including a review of recurrence rates for patients with one to three positive nodes and another based on receptor status. Caution should be used when interpreting results gleaned from post hoc subset analysis, as these factors were not controlled for in the initial randomization and may be subject to uncontrolled bias.

There is some controversy regarding the impact of postmastectomy radiation for patients with more limited disease. The main critique of the aforementioned studies is that the locoregional recurrence rates seen in the control groups were unusually high ($\geq$ 30 %). Retrospective series from ECOG [68], MD Anderson [69], and the NSABP [70] published in response to these studies demonstrated comparatively lower locoregional recurrence rates in patients with one to three positive nodes treated with surgery and chemotherapy alone (<15 %). The variation in control rates has been attributed to more limited axillary nodal dissection in the randomized studies. However, a follow-up analysis of the Danish studies controlling for number of nodes dissected continued to find high rates of local recurrence in the control arm [71]. As such, the reason for the differences in control rates remains unexplained and a matter of debate.

A SWOG study was designed to address the role of postmastectomy radiation therapy in women with one to three positive nodes. These women were required to have tumors less than 5 cm, negative margins, and at least ten nodes removed at the time of axillary dissection. Unfortunately, this trial failed to accrue an adequate number of patients and was closed in 2003. There is broad consensus that patients with locally advanced disease (T4, T3 and node positive inflammatory) require adjuvant radiation therapy [63–65]. In patients who fall within an intermediate-risk group (T1–2, N1 patients with one to three positive nodes or T3, N0 disease), the extent of additional risk factors must be considered when deciding to offer adjuvant chest wall radiation. Risk factors associated with increased risk of recurrence include receptor status [72, 73], young age [70, 74], lymph-vascular space invasion [75], multicentricity [76], and margin status [77, 78]. Each of these risk factors have mixed data regarding the degree of significance that they may hold regarding the risk of local regional relapse and therefore should be considered collectively [79, 80] when estimating risk and benefit from adjuvant radiation therapy.

Radiation After Neoadjuvant Chemotherapy

Neoadjuvant chemotherapy can facilitate the conversion of a patient who may have required a mastectomy upfront to breast conservation and is considered the standard initial treatment for patients with inflammatory breast cancer. There is randomized data that shows no improvement in survival compared to adjuvant chemotherapy [39, 40] and does not obviate postoperative radiation therapy. In the setting of breast conservation, women who have had neoadjuvant chemotherapy and then a lumpectomy require breast radiation therapy regardless of a partial or complete response to therapy. Data from the neoadjuvant chemotherapy studies suggest that patients who have undergone neoadjuvant chemotherapy have a higher risk of local recurrence particularly when converted to a lumpectomy from requiring a mastectomy [39]. Several retrospective series have been performed on patients who have received neoadjuvant chemotherapy prior to mastectomy to determine based on pathologic factors which patients face a higher risk of local regional relapse.

Studies at the MD Anderson Cancer Center compared patients who were treated adjuvantly and neoadjuvantly and found that patients who presented in clinical stage III, who had disease involving more than four nodes or T3 disease were at significantly higher risk of local regional failure compared to their matched cohort [81]. Additional series specifically reviewing patients who had a complete response to chemotherapy demonstrated increased rates of local relapse [82] and general guidelines state that patients with stage III will likely benefit from therapy [64]. Chest wall radiation has not been clearly defined in a prospective study. Given the available data, patients with stage III disease, T3 tumors, four or more nodes at presentation, and residual nodal disease will likely benefit from therapy to reduce the likelihood of recurrence [83, 84].

Postmastectomy Radiation Therapy and Breast Reconstruction

Patients who are interested in breast reconstruction but also require adjuvant radiation after their mastectomies have some challenges regarding sequencing. From the radiation oncology perspective, there are issues with meeting the therapeutic goals and minimizing treatment to the adjacent normal organs. This can be difficult in patients who have undergone immediate breast reconstruction with either tissue expanders or permanent implants. Several analyses of these patients have found differing results. Two large retrospective studies performed at MD Anderson [85] and Memorial Sloan Kettering [86] reviewed the dosimetric outcomes for patients treated postoperatively with either immediate or no reconstruction. The MD Anderson study found that patients treated with immediate reconstruction were more likely to have inferior coverage of the target volumes and greater doses to the heart and underlying lung tissue. The difference in immediate reconstruction patients was largely attributed to the attempt to treat the internal mammary nodes (IMNs).

In Memorial's review, they also found that coverage of the IMNs resulted in higher heart and lung doses but found that reconstruction allowed for improved coverage of the IMNs due to a modification in the technique used for treatment. Fundamentally, the decision for immediate reconstruction changes the anatomy and as such a change in radiation technique is required. Awareness of the appropriate radiation techniques and understanding of the therapeutic trade-offs are essential in planning the postmastectomy patient.

The data regarding cosmetic outcome and complication rates for patients who undergo reconstruction consistently demonstrate a balance between techniques and outcomes. Patients who are treated with radiation therapy followed by reconstruction have a higher rate of early complications related to wound healing and seroma formation. Patients who receive postmastectomy radiation after reconstruction have a higher rate of late complications such as capsular contraction or malposition of the implant. Patient-reported satisfaction with their reconstruction is generally high but still lower than those who do not require radiation therapy [87]. Current NCCN guidelines regarding reconstruction suggest that delayed reconstruction is favored in patients who require autologous reconstructions so as to avoid radiating transposed tissues [64]. Patients who require implant reconstruction are usually well served by a temporary tissue expander placed and partially inflated prior to radiation therapy as the ability to expand irradiated tissue is difficult.

Radiation Techniques

Treatment techniques are similar to those used in breast conservation. The simulation is the first step in the process when the patient is setup in the treatment position. This is the patient alignment that will be duplicated on a daily basis through the course of therapy and requires care and consideration with regard to reproducibility. Of particular concern in patients who have had mastectomies is the change in range of motion and the increased likelihood of surgery-related lymphedema. Occasionally, patients who have been guarding their ipsilateral upper extremity may have developed reduced passive and active range of motion in the shoulder [88] and may require physical therapy to help them to regain function prior to attempting a simulation. The most common treatment position is supine at a slight incline with an armrest to hold either the ipsilateral or both upper extremities above the head. Wires are often used on the chest wall to mark the mastectomy scar as well as the inferior, superior, medial, and lateral aspects of the chest wall that require therapy.

As 3D conformal planning is now considered a standard approach, patients have a CT scan for treatment planning that is then transferred into the treatment planning computer for reconstruction. The normal anatomy and target tissues are identified and beams are created in the treatment computer. A variety of treatment techniques have been described to treat the chest wall after mastectomy including opposed tangents fields similar to those used in whole-breast radiation, electron fields, or a combination of the two [89].

It is often the patient's anatomy that dictates which technique will provide the best target coverage. Knowledge and technical prowess in the use of varied techniques can allow for individualized treatment optimization.

Regional Nodal Radiation

Radiation can be used to address regional disease in addition to improving local control within the breast itself. The role of radiation to control regional disease has evolved significantly as has the surgical management of the axilla. Adjuvant radiation is considered appropriate for patients with four or more positive nodes after dissection. The role of radiation is evolving in patients with one to three positive nodes or who have had neoadjuvant chemotherapy, incomplete dissections, no lymph node sampling, or undissected axillae with positive sentinel nodes.

After Positive Sentinel Node

The role of axillary surgery after sentinel lymph node biopsy is an area of active investigation. The ACOSOG Z11 [90] study has questioned if additional surgery is required after a positive sentinel node. While this trial closed early after accruing 856 of a planned 1,900 patients, an analysis of the available patients has been published with a median follow-up of 6.3 years. The results demonstrated no significant difference in overall or disease-free survival at 5 years despite a median of 17 nodes vs. 2 nodes removed. The radiation delivered on this study was tangent radiation therapy to the breast only. Radiation to the regional nodes was specifically excluded. Of note, the women included in this study generally were in a more favorable disease category. Most had receptor-positive T1 disease without lymph-vascular space invasion, and most had only one or two positive nodes.

Therefore, it is necessary to choose carefully the patients in whom further axillary intervention is planned. This philosophy is reflected in the most current NCCN recommendations where only patients with T1 or T2 disease, one to two positive nodes who have not had neoadjuvant therapy and in whom adjuvant whole breast radiation therapy is planned can avoid further nodal treatment. For patients with more advanced disease, radiation may serve as an alternative to nodal dissection. Recent release of interim findings of the AMAROS study [91] in abstract revealed that women with positive sentinel nodes treated with either axillary dissection or regional nodal radiation had acceptably low recurrence rates of 0.54 and 1.03 %, respectively. This study allowed for women with T1–2 disease and one to three nodes. The risk of lymphedema was higher in the surgical group. These findings have not been published in a peer review journal and as such should be considered preliminary particularly as the breakdown of disease characteristics has not been fully analyzed. However, it may represent an alternative to surgery or observation as in the Z-11 study.

One to Three Nodes After Complete Dissection

The role of regional radiation therapy for women with four or more nodes positive in the axilla is widely considered an adequate indication for regional nodal irradiation. However, controversy remains in women with one to three positive nodes. The ASCO 2011 release of preliminary data from the MA-20 [92] study demonstrated an improvement in local regional control and a trend toward improvement in survival. The study randomized 1,832 women who had adverse features after surgery to breast only radiation therapy or breast and comprehensive regional nodal radiation therapy. The women in this study were by design in a higher-risk category than the women in the Z-11 or AMAROS studies. Inclusion criteria for this study required N1 disease or high-risk primary features such as T3 primary, less than ten nodes dissected or high-risk pathologic features including ER negativity, lymph-vascular space invasion, and grade 3 disease. This study has not been presented in a peer-reviewed journal and therefore should be considered carefully before adopting as standard practice.

After Neoadjuvant Chemotherapy

For women who have undergone neoadjuvant chemotherapy, yet who choose to pursue breast conservation, there are no prospective studies that specifically address nodal radiation therapy in a randomized fashion. There is data from the NSABP B-18 and B-27 which are prospective, randomized studies looking at preoperative and postoperative chemotherapy [39] and if taxane-based chemotherapy added to standard chemotherapy improved outcomes [40]. A recent analysis of these two studies by Mamounas [93] in regard to locoregional recurrence rates after neoadjuvant chemotherapy found that age, tumor size, presenting nodal status and response to therapy were the most important predictors of relapse. Regional relapses were highest (4.8 – 8.7 %) for women who failed to achieve a complete response in the lymph nodes. Patients on these studies treated with breast conservation were only allowed tangent radiation therapy per the protocol. A retrospective study of a French experience of 248 cN0-N2 patients who achieved pCR after neoadjuvant chemotherapy demonstrated equal outcomes for patients who did or did not receive lymph node irradiation [94]. However, the patients were not balanced as those who received adjuvant radiation were more likely to be young, have more extensive nodal disease at presentation, and have a centrally or medially located primary. Further study is required and adjuvant nodal radiation should be considered for women of younger age who do not achieve pathologic complete response [82, 83].

Internal Mammary

Irradiation of the internal mammary chain is a highly controversial issue when considering regional nodal therapy. The concern regarding internal mammary chain radiation includes a higher risk of long-term toxicity, particularly of underlying lung and cardiac tissue. However, true rates of these toxicities may take over 10 years to be fully realized. Patients with medial tumor location and positive axillary nodes are considered at higher risk for internal mammary involvement. Several studies have been completed regarding this issue but have yet to be published in peer review journals. The MA-20 study [92] has been presented in abstract form with a 5-year median follow-up and has demonstrated a statistically significant improvement in local, regional, distant, and combined disease-free survival with a trend for improvement in overall survival. This study took women who had breast-conserving therapy and level one to two axillary node dissections who were considered high risk (85 % had one to three positive nodes) and randomized them to either breast radiation or breast plus regional nodal irradiation including the internal mammary chain.

The EORTC 22922 [95] study randomized 4,004 women to either breast radiation or additional medial supraclavicular and internal mammary node irradiation if they had breast conservation (76 % of patients enrolled). Short-term toxicity data has been published and demonstrated an increased rate of pulmonary fibrosis without a corresponding decrease in performance status. An interval analysis of disease control is expected. A randomized French study in the postmastectomy setting has also been presented with an 11-year median follow-up and demonstrated no significant change in disease control or toxicity when including the internal mammary chain compared to chest wall and supraclavicular radiation alone [96]. This study only included women with stage I or II disease and the lack of benefit may reflect the low risk nature of the group as a whole.

Techniques for Nodal Irradiation

Tangent radiation therapy, as described, can adequately treat the level one axilla by raising the superior edge of the tangent field with a technique referred to as "high tangents." Alternatively, particularly if high tangents are dosimetrically unfavorable or if the higher levels require treatment as well, a posterior axillary boost field may be paired with a supraclavicular field. A supraclavicular field is employed to treat the level two and three lymph nodes of the axilla. The classic two-dimensional field description is constructed from a direct or 15° offset field that extends inferiorly from the cricoid cartilage to the clavicular head where it abuts the tangent fields and medially from the transverse processes of the cervical spine to the coracoid process. It may be extended further laterally beneath the humeral head if the level one nodes require treatment and have not been included in the tangents. This field is conventionally prescribed to a depth of 3 cm. However, with modern CT-guided 3D conformal techniques, a more accurate field can be constructed by contouring the appropriate nodal volumes and prescribing to cover this volume. An arbitrary depth of 3 cm is frequently inadequate, particularly in patients with greater BMIs [97, 98]. The dose prescription and fractionation pattern is typically the same as that prescribed to the tangent fields.

Irradiation of the internal mammary nodes may be achieved either by extending the deep margin of the tangent fields or by using a matched anterior electron field. The depth of the internal mammary nodal chain and the goal to minimize dose to the underlying lung are typically the factors that most influence the chosen technique.

Complications of Radiation Therapy for Breast Cancer

While radiation clearly has a place in the management of breast cancer, there are associated risks as with any therapy. Risk of complication can be substantially minimized through thoughtful application of appropriate treatment techniques and patient selection. Unfortunately, despite best efforts, some percentage of patients will develop sequelae from therapy. Understanding these complications is the first step in management. The incidence of lung injury with standard breast techniques is low. Even when adding comprehensive nodal radiation therapy, the risk remains less than 5 % [95, 96]. Rib injury or fracture is also an uncommon occurrence with incidences of less than 1 % with modern techniques [99, 100].

Likely the most discussed complication in breast cancer management is lymphedema. Traditionally described as a complication related to Halstedian surgical technique [101], lymphedema is known to be closely associated with the degree of axillary dissection. This is supported by the data demonstrating a lower incidence of lymphedema associated with sentinel lymph node biopsy or with radiation therapy alone [91, 102]. Radiation added to axillary surgery is also associated with an increased risk of both upper extremity and breast lymphedema. The etiology remains the same as the lymphatic channels draining the upper extremity and breast are interrupted by both techniques, although alteration of the lymph node architecture by radiation has also been a proposed mechanism [103]. Axillary radiation in combination with axillary surgery carries the highest risk of lymphedema. Breast only radiation has a lower rate of symptomatic upper extremity lymphedema.

Apart from very selective use of axillary radiation, early counseling and education of at-risk patients can help to reduce the incidence of symptomatic lymphedema [104]. Patients who develop lymphedema of the upper extremity and breast are best managed by referral to a qualified physical therapist with specialized training in lymphedema management. Often treatment courses include manual lymphatic massage, instruction on precautions and risk factors for exacerbation, and evaluation and fitting of compression garments [105].

Chronic lymphedema puts a patient at risk for another feared complication of radiation, which is the secondary malignancy. Like lymphedema, it was first described as a complication from mastectomy; Stewart-Treves syndrome is a lymphangiosarcoma arising in a patient afflicted with chronic lymphedema [106]. A rare, but frequently fatal complication, lymphangiosarcoma of the breast or chest wall is typically managed with definitive surgery [107]. Due to improved surgical and radiation techniques, the incidence of lymphedema and secondarily this disease is declining. The Early Breast Cancer Trialists' Collaborative Group analysis in 2005 found a small but real incremental increase risk of secondary malignancies, predominantly lung and contralateral breast cancers [29]. Secondary malignancies contributed to a reduced overall survival benefit compared to the improvement seen in breast cancer mortality. This reduction in survival benefit increased with increasing length of follow-up. It is not clear if the increased risk of malignancy with longer follow-up is related to the natural history of secondary malignancy or that the patients with the longest follow-up were more likely to have been treated with less precise and more comprehensive radiation therapy techniques. Analysis by the NCI of large tumor registries found that patients who smoke and have radiation have an increased risk of both lung [108, 109] and esophageal cancers [110]. Two large SEER population analysis studies looking at the risk of contralateral breast cancer found fewer contralateral malignancies in patients treated with more contemporary techniques [111, 112]. In general the overall risk of a second malignancy from radiation is statistically real but low enough that primary consideration should focus on treating the disease at hand [113] and no additional screening measures are required. Reducing lifestyle factors that may also contribute to second cancers is always a prudent measure.

Cardiac injury from radiation therapy encompasses a variety of clinical syndromes. Data from patients treated for Hodgkin's lymphoma at a young age demonstrated significant long-term risk of coronary artery disease, valvular disease, congestive heart failure and pericarditis, and fibrosis. These complications correlate strongly with dose and volume used to treat the mediastinum [114]. Breast patients rarely require such extensive therapy, and data regarding the clinical effects of radiation in these patients is largely related to the incidence of coronary artery disease. Numerous registry studies have been performed reviewing the impact of breast radiation therapy on risk of cardiac disease [115, 116]. Unfortunately, most of these registry studies span decades of evolving treatment techniques and limited true dosimetric data on heart doses. While they can reinforce the proof of concept that increasing heart doses are detrimental, the true impact and degree of risk presented to patients treated in a contemporary clinical setting is likely small. As with secondary malignancies, risk reduction through alteration of lifestyle factors associated with cardiac disease is as prudent a patient counseling point as the impact of radiation.

In summary, the judicious use of radiation therapy in patients with breast cancer can greatly improve local regional disease control and modestly improve long-term survival. These benefits can be further enhanced by the application of modern computer-based planning with appropriate technique and multidisciplinary coordination.

References

1. Hodges PC. The life and times of Emil H. Grubbe. Chicago: The University of Chicago Press; 1964.
2. Fisher B, Anderson S, Bryant J, Margolese RG, Deutsch M, Fisher ER, et al. Twenty-year follow-up of a randomized trial comparing total mastectomy, lumpectomy, and lumpectomy plus irradiation for the treatment of invasive breast cancer. N Engl J Med. 2002;347:1233–41. PubMed PMID: 12393820.
3. Overgaard M, Jensen MB, Overgaard J, Hansen PS, Rose C, Andersson M, et al. Postoperative radiotherapy in high-risk postmenopausal breast-cancer patients given adjuvant tamoxifen: Danish Breast Cancer Cooperative Group DBCG 82c randomised trial. Lancet. 1999;353(9165):1641–8. PubMed PMID: 10335782.
4. Beadle GF, Silver B, Botnick L, Hellman S, Harris JR. Cosmetic results following primary radiation therapy for early breast cancer. Cancer. 1984;54(12):2911–8. PubMed PMID: 6498767.
5. Early Breast Cancer Trialists' Collaborative Group (EBCTCG). Effect of radiotherapy after breast-conserving surgery on 10-year recurrence and 15-year breast cancer death: meta-analysis of individual patient data for 10,801 women in 17 randomised trials. Lancet. 2011;378(9804):1707–16. PubMed PMID: 22019144.
6. Karzmark CJ, Pering NC. Electron linear accelerators for radiation therapy: history, principles and contemporary developments. Phys Med Biol. 1973;18(3):321–54. PubMed PMID: 4610600.
7. Khan F. The physics of radiation therapy. 2nd ed. Philadelphia: Lippincott Williams & Wilkins; 1994.
8. Ward JF. DNA damage produced by ionizing radiation in mammalian cells: identities, mechanisms of formation and repairability. Prog Nucleic Acid Res Mol Biol. 1988;35:95–125. PubMed PMID: 3065826.
9. Elkind MM, Sutton H. Radiation response of mammalian cells grown in culture; 1. Repair of x-ray damaging in surviving Chinese hamster cells. Radiat Res. 1960;13:556–93. PubMed PMID: 13726391.
10. Hall EJ. Radiobiology for the radiologist. 5th ed. Philadelphia: Lippincott Williams & Wilkins; 2000.
11. Beriwal S, Schwartz GF, Komarnicky L, Garcia-Young JA. Breast-conserving therapy after neoadjuvant chemotherapy: long-term results. Breast J. 2006;12(2):159–64. PubMed PMID: 16509842.
12. Aref I, Cross P. Conservative surgery and radiation therapy for early stage breast cancer after previous mantle radiation for Hodgkin's disease. Br J Radiol. 2000;73(872):905–6. PubMed PMID: 11026871.
13. Deutsch M, Gerszten K, Bloomer WD, Avisar E. Lumpectomy and breast irradiation for breast cancer arising after previous radiotherapy for Hodgkin's disease or lymphoma. Am J Clin Oncol. 2001;24(1):33–4. PubMed PMID: 11232946.
14. Deutsch M. Repeat high-dose external beam irradiation for in-breast tumor recurrence after previous lumpectomy and whole breast irradiation. Int J Radiat Oncol Biol Phys. 2002;53(3):687–91. PubMed PMID: 12062613.

15. Trombetta M, Julian TB, Werts DE, McWilliams W, Kim Y, Miften M, et al. Long-term cosmesis after lumpectomy and brachytherapy in the management of carcinoma of the previously irradiated breast. Am J Clin Oncol. 2009;32(3):314–8. PubMed PMID: 19451803.
16. Martin DD. Review of radiation therapy in the pregnant cancer patient. Clin Obstet Gynecol. 2011;54(4):591–601. PubMed PMID: 22031249.
17. Meisel JL, Economy KE, Calvillo KZ, Schapira L, Tung NM, Gelber S, et al. Contemporary multidisciplinary treatment of pregnancy-associated breast cancer. Springerplus. 2013;2(1):297. PubMed PMID: 23888269.
18. Loibl S, Han SN, von Minckwitz G, Bontenbal M, Ring A, Giermek J, et al. Treatment of breast cancer during pregnancy: an observational study. Lancet Oncol. 2012;13(9):887–96. PubMed PMID: 22902483.
19. Chen AM, Obedian E, Haffty BG. Breast-conserving therapy in the setting of collagen vascular disease. Cancer J. 2001;7(6):480–91. PubMed PMID: 11769860.
20. Sakorafas GH, Tsiotou AG. Selection criteria for breast conservation in breast cancer. Eur J Surg. 2000;166(11):835–46. PubMed PMID: 11097148.
21. Wapnir IL, Dignam JJ, Fisher* B, Mamounas EP, Anderson SJ, Julian TB, et al. Long-term outcomes of invasive ipsilateral breast tumor recurrences after lumpectomy in NSABP B-17 and B-24 randomized clinical trials for DCIS. J Natl Cancer Inst. 2011;103:478–88. PubMed PMID: 21398619.
22. Donker M, Litière S, Werutsky G, Julien JP, Fentiman IS, Agresti R, et al. Breast-conserving treatment with or without radiotherapy in ductal carcinoma in situ: 15-year recurrence rates and outcome after a recurrence, from the EORTC 10853 randomized phase III trial. J Clin Oncol. 2013;31(32):4054–9. PubMed PMID: 24043739.
23. Holmberg L, Garmo H, Granstrand B, Ringberg A, Arnesson L, Sandelin K, et al. Absolute risk reductions for local recurrence after postoperative radiotherapy after sector resection for ductal carcinoma in situ of the breast. J Clin Oncol. 2008;26:1247–52. PubMed PMID: 18250350.
24. Houghton J, George WD, Cuzick J, Duggan C, Fentiman IS, Spittle M, et al. Radiotherapy and tamoxifen in women with completely excised ductal carcinoma in situ of the breast in the UK, Australia, and New Zealand: randomised controlled trial. Lancet. 2003;362(9378):95–102. PubMed PMID: 12867108.
25. Wong JS, Kaelin CM, Troyan SL, Gadd MA, Gelman R, Lester SC, et al. Prospective study of wide excision alone for ductal carcinoma in situ of the breast. J Clin Oncol. 2006;24(7):1031–6. PubMed PMID: 16461781.
26. Hughes LL, Wang M, Page DL, Gray R, Solin LJ, Davidson NE, et al. Local excision alone without irradiation for ductal carcinoma in situ of the breast: a trial of the Eastern Cooperative Oncology Group. J Clin Oncol. 2009;27(32):5319–24. PubMed PMID: 19826126.
27. McCormick B. RTOG 9804: a prospective randomized trial for "good risk" ductal carcinoma in situ (DCIS), comparing radiation (RT) to observation (OBS). J Clin Oncol. 2012;30(15):1004. 2012 ASCO Annual Meeting Abstracts.
28. Early Breast Cancer Trialists' Collaborative Group (EBCTCG). Overview of the randomized trials of radiotherapy in ductal carcinoma in situ of the breast. J Natl Cancer Inst Monogr. 2010;2010(41):162–77. PubMed PMID: 20956824.
29. Clarke M, Collins R, Darby S, Davies C, Elphinstone P, Evans E. Effects of radiotherapy and of differences in the extent of surgery for early breast cancer on local recurrence and 15-year survival: an overview of the randomised trials. Lancet. 2005;366(9503):2087–106. PubMed PMID: 16360786.
30. Veronesi U, Cascinelli N, Mariani L, Greco M, Saccozzi R, Luini A, et al. Twenty-year follow-up of a randomized study comparing breast conserving surgery with radical mastectomy for early breast cancer. N Engl J Med. 2002;347:1227–32. PubMed PMID: 12393819.
31. Blichert-Toft M, Nielsen M, Düring M, Møller S, Rank F, Overgaard M, et al. Long-term results of breast conserving surgery vs. mastectomy for early stage invasive breast cancer: 20-year follow-up of the Danish randomized DBCG-82TM protocol. Acta Oncol. 2008;47(4):672–81.
32. Arriagada R, Lê MG, Rochard F, Contesso G. Conservative treatment versus mastectomy in early breast cancer: patterns of failure with 15 years of follow-up data. Institut Gustave-Roussy Breast Cancer Group. J Clin Oncol. 1996;14(5):1558–64. PubMed PMID: 8622072.
33. Jacobson JA, Danforth DN, Cowan KH, D'Angelo T, Steinberg SM, Pierce L, et al. Ten-year results of a comparison of conservation with mastectomy in the treatment of stage I and II breast cancer. N Engl J Med. 1995;332:907–11. PubMed PMID: 7877647.
34. van Dongen JA, Voogd AC, Fentiman IS, Legrand C, Sylvester RJ, Tong D, et al. Long-term results of a randomized trial comparing breast conserving therapy with mastectomy: European Organization for Research and Treatment of Cancer 10801 trial. J Natl Cancer Inst. 2000;92(14):1143–50. PubMed PMID: 10904087.
35. Fisher B, Bryant J, Dignam JJ, Wickerham DL, Mamounas EP, Fisher ER, et al. Tamoxifen, radiation therapy, or both for prevention of ipsilateral breast tumor recurrence after lumpectomy in women with invasive breast cancers of one centimeter or less. J Clin Oncol. 2002;20(20):4141–9. PubMed PMID: 12377957.
36. Hughes KS, Schnaper LA, Bellon JR, Cirrincione CT, Berry DA, McCormick B, et al. Lumpectomy plus tamoxifen with or without irradiation in women age 70 years or older with early breast cancer: long-term follow-up of CALGB 9343. J Clin Oncol. 2013;31(19): 2382–7. PubMed PMID: 23690420.
37. Fyles AW, McCready DR, Manchul LA, Trudeau ME, Merante P, Pintilie M, et al. Tamoxifen with or without breast irradiation in women 50 years of age or

older with early breast cancer. N Engl J Med. 2004;351(10):963–70. PubMed PMID 15342804.
38. Pötter R, Gnant M, Kwasny W, Tausch C, Handl-Zeller L, Pakisch B. Lumpectomy plus tamoxifen or anastrozole with or without whole breast irradiation in women with favorable early breast cancer. Int J Radiat Oncol Biol Phys. 2007;68(2):334–40. PubMed PMID: 17363187.
39. Wolmark N, Wang J, Mamounas E, Bryant J, Fisher B. Preoperative chemotherapy in patients with operable breast cancer: nine-year results from National Surgical Adjuvant Breast and Bowel Project B-18. J Natl Cancer Inst Monogr. 2001;(30):96–102. PubMed PMID: 11773300.
40. Bear HD, Anderson S, Smith RE, Geyer Jr CE, Mamounas EP, Fisher B, et al. Sequential preoperative or postoperative docetaxel added to preoperative doxorubicin plus cyclophosphamide for operable breast cancer: National Surgical Adjuvant Breast and Bowel Project Protocol B-27. J Clin Oncol. 2006;24(13):2019–27. PubMed PMID: 16606972.
41. Bartelink H, Horiot JC, Poortmans PM, Struikmans H, Van den Bogaert W, Fourquet A, et al. Impact of a higher radiation dose on local control and survival in breast-conserving therapy of early breast cancer: 10-year results of the randomized boost versus no boost EORTC 22881-10882 trial. J Clin Oncol. 2007;25(22):3259–65. PubMed PMID : 17577015.
42. Romestaing P, Lehingue Y, Carrie C, Coquard R, Montbarbon X, Ardiet JM, et al. Role of a 10-Gy boost in the conservative treatment of early breast cancer: results of a randomized clinical trial in Lyon, France. J Clin Oncol. 1997;15(3):963–8. PubMed: PMID 9060534.
43. Polgár C, Fodor J, Orosz Z, Major T, Takácsi-Nagy Z, Mangel LC, et al. Electron and high-dose-rate brachytherapy boost in the conservative treatment of stage I-II breast cancer first results of the randomized Budapest boost trial. Strahlenther Onkol. 2002;178(11):615–23. PubMed PMID: 12426672.
44. Omlin A, Amichetti M, Azria D, Cole BF, Fourneret P, Poortmans P. Boost radiotherapy in young women with ductal carcinoma in situ: a multicentre, retrospective study of the Rare Cancer Network. Lancet Oncol. 2006;7(8):652–6. PubMed PMID 16887482.
45. Wong P, Lambert C, Agnihotram RV, David M, Duclos M, Freeman CR. Ductal carcinoma in situ–the influence of the radiotherapy boost on local control. Int J Radiat Oncol Biol Phys. 2012;82(2):e153–8. PubMed PMID: 21664063.
46. Singletary SE. Surgical margins in patients with early-stage breast cancer treated with breast conservation therapy. Am J Surg. 2002;184(5):383–93. PubMed PMID: 12433599.
47. Houssami N, Macaskill P, Marinovich ML, Dixon JM, Irwig L. Brennan ME Meta-analysis of the impact of surgical margins on local recurrence in women with early-stage invasive breast cancer treated with breast-conserving therapy. Eur J Cancer. 2010;46(18): 3219–32. PubMed PMID: 20817513.
48. DiBiase SJ, Komarnicky LT, Heron DE, Schwartz GF, Mansfield CM. Influence of radiation dose on positive surgical margins in women undergoing breast conservation therapy. Int J Radiat Oncol Biol Phys. 2002;53(3):680–6. PubMed PMID: 12062612.
49. Vicini FA, Recht A, Abner A, Boyages J, Cady B, Connolly JL, et al. Recurrence in the breast following conservative surgery and radiation therapy for early-stage breast cancer. J Natl Cancer Inst Monogr. 1992; 11:33–9.
50. Fisher ER, Anderson S, Tan-Chiu E, Fisher B, Eaton L, Wolmark N. Fifteen-year prognostic discriminants for invasive breast carcinoma: National Surgical Adjuvant Breast and Bowel Project Protocol-06. Cancer. 2001;91(8 Suppl):1679–87. PubMed PMID: 11309768.
51. Arthur DW, Vicini FA. Accelerated partial breast irradiation as a part of breast conservation therapy. J Clin Oncol. 2005;23(8):1726–35.
52. American Society of Breast Surgeons. Consensus statement for accelerated partial breast irradiation. Updated 15 Aug 2011 cited 13 Nov, 2013 www.breastsurgeons.org/statements/index.php.
53. Shah C, Vicini F, Wazer DE, Arthur D, Patel RR. The American Brachytherapy Society consensus statement for accelerated partial breast irradiation. Brachytherapy. 2013;12(4):267–77. PubMed PMID: 23619524.
54. Smith BD, Arthur DW, Buchholz TA, Haffty BG, Hahn CA, Hardenbergh PH, et al. Accelerated partial breast irradiation consensus statement from the American Society for Radiation Oncology (ASTRO). Int J Radiat Oncol Biol Phys. 2009;74(4):987–1001. PubMed PMID: 19545784.
55. Whelan T, MacKenzie R, Julian J, Levine M, Shelley W, Grimard L, et al. Randomized trial of breast irradiation schedules after lumpectomy for women with lymph node-negative breast cancer. J Natl Cancer Inst. 2002;94(15):1143–50. PubMed PMID: 12165639.
56. START Trialists' Group. The UK Standardisation of Breast Radiotherapy (START) Trial A of radiotherapy hypofractionation for treatment of early breast cancer: a randomized trial. Lancet Oncol. 2008;9(4):331–41. PubMed PMID: 18356109.
57. START Trialists' Group. The UK Standardisation of Breast Radiotherapy (START) trials of radiotherapy hypofractionation for treatment of early breast cancer: 10-year follow-up results of two randomised controlled trials. Lancet Oncol. 2013;14(11):1086–94. PubMed PMID 24055415.
58. START Trialists' Group. The UK Standardisation of Breast Radiotherapy (START) Trial B of radiotherapy hypofractionation for treatment of early breast cancer: a randomized trial. Lancet. 2008;371(9618):1098–107. PubMed PMID: 18355913.
59. FAST Trialists Group. First results of the randomised UK FAST Trial of radiotherapy hypofractionation for treatment of early breast cancer (CRUKE/04/015). Radiother Oncol. 2011;100(1):93–100. PubMed PMID: 21752481.

60. Smith BD, Bentzen SM, Correa CR, Hahn CA, Hardenbergh PH, Ibbott GS. Fractionation for whole breast irradiation: an American Society for Radiation Oncology (ASTRO) evidence-based guideline. Int J Radiat Oncol Biol Phys. 2011;81(1):59–68. PubMed PMID: 20638191.
61. Shah AP, Strauss JB, Kirk MC, Chen SS, Dickler A. A dosimetric analysis comparing electron beam with the MammoSite brachytherapy applicator for intact breast boost. Phys Med. 2010;26(2):80–7. PubMed PMID: 19836283.
62. Fastner G, Sedlmayer F, Merz F, Deutschmann H, Reitsamer R, Menzel C, et al. IORT with electrons as boost strategy during breast conserving therapy in limited stage breast cancer: long term results of an ISIORT pooled analysis. Radiother Oncol. 2013; 108(2):279–86. PubMed PMID: 23830467.
63. Eifel P, Axelson JA, Costa J, Crowley J, Curran Jr WJ, Deshler A, et al. National Institutes of Health Consensus Development Conference Statement: adjuvant therapy for breast cancer, November 1–3, 2000. J Natl Cancer Inst. 2001;93(13):979–89. PubMed PMID: 11438563.
64. Theriault RL, Carlson RW, Allred C, Anderson BO, Burstein HJ, Edge SB. Breast cancer, version 3.2013: featured updates to the NCCN guidelines. J Natl Compr Canc Netw. 2013;11(7):753–60. PubMed PMID 23847214.
65. Taylor ME, Haffty BG, Rabinovitch R, Arthur DW, Halberg FE, Strom EA, et al. ACR appropriateness criteria on postmastectomy radiotherapy expert panel on radiation oncology-breast. Int J Radiat Oncol Biol Phys. 2009;73(4):997–1002. PubMed PMID 19251087.
66. Ragaz J, Olivotto IA, Spinelli JJ, Phillips N, Jackson SM, Wilson KS, et al. Locoregional radiation therapy in patients with high-risk breast cancer receiving adjuvant chemotherapy: 20-year results of the British Columbia randomized trial. J Natl Cancer Inst. 2005;97(2):116–26. PubMed PMID: 15657341.
67. Overgaard M, Hansen PS, Overgaard J, Rose C, Andersson M, Bach F, et al. Postoperative radiotherapy in high-risk premenopausal women with breast cancer who receive adjuvant chemotherapy. Danish Breast Cancer Cooperative Group 82b Trial. N Engl J Med. 1997;337(14):949–55.
68. Recht A, Gray R, Davidson NE, Fowble BL, Solin LJ, Cummings FJ, et al. Locoregional failure 10 years after mastectomy and adjuvant chemotherapy with or without tamoxifen without irradiation: experience of the Eastern Cooperative Oncology Group. J Clin Oncol. 1999;17(6):1689–700. PubMed PMID: 10561205.
69. Katz A, Strom EA, Buchholz TA, Thames HD, Smith CD, Jhingran A, et al. Locoregional recurrence patterns after mastectomy and doxorubicin-based chemotherapy: implications for postoperative irradiation. J Clin Oncol. 2000;18(15):2817–27. PubMed PMID: 10920129.
70. Taghian A, Jeong JH, Mamounas E, Anderson S, Bryant J, Deutsch M, et al. Patterns of locoregional failure in patients with operable breast cancer treated by mastectomy and adjuvant chemotherapy with or without tamoxifen and without radiotherapy: results from five National Surgical Adjuvant Breast and Bowel Project randomized clinical trials. J Clin Oncol. 2004;22(21):4247–54. PubMed PMID: 15452182.
71. Overgaard M, Nielsen HM, Overgaard J. Is the benefit of postmastectomy irradiation limited to patients with four or more positive nodes, as recommended in international consensus reports? A subgroup analysis of the DBCG 82 b&c randomized trials. Radiother Oncol. 2007;82(3):247–53. PubMed PMID: 17306393.
72. Voduc KD, Cheang MC, Tyldesley S, Gelmon K, Nielsen TO, Kennecke H. Breast cancer subtypes and the risk of local and regional relapse. J Clin Oncol. 2010;28(10):1684–91. PubMed PMID: 20194857.
73. Kyndi M, Sørensen FB, Knudsen H, Overgaard M, Nielsen HM, Overgaard J. Estrogen receptor, progesterone receptor, HER-2, and response to postmastectomy radiotherapy in high-risk breast cancer: the Danish Breast Cancer Cooperative Group. J Clin Oncol. 2008;26(9):1419–26. PubMed PMID: 18285604.
74. Truong PT, Olivotto IA, Kader HA, Panades M, Speers CH, Berthelet E. Selecting breast cancer patients with T1-T2 tumors and one to three positive axillary nodes at high postmastectomy locoregional recurrence risk for adjuvant radiotherapy. Int J Radiat Oncol Biol Phys. 2005;61(5):1337–47. PubMed PMID: 15817335.
75. Floyd SR, Buchholz TA, Haffty BG, Goldberg S, Niemierko A, Raad RA. Low local recurrence rate without postmastectomy radiation in node-negative breast cancer patients with tumors 5 cm and larger. Int J Radiat Oncol Biol Phys. 2006;66(2):358–64. PubMed PMID: 16887288.
76. Katz A, Strom EA, Buchholz TA, Theriault R, Singletary SE, McNeese MD. The influence of pathologic tumor characteristics on locoregional recurrence rates following mastectomy. Int J Radiat Oncol Biol Phys. 2001;50(3):735–42. Pub Med PMID 11395242.
77. Childs SK, Chen YH, Duggan MM, Golshan M, Pochebit S, Wong JS, et al. Surgical margins and the risk of local-regional recurrence after mastectomy without radiation therapy. Int J Radiat Oncol Biol Phys. 2012;84(5):1133–8. PubMed PMID: 22543200.
78. Rowell NP. Are mastectomy resection margins of clinical relevance? A systematic review. Breast. 2010;19(1):14–22. PubMed PMID: 19932025.
79. Abi-Raad R, Boutrus R, Wang R, Niemierko A, Macdonald S, Smith B, et al. Patterns and risk factors of locoregional recurrence in T1-T2 node negative breast cancer patients treated with mastectomy: implications for postmastectomy radiotherapy. Int J Radiat Oncol Biol Phys. 2011;81(3):e151–7. PubMed PMID: 21420245.
80. Wallgren A, Bonetti M, Gelber RD, Goldhirsch A, Castiglione-Gertsch M, Holmberg SB, et al. Risk factors for locoregional recurrence among breast cancer patients: results from International Breast Cancer Study Group Trials I through VII. J Clin Oncol. 2003;21(7):1205–13. PubMed PMID: 12663706.
81. Buchholz TA, Katz A, Strom EA, McNeese MD, Perkins GH, Hortobagyi GN, et al. Pathologic tumor

size and lymph node status predict for different rates of locoregional recurrence after mastectomy for breast cancer patients treated with neoadjuvant versus adjuvant chemotherapy. Int J Radiat Oncol Biol Phys. 2002;53(4):880–8. PubMed PMID: 12095553.
82. McGuire SE, Gonzalez-Angulo AM, Huang EH, Tucker SL, Kau SW, Yu TK, et al. Postmastectomy radiation improves the outcome of patients with locally advanced breast cancer who achieve a pathologic complete response to neoadjuvant chemotherapy. Int J Radiat Oncol Biol Phys. 2007;68(4):1004–9. PubMed PMID: 17418973.
83. Hoffman KE, Mittendorf EA, Buchholz TA. Optimising radiation treatment decisions for patients who receive neoadjuvant chemotherapy and mastectomy. Lancet Oncol. 2012;13(6):e270–6. PubMed PMID: 22652235.
84. Fowble BL, Einck JP, Kim DN, McCloskey S, Mayadev J, Yashar C, et al. Role of postmastectomy radiation after neoadjuvant chemotherapy in stage II-III breast cancer. Int J Radiat Oncol Biol Phys. 2012;83(2):494–503. PubMed PMID: 22579377.
85. Motwani SB, Strom EA, Schechter NR, Butler CE, Lee GK, Langstein HN, et al. The impact of immediate breast reconstruction on the technical delivery of postmastectomy radiotherapy. Int J Radiat Oncol Biol Phys. 2006;66(1):76–82. PubMed PMID: 16765534.
86. Ohri N, Cordeiro PG, Keam J, Ballangrud A, Shi W, Zhang Z, et al. Quantifying the impact of immediate reconstruction in postmastectomy radiation: a large, dose-volume histogram-based analysis. Int J Radiat Oncol Biol Phys. 2012;84(2):e153–9. PubMed PMID: 22560544.
87. Lee BT, A Adesiyun T, Colakoglu S, Curtis MS, Yueh JH, E Anderson K, et al. Postmastectomy radiation therapy and breast reconstruction: an analysis of complications and patient satisfaction. Ann Plast Surg. 2010;64(5):679–83. PubMed PMID: 20395800.
88. Mansel RE, Fallowfield L, Kissin M, Goyal A, Newcombe RG, Dixon JM, et al. Randomized multicenter trial of sentinel node biopsy versus standard axillary treatment in operable breast cancer: the ALMANAC Trial. J Natl Cancer Inst. 2006;98(9):599–609. PubMed PMID 16670385.
89. Pierce LJ, Butler JB, Martel MK, Normolle DP, Koelling T, Marsh RB, et al. Postmastectomy radiotherapy of the chest wall: dosimetric comparison of common techniques. Int J Radiat Oncol Biol Phys. 2002;52(5):1220–30. PubMed PMID: 11955732.
90. Giuliano AE, Hunt KK, Ballman KV, Beitsch PD, Whitworth PW, Blumencranz PW, et al. Axillary dissection vs no axillary dissection in women with invasive breast cancer and sentinel node metastasis: a randomized clinical trial. JAMA. 2011;305(6):569–75. PubMed PMID: 21304082.
91. Rutgers EJ, Donker M, Straver EM, Meijnen P, Van De Velde C, Robert E, Mansel RE, et al. Radiotherapy or surgery of the axilla after a positive sentinel node in breast cancer patients: final analysis of the EORTC AMAROS trial. ASCO Annual Meeting Abstracts. J Clini Oncol. 2013;31(15 suppl) (May 20 Supplement), 2013: LBA1001.
92. Whelan TJ, Olivotto I, Ackerman I, Chapman JW, Chua B, Nabid A, et al. NCIC-CTG MA.20: an intergroup trial of regional nodal irradiation in early breast cancer. ASCO Annual Meeting Abstracts. J Clin Oncol. 2011;29(18 suppl) (June 20 Supplement), 2011: LBA1003.
93. Mamounas EP, Anderson SJ, Dignam JJ, Bear HD, Julian TB, Geyer Jr CE, et al. Predictors of locoregional recurrence after neoadjuvant chemotherapy: results from combined analysis of National Surgical Adjuvant Breast and Bowel Project B-18 and B-27. J Clin Oncol. 2012;30(32):3960–6. PubMed PMID: 23032615.
94. Daveau C, Stevens D, Brain E, Berges O, Villette S, Moisson P, et al. Is regional lymph node irradiation necessary in stage II to III breast cancer patients with negative pathologic node status after neoadjuvant chemotherapy? Int J Radiat Oncol Biol Phys. 2010;78(2):337–42. PubMed PMID: 20171795.
95. Matzinger O, Heimsoth I, Poortmans P, Collette L, Struikmans H, Van Den Bogaert W, et al. Toxicity at three years with and without irradiation of the internal mammary and medial supraclavicular lymph node chain in stage I to III breast cancer (EORTC trial 22922/10925). Acta Oncol. 2010;49(1):24–34. PubMed: PMID 20100142.
96. Hennequin C, Bossard N, Servagi-Vernat S, Maingon P, Dubois JB, Datchary J, et al. Ten-year survival results of a randomized trial of irradiation of internal mammary nodes after mastectomy. Int J Radiat Oncol Biol Phys. 2013;86(5):860–6. PubMed PMID: 23664327.
97. Goodman RL, Grann A, Saracco P, Needham MF. The relationship between radiation fields and regional lymph nodes in carcinoma of the breast. Int J Radiat Oncol Biol Phys. 2001;50(1):99–105. PubMed PMID: 11316551.
98. Jephcott CR, Tyldesley S, Swift CL. Regional radiotherapy to axilla and supraclavicular fossa for adjuvant breast treatment: a comparison of four techniques. Int J Radiat Oncol Biol Phys. 2004;60(1): 103–10. PubMed PMID: 15337545.
99. Pierce SM, Recht A, Lingos TI, Abner A, Vicini F, Silver B, et al. Long-term radiation complications following conservative surgery (CS) and radiation therapy (RT) in patients with early stage breast cancer. Int J Radiat Oncol Biol Phys. 1992;23(5): 915–23. PubMed PMID: 1639653.
100. Overgaard M. Spontaneous radiation-induced rib fractures in breast cancer patients treated with post-mastectomy irradiation. A clinical radiobiological analysis of the influence of fraction size and dose-response relationships on late bone damage. Acta Oncol. 1988;27(2):117–22. PubMed PMID: 3390342.
101. Britton RC, Nelson PA. Causes and treatment of post-mastectomy lymphedema of the arm. Report of 114 cases. JAMA. 1962;180:95–102. PubMed PMID: 13873187.
102. Golshan M, Martin WJ, Dowlatshahi K. Sentinel lymph node biopsy lowers the rate of lymphedema

when compared with standard axillary lymph node dissection. Am Surg. 2003;69(3):209–11. PubMed PMID: 12678476.

103. Meek AG. Breast radiotherapy and lymphedema. Cancer. 1998;83(12 Suppl American):2788–97. PubMed PMID: 9874399.

104. Box RC, Reul-Hirche HM, Bullock-Saxton JE, Furnival CM. Physiotherapy after breast cancer surgery: results of a randomised controlled study to minimise lymphoedema. Breast Cancer Res Treat. 2002;75(1):51–64. PubMed PMID: 12500934.

105. Ko DS, Lerner R, Klose G, Cosimi AB. Effective treatment of lymphedema of the extremities. Arch Surg. 1998;133(4):452–8. PubMed PMID: 9565129.

106. Stewart FW, Treves N. Classics in oncology: lymphangiosarcoma in postmastectomy lymphedema: a report of six cases in elephantiasis chirurgica. CA Cancer J Clin. 1981;31(5):284–99. PubMed PMID: 6793218.

107. Sharma A, Schwartz RA. Stewart-Treves syndrome: pathogenesis and management. J Am Acad Dermatol. 2012;67(6):1342–8. PubMed PMID: 22682884.

108. Inskip PD, Stovall M, Flannery JT. Lung cancer risk and radiation dose among women treated for breast cancer. J Natl Cancer Inst. 1994;86(13):983–8. PubMed PMID: 8007020.

109. Kaufman EL, Jacobson JS, Hershman DL, Desai M, Neugut AI. Effect of breast cancer radiotherapy and cigarette smoking on risk of second primary lung cancer. J Clin Oncol. 2008;26(3):392–8. PubMed PMID: 18202415.

110. Morton LM, Gilbert ES, Hall P, Andersson M, Joensuu H, Vaalavirta L, et al. Risk of treatment-related esophageal cancer among breast cancer survivors. Ann Oncol. 2012;23(12):3081–91. PubMed PMID: 22745217.

111. Storm HH, Andersson M, Boice Jr JD, Blettner M, Stovall M, Mouridsen HT, et al. Adjuvant radiotherapy and risk of contralateral breast cancer. J Natl Cancer Inst. 1992;84(16):1245–50. PubMed PMID: 1640483.

112. Boice Jr JD, Harvey EB, Blettner M, Stovall M, Flannery JT. Cancer in the contralateral breast after radiotherapy for breast cancer. N Engl J Med. 1992;326(12):781–5. PubMed PMID: 1538720.

113. BerringtondeGonzalez A, Curtis RE, Gilbert E, Berg CD, Smith SA, Stovall M, et al. Second solid cancers after radiotherapy for breast cancer in SEER cancer registries. Br J Cancer. 2010;102(1):220–6. PubMed PMID: 19935795.

114. Ng AK, Abramson JS, Digumarthy SR, Reingold JS, Stone JR. Case records of the Massachusetts General Hospital. Case 24-2010. A 56-year-old woman with a history of Hodgkin's lymphoma and sudden onset of dyspnea and shock. N Engl J Med. 2010;363(7):664–75.

115. Henson KE, McGale P, Taylor C, Darby SC. Radiation-related mortality from heart disease and lung cancer more than 20 years after radiotherapy for breast cancer. Br J Cancer. 2013;108(1):179–82. PubMed PMID: 23257897.

116. Darby SC, Ewertz M, McGale P, Bennet AM, Blom-Goldman U, Brønnum D, et al. Risk of ischemic heart disease in women after radiotherapy for breast cancer. N Engl J Med. 2013;368(11):987–98. PubMed PMID 23484825.

27 Partial Breast Radiation Therapy

Peter D. Beitsch and J. Ben Wilkinson

Introduction

Breast cancer treatment over the past 40 years has moved from surgically dominated, one-size-fits-all to a multidisciplinary, targeted approach. Breast (local) surgical care has evolved from radical mastectomy to modified radical mastectomy to lumpectomy in appropriate candidates. Similarly, regional treatment of the draining lymph node basin has evolved from ultraradical axillary, internal mammary, and supraclavicular removal to now targeted removal of the first (sentinel) draining lymph nodes. In the early 1980s, the importance of radical surgery was brought into question with the initial publication of the National Surgical Adjuvant Breast and Bowel Project (NSABP) B-06 and the Italian National Cancer Institute (Milan) trials demonstrating equivalence between modified radical mastectomy and breast conserving surgery combined with whole breast radiotherapy. These results have been updated by the original authors [1, 2] and verified in other trials including studies from the Institut Gustave-Roussy Breast Cancer Group and the Danish Breast Cancer Cooperative Group [3, 4]. Whole breast irradiation (WBI) was chosen as the adjuvant radiation to mimic a mastectomy – treating the entire breast by either removing it or radiating it. This was not based on any prospective randomized trials but was considered by many as essentially the only available method for radiating the breast (tangential fields).

As breast conservation became more widespread, local recurrences in the breast began to occur. Data emerged demonstrating that the highest risk for local recurrence following lumpectomy, plus WBI, lies near the original tumor bed. This led to the addition of a "boost dose" to WBI in an attempt to lower tumor bed recurrences, especially in women with higher-risk disease including younger age, close margins, and pathologic factors such as high-grade, estrogen receptor-negative, lymphovascular space invasion (LVSI) or an extensive intraductal component (EIC). This concept led to the development of tailored adjuvant radiation therapy to just the lumpectomy cavity walls with internal radiation – brachytherapy (treatment at a short distance). Patient selection was very conservative in the early stages of use, choosing only those older patients with small primary breast cancers and with node-negative disease. Although current outcome data is primarily in the form of

P.D. Beitsch, MD, FACS (✉)
Dallas Breast Center,
7777 Forest Lane, Suite C760,
Dallas, TX 75230, USA
e-mail: beitsch@aol.com

J.B. Wilkinson, MD
Department of Radiation Oncology,
Willis-Knighton Health System,
LSU Feist-Weiller Cancer Center,
2600 Kings Highway, Shreveport, LA 71103, USA
e-mail: j.ben.wilkinson@gmail.com

A.I. Riker (ed.), *Breast Disease: Comprehensive Management*,
DOI 10.1007/978-1-4939-1145-5_27, © Springer Science+Business Media New York 2015

retrospective analyses, ongoing phase III clinical trials including the NSABP B-39/Radiation Therapy Oncology Group (RTOG) 0413 study will assist in answering the effectiveness and safety of limited radiotherapy to the lumpectomy cavity alone.

Efficacy of Adjuvant Radiotherapy

Adjuvant radiation therapy is critically important following breast conservation surgery. NSABP B-06 demonstrated this with patients who received breast conserving surgery followed by radiation having a local control rate of 86 % at 20 years vs. 61 % for women who received surgery alone [1]. It is also clear that local control after adjuvant WBI can be further improved by adding a "boost" to the lumpectomy bed. Both the EORTC and Lyon trials have shown that additional radiation delivered to the peri-lumpectomy tissues will decrease absolute rates of local failure following traditional breast conserving therapy [5, 6]. In addition to improved local control, adjuvant radiation therapy has been shown to have a positive impact on overall survival. The meta-analysis by the Early Breast Cancer Trialists Collaborative Group (EBCTCG) showed improved survival at 15 years when local recurrences are prevented by adjuvant radiotherapy [7].

Although breast conservation therapy (BCT) has garnered widespread support, many women eligible for BCT receive either a mastectomy or lumpectomy without radiation therapy. This may be due in part to the lengthy course of whole breast radiotherapy or even their proximity to a radiation facility. A study by Athas et al. confirmed this by showing an increased rate of complete breast conservation for patients who live close to a radiation center [8]. Despite strong data in support of adjuvant radiation therapy, approximately 20 % of patients with early-stage breast cancer who receive BCT forgo radiation treatments [9, 10], which places them at a significantly increased risk of local recurrence (and death) when compared to patients who receive proper adjuvant therapy [1, 2].

History of Accelerated Partial Breast Irradiation

Radiation was first used to treat breast cancer 2 years after Marie and Pierre Curie's discovery of radium in 1898. A vial of radium salt was placed on the skin surface of a woman with breast cancer and the tumor was observed to decrease in size [11]. Implantation of radium needles into palpable breast cancers was the next development in the early 1900s with further refinement through the 1930s until they were supplanted by cobalt and cesium sources of low-voltage external X-rays. Although the current technique has been significantly refined and the pathological basis for accelerated partial breast irradiation (APBI) is different, credit for initial percutaneous implantation of radiation within a limited segment of the breast belongs to some of the earliest radiotherapists including Geoffrey Keynes.

Radiating only part of the breast did not reemerge until breast conservation became more acceptable. In the United States, modern APBI was initially begun in 1991 at the Ochsner Clinic in New Orleans, Louisiana, and William Beaumont Hospital in Royal Oak, Michigan. At both locations, radiation treatment to a limited portion of the breast over a shortened course was designed for women who had logistical reasons for not receiving the traditional 5 weeks of whole breast irradiation (WBI). Each dose (fraction) was larger and given twice a day over 5 days and designed to be radiobiologically equivalent to 5 weeks of WBI while maintaining minimal normal tissue toxicity.

Oncologic Basis for APBI

In addition to the obvious logistical benefits of shortening the length of treatment for patient convenience, there is oncologic support for concentrating the radiation to the breast tissue surrounding the lumpectomy cavity. Vicini et al. found that lumpectomies that initially met NSABP criteria for negative microscopic margins (no tumor on ink) had residual carcinoma almost 40 % of the time after re-excision. However, the residual disease was limited to the first one centimeter beyond a lumpectomy margin in over 90 % of cases [12]. In a study of 1,598 patients treated with BCT by Kurtz et al., 179 had an ipsilateral breast tumor recurrence (IBTR), of which 86 % occurred within close proximity to the lumpectomy bed [13]. Many other reports support the finding of local recurrence being predominantly in the tumor bed and that recurrences elsewhere in the breast occur at the same rate whether the patient receives WBI or not [1, 14–16]. Since the vast majority of IBTR occur within close proximity of the tumor bed and radiation therapy does not appear to "prevent" new elsewhere primaries, it makes sense to treat the area at highest risk with targeted radiation. This is the oncologic basis of partial breast irradiation.

Patient Selection for APBI

Not all breast conservation patients are candidates for APBI but obviously all APBI patients are having breast conservation (lumpectomy). Both the American Society of Breast Surgeons (ASBrS) and the American Brachytherapy Society (ABS) have issued criteria for appropriate patient selection for APBI (Table 27.1) [17, 18].

Table 27.1 ASBrS and ABS patient selection criteria for APBI [17, 18]

ASBrS [17]	ABS [18]
Age ≥45 (IDC), ≥50 (DCIS)	Age ≥50
Size ≤3 cm	≤3 cm
Histology: IDC, DCIS	All invasive subtypes and DCIS
Negative microscopic margins	Negative surgical margins
LN negative	LN negative
	No LVSI
	ER positive or ER negative

LVSI lymphovascular space invasion, *ER* estrogen receptor

In 2009, the American Society for Radiation Oncology (ASTRO) issued consensus statement (CS) recommendations, which identified the amount of scientific data in the literature for groups of patients treated with APBI subdivided by various clinical and pathologic parameters [19]. Patients were grouped into three categories: suitable, cautionary, and unsuitable (Table 27.2). The word "unsuitable," as it is used in the ASTRO guidelines, only refers to the paucity of scientific data that is presently available for patients with these pathologic features. This designation does not necessarily indicate that it is inappropriate to treat patients with these features as part of a clinical trial or even off-trial in a properly informed patient. In addition, the "cautionary" designation only refers to the fact that limited data existed at the time the guidelines were published for the use of APBI in this subgroup of patients. Since publication, additional data have emerged (see below) which would potentially alter these guidelines for selecting patients for APBI.

Several studies have retrospectively categorized patients treated with APBI into the ASTRO groupings and analyzed for rates of local recurrence, axillary failure, and distant metastasis. These studies have demonstrated similar clinical outcomes following partial breast irradiation regardless of category, with similar rates of local recurrence, axillary failure, and distant metastasis for patients with pure ductal carcinoma in situ, invasive lobular carcinoma, triple-negative histology, and node-positive disease [20–23]. In a review of the ASBrS MammoSite® Registry Trial, the only factor on multivariate analysis that showed an increased propensity for local recurrence was estrogen receptor (ER)-negative status ($p=0.002$), which is also true of ER-negative tumors treated with WBI [24]. Although there has been recent discussion regarding revision of these groups, no definitive plans have yet been made to change the current ASTRO CS guidelines for APBI. Results from NSABP B-39/RTOG 0413 phase III trial are not expected until at least 2015, and until that time, appropriate patient selection will continue to be on an individual basis.

Table 27.2 ASTRO consensus statement groups for APBI [19]

Factor	Suitable	Cautionary	Unsuitable
Age	60 y/o	50–59	<50
BRCA 1 or 2 mutation	Not present	–	Present
Tumor size	≤2 cm	>2 cm, ≤3 cm	>3 cm
T stage	T1	T0 or T2	T3 or T4
Margin status	Negative by ≥2 mm	Close (<2 mm)	Positive
Grade	Any	–	–
LVSI	No	Limited/focal	Yes
ER status	Positive	Negative	–
Multicentricity	Unicentric only	–	Present
Multifocality	Clinically unifocal with total size ≤2 cm	Clinically unifocal with total size 2.1–3.0 cm	Multiple foci >3 cm apart
Histology	Invasive ductal or other favorable subtype	Invasive lobular	
Pure DCIS	Not allowed	≤3 cm	If >3 cm
EIC	Not allowed	≤3 cm	If >3 cm
Associated LCIS	Allowed	–	–
N stage	pN0 (i^-,i^+)	–	pN1, pN2, pN3
Nodal surgery	SLN Bx or ALND	–	None performed
Neoadjuvant therapy	Not allowed	–	If used

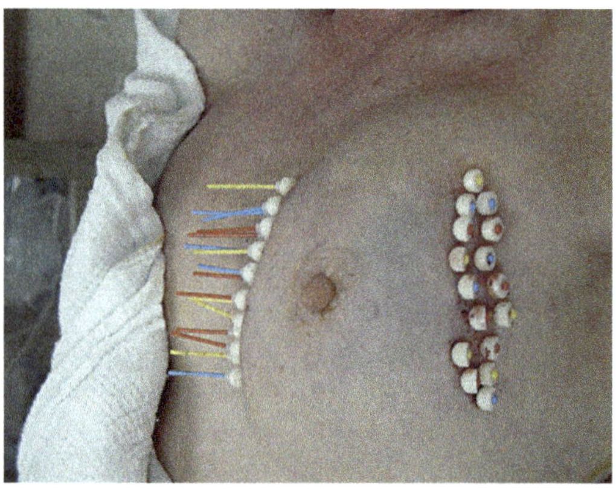

Fig. 27.1 Patient with multiple interstitial brachytherapy catheters in her breast (Image appears courtesy of Dr. L. Cuttino)

Techniques for Partial Breast Irradiation

The first technique of partial breast irradiation and the one with the longest follow-up is the multi-catheter interstitial technique (Fig. 27.1). Developed as a method of boosting the lumpectomy cavity, this approach was then applied to the treatment of the peri-lumpectomy tissues alone, first with low-dose rate seeds (LDR brachytherapy) and subsequently with a high-dose rate iridium source (HDR brachytherapy) [25–28]. Most interstitial implants require 15–20 catheters and are typically arranged in two to three planes. This technique is a very versatile form of APBI, with the ability to sculpt the radiation dose as needed to treat the lumpectomy cavity and minimize radiation to other tissues (skin, normal breast, chest wall/rib, heart, lung). The most common dose and fractionation scheme for interstitial HDR brachytherapy is 3.4 Gy for ten fractions delivered twice a day with 6 h between fractions.

The MammoSite® Radiation Therapy System (RTS) (Hologic, Inc, Bedford, MA) was cleared by the United States FDA in 2002, dramatically changing the adoption of partial breast irradiation for breast cancer patients. Since 2002, the MammoSite® RTS (Fig. 27.2) has been used to treat over 60,000 women with early-stage breast cancer. Hattangadi has showed a dramatic 16-fold increase in the use of APBI from 2000 to the end of 2007 [29]. The main reason for this increase is the ease of insertion of the single balloon catheter and the simplicity of treatment planning.

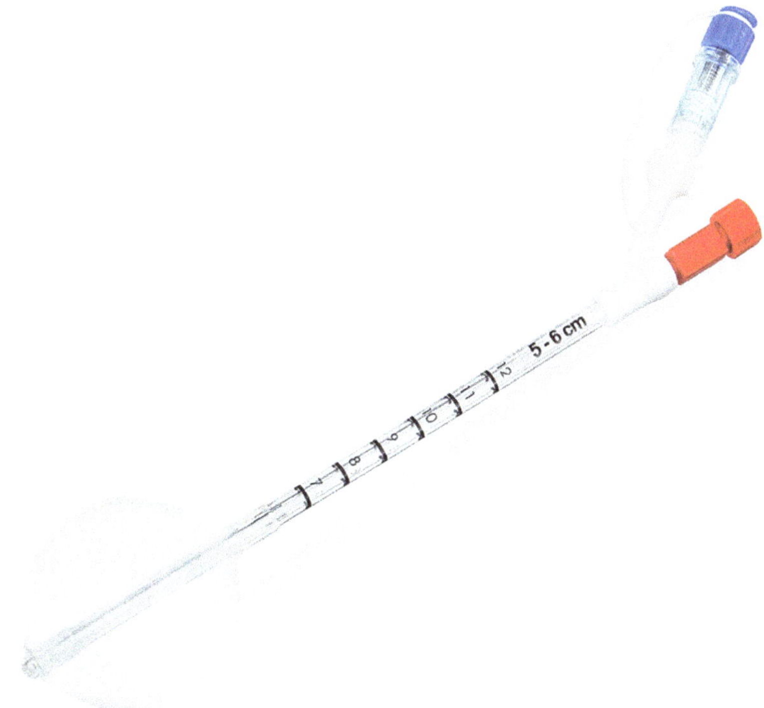

Fig. 27.2 MammoSite® single-lumen balloon brachytherapy device (Image provided courtesy of Hologic, Inc.)

However, some patients treated with the MammoSite® balloon catheter had a problem with cosmesis. Decreased cosmetic outcome after single-channel applicator-based brachytherapy was most notable in patients with decreased amount of tissue (<7 mm) from their skin to the balloon, resulting in an unwanted increase in the radiation dose to the skin. This problem was overcome by the development of second-generation multi-lumen devices that allowed for a more tailored treatment plan which could selectively adjust and minimize the radiation dose to the adjacent normal structures. The first multi-lumen device cleared by the FDA in May 2007 was the Contura® multi-lumen balloon (MLB) (Bard Biopsy Systems, Irvine, CA) (Figs 27.3a, b). The Contura® MLB has a central catheter and four offset catheters that are flexed away from the central catheter by 0.5 cm. These additional catheters allow shaping of the dose away from critical structures (skin, chest wall, lung, heart) that may be in close proximity to the lumpectomy cavity [30].

Hologic developed an improved MammoSite® with multi-lumens, named the MammoSite® Multi-Lumen (ML) (Fig. 27.4) that is designed with three additional lumens offset from the central lumen by 3 mm, which also offers improved flexibility in treatment design. Prior to the introduction of multi-lumen devices, the optimal distance between the skin and balloon surface was 7 mm, which made many women ineligible for APBI. The improved dosimetric flexibility of multi-lumen balloon applicators allows the treatment of patients down to 3 mm of skin spacing (skin to balloon distance).

The first single insertion multi-lumen applicator that does not use a balloon is the Strut Adjusted Volumetric Implant® (SAVI®) (Cianna Medical, Aliso Viejo, CA) which received FDA approval in 2006 (Fig. 27.5). Unlike the balloon applicators, the SAVI® has multiple struts that project outward to create a whisk-like apparatus with each of the exterior struts in direct contact with breast tissue (similar to multiple catheter interstitial implants) [31]. This device comes in a variety of sizes with the smallest, a SAVI Mini-6, allowing brachytherapy treatment of women with small breasts or with breast augmentation (very difficult with a balloon-based device) [32].

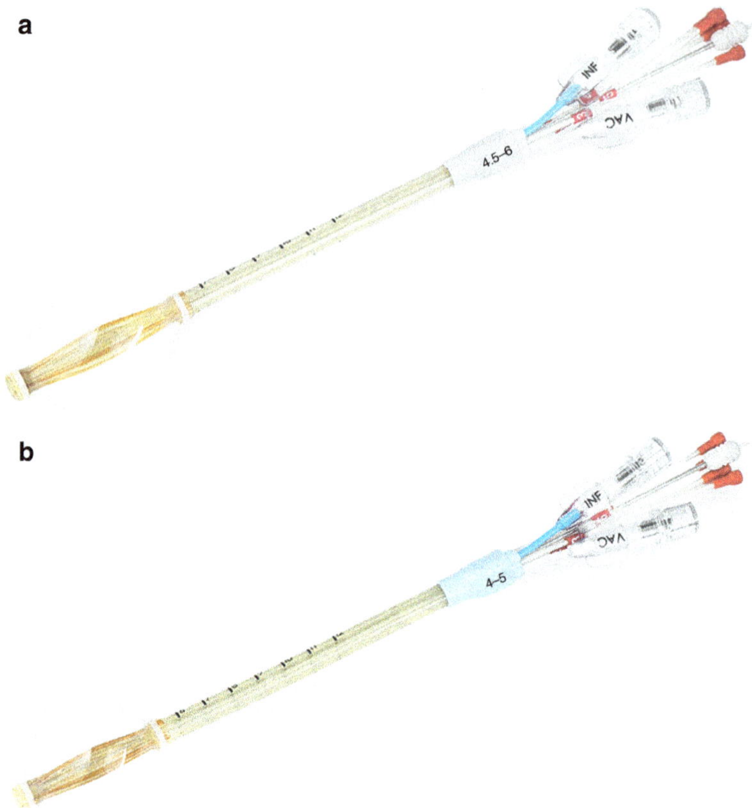

Fig. 27.3 (**a**, **b**) Contura® multi-lumen balloon brachytherapy device (Image provided courtesy of Hologic, Inc.)

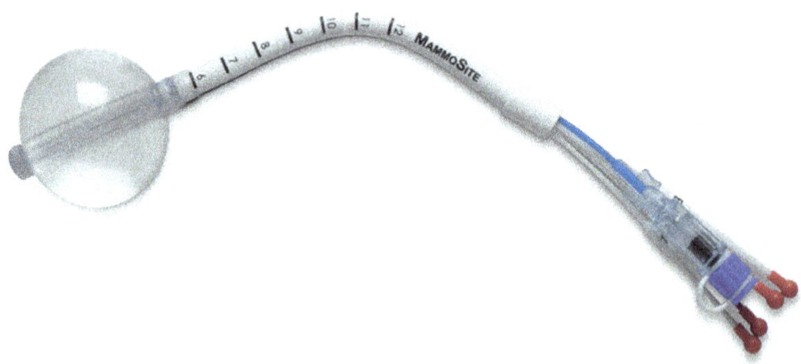

Fig. 27.4 MammoSite® ML multi-lumen balloon brachytherapy device (Image provided courtesy of Hologic, Inc.)

Outpatient-based APBI utilizing brachytherapy is most commonly delivered via a high-dose rate (HDR) source administered using a robotic afterloader in a standard radiation vault (Fig. 27.6). An alternative to high-dose rate brachytherapy is electronic brachytherapy which is delivered with a miniaturized high-dose rate 50 kV X-ray source (Fig. 27.7) via the Axxent® brachytherapy applicator (Xoft, a subsidiary of iCAD, Inc, San Jose, CA) [33] (Fig. 27.8). An advantage of electronic brachytherapy is the reduced shielding requirements for brachytherapy treatment rooms (can be done in physician office with a lead drape over the patient). However, this system only has a single lumen and therefore minimal ability to shape the dose away from normal tissue, with

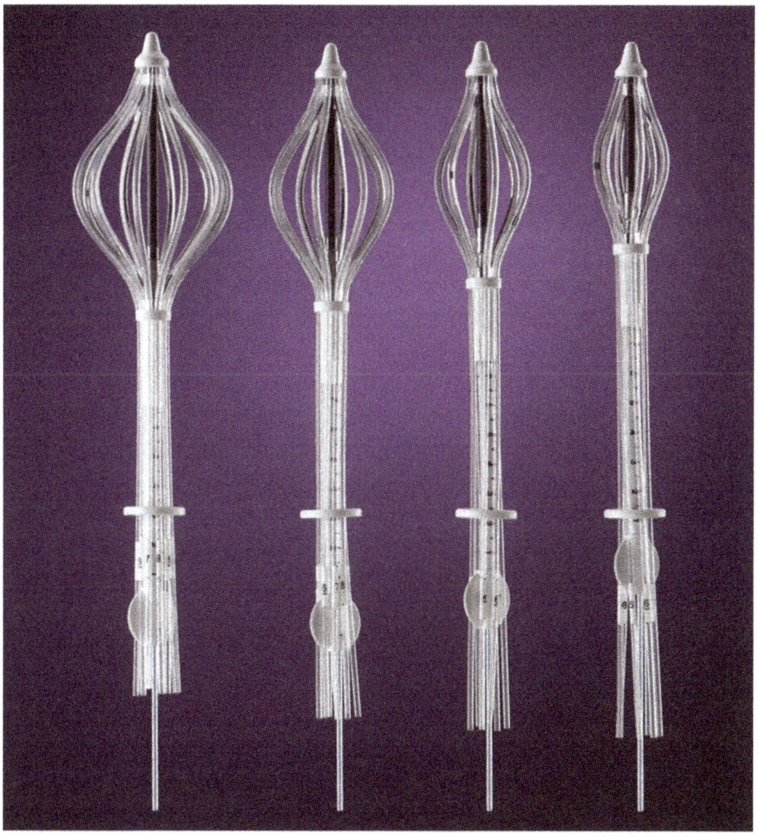

Fig. 27.5 SAVI® multi-lumen brachytherapy device (Image courtesy of Cianna medical)

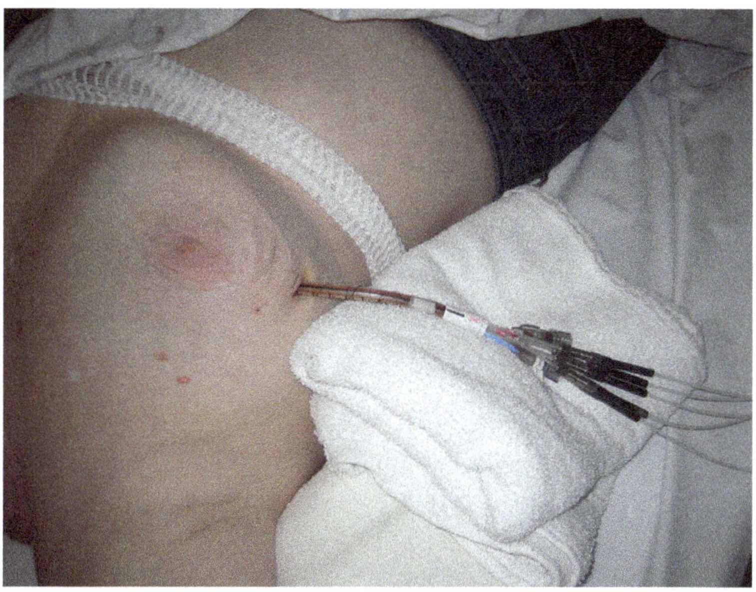

Fig. 27.6 Afterloader connected to a multi-lumen applicator for high dose rate brachytherapy (Image appears courtesy of Dr. L. Cuttino)

further theoretical concerns about the radiobiologic effect (RBE) of low-energy X-rays. This will need to be closely monitored as radiation centers gain experience with this system. The Xoft Axxent balloon-based system is also used for another APBI technique, intraoperative radiotherapy (IORT), as discussed in the following section.

The most widely used method of accelerated partial breast irradiation is three-dimensional conformal radiotherapy or 3D-CRT. Initially introduced in 2003 [34], this method uses a standard linear accelerator with between three and five noncoplanar external radiotherapy segments to deliver the accelerated course of radiotherapy to the area surrounding the lumpectomy cavity (Fig. 27.9). There are limitations to the 3D-CRT technique including the need to treat a larger volume of breast (and normal) tissue surrounding the lumpectomy cavity due to variability with setup and respiration (neither of which are an issue with internal/HDR brachytherapy) as well as an increased dose to the contralateral breast, heart, and lungs. The treatment is delivered two times per day, similar to conventional brachytherapy, but with a slightly larger dose per fraction (3.85 Gy) to a total prescription dose of 38.5 Gy to account for the lack of heterogeneity using this technique.

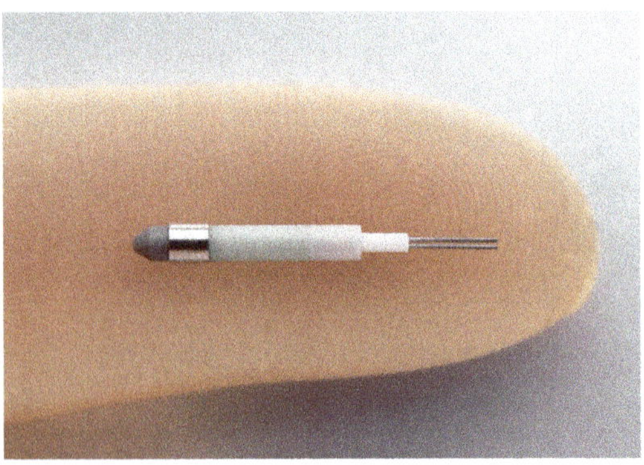

Fig. 27.7 X-ray source for Xoft brachytherapy system (Courtesy of Xoft, a subsidiary of iCAD, Inc.)

Intraoperative APBI

In Europe, several centers have developed intraoperative radiation therapy (IORT), which delivered a single dose of radiation immediately following lumpectomy but prior to wound closure. One technique utilizes a standard linear accelerator built into the operating room to deliver a single 21 Gy dose of electrons [35]. Intraoperative partial breast irradiation has the distinct advantage of visualizing the tumor bed at the time of surgery; however, final pathologic assessment of the margins and lymph nodes is not available at the time of treatment. Advocates for IORT promote the potential benefit of treating residual tumor cells prior to the onset of hypoxia, which can occur following breast surgery. In addition to the Xoft® Axxent® balloon-based system, another form of intraoperative RT uses a high-dose rate,

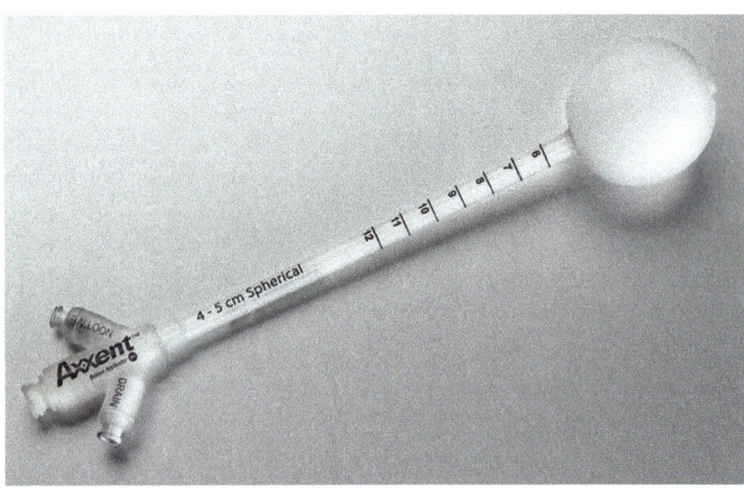

Fig. 27.8 Axxent single-lumen balloon catheter (Courtesy of Xoft, a subsidiary of iCAD, Inc.)

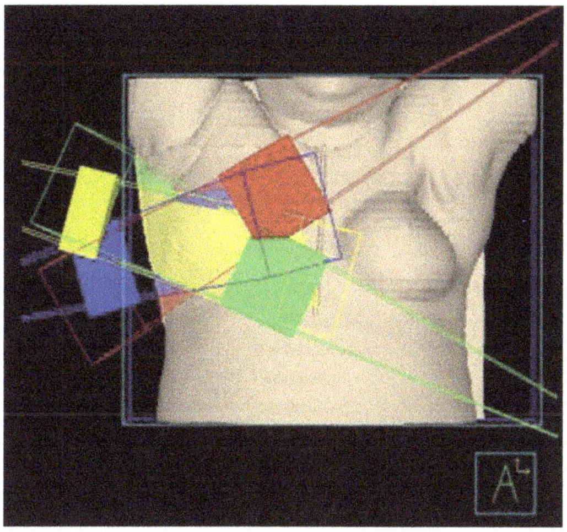

Fig. 27.9 Example of four-field three-dimensional conformal radiation therapy (3D-CRT) (Image appears courtesy of Beaumont Health System)

low-energy X-ray source (50 kV) placed directly into the lumpectomy via a collimator with a sphere on the end (INTRABEAM® System). There is a randomized, phase III clinical trial of targeted intraoperative radiotherapy versus whole breast radiotherapy (TARGIT-A trial) that has accrued to completion and awaits long-term follow-up data on these patients. Preliminary results, published in 2010, showed non-inferiority of the IORT arm as compared with whole breast irradiation; however, an update provided at the 2012 San Antonio Breast Cancer Symposium suggested an increased rate of ipsilateral recurrence for patients treated with IORT [36]. The most recent publication of the TARGIT data suggests that excess local recurrences may primarily occur when the single-fraction technique is used at an extended time from the original surgery [37]. Xoft has also initiated a prospective, multicenter, non-inferiority study utilizing the Xoft® Axxent® System for IORT which will enroll 600 patients; the results of this study are pending at this time.

Other APBI Techniques

Novel concepts that are being studied in partial breast irradiation include LDR seed implantation into the breast [38], intraoperative pre-lumpectomy radiation therapy [39], stereotactic radiation therapy utilizing a CyberKnife® [40], and proton therapy. Proton therapy for partial breast irradiation has been investigated at several centers including Massachusetts General Hospital, M.D. Anderson Cancer Center, and Loma Linda University [41, 42]. An initial publication from Massachusetts General by Kozak et al. suggested a higher than expected acute skin toxicity with proton-based APBI; however, a separate phase II trial conducted at Loma Linda University did not report this same toxicity pattern. The unexpected toxicity produced within the protocol at Massachusetts General was likely due to the use of a single gantry angle as opposed to two to three tangents. Ongoing prospective study of particle therapy for partial breast irradiation with long-term follow-up is needed.

Outcomes Following APBI

Several single-institution and collaborative series on APBI have been published and updated including reports by William Beaumont Hospital, Virginia Commonwealth University, Tufts Medical Center, New York University, and others (Table 27.3).

At this time, results for only two phase III trials are available that compare APBI to WBI. The National Institute of Oncology in Hungary conducted a randomized trial of 258 patients, reporting a 5-year interim analysis in 2007 showing equivalent control between the study arms with a local recurrence of 4.7 % in the partial breast irradiation arm and 3.4 % in the WBI arm (p=NS) [43]. Cosmesis was improved in the patients receiving HDR partial breast irradiation versus those who received standard WBI. The TARGIT-A trial, as discussed above, reported in 2010 a non-inferiority between their single-fraction partial breast and standard whole breast treatment arms, although the median follow-up was less than 3 years, and new data suggest the potential for increased treatment failure using this intraoperative technique, especially at an increased time from the initial surgery [36, 37]. Other groups have attempted to compare APBI and WBI through retrospective methods. A 12-year matched pair analysis was published by

Table 27.3 Interstitial and balloon-based APBI trials [26, 31, 43–49]

Institution	# Patients	Follow-up (years)	Local recurrence	Toxicity
National Institute of Oncology – Hungary [43]	45	12	9.3 %	<3 % grade III
William Beaumont Hospital [49]	199	12	5 %	
Ochsner Clinic [26]	71	6.25	8 %	Grade III (late) LDR: 3.8 % HDR: 7.7 %
Tufts Medical Center [44]	32	5	6 %	Fat necrosis, skin, and subcutaneous toxicity declined with additional follow-up
RTOG 95-17 [45]	99	5	3 % (HDR) 6 % (LDR)	Grade III (late) LDR 18 % HDR 4 %
ASBrS MammoSite® Registry [46]	1,449	5	3.8 %	
William Beaumont Hospital – MammoSite® [47]	80	3.5	2.9 %	
Multi-institutional (VCU) [48]	493	2	1.2 %	9 % infection rate (5 % if closed cavity technique used)
SAVI Collaborative Group [31]	100	2.1	1.0 %	First 100 patients treated as part of the SAVI registry trial

Shah et al. comparing 199 patients treated with APBI with a similar cohort of 199 patients treated with WBI. This study concluded that patients who received a limited radiation field had similar outcomes including local relapse ≤5.0 %, regional relapse ≤2.0 %, and disease-free survival >87 % at 12 years [49, 50].

Acute toxicities include skin irritation (pruritus, light erythema) and changes (more intense erythema and desquamation) and infection. Long-term complications include hypopigmentation, telangiectasia, symptomatic fat necrosis/fibrosis, late infection/abscess, and symptomatic seroma formation. The rates of each of acute and chronic complications vary by the APBI technique utilized; for example, for single-lumen MammoSite® balloon brachytherapy, the acute infection rate is ~9 % (all resolved with oral antibiotics). The overall rate of fat necrosis and tissue fibrosis was 2.5 %, with a symptomatic seroma rate was 13.4 % at any time and 0.6 % beyond 2 years. The percentage of breasts with excellent/good cosmetic results at 60, 72, and 84 months was 91.3 %, 90.5 %, and 90.6 % [51].

Future Directions

We stand ready to enter an era of personalized medicine where adjuvant therapy will no longer be offered to groups of women in particular disease categories or stages, but instead will be risk appropriate to an individual based upon patterns of genetic expression. Although radiotherapy recommendations are not presently based on tumor gene expression, there is emerging data on local/regional recurrence rates and gene expression that may allow personalization of the type and extent of radiation treatment based on the risk and potential pattern for tumor recurrence [52].

Another area of continued research involves shortening of APBI fractionation schedules to improve convenience of and compliance with adjuvant radiation therapy. At least two of the companies that manufacture brachytherapy applicators have sponsored phase II trials using 2-day dose fractionation schedules in the United States. As results from these trials mature, consideration of a phase III trial to compare various fractionation patterns should be discussed.

Future challenges to this segment of breast cancer care will be defining the appropriate management for recurrences/new primaries following whole breast irradiation or APBI. Lastly, there will be continued refinement of appropriate guidelines for APBI as additional data become available, including the publication of the ongoing phase III trials.

References

1. Fisher B, Anderson S, Bryant J, et al. Twenty-year follow-up of a randomized trial comparing total mastectomy, lumpectomy, and lumpectomy plus irradiation for the treatment of invasive breast cancer. N Engl J Med. 2002;347(16):1233–41.
2. Veronesi U, Cascinelli N, Mariani L, et al. Twenty-year follow-up of a randomized study comparing breast-conserving surgery with radical mastectomy for early breast cancer. N Engl J Med. 2002;347(16):1227–32.
3. Arriagada R, Lê MG, Rochard F, et al. Conservative treatment versus mastectomy in early breast cancer: patterns of failure with 15 years of follow-up data. Institut Gustave-Roussy Breast Cancer Group. J Clin Oncol. 1996;14(5):1558–64.
4. Blichert-Toft M, Rose C, Andersen JA, et al. Danish randomized trial comparing breast conservation therapy with mastectomy: six years of life-table analysis. Danish Breast Cancer Cooperative Group. J Natl Cancer Inst Monogr. 1992;11:19–25.
5. Bartelink H, Horiot JC, Poortmans PM, et al. Impact of a higher radiation dose on local control and survival in breast-conserving therapy of early breast cancer: 10-year results of the randomized boost versus no boost EORTC 22881-10882 trial. J Clin Oncol. 2007;25(22):3259–65.
6. Polgár C, Fodor J, Orosz Z, et al. Electron and high-dose-rate brachytherapy boost in the conservative treatment of stage I-II breast cancer first results of the randomized Budapest boost trial. Strahlenther Onkol. 2002;178(11):615–23.
7. Clarke M, Collins R, Darby S, et al. Effects of radiotherapy and of differences in the extent of surgery for early breast cancer on local recurrence and 15-year survival: an overview of the randomised trials. Lancet. 2005;366(9503):2087–106.
8. Athas WF, Adams-Cameron M, Hunt WC, et al. Travel distance to radiation therapy and receipt of radiotherapy following breast-conserving surgery. J Natl Cancer Inst. 2000;92(3):269–71.
9. Nattinger AB, Hoffman RG, Kneusel RT, et al. Relation between appropriateness of primary therapy for early-stage breast carcinoma and increased use of breast conserving surgery. Lancet. 2000;356:1148–53.
10. Baxter NN, Virning BA, Durham SB, et al. Trends in treatment of ductal carcinoma in situ of the breast. J Natl Cancer Inst. 2004;96:443–8.
11. Kuske R, Quiet C. The history of brachytherapy. http://www.arizona-breast-cancer-specialists.com/brachytherapy/brachytherapy-history.html Updated 2007. Accessed 1 Oct 2011.
12. Vicini FA, Kestin LL, Goldstein NS, et al. Defining the clinical target volume for patients with early-stage breast cancer treated with lumpectomy and accelerated partial breast irradiation: a pathologic analysis. Int J Radiat Oncol Biol Phys. 2004;60:722–30.
13. Kurtz JM, Spitalier JM, Amalric R, et al. The prognostic significance of late local recurrence after breast-conserving therapy. Int J Radiat Oncol Biol Phys. 1990;18(1):87–93.
14. Veronesi U, Marubini E, Marinani L, et al. Radiotherapy after breast conserving therapy in small breast carcinoma: long-term results of a randomized trial. Ann Oncol. 2001;12:1075–80.
15. Clark RM, McCulloch PB, Boolbol S, et al. Randomized clinical trial to assess the effectiveness of breast irradiation following lumpectomy and axillary dissection for node-negative breast cancer. J Natl Cancer Inst. 1992;84:683–9.
16. Uppsala-Oreboro Breast Cancer Study Group. Sector resection with or without postoperative radiotherapy for stage I breast cancer: a randomized trial. J Natl Cancer Inst. 1990;82:277–82.
17. American Society of Breast Surgeons. Consensus statement for accelerated partial breast irradiation 2011. http://www.breastsurgeons.org/statements.
18. Shah C, Vicini F, Wazer D, et al. The American Brachytherapy Society consensus statement for accelerated partial breast irradiation. Brachytherapy. 2013; 12(4):267–77.
19. Smith BD, Arthur DW, Buchholz TA, et al. Accelerated partial breast irradiation consensus statement from the American Society for Radiation Oncology (ASTRO). Int J Radiat Oncol Biol Phys. 2009;74(4):987–1001.
20. Park SS, Grills IS, Chen PY, et al. Accelerated partial breast irradiation for pure ductal carcinoma in situ. Int J Radiat Oncol Biol Phys. 2011;81(2):403–8.
21. Shah C, Wilkinson JB, Shaitelman S, et al. Clinical outcomes using accelerated partial breast irradiation in patients with invasive lobular carcinoma. Int J Radiat Oncol Biol Phys. 2011;81(4):e547–51.
22. Shah C, Wilkinson JB, Shaitelman S, et al. Impact of lymph node status on clinical outcomes after accelerated partial breast irradiation. Int J Radiat Oncol Biol Phys. 2012;82(3):e409–14.
23. Wilkinson JB, Reid RE, Shaitelman SF, et al. Outcomes of breast cancer patients with triple negative receptor status treated with accelerated partial breast irradiation. Int J Radiat Oncol Biol Phys. 2011;81(3):e159–64.
24. Beitsch P, Vicini F, Keisch M, et al. Five-year outcome of patients classified in the "unsuitable" category using the American Society of Therapeutic Radiology and Oncology (ASTRO) Consensus Panel guidelines for the application of accelerated partial breast irradiation: an analysis of patients treated on the American Society

of Breast Surgeons MammoSite® Registry trial. Ann Surg Oncol. 2010;S3:219–25.
25. Vicini F, White J, Gustafson G, et al. The use of iodine-125 seeds as a substitute for iridium-192 seeds in temporary interstitial breast implants. Int J Radiat Oncol Biol Phys. 1993;27(3):561–6.
26. King TA, Bolton JS, Kuske RR, et al. Long-term results of wide-field brachytherapy as the sole method of radiation therapy after segmental mastectomy for T(is,1,2) breast cancer. Am J Surg. 2000;180(4): 299–304.
27. Vicini FA, Chen PY, Fraile M, et al. Low-dose-rate brachytherapy as the sole radiation modality in the management of patients with early-stage breast cancer treated with breast-conserving therapy: preliminary results of a pilot trial. Int J Radiat Oncol Biol Phys. 1997;38(2):301–10.
28. Baglan KL, Martinez AA, Frazier RC, et al. The use of high-dose-rate brachytherapy alone after lumpectomy in patients with early-stage breast cancer treated with breast-conserving therapy. Int J Radiat Oncol Biol Phys. 2001;50(4):1003–11.
29. Hattangadi JA, Taback N, Neville BA, et al. Accelerated partial breast irradiation using brachytherapy for breast cancer: patterns in utilization and guideline concordance. J Natl Cancer Inst. 2012;104(1):29–41.
30. Arthur DW, Vicini FA, Todor DA, et al. Improvements in critical dosimetric endpoints using the contura multilumen balloon breast brachytherapy catheter to deliver accelerated partial breast irradiation: preliminary dosimetric findings of a phase IV trial. Int J Radiat Oncol Biol Phys. 2011;79(1):26–33.
31. Yashar CM, Scanderbeg D, Kuske R, et al. Initial clinical experience with the Strut-Adjusted Volume Implant (SAVI) breast brachytherapy device for accelerated partial-breast irradiation (APBI): first 100 patients with more than 1 year of follow-up. Int J Radiat Oncol Biol Phys. 2011;80(3):765–70.
32. Bloom ES, Kirsner S, Mason BE, et al. Accelerated partial breast irradiation using the strut-adjusted volume implant single-entry hybrid catheter in brachytherapy for breast cancer in the setting of breast augmentation. Brachytherapy. 2011;10(3):178–83.
33. Mehta VK, Algan O, Greim KL, et al. Experience with an electronic brachytherapy technique for intracavitary accelerated partial breast irradiation. Am J Clin Oncol. 2010;33(4):327–35.
34. Baglan KL, Sharpe MB, Jaffray D, et al. Accelerated partial breast irradiation using 3D conformal radiation therapy (3D-CRT). Int J Radiat Oncol Biol Phys. 2003;55(2):302–11.
35. Veronesi U, Orecchia R, Luini A, et al. Intraoperative radiotherapy during breast conserving surgery: a study on 1,822 cases treated with electrons. Breast Cancer Res Treat. 2010;124(1):141–51.
36. Vaidya JS, Joseph DJ, Tobias JS, et al. Targeted intraoperative radiotherapy versus whole breast radiotherapy for breast cancer (TARGIT-A trial): an international, prospective, randomised, non-inferiority phase III trial. Lancet. 2010;376(9735):91–102.
37. Vaidya JS, Wenz F, Bulsara M, et al. Risk-adapted targeted intraoperative radiotherapy versus whole-breast radiotherapy for breast cancer: 5-year results for local control and overall survival from the TARGIT-A randomised trial. Lancet. 2014;383(9917):603–13.
38. Pignol JP, Keller B, Rakovitch E, et al. First report of a permanent breast 103Pd seed implant as adjuvant radiation treatment for early-stage breast cancer. Int J Radiat Oncol Biol Phys. 2006;64(1):176–81.
39. VanderWalde NA, Ollila DW, DeMore NK, et al. Local recurrence outcomes in phase II clinical trial using single dose Intraoperative Radiotherapy (IORT) before surgical excision of early-stage breast cancer. Int J Radiat Oncol Biol Phys. 2011;81(2):S10–1.
40. Vermeulen S, Cotrutz C, Morris A, et al. Accelerated partial breast irradiation: using the CyberKnife as the radiation delivery platform in the treatment of early breast cancer. Front Oncol. 2011;1:43.
41. Kozak KR, Smith BL, Adams J, et al. Accelerated partial-breast irradiation using proton beams: initial clinical experience. Int J Radiat Oncol Biol Phys. 2006;66(3):691–8.
42. Bush DA, Slater JD, Garberoglio C, et al. Partial breast irradiation delivered with proton beam: results of a phase II trial. Clin Breast Cancer. 2011;11(4): 241–5.
43. Polgár C, Major T, Fodor J, et al. Accelerated partial-breast irradiation using high-dose-rate interstitial brachytherapy: 12-year update of a prospective clinical study. Radiother Oncol. 2010;94(3):274–9.
44. Kaufman SA, DiPetrillo TA, Price LL, et al. Long-term outcome and toxicity in a Phase I/II trial using high-dose-rate multicatheter interstitial brachytherapy for T1/T2 breast cancer. Brachytherapy. 2007;6(4): 286–92.
45. Arthur DW, Winter K, Kuske RR, et al. A Phase II trial of brachytherapy alone after lumpectomy for select breast cancer: tumor control and survival outcomes of RTOG 95–17. Int J Radiat Oncol Biol Phys. 2008;72(2):467–73.
46. Vicini F, Beitsch P, Quiet C, et al. Five-year analysis of treatment efficacy and cosmesis by the American Society of Breast Surgeons MammoSite breast brachytherapy registry trial in patients treated with accelerated partial breast irradiation. Int J Radiat Oncol Biol Phys. 2011;79(3):808–17.
47. Chao KK, Vicini FA, Wallace M, et al. Analysis of treatment efficacy, cosmesis, and toxicity using the MammoSite breast brachytherapy catheter to deliver accelerated partial-breast irradiation: the William Beaumont Hospital experience. Int J Radiat Oncol Biol Phys. 2007;69(1):32–40.
48. Cuttino LW, Keisch M, Jenrette JM, et al. Multi-institutional experience using the MammoSite Radiation Therapy System in the treatment of early-stage breast cancer: 2-year results. Int J Radiat Oncol Biol Phys. 2008;71:107–14.
49. Shah C, Antonucci JV, Wilkinson JB, et al. Twelve-year clinical outcomes and patterns of failure with accelerated partial breast irradiation versus whole-breast

irradiation: results of a matched-pair analysis. Radiother Oncol. 2011;100(2):210–4.
50. Benitez PR, Chen PY, Vicini FA, et al. Partial breast irradiation in breast conserving therapy by way of interstitial brachytherapy. Am J Surg. 2004;188(4):355–64.
51. Vicini FA, Keisch M, Shah C, et al. Factors associated with optimal long-term cosmetic results in patients treated with accelerated partial breast irradiation using balloon-based brachytherapy. Int J Radiat Oncol Biol Phys. 2012;83(2):512–8.
52. Mamounas EP, Tang G, Fisher B, et al. Association between the 21-gene recurrence score assay and risk of locoregional recurrence in node-negative, estrogen receptor-positive breast cancer: results from NSABP B-14 and NSABP B-20. Clin Oncol. 2010;28(10):1677–83.

28 The Emerging Role of Intraoperative Radiation Therapy [IORT] in Breast Cancer

Donald A. Goer and Melvin J. Silverstein

Introduction

Intraoperative radiation treatment (IORT) is the application of radiation directly to the residual tumor or tumor bed during surgery, after the surgical removal of the tumor. IORT has long been used to treat a variety of locally advanced and recurrent cancers. Studies have demonstrated that when used as a component of multidisciplinary treatment, IORT improves local control and survival for a number of tumors. IORT's use in breast cancer treatment is more recent, but has shown a remarkable rate of adoption in the last decade, with more than 20,000 women receiving IORT treatment. For breast cancer, IORT can be used to provide either a precision boost to the tumor bed, replacing the traditional external beam radiation therapy (EBRT) boost, or as the only radiation treatment the patient will receive. This chapter will discuss the evolution of radiation treatment in breast cancer that has led to the rapid adoption of IORT, the rationale for its use, the various IORT approaches that have been employed, the clinical results of IORT treatment, and the future potential of IORT as it is applied to breast cancer.

D.A. Goer, PhD (✉)
Intraop Medical Corporation,
570 Del Rey Avenue, Sunnyvale, CA 94085, USA
e-mail: dagoer@intraopmedical.com

M.J. Silverstein, MD
Gross Family Foundation Endowed Chair in Oncoplastic Surgery, Hoag Breast Program, Hoag Memorial Hospital Presbyterian, Newport Beach, CA, USA

Clinical Professor of Surgery, Keck School of Medicine, University of Southern California, Los Angeles, CA, USA

Evolution of IORT in Breast-Conserving Treatment

Multiple clinical trials have established that breast-conserving therapy (BCT) is equivalent to mastectomy in terms of overall survival [1–4]. While mastectomy patients in these early series had better local control than BCT patients, the radiation treatments used in these studies did not employ modern radiotherapy technology nor utilize the postoperative imaging techniques available today. More modern BCT series have demonstrated that BCT has equivalent local control when compared to mastectomy [5, 6]. Even without today's improvements in radiotherapy delivery, the BCT patients in these earlier series had higher breast preservation with equivalent overall survival. BCT is recommended by the National Comprehensive Cancer Network (NCCN) in their guidelines as an excellent treatment option for early-stage breast cancer. Furthermore, BCT is superior to breast-conserving surgery (BCS) alone, in terms of local control and breast preservation [7–9], and a recent study showed that BCT had improved disease-specific survival compared to mastectomy for early-stage breast cancer [10]. Since it is now established that improved local control at 5 years translates into a survival advantage at 15 years [11], BCT should be the clear treatment of choice for early-stage breast cancer.

A.I. Riker (ed.), *Breast Disease: Comprehensive Management*,
DOI 10.1007/978-1-4939-1145-5_28, © Springer Science+Business Media New York 2015

Table 28.1 Effect of travel distance and age on BCT compliance
Travel distance data from Athas et al. [13]. Age data from Ballard-Barbash et al. [14]

Travel Distance (miles)	Completion of BCT	Patient Age (years)	Use of Radiotherapy
0-24.9	84%	65-69	76%
25-49.9	78%	70-74	68%
50-74.9	69%	75-79	56%
75-99.9	57%	≥80	24%
> 100	42%		

The "gold standard" of BCT involves surgical removal of the tumor and sufficient adjacent tissue to the tumor in order to achieve clear margins, usually followed by 5–7 weeks of external beam radiation therapy (EBRT) after the breast has healed. Studies have also validated that most women benefit from an additional five to eight treatments of radiation, called a "boost," directed to the tumor bed [5, 12]. Radiation treatment generally begins 4–5 weeks after surgery – once the final margins have been determined to be negative and after the breast has healed from the operation. For those patients who will require chemotherapy, the start of EBRT is delayed for up to 6 months.

Even though BCT is an excellent choice, many women in the United States who are eligible for BCT opt for mastectomy or undergo only BCS but not the additional radiation treatment that is needed. This may occur for several reasons. BCT requires daily radiation treatments for 5–7 weeks. Women who live far from radiation treatment centers often find it difficult to travel long distances for their daily treatments; BCT compliance is inversely proportional to the distance of the closest radiation center [13]. Women who work, even if they live close to radiation centers, may find that the requirement for daily BCT treatments interferes with their work schedules. Elderly patients, especially those older than 70, also show a very low compliance rate with BCT [14, 15] (see Table 28.1). Finally, some women choose mastectomy because they have concerns about radiation toxicity.

Changes in BCT

The inconvenience of protracted BCT radiation schedules has led several investigators to explore whether it is possible to deliver the needed radiation treatment over a shorter period of time. Whelan [16] and the Start B Trial [6] have demonstrated that 3 weeks of EBRT, with or without a boost, is equivalent to 5 weeks of EBRT for women with moderate-sized breasts (<1,800 ml for the radiation planning volume) in terms of both local control and cosmesis. This 3-week EBRT approach is gradually replacing the standard 5-week EBRT regimen for women who qualify for BCT and are ≥35 years old and who have tumor stage ≤ T2 and nodal status ≤ N1.

Since 3 weeks of EBRT can still be a hardship for many women, researchers are investigating whether the radiation treatment for some women might be reduced even further. Based upon the observation that 80–85 % of breast cancer recurrences happen within the index quadrant in postmenopausal women, a number of investigators are exploring whether partial breast irradiation (PBI) can further shorten the course of radiotherapy. The concept behind PBI is that treating the entire breast (whole breast irradiation or WBI) may result in overtreating some women, thereby increasing toxicity. If equivalent local control in these women can be achieved by irradiating a smaller volume of tissue, the dose to the normal tissues, and thus the toxicities of the treatments, will be reduced.

These efforts have resulted in a variety of different techniques for PBI that employ different geometries in treatment delivery, irradiate different volumes, and have different fractionation schedules. Most of the current PBI approaches are delivered postsurgically, as is the case with standard WBI and hypofractionated treatment, but reduce the overall time of the radiation treatment to a week or less. Due to a shorter course of treatment, these PBI techniques are usually referred to as *accelerated* PBI or APBI. With IORT APBI, all of the radiation treatment is delivered in one treatment during the lumpectomy.

Non-IORT APBI in Early-Stage Breast Cancer

The oldest APBI method, and one that has the longest follow-up, is multi-plane high-dose-rate (HDR) brachytherapy, pioneered by Polgar in Europe [17] and several centers in the United States [18–21]. This approach involves inserting 14–20 catheters at 1–1.5 cm spacing to cover the lumpectomy cavity in more than one plane. Patients receive between 30 and 36 Gy given over 4–5 days in seven to ten fractions. In highly selected women, in small single-institutional studies, this APBI approach has shown comparable results to WBI, with a 5-year local recurrence rate of 4–5 %. For example, in a single-institution, nonrandomized study of 45 consecutively treated patients, Polgar et al. [22] showed 5- and 10-year local recurrence rates of 4.4 and 9.3 %, respectively, with an overall survival at 12 years of 88.9 %. Of note, all patients had T1 tumors and were node negative. In another randomized trial, Polgar et al. [23] assigned low-risk women (median age 59 years, T $\leq$ 2.0 cm, pN0, G1 or G2, ER/PR+, negative margins $\geq$2 mm, DCIS and lobular carcinoma excluded) to either APBI (128 women) or conventional BCT (130 women). The study was stopped prematurely in 2004, before it accrued the necessary 570 patients to determine non-inferiority of this APBI approach with BCT, in order to participate in the larger randomized GEC-ESTRO study [24] of 1,170 women treated with either brachytherapy PBI or conventional BCT. Though underpowered when it was stopped, the difference in LR in the arms proved non-significant (4.7 % for PBI vs. 3.1 % for BCT) with a median follow-up of over 5 years,

Multi-plane brachytherapy requires a high level of skill to deliver, and it is also uncomfortable for many patients. For these reasons, this approach to APBI has not gained as wide an overall acceptance as originally anticipated. A simpler HDR brachytherapy technique, based on a double-lumen balloon catheter that can be inserted into excision cavity, was developed by Mammosite® (Hologic, Marlborough, MA). The balloon catheter technique is discussed in detail elsewhere in this book (Beitsch, "Partial Breast Radiation Therapy"). The ease of use of this device and its relatively high reimbursement led to a rapid adoption of its use in the United States, despite limited evidence of clinical efficacy. While balloon brachytherapy is technically easier, its radiation technique has significantly less volume coverage than either multi-plane brachytherapy or 3D conformal APBI. Holland et al. [25] and Faverly et al. [26] have shown that disease extends up to 2 cm beyond the tumor in more than 20 % of patients. If the APBI volume of breast tissue irradiated is reduced too severely, it is arguable whether limiting the radiation coverage to the excision cavity plus less than 2 cm of adjacent tissue will prove effective in the long term.

Smith et al. [27] analyzed Medicare billing claims for women $\geq$67 years for IDC diagnosed between 2000 and 2007, treated with BCS, and followed by either Mammosite brachytherapy or WBI. Subsequent mastectomy was used as a surrogate for recurrence and was compared between the two groups. Risks of acute complications (hospitalization or infection within 120 days of treatment) and long-term toxicities (rib fractures, necrosis, breast pain, and pneumonitis) were also compared. A total of 7,291 women received APBI brachytherapy, vs. 123,244 who had WBI. The median FU was 3.84 years for the Mammosite group, and the median age was 75. At 5 years, the cumulative incidence of subsequent mastectomy was 4.0 % in the Mammosite group vs. 2.2 % in the WBI group (p<0.001). In addition, Mammosite therapy generated more acute complications and toxicities, including hospitalizations (9.6 % vs. 5.7 %, p<0.001), infections (8.1 % vs. 4.5 %, p<0.001), rib fractures (4.2 % vs. 3.6 %, p<0.0010), fat necrosis (9.1 % vs. 3.7 %, p<0.001), and breast pain (14.9 vs. 11.7 %, p<0.001). The incidence of radiation pneumonitis was lower in the Mammosite group (0.1 % vs. 0.8 %, p<0.001). It is possible that the Smith study indicates that inadequate coverage of residual breast disease by the smaller target volume used in balloon brachytherapy can have consequences, but it is also useful because it points out the pitfalls of the rapid acceptance of a breast technique in the absence of adequate long-term clinical data. This is especially true since most women today routinely receive adjuvant hormonal therapy, which will delay recurrences rather than eliminate them.

A third nonoperative APBI approach involves twice daily treatment of the breast using either 3D conformal radiation or intensity-modulated radiation therapy (IMRT). A total of 38.5 Gy is the usual dose prescription delivered twice a day over a 5-day period, though other dose formulations are also being tested. This schedule was deemed equivalent to the conventional approach because it used the linear-quadratic formula, which called for waiting 6 h between fractions. This is an attractive method to explore, because most radiotherapy centers have the ability to provide this APBI approach. However, two recent publications have indicated high levels of unacceptable moderate-to-severe late toxicity (pronounced subcutaneous fibrosis, retraction, telangiectasia) with relatively short median follow-ups of 15 and 30 months, respectively, Jagsi et al. [28] and Hepel et al. [29], but these complications have not been universally reported by other centers [30]. This discrepancy has not yet been reconciled, with further investigation into this approach with an ongoing randomized trial.

In 2005, the NSABP initiated a prospective, randomized trial in the United States to comparatively evaluate these three methods of APBI delivery against conventional WBI [31]. In addition to the NSABP B-39 trial, there is the GEC-ESTRO trial for APBI with multi-plane brachytherapy and two randomized trials in Europe testing 3D conformal ABPI with WBI, called the RAPID trial [32] and the IMPORT trial [33]. These began in 2006 and 2007, respectively. These trials are not yet closed to accrual, and it will be several more years before the data matures sufficiently to evaluate them. Even though the target volumes differ in these studies, they should be very helpful in defining the role of APBI in the management of early-stage breast cancer, further identifying the most suitable patients for these nonsurgical APBI approaches.

Treatment guidelines for radiation oncologists in the United States and Europe have been published by ASTRO [34] and ESTRO [35] in an attempt to identify which patients may be best suited to treat with APBI. However, neither ASTRO nor ESTRO has considered including a single dose of IORT when formulating their guidelines, as the clinical results from trials of IORT were immature and insufficient at the time of their respective publications.

Intraoperative Radiation Therapy Use in Breast Conservation Treatment

IORT using electron beams of radiation (IOERT) was first utilized for breast cancer treatment in the early 1990s attempting to replace the traditional EBRT boost. EBRT boost, given in five to eight fractions, is delivered after 5 weeks of WBI and several months after the lumpectomy. The EBRT boost needs to irradiate the excision cavity, but there can be some uncertainty as to exactly where that cavity is located. There is a potential of the radiation boost missing all or part of the cavity. The rationale for using an IOERT boost is that direct visualization of the tumor bed during IOERT best eliminates any possibility of this geometric miss. Previously, boosting the tumor bed postsurgically was difficult to do well, because it was hard for the radiation oncologist to direct the radiation boost beam to the excision cavity using the less sophisticated imaging systems available. This often required the surgeon to place titanium clips outlining the periphery of the lumpectomy site to aid the radiation oncologist in viewing the excision cavity. In addition to better targeting of the excision cavity, IOERT irradiation delivers a very high biological dose at the time of the surgery, coinciding with the time that residual tumor cells are more rapidly proliferating. IORT also reduces the skin dose (as the radiation is delivered subcutaneously) and saves about 1 week of fractionated EBRT treatments. Finally, with an EBRT boost, the radiation fields used must be larger than with IOERT to account for patient motion (breathing) and for positioning errors that might occur during the multiple patient setups needed to deliver the EBRT boost. The IOERT boost volume is significantly smaller than the EBRT boost volume,

Table 28.2 Comparison of IORT/IOERT boost vs. EBRT boost

Feature	IOERT/IORT boost	EBRT boost	Advantages of IOERT boost
Skin dose	None with IOERT; negligible with IORT if 1 cm spacing from applicator to skin	Substantial	Subcutaneous delivery of IORT/IOERT eliminates skin boost dose
Size of boost volume	Typically 25 mm^3 for a 1.5 cm tumor with IOERT[a]	Typically 50 mm^3 for a 1.5 cm tumor	Smaller CTV should result in less toxicity
# of fractions	1 treatment; IOERT adds 15–20 min to the surgical time. IORT adds about 40–60 min	5–8 treatments; does not impact surgical time	IOERT/IORT eliminates 1+ week of treatment
Accuracy of radiation delivery	No chance for geometric miss of CTV[b]	Depends on imaging and varies center to center	Direct visualization of target makes IOERT/IORT superior method
Time of radiation boost	During surgery	9–40 weeks postsurgery[c]	IOERT boost provides 1–2 log cell kill, reducing tumor burden for the postoperative radiation
Breast size	Irrelevant with IOERT, as delivered directly to tumor bed; IORT challenging for small-breasted women	Large-breasted women more challenging to boost	If volume to boost is deep-seated, more normal tissue must be irradiated, compromising cosmesis
Dose uniformity	Excellent with IOERT[d], poor with IORT	Excellent	Excellent
Ipsilateral recurrence	IOERT: <0.5 % at 6 years; <1 % at 10 years IORT: 1.73 % at 5 years	Typically 3–4 % at 5 years Typically 7–8 % at 10 years	Both IOERT and IORT have lower recurrence rate than EBRT boost
Cosmesis	90 % good to excellent at 5 years+	70–85 % long-term good to excellent cosmesis	30 %+ of EBRT women unhappy with breast appearance after BCT

[a]With IORT, CTV is smaller than with EBRT boost. With IOERT, 2–3 cm of tissue adjacent to the tumor is included, but still has slightly smaller CTV than with EBRT. See technical discussion

[b]Postoperative pathology administration of IORT requires reoperation and insertion of applicator into the residual seroma from the excision cavity

[c]WBI precedes EBRT boost

[d]See discussion in technical section, below

resulting in less dose to normal tissues, and, theoretically, should result in less normal tissue toxicity. Table 28.2 compares the advantages of an IOERT boost over that of an EBRT boost.

Despite numerous advantages, IOERT boost for breast cancer was impractical prior to the development of mobile IORT technology. Patients had to either be transported from the operating room to the radiation oncology department, adding an hour or more to the surgical time, or a shielded bunker had to be constructed within the operating room. Such cost was often prohibitively expensive for most hospitals. Mobile IORT technology, using either electron beams or 50 kV X-rays, has now made IOERT boost practical, with more than 10,000 women (mostly in Europe) with breast cancer already receiving IOERT boost. More recently, thousands of women each year now receive IOERT boost, with several more centers realizing the advantages of such technology for the breast cancer patient. Even though improvements in EBRT boost technology and technique have occurred, IORT boost still has advantages as it is now widely recognized that the size and shape of the excision cavity changes over time [36–39]. In fact, the excision cavity imaged many weeks later at the time of the EBRT boost can be quite different from the excision cavity created by the surgeon at the time of the tumor removal. This begs the question of which is the "correct" volume to boost in the first place. Additionally, the increasing trend in oncoplastic reconstruction at the time of BCS compromises the ability of the radiation oncologist to target the lumpectomy cavity, even when surgical clips have been added to guide the boost delivery.

The data collected worldwide utilizing IOERT points to the likely most accurate method of boosting the tumor bed, appearing to be synergistic with the modern surgical and medical oncology approaches for the treatment of breast cancer. As we will see when we discuss clinical results, for patients eligible for BCT, IOERT boost results in 10-year local control rates of 99 %, a figure that is just not achievable with EBRT boost approaches. This higher local control rate should result in improved long-term survival rates [11], with the added advantage of higher rates of breast preservation.

While extending the principles of a radiation boost to IORT, APBI was conceived and initiated before IORT boost results were sufficiently mature. If IORT APBI were proven safe and effective, all of the purported benefits of IORT boost could be achieved with the added bonus of a 1-day treatment. Results to date for IORT APBI have not been an unequivocal success. Nevertheless, IORT APBI will likely continue to be explored in an effort to optimize the technique and to find the select low-risk patients for whom the benefits of a single-day treatment might be appropriate.

Technical Aspects of IORT

Before we discuss the clinical results of IORT, it is important to understand the technical differences in the various approaches that have been used, because they can influence the outcome. There are three IORT techniques that provide APBI at the time of surgery: A single HDR treatment using a specially developed HDR breast applicator (HDR-IORT); 50 kV low-energy X-rays delivered through spherical plastic applicators or balloon catheters of varying diameters from 1 to 5 cm; and intraoperative electron beam treatments from linear accelerators delivered through cylindrical applicator tubes varying in diameter from 3 to 10 cm and ranging in energy from 4 to 12 MeV. Electron IORT is often designated as IOERT to distinguish it from 50 kV IORT approaches. Both 50 kV IORT and IOERT have been used to boost the tumor bed during surgery and also for single-fraction APBI treatment. One 50 kV device that uses a double-lumen balloon applicator has also been used to replace the Ir^{192} source used in balloon APBI, delivering the radiation treatment postsurgically in ten fractions over 1 week.

It is important to understand that each IORT technique generates different energies and utilizes a different applicator system, thus is associated with very different radiation target volumes and dose distributions. It is therefore not possible to extrapolate the results from one IORT technique to another. Required surgical techniques for performing a lumpectomy differ among surgeons with several technical restrictions, such as margin positivity, size of the tumor, and receptor analysis. It therefore may not even be appropriate to extrapolate the results from the same IORT technique and assume it still applies if the surgical approach and restrictions differ widely.

HDR-IORT [40]

Applicator: HDR-IORT uses a modified quadrangular Silastic breast applicator (HAM applicator, Mick Radio-Nuclear Instruments, Mt, Vernon, NY). The HAM applicator for breast IORT is a 2 cm thick, rectangular block of tissue-equivalent material with catheters running the length of the block through its center, spaced 1 cm apart. The catheters accept Ir^{192} sources from an HDR afterloader (Fig. 28.1b). The width of the HDR applicator and the number of catheters can be varied depending on tumor size. The length of the HDR applicator block varies from 4 to 6 cm, which is sufficient to provide radiation down to the level of the muscular fascia.

Surgical Approach: The radiation from this approach has very limited penetration beyond the lumpectomy cavity, so it is especially important to achieve negative margins upon final pathologic

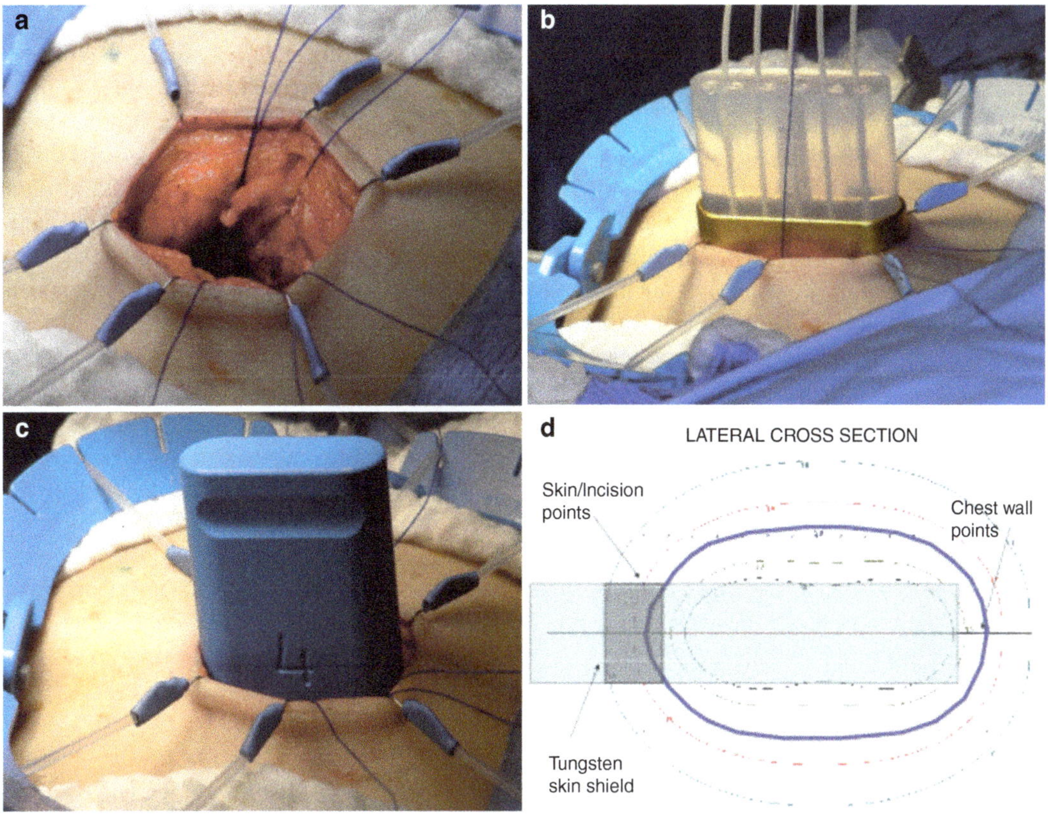

Fig. 28.1 HDR-IORT Technique: (**a**) Skin retraction; (**b**) use of *blue* plastic simulation applicator to obtain best applicator fit; (**c**) HAM applicator placed in the surgical cavity reaching the pectoralis major muscle. Note that the breast parenchyma is flush with the applicator and that a tungsten shield protects the skin; (**d**) cross-sectional display of dose distribution, optimized by computerization of dwell times of the Ir^{192} source in each of the catheters (Photos courtesy of G. Cohen, Memorial Sloan Kettering Cancer Center, New York City)

analysis. The tumor is excised with the objective of achieving a grossly free margin of at least 15 mm. The surgical specimen is examined radiographically and then sent to the pathologist for further gross margin analysis. Immediate re-excision is then performed for a margin that appears positive or even close. All patients receive a sentinel lymph node biopsy (SNLB). The breast parenchyma must be detached from the skin and the skin edges retracted to avoid excessive radiation exposure (Fig. 28.1a). After the tumor is removed, the applicator is inserted into the excision cavity.

Radiation Treatment: The catheters are attached to a remote afterloader. An Ir^{192} source is sequentially inserted into each catheter of the applicator and moved over its length under computer guidance. The computer then determines the dwell time of the radioactive source at each point along the catheter in an attempt to achieve a homogeneous distribution of radiation. The resultant radiation distribution is in the form of an elliptic cylinder, with the maximum dose delivered at the surface of the cylinder. The dose rapidly decreases as the distance from the applicator surface increases. Figure 28.1c shows the special HDR applicator and its placement in the lumpectomy cavity. It is important that the breast tissue to be irradiated is in direct contact with the applicator. This is typically not an issue, since any space between the applicator and the surrounding breast parenchyma is filled with fluid. A single fraction of 20 Gy was initially prescribed 1 cm from the surface of the applicator; however, after the first 18 patients had significant acute toxicity, the dose prescription was reduced to 18 Gy to the lateral margin of the surgical cavity.

Other Factors: A shielded operating room (OR) is required for the treatment. The placement of the applicator and the treatment planning takes about 10 min, and irradiation times are approximately 40 min, for a total additional operative time of about 1 h. All personnel must leave the OR during the treatment, so provisions for remote anesthesia monitoring and patient observation are required. Subsequent to the initial published trial, the HAM breast applicator was modified to have a curved surface on the short side of the applicator to promote better conformation of the breast tissue to the applicator. There is also now a tungsten shield at the top of the applicator to provide greater protection to the skin.

50 kV IORT

There are currently two 50 kV systems being used for IORT breast cancer treatment: Intrabeam (Carl Zeiss, Saarbrucken Germany) (Fig. 28.2) and Xoft (iCad, Burlington, MA) (Fig. 28.3). Both systems use miniature X-ray generators that attach to X-ray tubes with diameters of approximately 3.2 mm (Zeiss) or 2.5 mm (iCad). The target of these X-ray tubes, located at the distal end of the tube, generates low-energy X-rays of approximately 25 kV energy. The X-ray tubes are inserted into applicators that can be sterilized and then used for treatment in the OR. Prior to the introduction of these devices, there was little clinical experience with X-rays of such low energy. ASTRO has issued an Emerging Technology Committee Report on "electronic brachytherapy" devices [41] and the American Association of Physicists in Medicine (AAPM) established Task Group 146 to provide a standard for calibration and quality assurance of these low-energy devices. The AAPM was not charged with addressing the radiobiological equivalence (RBE) issues associated with these low-energy devices. This is an important, unresolved issue in the clinical use of these devices, since the effectiveness of this low-energy radiation changes as a function of applicator size and distance from the applicator surface, resulting in different equivalent biological doses delivered at a 1 cm distance from the applicator. Clinically, this means that because the same dose is applied to the applicator surface, patients with smaller tumors might have different clinical outcomes than those with slightly larger tumors, since they are treated with different-sized applicators and thus receive different biological doses.

Applicator – Intrabeam: The Intrabeam applicator consists of different-sized plastic spheres ranging in diameters from 1.5 up to 5 cm, with 5 mm increments in size that fit over a rigid X-ray tube.

Applicator – Xoft: The Xoft applicator is the double-lumen balloon used with the Mammosite system. Four balloons are currently available, depending on the tumor size and shape: 3–4 cm, 4–5 cm, 5–6 cm, and a 5×7 cm elliptical balloon. The Xoft X-ray tube is on a flexible cable that can be inserted into the catheter of the double-lumen balloon.

Surgical Approach – Intrabeam: [42–46]. The tumor is excised with an attempt to achieve negative margins of at least 10 mm. Radiographic examination of the tumor specimen and additional excision is recommended until the margins achieve this clearance. It is important to achieve complete hemostasis since the radiation treatment time can range from 25 to 50 min, and even a small amount of bleeding can cause inaccurate dose delivery. After tumor removal, the various applicator sizes are positioned within the lumpectomy cavity until there appears to be a snug fit of surrounding tissue around the applicator. The breast parenchyma is sutured with a purse string to hold the breast tissues snugly against the applicator. It is important to insure that the skin is not brought closer than 1 cm from the applicator surface. This can be achieved by undermining the skin edges and retracting the skin away from the applicator. When this is not possible, radiopaque, tungsten-filled polyurethane protector sheets can be inserted under the skin surface. Alternatively, saline-soaked surgical gauze, 5–9 mm thick, can

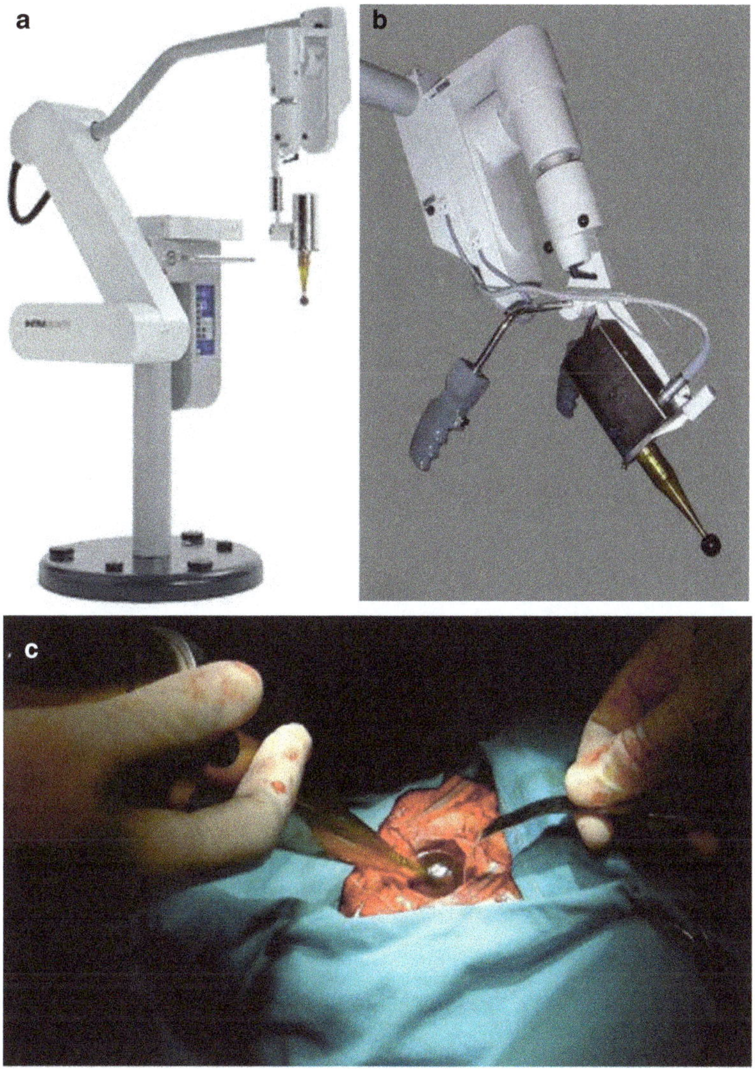

Fig. 28.2 Intrabeam System (Carl Zeiss, Saarbrucken, Germany): (**a**) Intrabeam System; (**b**) X-ray generator with applicator inserted over X-ray tube; (**c**) applicator in excision cavity and being purse-string sutured into place

be inserted deep to the skin to lift the dermis off the applicator in order to protect the surrounding skin. The radiopaque tungsten-filled polyurethane protector sheets can also be fitted like a cap on the applicator to protect the chest wall, sometimes necessary to reduce the dose to the thoracic structures by 95 %. It is also possible to deliver the IORT radiation during a second surgical procedure, several weeks after the original operation once the final pathology is available.

Surgical Approach – Xoft [47, 48]*:* The surgical approach does not differ markedly from that used in postoperative balloon catheter placement, except that with IORT, the balloon is implanted during the lumpectomy procedure, the radiation is delivered, and then the balloon is removed before closure. All patients undergo SLNB for node assessment, which must be negative for IORT to be administered. Margins also need to be negative, though no special assessments during surgery have been reported, other than selecting low-risk women, using preoperative MRI to eliminate multicentric or multifocal disease, and careful attention to procedure. (Note: If final pathology reveals positive margins, the patients are re-excised. If the re-excision is clear, no further treatment is given. If the re-excision is still positive, the patient is referred for WBI.)

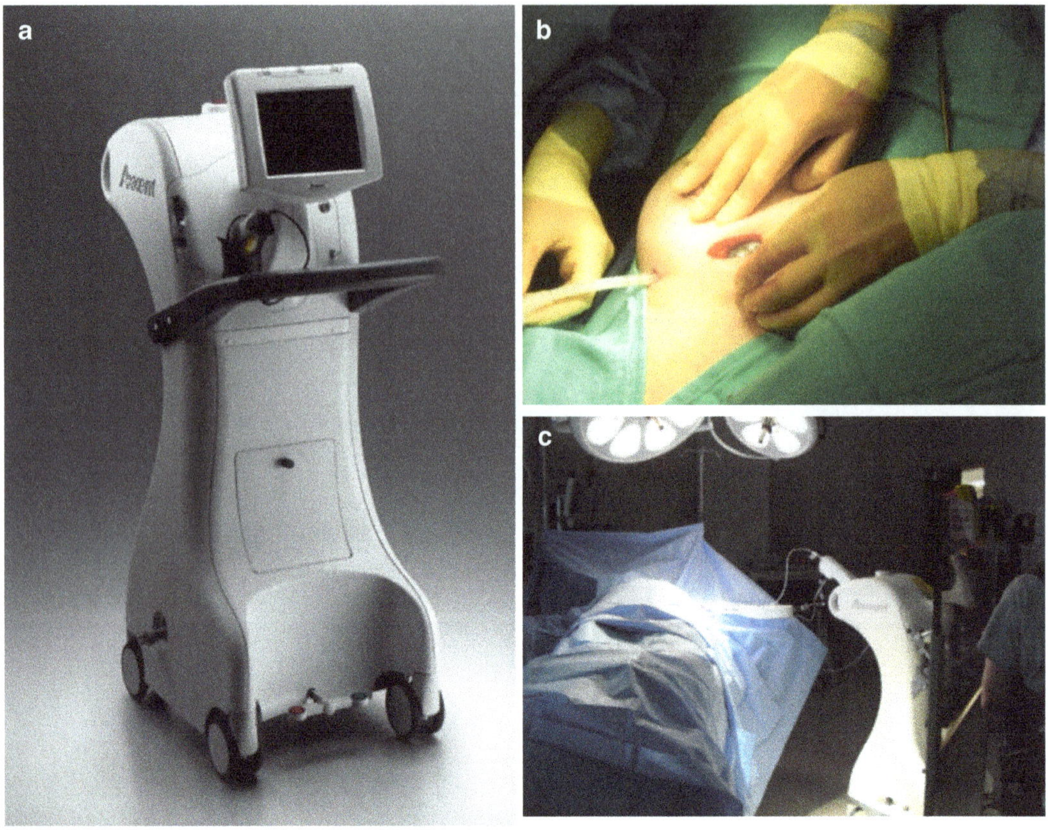

Fig. 28.3 Xoft Axxent System: (**a**) Xoft Controller; (**b**) balloon catheter insertion; (**c**) IORT delivery. Note the operator is standing behind a shielding screen (Photos courtesy of Xoft, Inc., an *i*Cad company, Burlington, Massachusetts, USA)

The minimum skin spacing must be at least 1 cm. If the skin spacing is between 7 mm and 1 cm, the patient is not a candidate for IORT but can still receive 5 days of postoperative APBI. If the skin spacing is less than 7 mm, the patient is not a candidate for either technique. The breast tissue is dissected to the level of the superficial pectoralis fascia so that a flexible lead shield can be inserted to protect the chest wall. A cavity evaluation device (CED) is inserted into the lumpectomy cavity through a small incision made within the lateral aspect of the breast and filled with saline solution until the correct size balloon for treatment is determined. The CED is replaced with the appropriately sized balloon for the procedure. Temporary retention sutures are used to hold the balloon into place and to build up subcutaneous tissue to increase the skin spacing from the balloon. Ultrasound is used to assure conformance of the surgical cavity to the balloon surface and to assess the balloon to skin distance.

Radiation Approach – Intrabeam [42–46]*:* A dose of 20 Gy to the surface of the sphere is prescribed, falling to 5 Gy at 1 cm from the surface of the sphere. Typical irradiation times using this approach are 30–50 min. The advocates of 50 kV treatments maintain that, despite the sharp falloff in dose, there is an increase in RBE as a function of distance from the sphere as the energy decreases. Even if one were to accept this concept, the equivalent dose at 1 cm could at most be only 18 Gy, with the dose at 2 cm only 6.3 Gy [49]. The rapid falloff in dose, even with an increase in RBE, may not adequately irradiate the microscopic disease that is known to extend at least 2 cm in some cases beyond the tumor proper. If the IORT is delivered in a second procedure, the applicator is reinserted into the excision site. However, the diameter of the applicator used in a second procedure is considerably smaller than if the IORT was given at the time of the tumor excision, e.g., 2.5 cm vs. 4.5 cm [42]. The reduction in applicator size and the delay in delivery will irradiate a different volume to a different dose and at a different time with respect to the microscopic tumor environment, than if the IORT was delivered during the initial surgery. This difference in timing of IORT delivery apparently impacts clinical outcomes for APBI [50, 51], but has not yet shown to affect the outcomes for IORT kV boost.

Radiation Treatment – Xoft [47, 48]*:* While the surgeon is inserting and checking the placement of the balloon, the physicist calibrates the Xoft X-ray source using a modified well chamber, similar to those used in the calibration of brachytherapy sources. During calibration, the X-rays are turned on for about 15 s and the entire calibration process takes less than 15 min. A flexible lead-equivalent shield is draped over the breast to protect the patient, with the anesthesiologist, physicist, and radiation oncologist standing behind protective shields. The rest of the OR staff leaves the room for the radiation delivery, which lasts 22 min and varies only slightly with balloon diameter (20–24 min). A dose of 20 Gy is delivered to the surface of the balloon falling to about 5 Gy at 1 cm. Due to the design of the Xoft balloon applicators, it can also be used to provide postoperatively APBI in ten fractions over 5 days.

Other Factors: Before each day's treatment, the physicist must calibrate and conduct quality assurance (QA) testing on the Intrabeam system to assure proper performance. It takes about 2 h to perform calibration and QA [46] using the Intrabeam supplied equipment calibration and QA equipment. With the Xoft system, calibration is performed concurrently with the surgery and takes less than 15 min. During the radiation procedure, for both systems, everyone leaves the OR, except the radiation oncologist, physicist, and anesthesiologist who stay behind protective shields. It is recommended that patients receive prophylactic antibiotics to reduce the risk of infection. Both systems recommend that the patient be draped with protective radiation shields. Utilization of the Intrabeam adds about one additional hour to the surgical procedure, excluding the 2 h of physics calibration. Total time for a Xoft IORT procedure, including the lumpectomy, SLNB, balloon placement, radiation treatment and closure, is about 2 h.

IOERT [52–56]

There are currently two types of electron generators that can deliver IOERT: conventional radiotherapy accelerators operating in the electron mode and mobile IOERT units, Mobetron® (Intraop Medical, Sunnyvale, California USA), Liac (Sordina, Padova, Italy), and Novac (NRT, Aprilla, Italy). Conventional accelerators have higher electron energy ranges (4–20 MeV) compared to the mobile units (3–12 MeV), but for breast IOERT, 12 MeV is sufficient penetration. A conventional accelerator weighs 8–10 tons and requires substantial radiation shielding of 100 tons or more in order to limit stray radiation to the surrounding areas. The mobile units can be used in unshielded ORs, though some require about 1 ton of mobile shielding be positioned around the surgical bed before treatment to protect surrounding areas from excessive stray radiation. Figure 28.4 shows the IOERT units currently available.

Applicators: All IOERT units use cylindrical applicators for breast treatment. Both acrylic applicators and metallic applicators are in use. Metallic applicators can be steam sterilized quickly using an autoclave, while acrylic applicators need to be gas sterilized or sterilized with a liquid process, both of which take a day or more to complete. The sterilization process can be an issue if multiple IOERT cases are planned for the same day or for consecutive days. Acrylic applicators have diameters that range from 3 to 10 cm in 1 cm increments, with a wall thickness of 5 mm. Metallic applicators have the same range

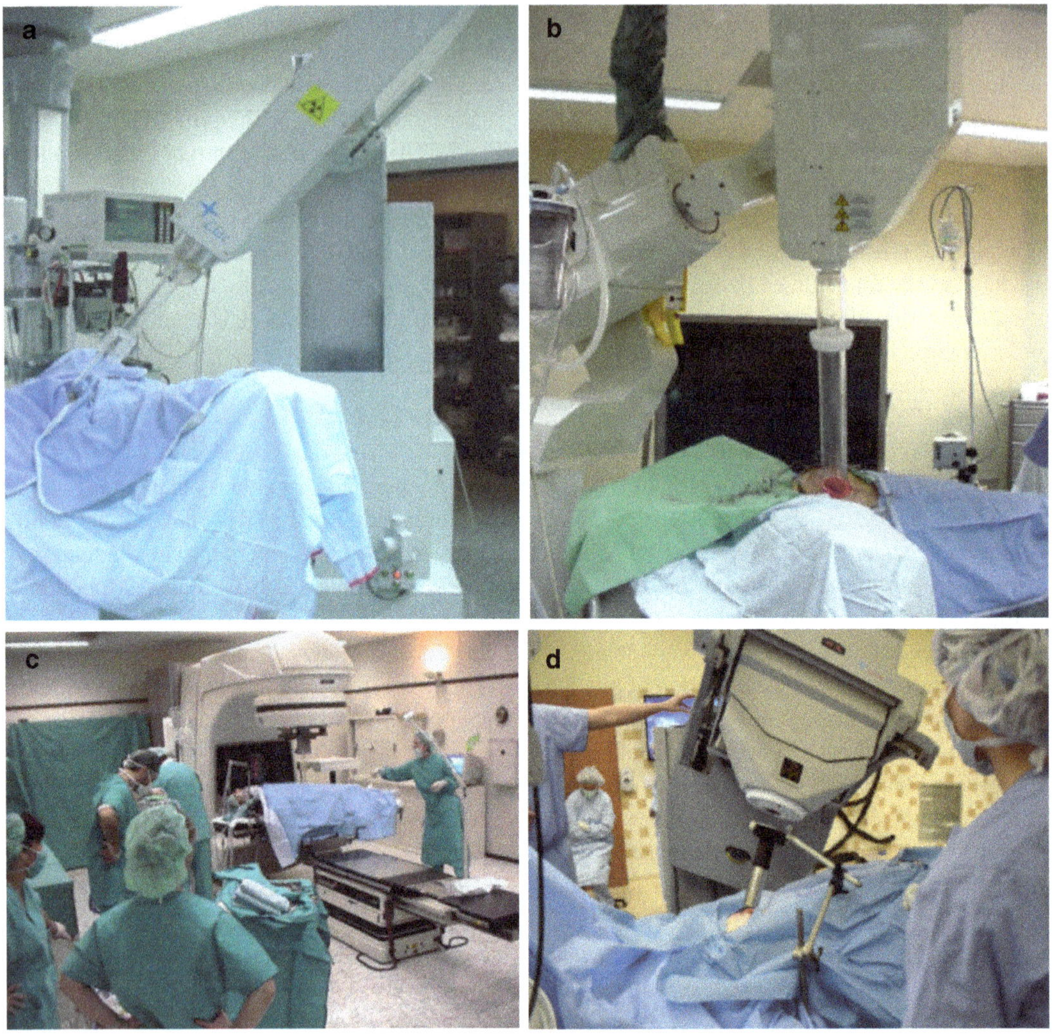

Fig. 28.4 Mobile IOERT linacs: (**a**) Novac 7; (**b**) Liac; (**c**) Mobetron; and (**d**) conventional linac being used for IOERT. Conventional linacs used in IOERT require shielded bunker. Mobile linacs can be used in ORs with little or no additional shielding. Novac and Liac usually require about 1 ton of mobile shielding to be placed around and under surgical bed for radiation protection of surrounding areas

of diameters, but with 5 mm increments and 2 mm wall thickness. IOERT applicators must be in direct contact with the breast parenchyma surface before irradiation. Acrylic applicators used with the Liac and Novac are 60–100 cm in length and are directly connected to the head of the accelerator for treatment. The metallic applicators used with the Mobetron are held in place by a special clamp that attaches to the rails of the surgical bed.

Conventional accelerators use both acrylic and metallic applicators of varying lengths, depending on the attachment mechanism they employ. The Mobetron also provides 5 and 10 mm acrylic bolus disks that can be used either to increase the surface dose or to provide protection to deep-seated tissues. To facilitate contact for tumors located over the curvature of the CW, applicators come with bevel angles of 0°, 15°, 30°, and 45°. The smaller the bevel angle, the more uniform the radiation is across the applicator diameter. It is inadvisable to use 45° bevels, as the homogeneity across the field is inadequate to provide for sufficient dose coverage of the tissue

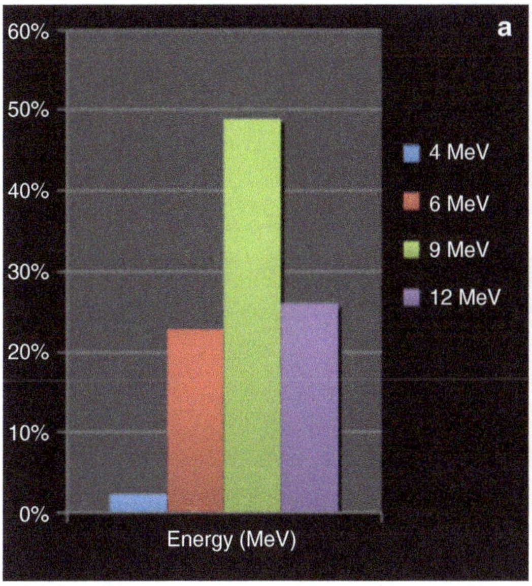

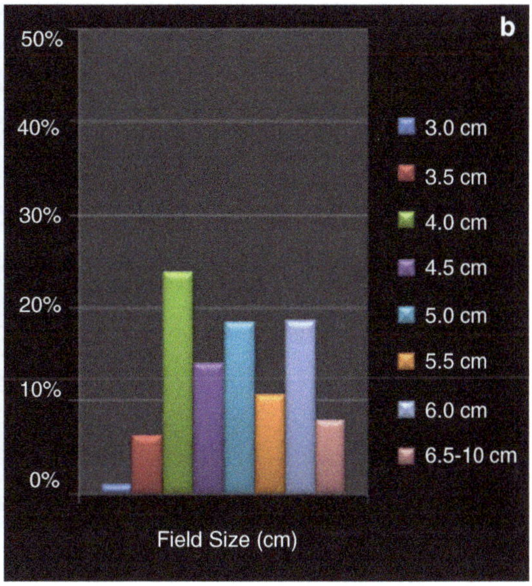

Fig. 28.5 Typical energy (**a**) and field size (**b**) use for breast IOERT. Median field size used was 5.5 cm; bolus was used in 40 % of patients to either increase the surface dose or reduce the depth of penetration; beveled applicators were used in 45 % of patients, and ½ cm rather than integral field size applicators were used in 40 % of patients (Data from March 2011 customer survey involving 2,200 breast IOERT boost and IOERT APBI patients, courtesy of Intraop Medical Corporation, Sunnyvale, California)

at risk, especially at the applicator perimeter. Typical energy and field size use for a mobile IOERT unit used in breast cancer treatment is shown in Fig. 28.5.

Surgical Approach: The surgical approach is identical, irrespective of which electron generator is used, and is similar whether boost or APBI is planned, with the exception that the chest wall (CW) protector is always used in IOERT APBI and is not usually employed for IOERT boost. The tumor is removed as usual with an attempt to achieve free margins. If oncoplasty is planned for the patient, an oncoplastic approach suitable for the breast in question is used to remove the tumor. There is no consistently reported method of margin clearance, with some centers relying only on good technique and wide excision surgery and others on the wider surgery of quandrantectomy. In some centers, intraoperative frozen section is performed of the margins in order to assess margin clearance. After the tumor is excised, in IOERT boost, the breast parenchyma is loosely approximated so that the sides of the excision cavity can be temporarily sutured to form a flat surface for the IOERT radiation. In IOERT APBI, the breast parenchyma is also lifted off the CW and is remodeled. The remodeling of the breast parenchyma, together with the temporary re-approximation, morphologically transforms the breast tissue at risk, irrespective of the tumor shape, so that it is compactly positioned directly beneath the electron applicator (Fig. 28.6). This surgical approach positions all of the tumor margins at the center of the radiation field and irradiates several centimeters of tissue from the center in all directions. The amount of peripheral circumferential extension of the radiation field depends upon the size of the applicator chosen. The clinical treatment volume (CTV) irradiated with IOERT is comparable to that used in 3D conformal APBI, but can be slightly smaller while covering the same tissue at risk, since no additional tissue volume needs to be included to allow for patient motion and errors in patient setup. Furthermore, because more normal tissue can be excluded from the radiation field with IOERT, the dose-volume histograms (a measure

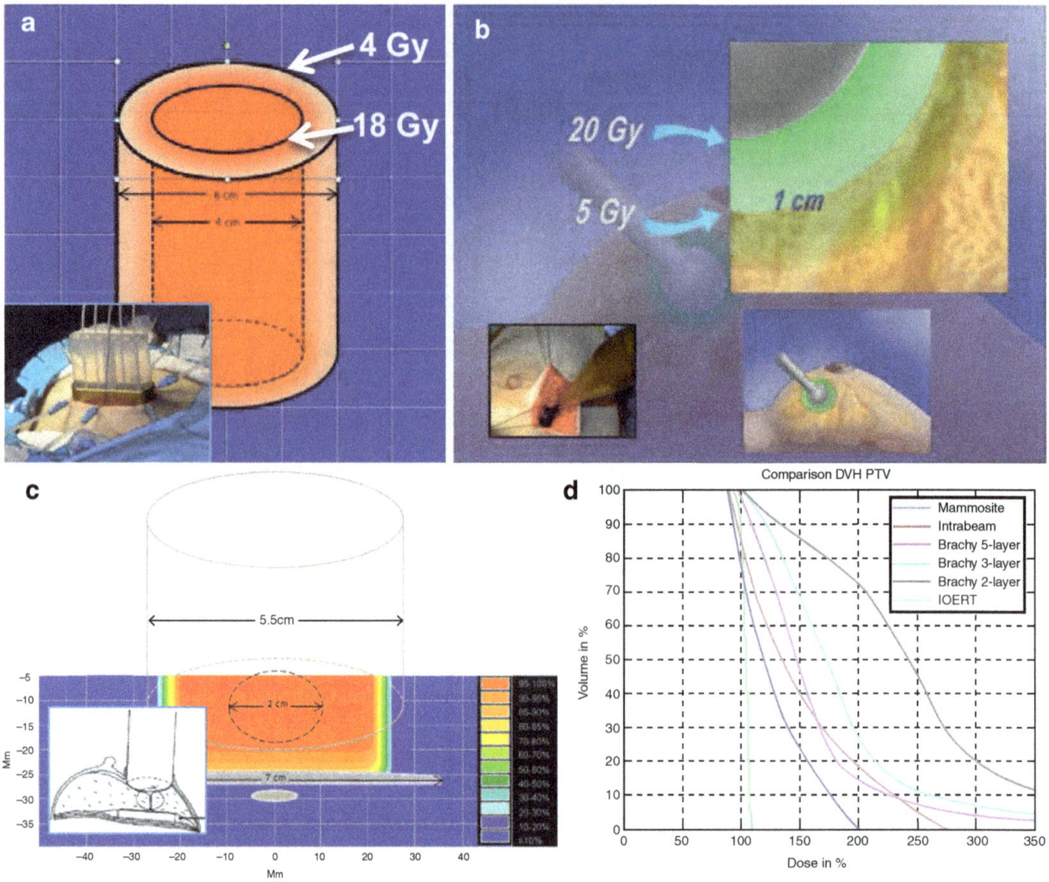

Fig. 28.6 Volumes treated and dose distributions resulting from the different IORT approaches. (**a**) HDR-IORT: The volume irradiated is an elliptic cylindrical shell extending down to the CW, with 18 Gy delivered at the inside surface of the cylinder, dropping to about 4 Gy at 1 cm from the inside surface. (**b**) Intrabeam: The volume irradiated is a spherical shell, with 20 Gy at the applicator surface (inside shell) dropping to 5 Gy at 1 cm. (**c**) IOERT: The surgical approach morphologically transforms the breast tissue, irrespective of the tumor shape, so that several centimeters of tissue originally adjacent to the tumor is compactly positioned under the applicator (see *inset*). Radiation is uniform across the applicator and extends to the CW. (**d**) Dose-volume histograms from [57] showing uniformity of tumor volume coverage of the various approaches used in IORT

of homogeneity of tumor coverage and normal tissue exposure) with IOERT APBI appears to be more precise compared to those generated with any of the EBRT APBI techniques.

For IOERT APBI, a shielding disk must be inserted between the remodeled breast parenchyma and the CW (Fig. 28.7c). Shielding disks are usually comprised of a lead and aluminum sandwich of 6–9 mm in thickness, though disks with other shielding materials are in use, such as acrylic disks with and without metal inserts. It is important to select a CW shield with a diameter at least 1 cm circumferentially larger than the applicator for the treatment. Validation of the correct placement of the shielding disk by U/S or a physical probe should be made prior to radiation delivery. For IOERT boost, a CW shield is generally not required, providing the dose to the rib from the IOERT boost will be <5 Gy. If acrylic applicators are used, the skin must be retracted, so it is not in contact with the applicator (Fig. 28.7a). This is not necessary with metallic applicators, but provision must be made so that the skin cannot fall into the radiation field. This is usually accomplished by tying sutures from the skin to the clamping system holding the metallic

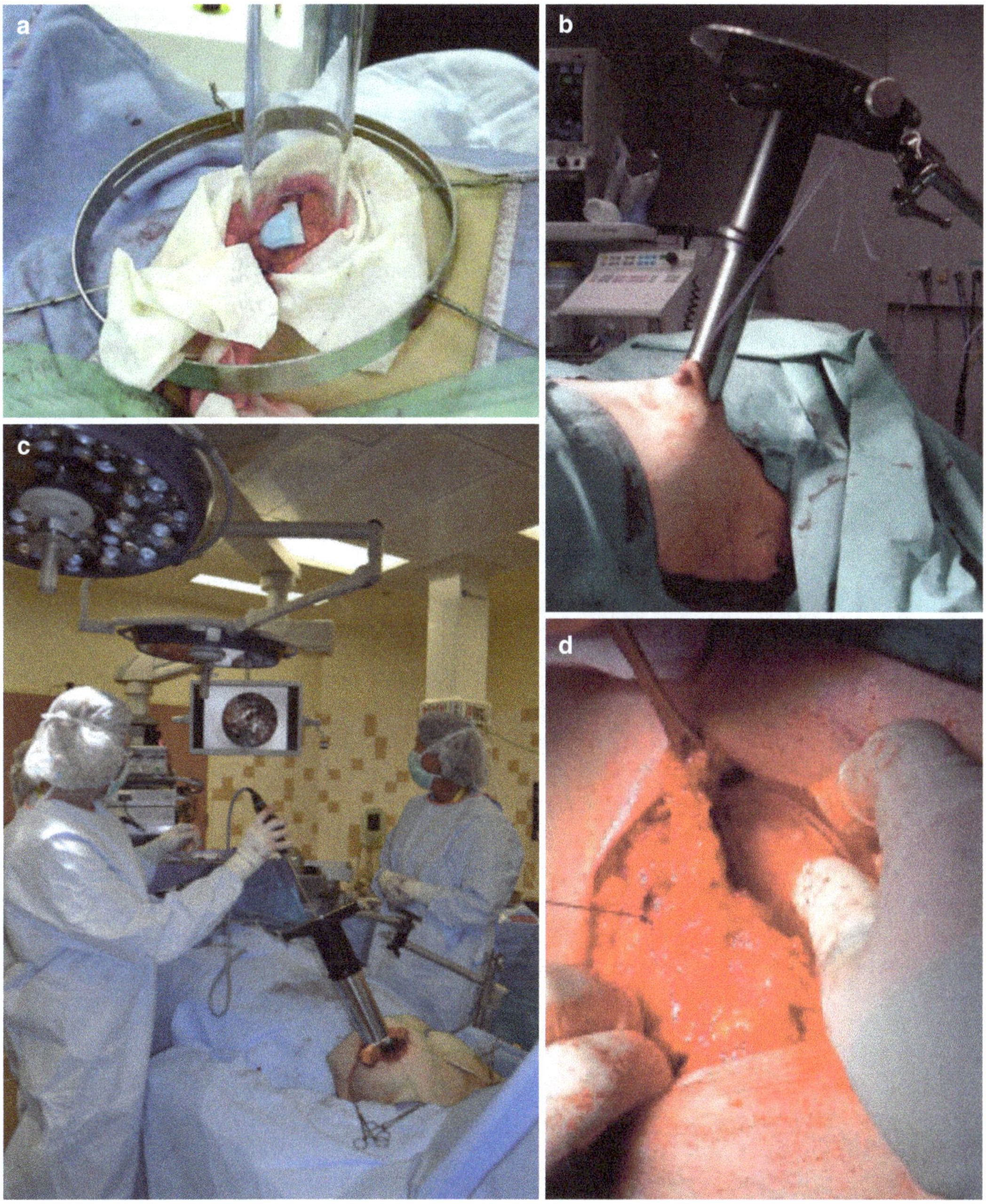

Fig. 28.7 IOERT Technical Aspects-Part I: (**a**) skin retraction needed with acrylic applicators; (**b**) suturing skin to applicator clamp to prevent from falling into radiation field with metal applicators; (**c**) visualizing and imaging the treatment field to assure proper coverage of boost or APBI; (**d**) inserting shielding disk to protect CW

applicator in place (Fig. 28.7b). After the IOERT treatment, the temporary sutures and the protective CW plate, if used, are removed. The breast parenchyma is remodeled, and closure is performed in the usual fashion. If an oncoplasty was planned, the breast remodeling needed for the IOERT will have already accomplished a large portion of that procedure.

If the final pathology reveals positive margins, IOERT boost patients are re-excised and receive

EBRT after their breast has healed (typically 3–4 weeks). If the nodes are positive, EBRT is delayed so that the patient can receive chemotherapy first, if necessary. For IOERT APBI patients with positive margins on final pathology, there is no standard consensus for margin treatment. Some centers do nothing, reasoning that because of the re-approximation technique, all the margins in IOERT APBI patients have already received a minimum dose of at least 18 Gy (i.e., surface dose for 21 Gy) for APBI and that margin positivity is less of a factor. This may be especially true in the older, low-risk group of women being treated with IOERT APBI [58]. Other centers re-excise and give no further radiation treatment.

Radiation Treatment: The radiation oncologist selects the applicator that is needed to cover the tissue at risk and positions and centers it on the re-approximated tumor bed. The applicator should be chosen with a diameter 1.0–1.5 cm larger than the maximum tumor dimension for IOERT boost and 1.5–2.0 cm larger for IOERT APBI. With IOERT boost, additional radiation is delivered through EBRT to adequately treat the microscopic disease that might extend a few cm beyond the tumor. For APBI, it is important to choose an applicator large enough to adequately treat this tissue at risk, because there is a "cold" radiation gap at the walls of the applicator (Fig. 28.6c). The 90 % radiation level – the usual prescription dose for IOERT – reaches only to within 4–5 mm of the inside wall of the applicator, depending on the design of the accelerator and applicator system. This "cold" gap is amplified when beveled applicators have to be used. Fortunately, the use of IOERT applicators that are sufficiently sized to adequately treat the tissue at risk does not appear to clinically result in increased fibrosis or poorer scar healing.

The 0° bevel applicator results in the best radiation coverage for all applicator sizes. Figure 28.8a shows a technique that allows a 0° bevel applicator to be used even when on a CW curvature, improving the homogeneity of the treatment. An acrylic bolus disk holds the remodeled breast parenchyma, and sterile gauze is wedged between the CW and the disk to present a 0° bevel angle for the IOERT. The depth from the surface to the shield plate or CW can be determined by utilizing intraoperative ultrasound or a mechanical probe (Fig. 28.8b). The depth measurement determines the energy of the treatment, with the 90 % depth having a variation from 11.0 to 35.0 mm for energies ranging from 4 to 12 MeV.

The applicator, now positioned in the patient, and the accelerator that is used to deliver the IOERT, must be aligned before treatment. For units that require physical connection of the applicator to the head of the treatment unit ("hard docking"), either the patient bed is moved under the treatment unit (e.g., in all conventional units) or the mobile accelerator is moved to the surgical bed. The head of the treatment unit is rotated and positioned so that the mechanical connection can be made. Care must be used to ensure that the applicator that is being handheld in the patient by one of the surgeons or radiation oncologists does not shift position during the attachment process (Fig. 28.8c).

In systems that do not directly connect the applicator to the treatment head ("soft docking"), alignment is achieved through the use of lasers to guide the orientation (Fig. 28.8d). Both docking systems are relatively quick, once some experience is gained. For units that use "soft docking," it is possible to document the tumor bed site using a small handheld TV camera (Fig. 28.7d). If the surgical bed needs to be moved for docking, the anesthesia equipment must also be moved or needs hoses long enough to accommodate the move. For some mobile units (the Liac and Novac), mobile shields must be positioned around the table and under the treatment bed for radiation protection to the surrounding areas.

The physicist calculates the amount of radiation units needed to deliver the prescription dose. Some centers use in vivo dosimetry to validate and/or monitor the IOERT dose (Fig. 28.7a). The Novac and Liac generally divide the treatment into two parts and adjust the dose delivered in the second half to improve the accuracy of dose delivery. This is not necessary with conventional IOERT units or the Mobetron. For IOERT boost, the dose prescription is usually 10 Gy to the 90 % depth. For IOERT APBI, it is predominantly 21 Gy to the 90 % depth.

Everyone leaves the room during the time that the radiation is being delivered. The patient and anesthesia must be monitored by video or

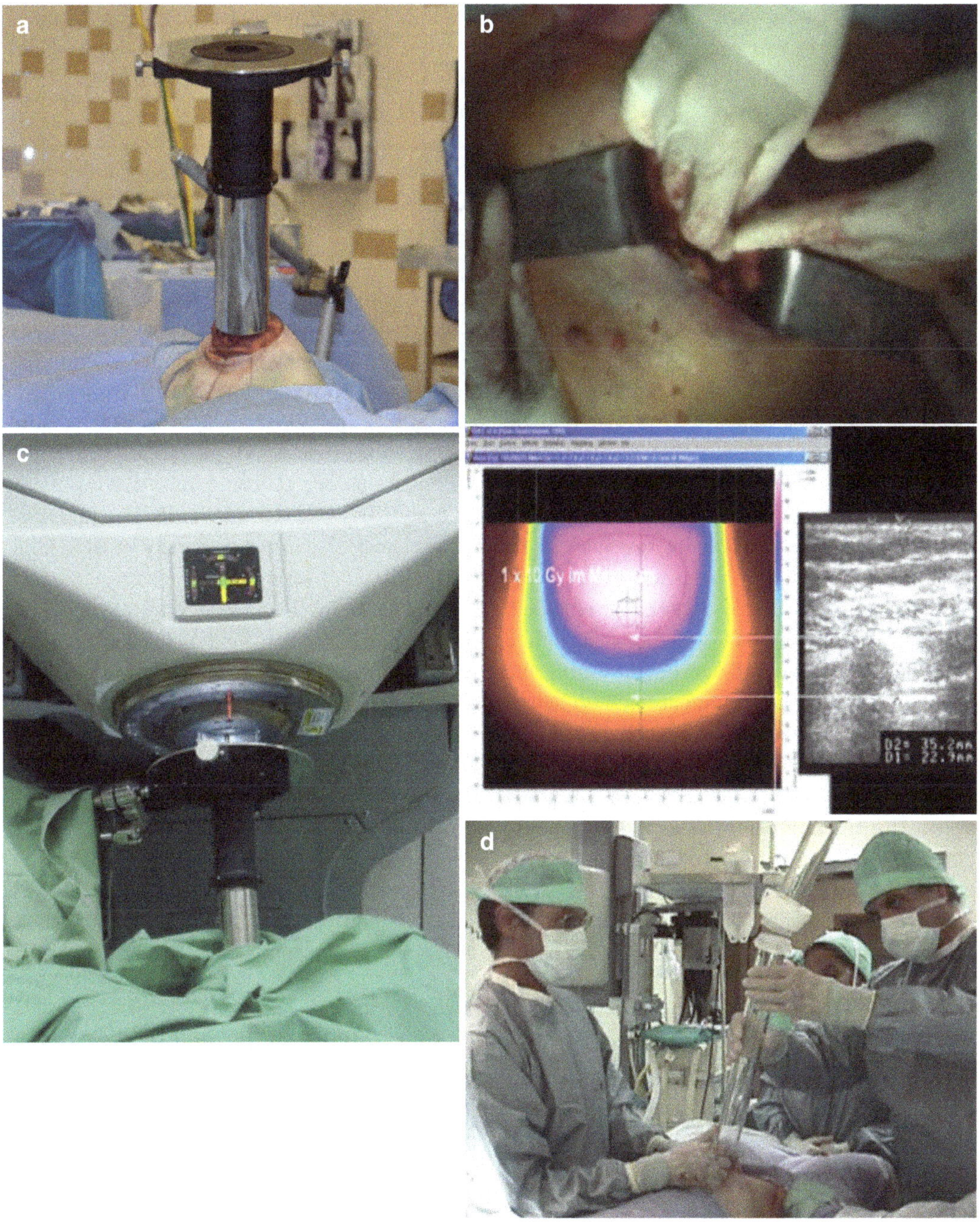

Fig. 28.8 IOERT Technical Aspects-Part II: (**a**) Flat surface created by wedging sterile gauze between the CW and an inserted bolus plate, allowing 0° bevel applicator to be used on sloping CW surface; (**b**) measuring the depth of the gland, either with a mechanical probe or with U/S; (**c**) soft docking; (**d**) hard docking

remotely. Treatment typically takes 1–5 min, depending on whether the treatment is a boost or APBI. Mobile IOERT units have treatment times of only 1–2 min, as the dose rate for mobile units is at least a factor of two higher than that of conventional units. Total time added to the surgical procedure for breast IOERT is 15–25 min.

Other Factors: The large dose of radiation delivered by IOERT in a single treatment makes the calibration and QA of each unit critically important to assuring proper treatment. Calibration and QA procedures for IOERT for conventional accelerator units was developed by the American Association of Physicists in Medicine (AAPM) and published in their Task Group 48 report [59]. Similar procedures for mobile IOERT units are published in Task Group 72 report [60]. The latter report recommends daily validation before treatment of both output and energy. For the Mobetron, these daily QA measurements can be made with 12 Gy exposure for all energies and outputs (about the amount of one IOERT boost treatment). With the Novac and Liac units, due to their unique method of generating the radiation, 60–100 Gy of exposure is required for output measurements.

This high level of exposure dose generated by these units for QA may require that the QA be taken when the adjacent areas are unoccupied, since the ORs for mobile units are unshielded. Alternatively, some of their users now use online in vivo dosimetry to validate output during the treatment, dividing the treatment into two halves and adjusting the remaining dose based on the output of the first [61–63]. Radiation QA is an important element for any multi-institutional study. The HIOB protocol (see Future applications) has developed QA procedures that allow all IOERT units to participate in multi-institutional studies with a high level of confidence.

The main technical difference between the IORT and IOERT approach is shown in Table 28.3. Nairz et al. [57] has evaluated the dose distributions from Intrabeam, IOERT, and brachytherapy and devised a "dose inhomogeneity index," or "Dii," to evaluate the mean deviation of the dose inside the PTV from the prescribed dose. A Dii of 0 indicates completely homogeneous irradiation. For IOERT, the Nairz Dii = 0.047, but rises to 0.505 for 50 kV treatments (Fig. 28.6d).

IORT Clinical Results: IORT as a Boost

IORT kV boost (when delivered at the time of the tumor removal) and IOERT boost have several similarities, despite very different radiation distributions and volumes irradiated by the two approaches. In both IORT approaches, radiation is given under direct visualization, eliminating the possibility of a geometric miss that is possible with an EBRT boost. Both the IORT and IOERT boosts can be used in wide variety of BCT eligible patients, delivering the dose subcutaneously, which should result in lower skin toxicity. They both eliminate approximately 1 week of EBRT boost treatment and start the radiation treatment at the time during the surgery when residual tumor cells are hypothesized to be rapidly proliferating. Because both IORT boosts are combined with several weeks of WBI to complete the BCT treatment, the differences in the volumes and dose distributions of the two approaches may be less important in IORT boost than in IORT APBI, since the WBI can partially compensate for the differences in the approaches.

Boost Clinical Results: 50 kV

Vaidya et al. [64] reports on long-term results of IORT boost with 50 kV using the Intrabeam sys-

Table 28.3 IORT vs. IOERT

Method	Meets TV concept of Holland	Homogeneity of radiation distribution	Can treat asymmetric PTV	Treatment time	Added OR time	Shielded OR needed
IORT	No	Poor[a]	No[b]	25–50 min[c]	~1 h	No
IOERT	Yes	Excellent	Yes	1–3 min[d]	15–30 min	No[e]

TV treatment volume, *PTV* planning treatment volume, *OR* operating room

[a]20 Gy dose at surface of applicator falls to 5 Gy at 1 cm from the applicator surface

[b]iCad Xoft has elliptical balloon available that can account for some asymmetry

[c]Treatment time is a function of applicator size

[d]Treatment time is about 1 min for boost and about 2 min for APBI. Conventional units take about twice as long

[e]Depending on the OR, Liac and Novac often require about 1 ton of mobile shields to be positioned around and under the surgical bed prior to treatment. Conventional units always require a heavily shielded OR

tem. Three hundred cancers (299 patients) underwent BCS and 20 Gy as a boost to the tumor bed. After wide excision of the breast cancer, the Intrabeam applicator that best fit the excision cavity was inserted into the cavity, and a purse-string suture was made to adapt the breast tissue to the applicator surface. A dose of 20 Gy to the surface of the applicator was administered, delivering 5–7 Gy of radiation 1 cm from the applicator surface. In this study, all tumors were unifocal on mammography, and none of the tumors exceeded 4 cm in diameter. There was no restriction on tumor type, tumor grade, receptor status, or axillary node involvement. The median patient age was 57 (range 28–83 years), 79 % of the tumors were 2 cm or less, and 29.9 % had Grade 3 tumors. Of the 242 patients in whom systemic therapy was analyzed, 94 patients (31 %) required adjuvant chemotherapy, and 195 patients (81 %) received adjuvant hormonal therapy. Patients with positive margins on final pathology that required re-excision either went on to receive a completion mastectomy or were excluded from the analysis. In one cohort of patients, IORT was delivered postoperatively in a second operation, after a median time of 4.9 weeks from the initial operative removal of the tumor. The additional time required for IORT setup and delivery was 30–50 min. All patients received 45–50 Gy of EBRT in 25 fractions over 5 weeks. If adjuvant chemotherapy was required, EBRT was delivered at its completion. With a median follow-up of 60.5 months (range 10–122 months), eight patients have had an ipsilateral recurrence. The 5-year Kaplan-Meier estimate for recurrence is 1.73 %, with five of eighth recurrences identified within the tumor bed, thus reducing the true local recurrence (TLR) rate at 5 years to 1.04 %.

Wenz et al. [65] reports on his own Intrabeam boost experience of 155 breast cancers in 154 women treated with Intrabeam as an anticipated boost. The median age was 63 years (range 30–83 years), 65 % of the patients had T1 tumors, and 35 % had T2 tumors. The median applicator size used was 4.5 cm (range 2.5–5 cm), resulting in treatment times of 7.5–51.1 min (median 36.6 min). A complete axillary lymph node dissection (CALND) was performed if the SNB was positive; 70 % of patients were N0, 22 % N1, and 8 % N2 or N3. EBRT was initiated after either wound healing or completion of chemotherapy (median 40 days, range 13–226 days). Adjuvant chemotherapy was given to 46 (29.9 %) patients and adjuvant hormonal therapy to 129 (83.8 %) patients. WBI using standard tangential treatment portals was delivered using a 6 MeV linear accelerator to a dose of 46 Gy in 23 fractions. The EBRT dose was increased to 50 Gy to the breast and to supra- or infraclavicular fossa in 26 patients with involved nodal areas.

With a median follow-up of 34 months (maximum 80 months), there were a total of ten deaths – eight due to distant metastases – and two ipsilateral breast tumor recurrences (IBTR), resulting in a 5-year Kaplan-Meier OS of 87 %, and a relapse-free survival rate of 98.5 %. Chronic toxicity after 3 years was mild, with two-thirds of patients experiencing none or barely palpable fibrosis. Five patients had a marked increase in breast density, with one patient with Grade 3 fibrosis requiring a mastectomy. Breast edema was seen in 8 % of patients, and skin toxicity was mild, with only 6 % experiencing telangiectasia and 6 % hyperpigmentation.

Wenz et al. [66] cautions that starting EBRT too soon after IORT could lead to increased toxicity. The toxicity analysis involved 48 patients with a median follow-up of 36 months (range 30–56 months). The median time between IORT delivery and the initiation of EBRT was 36 days. In general, the toxicity was mild, with 30/48 (63 %) experiencing either no change or only minor changes. However, a statistically significant and clinically relevant tendency for late toxicity occurred when the time interval between IORT and EBRT was too short: 8/12 higher-grade fibroses, 5/6 retractions, and 4/5 breast pains occurred in patients with an IORT-EBRT interval less than the median of 36 days. The recommended 5–6-week interval between IORT boost and initiating EBRT is 1–2 weeks longer than is needed with an IOERT boost or standard BCT treatment. While Wenz cautions that the impact of this longer gap between IORT and EBRT on recurrences is not known, it may not be significant, as longer time gaps occur with both IOERT and Intrabeam boost patients who have EBRT delayed due to adjuvant chemotherapy [56, 64, 67–70].

Most of the studies to date show that IORT boost with Intrabeam appears to provide an acceptable local control rate when compared with standard

BCT. The treatment toxicity is also considered acceptable, providing that attention is paid to proper technique and patient selection when using this device. For optimal cosmetic results, maintaining proper skin spacing and avoiding the Intrabeam's use in larger T2 tumors and small-breasted women, as well as waiting 5–6 weeks to initiate the EBRT, seem to be important factors. Long-term data, requiring further follow-up, is still needed in order to adequately assess cosmetic results. There is currently no long-term data or follow-up from the iCad Xoft system when used as a boost.

Boost Clinical Results: IOERT

The first reported use of IOERT for early-stage breast cancer was a combined study of the Medical College of Ohio and the Centre Regional de Lutte Contre le Cancer (Montpellier, France) [71]. In this study, 72 patients (Stage I – 43 %, Stage II – 57 %), between the age of 33 and 81 years, were given a 10 Gy IOERT boost following segmental mastectomy, with temporary re-approximation of the breast parenchyma to bring the margins of the cavity together. All patients underwent an axillary lymph node dissection. The field size was chosen to encompass the tumor bed with at least a 10 mm margin. After wound healing (typically 1–3 weeks), patients received an additional 45–50 Gy of radiation over 5–6 weeks with external X-ray radiation (6 MV or cobalt therapy). With follow-up of 2–17 years, only one patient developed a recurrence, and cosmesis was reported as excellent.

In 2006, Montpelier [72] updated results for the 50 patients it treated. Margins were assessed during the operation by frozen section, and all patients underwent a CALND. The median dose delivered was 10 Gy to the 90 % line (range 9–20). After IOERT, the temporary retaining sutures were removed, and the tumor cavity was remodeled. The EBRT dose was 50 Gy in 25 fractions, delivered with cobalt radiation. Nodal irradiation was given as required. For the two patients who required chemotherapy, EBRT began 3 weeks after its completion, with the others undergoing EBRT typically 4 weeks postsurgery. With a median follow-up of 9.1 years (range 5–15 years), they observed two local recurrences, one at 8 years and one at 14 years. Six additional patients had distant metastases, and 45 patients are alive, 1 with disease, giving a 10-year OS of 94 %. All patients in their series had good to excellent cosmesis, despite the fact that all had a CALND rather than SNB for nodal assessment. The high level of good cosmesis reported in this study might be a result of the skin and normal tissue sparing that occurs when using the IOERT boost as compared with the conventional EBRT external beam boost, as well as to the breast remodeling they employed at the time of surgery.

The University of Salzburg treated two consecutive series of patients with Stages I and II breast cancer [68]. Group I consisted of 188 patients treated with breast-conserving surgery and postoperative irradiation to the whole breast, followed by a postoperative external beam boost to the tumor bed. Group 2 was 190 patients treated with breast-conserving surgery, IOERT boost directly to the tumor bed, and postoperative irradiation to the whole breast. The groups were comparable in regard to age, menopausal status, tumor size, histological type, grading, and axillary lymph node status. Exclusion criteria were neoadjuvant chemotherapy, tumors > pT2, multicentricity, and ductal carcinoma in situ. For the IOERT boost patients, if margins were not clear with a minimum of 3–5 mm in the intraoperative pathologic assessment, re-excision was performed in the same surgical procedure prior to IORT. If margins were not clear in the final pathological report (minimum 3 mm), a secondary re-excision was performed before the patients had their EBRT. Margins were negative in all patients included in this study. Axillary surgery in Group 2 was confined to sentinel lymph node biopsy only, if sentinel lymph nodes were negative. Complete axillary clearance of levels I and II was performed, if sentinel lymph nodes were positive. After complete tumor resection and axillary surgery, the tissue surrounding the tumor bed was mobilized and temporarily approximated by sutures. Ultrasound was used to determine the depth dose, which ranged from 0.6 cm to 3.9 cm (median 1.9 cm). Applicators with diameters of 50–60 mm were used, and a dose of 9 Gy was delivered to the 90 % reference isodose, using the appropriate energy for the tumor thickness.

After wound healing, 51 Gy of EBRT for patients with IDC and 56.1 Gy for patients with

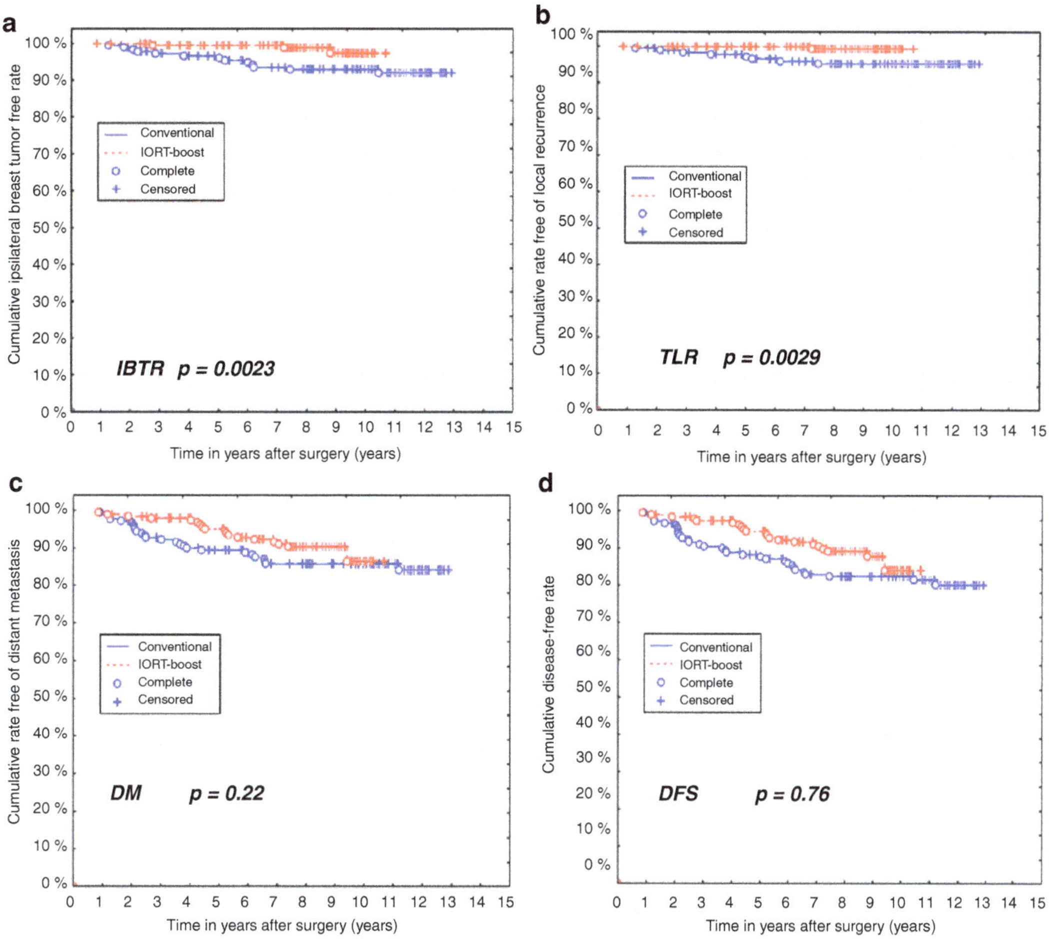

Fig. 28.9 Long-term results of the University of Salzburg matched-pair analysis comparing IOERT boost (median FU 10.7 years) with EBRT boost (median FU 12.6 years). IOERT boost has a 10-year true local recurrence (*TLR*) of only 0.6 %, and an IBTR of 1.6 %, both significantly better than the EBRT boost. IOERT also results in fewer distant metastases, though at the time of the analysis the difference was not statistically significant

ILC were delivered in daily fractions of 1.7 Gy to the whole breast. For the IOERT boost patients, 18.9 % received adjuvant chemotherapy, and an additional 4.7 % received combined chemotherapy and endocrine therapy. For these patients, EBRT was sequenced after completion of chemotherapy, with a time delay after IORT of up to 20 weeks. After median follow-ups of 81.0 months and 51.1 months in Group 1 and Group 2, respectively, no IBTR was observed in the IOERT boost patients, while 12 IBTRs (6.4 %) occurred in Group 1. The 5-year actuarial rates of IBTR were 4.3 and 0.0 %, respectively ($p=0.0018$). Distant metastases occurred in 24 patients (12.8 %) and 8 patients (4.2 %) in Group 1 and Group 2, respectively, for 5-year actuarial rates of distant recurrence of 8.6 % and 4.2 % ($p=0.08$). The 5-year disease-free survival in Group 1 was 90.9 % and was 95.8 % in Group 2 ($p=0.064$). The only serious complications reported were three rib fractures that occurred early on in the IOERT group. This complication was eliminated when the IOERT dose to the ribs was limited to 5 Gy or less.

Salzburg has recently updated this "matched-pair" analysis [67] with a very mature median follow-up period of 12.6 years for the patients treated with conventional BCT (Group 1), and 10.7 years for those receiving the IOERT boost (Group 2). Figure 28.9 shows the results of this study for IBTR, True Local Recurrence (TLR), distant metastases, and DFS at 10 years. The excellent results and advantage reported at 5 years of IOERT boost when combined with WBI over conventional BCT with EBRT boost have been maintained, with an TLR of 0.5 % vs. 4.4 % ($p=0.0029$) and an IBTR of 1.6 % vs. 7.2 % ($p=0.0023$). IOERT also has more favorable results for distant metastases and DFS, though with the small numbers in the study, it did not achieve statistical significance. It will be interesting to follow this study further to see if, as Clarke pointed out in his meta-analysis [11], the improved local control at 5 years translates into a survival advantage at 15 years.

A pooled analysis [69, 70] from seven European centers combined and analyzed patients who were treated using IOERT boost plus 5 weeks of postoperative EBRT. There were 1,109 patients treated between October 1998 and October 2005, 52 % of whom had one or more risk factors for recurrence: young age (<40 years), positive nodes, high grade of tumor (G3), or larger tumors (T3). The patients in the study were all treated similarly to those in the Salzburg approach. With a median follow-up of 72.4 months, there were just 16 IBTR (1.44 %) and only 8 TLR (0.8 %). DFS, DSS, and OS were 88.6, 94.0, and 91.3 %, respectively. Young age is clearly a risk factor (Table 28.4), but the 5-year recurrence rate of 3.8 % for the 53 women under the age of 40 still compares very favorably with historical rates of 10 % for this age group. In fact, IOERT boost results in lower recurrence rates in every age group, compared to historic controls (Fig. 28.10, Table 28.5).

One possible explanation for the lower recurrence rate with IOERT boost in younger women is that generally these women are considered higher risk and undergo many weeks of chemotherapy before adjuvant radiation is initiated. An IOERT boost at the time of their lumpectomy provides one to two log cell kill rate to the microscopic tumor burden that may remain in the surgical site, reducing the tumor burden for the delayed adjuvant radiation. There was no increased recurrence risk for delaying EBRT due to chemotherapy, providing EBRT was administered within 140 days of the surgery. It is also important to note that the median time for TLR was 71 months (range 12.5–151 months) and 62 months for "elsewhere" recurrences (range 17–103 months). IORT patients need a long follow-up to assess recurrence, especially since so many women are now receiving adjuvant hormonal therapy.

Table 28.4 Risk factors for IOERT

Factor	IOERT boost	IOERT APBI
Age	<40 years	<50 years
Tumor size	Any BCS tumor OK	>2.0 cm
Time between surgery and EBRT	>140 days	NA. No EBRT is given
Positive margins on final pathology	Re-excise	Re-excise, ignore
Tumor grade	G3	G3
Hormonal status	Any OK	Negative
Dose to ribs	≤5 Gy	NA. Shield plate protects ribs
Histology	No EIC	IDC and other low-risk histologies
Multicentric	No, if close together to allow BCS	Yes
Molecular subtype	Any OK	Non-Luminal A

Boost risk factors from the ISIORT-Europe pooled analysis. APBI risk factors are from Veronesi [93], Leonardi [88, 95], and Dall'Oglio [98]

Comment: In IOERT boost, women with high-risk factors still do very well. For example, the 5-year recurrence rate in women <40 years was only 3.8 % with IOERT boost, more than a factor of 2 better than achieved with either EBRT boost or mastectomy. And while > 140 days to start EBRT is a higher risk than <140 days, the 5-year recurrence rate was only 1.85 % (2 of 108 patients). For IOERT APBI, careful attention needs to be paid to proper patient selection: age ≥ 50 years, tumor size ≤2.0 cm, ER/PgR positive. High tumor grade (G3) is a risk factor for recurrence but can be compensated by favorable biology (Luminal A)

There are numerous other IOERT boost studies that have produced similar results to Salzburg, Montpellier, and the ISIORT pooled analysis. We will mention only the study from San Felipe Neri Hospital [73], because it is the only randomized trial reported comparing IOERT boost with EBRT boost. In this study, women with T1–T2 breast cancer underwent conservative surgery and were randomly assigned to receive IOERT boost (10 Gy) and postoperative EBRT (50 Gy) or postoperative EBRT (50 Gy) plus a 10 Gy external beam boost. Patients with DCIS, ILC, or EIC were excluded. IOERT was delivered using a single dose of 10 Gy with a radial margin of 2 cm,

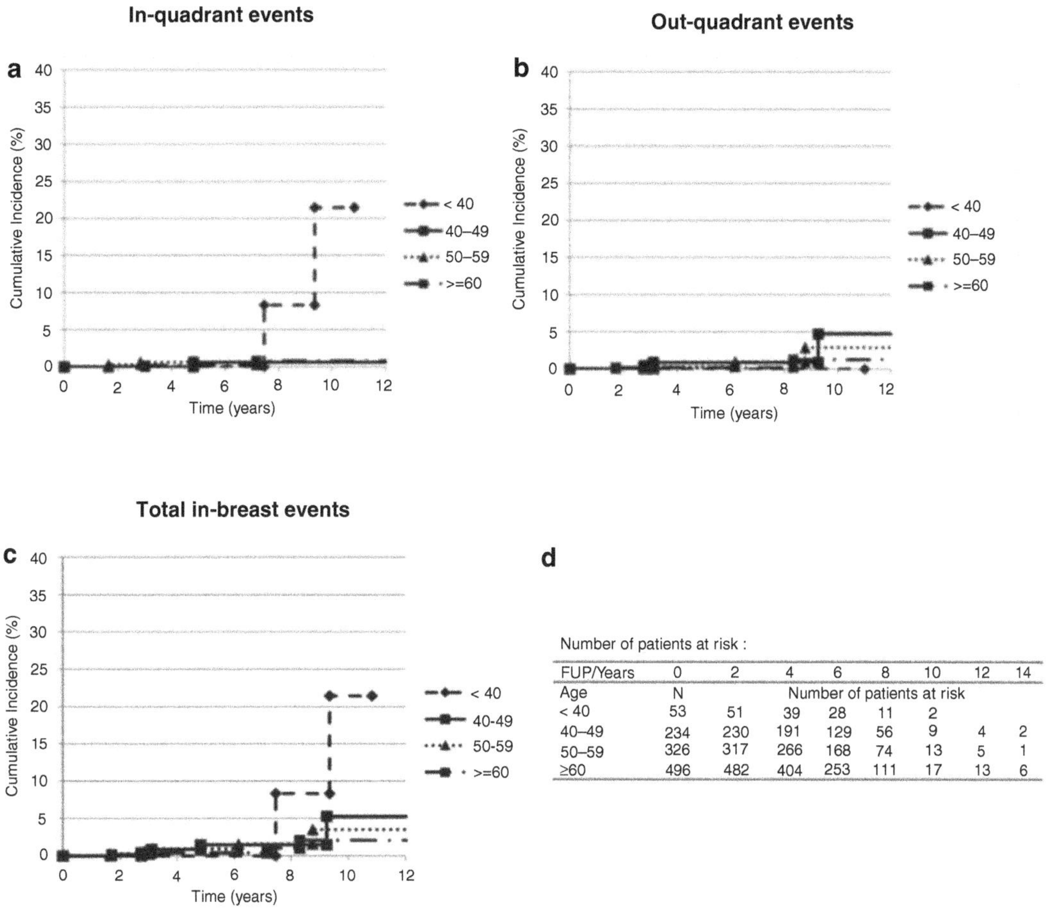

FUP/Years	0	2	4	6	8	10	12	14
Age	N	Number of patients at risk						
< 40	53	51	39	28	11	2		
40–49	234	230	191	129	56	9	4	2
50–59	326	317	266	168	74	13	5	1
≥60	496	482	404	253	111	17	13	6

Fig. 28.10 Cumulative incidence of local recurrence by age after IOERT boost, showing in quadrant, out quadrant and total breast events. From the ISIORT-Europe pooled analysis of IOERT boost [69]. Note that IOERT boost results in reduced local recurrence in every age group (see also Table 28.5)

Table 28.5 Local recurrences by age of patient after IOERT boost

LR	Age (years)	# of Pats.	Follow-up (mos and range)	LR: # of Pats.	Annual rate	Best EBRT annual rate
IB	<40	53 (4.8 %)	74.5 (16.5–126.0)	2 (3.7 %)	0.64 %	1.8 %
	40–49	234 (21.1 %)	75.9 (4.8–187.9)	5 (2.1 %)	0.34 %	1.5 %
	50–59	326 (29.4 %)	72.9 (3.8–208.5)	4 (1.2 %)	0.21 %	1.0 %
	≥60	496 (44.7 %)	73.0 (3.5–215.0)	5 (1.0 %)	0.16 %	0.6 %
IQ	<40			2 (3.7 %)	0.64 %	
	40–49			2 (0.9 %)	0.14 %	
	50–59			2 (0.6 %)	0.10 %	
	≥60			2 (0.4 %)	0.06 %	
OQ	<40			0 (0 %)	0 %	
	40–49			3 (1.3 %)	0.21 %	
	50–59			2 (0.6 %)	0.10 %	
	≥60			3 (0.6 %)	0.09 %	

From ISIORT boost pooled analysis, modified from Fastner et al. [69]. Best EBRT rate is taken from data cited in Fastner et al. Note that IOERT boost provides lower local recurrence rates for every age group compared to EBRT and, to a target depth of between 1.4 and 1.9 cm, using applicators with 4–8 cm diameter. Surgical clips were positioned at the edge of irradiated areas in all patients. Following wound healing, patients received an additional 50 Gy EBRT to the whole breast, with 6–10 MeV photon energy. In the non-IOERT arm, a boost of 10 Gy in five fractions (to the 90 % reference isodose) with a 6–12 MeV electron beam was administered.

From April 1999 to December 2004, 234 patients were randomized, 126 in the IOERT arm (with 131 treatments due to five bilateral neoplasms), and 118 in the non-IOERT arm. The mean age was 56.3 years (range, 29–75 years) in the IOERT arm and 56.2 years (range, 34–75 years) in the non-IORT arm; 88 patients in the IOERT arm and 79 in the non-IOERT arm were premenopausal. Margins were negative in all patients. One local recurrence was observed in the IOERT arm (0.8 %) and four in the non-IOERT arm (3.4 %). Patients were salvaged with mastectomy. Beginning in 2005, all patients eligible for BCT received IOERT boost. Ciabattoni et al. [74] updated the Felipe Neri IOERT boost experience at the GEC-ESTRO Meeting in 2009. With a median follow-up of 68.8 months (range 4–124 months), 223 patients had received IOERT boost. There was one local failure (0.4 %). DFS, DSS, and OS were 87.8, 96.4, and 94.6 %, respectively. Distant metastases occurred in 16 patients (7.2 %). Cosmetic evaluation was excellent or good in 88.3 % of patients. Both acute and late toxicities were low (6.5 % and 4.5 %, respectively), and five patients (2.4 %) experienced liponecrosis, two of whom required surgical aspiration to correct.

IORT Clinical Results: IORT as APBI

IOERT as APBI was first proposed by Veronesi in 2001 [52]. He observed that for postmenopausal women with small tumors, most recurrences were in the index quadrant. The percentage of women who developed ipsilateral recurrences elsewhere in the breast was about the same as women who developed contralateral breast cancer (~15 %). Veronesi reasoned that it made as little sense as to irradiate the entire breast for these women as it did to prophylactically irradiate the contralateral breast. He therefore began a randomized study, called ELIOT, to determine whether, for these postmenopausal women with small tumors, it was possible to deliver a single dose of radiation to a smaller volume of the breast, replacing the standard 6 weeks of whole breast radiation. Also in 2001, Vaidya, Baum, and Tobias [43, 75] proposed the use of 50 kV X-rays to treat early-stage, low-risk breast cancer with an APBI IORT technique called "TARGIT."

When Veronesi and the TARGIT group proposed their studies, neither ASTRO nor ESTRO had yet issued guidelines for which women were most suitable for APBI breast treatments. Both studies had less stringent inclusion criteria than is generally recommended for APBI studies today. In the ELIOT study, only 22 % of the patients met the ASTRO criteria of "suitable" for APBI, while in the TARGIT-A Trial, over one-third of the patients met the ASTRO low-risk criteria and over one-half met the ESTRO "good" low-risk criteria. The difference in the percentage of low-risk patients in these two trials is not surprising even though they began at about the same time. The ELIOT study was completed in December 2007, just after ASTRO or ESTRO issued their low-risk guidelines for APBI. The TARGIT-A Trial continued through 2012 and more than half of their patients were entered after the guidelines for low-risk women were issued. When evaluating the efficacy of these trials, the suitability of patients to receive APBI should be considered.

APBI Clinical Results: HDR-IORT

Only one center is currently using HDR as a single-dose APBI treatment during surgery. Sacchini et al. [40] reports on 52 patients with a median age of 76.2 (range 60–87 years, excluding 2 off-protocol patients younger than 60) and with tumors <2 cm that were treated with HDR using the HAM applicator in a shielded OR room. A single fraction of 20 Gy was initially prescribed one cm from the surface of the applicator. After the first 18 patients had significant acute toxicity, the dose prescription was reduced to

18 Gy to the lateral margin of the surgical cavity, falling to about 7 Gy at 1 cm from the applicator surface. The irradiation time was about 40 min. There were 63 complications reported in the 52 women treated, with 4 % requiring reoperation for poor wound healing. There were no recurrences reported at 31.4 months' median follow-up, but, in a recent update at the ASTRO 2011 Meeting, a 7.7 % recurrence rate was cited at 68 months' median follow-up [76]. The hospital has now treated a total of about 150 patients with this APBI approach (Cohen G, Brachytherapy physicist, Memorial Sloan Kettering Cancer Center, 2012, private communication). This HDR-IORT APBI approach is not likely to gain widespread acceptance, as the OR needs to be shielded to deliver the radiation; exposure times are very long, subjecting elderly women to prolonged anesthesia; the toxicity and recurrence rates seem to be higher than reported using other IORT techniques; and the dose homogeneity is suboptimal with this brachytherapy approach.

APBI Clinical Results: Orthovoltage (50 kV X-rays), Prospective Randomized Results

The TARGIT-A Trial [77] is an intent-to-treat, non-inferiority trial in which 2,232 patients from 28 centers in ten countries were randomized to either TARGIT or 5 weeks of EBRT with or without an EBRT boost, depending on the treatment policy of the individual treatment center. The TARGIT arm allowed conversion from IORT APBI to IORT boost if the patient presented with adverse factors after randomization. They call this approach "risk-adapted IORT." Each center was empowered to determine which adverse factors would necessitate converting a TARGIT APBI patient to a TARGIT boost patient. Interestingly, the prescribed doses for TARGIT APBI and TARGIT boost were both 20 Gy at the surface of the applicator sphere. The predefined non-inferiority margin was an absolute difference of 2.5 % in recurrences.

The TARGIT arm randomized 1,123 women, excluding 117 patients (10.4 %) for various reasons. Only 996 women actually received TARGIT, 142 (14 %) as TARGIT boost and 854 (86 %) as TARGIT APBI. Of the 854 women receiving TARGIT APBI, about 31 % received the IORT as a second procedure, post final pathology. The EBRT arm randomized 1,119 women and excluded 94 patients (8.4 %). The TARGIT Trial profile is shown in Fig. 28.11. They reported results only 3 months after completion of accrual, when the median follow-up was just 25 months. There were six local recurrences in the TARGIT group and five in the EBRT group, resulting in a Kaplan-Meier estimate at 4 years of 1.2 % recurrence for the TARGIT group and 0.95 % for the EBRT group. The authors assert that the peak time for ipsilateral breast recurrence is in the 2–3-year range, so the difference in projected 5-year recurrence in their study is well within the predefined non-inferiority margin of 2.5 %. They conclude that a single dose of TARGIT should be considered as an alternative for EBRT for select low-risk women. With a median follow-up of 25 months, complications in both groups were modest and similar, with TARGIT patients experiencing more seromas and needing three or more aspirations (2.1 % vs. 0.8 %, $p=0.012$) and the EBRT patients experiencing more RTOG Grade 3 or 4 toxicities (0.5 % vs. 2.1 %, $p=0.002$).

The authors updated the TARGIT-A Trial in a poster presentation at the San Antonio Breast Cancer Symposium (SABCS) in 2011 [78]. They reported a total of 23 recurrences, but did not identify in which arm they occurred. The median follow-up was less than 3 years. They concluded: *"The overall recurrence rate of the TARGIT-A trial have remained stable with a longer follow-up and it is therefore statistically implausible that one particular arm has a significantly higher local recurrence."* The latest TARGIT-A updates, presented at the 2012 SABCS [50] and published in Lancet [51], showed that the earlier optimism expressed in the 2010 Lancet publication and the 2011 SABCS poster was likely unfounded. An additional 1,219 patients were added to TARGIT-A since the 2010 Lancet publication, for a study total of 3,442 patients. This trial now has more than a 12-year accrual of patients from 33 centers in 11 countries. The original 2,232

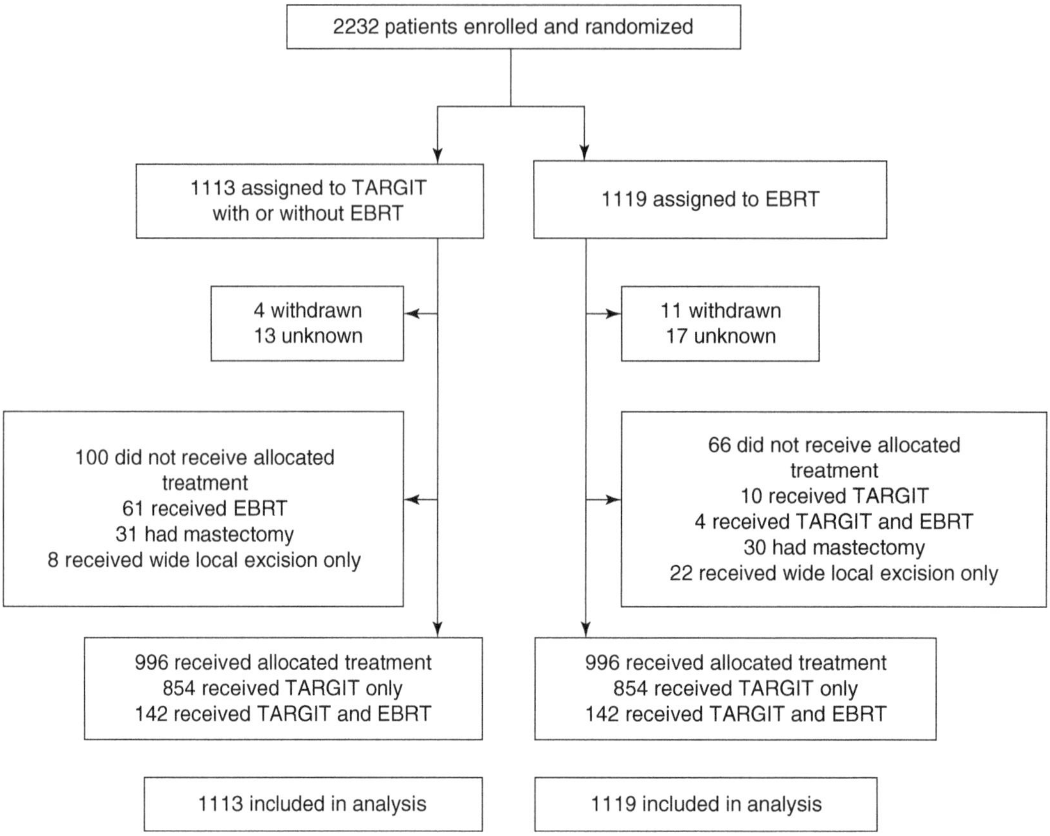

Fig. 28.11 TARGIT-A Trial profile [77]. All patients entered into this "intent-to-treat" study are included in the analysis, even if they were excluded from the treatment. In the Lancet publication, 10.4 % and 8.4 % of the TARGIT and EBRT arms, respectively, were not treated. In addition, 15 % of patients entered and treated in the TARGIT arm were converted to TARGIT boost and also received 5-weeks of EBRT. Approximately 30 % of patients received TARGIT in a second operation after final pathology was known

patients in the TARGIT-A study had sufficient power to distinguish non-inferiority in recurrences, the primary end point. The additional patients were needed to analyze sub-protocols that were not identified, but had the impact of loading the study with more women with short follow-up, keeping the study results immature. The Lancet publication had a median follow-up of 25 months, and the updated report has a median follow-up of only 29 months, even though more than 2 years had elapsed. Just 18 % of the total patients have 5 years of follow-up, and only 29 % have even 4 years of follow-up.

The local failure rate in the TARGIT group was now reported to be 2 % higher than in the EBRT group, and this difference is statistically significant ($p=0.042$, HR=2.05). The TARGIT group also did worse than the EBRT group for local-regional recurrence ($p=0.02$, HR=2.2) and showed a worsening trend for overall recurrences (ipsilateral, contralateral, axilla, and distant). There were 69 breast events in the TARGIT arm vs. 48 in the standard arm, though the difference in overall recurrence has not yet reached statistical significance ($p=0.053$, HR=1.44). Post-pathology TARGIT patients had worse local recurrence than pre-pathology TARGIT patients, compared to their respective EBRT group (5.4 % vs. 1.7 % for post-pathology TARGIT and 2.1 % vs. 1.0 % for pre-pathology TARGIT). The local recurrence for post-pathology patients was not yet statistically significant ($p=0.069$) but was greater than the preset non-inferiority margin of 2.5 %. The results and authors' conclusions from their original pub-

Table 28.6 TARGIT-A Trial results as reported over time

STUDY	Median Follow-up	Local Recurrences					Any Breast Event			
		Targit	EBRT	Total	% Diff.	p-value	Targit	EBRT	% Diff.	p-value
Lancet 2010	25 months	6	5	11	0.25	NS	10	8	NS	NS
LANCET 2010 Conclusion: "For selected patients with early breast cancer, a single dose of radiotherapy delivered at the time of surgery by use of targeted intraoperative radiotherapy should be considered as an alternative to external beam radiotherapy delivered over several weeks."										
SABCS 2011	32 months	NS	NS	23	NS	NS	Not Stated			
SABCS 2011 Conclusion: "The overall recurrence rate of the TARGIT-A trial have remained stable with a longer follow-up, and it is therefore statistically implausible that one particular arm has a significantly higher recurrence."										
SABCS 2012	29 months	23	11	34	2.01	0.042	69	48	2.5	0.053
SABCS 2012 Conclusion: "The risk-adapted approach using single dose Targit has a slightly higher recurrence rate than EBRT for the primary endpoint of IBR, but was within the present non-inferiority boundary, with the pre-pathology apparently performing better that the post-pathology stratum."										

Lancet 2013	29 months									
All recurrence rates are 5-year Kaplan-Meir projections.	Local Recurrences: Total Cohort					Any Other Breast Event: Total Cohort				
	Targit	%	EBRT	%	p-value	Targit	%	EBRT	%	p-value
	23	3.3	11	1.3	0.042	46	4.9	37	4.4	NS
	Local Recurrences: Pre-pathology Group					Any Other Breast Event: Pre-pathology Group				
	Targit	%	EBRT	%	p-value	Targit	%	EBRT	%	p-value
	10	2.1	6	1.1	0.31	29	4.8	25	4.7	0.72
	Local Recurrences: Post-pathology Group					Any Other Breast Event: Post-pathology Group				
	Targit	%	EBRT	%	p-value	Targit	%	EBRT	%	p-value
	13	5.4	5	1.7	0.069	17	5.2	12	3.7	NS

	Total Target	Total EBRT	Targit Pre-Pathology	EBRT Pre-pathology	Targit Post-Pathology	EBRT Post-pathology
Loco-regional Recurrences (p values not stated in Lancet 2013, but given as 0.02, HR =2.2 at SABCS 2012 for total cohort).	4.2% n = 31	2.0% n = 17	3.1%	2.0%	6.2%	2.0%
All recurrences (p values not stated in Lancet 2013, but given as 0.053, HR =1.44 at SABCS 2012 for total cohort)	8.2% 69	5.7% 48	6.9% 39	5.8% 31	10.4% 30	5.4% 17

Lancet 2013-Appendix	Pre-Pathology Targit Only (N = 793)	Pre-pathology Targit + EBRT (N = 219)	Post-Pathology Targit Only (N = 539)
5-year projected recurrence	2.7%	0.9%	5.9%
LANCET 2013 Conclusion: "Targit concurrent with lumpectomy within a risk-adapted approach should be considered as an option for eligible patients with breast cancer carefully selected as per the Targit-A trial protocol, as an alternative to postoperative external beam breast radiotherapy."			

NS = Not Stated

Lancet **2010: No metastatic events reported. Seven LRR reported**

SABCS **2011 Poster: Results kept blinded. Only total number of local recurrences reported**

SABCS **2012 Presentation: TARGIT recurrence was 3.3 % (HR = 2.07)**

Lancet **2013: Distant recurrences not reported separately. Total TARGIT plus EBRT metastases = 62 from SABCS 2012 Presentation**

NS **not stated**

lication [77] and three updates [50, 51, 78] are summarized in Table 28.6 and in Fig. 28.12.

Despite the fact that the post-pathology patients were presumably lower risk as the treatment was delivered in a second operation after final pathology, they had more than twice the recurrence rate of the pre-pathology group. The authors attribute this to possibly delay in wound fluid suppression of tumor cells since there is a delay of TARGIT radiation in post-pathology patients by about 30 days or to a geometric miss when inserting the applicator postsurgery. While this might partially explain the results, it is not the likely major cause of their finding. In the published IORT Intrabeam boost study of 299 patients [64], there was absolutely no difference in recurrences between the pre- and post-pathology patients. The true 5-year recurrence rate for all patients was <2 %. The explanation for the difference in the TARGIT A Trial probably lies in the fact that in post-pathology patients, there is a reduction in the size of the seroma, and so smaller spherical applicators are employed for tumors of the same size than in pre-pathology TARGIT patients. Thus, the volume-

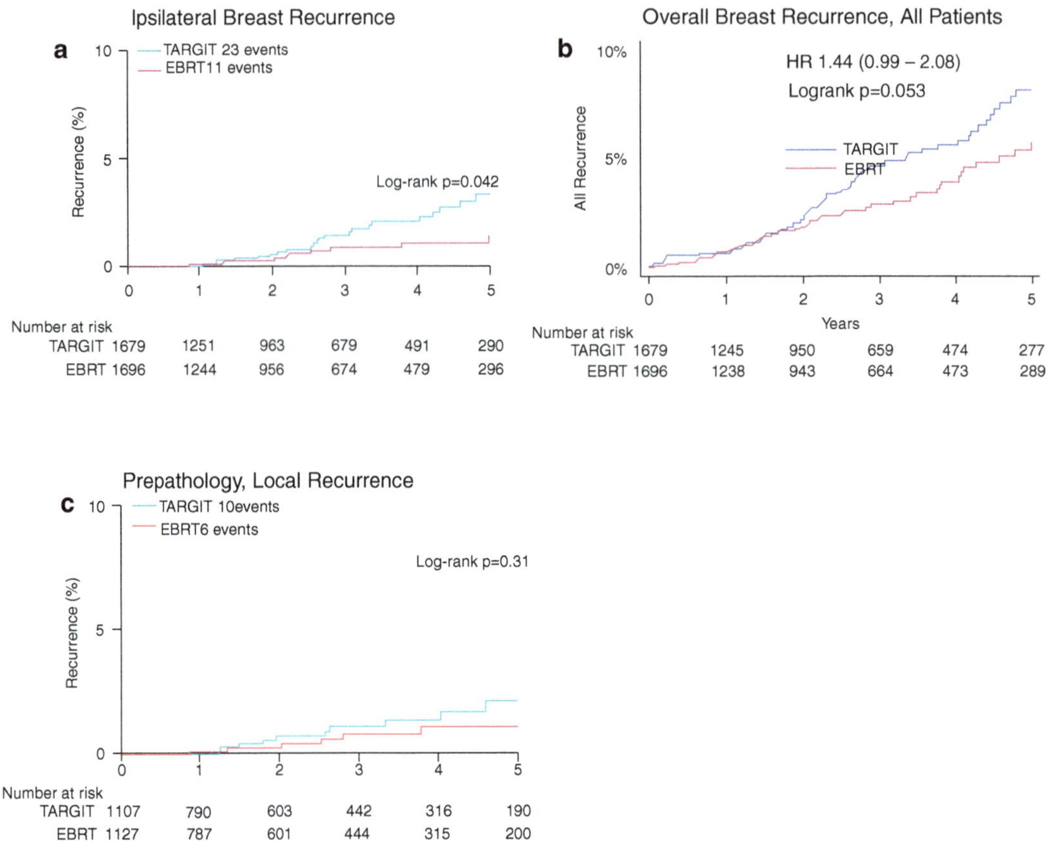

Fig. 28.12 5-year Kaplan-Meier projections for recurrences from TARGIT-A-treated patients vs. EBRT-treated patients: (**a**) Ipsilateral breast recurrences [51]; (**b**) all breast recurrences (ipsilateral, regional, contralateral, and distant) [50]; (**c**) pre-pathology only TARGIT-A ipsilateral recurrences [51]

irradiated post-pathology is much smaller than the volume irradiated when TARGIT is given concurrently with surgery. In boost, EBRT can compensate for the smaller volume irradiated. One can also see this trend in the pre-pathology TARGIT patients since TARGIT plus EBRT has three times fewer local recurrences than TARGIT alone (Tables 28.6 and 28.7).

The authors noted that the difference in ipsilateral breast failure for all patients is still within their absolute non-inferiority margin of 2.5 %. However, as the Ipsilateral Recurrences in Fig. 28.12a shows, the TARGIT group recurrences are diverging from the EBRT group with a slope two or three times greater than that of the EBRT group. There is little doubt that the 2.5 % criteria for non-inferiority will soon be surpassed for the entire cohort. The still immaturity of the data also makes suspect the claim of equivalent ipsilateral breast recurrence for their favorable cohort of pre-pathology TARGIT patients. This favorable group also shows a higher divergence of local recurrence for TARGIT patients compared to EBRT patients (see Fig. 28.12c). The difference between this favorable TARGIT cohort and the EBRT group is 1.0 %, with a median follow-up of 29 months. The initial Lancet publication, with a median follow-up of 25 months, had a difference of only 0.25 % between the TARGIT group and the EBRT group. Therefore, there is simply not sufficient follow-up to draw solid conclusions about possible favorable cohorts.

One potential problem for the TARGIT technique is overall breast recurrence (Fig. 28.12b) which was presented at the SABCS but not shown in the Lancet publication. The nearly statistically

Table 28.7 TARGIT-A local recurrence summary by treatment strata

Cohort	# of recurrences	Percent	P-Value
Pre-Pathology Targit	10	2.1%	0.31
Pre-Pathology EBRT	6	1.1%	
Post Pathology Targit	13	5.4%	0.069
Post Pathology EBRT	5	1.7%	
Pre-Pathology Targit Alone (N = 793)	~ 7[a]	2.7%	**Not stated**
Pre-Pathology Targit + Boost (N = 219)	~ 3[a]	0.9%	

[a]*Number of recurrences extrapolated from presented data in Lancet Appendix;* **approximately 20 % of women who receive an Intrabeam treatment will subsequently also require 5 weeks of EBRT [51]**

significant difference in overall breast recurrences in the two groups ($p = 0.053$) is a reason for concern, especially since the breast cancer deaths are already, even at 29 months median follow-up, higher with TARGIT (20 deaths, 2.6 %) than with EBRT (16 deaths, 1.9 %), though not yet statistically significant ($p = 0.56$).

In their favorable cohort of pre-pathology TARGIT patients, patients that receive TARGIT only vs. those that receive TARGIT plus 5 weeks of EBRT [51, Appendix] have a higher Kaplan-Meier 5-year local recurrence rate (2.7 % vs. 0.9 %). The authors' state that these rates of local recurrence did not differ (i.e., statistically), despite the fact that the recurrence rate for TARGIT alone is three times that of TARGIT boost. Strangely, the authors claim that the TARGIT boost patients had a 5-year risk of breast cancer death of 8 % vs. only 1.8 % for those that received TARGIT alone. This result appears inconsistent with the IORT boost results discussed previously.

Several issues were raised with this trial very early on [49, 79–82], primarily highlighting the immaturity of the data and the nonhomogeneous nature of the patient population, together with the fact that 75 % of the women had adjuvant hormonal treatment known to delay recurrences. The TARGIT group consists of three different clinical cohorts: pre-pathology patients, post-pathology patients, and patients who were found at high risk after final pathology or at the time of surgery who were treated with 5 weeks of WBI, in addition to an IORT boost of 20 Gy. These cohorts have potentially different clinical outcomes, and attempting to analyze them as one group can only lead to inaccurate assessments of the efficacy of the treatment. Table 28.7 is a summary of local recurrences by treatment strata.

The TARGIT study had 33 centers in 11 countries and lasted more than 12 years. One-third of these centers contributed less than 25 patients, less than 50 % of the centers contributed as many as 50 patients, and only 8 centers contributed more than 100 patients. The large number of centers and the relatively few patients contributed by many of the centers demanded a high level of control. However, *the study did not impose standard inclusion/exclusion criteria*. Each center was permitted to treat the EBRT group according to its own institutional guidelines, including the decision of whether to incorporate an EBRT boost. Each center was also free to impose its own criteria for high-risk patients who would go on to receive TARGIT boost rather than TARGIT APBI. This lack of discipline in imposing standard criteria can only throw into question the results of the trial.

The importance of standardization in selection criteria in a randomized trial cannot be overemphasized. Sperk [83] analyzes the Mannheim cohort of TARGIT-A patients for recurrence and toxicity. In their cohort of 54 TARGIT-A patients, a much larger percentage of patients (37 %, not the 15 % reported in TARGIT-A) were converted from TARGIT APBI to TARGIT boost because of the risk factors they chose for conversion, which included tumors > 2 cm and margins <10 mm. With a median follow-up of 40 months, they report no recurrences, but 40 months is still early, since 80 % of their patients received adjuvant endocrine therapy. Despite the fact that the number of TARGIT APBI patients at Mannheim was small (34), if these good results are sustained over the passage of time, it is possible that there may yet be a small subset of women for whom "risk-adjusted" TARGIT treatment is a reasonable option. However, due to the lack of discipline in TARGIT-A selection and exclusion criteria, it is questionable whether the larger TARGIT-A Trial will be able to discover whether there is a suitable cohort of women who might benefit from TARGIT-A. This makes the results of this study difficult for clinicians to interpret as there are likely to be no risk criteria that will be proven.

APBI Clinical Results: Orthovoltage (50 kV X-Rays), Nonrandomized Results

There have been a few reports of single-institutional studies outside of the TARGIT-A Trial using "risk-adjusted" Intrabeam for APBI IORT [84, 85]. These studies used the TARGIT-A technique, but treated a lower-risk population of patients than the TARGIT-A study did, and converted slightly more patients from TARGIT APBI to TARGIT boost (17 and 19 %, respectively). However, they involve too few patients and still have too short of a follow-up to determine whether treating these lower-risk patients will lead to better results than in the TARGIT-A study.

There have been no randomized studies using the iCad Xoft system, with no ongoing trials for IORT breast treatments and very limited published breast data (studies totaling less than 25 patients) on the use of this device for APBI IORT [47, 48]. Unlike the rigid Intrabeam spherical applicators, newer balloon technology applicators allow the Xoft balloon-based applicator to more accurately conform to nonspherical tumor volumes, theoretically providing them a technical advantage over Intrabeam.

However, without a large and mature base of clinical data, it is impossible to predict whether this theoretical advantage will lead to an improvement in clinical results compared to those of Intrabeam or if Xoft is even an acceptable alternative. Most of the issues associated with Intrabeam in terms of skin spacing and breast size, uncertainty in RBE, limited target coverage, and inhomogeneous delivery of radiation to the target apply to the iCad Xoft system as well. Since the TARGIT-A Trial has not shown to be equivalent to standard BCT, Xoft will need to find for what patient cohort its device is suited to treat. Xoft does have the advantage over the Intrabeam device in that, similar to balloon brachytherapy devices, it can be used postoperatively in APBI treatments.

A new Phase II trial for a low-risk group of women 70 years and older, TARGIT-E, is now recruiting patients [86]. It is based on the TARGIT-A Trial and allows both pre- and post-pathology patients and conversion of pre-pathology patients from IORT APBI to IORT boost. Since each participating institution has the option to modify the entry criteria and the criteria to convert patients to IORT boost, this study contains the same design flaws already pointed out in the TARGIT-A analysis. The study intends to accrue patients through 2015 and expects 10 years of follow-up. The primary end point is local recurrence, and the stopping point at 5 years is 4 % (which, interestingly, is the same recurrence that has been obtained in the trial of BCS + tamoxifen, with or without radiotherapy [87]). Though it is meant as a Phase II study, it is unclear what new information will be gained that could not be found from evaluating women over 70 in the TARGIT-A Trial who have already received this treatment. Such an analysis might justify a randomized trial for women over 70 to determine whether APBI IORT treatment plus adjuvant hormonal therapy has better local control than BCS and adjuvant hormonal therapy without radiotherapy.

IOERT as APBI

IOERT has some technical advantages over 50 kV IORT (see Table 28.3). The surgical remodeling of the breast parenchyma in IOERT morphologically transforms the at-risk breast tissue so that it is compactly placed under the electron applicator. Together with the temporary re-approximation of the tumor bed, which also places all of the tumor margins in the center of the radiation field, this approach allows irradiation of the microscopic disease that may extend 2–3 cm beyond the original tumor. This is consistent with the work of Holland and Faverly [25, 26] and assures that all margins receive a minimum dose of 18 Gy. This should be sufficient to sterilize any microscopic disease that remains [57, 88]. IOERT adequately covers the tumor and tissue at risk, irrespective of the tumor shape. The CTV irradiated with IOERT is comparable to that used in 3D conformal APBI [89], but can be slightly smaller while covering the same tissue at risk, since no additional tissue volume need be included to allow for patient motion and errors in patient setup.

Furthermore, because more normal tissue can be excluded from the radiation field with IOERT, the dose-volume histograms (a measure of homogeneity of tumor coverage and normal tissue exposure) with IOERT APBI will be superior to those generated with any of the EBRT APBI techniques. The high quality of electron beam radiation generates substantially more uniform dose distributions than those produced with 50 kV X-rays or brachytherapy. Treatment times are very short, only 1–2 min, compared to 30 or more minutes with 50 kV X-rays or brachytherapy. IOERT is independent of breast size and tumor location, providing the tumor location has sufficient breast tissue beneath it to insert a protective chest wall disk. IOERT is the only APBI method that lends itself to immediate oncoplastic reconstruction, as the target volume receives all radiation in the one treatment. The mobilization of the breast tissue required to prepare the target gland for IOERT is a necessary step in any oncoplastic reconstruction procedure, so the oncoplastic reconstruction time is significantly shortened. A 1 day, single-dose IOERT treatment, with or without oncoplastic reconstruction, might convert some women from unnecessary mastectomies to BCS.

APBI Clinical Results: IOERT Randomized Results

A single dose of IOERT, called "ELIOT," was first proposed by Veronesi et al. [9]. After a toxicity study which began in 1999 of 22 women to determine the safe single IOERT dose of radiation to the breast, they decided that 21 Gy delivered to a 90 % depth was safe. Their randomized study [90] had a very simple stratification: women over 48 with tumors <2.5 cm were randomized to either a single IOERT dose of 21 Gy prescribed to the 90 % point (ELIOT) or 5 weeks of WBI with a 10 Gy EBRT boost. Both IDC and lobular carcinoma were allowed. All patients received wide excision (quandrantectomy) surgery. For ELIOT patients, a 9 mm thick protective metallic disk, consisting of lead and aluminum plates, was inserted below the gland to protect the chest wall. The trial closed on December 2007, with 1,305 patients randomized: 651 to ELIOT and 654 to EBRT. Analysis began 5 years after the last patient was accrued. The median FU was 5.9 years for the EBRT patients and 5.5 years for the IOERT patients. The data was analyzed using both "intent to treat" and "per protocol." The ELIOT Trial profile is shown in Fig. 28.13. The ELIOT and EBRT patients achieved 5-year recurrence rates of 4.4 and 0.4 %, respectively, $p<0.0001$. The ELIOT patients had lower recurrences than their initial projections, but the conventional patients did exceptionally well and are one of the best reported in any conventionally treated BCT series.

The ELIOT arm had less skin damage (i.e., erythema, dryness, hyperpigmentation, or itching) than the conventional arm, $p=0.0002$. There were no differences for fibrosis, retraction, pain, or burning, but there was a higher incidence of radiological determined fat necrosis in the ELIOT group, 5 %, vs. 2 % for the EBRT group, $p=0.04$. In addition, ELIOT showed less pulmonary toxicity than the EBRT arm [91] as diagnosed by follow-up spiral CT (4 in the ELIOT arm and 38 in the EBRT arm). These differences in skin and pulmonary toxicity are not unexpected given the differences in IOERT vs. EBRT radiation techniques. The authors point out that less skin damage through use of IOERT might be important in the event of a salvage mastectomy for recurrence. The integrity of the skin, they say, is important to the success of skin-sparing and nipple-sparing mastectomies, which are rapidly becoming standard procedure.

When analyzing for risk of relapse, the 5-year IBTR exceeded 10 % for patients who had tumors

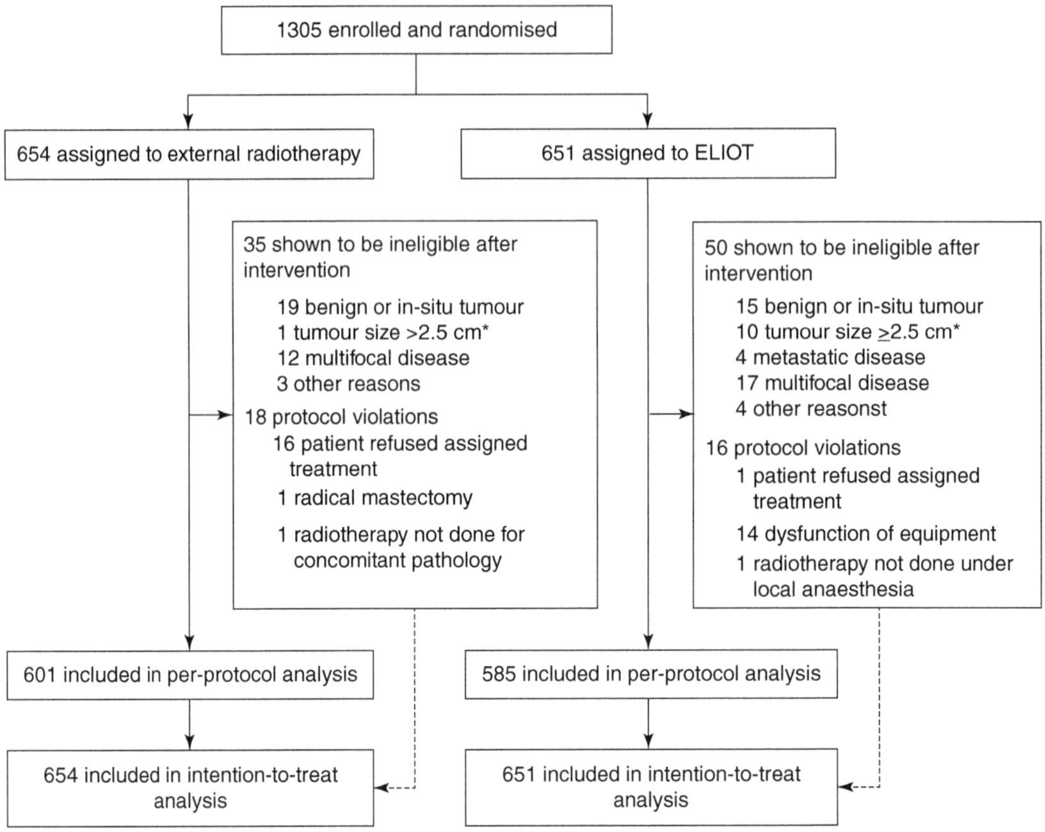

Fig. 28.13 ELIOT Trial profile [90]. Both "intent-to-treat" and "per-protocol" strata are identified. * At pathological examination

> 2 cm (10/83 = 10.9 %), or four or more positive nodes (4/31 = 15.0 %), those with poorly differentiated tumors, i.e., G3 (15/129 = 11.9 %), or with ER-tumors (8/63 = 14.9 %), or with triple-negative disease (7/43 = 18.9 %). Patients with a high proliferative index, i.e., Ki-67 > 20 %, also trended to a high IBTR rate (22/244 = 9.1 %) but was not used in their risk factor analysis since it did not reach their imposed 10 % threshold. The 5-year IBTR was 11.3 % for the 199 (30.6 %) women with one or more of these risk factors vs. only 1.5 % for the remaining 452 (69.4 %) women who had none of these factors.

The per-protocol results, which analyzed just the 585 women who actually received ELIOT and the 601 who actually received EBRT, are reported in an Appendix to the publication. It had very similar results to the intent-to-treat analysis. The IBTR was 4.7 % for ELLIOT vs. 0.5 % for the EBRT arm, and the 5-year IBTR was 11.8 % for the 178 (30.4 %) women with one or more of these risk factors vs. 1.7 % for the remaining 407 (69.6 %) women who had none of these factors.

There was a slightly greater regional (nodal) failure with ELIOT (nine patients, 1.0 %) vs. the EBRT arm (two patients, 0.3 %), $p = 0.03$, raising the concern that the lower regional recurrence in the EBRT arm is due in part to the axillary 1 coverage by the tangential breast radiation. However, the recurrences were too low in either arm to allow statistical analysis. Patients with four or more nodes in either arm received additional EBRT of 50 Gy to the axilla, the EBRT patients concurrently with their WBI, and the IOERT patients delayed 8–12 weeks from the surgery. Adjuvant chemotherapy must have been administered to these patients, but the timing of the administration is not specified in the publication.

The contralateral breast cancer rate was 50 % higher in the EBRT group (13 patients vs. 8

patients in the ELIOT group), but was not statistically significant. Metastases, other primary cancers, breast cancer death, and other deaths were very similar in the two groups. Importantly, the OS at 5 years was identical (96.8 % for ELIOT and 96.9 % for the EBRT patients), and the survival so far at 10 years was also the same (89.8 % for ELIOT and 92.0 % for EBRT patients).

The authors conclude that IOERT with electrons should be restricted to suitable patients, once the characteristics for suitability have been defined. They note that the risk factors identified in their study need further validation. They suggest that one can use preoperative criteria (tumor size, age, and pathological and biological examination of the biopsy specimen) to identify suitable patients. A second option would be to treat all low-risk patients with IOERT and, after post-surgical categorization, give additional WBI to patients at high risk for recurrence. The current reported guidelines used for low-risk ELIOT patients at the EIO are listed in Table 28.8.

Table 28.8 EIO criteria for low-risk ELIOT patients

Age ≤ 60 years
Tumor size ≤2.0 cm
Nodal status: N0–N1
Grade: G1/G2
Hormone status: ER+
Biology: Luminal A preferred. No triple negative
Proliferation index: Ki-67 < 20
Lobular cancer – only after MRI evaluation

Modified from EIO presentations at ESTRO
Patients found with higher risk factors post-IOERT will also receive eight fractions of 3.6–4.0 Gy of EBRT, excluding the volume treated with IOERT. Minimum field size now used for ELIOT is 6 cm with the occasional use of 5 cm

A second randomized IOERT study, begun in 2003, is being conducted by a consortium of seven Italian cancer centers [92]. At the time of their last report in June 2008, they had randomized 451 patients, 229 of whom received IOERT. The study is enrolling postmenopausal patients between the ages of 48 and 75 years, who have unifocal tumors ≤ 2.5 cm and less than four positive axillary nodes. The surgical and radiation approach used in the Italian multicenter study is identical to that used by the EIO. Though the study is still open, the consortium reported that, with a median follow-up of 34 months (range 7–61 months), there had been no recurrences in either arm, and one woman in each arm had progression of disease in the lymph nodes. Significantly, 94 % of the IOERT patients were reported to have no late-term toxicity from the treatment, compared to only 38 % in the BCT arm.

APBI Clinical Results: IOERT (Electrons), Nonrandomized Results

In addition to the ELIOT trial, there are a number of single-institutional studies using IOERT APBI. The largest published study involves 1,822 patients treated with IOERT at the European Institute of Oncology by the ELIOT technique [93]. The median age of these patients was 58 years (range 33–83), and while patients were limited to tumors with a maximum dimension of 2.5 cm (determined by preoperative imaging), at the time of surgery, 5 % had tumors larger than 2.5 cm, and two women had tumors larger than 5 cm. The histology was mostly IDC (1,381 women or 78.3 %), but 202 women (11.1 %) had invasive lobular carcinoma (ILC). Grade 3 tumors were found in 459 women (25.2 %), and 146 (8 %) had three or more positive nodes. Most were ER+ and PgR+ (89.2 and 77.9 %, respectively). As for adjuvant treatment, 75.8 % received endocrine therapy, 9.6 % chemotherapy alone, and 10.9 % both endocrine and chemotherapy.

With a median follow-up of 36 months, 42 patients (2.3 %) had a true recurrence, and another 24 (1.2 %) patients had an elsewhere recurrence, for a total ipsilateral breast recurrence rate of 3.6 %. The median time for LR was 29.2 months (range 10–92.5 months). All patients were salvaged by either a second BCS or mastectomy, of which 34 are alive without evidence of disease, and 3 died of disease progression. The time for elsewhere recurrences was not reported, but all patients were salvaged with either BCS or mastectomy, and four patients in that group have died of disease progression. The positive or close margin rates were low (6 positive margins and 48 close margins). These patients had no further treatment, and none of them have recurred so far with a follow-up of 1.2–28.1 months. Total deaths due to breast cancer were 28 (1.5 %), for a 10-year overall survival and breast cancer-specific survival of 89.7 and 94.6 %, respectively. In a multivariate analysis, age <50 years, tumor size > 2 cm, and unfavorable biology (non-Luminal A) were independent indicators of local relapse.

Toxicity was judged to be low, with 78.7 % experiencing no side effects, 16 % only one side effect, and 5.3 % two or more side effects. The greatest toxicities were fibrosis and liponecrosis. Two patients developed severe fibrosis, and 32 (1.8 %) had mild fibrosis, most of whom resolved after 36 months. They observed 78 (4.2 %) cases of liponecrosis, which is a localized collection of brown fluid with skin erythema appearing 2–4 weeks postsurgery that appears to be more frequent with women with fatty breasts. This resolved in most cases with conservative management, though a few patients required aspiration of the fluid. Of interest, liponecrosis has not been reported at centers that use conventional linacs or other mobile IOERT units (Mobetron) to deliver IOERT.

Late toxicity in 119 women randomly selected from the 1,822 out-trial patients has been assessed by Leonardi et al. [94]. After a median follow-up of 71 months, 38 patients (31.9 %) had Grade II fibrosis and 7 patients (5.9 %) had Grade III. Grade II or greater pain was experienced by 11 patients (9.3 %), but there was no correlation between pain and the grade of fibrosis. Cosmesis was independent of the location of the tumor in the breast and whether the patient experienced any postoperative complications. Physician-scored cosmesis was good or excellent in 84 % of the patients, compared to 74 % when patients' evaluated results, but patient satisfaction with the procedure still exceeded 90 %. Late toxicity was significantly correlated with tumor size > 1.5 cm and applicator diameter. Cosmetic evaluation was significantly worse in patients who received adjuvant hormonal therapy rather than adjuvant chemotherapy (+/− hormonal therapy).

This cohort of 1,822 patients has been analyzed according to the ASTRO [95] and ESTRO [88] guidelines for patients "suitable" or "good" for APBI treatment. For the 294 patients that fell into the ASTRO-suitable category and the 573 patients that were in the ESTRO-good group, the 5-year rate of ipsilateral breast recurrence was 1.5 and 1.9 %, respectively (Table 28.9). These APBI favorable groups also did significantly better than the less favorable APBI category patients in terms of distant metastases, any breast-related event, cause-specific survival, and overall survival (Figs. 28.14 and 28.15). There was no difference in regional lymph node failures among these categories of patients. Tumor grade, however, though not a selection criteria by either ASTRO or ESTRO, was a significant factor for ipsilateral breast recurrence, regional node failure, and distant metastases. While neither ASTRO nor ESTRO considered IOERT in their criteria selections for suitable or good APBI patients, applying these guidelines to the 1,822 out-trial patients suggests that they might also form reasonable selection criteria for IOERT APBI patients, too.

For all of the 1,822 out-trial patients, the ipsilateral breast recurrence rate at 5 years was 6 %. As the authors point out, this is higher than would be expected with conventional BCT, leading them to examine whether the tumor bed in their study was properly covered in terms of volume and dosage. IOERT is delivered to the tumor bed under direct visualization, so a geometric miss, as might occur with EBRT, is not possible. The linear-quadratic model used to establish equivalency of different fractionation schedules is valid for single doses of 10 Gy and probably can be extended at least up to 18 Gy [96], so their dose of 21 Gy should have been sufficient to sterilize microscopic disease surrounding the tumor. However, the median applicator size of 4 cm may have been too small to adequately cover larger tumors. When using a 4 cm applicator, even though the IOERT surgical preparation brings almost 2 cm of surrounding tissue within the applicator, only about 1.5 cm of surrounding tissue is irradiated to the prescription dose of 90 %. Tissue 4–5 mm from the walls of the applicator receives less radiation (see Fig. 28.6c). To assure uniform coverage of the tissues at risk, the applicator should be chosen 1.5–2 cm larger than the maximum tumor dimension, as discussed in the technical aspects of IOERT. The authors

Table 28.9 Analysis of 1,822 patients by ASTRO and ESTRO guidelines for PBI

ASTRO GUIDELINES					
	All	**Suitable**	**Cautionary**	**Unsuitable**	**Not Accessible**
Patients	1822	295 (16%)	690 (38%)	812 (45%)	25 (1.0%)
Local Relapses	76	3	21	50	2
5-year rate	6.0%	1.5%	4.4%	8.8%	9.9%
Luminal A	648	118	271	251	8
Local-regional relapse	8	2	3	3	0
5-year rate	1.7%	2.3%	1.6%	1.6%	-

ESTRO GUIDELINES					
	All	**Good**	**Possible**	**Unsuitable**	**Not Accessible**
Patients	1822	572 (31%)	268 (15%)	965 (53%)	17 (1.0%)
Local Relapses	76	7	12	56	1
5-year rate	6.0%	1.9%	7.1%	7.8%	6.6%
Luminal A	648	206	129	306	8
Local-regional relapse	8	0	2	6	0
5-year rate	1.7%	0%	2.5%	2.4%	-

The analysis of the 1,822 patients treated with ELIOT off-trial produces very low local recurrence rates for ASTRO-suitable and ESTRO-good patients, and Luminal A patients do well with APBI irrespective of the ASTRO/ESTRO category. Age, tumor size, and biology remain independent prognosticators for recurrence with IOERT APBI (Adapted from Leonardi et al. [88, 95])

acknowledge that tissues at the periphery of these smaller applicators might have been inadequately irradiated.

The second-largest nonrandomized study of IOERT APBI is of 226 women from the University of Verona, which began in 2006 [55]. Patient selection criteria were restricted to only very low-risk patients. The initial patients were women ≥50 years with biopsy-proven IDC, who had low-grade G1 and G2 tumors ≤ 2 cm, and were N0, ER+, and PgR+. When ESTRO/ASTRO released their guidelines for APBI-suitable and good patients, they expanded inclusion criteria to be consistent with these recommendations. All patients still had quandrantectomy and axillary node management, including sentinel node evaluation and completion axillary node dissection for positive sentinel nodes, but the radiation technique was modified from the ELIOT approach.

The prescribed dose was reduced by about 10 %, so the maximum dose to the gland was 21 Gy with the energy selected to assure that the entire gland was covered to at least the 80 % dose line. Using the linear-quadratic model, both dose regimens gave an adequate dose for tumor control when compared to 6 weeks of EBRT. Verona used a 10 mm thick acrylic disk to protect the CW, rather

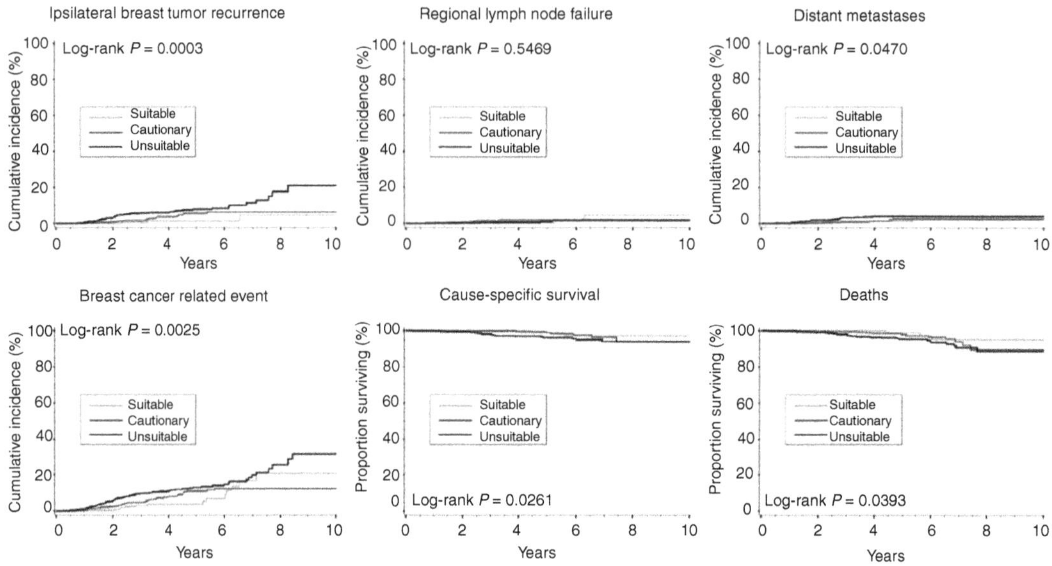

Fig. 28.14 Cumulative incidence of breast-related events and survival for the ELIOT out-trial patients categorized by the ASTRO guidelines for APBI [95]. The 5-year local recurrence rate for ASTRO "suitable" patients was 1.5 %, vs. 4.4 % and 8.8 % for ASTRO "cautionary" and ASTRO "unsuitable" patients, respectively. For patients with Luminal A biology, the 5-year recurrence rate is about 2 % irrespective of the ASTRO category

than the metallic plates used with ELIOT. The use of the acrylic disk eliminated any dose uncertainty from backscatter caused by metallic disks. They could use acrylic in their study because they treated to the 80 % dose line, so most patients (95.5 %) were able to be treated with electron energies of 6 MeV or less. At these energies the transmitted dose is, at most, only 15 % of the maximum dose, or 3.2 Gy, which is of no consequence clinically.

Of the 50 patients (22.1 %) that had a positive SNB and underwent a CALND, 38 had one positive lymph node, and 12 had two, with all receiving IOERT. After final pathology, 16 patients (7.1 %) were determined to have positive margins and underwent re-excision. An additional 17 patients (7.5 %) had close margins (<2 mm clearance), but received no further treatment. No additional radiation was given to either patients with positive nodes or positive margins. With a mean FU of 46 months, only one recurrence in a quadrant outside the index quadrant was observed. The treatment toxicity was very low, with only 15 patients experiencing various Grade 1 complications (on the SOMA-Lent scale) and 1 patient experiencing Grade 3 complications.

At the 2012 ASCO San Francisco Meeting [97] and at the SABCS Meeting [98], the results were updated. With a mean follow-up now of 51 months (33–68 months), they reported four recurrences (Table 28.10), with a median time to recurrence of 41 months. One recurrence was a 2.8 cm tumor, and other recurrences were high grade (Grade 3), with one triple-negative breast cancer. All recurrences were salvaged with mastectomy. All patients in the study are alive and free of disease. The key technical factors of the Verona treatment are shown in Table 28.11. In contrast to the 1,822 out-trial ELIOT study, the applicator size chosen was approximately 2 cm greater radially than the largest tumor dimension. The median applicator size used was 6 cm, assuring good coverage to the tumor bed, with 87 % of the field sizes ≥5 cm and 31 % >6 cm.

Publications and presentations at scientific meetings from other Italian centers that have used IOERT APBI on more than 1,000 patients combined also show excellent short-term oncologic, toxicity, and cosmetic results, though the follow-up is still early. These Italian centers have mostly followed the ELIOT approach, but often use a lower-risk patient profile similar to that of

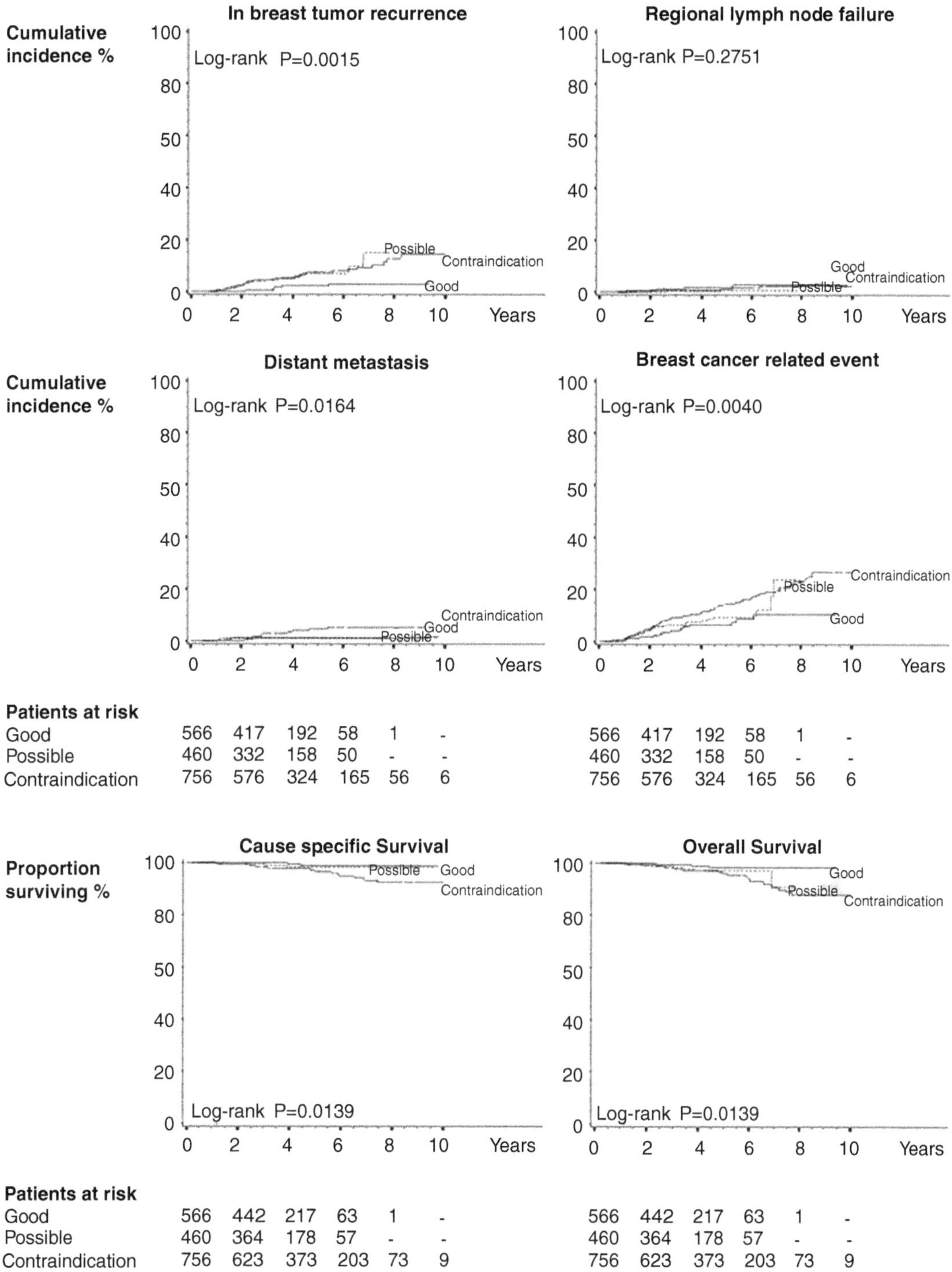

Fig. 28.15 Cumulative incidence of breast-related events and survival for the ELIOT out-trial patients categorized by the GEC-ESTRO guidelines for APBI [88]). The 5-year local recurrence rate for GEC-ESTRO "good" patients was 1.9 %, vs. 7.1 % and 7.8 % for GEC-ESTRO "possible" and GEC-ESTRO "unsuitable" patients, respectively. For patients with Luminal A biology, the 5-year recurrence rate is about 2.5 % irrespective of the GEC-ESTRO category

Table 28.10 U. of Verona recurrences after APBI compared to ASTRO/ESTRO low-risk women

Factor	Patient 1	Patient 2	Patient 3	Patient 4	ASTRO Suitable	ESTRO Good
Age	55	62	68	75	≥ 60	≥ 50
Histology	IDC	IDC	IDC	IDC	IDC[(2)]	IDC[(2)]
Tumor Size	2.0 cm	2.8 cm	1.5 cm	1.8 cm	≤ 2.0 cm	≤ 3.0 cm
Grade	G2	G2	G3	G3	Any	Any
Nodal Status	pN0	pN0	pN0	pN0	pN0	pN0
ER Status	Positive	Positive	Positive	Negative	Positive	Any
PR Status	Positive	Positive	Positive	Negative	Positive	Any
Her 2- Status	Negative	Unknown	Negative	Unknown	NS	NS
LVI Status	Absent	Absent	Absent	Present	Not allowed	Not allowed
Margin Status	Negative	Negative	Negative	Negative	Negative	Negative
Adjuvant HT/CT	HT	HT	HT	None[(1)]		
Time to relapse	28 months	36 months	40 months	60 months		
Salvage	Mastectomy	Mastectomy	Mastectomy	Mastectomy		

[a]No CT was given due to patient's age. Note that three of four failures did not meet ASTRO-suitable guidelines for APBI, while all but the triple negative met the ESTRO-good guidelines for APBI. If G3 and tumors > 2.0 cm are excluded, there is only one recurrence in the U, of Verona cohort with a mean FU of 51 months

[b]Other low-risk histologies also permitted

Table 28.11 Technical factors in the U. of Verona APBI Study

Tumor size	5 mm (*n*=0)	5–10 cm (*n*=38)	10–20 cm (*n*=159)	20–30 cm (*n*=49)
Field size used (cm)				
4.0	–	–	12	–
4.5	–	4	18	–
5.0	–	7	35	13
5.5	–	–	25	6
6.0	–	4	49	21
>6.0	–	3	20	9
Energy used (80 % depth in mm)				
4 MeV (11 mm)	–	18	48	–
6 MeV (20 mm)	–	–	111	39
9 MeV (29 mm)	–	–	–	10
12 MeV (39 mm)	–	–	–	–

As presented at the ASCO San Francisco Breast Meeting, September 2012 (Dall'Oglio 97]). Note that applicator size covers the tumor with sufficient margins to ensure proper radiation coverage

Verona. All of these centers performed a quandrantectomy to remove the tumor, so the question remains whether lesser surgeries, such as a standard lumpectomy, can lead to similar outcomes when combined with IOERT APBI.

IOERT APBI published studies, using lesser surgeries, come from Montpellier [99], Brussels [100], Nagoya [101], and Chapel Hill [102].

Lemanski et al. [99] reports on 53 patients over the age of 65 with T1N0M0 disease treated using the ELIOT dose prescription of 21 Gy to the 90 % isodose. The study does not indicate the use of protective disk, but doctors used in vivo dosimetry to measure the delivered dose, to confirm that it was within 10 % of the planned dose. The researchers focused on elderly women since, in their experience, compliance with 6 weeks of BCT in this age group is poor and gets worse with increasing age. Nodal assessment was done intraoperatively through SNB, and frozen section analysis was used to reduce positive margins. The median tumor size was 1.0 cm, 86 % had Grade 1 or 2 tumor, and all patients were ER+. Eleven patients received IORT, but were excluded from the analysis, since final pathology showed that they did not strictly meet the inclusion criteria: six had positive nodes, two had lobular carcinoma, one had bifocality, and two patients had margins <2 mm. The patients with close margins underwent a completion mastectomy. The rest were followed, but were not part of the protocol analysis. In this 11 patient subgroup, there were no local, regional, or distant relapses observed. In the remaining 42 patients, with a median follow-up of 30 months (range 12–49 months), 2 patients recurred: a true recurrence at 20 months and an elsewhere recurrence at 24 months. These patients had salvage mastectomies and are still alive. They did not observe any Grade 3 side effects, and there were only four cases of Grade 2 subcutaneous fibrosis. Cosmetic outcomes were judged to be good to excellent. Montpellier updated their results at the 2011 San Antonio Breast Conference [103] with a longer follow-up of 54 months, with still only two recurrences reported. All patients were alive, and the 4-year disease-free survival was 97 %. Cosmesis continued to be good to excellent. A further Montpellier update [104] with a median follow-up of 72 months found a total of four patients (9.5 %) had recurred. All patients that recurred underwent salvage mastectomy and are still alive. While this unexpectedly high local recurrence rate for such a low-risk population could just be the result of too few patients in the study, the radiation technique used for APBI by Montpellier has been criticized. Dall'Oglio [105] points out that the radiation approach used by Montpellier may not have adequately irradiated the tissues at risk to the proper depth and that too small a field size might have been used.

The Institut Jules Bordet in Belgium has treated more than 200 women with single-fraction IOERT (Philippson C, Radiation oncologist, Institut Jules Bordet, 2012, private communication). All prospective patients received preoperative MRI and SNB and frozen margin assessment during surgery. Only IDC patients with T1 tumors were eligible; patients with LVI and EIC were not. Of the first 113 patients entered into the study, 30 were excluded after preoperative MRI or during surgery due to involved lymph nodes or tumor size. The results for the first 83 patients who received IOERT were presented at the French Radiotherapy Meeting in March 2011 [100]. Patients received 21 Gy prescribed to the 90 % isodose using a protective metallic CW shield (7 mm of aluminum and lead). If the patient had a positive sentinel node or lobular carcinoma, she received a 9 Gy IOERT boost followed by 5 weeks of WBI instead of 21 Gy APBI. The early cosmetic results were good or excellent in 87.5 % of the patients. Only two of the IOERT APBI patients had positive margins on final pathology. Those patients had re-excision and no further treatment.

Sawaki et al. [101] has treated 32 patients, 88 % with IDC, with IOERT APBI at Nagoya. Though the numbers are small, and the study was primarily designed to assess the toxicity of the procedure, it is the first report of single-fraction IOERT in the Asian population, which has smaller, denser breasts than those of other ethnic groups. It is also technically interesting, as the breast shield they use sandwiches a copper metallic plate between acrylic disks, resulting in virtually no transmission or backscatter. Patients had a median age of 65 years (range 55–80), and while the maximum allowed tumor size was 2.5 cm, 66 % were 1 cm or smaller, and only one tumor was more than 2 cm. Only 12 % of the patients had Grade 3 disease, and 91 % of the patients were ER and/or PgR positive. Patients were N0 as assessed by SNB and had free margins of at least 10 mm, assessed intraoperatively. A single dose of 21 Gy was delivered to the 90 % depth, following the ELIOT prescription, with an acrylic resin-copper disk used to protect the chest wall. Four patients were excluded from the analysis because of positive margins on final pathology. With a median follow-up of 26 months (range 11–39.5 months), there have been no recurrences. No Grade 3 or greater toxicities were reported, and only seven Grade 2 toxicities were seen.

The University of North Carolina at Chapel Hill ("UNC") has used an IOERT dose of only 15 Gy to treat the tumor in situ, prior to surgical removal, with a 20 mm circumferential radiation margin with the 90 % isodose line covering a depth 10 mm posterior to the tumor [102, 106, 107]. The protocol was open to patients aged older than 55 with ultrasonographically defined tumors $\leq$ 3 cm and invasive ductal carcinoma confirmed by core biopsy. Preoperative ultrasound was performed at the time of needle localization and radiocolloid injection. IOERT treatment planning was performed prior to surgery using ultrasound for tumor definition and selecting the applicator size and electron energy to optimize dose distribution. In the operating room, the surgeon retracted the skin over the tumor, positioned the applicator, and 15 Gy of IOERT was delivered. No chest wall shield was employed, in order to manipulate the tumor as little as possible prior to irradiation. The dose to the chest wall was limited to less than 10 Gy. Patients with tumors close to the chest wall did not receive IOERT. Once the radiation phase of the procedure was complete, segmental resection (partial mastectomy) was performed in the standard fashion. Between March 2003 and July 2007, a total of 71 patients received IOERT – 53 patients as a single-dose treatment; 11 as a postoperative boost (tumor larger than 3 cm, EIC component, lobular carcinoma, positive nodes, patient choice); and 7 went on to mastectomy based on the final histological results (positive margins, multicentricity, patient choice). There were no Grade 3 or 4 toxicities, and only 6 % (4/71) experienced any Grade 1 or 2 toxicity.

With a median follow-up of 3.1 years, 83 % patients who received IOERT alone had good or excellent cosmesis, and 95 % were totally satisfied or would choose IOERT again [107]. Unfortunately, the recurrence rate with this approach was higher than expected, with four recurrences in the patients who received IOERT alone, and none in the IOERT patients who also received WBI [107]. Actuarial local control was 92 %. Three of the recurrences were true/marginal recurrences, and one was an elsewhere failure. Two of the recurrences were patients with triple-negative disease. The median time to recurrence was 2.7 years. The true recurrences were salvaged with BCT, and the elsewhere recurrence was salvaged with mastectomy, resulting in an actuarial mastectomy-free survival of 98 % (52/53). No breast cancer deaths have been observed, though one patient died from other causes. Due to the unexpectedly high ipsilateral breast cancer recurrence rate (8 % at 3 years), the study was discontinued.

Whether in situ IOERT would have developed further had the recurrence rate been more acceptable cannot be known. Better patient selection, for example, only allowing smaller tumors (T1) and excluding high-risk triple-negative patients, could have improved the study's outcome. However, technically, there are some problems with the study's in situ technique, which Kimple points out [107]. The dose of 15 Gy used was probably too low. Using the linear-quadratic model and an α/β of 4, Kimple calculates that 15 Gy of IOERT is comparable to the 2 Gy × 25 fractions used in conventional BCT. However, this overlooks the additional EBRT boost dose of 10–16 Gy that has been used by all other IOERT investigators in establishing 21 Gy as the BED equivalent IOERT dose.

More importantly, all other IOERT studies have 21 Gy delivered to the CW, emulating the dose coverage of EBRT to the index quadrant. In the UNC study, the dose to the chest wall was limited to 10 Gy or less, since they did not use a CW protector. Thus, dose to the target tissues beneath the tumor was probably suboptimal. Finally, while they did use an applicator 2 cm larger than the tumor, citing the data of Holland, radiation coverage to the prescribed dose level does not fully extend to the applicator walls, so perhaps they under-radiated the peripheral tissues at risk. In the usual IOERT approach, after removing the tumor and temporarily re-approximating the breast parenchyma, an applicator with a circumferential margin 2 cm larger than the excised tumor will irradiate a larger volume of tissue than in the in situ approach.

From all of the studies to date, there appears to be a group of women for whom IOERT APBI could be an appropriate procedure. ASTRO-suitable patients, perhaps with G3 tumors excluded, appear to have very low recurrence rates when treated with IOERT APBI. However, many questions about the technical aspects and patient selection remain open, and further studies will be required to resolve these issues.

Future Applications

IOERT Boost Combined with Hypofractionated EBRT

Just as EBRT treatment in BCT is trending towards standardizing to 3 weeks of treatment for eligible women (based on the excellent long-term results of Whelan et al. [16] and the Start B Trial [6]), IOERT boost is also being investigated with this accelerated EBRT schedule. Between June 2004 and March 2007, 211 women were treated at the EIO with BCS, and an IOERT boost of 12 Gy delivered to the tumor bed at the time of surgery

[108]. Adjuvant EBRT consisted of 13 daily fractions of 2.85 Gy to the whole breast, to a total dose of 37 Gy. The protocol required patients to start EBRT within 4 weeks of surgery. The median interval between surgery and the start of EBRT was 22 days (range 15–80 days); 88.3 % of the patients started their EBRT within 4 weeks, 10.6 % within 6 weeks, and 1 % after 6 weeks. EBRT did not start within the required 4 weeks, mainly due to delay in wound healing. Acute toxicity was evaluated at the end of the accelerated EBRT and after 1 month of follow-up. Late toxicity was recorded at 6 and 12 months of follow-up. Acute skin reactions of 7 % Grade 3 and 28.6 % Grade 2 were observed. As for late toxicity, 1 patient had Grade 4 and 1 patient Grade 3 toxicity, while 98.2 % of the patients had Grade 2 toxicity or less.

A multi-institutional, international trial of IOERT boost, combined with 3 weeks of EBRT, is currently being conducted by the ISIORT under the direction of the University of Salzburg for women over the age of 35 years with histologically confirmed invasive breast cancer (ClinicalTrials.gov Identifier: NCT01343459).

The trial is called HIOB for **H**ypofractionated Whole-Breast Irradiation preceded by Intra**O**perative Radiotherapy with Electrons as anticipated **B**oost Treatment. The HIOB schedule consists of an IOERT boost of 11.1 Gy to Dmax (10 Gy to the 90 % dose level), followed by WBI of 15 fractions × 2.7 Gy/fraction in 3 weeks. Three separate age cohorts are stratified: women ≥ 50 years, women ≥ 40 years but <50 years, and women ≥ 35 years but <40 years. The primary end point is proof of superiority in terms of in-breast tumor control rates, by benchmarking with the best published results that use "gold standard" RT. Secondary end points are acute and late toxicity, cosmetic results, DFS, and OS. Exclusion criteria are tumor stage T3 or T4, nodal status > N1, regional irradiation of lymphatics required, neoadjuvant chemotherapy required, pure DCIS, surgical margins <2 mm, re-excision after IOERT, distant metastases, multicentricity, breast size ≥ 1,800 ml, and previous radiotherapy to the involved breast. Patients that require re-excision or have breasts too large to participate are eligible for IOERT boost and 5 weeks of WBI. Accrual to HIOB began in January of 2011, and, as of December 2012, 322 women have been treated, with an ultimate accrual goal of 1,000.

IOERT Boost After Neoadjuvant Chemotherapy

Mastectomy is the most frequent surgical approach for locally advanced breast cancer, due to the high probability of micrometastases remaining in the intact breast. Recently, studies on neoadjuvant chemotherapy have shown that it can shrink larger tumors and reduce the probability of early metastatic spread. The University of Salzburg initiated a Phase II trial [109] to examine whether an IOERT boost after neoadjuvant chemotherapy could improve ipsilateral breast recurrence in locally advanced patients, as it has done in early breast cancer patients. In their study, between 2002 and 2007, 83 patients with Stage II and III breast cancer were entered. The median age was 48 years (range 24–74 years), 59 % were premenopausal, and 49 % had G3 tumors. The median primary tumor size was 3.4 cm (range 1.6–8.6 cm), and the axilla was positive in 60 % of the patients. All patients received 6 cycles of neoadjuvant chemotherapy, followed by surgical resection of the residual tumor with CALND. Pathological complete response was obtained in 17 (21 %) patients, and partial response in 60 (76 %) patients. Six patients also received adjuvant chemotherapy postsurgery, and 52 patients (62 %) received adjuvant hormonal therapy. IOERT was delivered at a dose of 10 Gy to Dmax, mostly with 6 cm diameter applicators and energies of 6 MeV. Following breast healing, with a median time of 6 weeks (range 4–24 weeks), EBRT of 54 Gy was delivered in daily fractions of 1.8 Gy.

With a median follow-up of 59 months, only 2 patients experienced a breast recurrence, 2 patients had regional recurrences in the axilla, and 11 patients had distant metastases. The LC, local-regional control (LRC), DFS, OS, and freedom from metastases (FFM) at 59 months were 98.5, 94.9, 80.7, 86.4, and 86.8 %, respectively. The LC in this Phase II study compares favorably with 5-year rates in other studies of BCT for LABC.

This has prompted consideration of starting a prospective randomized trial for LABC comparing IOERT boost to EBRT boost after neoadjuvant chemotherapy. The trial is expected to begin in 2014.

IOERT for Nipple-Sparing Mastectomy (NSM)

The EIO reports on 801 patients with 16 Gy of IOERT to preserve the nipple-areola complex (NAC) during NSM [110]. An additional 200 patients were treated with EBRT to the NAC postsurgically due to poor vascularization of the NAC, which required several hours of observation. Tumor histology was invasive carcinoma in 819 (82 %) of the patients and intraductal carcinoma in 182 (18 %) patients. None of the mastectomies were prophylactic. The technique requires that the tissue underlying the NAC be biopsied during the surgery. If the NAC is negative, the patient was given 16 Gy of IOERT through the NAC. The EBRT patients received the same 16 Gy to the NAC, delayed by a few days. With a median follow-up of 20 months (range 1–69 months), 14 patients (1.4 %) had local-regional recurrences, and 36 patients (3.6 %) had distant recurrences. Four patients died. Despite the frozen section analysis of the NAC during surgery, final pathology revealed the presence of disease in 86 (8.6 %) of the patients, 61 of whom had in situ disease. The NAC was preserved in 79 of these patients, none of whom developed recurrences.

The functional and aesthetic appearance of the breast was judged to be good in 78 % of the patients. Partial or global return of NAC sensitivity was present in about 20 % of patients at the time of the analysis. The rate of necrosis or partial necrosis of the NAC was 9, and 5 % of the patients subsequently had the NAC removed. The rate of NAC necrosis and recurrence is comparable to that reported in NSM without IOERT, typically 90–95 % tumor control with NAC necrosis on the order of 8–15 % [111]. However, reported series without IOERT usually include a substantial number of prophylactic mastectomies, and usually NSM is not attempted if the disease is closer than 2 cm from the edge of the areola. In the EIO series, there were no prophylactic mastectomies, and 160 patients had tumor reaching the retro areola area close to the areola dermis. With a follow-up of 23 months, none of these patients had recurred. These results are encouraging, but it is still unclear whether IOERT has a major role to play in NSM as compared to surgery alone. A prospective randomized trial for NSM, with and without IOERT, could decide the question.

IOERT as Salvage Therapy After BCT Recurrence

After BCT failure, the usual salvage for breast recurrence is a completion mastectomy. However, if the recurrence is in a different quadrant than the original tumor, is it possible to use IORT APBI as salvage and still preserve the breast? This is a rational concept, but it may be difficult to obtain evidence of its efficacy. There have been several anecdotal references in IORT and IOERT APBI studies of patients who fail and are salvaged with IOERT boost or IOERT or IORT APBI. There have been no subsequent reports on these salvaged patients, so it is not possible to draw a conclusion as to whether this really is an effective salvage option. Since the number of such patients at any one institution is likely to be small, the formation of an IORT registry may enable information on IORT salvage to be gathered for evaluation.

IOERT in DCIS

Only a handful of patients have been treated with IORT or IOERT for DCIS. Most IORT protocols restrict the amount of DCIS in IORT patients and exclude patients who have more than a small DCIS component. Both ASTRO and ESTRO guidelines for APBI exclude DCIS for their low-risk patient categories. ESTRO does allow DCIS for their intermediate risk patient group who are classified as possible candidates for APBI, while ASTRO classifies DCIS histology as unsuitable for APBI. It is possible that DCIS patients with favorable biology might be candidates for IORT, but, until there are more long-term results on the use of IORT in invasive cancer, it is unlikely there will be any serious effort to study IORT in this higher-risk patient cohort.

IOERT Combined with Oncoplastic Reconstruction

While BCT preserves the woman's breast, approximately 30 % of those receiving BCT are unhappy with the breast appearance upon completion of treatment [112]. This has led to the rise in the use of oncoplasty at the time of the initial breast surgery. Oncoplastic surgery incorporates plastic surgery techniques into the removal of breast cancer, focusing on tumor excision with the best possible cosmetic result.

Oncoplasty at the time of surgery has the potential advantage of improving cosmesis over standard operative approaches. At the same time, especially when the procedure leads to a reduction of breast size, as is often the case, oncoplasty results in a smaller breast radiation volume, which should provide a more homogeneous distribution of the whole breast radiation, and thus a lower risk of radiation toxicity. However, with conventional BCT, oncoplasty makes targeting the boost volume more uncertain, even when the surgeon places clips to assist with postoperative radiation field planning. The boost volume after oncoplasty appears much larger than boost volumes without oncoplasty, requiring the radiation oncologist to design much larger boost radiation fields than would otherwise be done for patients without oncoplasty.

The larger the boost volume is, the higher the risk of radiation toxicity. IOERT combined with oncoplasty solves the issue of the larger postoperative boost volume, since IOERT is given to the target volume at the time of surgery and before the oncoplasty, with no external beam boost required. If the IOERT is given as APBI, no further radiation treatment at all is required. Furthermore, in preparing the target volume for IOERT, much of what one would normally do in an oncoplastic procedure has already been accomplished, so only an additional 5–10 min is typically needed to complete the oncoplasty after the IOERT has been delivered. To date, there have only been a few feasibility reports of surgeons combining oncoplasty and IOERT [113, 114]. However, as more breast surgeons begin to offer oncoplasty to their patients, and as IOERT becomes more widely available, shortening the treatment time using IOERT while enhancing the breast appearance through oncoplasty is likely to become common.

Summary and Conclusions

IORT boost has mature and compelling clinical results, whether delivered with IOERT or 50 kV X-rays. While the electron data for boost is more mature (10-year data) and robust (10,000 patients) than the 50 kV data (5-year data and 750 patients), both would seem to provide advantages over EBRT boost. The comparison of IOERT boost by age groups with the EORTC boost data is compelling. If the current HIOB trial proves superiority, IOERT boost could become the treatment of choice for the majority of early-stage breast cancer patients.

IORT APBI is on less firm ground. A thorough analysis of the data suggests that it is unlikely that the Intrabeam or Xoft systems will find a major role in APBI. The volume of tissue irradiated and the homogeneity of the radiation generated with these 50 kV devices is simply inadequate for the majority of APBI-suitable patients. The studies to date have serious flaws, making it very difficult to assess what subset of women, if any, might be suitable candidates for APBI. It is possible that further studies might find a group of women for whom APBI with 50 kV is an acceptable alternative to other techniques, but with the current information available, clinicians should use these devices, outside of well-designed clinical trials, with caution.

On the other hand, IOERT APBI *appears* to have a subset of low-risk women for whom IOERT will be effective (e.g., ASTRO suitable for APBI, perhaps with G3 excluded), but many open questions still remain.

- Can that low-risk cohort be expanded to younger women or to larger tumors if the biology is favorable?
- Will the lesser surgeries used outside of Italy produce equivalent results to quandrantectomy?

- Is 21 Gy to the 90 % dose level the optimal dose, or can a lower dose be used?
- What is the best way to handle positive margins on final pathology?
  - Ignore them?
  - Re-excise them?
  - Require these patients undergo a mastectomy?
- What is the best way to handle positive nodes? (Positive nodes are not allowed in other post-op APBI trials.) With IOERT, are one to two positive nodes after SNB and CALND an important factor in ipsilateral recurrence, since the radiation treatment to the tissue at risk for local recurrence has already been delivered?
- What is the optimal screening approach for IORT APBI? Should MRI be used in all patients to assure unicentric disease?
- Can IOERT APBI be safely extended to DCIS and/or some lobular Cancer?
- Can IOERT be used a salvage therapy for recurrences outside the index quadrant?
- Will IOERT APBI improve results when used in NSM?
- Will IOERT boost prove valuable in LABC?

IORT is a modality that is extremely promising and could have an expanding and important role in breast cancer management both now and in the future. We are just at the beginning of learning how best to use this technique; it will take many more years of study and many thousands of patients willing to participate in those studies to bring its potential to fruition.

Acknowledgement We would like to thank Amy Evans and Bryce Dehring for their help in preparing the figures that appear in this chapter.

References

1. Veronesi U, Cascinelli N, Mariani L, Greco M, Saccozzi R, Luini A, et al. Twenty-year follow-up of a randomized study comparing breast-conserving surgery with radical mastectomy for early breast cancer. N Engl J Med. 2002;347(16):1227–32.
2. van Dongen JA, Voogd AC, Fentiman IS, Legrand C, Sylvester RJ, Tong D, et al. Long-term results of a randomized trial comparing breast-conserving therapy with mastectomy: European Organization for Research and Treatment of Cancer 10801 trial. J Natl Cancer Inst. 2000;92(14):1143–50.
3. Arriagada R, Lê MG, Guinebretière JM, Dunant A, Rochard F, Tursz T. Late local recurrences in a randomized trial comparing conservative treatment with total mastectomy in early breast cancer patients. Ann Oncol. 2003;14(11):1617–22.
4. Fisher B, Anderson S, Redmond CK, Wolmark N, Wickerham DL, Cronin WM. Reanalysis and results after 12 years of follow-up in a randomized clinical trial comparing total mastectomy with lumpectomy with or without irradiation in the treatment of breast cancer. N Engl J Med. 1995;333(22):1456–61.
5. Bartelink H, Horiot JC, Poortmans PM, Struikmans H, Van den Bogaert W, Fourquet A, et al. Impact of a higher radiation dose on local control and survival in breast-conserving therapy of early breast cancer: 10-year results of the randomized boost versus no boost EORTC 22881-10882 trial. J Clin Oncol. 2007;25(22):3259–65.
6. START Trialists' Group, Bentzen SM, Agrawal RK, Aird EG, Barrett JM, Barrett-Lee PJ, Bentzen SM, et al. The UK Standardization of Breast Radiotherapy (START) Trial B of radiotherapy hypofractionation for treatment of early breast cancer: a randomized trial. Lancet. 2008;371(9618):1098–107.
7. Liljegren G, Holmberg L, Bergh J, Lindgren A, Tabár L, Nordgren H, et al. Ten year results after sector resection with or without postoperative radiation therapy for stage I breast cancer: a randomized trial. J Clin Oncol. 1999;17(8):2326–33.
8. Clark RM, Whelan T, Levine M, Roberts R, Willan A, McCulloch P, et al. Randomized clinical trial of breast irradiation following lumpectomy and axillary dissection for node-negative breast cancer: an update. Ontario Clinical Oncology Group J Natl Cancer Inst. 1996;88(22):1659–64.
9. Veronesi U, Marubini E, Mariani L, Galimberti V, Luini A, Veronesi P, et al. Radiotherapy after breast-conserving surgery in small breast carcinoma: long-term results of a randomized trial. Ann Oncol. 2001; 12(7):997–1003.
10. Hwang ES, Lichtensztain DY, Gomez SL, et al. Survival after lumpectomy and mastectomy for early stage invasive breast cancer: the effect of age and hormone receptor status. Cancer. 2013;119(7): 1402–11.
11. Clarke M, Collins R, Darby S, Davies C, Elphinstone P, Evans E. Early Breast Cancer Trialists' Collaborative Group (EBCTCG), et al. Effects of radiotherapy and of differences in the extent of surgery for early breast cancer on local recurrence and 15-year survival: an overview of the randomized trials. Lancet. 2005;366(9503):2087–106.
12. Early Breast Cancer Trialists' Collaborative Group (EBCTCG). Effects of chemotherapy and hormonal therapy for early breast cancer on recurrence and 15-year survival: an overview of the randomised trials. Lancet. 2005;365(9472):1687–717.

13. Athas WF, Adams-Cameron M, Hunt WC, Amir-Fazli A, Key CR. Travel distance to radiation therapy and receipt of radiotherapy following breast-conserving surgery. J Natl Cancer Inst. 2000;92:269–71.
14. Ballard-Barbash R, Potosky AL, Harlan LC, Nayfield SG, Kessler LG. Factors associated with surgical and radiation therapy for early stage breast cancer in older women. J Natl Cancer Inst. 1996;88(11):716–26.
15. Mandelblatt JS, Hadley J, Kerner JF, Schulman KA, Gold K, Dunmore-Griffith J, et al. Patterns of breast carcinoma treatment in older women: patient preference and clinical and physical influences. Cancer. 2000;89:561–73.
16. Whelan T, Pignol JP, Julian J, Levine MN, MacKenzie R, Parpia S, et al. Long-term results of a randomized trial of accelerated hypofractionated whole breast irradiation following breast conserving surgery in women with node negative breast cancer. Breast Cancer. 2007;106 Suppl 1:S6.
17. Polgár C, Sulyok Z, Fodor J, Orosz Z, Major T, Takácsi-Nagy Z, et al. Sole brachytherapy of the tumor bed after conservative surgery for T1 breast cancer: five-year results of a phase I-II study and initial findings of a randomized phase III trial. J Surg Oncol. 2002;80(3):121–8. discussion 129.
18. King TA, Bolton JS, Kuske RR, Fuhrman GM, Scroggins TG, Jiang XZ. Long-term results of wide field brachytherapy as the sole method of radiation therapy after segmental mastectomy for t(is,1,2) breast cancer. Am J Surg. 2000;180:299–304.
19. Baglan KL, Martinez AA, Frazier RC, Kini VR, Kestin LL, Chen PY, et al. The use of high-dose-rate brachytherapy alone after lumpectomy in patients with early-stage breast cancer treated with breast conserving therapy. Int J Radiat Oncol Biol Phys. 2001;50(4):1003–11.
20. Mele E, Jaffray D, Vicini FA. The use of high-dose-rate brachytherapy alone after lumpectomy in patients with early-stage breast cancer treated with breast-conserving therapy. Int J Radiat Oncol Biol Phys. 2001;50(4):1003–11.
21. Wazer DE, Berle L, Graham R, Chung M, Rothschild J, Graves T, et al. Preliminary results of a phase I/II study of HDR brachytherapy alone for T1/T2 breast cancer. Int J Radiat Oncol Biol Phys. 2002;53(4):889–97.
22. Polgár C, Major T, Fodor J, Sulyok Z, Somogyi A, Lövey K, et al. Accelerated partial-breast irradiation using high-dose-rate interstitial brachytherapy: 12-year update of a prospective clinical study. Radiother Oncol. 2010;94(3):274–9.
23. Polgár C, Fodor J, Major T, Németh G, Lövey K, Orosz Z, Sulyok Z, et al. Breast-conserving treatment with partial or whole breast irradiation for low-risk invasive breast carcinoma–5-year results of a randomized trial. Int J Radiat Oncol Biol Phys. 2007;69(3):694–702.
24. Strnad V, Polgar C, On behalf of the European Brachytherapy Breast Cancer GEC-ESTRO Working Group. GEC-ESTRO APBI trial: interstitial brachytherapy alone versus external beam radiation therapy after breast conserving surgery for low risk invasive carcinoma and low risk duct carcinoma in-situ (DCIS) of the female breast, 2006. Available from: http://www.apbi.uni-erlangen.de/outline/outline.html.
25. Holland R, Veling SHJ, Mravunac M, Hendriks JHCL. Histologic multifocality of tis, T1–2 breast carcinomas implications for clinical trials of breast-conserving surgery. Cancer. 1985;56(5):979–90.
26. Faverly DR, Hendricks JH, Holland R. Breast carcinomas of limited extent: frequency, radiologic-pathologic characteristics, and surgical margin requirements. Cancer. 2001;91(4):647–59.
27. Smith GL, Xu Y, Buchholz TA, Giordano SH, Jiang J, Shih YC, et al. Association between treatment with brachytherapy vs. whole-breast irradiation and subsequent mastectomy, complications, and survival among older women with invasive breast cancer. JAMA. 2012;307:1827–37.
28. Jagsi R, Ben-David MA, Moran JM, Marsh RB, Griffith KA, Hayman JA, et al. Unacceptable cosmesis in a protocol investigating intensity-modulated radiotherapy with active breathing control for accelerated partial-breast irradiation. Int J Radiat Oncol Biol Phys. 2010;76:71–8.
29. Hepel JT, Tokita M, MacAusland SG, Evans SB, Hiatt JR, Price LL, et al. Toxicity of three-dimensional conformal radiotherapy for accelerated partial breast irradiation. Int J Radiat Oncol Biol Phys. 2009;75:1290–6.
30. Vicini FA, Chen P, Wallace M, Mitchell C, Hasan Y, Grills I, et al. Interim cosmetic results and toxicity using 3D conformal external beam radiotherapy to deliver accelerated partial breast irradiation in patients with early-stage breast cancer treated with breast conserving therapy. Int J Radiat Oncol Biol Phys. 2007;69(4):1247–53.
31. NSABP B-39, RTOG 0413. A randomized phase III study of conventional whole breast irradiation versus partial breast irradiation for women with stage 0, I, or II breast cancer. Clin Adv Hematol Oncol. 2006;4:719–21.
32. Ontario Clinical Oncology Group (OCOG), Canadian Institutes of Health Research (CIHR), Canadian Breast Cancer Research Alliance. RAPID: Randomized Trial of Accelerated Partial Breast Irradiation, 2008. Available from: http://clinicaltrials.gov/ct2/show/NCT00282035.
33. Yarnold J, Coles C. On behalf of the IMPORT LOW Trial Management Group: Intensity Modulated and Partial Organ Radiotherapy. Randomised trial testing intensity modulated and partial organ radiotherapy following breast conservation surgery for early breast cancer. Trial Protocol, Version 4. Sutton: The Institute of Cancer Research, Royal Cancer Hospital; 2008. pp. 1–74.
34. Smith BD, Arthur DW, Buchholz TA, Haffty BG, Hahn CA, Hardenbergh PH, et al. Accelerated partial breast irradiation consensus statement from the American Society for Radiation Oncology (ASTRO). J Am Coll Surg. 2009;209:269–77.
35. Polgár C, Van Limbergen E, Pötter R, Kovács G, Polo A, Lyczek J. GEC-ESTRO breast cancer working

group, et al. Patient selection for accelerated partial-breast irradiation (APBI) after breast-conserving surgery: recommendations of the Groupe Européen de Curiethérapie-European Society for Therapeutic Radiology and Oncology (GEC-ESTRO) breast cancer working group based on clinical evidence (2009). Radiother Oncol. 2010;94:264–73.
36. Machtay M, Lanciano R, Hoffman J, Hanks G. Inaccuracies in using the lumpectomy scar for planning electron boosts in primary breast carcinoma. Int J Radiat Oncol Biol Phys. 1994;30:43–8.
37. Hepel JT, Evans SB, Hiatt JR, Price LL, DiPetrillo T, Wazer DE, et al. Planning the breast boost: comparison of three techniques and evolution of tumor bed during treatment. Int J Radiat Oncol Biol Phys. 2009;74(2):458–63.
38. Tersteeg RJ, Roesink JM, Albregts M, Wárlám-Rodenhuis CC, van Asselen B. Changes in excision cavity volume: prediction of the reduction in absolute volume during breast irradiation. Int J Radiat Oncol Biol Phys. 2009;74(4):1181–5.
39. Kim LH, DeCesare S, Vicini F, Yan D. Effect of lumpectomy cavity volume change on the clinical target volume for accelerated partial breast irradiation: a deformable registration study. Int J Radiat Oncol Biol Phys. 2010;78(4):1121–6.
40. Sacchini V, Beal K, Goldberg J, Montgomery L, Port E, McCormick B. Study of quadrant high-dose intraoperative radiation therapy for early-stage breast cancer. Br J Surg. 2008;95:1105–10.
41. Park CC, Yom SS, Podgorsak MB, Harris E, Price Jr RA, Bevan A. Electronic Brachytherapy Working Group, et al. American Society for Therapeutic Radiology and Oncology (ASTRO) Emerging Technology Committee report on electronic brachytherapy. Int J Radiat Oncol Biol Phys. 2010;76(4):963–72.
42. Joseph DJ, Byddar S, Jackson LR, Corica T, Hastrich DJ, Oliver DJ, et al. Prospective trial of intraoperative radiation treatment for breast cancer. ANZ J Surg. 2004;74:1043–8.
43. Vaidya JS, Baum M, Tobias JS, Morgan S, D'Souza D. The novel technique of delivering targeted radiotherapy (Targit) for early breast cancer. Eur J Surg Oncol. 2002;28(4):447–54.
44. Vaidya JS, Tobias JS, Baum M, Wenz F, Kraus-Tiefenbacher U, D'souza D, et al. TARGeted Intraoperative radiotherapy (TARGIT): an innovative approach to partial-breast irradiation. Semin Radiat Oncol. 2005;15(2):84–91.
45. Holmes DR, Baum M, Joseph D. The TARGIT trial: targeted intraoperative radiation therapy versus conventional postoperative whole-breast radiotherapy after breast-conserving surgery for the management of early-stage invasive breast cancer (a trial update). Am J Surg. 2007;194(4):507–10.
46. Kraus-Tiefenbacher U, Scheda A, Steil V, Hermann B, Kehrer T, Bauer L, et al. Intraoperative radiotherapy (IORT) for breast cancer using the Intrabeam system. Tumori. 2005;91(4):339–45.
47. Ivanov O, Dickler A, Lum BY, Pellicane JV, Francescatti DS. Twelve-month follow-up results of a trial utilizing Axxent electronic brachytherapy to deliver intraoperative radiation therapy for early-stage breast cancer. Ann Surg Oncol. 2011;18(2):453–8.
48. Dickler A, Ivanov O, Francescatti D. Intraoperative radiation therapy in the treatment of early-stage breast cancer utilizing xoft axxent electronic brachytherapy. World J Surg Oncol. 2009;7:24.
49. Sautter-Bihl ML, Sedlmayer F, Budach W, Dunst J, Engenhart-Cabillic R, Fietkau R, et al. Intraoperative radiotherapy as accelerated partial breast irradiation for early breast cancer : beware of one-stop shops? Strahlenther Onkol. 2010;186(12):651–7.
50. Vaidya JS, Wenz F, Bulsara M, Joseph DJ, Tobias JS, Keshtgar M, et al. Targeted intraoperative radiotherapy for early breast cancer: TARGIT-A trial-updated analysis of local recurrence and first analysis of survival. Oral presentation, Abstract S4-2, San Antonio Breast Cancer symposium, Dec 2012.
51. Vaidya JS, Wenz F, Bulsara M, Tobias JS, Joseph DJ, et al. Risk-adapted targeted intraoperative radiotherapy versus whole-breast radiotherapy for breast cancer: 5-year results for local control and overall survival from the TARGIT-A randomized trial. Lancet. 2014;383:603–13.
52. Veronesi U, Orecchia R, Luini A, Gatti G, Intra M, Zurrida S, et al. Preliminary report of intraoperative radiotherapy (IORT) in limited-stage breast cancers that are conservatively treated. Eur J Cancer. 2001;37(17):2178–83.
53. Intra M, Leonardi C, Luini A, Veronesi P, Gennari R, Gatti G, et al. Full-dose intraoperative radiotherapy with electrons in breast surgery: broadening the indications. Arch Surg. 2005;140(10):936–9.
54. Intra M, Luini A, Gatti G, Ciocca M, Gentilini OD, Viana AA, et al. Surgical technique of intraoperative radiation therapy with electrons (ELIOT) in breast cancer: a lesson learned by over 1000 procedures. Surgery. 2006;140(3):467–71.
55. Maluta S, Dall'oglio S, Marciai N, Gabbani M, Franchini Z, Pietrarota P, et al. Accelerated partial breast irradiation using only intraoperative electron radiation therapy in early stage breast cancer. Int J Radiat Oncol Biol Phys. 2012;84(2):145–52.
56. Reitsamer R, Sedlmayer F, Kopp M, Kametriser G, Menzel C, Deutschmann H, et al. The Salzburg concept for intraoperative radiotherapy for breast cancer: results and considerations. Int J Cancer. 2006;118:2882–7.
57. Nairz O, Deutschmann H, Kopp M, Wurstbauer K, Kametriser G, Fastner G, et al. A dosimetric comparison of IORT techniques in limited-stage breast cancer. Strahlenther Onkol. 2006;182(6):342–8.
58. Jobsen JJ, van der Palen J, Ong F, Meerwaldt JH. The value of a positive margin for invasive carcinoma in breast-conservative treatment in relation to local recurrence is limited to young women only. Int J Radiat Oncol Biol Phys. 2003;57(3):724–31.
59. Palta JR, Biggs PJ, Hazle JD, Huq MS, Dahl RA, Ochran TG, et al. Intraoperative electron beam radiation therapy:

technique, dosimetry, and dose specification: report of task force 48 of the Radiation Therapy Committee, American Association of Physicists in Medicine. Int J Radiat Oncol Biol Phys. 1995;33(3):725–46.
60. Beddar AS, Biggs PJ, Chang S, Ezzell GA, Faddegon BA, Hensley FW, et al. Intraoperative radiation therapy using mobile electron linear accelerators: report of AAPM Radiation Therapy Committee Task Group No. 72. Med Phys. 2006;33(5):1476–89.
61. Consorti R, Petrucci A, Fortunato F, Soriani A, Marzi S, Iaccarino G, et al. In vivo dosimetry with MOSFETs: dosimetric characterization and first clinical results in intraoperative radiotherapy. Int J Radiat Oncol Biol Phys. 2005;63(3):952–60.
62. Ciocca M, Piazzi V, Lazzari R, Vavassori A, Luini A, Veronesi P, et al. Real-time in vivo dosimetry using micro-MOSFET detectors during intraoperative electron beam radiation therapy in early-stage breast cancer. Radiother Oncol. 2006;78(2):213–6.
63. Agostinelli S, Gusinu M, Cavagnetto F, Garelli S, Zeverino M, Guenzi M, et al. On-line optimization of intraoperative electron beam radiotherapy of the breast. Radiother Oncol. 2012;103(2):188–9.
64. Vaidya JS, Baum M, Tobias JS, Wenz F, Massarut S, Keshtgar M, et al. Long-term results of targeted intraoperative radiotherapy (targit) boost during breast-conserving surgery. Int J Radiat Oncol Biol Phys. 2011;81(4):1091–7.
65. Wenz F, Welzel G, Blank E, Hermann B, Steil V, Sütterlin M, et al. Intraoperative radiotherapy as a boost during breast-conserving surgery using low-kilovoltage x-rays: the first 5 years of experience with a novel device. Int J Radiat Oncol Biol Phys. 2010;77(5):1309–14.
66. Wenz F, Welzel G, Keller A, Blank E, Vorodi F, Herskind C, et al. Early initiation of external beam radiotherapy (EBRT) may increase the risk of long-term toxicity in patients undergoing intraoperative radiotherapy (IORT) as a boost for breast cancer. Breast. 2008;17(6):617–22.
67. Fastner G, Reitsamer R, Kopp M, Menzel C, Gluck S, Merz F, et al. IOERT versus conventional boost during breast conserving therapy: 10 year results of a matched pair analysis. Scottsdale: Presented at the ISIORT meeting; 2010 (in publication).
68. Reitsamer R, Peintinger F, Kopp M, Menzel C, Kogelnik HD, Sedlmayer F. Local recurrence rates in breast cancer patients treated with Intraoperative electron-boost radiotherapy versus postoperative external-beam electron-boost irradiation. A sequential intervention study Strahlenther Onkol. 2004;180(1): 38–44.
69. Fastner G, Sedlmayer F, Merz F, Deutschmann H, Reitsamer R, et al. IORT with electrons as boost strategy during breast conserving therapy in limited stage breast cancer: long term results of an ISIORT pooled analysis. Radiother Oncol. 2013;108(2):279–86.
70. Sedlmayer F, Fastner G, Merz F, Deutschmann H, Reitsamer R, Menzel C, et al. on behalf of the ISIORT Europe. ISIORT pooled analysis on LINAC-based IORT as boost strategy during breast conserving therapy. Presented at the GEC-ESTRO meeting, May 2011, London; 2011 (in publication).
71. Merrick 3rd HW, Hager E, Dobelbower Jr RR. Intraoperative radiation therapy for breast cancer. Surg Oncol Clin N Am. 2003;12(4):1065–78.
72. Lemanski C, Azria D, Thezenas S, Gutowski M, Saint-Aubert B, Rouanet P, et al. Intraoperative radiotherapy given as a boost for early breast cancer: long-term clinical and cosmetic results. Int J Radiat Oncol Biol Phys. 2006;64(5):1410–5.
73. Ciabattoni A, Petrucci A, Palloni T, Siniscalchi A, Vidiri F, Consorti R, et al. IORT in breast cancer as boost: preliminary results of a pilot randomized study. Suppl Tumori. 2005;4(6):S53–8.
74. Ciabattoni A, Ciccone V, Palloni T, Siniscalchi A, Vidiri F, Di Marzo A, et al. IORT as anticipated boost in Stage I and II breast cancer: long term follow-up results. Barcelona: Presented at the GEC ESTRO meeting; 2009 (in publication).
75. Vaidya JS, Baum M, Tobias JS, D'Souza DP, Naidu SV, Morgan S, et al. Targeted intra-operative radiotherapy (Targit): an innovative method of treatment for early breast cancer. Ann Oncol. 2001;12(8):1075–80.
76. Beal K, Sacchini V, Zelefsky M, et al. 5 year update on intraoperative radiation therapy for breast cancer. Int J Radiat Oncol Biol Phys Suppl to Annual Meeting. 2011;S241–42 (Abstract 2061).
77. Vaidya JS, Joseph DJ, Tobias JS, Bulsara M, Wenz F, Saunders C, et al. Targeted intraoperative radiotherapy versus whole breast radiotherapy for breast cancer (TARGIT-A trial): an international, prospective, randomised, non-inferiority phase 3 trial. Lancet. 2010;376(9735):91–102.
78. Vaidya JS, Baum M, Wenz F, Bulsara M, Tobias JS, Alvarado M, et al., on behalf of the TARGIT Trialists Group. The TARGIT-A Trial-Update confirms no increase in Local recurrence. Poster presentation, Abstract P3-13-07. San Antonio Breast Cancer symposium, Dec 2011.
79. Haviland JS, A'Hern R, Bliss JM. Intraoperative radiotherapy for early breast cancer. Lancet. 2010;2(376(9747)):1142.
80. Smith BD, Buchholz TA, Kuerer HM. Intraoperative radiotherapy for early breast cancer. Lancet. 2010;376(9747):1141.
81. Cameron D, Kunkler I, Dixon M, Jack W, Thomas J, Kerr G. Intraoperative radiotherapy for early breast cancer. Lancet. 2010;376(9747):1142.
82. Reitsamer R, Fastner G, Kopp M, Menzel C, Sedlmayer F. Intraoperative radiotherapy for early breast cancer. Lancet. 2010;376(9747):1141.
83. Sperk E, Welzel G, Keller A, Kraus-Tiefenbacher U, Gerhardt A, Sutterlin M, et al. Late radiation toxicity after intraoperative radiotherapy (IORT) for breast cancer: results from the randomized phase III trial Targit A. Breast Cancer Res Treat. 2012;135:253–60.
84. Elliott RL, DeLand M, Head JC, Elliott MC. Accelerated partial breast irradiation: initial experi-

ence with the intrabeam system. Surg Oncol. 2011;20(2):73–9.
85. Deneve JL, Hoefner Jr RA, Harris ER, Laronga C. Accelerated partial breast irradiation: a review and description of an early north American surgical experience with the intrabeam delivery system. Cancer Control. 2012;19(4):295–308.
86. Neumaier C, Sperk E, Welzel G, Yasser AM, Kraus-Tiefenbacher U, Keller A, et al. Trait-E(lderly)-Prospective phase II study of intraoperative radiotherapy (IORT) in elderly patients with small breast cancer. BMC Cancer. 2012;12:171.
87. Hughes KS, Schnaper LA, Berry D, Cirrincione C, McCormick B, Shank B. Cancer and Leukemia Group B, Radiation Therapy Oncology Group, Eastern Cooperative Oncology Group, et al. Lumpectomy plus Tamoxifen with or without irradiation in women 70 years of age or older with early breast cancer. N Engl J Med. 2004;351(10):971–7.
88. Leonardi MC, Maisonneuve P, Mastropasqua MG, Morra A, Lazzari R, Dell'acqua V, et al. Accelerated partial breast irradiation with intraoperative electrons: using GEC-ESTRO recommendations as guidance for patient selection. Radiother Oncol. 2013;106(1):21–7.
89. Guenzi M, Fozza A, Blandino G, Timon G, Belgioia L, Vidano G, et al. Focus on the actual clinical target volume irradiated with intraoperative radiotherapy for breast cancer. Anticancer Res. 2012;32:4945–50.
90. Veronesi U, Orecchia R, Maisonneuve P, Viale G, Rotmensz N, et al. Intraoperative radiotherapy versus external radiotherapy for early breast cancer (ELIOT): a randomized controlled equivalence trial. Lancet Oncol. 2013;14(13):1269–77.
91. Rampinelli C, Bellomi M, Ivaldi GB, Intra M, Raimondi S, Meroni S, et al. Assessment of pulmonary fibrosis after radiotherapy (RT) in breast conserving surgery: comparison between conventional external beam RT (EBRT) and intraoperative RT with electrons (ELIOT). Technol Cancer Res Treat. 2011;10(4):323–9.
92. Arcangeli G, for the collaborative breast IORT group of the Italian Association of radiation Oncology (AIRO). Intraoperative (IORT) versus standard radiotherapy (EBRT) in breast cancer: an update of an ongoing Italian multicenter, randomized study. Presented at: the fifth international conference of International Society of Intraoperative Radiation Therapy (ISOIRT) held in Madrid, 10–13 June 2008.
93. Veronesi U, Orecchia R, Luini A, Galimberti V, Zurrida S, Intra M, et al. Intraoperative radiotherapy during breast conserving surgery: a study on 1,822 cases treated with electrons. Breast Cancer Res Treat. 2010;124(1):141–51.
94. Leonardi MC, Ivaldi GB, Santoro L, Lazzari R, Ferrari A, Morra A, et al. Long-term side effects and cosmetic outcome in a pool of breast cancer patients treated with intraoperative radiotherapy with electrons as sole treatment. Tumori. 2012;98:324–30.
95. Leonardi MC, Maisonneuve P, Mastropasqua MG, Morra A, Lazzari R, Rotmensz N, et al. How do the ASTRO consensus statement guidelines for the application of accelerated partial breast irradiation fit intraoperative radiotherapy? A retrospective analysis of patients treated at the European Institute of Oncology. Int J Radiat Oncol Biol Phys. 2012;83(3): 806–13.
96. Brenner DJ. Point: the linear-quadratic model is an appropriate methodology for determining iso-effective doses at large doses per fraction. Semin Radiat Oncol. 2008;18(4):234–9.
97. Dall'Oglio S, Maluta S, Marcial N, Gabbani M, Franchini Z, Pietrarota P, et al. Accelerated Partial Breast Irradiation (APBI) using only Intraoperative Electron Radiation Therapy (IOERT) in early-stage breast cancer. Oral Presentation BRD A5, San Francisco Breast Cancer symposium, Sept 2012.
98. Dall'Oglio S, Maluta S, Marcial N, Gabbani M, Franchini Z, Pietrarota P, et al. Intraoperative electron radiotherapy in early-stage breast cancer: a mono-institutional experience. Poster presentation, Abstract P3-13-07. San Antonio Breast Cancer symposium, Dec 2012.
99. Lemanski C, Azria D, Gourgon-Bourgade S, Gutowski M, Rouanet P, Saint-Aubert B, et al. Intraoperative radiotherapy in early-stage breast cancer: results of the Montpellier phase II trial. Int J Radiat Oncol Biol Phys. 2010;76(3):698–703.
100. Philippson C, Nogales JM, Simon S, Vanderkerkhove C, Hertens D, Veys I, et al. Intraoperative radiotherapy (IORT) with electrons during breast conserving surgery in early stage breast cancer: review of our first 85 cases. Poster 261, Poster presentation at the French Radiotherapy meeting, 18 Mar 2011.
101. Sawaki M, Sato S, Noda S, Idota A, Uchida H, Tsunoda N, et al. Phase I/II study of intraoperative radiotherapy for early breast cancer in Japan. Breast Cancer. 2012;19(4):353–9.
102. Ollila DW, Klauber-DeMore N, Tesche LJ, Kuzmiak CM, Pavic D, Goyal LK, et al. Feasibility of breast preserving therapy with single fraction in situ radiotherapy delivered intraoperatively. Ann Surg Oncol. 2007;4(2):660–9.
103. Lemanski C, Dubois JB, Gutowski M, Gourgon-Bourgade S, Ailleres N, Azria D. Electrons for Intraoperative breast radiotherapy in selected patients: long-term results of the Montpellier Phase II Trial. Poster presentation, Abstract P3-13-12. San Antonio Breast Cancer symposium, Dec 2011.
104. Lemanski C, Azria D, Gourgou-Bourgade S, Ailleres N, et al. Electrons for intraoperative radiotherapy in selected breast-cancer patients: late results of the Montpellier phase II trial. Radiat Oncol. 2013; 8(1):191.
105. Dall'Oglio S. In reply to: Lemanski C, et al. Radiat Oncol. 2013;8:191.
106. Kimple RJ, Klauber-DeMore N, Kuzmiak CM, Pavic D, Lian J, Livasy CA, et al. Local control following single-dose intraoperative radiotherapy prior to surgical excision of early-stage breast cancer. Ann Surg Oncol. 2011;18(4):939–45.

107. Kimple RJ, Klauber-DeMore N, Kuzmiak CM, Pavic D, Lian J, Livasy CA, et al. Cosmetic outcomes for accelerated partial breast irradiation before surgical excision of early stage breast cancer using single-dose intraoperative radiotherapy. Int J Radiat Oncol Biol Phys. 2011;79(2):400–7.
108. Ivaldi GB, Leonardi MC, Orecchia R, Zerini D, Morra A, Galimberti V, et al. Preliminary results of electron intraoperative therapy boost and hypofractionated external beam radiotherapy after breast-conserving surgery in premenopausal women. Int J Radiat Oncol Biol Phys. 2008;72(2):485–93.
109. Fastner G, Reitsamer R, Menzel C, Fischer T, Kopp M, Ziegler I, et al. Ipsilateral recurrence rates in breast cancer patients after preoperative chemotherapy, breast conserving surgery and intraoperative radiotherapy with electrons-updated results. Scottsdale: Presented at the ISIORT meeting; 2010 (in publication).
110. Petit JY, Veronesi U, Orecchia R, Rey P, Martella S, Didier F, et al. Nipple sparing mastectomy with nipple areola intraoperative radiotherapy: one thousand and one cases of a five year experience at the European institute of oncology of Milan (EIO). Breast Cancer Res Treat. 2009;117(2):333–8.
111. Rusby JE, Smith BL, Gui GP. Nipple sparing mastectomy. Br J Surg. 2010;97:305–16.
112. Urban C, Lima R, Schunemann E, Spautz C, Rabinovich I, Anselmi K. Oncoplastic principles in breast conserving surgery. Breast. 2011;20 Suppl 3:S92–5.
113. Rietjens M, De Lorenzi F, Veronesi P, Intra M, Venturino M, Gatti G, et al. Breast conservative treatment in association with implant augmentation and intraoperative radiotherapy. J Plast Reconstr Aesthet Surg. 2006;59(5):532–5.
114. Franchelli S, Meszaros P, Guenzi M, Corvó R, Pertile D, Massa M, et al. Preliminary experience using oncoplastic techniques of reduction mammaplasty and intraoperative radiotherapy: report of 2 cases. Aesthetic Plast Surg. 2011;35(6):1180–3.

Triple-Negative Breast Cancer

29

Roohi Ismail-Khan, Susan Minton, and Nazanin Khakpour

Introduction

Breast cancer is the most common cancer for females in the United States, the second most common cause of cancer-related death in women, and the main cause of death in women ages 45–55 years. In 2013, approximately 234,580 women in the United States will be diagnosed with breast cancer, with 39,620 women predicted to die from the disease [1]. Breast cancer affects women all over the globe, accounting for 23 % of all cancers worldwide (excluding nonmelanoma skin cancers) in women [2].

A search of oncology publications reveals that the first mention of "triple-negative" breast cancer was in 2005, and, since then, this term has appeared in more than 600 publications [3]. Triple-negative breast cancer (TNBC) accounts for approximately 15 % of breast cancer cases [4, 5]. Although it has only appeared recently in the limelight and is now frequently discussed, triple-negative breast cancer is not a new type of breast cancer. In fact, the term has been recently coined to describe a subtype of breast cancer that is defined by the lack of protein expression of estrogen receptor (ER) and progesterone receptor (PR) and absence of HER2 overexpression. Triple-negative breast cancer is an important area of interest for both researchers and clinicians because of the following five important facts:

1. Triple-negative breast cancer is a poor prognostic factor for disease-free survival and overall survival.
2. As of today, there is no effective specific targeted therapy readily available for triple-negative breast cancer.
3. There is clustering of triple-negative breast cancer cases in premenopausal women and in women of African descent.
4. There is a significant overlap of "basal-like" breast cancers with the triple-negative breast cancer phenotype.
5. There is a significant overlap of BRCA1-associated breast cancers with the triple-negative breast cancer phenotype.

Epidemiology

It has been estimated that one million cases of breast cancer are diagnosed annually worldwide [6]. Of these, approximately 170,000 are of the triple-negative (ER-/PR-/HER2-negative) phenotype with approximately 75 % considered basal like [7]. The prevalence of triple-negative breast cancer is highest in premenopausal African-

R. Ismail-Khan, MD, MS (✉) • S. Minton, DO
Division of Breast Oncology and Experimental Therapeutics, H. Lee Moffitt Cancer Center and Research Institute, 12902 Magnolia Drive, Tampa, FL 33612, USA
e-mail: roohi.ismail-khan@moffitt.org; susan.minton@moffitt.org

N. Khakpour, MD, FACS
Department of Women's Oncology, H. Lee Moffitt Cancer Center and Research Institute, 12902 Magnolia Drive, Tampa, FL 33612, USA
e-mail: nazanin.khakpour@moffitt.org

A.I. Riker (ed.), *Breast Disease: Comprehensive Management*,
DOI 10.1007/978-1-4939-1145-5_29,

American women. It has recently been reported that 39 % of all African-American premenopausal women diagnosed with breast cancer are diagnosed with triple-negative breast cancer [8]. The prevalence of this disease in the same age group in non-African-American females is much less, at approximately 15 %. These ethnic or menopausal differences are not seen in the ER-positive/HER2-positive breast cancer subgroup, nor is it seen in the ER+/HER2-negative subgroup [8].

A recent study examined the racial differences related to the prevalence of triple-negative invasive breast tumors, which was initially presented at the San Antonio Breast Symposium in 2006 and later published in 2009 [5]. The group found that the incidence of triple-negative disease in African-American women was more than twice that of Caucasian women. Furthermore, they showed that 47 % of breast cancers in black women were "triple negative," compared to only 22 % in Caucasians. After adjusting for age and stage at diagnosis, black women were almost threefold more likely than white women to have triple-negative tumors [4, 5].

Unlike hormone receptor-positive cancers that more commonly develop in nulliparous women, women who have never given birth are 39 % less likely to develop TNBC compared to women with children. In fact, women with two or more children are 50 % more likely to develop TNBC compared to women with 1 child. This suggests a pathophysiology that may not be dependent upon the menstrual cycles or lack thereof in women [8].

The stark differences in incidence between various racial groups have led oncologists and researchers to further examine possible genetic or environmental factors that may predispose these women to develop TNBC breast cancer and, in particular, premenopausal African-American women. Studies have also shown that breast cancers in women with germline BRCA1 mutations are more likely to have TNBC in addition to a high-grade tumor [9]. Gene expression studies have confirmed this phenomenon, and BRCA-1-associated breast cancer appears to cluster in the basal-like subtype [10]. It is very important to review the differences and similarities between the phenotype (triple-negative breast cancer) and the molecular genotype (basal-like breast cancer) because we cannot assume that the different subtypes of TNBC behave similarly.

Molecular Features of Triple-Negative Breast Cancers

The management of breast cancer has improved with the advent of widespread screening programs, with striking advances in treatment due to the research and development of hormonal and targeted therapies and improved regimens of chemotherapy. These changes have had a major impact on outcome and have significantly increased overall survival. Fortunately, despite an overall increased incidence of breast cancer in the United States, the mortality appears to be decreasing. Possible reasons include better therapies as outlined above or a national screening program for breast cancer that identifies a majority of early-stage disease, such as DCIS and stage I tumors. Tamoxifen, a serum estrogen receptor modulator (SERM), has a confirmed benefit in patients with ER-positive disease; thus, tamoxifen and aromatase inhibitors are excellent targeted treatments for hormone receptor-positive breast cancers. In addition, the prognosis of women with HER2-positive tumors has greatly improved with trastuzumab and other HER2-targeted therapies [11].

These examples, and several other lines of evidence, clearly show us that breast cancer represents a very *heterogeneous group of breast diseases*. Molecular profiling of breast cancers using array technology has allowed us to examine the biologic and clinical heterogeneity of breast cancer [12]. Multiple studies have revealed that the differences in clinical outcome can be explained by differences in the genetic profile of the primary breast cancer.

Perou et al. were considered the first group to provide an in-depth analysis of the various molecular subtypes of breast cancer based upon their distinct gene profiles. They described subtypes of breast cancer based upon cDNA microarrays, including a "basal-like" subtype. It was also shown that most triple-negative breast cancers cluster in the basal-like subtype [12]. The other subtypes included luminal A and B subtypes, a normal-like subtype, as well as an HER2-enriched subtype. Since then, multiple studies of gene expression profiling have advanced our understanding of the molecular diagnosis of breast cancer, providing the background for oncologists to use the triple-negative phenotype to describe the basal-like molecular subtype [10, 13–15].

Pathological Features of Triple-Negative Breast Cancers

Although the terms “triple-negative breast cancer” and “basal-like breast cancer” are often used interchangeably, they are not the same. Triple-negative breast cancer refers to the immunophenotype of the breast cancer, which is immunologically negative to ER, PR, and HER2, as shown in immunological studies conducted with formalin-fixed and paraffin-embedded tumor sections. Basal-like breast cancer refers to the molecular phenotype [the over-and under-expression of the genes within the tumor cells], as defined by cDNA microarray analysis and other gene expression analyses. As noted above, about 75 % of TNBC have been correlated to have a basal-like expression pattern (Fig. 29.1).

The luminal subtypes of breast cancer express high amounts of luminal cytokeratins and express genetic markers of luminal epithelial cells and normal breast cells [16, 17]. In contrast, “basal-like” breast cancers are so named because they tend to express cytokeratins associated with “basal” types of cancers, as they arise from the outer basal layer. Basal-like breast cancers are typically high grade and poorly differentiated when examined morphologically. Whereas the TNBC phenotype is defined by immunohistochemistry, there are no established diagnostic criteria for basal-like breast cancer on a morphological basis. In general, basal-like breast cancers are morphologically consistent with a high nuclear grade, high mitotic count, and necrosis (Fig. 29.2a), such as a grade 3, invasive ductal carcinoma, not otherwise specified. Some have

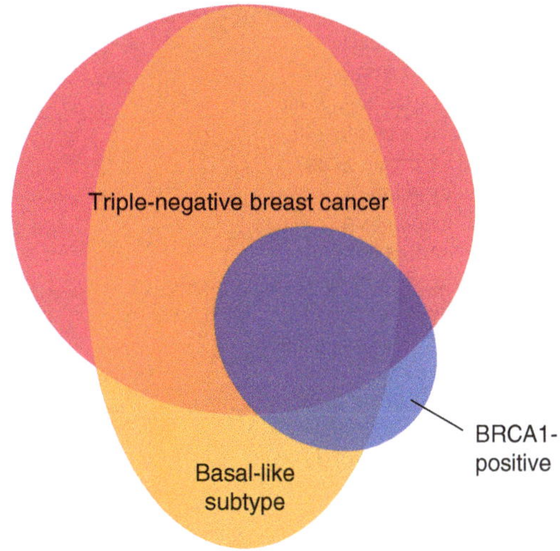

Fig. 29.1 This is a Venn diagram depicting the overlap patterns between TNBC, basal-like breast cancer, and BRCA-1-associated breast cancers

the histomorphology of medullary carcinoma or metaplastic carcinoma. It has also been described that almost 82 % of basal-like breast cancers express p53, compared to only 13 % in the luminal A subgroup [14].

There is also a subset of triple-negative breast cancer and basal-like breast cancer that is of low histological grade, such as secretory, adenoid cystic, acinic cell, or apocrine breast carcinoma. Some of the useful immunohistochemical markers for characterizing basal-like carcinomas are CK5/CK6 (Fig. 29.2b), CK14, CK8/CK18, p63, p-cadherin, vimentin, EGFR1 (or HER1), c-kit, and other growth factors such as IGFR (insulin-like growth factor receptor) [7, 17, 18].

It is also worth mentioning that not all basal-like carcinomas are HER2 negative. A study found that 23 % of basal-like tumors are HER2 positive [19]. Therefore, HER2 immunoreactivity should not be used to rule out a basal-like carcinoma. In addition, because not all triple-negative breast cancers and basal-like breast cancers are of high histological grade, the clinical management strategies outlined for high-risk triple-negative carcinomas are not always applicable. Oncologists need to be aware of this when using triple negative to define a potentially aggressive group of breast cancers. Although the majority of triple-negative breast cancers are basal-like and

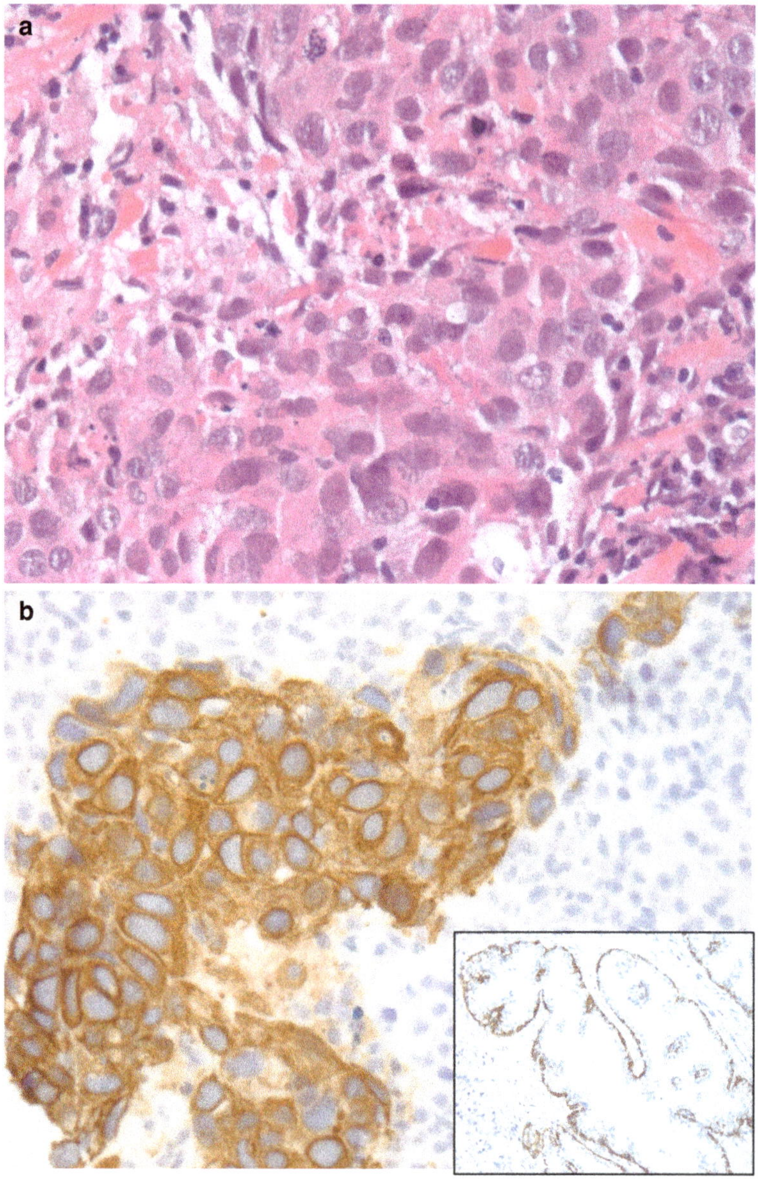

Fig. 29.2 (**a**) Shown is a high-grade breast cancer (invasive ductal carcinoma, not otherwise specified, grade 3), which is an example of a triple-negative breast cancer, basal-like carcinoma. Hematoxylin and eosin (H&E) staining, at ×400 magnification. (**b**) The above tumor showing CK5 positivity, which is typical for a basal-like cancer. Immunohistochemical CK5 staining, at ×400 magnification. *Inset*: CK5 stain of a normal control slide highlighting the basal cells, at ×200 magnification

the majority of basal-like breast cancers are triple negative, there is a about a 25 % discordance between the two descriptive subgroups [7].

Clinical Course and Prognosis

Triple-negative breast carcinomas are known to be biologically aggressive. Although it has been suggested that they respond better to chemotherapy than other types of breast cancers, prognosis remains very poor [20]. This can be explained by two clinical factors: shortened disease-free interval in the adjuvant and neoadjuvant setting and more aggressive clinical course in the metastatic setting.

Triple-negative tumors have a very good initial response to chemotherapy, particularly with anthracycline- and taxane-based therapies. Despite this initial sensitivity, they continue to exhibit a very short disease-free survival [5, 7]. Recent studies examining the effectiveness of neoadjuvant chemotherapy in TNBC reveal that

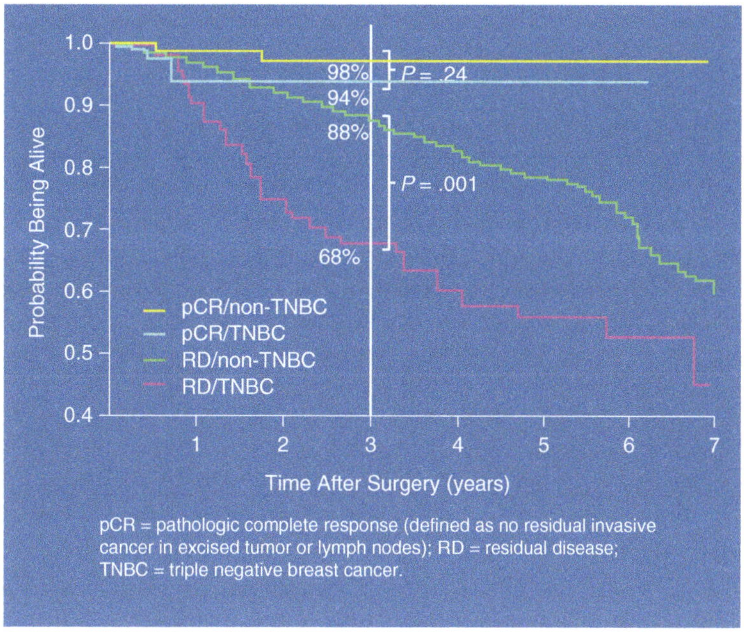

Fig. 29.3 This graph is taken from Lisa Carey's study describing the impact of complete pathological response (pCR) on overall survival in patients receiving neoadjuvant chemotherapy. Patients with TNBC who had a complete pathological response did significantly better than those with residual disease [22]

patients who have a good pathological outcome from surgery also have a good clinical response. However, those who have residual disease after completing their course of neoadjuvant chemotherapy have an overall worst prognosis compared to all other groups [21].

Carey and colleagues examined the relationship between the overall response to neoadjuvant chemotherapy and clinical outcome among three breast cancer subtypes. They used immunohistochemical profiles to classify each molecular subtype of breast cancer: group 1 was the HER2+/hormone receptor-negative (HER2 overexpressed), group 2 was hormone receptor-negative, and group 3 was HER2- (basal-like), hormone receptor-positive (luminal) subtypes. They followed a prospectively maintained dataset of patients with breast cancer treated with neoadjuvant, anthracycline-based (doxorubicin plus cyclophosphamide, AC) chemotherapy. They analyzed each subtype for clinical and pathological responses to neoadjuvant chemotherapy and examined the relationship of this response to distant disease-free survival and overall survival. After neoadjuvant AC, 75 % of patients received subsequent chemotherapy (physician dependent, but most revived a taxane) and all patients who were hormone receptor-positive received endocrine therapy [21].

Although the chemotherapy regimen administered and pretreatment stage did not differ by subtype, the clinical response to AC neoadjuvant therapy was higher among the HER2+/ER- group (70 %) and basal-like (85 %) subtypes (group 3) compared to the luminal subtypes (47 %; $P<0.0001$). Pathological complete responses occurred in 36 % of HER2+/ER-, 27 % of basal-like, and 7 % of luminal subtypes ($P=0.01$). Of interest, despite displaying initial chemosensitivity, patients with the basal-like and HER2+/ER- subtypes had a worse distant disease-free survival ($P=0.04$) and overall survival ($P=0.02$) than those with the luminal subtypes. This worse outcome among the basal-like and HER+/ER- subtypes was due to higher relapse among those patients with residual disease after completing neoadjuvant chemotherapy ($P=0.003$) (Fig. 29.3) [21].

In another study, triple-negative breast cancer was associated with an increased risk for visceral metastases ($P=0.0005$), lower risk for bone recurrence ($P=0.027$), and shorter post-recurrence survival ($P<0.0001$) [22]. If a pathological complete response rate was achieved, patients with triple-negative breast cancer and non-triple-negative breast cancer had a similar overall survival ($P=0.24$). In contrast, patients with residual disease after completing neoadjuvant chemotherapy had a worse overall survival if they had triple-negative breast cancer compared with non-triple-negative breast cancer ($P<0.0001$). It is clear that patients with triple-negative breast cancer have an increased pathological complete response rate compared with non-triple-negative breast cancer patients. However, although those with pathological complete response rate have an excellent overall survival, patients with residual disease after neoadjuvant chemotherapy have significantly worse survival if they have TNBC compared with non-TNBC, particularly within the first 3 years [22].

Even for those patients with an early-stage, triple-negative breast cancer, relapse is still quite common, as high as 20 % in stage I patients over 3–5 years posttreatment. It has been noted that there is a predilection for visceral metastasis, including lung, liver, and, notably, brain metastasis. Current estimates are that approximately 15 % of patients with triple-negative breast cancer develop brain metastasis. Patients with triple-negative breast cancer have a higher risk for developing cerebral metastasis than those with other types of breast cancer. Studies show that, even in patients with cerebral metastasis, TNBC patients have a poor prognosis, as metastasis to the brain occurred earlier [23].

According to the current NCCN treatment guidelines, the appropriate management of a T1N0 (stage 1) breast cancer is based upon both tumor size and cellular characteristics. However, many oncologists will tend to treat the same group of patients who are triple negative with a more aggressive regimen of chemotherapy, in both the neoadjuvant and the adjuvant setting with the knowledge that the risk of recurrence is higher stage for stage. When the number of patients treated and the type of adjuvant chemotherapy administered were both examined, triple-negative T1N0 patients had a greater recurrence risk despite this more aggressive therapy [5]. Unfortunately, treating more aggressively with chemotherapy does not seem to help. Researchers from the Swedish Cancer Institute from Seattle, Washington, report that patients with stage 1 [T1N0] TNBC have twice the risk of recurrence, despite having received much more aggressive treatment [5]. In addition to having a very short disease-free survival, triple-negative breast tumors are aggressive in the metastatic setting, significantly contributing to the shortened overall survival [6]. Progression-free survival is estimated to be 4 months at best in patients with triple-negative breast cancer for first-line therapy, even with bevacizumab-based therapy. Final results from the bevacizumab and paclitaxel study did not show an overall benefit in overall survival [24].

Platinum-based chemotherapy is the mainstay of treatment for patients with metastatic TNBC. Multiple studies have shown the benefit of carboplatin therapy in the neoadjuvant setting as well as the adjuvant setting. In fact, there are ongoing studies, such as the Hoosier study, currently being performed that are examining the benefit of adjuvant platinum therapy combined with a PARP inhibitor in women with BRCA gene mutations and TNBC who were found to have residual disease after neoadjuvant chemotherapy (*clinicalTrials gov*).

Surgical Considerations in the Multidisciplinary Era

Several important steps need to be evaluated to provide a patient with TNBC optimal care. The first step in management of TNBC patients is careful consideration of the timing of the operable disease with respect to systemic therapy. This decision is of paramount importance. The lack of targeted therapy leaves clinicians and patients with very little knowledge of the effectiveness of the current systemic therapy regimens. Since the early 1990s, neoadjuvant systemic therapy for operable breast cancer has been effectively used by clinicians and basic scientists to evaluate tumor response. Pathological complete response (pCR) has been shown by multiple studies to be a useful surrogate in determining overall survival in large trials including the B-18 and B-27. The timing of the systemic therapy in TNBC as discussed by the multidisciplinary team is very important in determining responders versus nonresponders.

The ability to achieve complete pathological response (pCR) varies in TNBC. However, due to high Ki-67 associated with most of these tumors, pCR can be achieved in about 22–45 % of patients, allowing for increased breast conservation rate.

Breast Conservation Therapy Versus Mastectomy in TNBC

Patients with TNBC who undergo breast conservation therapy (lumpectomy and whole breast radiation) have the same overall survival and local and regional recurrence (LRR) rates as patients who have a mastectomy [25–27]. The LRR in several studies were not significantly higher in TNBC patients than other breast cancer subtypes. The BCT was as effective as mastectomy. In a recent retrospective paper from Canada in the Journal of Clinical Oncology, TNBC patients undergoing BCT were found to have better outcome than mastectomy [28]. This was attributed to the use of radiation; however, further evaluation of this finding in prospective trials is warranted.

The issue of BRCA mutations in TNBC is very important in surgical decision making. Genetic counseling and testing in women (less than age 60) with TNBC is now the standard recommendation regardless of any family history. 75 % of BRCA1 mutation carriers diagnosed with breast cancer will have TNBC as opposed to 15–20 % (reflective of general population) of BRCA 2 carriers [29, 30]. Although local therapy for BRCA mutation carriers has shown the same LRR rates as non-mutation carriers, the risk of new primary tumors in ipsilateral and contralateral breast is four- to fivefold higher in BRCA mutation carriers [31, 32]. These patients are often counseled to consider bilateral mastectomy.

The multidisciplinary discussion of patient treatment options and screening for clinical trials are very important in our understanding of this subtype of breast cancer in hopes of finding better treatments in the future. The need for immediate surgical removal of the disease needs to be explained to the patient in the context of systemic disease processes and genetic counseling consideration to provide the patients with optimal outcome.

Hope for Targeted Therapy and Future Directions in Research

Although triple-negative breast cancer is sensitive to chemotherapy, early relapse is more likely than with other subtypes, as are visceral metastases, including the brain. Targeted agents that are currently being investigated include epidermal growth factor receptor (EGFR), vascular endothelial growth factor (VEGF), and poly (ADP-ribose) polymerase (PARP) inhibitors [24].

The anti-angiogenic agent bevacizumab (Avastin), a monoclonal antibody targeting VEGF, is active in many solid tumors including breast cancer. Miller et al. [24] demonstrated a significant improvement in progression-free survival (11.8 versus 5.9 months, HR = 0.60, $P<0.001$) when bevacizumab was added to paclitaxel-based combination chemotherapy versus paclitaxel alone as a first-line treatment for metastatic disease. Examining the triple-negative breast cancer subset of patients in this study confirmed the same improvement (HR = 0.53, 95 % confidence interval = 0.40–0.70) [24, 33]. Unfortunately, long-term follow-up of this trial was not able to demonstrate a benefit in overall survival. However, there was an increase in cardiac events within the bevacizumab group, leading the FDA to deny its use for the treatment of breast cancer.

The fact that the majority of BRCA1-associated breast cancers are also triple negative and basal like has lead researchers to examine the extent to which the BRCA1 pathway contributes to the behavior of "sporadic" basal-like breast cancers. It has been shown that basal-like breast carcinomas frequently harbor defects in DNA double-strand break repair through homologous recombinations, such as BRCA1 dysfunction. The DNA-repair defects characteristic of BRCA1-deficient cells confer sensitivity to PARP1 inhibition [34].

PARP1 is a gene that encodes a chromatin-associated enzyme that modifies various nuclear proteins. This gene is involved in the molecular events leading to cell recovery from DNA damage. When PARP1 is inhibited, double-strand DNA breaks accumulate. Under normal conditions, these double-strand DNA breaks would be repaired via homologous recombination. Both BRCA1 and BRCA2 are required for the homologous recombination pathway to function properly. Therefore, cells deficient in either BRCA1 or BRCA2 are very sensitive to PARP1 inhibition, resulting in cell death and apoptosis. Intuitively, inhibition of the PARP pathway should be of benefit to patients with BRCA-associated malignancies [35]. However, as stated above, not all TNBC are associated with BRCA mutations.

Several PARP1 inhibitors are currently under clinical investigation and hold promise in the treatment of basal-like and triple-negative breast cancers. Exciting results were presented at the plenary session of ASCO in 2009. Results of a randomized phase II study with BSI-201 (a PARP inhibitor) showed benefit in patients with triple-negative breast cancer who had two or less previous lines of chemotherapy. When BSI-201 was combined with gemcitabine and carboplatin, the clinical benefit rate improved to 62 % versus gemcitabine and carboplatin alone (control arm at only 21 %) ($P<0002$) [36].

The clinical benefit rate was defined as complete response rate plus partial response rate plus percentage of patients with stable disease greater than or equal to 6 months. In addition, the overall response rate was notably improved in the BSI-201 arm at 48 % compared to the control arm at 16 %. Progression-free survival was improved to 6.9 months in the BSI-201 arm versus 3.3 months in the control arm [36]. This initial positive study was followed by disappointing results in a larger phase III study, which has led clinical researchers to examine the use of PARP inhibitors in the treatment of triple-negative breast cancer with BRCA mutations. In addition, there are many new agents that are being investigated that may potentially provide promise in this subgroup of breast cancer patients.

The epidermal growth factor receptor (EGFR) is expressed in the basal cluster on cDNA arrays and approximately half of basal-like cancers express EGFR by immunohistochemistry. Basal-like cell lines are dependent on the EGFR pathway for proliferation and are sensitive to EGFR inhibitors. The phase II randomized trial of cetuximab, an anti-EGFR antibody, and carboplatin was not a positive study. Carboplatin was given either in combination or after progression on cetuximab. Of the 73 patients, 74 % had basal-like subtype upon molecular evaluation. However, responses were low at less than 20 %. Although the EGFR pathway was activated in most of the TNBCs, cetuximab was rarely able to block the pathway expression. Findings showed complex heterogeneity within the basal-like subtype and multiple pathways activating proliferation in addition to EGFR [37].

Joyce O'Shaughnessy presented very interesting data at SABCS last year investigating whole genome and transcriptome sequencing of TNBCs. Initial findings suggested that many of the tumors had co-activation of MAPK and PI3K/AKT pathway activation. Ongoing phase I trials are looking at combinations to inhibit the co-activation of these pathways after early findings showed some excellent responses in some but not all patients. Mesenchymal tumors appear to have frequent KRAS, BRAF, and RAS pathway activation. Some may have JAK-2/STAT3 activation [38]. These findings are being investigated further in ongoing trials. TNBCs are a heterogeneous group of tumors making treatment options extremely challenging. However, focusing on treatments geared toward the most commonly known activated pathways such as P53, MAPK, PI3K/AKT, Jak-2, and KRAS, BRAF, RAS and incorporating gene expression may help advance treatment for TNBCs.

Recently, The Cancer Genome Atlas (TCGA) Network made an interesting discovery using molecular profiling techniques, identifying a link between triple-negative breast cancer and serous ovarian cancer. Basal-like breast cancers revealed high mRNA expression correlations with serous ovarian cancers. They identified comparably high pathway activity of the HIF1-a/ARNT, MYC, and FOXM1 regulatory pathways in both ovarian and basal-like cancers. The common findings of TP53, RB1, and BRCA1 loss combined with MYC amplification strongly suggested that these are shared driving events for both TNBC and serous ovarian carcinoma [39].

The finding of a common pathway suggests that similar therapeutic approaches could and should be considered, which is supported by the activity of platinum analogues and taxanes in basal-like breast and serous ovarian cancers. Given that most basal-like breast cancers are of the triple-negative phenotype, finding new drug targets for this group is critical. Unfortunately, the somatic mutation repertoire for basal-like breast cancers has not provided a common target aside from BRCA1 and BRCA2. In their study, The Cancer Genome Atlas Network noted that 20 % of basal-like tumors had a germline and/or somatic BRCA1 or BRCA2 mutation, suggesting that only one in five patients with basal-like breast cancer may benefit from PARP inhibitors and/or platinum compounds [39]. This may partly explain the initial positive results of the phase II PARP trial followed by little further evidence of benefit in the later phase III study.

In this same study, the copy number landscape of basal-like cancers showed multiple amplifications and deletions, some of which may provide therapeutic targets in the future. Potential targets include knockout of PTEN and INPP4B, both of which have been shown to sensitize cell lines to PI3 kinase pathway inhibitors. They also found that many of the components of the PI3 kinase and RAS–RAF–MEK pathway were amplified, not mutated, in basal-like cancers including PIK3CA (49 %), KRAS (32 %), BRAF (30 %), and EGFR (23 %). Other receptor tyrosine kinases that are plausible drug targets and amplified in some basal-like cancers include FGFR1, FGFR2, IGFR1, KIT, MET, and PDGFRA. Finally, the identification of high HIF1-a/ARNT pathway activity suggests that these malignancies might be susceptible to angiogenesis inhibitors and/or bioreductive drugs that become activated under hypoxic conditions [39].

Expanding Testing of BRCA Mutations Based on Triple-Negative Status of Breast Cancers

Recently, the breast cancer community has been advocating testing for BRCA1 and BRCA2 mutations in women with triple-negative breast cancer due to the fact that this type of breast cancer is more often found in women who carry these mutations. A recent study revealed that testing women with triple-negative breast cancers who were younger than 50 years was cost effective, with an incremental cost-effectiveness ratio (ICER) of $8,027 per year of life gained ($9,084 per quality-adjusted life-year). The ICER is an equation used commonly in health economics to provide a practical approach to decision making regarding health interventions. It is typically used in cost-effectiveness analysis. ICER is the ratio of the change in costs to incremental benefits of a therapeutic intervention or treatment. By doing so, this could reduce the future incidence by effectively counseling these patients on their treatment options, with theoretical reductions in breast and ovarian cancer risks of 23 and 41 %, respectively [40]. Due to this rationale, many tertiary cancer centers are now incorporating genetic counseling and screening for TNBC patients through community outreach programs and from within their own breast cancer programs. It is important to educate others that a negative family history does not necessarily exclude women with TNBC from genetic counseling and testing for BRCA mutations.

References

1. Siegel R, Naishadham D, Jemal A. Cancer statistics, 2013. CA Cancer J Clin. 2013;63(1):11–30.
2. International Agency for Research on Cancer. 2008 http://www-dep.iarc.fr/. [cited 2012; International data on cancer statistics].
3. Foulkes WD, Smith IE, Reis-Filho JS. Triple-negative breast cancer. N Engl J Med. 2010; 363(20):1938–48.
4. Kaplan HG, Malmgren J, Atwood MK, Impact of triple negative phenotype on breast cancer prognosis. San Antonio Breast Cancer Symposium. 2006 (Dec 2006). p. poster session VI.
5. Kaplan HG, Malmgren JA, Atwood M. T1N0 triple negative breast cancer: risk of recurrence and adjuvant chemotherapy. Breast J. 2009;15(5):454–60.
6. Anders CK, Carey LA. Biology, metastatic patterns, and treatment of patients with triple-negative breast cancer. Clin Breast Cancer. 2009;9 Suppl 2:S73–81.
7. Rakha EA, Reis-Filho JS, Ellis IO. Basal-like breast cancer: a critical review. J Clin Oncol. 2008;26(15):2568–81.

8. Carey LA, et al. Race, breast cancer subtypes, and survival in the Carolina Breast Cancer Study. JAMA. 2006;295(21):2492–502.
9. Lakhani SR, et al. The pathology of familial breast cancer: predictive value of immunohistochemical markers estrogen receptor, progesterone receptor, HER-2, and p53 in patients with mutations in BRCA1 and BRCA2. J Clin Oncol. 2002;20(9):2310–8.
10. Sorlie T, et al. Repeated observation of breast tumor subtypes in independent gene expression data sets. Proc Natl Acad Sci U S A. 2003;100(14):8418–23.
11. Rocque G, et al. Adjuvant therapy for HER2+ breast cancer: practice, perception, and toxicity. Breast Cancer Res Treat. 2012;131(2):713–21.
12. Perou CM, et al. Molecular portraits of human breast tumours. Nature. 2000;406(6797):747–52.
13. Sorlie T, et al. Gene expression profiles do not consistently predict the clinical treatment response in locally advanced breast cancer. Mol Cancer Ther. 2006;5(11):2914–8.
14. Sorlie T, et al. Gene expression patterns of breast carcinomas distinguish tumor subclasses with clinical implications. Proc Natl Acad Sci U S A. 2001;98(19):10869–74.
15. Sorlie T, et al. Distinct molecular mechanisms underlying clinically relevant subtypes of breast cancer: gene expression analyses across three different platforms. BMC Genomics. 2006;7:127.
16. Rakha EA, et al. Prognostic markers in triple-negative breast cancer. Cancer. 2007;109(1):25–32.
17. Sotiriou C, Pusztai L. Gene-expression signatures in breast cancer. N Engl J Med. 2009;360(8):790–800.
18. Korsching E, et al. Basal carcinoma of the breast revisited: an old entity with new interpretations. J Clin Pathol. 2008;61(5):553–60.
19. Mallon E, et al. The basic pathology of human breast cancer. J Mammary Gland Biol Neoplasia. 2000;5(2):139–63.
20. De Giorgi U, et al. High-dose chemotherapy for triple negative breast cancer. Ann Oncol. 2007;18(1):202–3.
21. Carey LA, et al. The triple negative paradox: primary tumor chemosensitivity of breast cancer subtypes. Clin Cancer Res. 2007;13(8):2329–34.
22. Liedtke C, et al. Response to neoadjuvant therapy and long-term survival in patients with triple-negative breast cancer. J Clin Oncol. 2008;26(8):1275–81.
23. Heitz FP, Harter, Traut A, Lueck HJ, Beutel B, du Bois A. Cerebral metastases (CM) in breast cancer (BC) with focus on triple-negative tumors. Chicago: ASCO; 2008.
24. Miller K, et al. Paclitaxel plus bevacizumab versus paclitaxel alone for metastatic breast cancer. N Engl J Med. 2007;357(26):2666–76.
25. Freedman GM, et al. Locoregional recurrence of triple-negative breast cancer after breast-conserving surgery and radiation. Cancer. 2009;115(5):946–51.
26. Haffty BG, et al. Locoregional relapse and distant metastasis in conservatively managed triple negative early-stage breast cancer. J Clin Oncol. 2006;24(36):5652–7.
27. Voduc KD, et al. Breast cancer subtypes and the risk of local and regional relapse. J Clin Oncol. 2010;28(10):1684–91.
28. Abdulkarim BS, et al. Increased risk of locoregional recurrence for women with T1-2N0 triple-negative breast cancer treated with modified radical mastectomy without adjuvant radiation therapy compared with breast-conserving therapy. J Clin Oncol. 2011;29(21):2852–8.
29. Kandel MJ, ZS, Masciari S, Collins L, Schnitt S, Harris L, Miron A, Richardson A, Garber JE. Prevalence of BRCA1 mutations in triple negative breast cancer (BC) in 2006 ASCO annual meeting A.S.o.C. Oncology, Editor 2006.
30. Somer R, DF-C, Patel A, Schwarting R, Grana G, Rodler E. Screening for BRCA1 mutations in patients with triple negative breast cancer and basal phenotype. In: Research C editor. Thirty-second annual CTRC-AACR San Antonio Breast Cancer Symposium. San Antonio; 2009. p. Supplement 3.
31. Heemskerk-Gerritsen BA, et al. Prophylactic mastectomy in BRCA1/2 mutation carriers and women at risk of hereditary breast cancer: long-term experiences at the Rotterdam Family Cancer Clinic. Ann Surg Oncol. 2007;14(12):3335–44.
32. Kell MR, Burke JP. Management of breast cancer in women with BRCA gene mutation. BMJ. 2007;334(7591):437–8.
33. Siziopikou KP, Cobleigh M. The basal subtype of breast carcinomas may represent the group of breast tumors that could benefit from EGFR-targeted therapies. Breast. 2006;16:104.
34. Rottenberg S, et al. High sensitivity of BRCA1-deficient mammary tumors to the PARP inhibitor AZD2281 alone and in combination with platinum drugs. Proc Natl Acad Sci U S A. 2008;105(44):17079–84.
35. Farmer H, et al. Targeting the DNA repair defect in BRCA mutant cells as a therapeutic strategy. Nature. 2005;434(7035):917–21.
36. O'Shaughnessy J, Osborne C, Pippen J, Yoffe M, Patt D, Monaghan G, Rocha C, Ossovskaya V, Sherman B, Bradley C. Efficacy of BSI-201, a poly (ADP-ribose) polymerase-1 (PARP1) inhibitor, in combination with gemcitabine/carboplatin (G/C) in patients with metastatic triple-negative breast cancer (TNBC): results of a randomized phase II trial. Orlando: ASCO; 2009.
37. Carey LA, et al. TBCRC 001: randomized phase II study of cetuximab in combination with carboplatin in stage IV triple-negative breast cancer. J Clin Oncol. 2012;30(21):2615–23.
38. Craig DW, et al. Genome and transcriptome sequencing in prospective metastatic triple-negative breast cancer uncovers therapeutic vulnerabilities. Mol Cancer Ther. 2013;12(1):104–16.
39. Comprehensive molecular portraits of human breast tumours. Nature. 2012;490(7418):61–70.
40. Kwon JS, et al. Expanding the criteria for BRCA mutation testing in breast cancer survivors. J Clin Oncol. 2010;28(27):4214–20.

Management of Metastatic Breast Cancer

30

Sarah Keck, Melanie Majure, and Hope S. Rugo

Introduction

Metastatic breast cancer (MBC), or cancer that has spread beyond the breast and regional lymph nodes, is the primary cause of breast cancer mortality. In developed countries, only 5–10 % of breast cancers present with distant metastases at the time of diagnosis, but approximately one-third of patients with early-stage breast cancer will eventually develop distant metastases [1]. The timing of recurrence is dependent on tumor biology, with the more aggressive, highly proliferating breast cancers occurring within the first 5 years after diagnosis. In contrast, hormone receptor (HR)-positive breast cancers are equally as likely to recur with distant metastases after 5 years, even up to 20 years after initial diagnosis [1]. Breast cancer mortality has been decreasing in recent years, primarily due to the use of effective adjuvant therapies and to a lesser extent to increased utilization of screening mammography allowing diagnosis at an earlier stage [1, 2].

Evaluation of Suspected Metastatic Breast Cancer

After acute treatment for early-stage breast cancer has been completed, the American Society of Clinical Oncology (ASCO) recommends a regular history and physical examination in addition to mammographic evaluation as indicated by the patient's surgery [3]. Some clinicians routinely evaluate serum tumor markers and radiologic scans to screen for early signs of MBC. Serum tumor markers, such as CA 15-3, CA 27.29, and CEA (carcinoembryonic antigen), or radiographic imaging may diagnose MBC before it is clinically apparent [4], but prospective trials have failed to identify any survival benefit from this approach with distant recurrence just as likely to be diagnosed in between testing [5, 6]. Used as a screening tool, serum markers and routine imaging are costly and can result in false-positive results that further add to health-care expenses, potentially risky diagnostic evaluations, and anxiety on the part of the patient. Given insufficient prospective randomized data showing a

S. Keck, MD
Santa Rosa Medical Group, 3555 Round Barn Circle, Santa Rosa, CA 95403, USA
e-mail: skeck@rrmg.com

M. Majure, MD
Department of Medicine, University of California San Francisco, 505 Parnassus Avenue, Box 1270, San Francisco, CA 94143, USA
e-mail: melanie.majure@ucsf.edu

H.S. Rugo, MD (✉)
Department of Medicine, University of California San Francisco Helen Diller Family Comprehensive Cancer Center, 1600 Divisadero St., Box 1710, San Francisco, CA 94115, USA
e-mail: hrugo@medicine.ucsf.edu

A.I. Riker (ed.), *Breast Disease: Comprehensive Management*,
DOI 10.1007/978-1-4939-1145-5_30, © Springer Science+Business Media New York 2015

survival benefit, the American Society of Clinical Oncology (ASCO) and other international guidelines do not support routine screening for distant recurrence of breast cancer using serial serum tumor markers or radiologic studies [7].

When a breast cancer recurrence is detected, every effort should be made to obtain a pathologic diagnosis of metastatic disease. In addition to confirmation of the diagnosis, the standard markers, estrogen receptor (ER), progesterone receptor (PR), and human epidermal growth factor receptor 2 (HER2), must be evaluated so that appropriate treatment can be delivered. Occasionally, there is discordance in the expression of these markers between the primary tumor and metastatic sites, and this knowledge is critical to determining the appropriate course of treatment [8]. Baseline work-up of a metastatic diagnosis should include radiologic evaluation of the chest, abdomen, and pelvis as well as evaluation of the bones. An MRI of the brain should be obtained if there are suspicious neurologic symptoms. Basic blood work is necessary, such as a CBC, chemistries including calcium, and liver function tests. Serum tumor markers, such as CA 15-3, CA 27.29, and CEA, can be useful to follow response to treatment in conjunction with radiologic evaluation, if they are elevated at the time of metastatic diagnosis.

Although breast cancer metastases can involve any organ, there is tropism seen with specific subtypes. For instance, HR+ more indolent-type cancers tend to metastasize to the bones and soft tissues early in the course of disease, while the aggressive triple-negative and HER2+ breast cancers are more likely to involve visceral organs [9]. Brain metastases are seen more frequently early in the course of HER2+ and triple-negative breast cancers [9, 10].

Prognosis and General Approach to Management

MBC is not typically curable and most otherwise healthy patients diagnosed with MBC will eventually die of their disease. Median survival is determined by tumor biology, response to therapy, and patient tolerance of therapy as well as comorbid illnesses. The overall median survival for all subgroups is about 2.5 years, with the goal of management primarily focused on disease control to palliate symptoms and extend overall survival.

Inasmuch as the goal of treatment is to help patients live as long as possible with the best quality of life, evaluating effective therapies may be challenging in clinical trials. Although improved progression-free survival (PFS) and response rates (RR) are clearly desirable and are frequent primary endpoints of therapeutic trials, overall survival (OS) remains the gold standard of patient outcome in most oncology clinical trials. However, even significant improvements in PFS have not always correlated with improved OS [11–14], which is impacted by subsequent therapies, as well as disease subtype. In addition, measures of quality of life (QOL) have not historically been collected in a standardized fashion.

Although there is no recent evidence that systemic treatment of MBC improves overall survival, it is clinically evident that effective therapy results in longer survival. Population studies using time cohorts have demonstrated improved survival over the past two decades due to utilization of new therapies, namely, aromatase inhibitors, trastuzumab, and taxane-based chemotherapy [15–20]. Median OS is almost 2 years according to population studies and SEER statistics [15, 21, 22], but can be significantly longer in hormone-responsive ER+ and some HER2+ metastatic cancers. A systematic review incorporating 36 clinical trials from 1999 to 2009 found the median OS, from the time of chemotherapy initiation, to be 21.7 months [21].

Using survival curves from these studies, the authors created scenarios for estimating OS: worst-case mean OS of 6.3 months (range 4.8–7.5 months), lower-typical mean OS of 11.9 months (range 9.9–13.2 months), upper-typical mean OS of 36.2 months (range 31.1–41.3 months), and best-case mean OS of 55.8 months (range 47.5–60.2 months). Of note, these estimates are from the start of chemotherapy initiation and therefore do not include a potential significant number of years of hormone therapy or HER2-targeted therapy prior to chemotherapy. Poor prognostic features include HR-negative disease, visceral metastases, multiple sites of metastases, short disease-free interval, and poor performance status [15, 23, 24]. HER2+ breast cancer was previously associated with poor outcome, but this has markedly changed in the era of HER2-targeted therapies, particularly for those patients diagnosed with de novo MBC. Now that most patients with HER2+ MBC will have recurred after exposure to at least one if not two HER2-targeted therapies as well as chemotherapy and hormone therapy when appropriate, the prognosis for this decreasing number of patients may be worse over time. Longer survival can be predicted by ER+ and PR+ metastases, limited metastases, non-visceral disease, and overall good performance status [15, 19, 23, 25].

As MBC is considered a systemic disease, systemic therapies are the mainstay of treatment, including chemotherapy, hormone therapy, HER2-targeted therapy, and emerging molecularly targeted agents. Oligometastatic disease, or metastases limited to only a few isolated sites, can occasionally be managed with locally directed therapies, such as surgery and radiation techniques, in addition to systemic therapy [26]. These local therapies are discussed elsewhere. Current systemic management of MBC as well as the major studies that led to present recommendations will be presented here. Future directions for improving management will also be discussed.

Hormone Receptor-Positive Metastatic Breast Cancer

Initial management of HR+ MBC that does not involve life-threatening visceral metastases (visceral crisis) or rapidly progressing symptomatic metastases is typically hormone therapy. Oral therapy is well tolerated and does not require intravenous access, and achieving a faster tumor response with chemotherapy does not impact overall survival [27, 28]. The majority of women with a long disease-free interval from adjuvant hormone therapy will respond to first-line hormone therapy. A good response to first-line hormone therapy often predicts a number of years of disease control with the sequential use of hormonal agents. Despite a period of good response, virtually all HR+ MBC will eventually become refractory to hormone therapy alone.

For premenopausal women, selective estrogen receptor modulators (SERMs) are the primary hormone therapy unless ovarian suppression with luteinizing hormone-releasing hormone (LHRH) agonists or oophorectomy is utilized to induce a postmenopausal state. For postmenopausal women and for premenopausal women receiving ovarian suppression, several options for hormone therapy exist and the selection of agents may incorporate side effect profiles and logistical considerations (see Fig. 30.1).

Selective Estrogen Receptor Modulators

SERMs block estrogenic stimulation of breast tissue while having an estrogen-like effect in other organs. In the breast, competitive binding of the ER results in a cytostatic antitumor effect. Tamoxifen and toremifene are approved for use in HR+ MBC. Tamoxifen was approved for MBC in 1977 and was the accepted first-line hormone therapy for HR+ MBC for the next two decades. In the early clinical trials, over 50 % of patients with ER+ MBC responded to treatment with tamoxifen with fewer side effects compared with other hormonal manipulations used at that time [29]. Tamoxifen given orally at 20 mg daily (or 10 mg twice daily) is generally well tolerated, with the most common side effects being hot flashes, vaginal discharge, and gastrointestinal symptoms, with preservation of bone density. Rare side effects include venous thromboembolism and endometrial cancer. Tamoxifen is used to treat premenopausal women with or without ovarian suppression. It is also used in postmenopausal women who are diagnosed with MBC within 1 year of completing an adjuvant aromatase inhibitor, or after progression on an aromatase inhibitor for MBC.

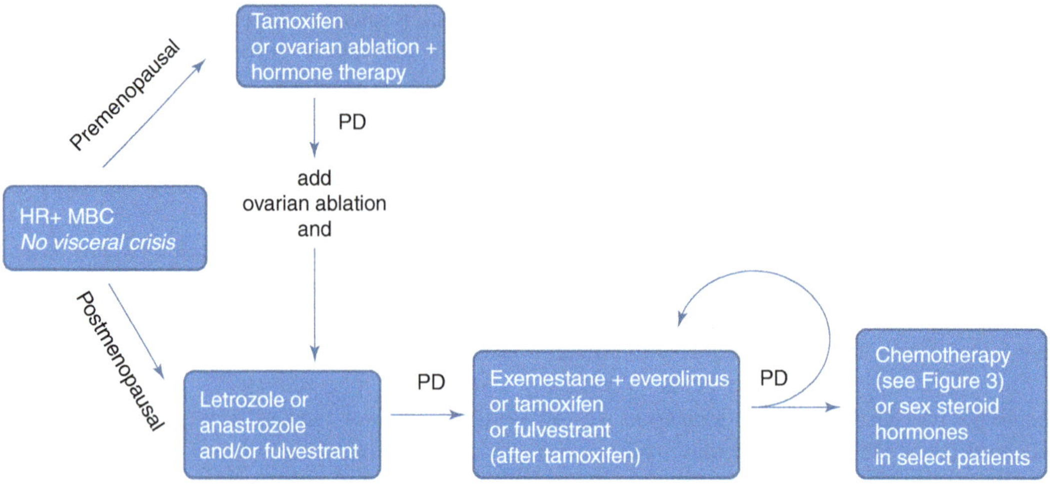

Fig. 30.1 Schema for initial management of HR+ metastatic breast cancer with no visceral crisis and with at least 12 months interval from completion of adjuvant hormone therapy. Many patients will receive sequential hormonal therapies with varying durations of response. Most patients will proceed to chemotherapy; select patients with indolent disease may be treated with sex-steroid hormones. Available clinical trials with novel agents to reverse hormone resistance should be considered. *HR+* hormone receptor positive, *PD* progressive disease

Other SERMs include toremifene and raloxifene. Toremifene has been compared with tamoxifen in MBC and a meta-analysis revealed no significant difference in efficacy and toxicity [30]. Cross-resistance exists, with no benefit from sequential treatment with different agents in this class. Raloxifene has demonstrated efficacy preventing invasive cancer in patients at high risk, but is a weak SERM that is not used to treat established breast cancer.

Aromatase Inhibitors

Aromatase inhibitors (AIs) block the aromatase enzyme, which converts androgens to estrogen in peripheral tissues such as the adrenal glands and adipose tissue. The result is a decrease in circulating estrogens, especially in postmenopausal women who have no other endogenous sources of estrogen. Third-generation AIs were developed to inhibit production of estrogen while sparing other adrenal hormones. Currently, approved agents include the irreversible steroidal AI, exemestane (25 mg orally daily), and the reversible nonsteroidal AIs, anastrozole (1 mg orally daily) and letrozole (2.5 mg orally daily). These agents are generally well tolerated with most common side effects being arthralgias, hot flashes, vaginal dryness, and accelerated loss of bone density. AIs as monotherapy are contraindicated in premenopausal women as these therapies do not affect ovarian production of estrogen and, in fact, increase gonadotropin stimulation of the ovary. AIs in combination with ovarian ablation may be used to treat premenopausal women with MBC as first-line therapy or after progression on tamoxifen; estradiol should be monitored to insure that the ovaries are suppressed. In postmenopausal women, an AI can be given alone or in combination with fulvestrant as first-line therapy, or in subsequent lines after PD on other hormonal therapies.

Several studies have demonstrated superior or equivalent outcomes with AIs compared with tamoxifen as first-line therapy in postmenopausal women [31–34]. A meta-analysis evaluating AIs versus tamoxifen or other hormonal therapies found a statistically significant survival benefit from third-generation AIs when used first line (11 % relative hazard reduction, 95 % CI 1–19 %, $p=0.03$) [35].

There is incomplete cross-resistance between steroidal and nonsteroidal AIs. In one study, patients with progressive MBC on one AI had a clinically beneficial response with an agent from the other class [36]. First-line therapy with either a steroidal or nonsteroidal AI is supported by current evidence. The first two studies compared tamoxifen to nonsteroidal AIs, and these two agents have become standard first-line therapy in clinical practice. The steroidal AI exemestane is approved for use with everolimus after progression on a nonsteroidal AI (discussed below), so exemestane may be reserved for this use.

Fulvestrant

In contrast to tamoxifen, fulvestrant is a pure ER antagonist and downregulates the receptor. It is given as a 500 mg intramuscular injection on days 0, 14, and 28 and then every 28 days. Initial dosing was 250 mg monthly, but this was proven inferior to 500 mg, which was equally well tolerated. The CONFIRM trial randomized women who had progressed on prior hormone therapy to either 250 mg or 500 mg and found a 20 % reduction in risk of progression with the higher dose without an increase in toxicity [37]. Final analysis of survival revealed a 4-month improvement in median OS with the higher dose [38]. Use of fulvestrant as first-line therapy was evaluated in a small phase II study (the FIRST trial) that randomized women to receive either fulvestrant 500 mg or anastrozole [39, 40]. Patients treated with fulvestrant arm had a longer time to progression (TTP) (23 versus 13 months, HR 0.66; 95 % CI, 0.47–0.92) and similar clinical benefit rate (CBR) and RR, with a suggestion of improved OS. There were no differences between the two arms regarding response to subsequent hormone therapy [40]. Although certainly encouraging, this trial does not provide definitive evidence of superiority of fulvestrant compared to AIs, and sequencing therapies is recommended.

The efficacy of fulvestrant in subsequent lines of therapy has been compared with AIs, but not at the currently recommended dose of 500 mg monthly. Mechanistically, fulvestrant may be able to overcome resistance to tamoxifen [41]. In tamoxifen-resistant MBC, fulvestrant (250 mg monthly) was similar in efficacy to anastrozole, including TTP, RR, and OS [42, 43]. Combined analysis of two phase III trials in tamoxifen-refractory MBC showed a longer duration of response with fulvestrant compared with anastrozole and fewer arthralgias [44]. In the EFECT, women with MBC that had progressed or recurred on treatment with a nonsteroidal AI were randomized to fulvestrant (at the suboptimal 250 mg monthly dose) or exemestane, and the treatments were found to be equivalent regarding TTP and RR [45].

The combination of fulvestrant (500 mg loading dose then 250 mg monthly) and anastrozole was compared with anastrozole monotherapy in the first-line setting in two different phase III clinical trials. In SWOG S0226, fulvestrant plus anastrozole resulted in an improved median OS of 47.7 months versus 41.3 months (HR 0.81; 95 % CI, 0.65–1.0, $p=0.05$), despite the majority of patients on anastrozole crossing over to fulvestrant after progression [46]. Median PFS was also better (15 months versus 13.5 months; HR 0.80; 95 % CI, 0.68–0.94, $p=0.007$). In contrast, the similarly designed and powered FACT showed equivalent TTP and OS [47]. One major difference between these trials was the number of patients with de novo metastatic disease (no prior treatment for breast cancer), which was more than threefold higher in the SWOG study than the FACT. Both trials used half of the currently approved dose of fulvestrant, raising the question of whether sequential therapy with the higher dose of fulvestrant would be as or more effective than the combination. There is currently no consensus regarding optimal first-line hormone therapy, but combination therapy could be considered in the specific setting of patients who have de novo metastatic disease.

Sex-Steroid Hormones

Subsequent-line therapies for patients with a low tumor burden and fairly asymptomatic disease include progestins, estrogen, and androgens. The progestin, megestrol acetate, has been shown to be effective in patients with tamoxifen-resistant MBC, but has not been prospectively studied after use of AIs or fulvestrant [48, 49]. Megestrol acetate is given as 40 mg four times daily and side effects include fluid retention, weight gain, vaginal bleeding, and thromboembolic events. After chronic estrogen deprivation with other hormone therapies, estrogen therapy may prove toxic to HR+ breast cancer cells [50]. Traditionally, high-dose estrogen has been used but a recent study compared estradiol 30 mg daily to 6 mg daily in patients who had progressed on an AI and found similar outcomes [51]. Side effects include breast tenderness, vaginal bleeding, pleural effusions, nausea and vomiting, and thromboembolic events. Both progestins and estrogen therapy are contraindicated in patients with significant risk factors for thromboembolism. Androgens, such as testosterone, fluoxymesterone, and danazol, have been used in MBC with some efficacy, but they are associated with more significant side effects.

Hormone Therapy in HER2-Positive MBC

In patients with MBC co-expressing HR and HER2 that is limited to non-visceral sites, hormone therapy along with HER2-targeted therapy is an effective therapy. The combination of AIs with either trastuzumab or lapatinib is approved in HR+, HER2+, and MBC. The TAnDEM trial randomized patients to first-line anastrozole plus trastuzumab versus anastrozole alone and found an improved median PFS with the combination. Similarly, the combination of trastuzumab and letrozole was superior to letrozole alone in terms of CBR [52]. Median OS was not statistically significant which is likely due to subsequent treatment with chemotherapy combined with trastuzumab [53]. The addition of lapatinib to letrozole improved PFS but not OS compared with letrozole [54]. A small proof-of-concept trial showed that a majority of patient's refractory to both AI monotherapy and trastuzumab monotherapy responded to the combination of trastuzumab and letrozole [55].

Biologic Agents in Hormone-Resistant MBC

When MBC has become refractory to one or more of the standard hormone therapies discussed above, treatment options include chemotherapy or a combination of hormone therapy with a targeted agent intended to reverse hormone resistance. Decisions about the type of treatment are based on prior response to hormone therapy, organ function, extent of disease, and performance status. Although combining biologically targeted agents with hormonal agents adds toxicity, the hope is that improving response or reversing resistance to hormone therapy will improve outcome with acceptable side effects.

Activation of the phosphatidylinositol-3-kinase (PI3K) pathway with subsequent upregulation of the mammalian target of rapamycin (mTOR), involved in growth and proliferation, is an important means of escaping responsiveness to hormone therapy. FDA approval of the mTOR inhibitor, everolimus, was granted in 2012 after results of the phase III randomized BOLERO-2 trial showed a significant benefit with the addition of everolimus to exemestane [56]. In 724 postmenopausal women with progression on a nonsteroidal AI, the addition of everolimus 10 mg daily to exemestane significantly improved PFS from 4.1 to 10.6 months compared to exemestane alone. An improvement in PFS was seen in subgroups with or without visceral metastases [57]. Although survival data is still maturing, preliminary analysis revealed more deaths in the control arm (22.6 % versus 17.3 %) [58]. Typical side effects from mTOR inhibitors include stomatitis, rash, fatigue, hematologic abnormalities, and hyperglycemia. Despite more grade 3 and 4 adverse effects, patients who remained on the combination treatment did not report a worse QOL [59].

Other combinations of hormone therapies and biologic agents are being studied and may be approved in the next few years. A phase II randomized trial compared 111 postmenopausal women with AI-resistant MBC to tamoxifen plus everolimus versus tamoxifen plus placebo [60]. Compared with tamoxifen alone, the combination improved CBR (61 % versus 42 %) and TTP (8.6 months versus 4.5 months). Risk of death was reduced by 55 % (HR 0.45; 95 % CI, 0.24–0.81). Side effects were similar to BOLERO-2; patients in the combination arm noted less grade 3/4 pain and fatigue.

The cyclin-dependent kinase inhibitor 4/6 (CDK 4/6 inhibitor) palbociclib has shown remarkable efficacy in HR+ breast cancer, based on an interim analysis of a phase II trial enrolling 165 women with treatment-naïve metastatic HR+ breast cancer, presented at the San Antonio Breast Cancer meeting in 2012 [61]. This agent prevents cellular DNA synthesis by blocking cell-cycle progression, and it was predicted in preclinical models to be of benefit in luminal breast cancer subtypes. Patients were randomized to receive letrozole alone or letrozole with palbociclib; those receiving combination therapy had a significant improvement in PFS (median 26.1 versus 7.5 months for the control arm). The combination was well tolerated, with the most commonly reported adverse events including neutropenia without an increase in neutropenic fever. Based on this data, a large, phase III trial with the same design was launched in 2013, and palbociclib was given "breakthrough" drug status by the FDA.

Antiangiogenic inhibitors have the potential to reverse hormone resistance. The addition of bevacizumab to hormone therapy in the first-line treatment of HR+ MBC in phase II trials showed tumor activity and safety, but a recent phase III trial showed no benefit from the addition of bevacizumab to first-line letrozole with increased toxicity [62–64]. Results from one additional cooperative group trial are pending.

The histone deacetylase inhibitor, entinostat, was evaluated in 130 heavily pretreated women with hormone-resistant MBC in the phase II clinical trial, ENCORE 301 [65]. Patients were randomized to exemestane with or without entinostat. The combination improved PFS from 2.3 to 4.3 months and was associated with more fatigue and neutropenia [66]. As an exploratory endpoint, median OS was improved from 19.8 to 28.1 months with the addition of entinostat (HR, 0.59; 95 % CI, 0.36–0.97; $P = .036$). A phase III registration trial will open in 2014 and entinostat has been given breakthrough drug status by the FDA.

Other promising combinations with hormone therapy include the addition of an insulin-like growth factor-1 receptor (IGF-1R) inhibitor to an mTOR inhibitor, AKT inhibitors, and PI3K inhibitors alone or in combination with other biologic agents including mTOR and CDK 4/6 inhibitors. An international phase III trial, BELLE-2, is underway to evaluate the addition of the pan-PI3K inhibitor BKM120 to fulvestrant in patients with progression on an AI [67]. A similar trial evaluates this combination in patients with progression on a combination of hormone therapy and mTOR inhibition [68]. An alpha-specific PI3K inhibitor, BYL719, is also being studied in combination with hormone therapy. Both agents appear to be effective with different side effect profiles.

Management of HER2-Positive MBC

Approximately 20–25 % of breast cancers are HER2+ [69], defined as 3+ overexpression by IHC or gene amplification by FISH, with 50 % also expressing hormone receptors. Unique features of HER2+ breast cancers include more aggressive tumor biology and a tropism for developing visceral and CNS metastases. Trastuzumab, a humanized monoclonal antibody (mAb) to the extracellular domain of HER2, has dramatically changed the way in which we approach and treat such patients. We now are able to specifically target HER2 (+) disease, resulting in significantly improved disease control and overall survival. Trastuzumab was approved by the US FDA for use in MBC in 1998, after a landmark randomized phase III trial as well as single-agent trials showed dramatic efficacy and minimal toxicity in women with HER2+ metastatic disease [70, 71]. The most significant side effect with trastuzumab is cardiotoxicity that is usually reversible with treatment interruption.

Other HER2-targeted agents have been developed with different mechanisms of action. Small molecule tyrosine kinase inhibitors that

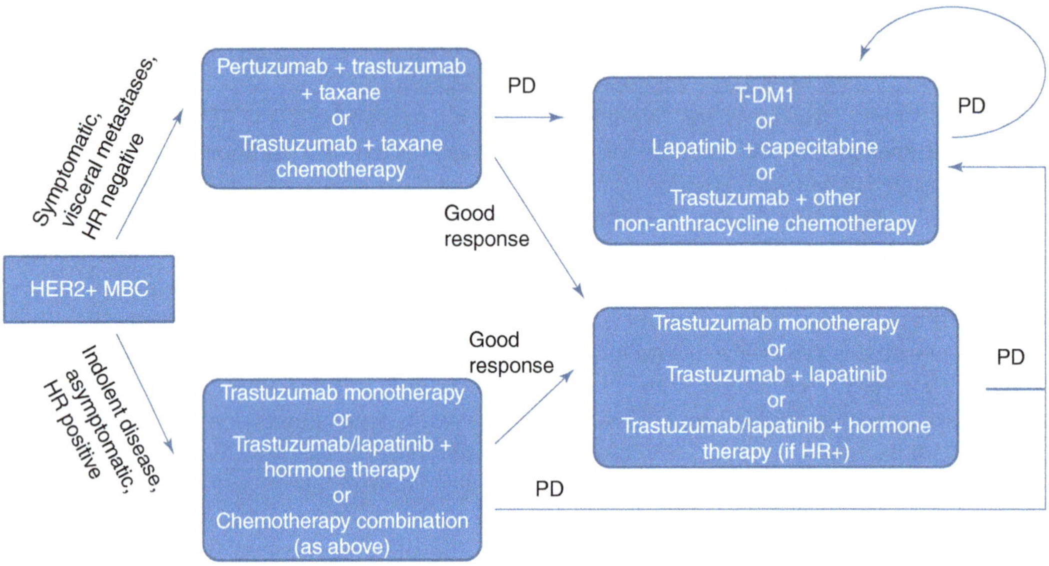

Fig. 30.2 Schema for management of HER2+ metastatic breast cancer. Initial treatment is chemotherapy plus a HER2-targeted agent for most patients, or the immunotoxin T-DM1. In certain situations, trastuzumab monotherapy or hormone therapy plus HER2 targeting may be used initially. Available clinical trials with novel agents should be considered. *HER2+* human epithelial growth factor receptor positive, *PD* progressive disease, *T-DM1* trastuzumab emtansine

target the intracellular kinase domain of HER2, such as lapatinib and neratinib, are effective in trastuzumab-refractory disease. Lapatinib is FDA approved in combination with capecitabine [72], and others, such as neratinib, are being studied. The combination of lapatinib and trastuzumab is relatively well tolerated and has demonstrated improved PFS and OS compared to lapatinib alone in trastuzumab-refractory disease [73]. Lapatinib causes diarrhea and rash that are usually manageable but have limited more widespread use of this agent. Recently, two agents were approved for the treatment of metastatic disease in 2012 and 2013, respectively. The first is pertuzumab, a HER2 mAb that prevents HER dimerization and in combination with trastuzumab causes minimal additional side effects. The second agent is trastuzumab emtansine (T-DM1), an antibody-drug conjugate that delivers a cytotoxic chemotherapy directly to HER2-overexpressing cells with tolerable side effects. The indications for use of each HER2-targeted agent, as well as ongoing studies of these and other agents, are discussed below.

First-Line Treatment of HER2+ MBC

Treatment of newly diagnosed, HER2-positive MBC should include either trastuzumab or lapatinib, as outcomes are consistently improved with their use [74–76]. Options for treating non-life-threatening metastases include trastuzumab or lapatinib in combination with hormone therapy, or chemotherapy with one or more HER2-targeted agents. Trastuzumab monotherapy is usually reserved for maintenance therapy after response to chemotherapy and trastuzumab combined. Rapidly progressing or symptomatic visceral metastases should be treated initially with a combination of HER2 targeting and chemotherapy (see Fig. 30.2). The recent data from the CLEOPATRA trial (see below) has changed the standard of care for first-line treatment of HER2+ breast cancer based due to the demonstrated survival advantage over the previous standard of care.

Single-agent trastuzumab has been evaluated in newly diagnosed HER2+ MBC. In a single-arm study of 114 women with MBC, first-line trastuzumab monotherapy was effective with an

RR of 26 % and a CBR of 38 % [77]. Few studies have compared trastuzumab monotherapy with trastuzumab plus chemotherapy. One phase III study looked at the upfront combination of trastuzumab and docetaxel versus trastuzumab monotherapy followed by trastuzumab plus docetaxel at the time of progression [78]. Median PFS and OS (HR 2.72; 95 % CI, 1.03–7.18) were significantly improved with the upfront combination therapy. Most of the 112 patients in this study had visceral metastases and multiple metastatic sites.

A similar phase II study in 101 patients compared first-line combination trastuzumab and docetaxel with first-line trastuzumab followed by single-agent docetaxel upon progression [79]. The two arms had similar PFS, but there was an improved RR and a nonstatistically significant improvement in OS with the combination. This trial design does not, however, reflect the current clinical practice of continuing trastuzumab along with chemotherapy after progression. Most clinicians treat newly diagnosed HER2+ MBC with HER2-targeting therapy plus taxane chemotherapy. Although there may be patients with nonvisceral, indolent disease and perhaps with other comorbidities that limit chemotherapy options who are appropriately treated with trastuzumab monotherapy, single-agent trastuzumab may be more appropriately reserved for maintenance therapy after response to chemotherapy. Indolent MBC that is both HER2+ and HR+ can be treated with a combination of hormone therapy and a HER2-targeted agent, as discussed above.

Studies have consistently shown the benefit of trastuzumab added to first-line chemotherapy. The pivotal phase III study by Slamon et al. randomized patients to first-line treatment with standard chemotherapy, either anthracycline-based or paclitaxel, versus chemotherapy plus trastuzumab [70]. The addition of trastuzumab improved OS (25 versus 20 months, $p=0.01$) as well as TTP and RR. Based on these results, trastuzumab plus paclitaxel was approved in the first-line setting. The combination of trastuzumab and doxorubicin resulted in unacceptably high rates of cardiomyopathy, so this approach was largely abandoned. A subsequent randomized, phase II study of docetaxel with or without trastuzumab also demonstrated a significant OS benefit of 31.2 months in the combination group versus 22.7 months for the group receiving docetaxel alone [80]. The majority of patients treated with docetaxel alone crossed over to receive trastuzumab, resulting in loss of a significant survival benefit with longer-term follow-up. The phase III, MA.31 trial compared trastuzumab versus lapatinib with first-line taxane chemotherapy [81]. An interim analysis found a significantly better PFS of 11.4 with trastuzumab-taxane versus 8.8 months for the lapatinib-taxane arm. The OS was similar in the two arms, but toxicity was significantly greater in the lapatinib arm.

The combination of pertuzumab with trastuzumab and taxane chemotherapy in the first-line setting was approved in 2012 based on the phase III, CLEOPATRA study [82], becoming the new standard of care in some parts of the world. In this study, 808 patients with newly diagnosed metastatic HER2+ breast cancer were randomized to trastuzumab and docetaxel with or without pertuzumab. The primary endpoint of median PFS was prolonged from 12.4 to 18.5 months with addition of pertuzumab (HR 0.62; 95 % CI, 0.51–0.75; $p<0.001$). Overall survival was significantly improved with the addition of pertuzumab as well, with a HR of 0.66 (95 % CI, 0.52–0.84, $p=0.0008$) [83]. Adding pertuzumab did not increase cardiac toxicity, but did increase rates of grade 3 febrile neutropenia and diarrhea. The combination of pertuzumab, trastuzumab, and docetaxel is a good, albeit expensive, option for untreated HER2+ MBC with the longest survival from any treatment available for this subtype of breast cancer. The majority of patients enrolled in the CLEOPATRA trial had not received adjuvant trastuzumab, bringing up the question of whether the dual targeting would be equally effective in patients whose disease recurs after exposure to adjuvant HER2-targeted therapy. A subset analysis of those patients relapsing after trastuzumab suggested similar efficacy.

Pertuzumab has also demonstrated improved rates of pathologic complete response in the neoadjuvant setting, with the same combination of agents. This finding led to the FDA-accelerated approval of pertuzumab as neoadjuvant therapy, with final approval pending the results from the phase III APHINITY adjuvant trial. APHINITY (BIG 4–11/BO25126/TOC 4939G) is a large randomized phase III, double-blind, placebo-controlled study that compares the efficacy and safety of chemotherapy plus trastuzumab and placebo with that of chemotherapy plus trastuzumab and pertuzumab as adjuvant therapy in 4,800 patients with operable, HER2-positive, primary breast cancer. The trial completed accrual in August of 2013, and results are eagerly anticipated.

For patients who develop a metastatic recurrence during, or within, 12 months after completing adjuvant trastuzumab, there are no rigorous studies to guide practice. Trastuzumab emtansine (T-DM1) is the most appropriate treatment based on current data (see below). Subsequent treatment could include lapatinib and trastuzumab, lapatinib and capecitabine, or trastuzumab and chemotherapy.

Subsequent-Line Treatment of HER2+ MBC

When MBC becomes refractory to first-line therapy that includes a HER2-targeted agent, there are several options for further management (see Fig. 30.2). Choice of treatment is often based on side effect profiles, sites of metastases, and patient preference. There is some evidence of benefit from continuing trastuzumab after disease progression. In a randomized, phase III study of 156 women with MBC that had progressed on trastuzumab, second-line treatment with capecitabine and continued trastuzumab improved PFS compared with capecitabine alone (8.2 versus 5.6 months; HR 0.69; 95 % CI, 0.48–0.97; $p=0.0338$) [84]. Overall survival showed a nonstatistically significant trend toward a benefit with continuing trastuzumab.

Options for subsequent treatment after progression on trastuzumab plus chemotherapy include changing to a different chemotherapy including T-DM1, switching to lapatinib plus capecitabine, or using the chemotherapy-free combination of trastuzumab plus lapatinib. Other chemotherapy options for use with trastuzumab are paclitaxel with or without carboplatin, docetaxel, nab-paclitaxel, vinorelbine, capecitabine, and gemcitabine. In general, trastuzumab is not combined with anthracyclines due to the higher risk of cardiomyopathy [70]. Lapatinib is approved for use with capecitabine after progression on a trastuzumab-taxane combination.

In the phase III EGF100151 clinical trial, patients with trastuzumab-refractory MBC were randomized to the addition of lapatinib and capecitabine versus capecitabine alone. At interim analysis, the median TTP was 8.4 months with the combination versus 4.4 months with capecitabine alone (HR 0.49; 95 % CI, 0.34–0.71, $p<0.001$) [72]. The addition of lapatinib did not increase the rates of serious adverse events or discontinuation of therapy due to toxicity. Early termination of the study after interim analysis and resultant crossover to the combination limited evaluation of OS, but final analysis failed to demonstrate a significant impact on survival [85].

T-DM1 was approved by the FDA in February 2013 for second- and subsequent-line treatment of HER2+ MBC. The antibody-drug conjugate was shown in phase II trials to have single-agent activity in heavily pretreated HER2+ MBC with only minimal toxicity [86, 87]. The phase III EMILIA trial randomized 991 patients with progression on trastuzumab and taxane chemotherapy to T-DM1 versus capecitabine plus lapatinib [88]. With less toxicity, T-DM1 improved median PFS from 6.4 months with lapatinib and capecitabine to 9.6 months (HR 0.65; 95 % CI, 0.55–0.77; $p<0.001$) and median OS from 25.1 to 30.9 months (HR 0.68; 95 % CI, 0.55–0.85; $p<0.001$).

Based on the OS benefit and tolerable side effects, T-DM1 has become many clinicians' choice for second-line treatment after progression on the combination of a taxane plus trastuzumab, with or without pertuzumab. The MARIANNE trial is a phase III trial that randomized 1,095 patients with treatment-naïve HER2+ metastatic breast cancer to receive trastuzumab and a taxane, T-DM1, or T-DM1 and pertuzumab. Accrual is completed with results expected in 2014. There are a number of studies planned with

T-DM1 examining its effectiveness in treating early-stage breast cancer as well, including the KATHERINE trial for patients with residual cancer after neoadjuvant chemotherapy plus HER2-targeted therapy.

The combination of dual HER2 targeting with an antibody and tyrosine kinase inhibitor was studied in a phase III clinical trial that randomized 296 heavily trastuzumab-pretreated patients to receive lapatinib or lapatinib plus trastuzumab [73]. The primary endpoint of median PFS was improved from 8.1 weeks with lapatinib alone to 11.1 weeks with the combination (HR 0.74; 95 % CI, 0.58–0.94; $p=0.011$). Overall survival improved significantly from 9.5 to 14 months with the combination (HR 0.74; 95 % CI, 0.57–0.97; $p=0.026$), despite half of the patients in the lapatinib arm crossing over to combination treatment. Exploratory analysis revealed a more significant survival benefit for patients with less heavily pretreated MBC, suggesting the benefit of this chemotherapy-free combination earlier in the course of treatment.

Future Directions for HER2+ MBC

The toolbox of effective HER2-targeted agents is rapidly growing, with much research underway to better understand and target mechanisms of resistance that develop to trastuzumab. As discussed above, pertuzumab was approved for first-line treatment in 2012, and results of the MARIANNE trial (see above) are expected to significantly impact treatment practice for both late- and early-stage disease. The combination of pertuzumab and trastuzumab was shown to be effective and well tolerated in trastuzumab-refractory MBC, with an RR of 24 % and a CBR of 50 %. However, pertuzumab is not yet approved in the subsequent-line setting [89]. Ongoing studies are evaluating pertuzumab in combination with alternate chemotherapy agents and trastuzumab in heavily pretreated patients. A phase II trial is evaluating the combination of T-DM1 and pertuzumab in early progressive MBC (NCT00943670).

Based on the results from the lapatinib and trastuzumab trial and encouraging responses in the neoadjuvant setting, this combination is being tested in the adjuvant setting in the ALTTO trial. This international phase III trial in women with early-stage, HER2-positive breast cancer is comparing chemotherapy combined with either lapatinib and trastuzumab, trastuzumab alone, or a sequencing approach. ALTTO is expected to report results in 2014.

Neratinib, an irreversible TKI, showed intriguing single-agent activity in trastuzumab-refractory MBC and even greater antitumor activity in trastuzumab-naïve MBC [90]. It is being evaluated in several different clinical trials, including a phase III, first-line comparison of paclitaxel with either neratinib or trastuzumab (NCT00915018), and a planned neoadjuvant trial.

The mTOR inhibitor, everolimus, is being evaluated in trastuzumab-refractory HER2+ MBC as the upregulation of the PI3K/mTOR pathway has been identified as an important mechanism for trastuzumab resistance. There have been two phase I/II single-arm studies that have demonstrated efficacy and tolerability with the combination of everolimus, trastuzumab, and chemotherapy in patients with heavily pretreated, advanced breast cancer [91–94]. Based on these intriguing results, two international, phase III, randomized trials were developed to further evaluate these combinations in HER2-overexpressing MBC. The BOLERO-1 (NCT00876395) trial is evaluating the addition of everolimus to trastuzumab and paclitaxel, and the BOLERO-3 (NCT01007942) trial examined the addition of everolimus to trastuzumab and vinorelbine. Preliminary results of BOLERO-3 revealed a modest improvement in PFS from 5.78 months without everolimus to 7 months with the addition of everolimus (HR 0.78; 95 % CI, 0.65–0.95, $p=0.0067$) [95]. Data from BOLERO-1 is expected in 2014.

Chemotherapy in MBC

Chemotherapy is the primary treatment for metastatic triple-negative breast cancer, as there are no identified targets at this time, and this subset of breast cancer does not respond to either HER2- or ER-targeted therapy. In addition, chemotherapy is the mainstay for the treatment of endocrine-refractory ER+ breast cancer and is given in combination with HER2-targeted therapy for HER2+ disease. There are several different chemotherapy agents with efficacy data for the treatment of MBC. Combinations of chemotherapy with molecularly targeted agents are discussed in other sections.

Combination Versus Sequential Single-Agent Chemotherapy

Chemotherapy can be given in a sequential single-agent fashion, moving from one to another at the time of disease progression, or as combination regimens. Historically, combination chemotherapy was the preferred strategy, as RR and TTP were higher with more intensive chemotherapy regimens, and it was previously thought that this would translate to an improved OS. A systematic review in the taxane era of all trials that compared a combination regimen with a single agent found that chemotherapy combinations were superior to single-agent chemotherapy, regarding RR, PFS, and OS (HR for OS 0.88; 95 % CI, 0.83–0.94, $p<0.0001$) [96], although with increased toxicity. This review did not answer the question of whether current, effective agents in combination are superior to these same agents in sequence. Surprisingly, few randomized controlled trials have effectively addressed this question.

The intergroup E1193 trial used a three-arm design to compare sequential doxorubicin followed by paclitaxel every 3 weeks, paclitaxel followed by doxorubicin, and the combination in 739 patients [97]. Despite an improved RR and longer time to treatment failure, the combination arm did not improve median OS (doxorubicin 18.9 months, paclitaxel 22 months, combination 22 months; p = not significant) nor QOL. Three other smaller clinical trials comparing an anthracycline-taxane combination and single agents in sequence found no significant benefit from the combination therapy [98–100].

Any potential benefits with combination chemotherapy come at the cost of significantly more toxicity, especially nausea, vomiting, alopecia, and neutropenia. The more common practice is to use sequential single-agent chemotherapy unless a rapid response is important for life-threatening disease. As the goal of chemotherapy for MBC is palliation of cancer-related symptoms and prolonging survival with an acceptable QOL, frequent assessment of symptoms, side effects, and tumor response is performed during chemotherapy and the treatment adjusted accordingly.

Choice of Chemotherapy

When choosing from a number of effective chemotherapy options, considerations may include previous treatment of breast cancer, side effect profiles, patient performance status, logistics regarding chemotherapy administration, and available targeted agents, such as trastuzumab (see Fig. 30.3). Metastatic recurrence during or shortly after adjuvant therapy suggests an aggressive cancer that is resistant to the recent treatment. Cancer that recurs beyond 12 months of adjuvant chemotherapy is generally considered chemotherapy sensitive, and re-treatment is often a reasonable approach. Prior exposure to anthracyclines must be considered when assessing the risk of cardiotoxicity. A patient's performance status, organ function, or comorbidities may limit the use of certain agents. To date, there has been no prospective, high-level evidence to support the use of the various chemotherapy sensitivity assays in development [101].

The majority of patients will respond to first-line chemotherapy treatment. There is no evidence that one agent, rather than another used first line, is associated with an improvement in OS. Anthracyclines and taxanes are considered to be the most effective classes of chemotherapy agents in breast cancer, and therefore, these are the most commonly used in the first-line setting. A randomized, controlled trial of first-line doxorubicin versus paclitaxel every 3 weeks, with crossover allowed at progression, found a higher RR and PFS with first-line doxorubicin, but no statistically significant difference in OS [102].

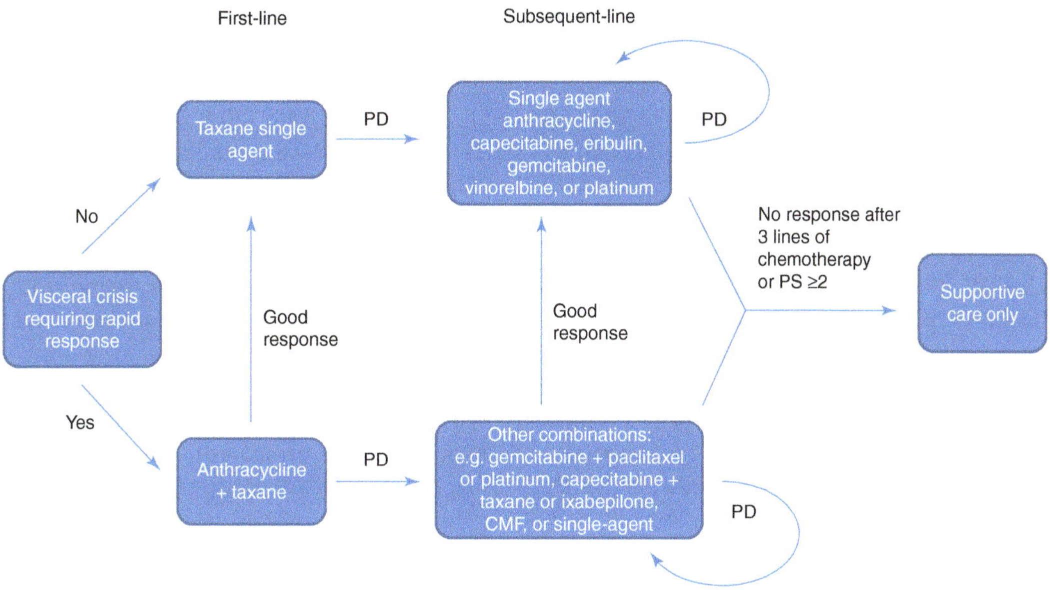

Fig. 30.3 Schema for the use of chemotherapy for metastatic breast cancer for triple-negative and hormone-resistant breast cancer. Life-threatening visceral crisis generally warrants combination chemotherapy, but generally sequential single agents are preferred to balance cancer control with chemotherapy toxicity. For patients with a short disease-free interval (<6–12 months) from adjuvant taxane-based chemotherapy, consider a subsequent-line chemotherapy. Available clinical trials should be considered. *PD* progressive disease, *PS* performance status, *CMF* cyclophosphamide/methotrexate/fluorouracil

Doxorubicin resulted in more toxicity but also better control of cancer-related symptoms.

In the E1193 clinical trial, the single-agent arms of doxorubicin and paclitaxel every 3 weeks showed equivalent RR, time to treatment failure, OS, and QOL [97]. A meta-analysis evaluated 919 patients in three randomized trials that compared first-line treatment with single-agent anthracycline versus a taxane given every 3 weeks [103]. The authors found a similar RR for anthracyclines and taxanes (33 % and 38 %, respectively, $p=0.08$) and no significant difference in OS (HR 1.01; 95 % CI, 0.88–1.16; $p=0.90$) but an advantage for anthracyclines regarding PFS (HR 1.19; 95 % CI, 1.04–1.36; $p=0.011$). Of note, no first-line studies have evaluated first-line anthracyclines versus the current weekly dosing of paclitaxel.

Single-Agent Chemotherapy Options

First-line chemotherapy is often a taxane given its efficacy and side effect profile. There is retrospective evidence that paclitaxel and docetaxel are not completely cross-resistant, so that progression on one taxane does not preclude use of a different taxane [104, 105]. In the phase III trial, CALGB 9840, weekly paclitaxel 80 mg/m2 doubled the median OS from 12 to 24 months, compared with paclitaxel 175 mg/m2 every 3 weeks (HR 1.28, $p=0.0092$) [106]. Unfortunately, grade 3 peripheral neuropathy was also increased from 12 % to 24 % ($p=0.0003$). Docetaxel every 3 weeks is superior to paclitaxel given every 3 weeks regarding PFS and OS but has not been compared to weekly paclitaxel [107]. In addition, continuing docetaxel for multiple cycles results in chronic side effects including loss of nails, eye tearing, and permanent hair loss.

Weekly docetaxel is not better than every-3-week docetaxel but resulted in more toxicity [108]. Nanoparticle albumin-bound paclitaxel (nab-paclitaxel) was developed to improve efficacy and decrease infusion reactions related to the solvent used with paclitaxel. Utilizing nab-paclitaxel (260 mg/m2) every 3 weeks resulted in superior efficacy outcomes when compared to every-3-week paclitaxel [109]. In a randomized, phase II study, nab-paclitaxel 150 mg/m2 given on days 1, 8, and 15 every 28 days improved PFS and was superior to every-3-week docetaxel [110]. Weekly nab-paclitaxel at this dose was not superior to paclitaxel in the first-line setting, when given in combination with bevacizumab in CALGB 40503, and resulted in more toxicity. Rates of peripheral neuropathy due to nab-paclitaxel are fairly similar to paclitaxel and docetaxel, but rates of neutropenia are lower with the every-3-week dosing schedule. Higher doses of nab-paclitaxel given weekly are associated with increased bone marrow suppression. Unlike solvent-bound paclitaxel and docetaxel, nab-paclitaxel does not require premedication to prevent allergic reactions, and it is significantly more expensive.

Anthracycline chemotherapy is also an option for first-line treatment. Consideration of cardiac risk factors and the lifetime anthracycline dose limit (450–500 mg/m2 for doxorubicin) are critically important to minimize the likelihood of cardiomyopathy. Doxorubicin can be given as 60–75 mg/m2 every 3 weeks or 20 mg/m2 weekly. Epirubicin can be given as 75–100 mg/m2 every 3 weeks or 20–30 mg/m2 weekly. Pegylated liposomal doxorubicin and liposome-encapsulated doxorubicin have been shown to be as effective as doxorubicin in the first-line setting with significantly less cardiotoxicity, alopecia, and nausea, but with more hand-foot syndrome and mucositis, as well as a higher cost [111–113].

Capecitabine, an antimetabolite oral prodrug of fluorouracil, is frequently used in MBC. It is active in the first-line setting and has the benefit of oral administration with generally tolerable side effects, including a minimal risk of alopecia [114, 115]. More often, capecitabine is utilized in anthracycline- and taxane-exposed patients where it has shown consistent efficacy [116–117]. A pooled analysis of individual patient data from trials of capecitabine monotherapy found a greater tumor response in patients with HR+ MBC and with a lower burden of disease [115]. Although the two starting doses, 2,500 mg/m2/day and 2,000 mg/m2/day, have not been compared head to head, the lower dose appears to be less toxic and yet remains equally effective as the higher dose [118, 120, 121]. It is common, therefore, to administer capecitabine as 2,000 mg/m2/day for 14 days followed by a 7-day break. Side effects include palmar-plantar erythrodysesthesia, diarrhea, and mucositis. Benefits of capecitabine include oral administration, little risk of alopecia, and generally tolerable side effects.

Eribulin mesylate, an inhibitor of tubulin polymerization, is approved for patients with anthracycline- and taxane-exposed MBC. In the phase III, EMBRACE trial, which randomized heavily pretreated patients to eribulin (1.4 mg/m2 days 1 and 8 every 21 days) or to chemotherapy (investigator's choice), eribulin improved median OS from 10.6 to 13.1 months (HR 0.81; 95 % CI, 0.66–0.99; $p=0.041$) [122]. Toxicities included grade 3/4 neutropenia in 45 % and peripheral neuropathy. There is also evidence for its activity earlier in the course of treatment. A phase III trial randomizing women, half of whom had received only one prior chemotherapy regimen, to eribulin or capecitabine found similar efficacy with a suggestion of benefit from eribulin in patients with HR- and HER2-negative (triple negative) disease [123].

Other effective subsequent-line chemotherapy options include gemcitabine, vinorelbine, ixabepilone, cisplatin, irinotecan, cyclophosphamide, methotrexate, and oral etoposide. Many patients will be exposed to a number of these chemotherapy agents over the course of their treatment.

Combination Regimen Options

For patients in whom combination chemotherapy seems indicated, either at the time of diagnosis or when symptomatic visceral crisis develops during treatment, there are several options. Chemotherapy regimens approved for use in the adjuvant and neoadjuvant settings as well as other combinations have been effective: anthracycline/cyclophosphamide with or without fluorouracil, anthracycline/taxane, cyclophosphamide/methotrexate/fluorouracil, gemcitabine/paclitaxel, gemcitabine/platinum, taxane/capecitabine, ixabepilone/capecitabine, epirubicin/cisplatin, and others. In some situations, single-agent chemotherapy can be initiated, and if progression occurs, then a second agent can be added, particularly if a response would improve a patient's cancer-related symptoms. Alternatively, combination chemotherapy can be initiated and narrowed down to only one of the agents after a response is obtained. The goal of using a combination regimen is to obtain a tumor response that translates into improvement of cancer-related symptoms or control of a life-threatening visceral crisis. Combination chemotherapy is generally more toxic and may not be an option for patients with a poor performance status.

Two meta-analyses comparing taxane-based combinations with non-taxane, anthracycline-based combinations found an improvement in RR and PFS but no significant improvement in OS with taxane combinations [103, 124]. In the more recent analysis, eight randomized trials including 3,034 patients compared taxane-anthracycline combinations to anthracycline-based combinations without taxanes [103]. Response rates were 57 % with taxanes versus 46 % without taxanes ($p<0.001$); PFS was modestly improved with taxane combinations (HR 0.92; 95 % CI, 0.85–0.99; $p=0.031$); and OS was not significantly different. Anthracycline-taxane combinations result in significant toxicity including febrile neutropenia, fatigue, cardiomyopathy, and neuropathy.

Non-anthracycline regimens are important due to the risk of cumulative cardiotoxicity with anthracyclines and frequent previous exposure either in the adjuvant or metastatic setting. Several combinations have been evaluated in phase III trials. These studies are limited by lack of complete crossover, such that the combination cannot be compared with sequential single agents. Docetaxel plus capecitabine improved RR and survival outcomes compared with docetaxel alone [125]. Paclitaxel every 3 weeks in combination with gemcitabine resulted in an improvement in all outcomes compared with paclitaxel alone. In contrast, when compared with weekly paclitaxel, the combinations of paclitaxel every 3 weeks plus carboplatin and docetaxel plus gemcitabine were inferior regarding OS without a significant difference in PFS [126]. Phase II studies of capecitabine (1,650 mg/m2/day) and weekly paclitaxel (80 mg/m2 days 1 and 8 every 21 days) show this to be an active and tolerable combination, even in patients who previously received paclitaxel every 3 weeks [127, 128].

For patients who relapse within 12 months of adjuvant anthracycline and taxane chemotherapy or with previous progression on these and other chemotherapies in the metastatic setting, there are still several other available chemotherapy options. Ixabepilone plus capecitabine improved RR and PFS, but not OS, when compared with capecitabine alone in heavily pretreated patients [129]. Ixabepilone use is limited by peripheral neuropathy and neutropenia. Gemcitabine combined with a platinum agent has activity in pretreated MBC [130, 131]. Vinorelbine combined with gemcitabine is also effective in pretreated MBC [132, 133].

Chemotherapy Duration

When MBC progresses on one regimen, then a different, non-cross-reactive chemotherapy is chosen based on preferences of both the patient and physician in regard to the side effect profile and logistics of treatment. The optimal duration of chemotherapy in the setting of a good response or stable disease is unclear and is a decision tailored to the individual patient. A meta-analysis including 2,269 patients found that giving first-line chemotherapy until progression, rather than for a predetermined number of cycles, resulted in an improved OS (HR 0.91; 95 % CI, 0.84–0.99; $p=0.046$) and PFS (HR 0.64; 95 % CI, 0.55–0.76; $p<0.001$) [134]. Many clinicians treat patients until progressive disease, as long as the chemotherapy is tolerated with an acceptable QOL. In patients with HER2+ or HR+ MBC, after a set number of cycles of chemotherapy or after a good response, a chemotherapy-free interval may be possible with the use of either HER2-targeted agents or hormone therapy.

For patients who have had a trial of three different sequential chemotherapy regimens and whose cancer has not at least stabilized with any of these, or for patients with an ECOG PS greater than 2, it is recommended to discontinue further attempts at chemotherapy and to discuss palliative and/or supportive care.

Other Molecularly Targeted Agents Combined with Chemotherapy in MBC

Vascular Endothelial Growth Factor Inhibition

Bevacizumab is a mAb directed against the vascular endothelial growth factor (VEGF) receptor, thereby inhibiting tumor angiogenesis. FDA approval for bevacizumab in combination with chemotherapy as first-line treatment of MBC was initially granted in 2008. The phase III, E2100 trial randomized 722 patients with untreated MBC, mostly HER2 negative, to the combination of bevacizumab (10 mg/kg every 2 weeks) and paclitaxel or to paclitaxel plus placebo [135]. The combination was found to be superior regarding PFS (11.8 versus 5.9 months) with no significant improvement in OS. Subsequent phase III first-line studies found similar results but with less of an impact on PFS and again no significant impact on OS. The AVADO trial showed an increase in PFS from 8.1 to 10 months with the addition of bevacizumab (15 mg/kg every 3 weeks) to docetaxel [136].

The RIBBON-1 trial randomized patients with HER2-negative, advanced breast cancer to chemotherapy of investigator's choice with or without bevacizumab (15 mg/kg every 3 weeks) and found a statistically significant increase in median PFS with the addition of bevacizumab to capecitabine, taxane, or anthracycline-based chemotherapy [137]. A meta-analysis of the above three trials in the first-line setting found no statistically significant difference in median OS (26.4 months without and 26.7 months with bevacizumab; HR 0.97; 95 % CI, 0.86–1.08, $p=0.056$) [138]. There was, however, a significant improvement in 1-year OS. The FDA withdrew approval of bevacizumab for MBC in the first-line setting in November 2011 as there was no significant OS benefit with its addition.

When evaluating the second-line setting in the RIBBON-2 trial, the addition of bevacizumab to chemotherapy, either capecitabine, taxane, gemcitabine, or vinorelbine, improved median PFS from 5.1 to 7.2 months, without a significant impact upon OS [139]. It is likely that certain subsets of patients are more sensitive to angiogenesis inhibition, but this information is not yet known. Based on this data, and the lack of FDA approval, bevacizumab is rarely used in the USA and used primarily in rapidly proliferative triple-negative disease in Europe. Use is complicated by lack of reimbursement of the drug, vascular-related side effects including hypertension and small vessel damage, as well as other potentially serious side effects.

Small molecule TKIs that target the VEGF receptor, sunitinib and motesanib, have been studied in MBC. In combination with chemotherapy, and compared with either placebo or bevacizumab, these TKIs have not shown clinically relevant activity, especially given their significant side effects [140–142].

Other Targeted Agents

Poly ADP-ribose polymerase (PARP) inhibitors are actively being studied, namely, in patients whose breast cancers have BRCA gene mutations. Mutated BRCA prevents repair of double-stranded DNA breaks by homologous repair. PARP inhibitors impair ability to repair single-stranded DNA damage, causing the accumulation of double-stranded DNA breaks. Without the ability to repair these double-stranded DNA breaks, BRCA-mutation breast cancers may be sensitive to treatment with PARP inhibitors, especially in combination with DNA-damaging chemotherapies such as platinum salts. Several clinical trials in selected patients are currently underway.

The epidermal growth factor receptor (EGFR) has been evaluated as a potential target especially in triple-negative MBC, where it is frequently overexpressed. Cetuximab, an anti-EGFR mAb, with or without carboplatin, was evaluated in the TBCRC001 study [143]. In 102 patients with triple-negative MBC, the combination had only modest antitumor activity, but 4 patients had responses lasting greater than 1 year. The BALI-1 phase II study found improved RR and PFS when cetuximab was added to cisplatin [144]. There may be biomarkers that can predict response to EGFR inhibition, with combinations of other targeted agents found to be more effective.

Special Situations

Bone Metastases

The bones are the most common site of breast cancer metastases and a frequent cause of morbidity including fractures, pain, spinal cord compression, and hypercalcemia. In conjunction with systemic antineoplastic therapy and appropriate local interventions, such as radiation and surgery, bone-targeted agents are an important part of management. In MBC, zoledronic acid reduced the risk of a skeletal-related event (SRE), mean time to SRE, and annual skeletal morbidity compared with both pamidronate and placebo [145, 146]. In a phase III trial, denosumab significantly delayed time to first and subsequent SRE compared with zoledronic acid, with no differences in OS, DFS, and serious adverse events [147]. Denosumab causes more hypocalcemia and is more costly but is associated with a quicker administration time, fewer acute-phase reactions, and fewer renal side effects. They appear to have similar rates of osteonecrosis of the jaw.

CNS Metastases

Metastases to the CNS occur in a small percentage of patients with MBC, but in HER2+ and triple-negative MBC, the incidence is approximately 30–45 % [9, 10, 148, 149]. There has been an increase in the incidence of brain metastases especially in HER2+ breast cancer, likely due to the improvement in systemic control with trastuzumab, which is unable to penetrate into the central nervous system [10]. In the pivotal trial that gained approval for the combination of capecitabine and lapatinib in MBC refractory to trastuzumab, the addition of lapatinib showed a trend toward decreased development of CNS metastases as first site of progression (4 versus 13 cases) [150].

Lapatinib alone, and in combination with capecitabine, has activity in progressive HER2+ brain metastases [151]. Lapatinib, neratinib, and other therapies targeted toward CNS metastases are being evaluated. Management of parenchymal brain metastases often involves a coordinated effort between neurosurgery, radiation oncology, and medical oncology. Leptomeningeal carcinomatosis is a devastating complication of MBC and often heralds the final stages of the patient's cancer. Treatment may include intrathecal chemotherapy, radiation, and supportive care with the involvement of hospice.

Summary

The heterogeneity of breast tumors and the uniqueness of each patient combined with a relative abundance of treatment options for MBC create a complex treatment landscape that the clinician must navigate on a case-by-case basis. Much progress has been made in the management of MBC that has resulted in improved survival over the past two decades. There is increasing consensus as to which treatments to use in specific settings of MBC, but there continue to be many unanswered questions.

While chemotherapy will likely always play a central role in the management of MBC for many years to come, it will become increasingly important to identify more specific targets that drive the metastatic process. We must also try to identify and block critical drivers with therapies that have tolerable side effects. Some of the more promising targets include PI3K inhibitors, which are being studied in several trials, Src TKIs such as dasatinib, and cyclin-dependent kinase inhibition of the MYC proto-oncogene signaling. There are exciting developments occurring in the areas of hormone- and trastuzumab-resistant MBC, combining targeted agents to overcome resistance.

Unfortunately, the molecular signaling environment within the cancer cell is quite complex, involving much redundancy and cross talk that allows for the development of resistance. Many of these pathways are common to nonmalignant cells, making some biologic therapies quite toxic to patients, especially when more than one targeted agent is needed to combat resistance. Antibody-drug conjugates deliver chemotherapy directly to the cancer cell that expresses the target of the antibody. These therapies are intriguing in that they may be highly effective and with minimal side effects. They rely on the presence of a cell-surface receptor, which limits their application to only certain cancers.

Triple-negative MBC is particularly challenging to manage. With no known targets, as there are in HR+ and HER2+, these patients rely only upon chemotherapy. Even when these cancers respond well to chemotherapy, resistance often develops quickly due to their inherent genetic instability. Novel treatments and identification of unique features that can be targeted are critically important. Other emerging trends include understanding the tumor microenvironment in an effort to target cells that support tumors and determining what triggers invasion and metastatic spread to prevent the development of late-stage disease.

References

1. Early Breast Cancer Trialists' Collaborative Group (EBCTCG). Effects of chemotherapy and hormonal therapy for early breast cancer on recurrence and 15-year survival: an overview of the randomised trials. Lancet. 2005;365(9472):1687–717.
2. Berry DA, Cronin KA, Plevritis SK, Fryback DG, Clarke L, Zelen M, et al. Effect of screening and adjuvant therapy on mortality from breast cancer. N Engl J Med. 2005;353(17):1784–92.
3. Khatcheressian JL, Wolff AC, Smith TJ, Grunfeld E, Muss HB, Vogel VG, et al. American Society of Clinical Oncology 2006 update of the breast cancer follow-up and management guidelines in the adjuvant setting. J Clin Oncol. 2006;24(31):5091–7.
4. Nicolini A, Anselmi L, Michelassi C, Carpi A. Prolonged survival by 'early' salvage treatment of breast cancer patients: a retrospective 6-year study. Br J Cancer. 1997;76(8):1106–11.
5. Impact of follow-up testing on survival and health-related quality of life in breast cancer patients. A multicenter randomized controlled trial. The GIVIO Investigators. JAMA 1994;271(20):1587–92.
6. Rosselli Del Turco M, Palli D, Cariddi A, Ciatto S, Pacini P, Distante V. Intensive diagnostic follow-up after treatment of primary breast cancer. A randomized trial. National Research Council Project on Breast Cancer follow-up. JAMA. 1994;271(20):1593–7.
7. Harris L, Fritsche H, Mennel R, Norton L, Ravdin P, Taube S, et al. American Society of Clinical Oncology 2007 update of recommendations for the use of tumor markers in breast cancer. J Clin Oncol. 2007;25(33):5287–312.
8. Pusztai L, Viale G, Kelly CM, Hudis CA. Estrogen and HER-2 receptor discordance between primary breast cancer and metastasis. Oncologist. 2010;15(11):1164–8.
9. Kennecke H, Yerushalmi R, Woods R, Cheang MC, Voduc D, Speers CH, et al. Metastatic behavior of breast cancer subtypes. J Clin Oncol. 2010;28(20):3271–7.
10. Brufsky AM, Mayer M, Rugo HS, Kaufman PA, Tan-Chiu E, Tripathy D, et al. Central nervous system metastases in patients with HER2-positive metastatic breast cancer: incidence, treatment, and survival in patients from registHER. Clin Cancer Res. 2011;17(14):4834–43.
11. Burzykowski T, Buyse M, Piccart-Gebhart MJ, Sledge G, Carmichael J, Luck HJ, et al. Evaluation of tumor response, disease control, progression-free survival, and time to progression as potential surrogate end points in metastatic breast cancer. J Clin Oncol. 2008;26(12):1987–92.
12. Osoba D. Health-related quality of life as a treatment endpoint in metastatic breast cancer. Can J Oncol. 1995;5 Suppl 1:47–53.
13. Geels P, Eisenhauer E, Bezjak A, Zee B, Day A. Palliative effect of chemotherapy: objective tumor response is associated with symptom improvement in patients with metastatic breast cancer. J Clin Oncol. 2000;18(12):2395–405.
14. Bruzzi P, Del Mastro L, Sormani MP, Bastholt L, Danova M, Focan C, et al. Objective response to chemotherapy as a potential surrogate end point of survival in metastatic breast cancer patients. J Clin Oncol. 2005;23(22):5117–25.
15. Chia SK, Speers CH, D'Yachkova Y, Kang A, Malfair-Taylor S, Barnett J, et al. The impact of new chemotherapeutic and hormone agents on survival in a population-based cohort of women with metastatic breast cancer. Cancer. 2007;110(5):973–9.
16. Gennari A, Conte P, Rosso R, Orlandini C, Bruzzi P. Survival of metastatic breast carcinoma patients over a 20-year period: a retrospective analysis based on individual patient data from six consecutive studies. Cancer. 2005;104(8):1742–50.

17. Dafni U, Grimani I, Xyrafas A, Eleftheraki AG, Fountzilas G. Fifteen-year trends in metastatic breast cancer survival in Greece. Breast Cancer Res Treat. 2010;119(3):621–31.
18. Mauri D, Polyzos NP, Salanti G, Pavlidis N, Ioannidis JP. Multiple-treatments meta-analysis of chemotherapy and targeted therapies in advanced breast cancer. J Natl Cancer Inst. 2008;100(24): 1780–91.
19. Giordano SH, Buzdar AU, Smith TL, Kau SW, Yang Y, Hortobagyi GN. Is breast cancer survival improving? Cancer. 2004;100(1):44–52.
20. Andre F, Slimane K, Bachelot T, Dunant A, Namer M, Barrelier A, et al. Breast cancer with synchronous metastases: trends in survival during a 14-year period. J Clin Oncol. 2004;22(16):3302–8.
21. Kiely BE, Soon YY, Tattersall MH, Stockler MR. How long have I got? Estimating typical, best-case, and worst-case scenarios for patients starting first-line chemotherapy for metastatic breast cancer: a systematic review of recent randomized trials. J Clin Oncol. 2011;29(4):456–63.
22. Dawood S, Broglio K, Gonzalez-Angulo AM, Buzdar AU, Hortobagyi GN, Giordano SH. Trends in survival over the past two decades among white and black patients with newly diagnosed stage IV breast cancer. J Clin Oncol. 2008;26(30):4891–8.
23. Clark GM, Sledge Jr GW, Osborne CK, McGuire WL. Survival from first recurrence: relative importance of prognostic factors in 1,015 breast cancer patients. J Clin Oncol. 1987;5(1):55–61.
24. Dawood S, Broglio K, Ensor J, Hortobagyi GN, Giordano SH. Survival differences among women with de novo stage IV and relapsed breast cancer. Ann Oncol. 2010;21(11):2169–74.
25. Greenberg PA, Hortobagyi GN, Smith TL, Ziegler LD, Frye DK, Buzdar AU. Long-term follow-up of patients with complete remission following combination chemotherapy for metastatic breast cancer. J Clin Oncol. 1996;14(8):2197–205.
26. Pagani O, Senkus E, Wood W, Colleoni M, Cufer T, Kyriakides S, et al. International guidelines for management of metastatic breast cancer: can metastatic breast cancer be cured? J Natl Cancer Inst. 2010; 102(7):456–63.
27. Wilcken N, Hornbuckle J, Ghersi D. Chemotherapy alone versus endocrine therapy alone for metastatic breast cancer. Cochrane Database Syst Rev. 2003;(2): CD002747.
28. Barrios CH, Sampaio C, Vinholes J, Caponero R. What is the role of chemotherapy in estrogen receptor-positive, advanced breast cancer? Ann Oncol. 2009;20(7):1157–62.
29. Jaiyesimi IA, Buzdar AU, Decker DA, Hortobagyi GN. Use of tamoxifen for breast cancer: twenty-eight years later. J Clin Oncol. 1995;13(2):513–29.
30. Pyrhonen S, Ellmen J, Vuorinen J, Gershanovich M, Tominaga T, Kaufmann M, et al. Meta-analysis of trials comparing toremifene with tamoxifen and factors predicting outcome of antiestrogen therapy in postmenopausal women with breast cancer. Breast Cancer Res Treat. 1999;56(2):133–43.
31. Bonneterre J, Thurlimann B, Robertson JF, Krzakowski M, Mauriac L, Koralewski P, et al. Anastrozole versus tamoxifen as first-line therapy for advanced breast cancer in 668 postmenopausal women: results of the Tamoxifen or Arimidex Randomized Group Efficacy and Tolerability study. J Clin Oncol. 2000;18(22):3748–57.
32. Nabholtz JM, Buzdar A, Pollak M, Harwin W, Burton G, Mangalik A, et al. Anastrozole is superior to tamoxifen as first-line therapy for advanced breast cancer in postmenopausal women: results of a North American multicenter randomized trial. Arimidex Study Group. J Clin Oncol. 2000;18(22):3758–67.
33. Vergote I, Bonneterre J, Thurlimann B, Robertson J, Krzakowski M, Mauriac L, et al. Randomised study of anastrozole versus tamoxifen as first-line therapy for advanced breast cancer in postmenopausal women. Eur J Cancer. 2000;36 Suppl 4:S84–5.
34. Thurlimann B, Robertson JF, Nabholtz JM, Buzdar A, Bonneterre J. Efficacy of tamoxifen following anastrozole ('Arimidex') compared with anastrozole following tamoxifen as first-line treatment for advanced breast cancer in postmenopausal women. Eur J Cancer. 2003;39(16):2310–7.
35. Mauri D, Pavlidis N, Polyzos NP, Ioannidis JP. Survival with aromatase inhibitors and inactivators versus standard hormonal therapy in advanced breast cancer: meta-analysis. J Natl Cancer Inst. 2006;98(18): 1285–91.
36. Lonning PE. Lack of complete cross-resistance between different aromatase inhibitors; a real finding in search for an explanation? Eur J Cancer. 2009;45(4): 527–35.
37. Di Leo A, Jerusalem G, Petruzelka L, Torres R, Bondarenko IN, Khasanov R, et al. Results of the CONFIRM phase III trial comparing fulvestrant 250 mg with fulvestrant 500 mg in postmenopausal women with estrogen receptor-positive advanced breast cancer. J Clin Oncol. 2010;28(30):4594–600.
38. Di Leo A, Jerusalem G, Petruzelka L, Torres R, Bondarenko I, Khasanov R, et al. Final analysis of overall survival for the Phase III CONFIRM trial: fulvestrant 500 mg versus 250 mg. Cancer Res. 2012;72(24 Supplement):S1–4.
39. Robertson JF, Llombart-Cussac A, Rolski J, Feltl D, Dewar J, Macpherson E, et al. Activity of fulvestrant 500 mg versus anastrozole 1 mg as first-line treatment for advanced breast cancer: results from the FIRST study. J Clin Oncol. 2009;27(27):4530–5.
40. Robertson JF, Lindemann JP, Llombart-Cussac A, Rolski J, Feltl D, Dewar J, et al. Fulvestrant 500 mg versus anastrozole 1 mg for the first-line treatment of advanced breast cancer: follow-up analysis from the randomized 'FIRST' study. Breast Cancer Res Treat. 2012;136(2):503–11.
41. Osborne CK, Coronado-Heinsohn EB, Hilsenbeck SG, McCue BL, Wakeling AE, McClelland RA, et al. Comparison of the effects of a pure steroidal

antiestrogen with those of tamoxifen in a model of human breast cancer. J Natl Cancer Inst. 1995;87(10): 746–50.
42. Howell A, Robertson JF, Quaresma Albano J, Aschermannova A, Mauriac L, Kleeberg UR, et al. Fulvestrant, formerly ICI 182,780, is as effective as anastrozole in postmenopausal women with advanced breast cancer progressing after prior endocrine treatment. J Clin Oncol. 2002;20(16):3396–403.
43. Osborne CK, Pippen J, Jones SE, Parker LM, Ellis M, Come S, et al. Double-blind, randomized trial comparing the efficacy and tolerability of fulvestrant versus anastrozole in postmenopausal women with advanced breast cancer progressing on prior endocrine therapy: results of a North American trial. J Clin Oncol. 2002;20(16):3386–95.
44. Robertson JF, Osborne CK, Howell A, Jones SE, Mauriac L, Ellis M, et al. Fulvestrant versus anastrozole for the treatment of advanced breast carcinoma in postmenopausal women: a prospective combined analysis of two multicenter trials. Cancer. 2003;98(2): 229–38.
45. Chia S, Gradishar W, Mauriac L, Bines J, Amant F, Federico M, et al. Double-blind, randomized placebo controlled trial of fulvestrant compared with exemestane after prior nonsteroidal aromatase inhibitor therapy in postmenopausal women with hormone receptor-positive, advanced breast cancer: results from EFECT. J Clin Oncol. 2008;26(10):1664–70.
46. Mehta RS, Barlow WE, Albain KS, Vandenberg TA, Dakhil SR, Tirumali NR, et al. Combination anastrozole and fulvestrant in metastatic breast cancer. N Engl J Med. 2012;367(5):435–44.
47. Bergh J, Jonsson PE, Lidbrink EK, Trudeau M, Eiermann W, Brattstrom D, et al. FACT: an open-label randomized phase III study of fulvestrant and anastrozole in combination compared with anastrozole alone as first-line therapy for patients with receptor-positive postmenopausal breast cancer. J Clin Oncol. 2012;30(16):1919–25.
48. Abrams J, Aisner J, Cirrincione C, Berry DA, Muss HB, Cooper MR, et al. Dose-response trial of megestrol acetate in advanced breast cancer: cancer and leukemia group B phase III study 8741. J Clin Oncol. 1999;17(1):64–73.
49. Ettinger DS, Allegra J, Bertino JR, Bonomi P, Browder H, Byrne P, et al. Megestrol acetate v tamoxifen in advanced breast cancer: correlation of hormone receptors and response. Semin Oncol. 1986;13(4 Suppl 4):9–14.
50. Lonning PE, Taylor PD, Anker G, Iddon J, Wie L, Jorgensen LM, et al. High-dose estrogen treatment in postmenopausal breast cancer patients heavily exposed to endocrine therapy. Breast Cancer Res Treat. 2001;67(2):111–6.
51. Ellis MJ, Gao F, Dehdashti F, Jeffe DB, Marcom PK, Carey LA, et al. Lower-dose vs high-dose oral estradiol therapy of hormone receptor-positive, aromatase inhibitor-resistant advanced breast cancer: a phase 2 randomized study. JAMA. 2009;302(7):774–80.
52. Huober J, Fasching PA, Barsoum M, Petruzelka L, Wallwiener D, Thomssen C, et al. Higher efficacy of letrozole in combination with trastuzumab compared to letrozole monotherapy as first-line treatment in patients with HER2-positive, hormone-receptor-positive metastatic breast cancer – results of the eLEcTRA trial. Breast. 2012;21(1):27–33.
53. Kaufman B, Mackey JR, Clemens MR, Bapsy PP, Vaid A, Wardley A, et al. Trastuzumab plus anastrozole versus anastrozole alone for the treatment of postmenopausal women with human epidermal growth factor receptor 2-positive, hormone receptor-positive metastatic breast cancer: results from the randomized phase III TAnDEM study. J Clin Oncol. 2009;27(33):5529–37.
54. Johnston S, Pippen Jr J, Pivot X, Lichinitser M, Sadeghi S, Dieras V, et al. Lapatinib combined with letrozole versus letrozole and placebo as first-line therapy for postmenopausal hormone receptor-positive metastatic breast cancer. J Clin Oncol. 2009;27(33):5538–46.
55. Koeberle D, Ruhstaller T, Jost L, Pagani O, Zaman K, von Moos R, et al. Combination of trastuzumab and letrozole after resistance to sequential trastuzumab and aromatase inhibitor monotherapies in patients with estrogen receptor-positive, HER-2-positive advanced breast cancer: a proof-of-concept trial (SAKK 23/03). Endocr Relat Cancer. 2011;18(2): 257–64.
56. Baselga J, Campone M, Piccart M, Burris 3rd HA, Rugo HS, Sahmoud T, et al. Everolimus in postmenopausal hormone-receptor-positive advanced breast cancer. N Engl J Med. 2012;366(6):520–9.
57. Campone M, Bachelot T, Gnant M, Deleu I, Rugo HS, Pistilli B, et al. Effect of visceral metastases on the efficacy and safety of everolimus in postmenopausal women with advanced breast cancer: Subgroup analysis from the BOLERO-2 study. Eur J Cancer. 2013;49:2621–32.
58. Hortobagyi GN, Piccart M, Rugo H, Burris H, Campone M, Noguchi S, et al. Everolimus for postmenopausal women with advanced breast cancer: updated results for the BOLERO-2 phase III trial. Cancer Res. 2011;71 Suppl 24:S3–7. abstr nr.
59. Burris 3rd HA, Lebrun F, Rugo HS, Beck JT, Piccart M, Neven P, et al. Health-related quality of life of patients with advanced breast cancer treated with everolimus plus exemestane versus placebo plus exemestane in the phase 3, randomized, controlled, BOLERO-2 trial. Cancer. 2013;119(10):1908–15.
60. Bachelot T, Bourgier C, Cropet C, Ray-Coquard I, Ferrero JM, Freyer G, et al. Randomized phase II trial of everolimus in combination with tamoxifen in patients with hormone receptor-positive, human epidermal growth factor receptor 2-negative metastatic breast cancer with prior exposure to aromatase inhibitors: a GINECO study. J Clin Oncol. 2012;30(22): 2718–24.
61. Finn RS, Crown JP, Lang I, et al. Results of a randomized phase 2 study of PD 0332991, a cyclin-dependent

kinase (CDK) 4/6 inhibitor, in combination with letrozole vs letrozole alone for first-line treatment of ER+/HER2- advanced breast cancer (BC). Presented at: 2012 CTRC-AACR San Antonio Breast Cancer Symposium; 2012. Abstract S1–6.
62. Yardley DA, Burris 3rd HA, Clark BL, Shipley D, Rubin M, Barton Jr J, et al. Hormonal therapy plus bevacizumab in postmenopausal patients who have hormone receptor-positive metastatic breast cancer: a phase II Trial of the Sarah Cannon Oncology Research Consortium. Clin Breast Cancer. 2011;11(3):146–52.
63. Martin M, Loibl S, von Minckwitz G, Morales S, Crespo C, Anton A, et al. Phase III trial evaluating the addition of bevacizumab to endocrine therapy as first-line treatment for advanced breast cancer – first efficacy results from the LEA study. Cancer Res. 2012;72(24 Supplement):S1–7.
64. Traina TA, Rugo HS, Caravelli JF, Patil S, Yeh B, Melisko ME, et al. Feasibility trial of letrozole in combination with bevacizumab in patients with metastatic breast cancer. J Clin Oncol. 2010;28(4): 628–33.
65. Yardley DA, Ismail-Khan R, Kelvin P. Results of ENCORE 301, a randomized, phase II, double-blind, placebo-controlled study of exemestane with or without entinostat in postmenopausal women with locally recurrent or metastatic estrogen-receptor-positive (ER+) breast cancer progressing on a nonsteroidal aromatase inhibitor (AI). J Clin Oncol. 2011;29(27s): abstr 268.
66. Yardley DA, Ismail-Khan RR, Melichar B, et al. Randomized phase II, double-blind, placebo-controlled study of exemestane with or without entinostat in postmenopausal women with locally recurrent or metastatic estrogen receptor-positive breast cancer progressing on treatment with a nonsteroidal aromatase inhibitor. J Clin Oncol. 2013;31: 2128–35.
67. Baselga J, Campone M, Cortes J, Iwata H, de Laurentiis M, Jonat W, et al. Phase III randomized study of the oral pan-PI3K inhibitor BKM120 with fulvestrant in postmenopausal women with HR+/HER2- locally advanced or metastatic breast cancer resistant to aromatase inhibitor – BELLE-2. Cancer Res. 2012;72(24 Supplement):OT2-3-09.
68. Di Leo A, Germa C, Weber D, Di Tomaso E, Dharan B, Massacesi C, et al. Phase III randomized study of the oral pan-PI3K inhibitor BKM120 with fulvestrant in postmenopausal women with HR+/HER2- locally advanced or metastatic breast cancer, treated with aromatase inhibitor, and progressed on or after mTOR inhibitor-based treatment – BELLE-3. Cancer Res. 2012;72(24 Supplement):OT2-3-08.
69. Slamon DJ, Clark GM, Wong SG, Levin WJ, Ullrich A, McGuire WL. Human breast cancer: correlation of relapse and survival with amplification of the HER-2/neu oncogene. Science. 1987;235(4785):177–82.
70. Slamon DJ, Leyland-Jones B, Shak S, Fuchs H, Paton V, Bajamonde A, et al. Use of chemotherapy plus a monoclonal antibody against HER2 for metastatic breast cancer that overexpresses HER2. N Engl J Med. 2001;344(11):783–92.
71. Cobleigh MA, Vogel CL, Tripathy D, Robert NJ, Scholl S, Fehrenbacher L, et al. Multinational study of the efficacy and safety of humanized anti-HER2 monoclonal antibody in women who have HER2-overexpressing metastatic breast cancer that has progressed after chemotherapy for metastatic disease. J Clin Oncol. 1999;17(9):2639–48.
72. Geyer CE, Forster J, Lindquist D, et al. Lapatinib plus capecitabine for HER2-positive advanced breast cancer. N Engl J Med. 2006;355:2733–43.
73. Blackwell K, Burstein HJ, Storniolo AM, et al. Overall survival benefit with lapatinib in combination with trastuzumab for patients with human epidermal growth factor receptor 2-positive metastatic breast cancer: final results from the EGF104900 Study. J Clin Oncol. 2012;30:2585–92.
74. Harris CA, Ward RL, Dobbins TA, Drew AK, Pearson S. The efficacy of HER2-targeted agents in metastatic breast cancer: a meta-analysis. Ann Oncol. 2011; 22(6):1308–17.
75. Dawood S, Broglio K, Buzdar AU, Hortobagyi GN, Giordano SH. Prognosis of women with metastatic breast cancer by HER2 status and trastuzumab treatment: an institutional-based review. J Clin Oncol. 2010;28(1):92–8.
76. Yip AY, Tse LA, Ong EY, Chow LW. Survival benefits from lapatinib therapy in women with HER2-overexpressing breast cancer: a systematic review. Anticancer Drugs. 2010;21(5):487–93.
77. Vogel CL, Cobleigh MA, Tripathy D, Gutheil JC, Harris LN, Fehrenbacher L, et al. Efficacy and safety of trastuzumab as a single agent in first-line treatment of HER2-overexpressing metastatic breast cancer. J Clin Oncol. 2002;20(3):719–26.
78. Inoue K, Nakagami K, Mizutani M, Hozumi Y, Fujiwara Y, Masuda N, et al. Randomized phase III trial of trastuzumab monotherapy followed by trastuzumab plus docetaxel versus trastuzumab plus docetaxel as first-line therapy in patients with HER2-positive metastatic breast cancer: the JO17360 Trial Group. Breast Cancer Res Treat. 2010;119(1): 127–36.
79. Hamberg P, Bos MM, Braun HJ, Stouthard JM, van Deijk GA, Erdkamp FL, et al. Randomized phase II study comparing efficacy and safety of combination-therapy trastuzumab and docetaxel vs. sequential therapy of trastuzumab followed by docetaxel alone at progression as first-line chemotherapy in patients with HER2+ metastatic breast cancer: HERTAX trial. Clin Breast Cancer. 2011;11(2):103–13.
80. Marty M, Cognetti F, Maraninchi D, Snyder R, Mauriac L, Tubiana-Hulin M, et al. Randomized phase II trial of the efficacy and safety of trastuzumab combined with docetaxel in patients with human epidermal growth factor receptor 2-positive metastatic breast cancer administered as first-line treatment: the M77001 study group. J Clin Oncol. 2005;23(19): 4265–74.

81. Gelmon KA, Boyle F, Kaufman B, Huntsman D, Manikhas A, Di Leo A, et al. Open-label phase III randomized controlled trial comparing taxane-based chemotherapy (Tax) with lapatinib (L) or trastuzumab (T) as first-line therapy for women with HER2+ metastatic breast cancer: interim analysis (IA) of NCIC CTG MA.31/GSK EGF 108919. ASCO meeting abstracts. 2012;30(15 suppl):LBA671.
82. Baselga J, Cortes J, Kim SB, Im SA, Hegg R, Im YH, et al. Pertuzumab plus trastuzumab plus docetaxel for metastatic breast cancer. N Engl J Med. 2012;366(2): 109–19.
83. Swain SM, Kim SB, Cortes J, Ro J, Semiglazov V, Campone M, et al. Pertuzumab, trastuzumab, and docetaxel for HER2-positive metastatic breast cancer (CLEOPATRA study): overall survival results from a randomised, double-blind, placebo-controlled, phase 3 study. Lancet Oncol. 2013;14(6):461–71.
84. von Minckwitz G, du Bois A, Schmidt M, Maass N, Cufer T, de Jongh FE, et al. Trastuzumab beyond progression in human epidermal growth factor receptor 2-positive advanced breast cancer: a German breast group 26/breast international group 03-05 study. J Clin Oncol. 2009;27(12):1999–2006.
85. Cameron D, Casey M, Oliva C, Newstat B, Imwalle B, Geyer CE. Lapatinib plus capecitabine in women with HER-2-positive advanced breast cancer: final survival analysis of a phase III randomized trial. Oncologist. 2010;15(9):924–34.
86. Burris 3rd HA, Rugo HS, Vukelja SJ, Vogel CL, Borson RA, Limentani S, et al. Phase II study of the antibody drug conjugate trastuzumab-DM1 for the treatment of human epidermal growth factor receptor 2 (HER2)-positive breast cancer after prior HER2-directed therapy. J Clin Oncol. 2011;29(4):398–405.
87. Krop IE, LoRusso P, Miller KD, Modi S, Yardley D, Rodriguez G, et al. A phase II study of trastuzumab emtansine in patients with human epidermal growth factor receptor 2-positive metastatic breast cancer who were previously treated with trastuzumab, lapatinib, an anthracycline, a taxane, and capecitabine. J Clin Oncol. 2012;30(26):3234–41.
88. Verma S, Miles D, Gianni L, Krop IE, Welslau M, Baselga J, et al. Trastuzumab emtansine for HER2-positive advanced breast cancer. N Engl J Med. 2012;367(19):1783–91.
89. Baselga J, Gelmon KA, Verma S, Wardley A, Conte P, Miles D, et al. Phase II trial of pertuzumab and trastuzumab in patients with human epidermal growth factor receptor 2-positive metastatic breast cancer that progressed during prior trastuzumab therapy. J Clin Oncol. 2010;28(7):1138–44.
90. Burstein HJ, Sun Y, Dirix LY, Jiang A, Paridaens R, Tan AR, et al. Neratinib, an irreversible ErbB receptor tyrosine kinase inhibitor in patients with advanced ErbB2-positive breast cancer. J Clin Oncol. 2010;28:1301–7.
91. Andre F, Campone M, O'Regan R, Manlius C, Massacesi C, Sahmoud T, et al. Phase I study of everolimus plus weekly paclitaxel and trastuzumab in patients with metastatic breast cancer pretreated with trastuzumab. J Clin Oncol. 2010;28(34):5110–5.
92. Dalenc F, Campone M, Hupperets P, O'Regan R, Manlius C, Vittori L, et al. Everolimus in combination with weekly paclitaxel and trastuzumab in patients (pts) with HER2-overexpressing metastatic breast cancer (MBC) with prior resistance to trastuzumab and taxanes: A multicenter phase II clinical trial. J Clin Oncol. 2010;28(15s):1013. abstr.
93. Jerusalem GH, Fasolo A, Massacesi C, M B, Manlius C, Sahmoud T, et al. Maintenance with everolimus (RAD001) and trastuzumab (T) after discontinuation of chemotherapy in patients (pts) with heavily pretreated HER2-positive metastatic breast cancer (MBC): Pooled data of extension cohorts of phase Ib/II studies. J Clin Oncol. 2010;28(15s):suppl; abstr 1041.
94. Jerusalem G, Fasolo A, Dieras V, Cardoso F, Bergh J, Vittori L, et al. Phase I trial of oral mTOR inhibitor everolimus in combination with trastuzumab and vinorelbine in pre-treated patients with HER2-overexpressing metastatic breast cancer. Breast Cancer Res Treat. 2011;125(2):447–55.
95. O'Regan RM, Ozguroglu M, Andre F, Toi M, Jerusalem G, Wilks S, et al., editors. Phase 3, randomized, double-blind, placebo-controlled multicenter trial of daily everolimus plus weekly trastuzumab and vinorelbine in trastuzumab-resistant, advanced breast cancer (BOLERO-3). ASCO annual meeting; Chicago, 2013.
96. Carrick S, Parker S, Wilcken N, Ghersi D, Marzo M, Simes J. Single agent versus combination chemotherapy for metastatic breast cancer. Cochrane Database Syst Rev. 2005;(2):CD003372.
97. Sledge GW, Neuberg D, Bernardo P, Ingle JN, Martino S, Rowinsky EK, et al. Phase III trial of doxorubicin, paclitaxel, and the combination of doxorubicin and paclitaxel as front-line chemotherapy for metastatic breast cancer: an intergroup trial (E1193). J Clin Oncol. 2003;21(4):588–92.
98. Cresta S, Grasselli G, Mansutti M, Martoni A, Lelli G, Capri G, et al. A randomized phase II study of combination, alternating and sequential regimens of doxorubicin and docetaxel as first-line chemotherapy for women with metastatic breast cancer. Ann Oncol. 2004;15(3):433–9.
99. Conte PF, Guarneri V, Bruzzi P, Prochilo T, Salvadori B, Bolognesi A, et al. Concomitant versus sequential administration of epirubicin and paclitaxel as first-line therapy in metastatic breast carcinoma: results for the Gruppo Oncologico Nord Ovest randomized trial. Cancer. 2004;101(4):704–12.
100. Alba E, Martin M, Ramos M, Adrover E, Balil A, Jara C, et al. Multicenter randomized trial comparing

sequential with concomitant administration of doxorubicin and docetaxel as first-line treatment of metastatic breast cancer: a Spanish Breast Cancer Research Group (GEICAM-9903) phase III study. J Clin Oncol. 2004;22(13):2587–93.
101. Burstein HJ, Mangu PB, Somerfield MR, Schrag D, Samson D, Holt L, et al. American Society of Clinical Oncology clinical practice guideline update on the use of chemotherapy sensitivity and resistance assays. J Clin Oncol. 2011;29(24):3328–30.
102. Paridaens R, Biganzoli L, Bruning P, Klijn JG, Gamucci T, Houston S, et al. Paclitaxel versus doxorubicin as first-line single-agent chemotherapy for metastatic breast cancer: a European Organization for Research and Treatment of Cancer Randomized Study with cross-over. J Clin Oncol. 2000;18(4):724–33.
103. Piccart-Gebhart MJ, Burzykowski T, Buyse M, Sledge G, Carmichael J, Luck HJ, et al. Taxanes alone or in combination with anthracyclines as first-line therapy of patients with metastatic breast cancer. J Clin Oncol. 2008;26(12):1980–6.
104. Yonemori K, Katsumata N, Uno H, Matsumoto K, Kouno T, Tokunaga S, et al. Efficacy of weekly paclitaxel in patients with docetaxel-resistant metastatic breast cancer. Breast Cancer Res Treat. 2005;89(3):237–41.
105. Sawaki M, Ito Y, Hashimoto D, Mizunuma N, Takahashi S, Horikoshi N, et al. Paclitaxel administered weekly in patients with docetaxel-resistant metastatic breast cancer: a single-center study. Tumori. 2004;90(1):36–9.
106. Seidman AD, Berry D, Cirrincione C, Harris L, Muss H, Marcom PK, et al. Randomized phase III trial of weekly compared with every-3-weeks paclitaxel for metastatic breast cancer, with trastuzumab for all HER-2 overexpressors and random assignment to trastuzumab or not in HER-2 nonoverexpressors: final results of Cancer and Leukemia Group B protocol 9840. J Clin Oncol. 2008;26(10):1642–9.
107. Jones SE, Erban J, Overmoyer B, Budd GT, Hutchins L, Lower E, et al. Randomized phase III study of docetaxel compared with paclitaxel in metastatic breast cancer. J Clin Oncol. 2005;23(24):5542–51.
108. Mauri D, Kamposioras K, Tsali L, Bristianou M, Valachis A, Karathanasi I, et al. Overall survival benefit for weekly vs. three-weekly taxanes regimens in advanced breast cancer: a meta-analysis. Cancer Treat Rev. 2010;36(1):69–74.
109. Gradishar WJ, Tjulandin S, Davidson N, Shaw H, Desai N, Bhar P, et al. Phase III trial of nanoparticle albumin-bound paclitaxel compared with polyethylated castor oil-based paclitaxel in women with breast cancer. J Clin Oncol. 2005;23(31):7794–803.
110. Gradishar WJ, Krasnojon D, Cheporov S, Makhson AN, Manikhas GM, Clawson A, et al. Significantly longer progression-free survival with nab-paclitaxel compared with docetaxel as first-line therapy for metastatic breast cancer. J Clin Oncol. 2009;27(22):3611–9.
111. O'Brien ME, Wigler N, Inbar M, Rosso R, Grischke E, Santoro A, et al. Reduced cardiotoxicity and comparable efficacy in a phase III trial of pegylated liposomal doxorubicin HCl (CAELYX/Doxil) versus conventional doxorubicin for first-line treatment of metastatic breast cancer. Ann Oncol. 2004;15(3):440–9.
112. Harris L, Batist G, Belt R, Rovira D, Navari R, Azarnia N, et al. Liposome-encapsulated doxorubicin compared with conventional doxorubicin in a randomized multicenter trial as first-line therapy of metastatic breast carcinoma. Cancer. 2002;94(1):25–36.
113. Batist G, Ramakrishnan G, Rao CS, Chandrasekharan A, Gutheil J, Guthrie T, et al. Reduced cardiotoxicity and preserved antitumor efficacy of liposome-encapsulated doxorubicin and cyclophosphamide compared with conventional doxorubicin and cyclophosphamide in a randomized, multicenter trial of metastatic breast cancer. J Clin Oncol. 2001;19(5):1444–54.
114. Oshaughnessy JA, Blum J, Moiseyenko V, Jones SE, Miles D, Bell D, et al. Randomized, open-label, phase II trial of oral capecitabine (Xeloda) vs. a reference arm of intravenous CMF (cyclophosphamide, methotrexate and 5-fluorouracil) as first-line therapy for advanced/metastatic breast cancer. Ann Oncol. 2001;12(9):1247–54.
115. Blum JL, Barrios CH, Feldman N, Verma S, McKenna EF, Lee LF, et al. Pooled analysis of individual patient data from capecitabine monotherapy clinical trials in locally advanced or metastatic breast cancer. Breast Cancer Res Treat. 2012;136(3):777–88.
116. Blum JL, Jones SE, Buzdar AU, LoRusso PM, Kuter I, Vogel C, et al. Multicenter phase II study of capecitabine in paclitaxel-refractory metastatic breast cancer. J Clin Oncol. 1999;17(2):485–93.
117. Blum JL, Dieras V, Lo Russo PM, Horton J, Rutman O, Buzdar A, et al. Multicenter, Phase II study of capecitabine in taxane-pretreated metastatic breast carcinoma patients. Cancer. 2001;92(7):1759–68.
118. Rossi D, Alessandroni P, Catalano V, Giordani P, Fedeli SL, Fedeli A, et al. Safety profile and activity of lower capecitabine dose in patients with metastatic breast cancer. Clin Breast Cancer. 2007;7(11):857–60.
119. Fumoleau P, Largillier R, Clippe C, Dieras V, Orfeuvre H, Lesimple T, et al. Multicentre, phase II study evaluating capecitabine monotherapy in

patients with anthracycline- and taxane-pretreated metastatic breast cancer. Eur J Cancer. 2004;40(4):536–42.
120. Hennessy BT, Gauthier AM, Michaud LB, Hortobagyi G, Valero V. Lower dose capecitabine has a more favorable therapeutic index in metastatic breast cancer: retrospective analysis of patients treated at M. D. Anderson Cancer Center and a review of capecitabine toxicity in the literature. Ann Oncol. 2005;16(8):1289–96.
121. Leonard R, Hennessy BT, Blum JL, O'Shaughnessy J. Dose-adjusting capecitabine minimizes adverse effects while maintaining efficacy: a retrospective review of capecitabine for metastatic breast cancer. Clin Breast Cancer. 2011;11(6):349–56.
122. Cortes J, O'Shaughnessy J, Loesch D, Blum JL, Vahdat LT, Petrakova K, et al. Eribulin monotherapy versus treatment of physician's choice in patients with metastatic breast cancer (EMBRACE): a phase 3 open-label randomised study. Lancet. 2011; 377(9769):914–23.
123. Kaufman P, Awada A, Twelves C, Yelle L, Perez E, Wanders J, et al. A Phase III, open-label, randomized, multicenter study of eribulin mesylate versus capecitabine in patients with locally advanced or metastatic breast cancer previously treated with anthracyclines and taxanes. Cancer Res. 2012;72(24 Supplement):S6.
124. Bria E, Giannarelli D, Felici A, Peters WP, Nistico C, Vanni B, et al. Taxanes with anthracyclines as first-line chemotherapy for metastatic breast carcinoma. Cancer. 2005;103(4):672–9.
125. O'Shaughnessy J, Miles D, Vukelja S, Moiseyenko V, Ayoub JP, Cervantes G, et al. Superior survival with capecitabine plus docetaxel combination therapy in anthracycline-pretreated patients with advanced breast cancer: phase III trial results. J Clin Oncol. 2002;20(12):2812–23.
126. Fountzilas G, Dafni U, Dimopoulos MA, Koutras A, Skarlos D, Papakostas P, et al. A randomized phase III study comparing three anthracycline-free taxane-based regimens, as first line chemotherapy, in metastatic breast cancer: a Hellenic Cooperative Oncology Group study. Breast Cancer Res Treat. 2009;115(1):87–99.
127. Blum JL, Dees EC, Chacko A, Doane L, Ethirajan S, Hopkins J, et al. Phase II trial of capecitabine and weekly paclitaxel as first-line therapy for metastatic breast cancer. J Clin Oncol. 2006;24(27):4384–90.
128. Blum JL, Dees EC, Vukelja SJ, Amare M, Gill DP, McMahon RT, et al. Phase II trial of capecitabine and weekly paclitaxel in patients with metastatic breast cancer previously treated with every-3-week taxane therapy. Clin Breast Cancer. 2007;7(6):465–70.
129. Thomas ES, Gomez HL, Li RK, Chung HC, Fein LE, Chan VF, et al. Ixabepilone plus capecitabine for metastatic breast cancer progressing after anthracycline and taxane treatment. J Clin Oncol. 2007; 25(33):5210–7.
130. Nagourney RA, Link JS, Blitzer JB, Forsthoff C, Evans SS. Gemcitabine plus cisplatin repeating doublet therapy in previously treated, relapsed breast cancer patients. J Clin Oncol. 2000;18(11):2245–9.
131. Burch PA, Mailliard JA, Hillman DW, Perez EA, Krook JE, Rowland KM, et al. Phase II study of gemcitabine plus cisplatin in patients with metastatic breast cancer: a North Central Cancer Treatment Group Trial. Am J Clin Oncol. 2005;28(2): 195–200.
132. Pallis AG, Boukovinas I, Ardavanis A, Varthalitis I, Malamos N, Georgoulias V, et al. A multicenter randomized phase III trial of vinorelbine/gemcitabine doublet versus capecitabine monotherapy in anthracycline- and taxane-pretreated women with metastatic breast cancer. Ann Oncol. 2012;23(5):1164–9.
133. Martin M, Ruiz A, Munoz M, Balil A, Garcia-Mata J, Calvo L, et al. Gemcitabine plus vinorelbine versus vinorelbine monotherapy in patients with metastatic breast cancer previously treated with anthracyclines and taxanes: final results of the phase III Spanish Breast Cancer Research Group (GEICAM) trial. Lancet Oncol. 2007;8(3):219–25.
134. Gennari A, Stockler M, Puntoni M, Sormani M, Nanni O, Amadori D, et al. Duration of chemotherapy for metastatic breast cancer: a systematic review and meta-analysis of randomized clinical trials. J Clin Oncol. 2011;29(16):2144–9.
135. Miller K, Wang M, Gralow J, Dickler M, Cobleigh M, Perez EA, et al. Paclitaxel plus bevacizumab versus paclitaxel alone for metastatic breast cancer. N Engl J Med. 2007;357(26):2666–76.
136. Miles DW, Chan A, Dirix LY, Cortes J, Pivot X, Tomczak P, et al. Phase III study of bevacizumab plus docetaxel compared with placebo plus docetaxel for the first-line treatment of human epidermal growth factor receptor 2-negative metastatic breast cancer. J Clin Oncol. 2010;28(20):3239–47.
137. Robert NJ, Dieras V, Glaspy J, Brufsky AM, Bondarenko I, Lipatov ON, et al. RIBBON-1: randomized, double-blind, placebo-controlled, phase III trial of chemotherapy with or without bevacizumab for first-line treatment of human epidermal growth factor receptor 2-negative, locally recurrent or metastatic breast cancer. J Clin Oncol. 2011;29(10):1252–60.
138. O'Shaughnessy J, Miles D, Gray RJ, Dieras V, Perez EA, Zon R, et al. A meta-analysis of overall survival data from three randomized trials of bevacizumab (BV) and first-line chemotherapy as treatment for patients with metastatic breast cancer (MBC). ASCO meeting abstracts. 2010;28(15 suppl):1005.
139. Brufsky AM, Hurvitz S, Perez E, Swamy R, Valero V, O'Neill V, et al. RIBBON-2: a randomized, double-blind, placebo-controlled, phase III trial evaluating the efficacy and safety of bevacizumab in combination with chemotherapy for second-line treatment of human epidermal growth factor receptor 2-negative metastatic breast cancer. J Clin Oncol. 2011;29(32):4286–93.

140. Bergh J, Bondarenko IM, Lichinitser MR, Liljegren A, Greil R, Voytko NL, et al. First-line treatment of advanced breast cancer with sunitinib in combination with docetaxel versus docetaxel alone: results of a prospective, randomized phase III study. J Clin Oncol. 2012;30(9):921–9.
141. Robert NJ, Saleh MN, Paul D, Generali D, Gressot L, Copur MS, et al. Sunitinib plus paclitaxel versus bevacizumab plus paclitaxel for first-line treatment of patients with advanced breast cancer: a phase III, randomized, open-label trial. Clin Breast Cancer. 2011;11(2):82–92.
142. Martin M, Roche H, Pinter T, Crown J, Kennedy MJ, Provencher L, et al. Motesanib, or open-label bevacizumab, in combination with paclitaxel, as first-line treatment for HER2-negative locally recurrent or metastatic breast cancer: a phase 2, randomised, double-blind, placebo-controlled study. Lancet Oncol. 2011;12(4):369–76.
143. Carey LA, Rugo HS, Marcom PK, Mayer EL, Esteva FJ, Ma CX, et al. TBCRC 001: randomized phase II study of cetuximab in combination with carboplatin in stage IV triple-negative breast cancer. J Clin Oncol. 2012;30(21):2615–23.
144. Baselga J, Gomez P, Awada A, editors. The addition of cetuximab to cisplatin increases overall response rate and progression-free survival in metastatic triple-negative breast cancer:results of a randomized phase II study (BALI-1). 35th European Society of Medical Oncology Congress. Milan; 2010.
145. Rosen LS, Gordon D, Kaminski M, Howell A, Belch A, Mackey J, et al. Long-term efficacy and safety of zoledronic acid compared with pamidronate disodium in the treatment of skeletal complications in patients with advanced multiple myeloma or breast carcinoma: a randomized, double-blind, multicenter, comparative trial. Cancer. 2003;98(8):1735–44.
146. Kohno N, Aogi K, Minami H, Nakamura S, Asaga T, Iino Y, et al. Zoledronic acid significantly reduces skeletal complications compared with placebo in Japanese women with bone metastases from breast cancer: a randomized, placebo-controlled trial. J Clin Oncol. 2005;23(15):3314–21.
147. Stopeck AT, Lipton A, Body JJ, Steger GG, Tonkin K, de Boer RH, et al. Denosumab compared with zoledronic acid for the treatment of bone metastases in patients with advanced breast cancer: a randomized, double-blind study. J Clin Oncol. 2010; 28(35):5132–9.
148. Lin NU, Claus E, Sohl J, Razzak AR, Arnaout A, Winer EP. Sites of distant recurrence and clinical outcomes in patients with metastatic triple-negative breast cancer: high incidence of central nervous system metastases. Cancer. 2008;113(10):2638–45.
149. Bendell JC, Domchek SM, Burstein HJ, Harris L, Younger J, Kuter I, et al. Central nervous system metastases in women who receive trastuzumab-based therapy for metastatic breast carcinoma. Cancer. 2003;97(12):2972–7.
150. Cameron D, Casey M, Press M, Lindquist D, Pienkowski T, Romieu CG, et al. A phase III randomized comparison of lapatinib plus capecitabine versus capecitabine alone in women with advanced breast cancer that has progressed on trastuzumab: updated efficacy and biomarker analyses. Breast Cancer Res Treat. 2008;112(3):533–43.
151. Lin NU, Dieras V, Paul D, Lossignol D, Christodoulou C, Stemmler HJ, et al. Multicenter phase II study of lapatinib in patients with brain metastases from HER2-positive breast cancer. Clin Cancer Res. 2009;15(4):1452–9.

Anesthetic Considerations for the Patient with Breast Disease

31

Maria A. Kimovec, Akram Abdoue, and Rebecca Grutsch

Abbreviations

BMI	Body mass index
COX-2	Cyclooxygenase-2
CPAP	Continuous positive airway pressure
CPET	Cardiac pulmonary exercise testing
ECHO	Echocardiograph
EKG	Electrocardiograph
EMLA	Eutectic mixture of local anesthetic
HIF	Hypoxia-inducible factor
NK	Natural killer
OSA	Obstructive sleep apnea
PONV	Postoperative nausea and vomiting
SPWC	Surgically placed wound catheters

Introduction

What makes anesthesia for breast cancer surgical patients special? In some ways, the anesthetic management is similar to other surgical cases. However, the wide range of ages of these patients in an anxious population with a large emotional component can be challenging for the anesthesiologist. Recently, both animal and human research has challenged the routine anesthetic care for breast cancer patients with an intriguing concept. The anesthetic techniques, anesthetic agent choices, and even the timing of surgery may affect the breast cancer patient's recurrence rate in future years. Will the anesthesia that is selected affect a surgeon's mortality results? This is a controversial area open for discussion.

Newer techniques for the intraoperative care and postoperative pain management are expanding the anesthesiologists' role in the perioperative care of these oncologic patients. These techniques include thoracic epidurals and paravertebral blocks, for both intraoperative and postoperative care. Aggressive management of postoperative pain and nausea and vomiting can increase patient satisfaction with their experience.

As newer genetic and cellular functions can be tested and anesthetic agents and techniques titrated to particular patients, the anesthetic management can then be individualized for the best outcome. This may play a vital role in the care of the patient as their prognosis and life may depend on it. By minimizing the physiologic and psychological stress of the perioperative experience, the patient can have an improved prognosis and long-term better quality of life.

M.A. Kimovec, MD (✉) • A. Abdoue, MD
Department of Anesthesia, Advocate Christ Medical Center, University of Illinois College of Medicine at Chicago, 4440 West 95th Street, Oak Lawn, IL 60453-2600, USA
e-mail: mkimovecgrutsch@yahoo.com; akramabdoue@att.net

R. Grutsch, MD
Department of Anesthesiology and Critical Care Medicine, The Johns Hopkins Hospital, Johns Hopkins University School of Medicine, 1800 Orleans St., Baltimore, MD 21287, USA
e-mail: rgrutsch@gmail.com

A.I. Riker (ed.), *Breast Disease: Comprehensive Management*,
DOI 10.1007/978-1-4939-1145-5_31, © Springer Science+Business Media New York 2015

Preoperative Assessment and Concerns

Patients come to the operating room with their own unique concerns and history. For the anesthesiologist, a huge challenge exists with each patient, from the very young woman with very aggressive disease to the very old patient with multiple comorbidities. Every case requires much skill and thought about patient safety and optimal patient care.

A preoperative assessment must include a detailed history from the patient about their medical problems, surgical history, and allergies. A focus on cardiac issues with an emphasis on the functional status of the patient and on pulmonary and airway issues is critical. A history of previous anesthetic experiences including difficult airway, postoperative nausea and vomiting, and family history of malignant hyperthermia will help shape the management of the patient through the perioperative period.

The ultimate goal of preoperative cardiovascular management is to safely deliver the anesthesia without complications during or after the case. It involves preoperative detection and management of cardiovascular disease and the prediction of both short- and long-term cardiovascular risk. It affects the choice of anesthetic drugs, type of monitoring, and postoperative care. Major noncardiac surgery is associated with an incidence of perioperative cardiac death of 0.5–1.5 %, and major cardiovascular complications include nonfatal cardiac arrest, nonfatal cardiac infarction, heart failure, arrhythmias, and stroke. Many patients, up to 5 %, of noncardiac surgeries may have an asymptomatic perioperative myocardial infarction [1]. As breast biopsies, mastectomies, and reconstructions are usually considered low risk for cardiac complications, the patient's actual cardiac status will dictate their cardiac risk and requirements for preoperative cardiac testing [2].

Active cardiac conditions, a high-risk surgical procedure, and poor exercise tolerance are the strongest independent predictors of adverse perioperative cardiac outcome. Active cardiac conditions such as heart failure, unstable angina, significant cardiac arrhythmias, symptomatic valvular disease, and recent myocardial infarction with residual ischemia are associated with poor outcome and must be evaluated and treated according to cardiac guidelines. The development of risk index, referred to as the Revised Cardiac Risk Index, has been validated as a measure of predicting cardiac risk in patients undergoing noncardiac surgery [3]. High-risk operations, ischemic heart disease, and a history of congestive heart failure were all identified as independent predictors of complications. Other predictors of cardiac risk include a history of stroke or transient ischemic attacks, diabetes mellitus treated with insulin, and renal insufficiency with creatinine values of >2 (Table 31.1).

Table 31.1 Cardiac risk factors (Revised Cardiac Risk Index)

High-risk type of surgery
Ischemic heart disease
History of congestive heart failure
History of cerebrovascular disease
Insulin therapy for diabetes
Preoperative serum creatinine >2.0 mg/dl

From Lee et al. [3]

Heart failure is a major independent predictor of adverse perioperative outcome in noncardiac surgery, even greater than that of ischemic heart disease [4]. These patients should be treated with beta-blockers, angiotensin converting enzyme inhibitors, angiotensin II receptor blockers, diuretics, and aldosterone antagonists with perioperative continuation of required therapy. Prior to proceeding with an operation that requires a general anesthetic, clinical and echocardiographic (ECHO) evaluation should be performed in all patients with any type of heart valve disease. For example, severe aortic stenosis, that is, an aortic valve area less than 1 cm^2, carries the highest perioperative cardiovascular morbidity and mortality in noncardiac surgery.

Preoperative functional status is probably the most important predictor of perioperative outcome. Low exercise tolerance is associated with poor perioperative outcome [5]. The main purpose of assessment is to predict the individual's ability to increase oxygen delivery in the perioperative period. Cardiac pulmonary exercise testing (CPET) assesses oxygen uptake and carbon dioxide elimination and can assess both cardiac and respiratory components of the exercise. This is correlated to electrocardiographic (EKG) changes during exercise. Testing for cardiac pathophysiology, such as left ventricular dysfunction, myocardial ischemia, and valve dysfunction, can be primarily evaluated with a thorough history and physical examination. Based upon this, other testing may be required, such as a resting EKG, ECHO, myocardial imaging, cardiac stress tests, and even cardiac catheterization with angiography. However, despite the high technology of several of these studies, they have quite a low overall positive predictive value in the range of 0–33 %.

If coronary angiography reveals abnormalities that will require further intervention such as coronary revascularization, the decision should be made to first address all relevant cardiac issues prior to an operative intervention. Guidelines have been established for the use of beta-blockers prior to a scheduled operation, with the goal of a heart rate of 60–80 beats per minute and a systolic arterial pressure >100 mmHg [5]. In addition to lipid-lowering effects, statins have pleiotropic effects that improve endothelial morphology and function and also stabilize coronary plaques [5]. Angiotensin II inhibitors or angiotensin receptor blockers are also used in these patients. Aspirin taken for secondary cardiac prevention should not be discontinued. Discontinuation of aspirin may be responsible for up to 15 % of all recent acute coronary syndromes in patients with documented stable coronary artery disease.

The combination of aspirin and adenosine diphosphate receptor antagonist therapy (such as clopidogrel, prasugrel, and ticagrelor) plays a significant role in patients with recent placement of coronary stents. Elective surgery should be postponed for at least 6 weeks after placement of a bare-metal stent and for at least 12 months after placement of a drug-eluting stent in order to guarantee a sufficient and adequate endothelialization. Premature discontinuation increases perioperative cardiac morbidity and mortality without significantly reducing the risk of bleeding. If a surgery cannot be delayed for such a long period of time, especially in those with a cancer, aspirin should be continued throughout the peri- and postoperative period.

Optimal preoperative cardiac management includes attention to several factors for a safe outcome. First, the individual stress response, for example, cardiovascular and endocrine, to a given stressor such as a surgical procedure or hematocrit value, must be considered. Secondly, one must address the individual reactions from pharmacological intervention, such as antiplatelet and cardiovascular medications. Third, intra- and postoperative risk factors, such as anemia, hypercoagulability, hypovolemia, inflammatory responses, and cardiovascular depression, must be taken into account [6]. Recognition of such factors and aggressive attempts at appropriate intervention may reduce overall risk more than preoperative management alone (e.g., hemodynamic, endocrine, metabolic, and inflammatory responses, duration of surgery, hypovolemia, hypothermia, pulmonary dysfunction, and pain). Such an approach may render the high-risk patient a lower risk and improve overall outcome [2, 5–7].

Airway difficulties and pulmonary issues have become an increasingly important and difficult area to address. Ventilation of the patient is key, and therefore, a thorough assessment of the patient's ability to open the mouth and move their head and neck and dentition is a crucial component of the preoperative exam. The Mallampati score is a widely used evaluation system used preoperatively to predict the view of the vocal cords with a laryngoscope blade and the difficulty of intubation [8–12].

The burgeoning phenomenon of surgical patients with an increased body mass index (BMI) has greatly increased the difficulty of airway management and operative approach for both the surgical and anesthetic management teams. Obese patients are complicated from many standpoints. They often have the metabolic syndrome with hypertension and diabetes that have to be medically controlled. Airway management and ventilation are a vital component of their safe care, with many obese patients often requiring such special equipment as fiberoptic bronchoscopy or video laryngoscopy in order to secure an airway. The increasing number of patients who present with sleep apnea has become a major concern for clinicians, with conservative estimates of up to a third of the United States population now have obstructive sleep apnea (OSA). Up to 24 % of males and 9 % of females have mild OSA, with another 11.4 % of males and 4.7 % of females diagnosed with moderate to severe OSA [13–15].

In obese patients, the percentage of OSA increases up to 50 % of men and 30 % of women, and up to 82 % of the men and 93 % of the women are undiagnosed [16, 17]. This diagnosis, whether known or not in a particular patient, has strong implications for the anesthesiologist and surgeon. These patients will have airways that are more difficult to manage, both at the beginning and end of surgery. In addition to often being overweight with a difficult airway, a certain subset is extremely sensitive to anesthetics and narcotics. Their sleep deprivation combined with anesthetic depressant effects can cause them to be sedated for an inordinately long time and even have a critical postoperative respiratory event. Their anesthetic requirements will be decreased and they will need postoperative monitoring of their respiratory and oxygen status to avoid severe respiratory depression and possible arrest secondary to the administration of postoperative pain medications. These patients definitely have a higher rate of postoperative complications and an overall increased morbidity and mortality [18].

The Stop-Bang Questionnaire was developed to help clinicians determine which patients are at a higher risk of sleep apnea [19]. The following table includes the simple eight questions that can be used preoperatively to assess each patient's risk of sleep apnea (Table 31.2). A high-risk patient may need to be tested preoperatively and taught to use the continuous positive airway pressure (CPAP) machine. They may further require a prolonged course of postoperative monitoring, especially with narcotic use. Many patients do not understand all of the adverse implications that sleep apnea has upon their operative risk and future health. A few such side effects include hypertension, pulmonary hypertension, daytime fatigue, depression, weight gain, diabetes, a compromised immune system, and disruption of circadian rhythms.

Methods

Classically, general anesthesia is the most common method used to care for breast surgical patients. Patients with breast cancer usually come to the operating room for biopsies, mastectomies, axillary node dissections with staging, and possible reconstructions. Whatever their operation, the patients can have many emotional issues that include concerns about the surgery and anesthesia, body image, and prognosis. Anxiety runs high and the anesthesiologist can play a vital role to minimize the psychological stress of the experience.

Anxiolytics given preoperatively, even orally, can help patients feel more comfortable with improved self-control over their situation. If patients have to go to the radiology department for needle localization before surgery, the patient can be given oral sedation for relaxation during the localization procedure. Oral hypnotics that are commonly used include benzodiazepines, such as alprazolam.

A short operative case that is often <1 h in total duration, such as a breast biopsy or lumpectomy, can often be accomplished with local anesthesia and intravenous sedation. Eutectic mixture of local anesthetic (EMLA) with lidocaine and prilocaine can also be used in minor breast surgery without any additional sedation [20]. Intraoperative sedation is often accomplished with a continuous infusion of propofol, an agent that has a short half-life and faster recovery for patients with few side effects, including a low incidence of postoperative nausea and vomiting (PONV) [21].

The anesthetic management has to take many factors into account for the breast surgery patient. General anesthesia is effective and safe, with newer anesthetic agents having a shorter half-life with faster recovery times. When the surgeon is performing a sentinel node biopsy or an axillary

Table 31.2 STOP-Bang Scoring Model Questionnaire

Adapted from: STOP Questionnaire: A Tool to Screen Patients for Obstructive Sleep Apnea
Frances Chung, et al. Anesthesiology 2008(May); 108:812-21. Copyright 2008, The American Society of Anesthesiologists, Inc. Lippincott Williams & Wilkins, Inc.

Height______inches/cm Weight_______lb/kg
Age_______ Male/Female BMI_______
Collar size of shirt: S, M, L, XL, or ______inches/cm
Neck circumference* _______cm

1. *S*noring
Do you snore loudly (louder than talking or loud enough to be heard through closed doors)?
Yes No

2. *T*ired
Do you often feel *t*ired, fatigued, or sleepy during daytime?
Yes No

3. *O*bserved
Has anyone *o*bserved you stop breathing during your sleep?
Yes No

4. Blood *p*ressure
Do you have or are you being treated for high blood *p*ressure?
Yes No

5. *B*MI
*B*MI more than 35 kg/m^2?
Yes No

6. *A*ge
*A*ge over 50 year old?
Yes No

7. *N*eck circumference
*N*eck circumference greater than 40 cm?
Yes No

8. *G*ender
*G*ender male?
Yes No

High risk of OSA: answering yes to three or more items
Low risk of OSA: answering yes to less than three items

From Chung F, Yegneswaran B, Liao P, Chung SA, Vairavanathan S, Islam S, Khajehdehi A, Shapiro CM. STOP Questionnaire: A tool to screen patients for obstructive sleep apnea. Anesthesiology 2008; 108(5):812-21.

Adapted from Chung et al. [19]

node dissection, paralytics should be avoided so that the surgeon is able to identify the functionality and prevent injury to the nerves in this area, particularly the thoracodorsal and long thoracic nerves. General anesthesia with a laryngeal mask airway (LMA) avoids the need for muscle relaxants in these cases, and patients often have less postoperative nausea and vomiting, sore throats, and pain as compared to the use of an endotracheal tube [22].

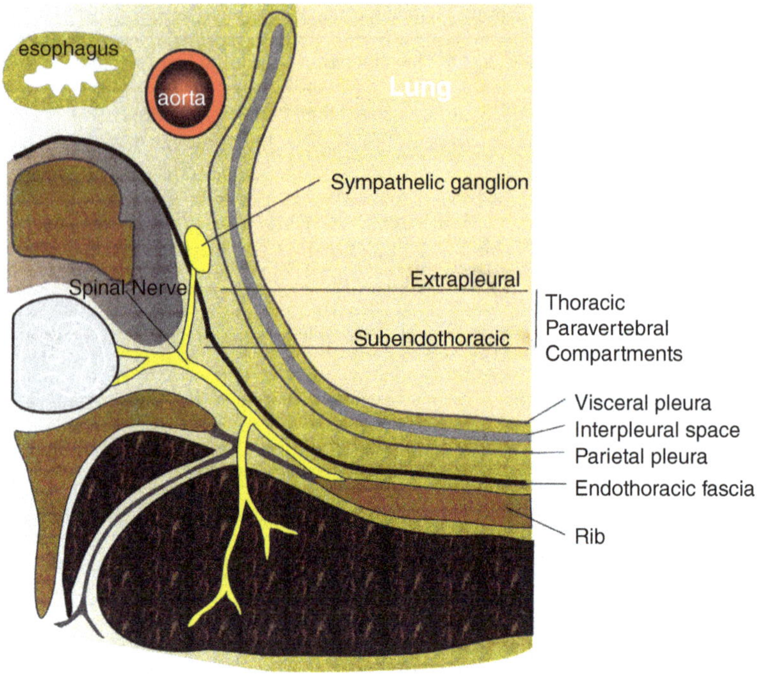

Fig. 31.1 A schematic representation of the thoracic paravertebral space and its structures of relevance to paravertebral block

Thoracic epidural and paravertebral blocks with sedation are becoming more popular in the last several years as their benefits have been increasingly recognized. These include improved postoperative pain relief, decreased narcotic requirements, and a decreased incidence of PONV [23, 24]. Increased patient satisfaction is also a benefit with a trend toward shorter hospital stays [25].

The thoracic paravertebral block is a technique where local anesthetic is injected into the paravertebral space, resulting in an ipsilateral somatic and sympathetic nerve blockade. This block will lead to a unilateral, band-like segmental distribution at the desired levels. It is indicated for the anesthesia and analgesia in patients having a mastectomy, cosmetic breast surgery, and thoracic surgery or in patients with rib fractures [26]. This technique can be done as a single needle injection or as a continuous block by placement of a catheter. The thoracic paravertebral space is a wedge-shaped area that lies on either side of the vertebral column (Fig. 31.1). The anterolateral wall is formed of parietal pleura and the posterior wall is the superior costotransverse ligament. The medial wall is formed from the vertebral body, intervertebral disk, and foramen. This space is continuous with the intercostal space laterally and epidural space medially. A local anesthetic agent can spread longitudinally along this space and even into the intercostal and epidural spaces.

The spinous processes are the main landmarks for the thoracic paravertebral block, with the C7 spinous process being the most prominent vertebra. Another landmark is the thoracic vertebra, T7, which is at the level of the tip of the scapula. The needle is inserted 2.5 cm lateral to the spinous process, often identifying these landmarks with the guidance of ultrasound (Fig. 31.2) [27–29]. Blockade of T2 through T6 will often be more than adequate for the successful anesthesia of this anatomic distribution. Local anesthetics work directly on the lateral extension of the spinal nerve along with the intercostal nerves and also a medial extension into the epidural space through the intervertebral foramina. This results in the ipsilateral anesthesia that correlates to the desired thoracic dermatome level.

The patient can be placed in a sitting, prone, or lateral decubitus position, with the site to be blocked at the uppermost location (Table 31.3) [29]. For a single paravertebral injection, 5–8 ml of local anesthetic can be used at each segmental level to be blocked, or 15–20 ml can be used as a single injection at one level. We utilize ropivacaine 0.5 %, which will provide analgesia for about 8–12 h. Another option is bupivacaine

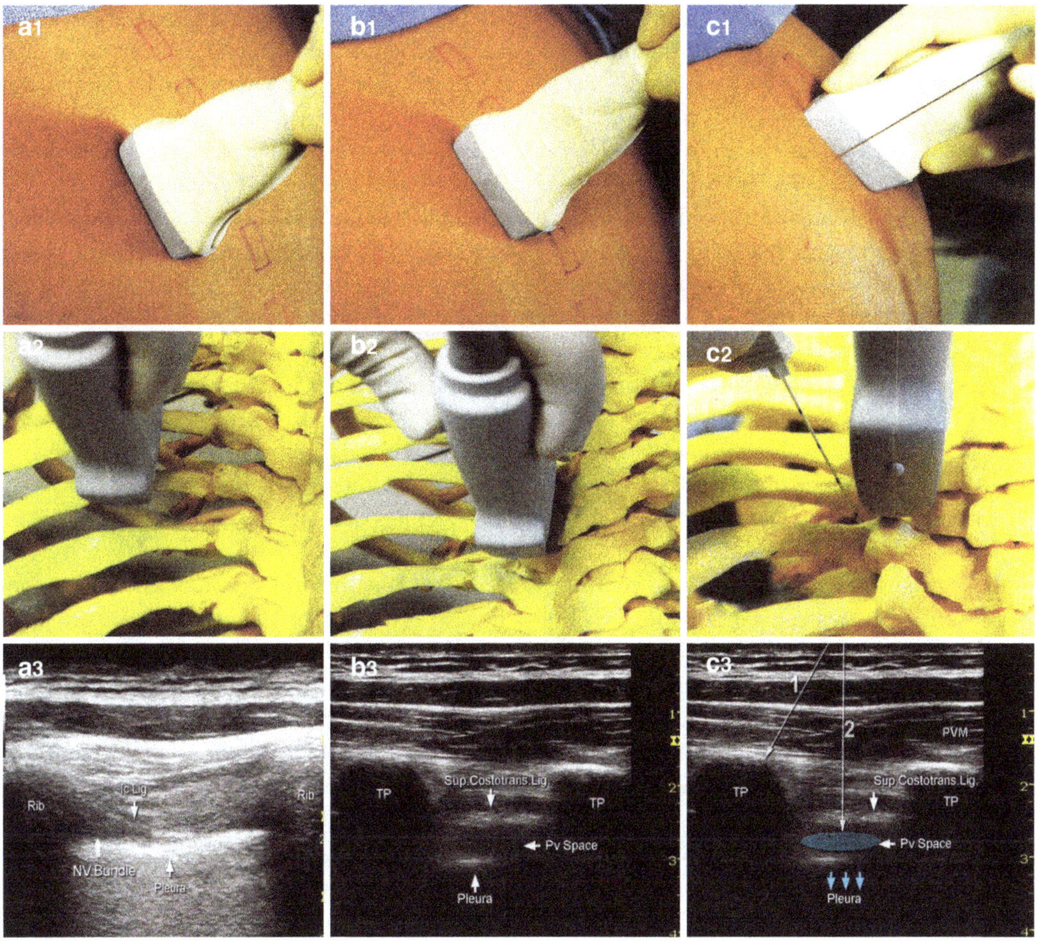

Fig. 31.2 Longitudinal out-of-plane approach to thoracic paravertebral block. The transducer is first placed 5–6 cm lateral to the spinous processes to identify the ribs, parietal pleura, and intercostal spaces (*A1–A3*). The transducer is then moved progressively medially to identify transverse processes (*B1–B3*). The transverse processes (TP) appear square and deeper than the ribs (round, superficial). The block needle is inserted out of plane to contact the TP (*C1–C2* and *C3*, *line 1*) and then walked off the TP (*C3*, *line 2*) inferior or superior to TP to enter the paravertebral space and for injection of local anesthetic (*blue*). Proper injection displaces the pleura (*blue arrows*). *PVM* paravertebral muscles

Table 31.3 Technique of paravertebral block

1. Adequate sedation and monitoring
2. Sterile technique
3. Local anesthetic infiltration of subcutaneous tissue and paravertebral muscles
4. The needle is inserted at 2.5 cm lateral to the spinous process with the intention to contact the transverse process (usually at a depth of 3–6 cm from the skin)
5. The needle is then withdrawn and redirected superiorly or inferiorly to walk off the transverse process
6. The needle is then advanced to a depth of 1–1.5 cm past the transverse process
7. The local anesthetic is then injected after negative aspiration
8. Ultrasound guidance can be used to help identify the paravertebral space, needle placement, and the spread of local anesthetic [27, 28] (a) Visualization of the needle tip and the control of its path and depth at all times are essential to avoid inadvertent pleural puncture or entry into the intervertebral foramen with epidural spread (b) Either a transverse in-line or longitudinal out-of-plane technique can be performed

Adapted from Hadzic and Vloka [29]

0.5 % with epinephrine, providing analgesia for up to 18 h. For a continuous block, a bolus injection of local anesthetic, e.g., 8 ml, can be placed and a continuous infusion of ropivacaine 0.2 % or bupivacaine 0.25 % at 10 ml/h started. If a patient-controlled regional analgesia (PCA) system is used, then the continuous infusion can run at 5 ml/h with an as needed bolus of 5 ml every hour. Paravertebral blocks do not result in an extremity motor block and do not impair the patient's ability to ambulate. This is very helpful in the postoperative setting and overall management of patients. Infection, hematoma, local anesthetic toxicity, nerve injury, total spinal anesthesia, and paravertebral muscle pain are possible complications, albeit quite uncommon.

A continuous epidural thoracic catheter technique is another alternative for pain control in breast surgery patients, especially for bilateral mastectomies and reconstruction. The major risk factor is a high total spinal level and associated respiratory depression. These patients may need postoperative monitoring to watch for hemodynamic changes, such as hypotension or respiratory complications. There is a risk of possible dural puncture and inadvertent total spinal anesthesia at this high thoracic level. Patients with thoracic epidurals, however, are discharged earlier and have less PONV than patients without them [24].

Postoperative Pain Control

Postoperative pain control can be quite complex in breast surgical patients, often with the need for a combination of different therapeutic approaches in order to maximize the benefit. Regional techniques that include paravertebral blocks and thoracic epidurals are now used to spare narcotic usage and provide for improved postoperative pain control.

For patients with breast lumps or any breast incision, local anesthetic such as bupivacaine 0.25–0.5 % with epinephrine 1:200,000 can be infiltrated into the wound to provide approximately 8–20 h of pain relief. The bupivacaine can be infiltrated preemptively into the area of the surgical incision. In one study, it was shown to decrease intraoperative and postoperative narcotic use and lower postoperative pain scores [30]. This, combined with oral or intravenous ketorolac in appropriate patients, can markedly decrease and often avoid completely the use of narcotics and the risk of PONV [31]. Ketorolac is a nonsteroidal anti-inflammatory agent that provides 4–9 h of pain relief. Its use may be contraindicated in patients with a history of renal insufficiency and gastric bleeding or in geriatric patients. Additionally, there is at least one study that has shown a decrease in the local recurrence rate in breast cancer patients when ketorolac is administered preoperatively [32].

Narcotics are often used for postoperative pain therapy. Patients can be given oral, intravenous, or intramuscular narcotics. Intravenous therapy is most commonly used in the perioperative period and inpatient care. To promote comfort, often a patient-controlled intravenous pump of morphine, hydromorphone, or fentanyl is used. The major drawback is the high incidence of postoperative nausea, vomiting, and drowsiness, and some patients are at an increased risk for respiratory depression.

An On-Q™ pain pump is a device that infuses pain medication directly into the wound site and can remain in place for several days postoperatively. A mixture of bupivacaine 0.5 % and ketorolac can be delivered directly to the wound via catheters to provide continuous pain relief. One meta-analysis of surgically placed wound catheters (SPWC) with local anesthetic infusion showed a trend toward improved pain relief and decreased opioid requirements [33].

Intercostal nerve blocks have also been used in patients for minor breast surgeries or for patients with significant comorbidities such as metastatic disease to the lungs [34–36]. The intercostal nerve blocks can be supplemented with an infraclavicular nerve block of the superficial cervical plexus branches that innervate the upper part of the breast and a subcutaneous infiltration of the midline to block the intercostal nerves that cross from the contralateral side [30]. Good outcomes have been reported for both, with decreased postoperative nausea and vomiting with a concomitant decrease in postoperative pain requirements [37].

When a patient has a unilateral or bilateral mastectomy, with or without breast reconstruction, the patient may experience a persistent chronic pain syndrome postoperatively [38]. Postmastectomy pain syndrome is neuropathic pain that persists beyond the normal 3-month healing period. The incidence has been shown to be as high as 52 % [39]. It is seen more commonly in younger patients, up to 65 % of patients [40], and in those who had an axillary lymph node dissection [41] and/or adjuvant radiotherapy [42]. In a recent study, local anesthetic wound infiltration decreased immediate postoperative pain for 90 min in patients undergoing breast cancer surgery. However, this wound infiltration did not appear to reduce the incidence or severity of chronic postoperative pain over the next year in these patients [37].

Regional anesthesia, such as paravertebral blocks or thoracic epidurals, is another method of decreasing the risk of chronic postoperative pain. In one meta-analysis of studies which looked at local anesthetics or regional anesthesia for the prevention of continued pain, the authors concluded that paravertebral blocks may decrease chronic pain after breast cancer surgery in approximately one of every five patients treated [43]. The paravertebral lamina technique performed with continuous catheters can spare opioid use both intraoperatively and postoperatively [23, 44]. Use of local and paravertebral blocks for surgery decreased PONV to 10 % of patients [45].

Postoperative Nausea and Vomiting

Postoperative nausea and vomiting (PONV) is a common and difficult problem to treat. It typically occurs in one third of postoperative patients but can be seen in as many as 80 % of patients. Many breast cancer patients are found to be within the highest risk categories to develop postoperative vomiting. These include the female gender, younger patients, patients with a history of PONV or motion and seasickness, and nonsmokers. Breast surgery itself is a risk factor for increased PONV [46–48].

Hormonal status may also affect the risk of PONV. Estrogen use has been implicated as a risk factor, with one study showing that older patients with estrogen receptor-positive breast cancer had a higher incidence of PONV, possibly due to an altered hormonal milieu [46].

Intraoperatively, both the duration of the operation and the length of the general anesthesia with the use of volatile agents and nitrous oxide were associated with anesthesia-related predictors of PONV [47, 48]. Other predictors include intraoperative and postoperative opioid use, longer-acting narcotics, and larger doses of narcotics [47]. These factors have paved the way for use of regional anesthesia or nonnarcotic alternatives for adequate pain relief.

Different approaches to the problem of PONV are prevention with prophylaxis medications given before or during surgery and the addition of rescue therapy as the symptoms occur. Intravenous treatment options for PONV include serotonin receptor 5HT3 antagonists like ondansetron and granisetron, glucocorticoids such as dexamethasone [49], benzamides such as metoclopramide, butyrophenones (droperidol), and phenothiazines (promethazine). The 5HT3 antagonists are very effective and seem to be somewhat superior to other pharmacological interventions to prevent PONV [50].

The scopolamine transdermal patch is also a great antiemetic agent for narcotic-induced PONV, whether due to intravenous or epidural narcotics. It is often used prophylactically in patients with a history of motion or seasickness that present to the operating room. This patch is effective for up to 3 days and has been shown to be additive to ondansetron in the prevention of PONV [51].

Anesthetic management also has an effect on the risk of PONV. Use of total intravenous anesthesia versus balanced anesthesia with a volatile agent can help prevent PONV [47]. Avoidance of a large dose of neostigmine to reverse muscle relaxation and limitation of narcotic use whether by infiltration of local anesthesia, a regional technique, or use of non-opioid pain medications can also be helpful. A small dose of the hypnotic, propofol, can be used as an antiemetic agent in itself [52].

A multimodal approach to the prevention and treatment of PONV helps to decrease the incidence of complications and increases patient overall satisfaction. Prophylaxis includes assessment of high-risk patients, avoidance of higher-risk agents, and then aggressive use of antiemetic agents. These agents can be given prophylactically or later for treatment as a rescue agent. Routine prophylaxis with ondansetron has been shown to increase patient satisfaction in breast surgery patients [53].

Anesthesia Effects on Outcomes of Breast Cancer Patients

Anesthetic technique and choice of anesthetic agents have been implicated in breast cancer recurrence rates, the development of metastatic disease, and long-term outcome and prognosis [54, 55]. This is a controversial area at present, with some clinicians asking whether the anesthetic management during primary cancer resection can cause, or correlate with, long-term patient outcome. Both the actual surgery and the inhalational anesthetic agents and narcotics can cause immunosuppression after the primary tumor resection. A regional anesthesia technique with decreased use of narcotics and anesthetic agents or use of intravenous agents instead of inhalational agents has been shown in some animal and human studies to decrease the recurrent cancer and metastases rates in oncologic patients [56–58].

A reduction of the surgical stress response and prevention of the decrease in perioperative immune activity could potentially attenuate tumor growth and spread at the time of primary resection of the tumor [59–62]. Surprisingly, this idea that certain anesthetic agents could affect recurrence rates and growth of primary breast cancer was considered more than 30 years ago [63]. At that time, in a study of breast cancer patients, survival rates of patients when halothane was used as the primary anesthetic agent were higher than when ether was used. This was explained by influences of the anesthetic agents both on the pituitary-adrenal cortical system with effects on carcinemia and on the immune system with effects on tumor implantation and metastatic growth. In a more recent study, the type of anesthetic agent used during the surgical procedure was correlated with a decreased risk of recurrence or metastases by fourfold, within the 2.5–4 years of patient follow-up [54]. At present, a clinical multicenter prospective trial has been generated to follow the outcome of patients receiving general versus regional anesthesia [64].

There are several human retrospective and prospective studies that have linked some of these findings to the immune response and even to specific immune regulators. Anesthetic drugs affect neutrophil and natural killer cell function (Table 31.4). In one study, ketamine, thiopental, and halothane, but not propofol, significantly reduced the natural killer cell activity and increased metastasis in rats. Natural killer cell activity helps prevent cancer dissemination and establishment [65]. Especially in the postoperative period, suppression of cell-mediated immunity can allow preexisting and new metastases to take hold [66]. As interferon can stimulate natural killer cell function, it may decrease the immunosuppression during the perioperative period.

The postoperative immune suppression that occurs can last for several days and is not well understood. However, the neuroendocrine and inflammatory systems, in addition to the hypothalamic-pituitary-adrenal axis, all play a role in the mechanism [67]. The neuroendocrine system takes into account the stress response and the release of catecholamines that can affect the beta-adrenergic receptors and tumor progression. The catecholamines can also influence cell migration and angiogenesis and decrease cell-mediated immunity. During the inflammatory response to surgery, cytokines, chemokines, prostaglandins, and cyclooxygenase (COX) all have the capacity to influence tumor progression, where tumor cells may proliferate and metastases take hold. Besides immunosuppression, a resis-

Table 31.4 Anesthetic drugs and host defenses

Drug	Potential effect on antitumor host defenses
Ketamine	Reduced NK cell activity and number in animal models
Thiopental	Reduced NK cell activity and number in animal models
Propofol	Reduced NK cell number in animal models
Volatile agents	Inhibits interferon stimulation of NK cell cytotoxicity in animal models
	Reduces NK cell number in humans; associated with worse outcome when compared with local anesthesia for melanoma excision
Nitrous oxide	Associated with acceleration in development of lung and liver metastases in animal model 0073
	No effect on cancer outcome after surgery for colorectal carcinoma in humans
	Inhibits formation of hematopoietic cells that may be important for tumor cells
Local anesthetic drugs	Lidocaine inhibits EGF receptor and tumor cell proliferation in vitro; ropivacaine inhibits growth of cancer cells
Morphine	Inhibits cellular immunity including NK cell activity in animal models
	Inhibits NK cell activity in humans
Fentanyl	Inhibits NK cell activity in humans
Tramadol	Stimulates NK cell activity in animal models
	Simulates NK cell activity in humans
COX-2 inhibitors	Display anti-angiogenesis and antitumor effects in animal models

From Snyder and Greenberg [57]

tance to apoptosis and promotion of angiogenesis increase tumor recurrence [68]. Pain stimulates the hypothalamic-pituitary-adrenal axis and the sympathetic nervous system that will lead to immunosuppression that includes suppression of natural killer cell activity [60]. Postoperative pain control, therefore, is very important in the management of breast cancer patients.

Specific anesthetics have also been shown to affect the production of angiogenic factors. Angiogenesis is a necessary process for a tumor or metastasis to grow beyond a certain size. Angiogenic mediators include vascular endothelial growth factor C and transforming growth factor *b*. The serum levels of these two factors differed in patients that received general anesthesia versus those having paravertebral block with propofol, suggesting a protective effect of the regional technique [69].

A variety of agents can affect angiogenesis and anesthetics. COX-2 antagonists, specifically ketorolac, given preoperatively or during the perioperative period, have been shown to decrease cancer recurrence rates. These agents have been shown to have both antitumor and anti-angiogenic activity [32, 57].

Besides the actual surgery itself and the concomitant use of anesthetic agents, other factors may also influence the recurrence rate of breast cancer and long-term outcome. These include the administration of blood transfusions, control of perioperative temperature, and the use of statins, beta-blockers, and COX-2 medications [54, 57, 60]. Anxiety and the psychological stress associated with surgery also contribute to perioperative immunosuppression [57].

During surgery, cancer cells can be released and disseminated into the circulation. It is hypothesized that the operation, general anesthesia, and the stress response can increase the ability of the cancer cells to implant and proliferate. Some have suggested that the choice of anesthetic agents and techniques like regional blocks can actually influence and decrease the effects on the cancer cells. Overall, regional anesthesia, by decreasing the noxious neural input from surgery, can decrease the surgical stress response, therefore resulting in decreased immunosuppression that may influence the possibility of a recurrence [54]. A study of patients that had paravertebral blocks and intravenous propofol for sedation during breast cancer surgery showed a decrease in several cytokines that promoted the growth of tumors and an increase of an antitumor cytokine IL-10 [57]. Another study showed that the anesthetic agent, propofol, has been examined as a potential treatment for breast cancer, through its ability to inhibit cellular adhesion, migration, and apoptosis in breast cancer cells [70].

Recently, anesthetic inhalational agents have been found to have an impact on tumor cell signaling pathways that can lead to an upregulation of hypoxia-inducible factor-1α (HIΦ1-**α**), a transcription factor that is ubiquitous and has many effects upon cancer cells [71]. This factor has pro-tumor effects on cancer cells and may allow residual cancer cells at the time of surgery to disseminate and develop into metastases. Again, certain anesthetic agents, such as propofol, may decrease the level of this factor and be more suitable for use during tumor resection.

Opioids are routinely used for management of postoperative pain, but morphine has been shown to be proangiogenic and promote breast tumor growth [57, 72]. Acute pain itself can affect the stress response and suppress natural killer cell activity [54, 57, 65].

Although the data is very limited, the use of ketorolac prior to surgery has resulted in a decrease in cancer recurrence rates. Prostaglandins have a large effect on immunity and inflammation in breast cancer, both capable of stimulating angiogenesis, epithelial cell proliferation, inhibition of apoptosis, immune suppression, and increased mutagen production [32]. When the prostaglandins are removed, their suppression of natural killer cell activity dissipates very quickly. COX-2 inhibitors have been shown to attenuate surgery's immunosuppression and prevent metastatic spread. Using ketorolac seems to prevent the early recurrence rates by up to fivefold [32, 73]. Adding a beta-blocker to decrease adrenergic activation with a COX-2 inhibitor can also be helpful in the prevention of developing metastatic disease [59, 74].

Timing of a primary tumor resection during certain phases of the menstrual cycle may affect breast cancer metastatic rate and overall outcome and cure rate of patients [75]. If an operation is performed during the diestrus phase of the menstrual cycle, rats have increased breast cancer growth, increased metastases, and lowered cure rates. Tumor angiogenesis and capillary permeability are affected by the cyclical change in sex hormones [76]. A recent study suggests that performing surgery during the luteal phase of the menstrual cycle might be beneficial for a patient's overall survival [77]. Premenopausal women may have increased survival rates if the surgical tumor resection is done in the luteal, rather than follicular, phase [78]. Certain candidate genes and pathways in mouse breast tumors have been discovered to have significant expression changes during various phases of the menstrual cycle and are associated with post resection breast cancer outcome [78].

The circadian clock also regulates cellular proliferation and the expression of cell cycle regulators. Breast cancer growth rate in mice has been shown to have two daily tumor growth peaks and is regulated by circadian clock-controlled genes [79]. The expressions of the genes can either enhance the circadian amplitude of the two daily growth peaks or suppress the tumor growth at those specific times during the day. Some have suggested to better time the operation to coincide with the circadian rhythms of the body during its peak ability to suppress tumor growth.

If the circadian clock is disrupted, cell proliferation may be deregulated and tumor growth rates increase [79, 80]. This has implications for cancer patients in that it may be better for them to maintain intact circadian rhythms. Patients that have circadian rhythms disrupted include the untreated sleep apnea patients, patients with poor night sleep quality, and patients exposed to light at night with decreased melatonin production. These patients may need circadian-based lifestyle interventions and therapies to improve their circadian rhythms, quality of life, and possibly overall prognosis [80].

In summary, avoidance of certain anesthetic and postoperative pain medications and an increased use of regional anesthesia techniques may decrease the perioperative stress response and immune depression. Many other perioperative factors may also affect the stress response, such as the operation itself, acute and chronic pain, hypothermia, blood transfusions, adrenergic activation, beta-blocker, and statin therapy. Eventually, further research into these areas may help to discern the effects of each anesthetic agent and technique on the physiology of stress, neuroendocrine, and immune responses of cancer patients. This may help us to elucidate the effects of certain anesthetics upon tumor cells and the patients overall outcome as it relates to the disease process.

Summary

For the breast surgical patient, the anesthetic management can be quite smooth throughout the operation and in the postoperative setting. Regional anesthesia and certain intravenous agents may improve a patient's immediate postoperative outcome without pain or nausea and also long-term prognosis without recurrence or metastasis. Basic studies in both animals and humans have linked these findings to the immune response and now even to specific immune regulators. In the future, each anesthetic agent used perioperatively may be specifically tailored to each individual patient using genetic and oncologic testing.

References

1. Devereaux PJ, Xavier D, Pogue J, Guyatt G, Sigamani A, Garutti I, et al. Characteristics and short-term prognosis of perioperative myocardial infarction in patients undergoing noncardiac surgery: a cohort study. Ann Intern Med. 2011;154(8):523–8.
2. Williams FM, Bergin JD. Cardiac screening before noncardiac surgery. Surg Clin North Am. 2009;89: 747–62.
3. Lee TH, Marcantonio ER, Mangione CM, Thomas EJ, Polanczyk CA, Cook EF, et al. Derivation and prospective validation of a simple index for prediction of cardiac risk of major noncardiac surgery. Circulation. 1999;100(10):1042–9.
4. Hammill BG, Curtis LH, Bennett-Guerrero E, O'Connor CM, Jollis JG, Schulman KA, Hernandez AF. Impact of heart failure on patients undergoing major noncardiac surgery. Anesthesiology. 2008;108(4):559–67.
5. Fleischmann KE, Beckman JA, Buller CE, Calkins H, Fleisher LA, Freeman WK, et al. ACCF/AHA focused update on perioperative beta blockade incorporated into the ACC/AHA 2007 guidelines on perioperative cardiovascular evaluation and care for noncardiac surgery: a report of the American College of Cardiology Foundation/American Heart Association Task Force on Practice Guidelines. J Am Coll Cardiol. 2009;120(21):e169–276.
6. Landesberg G, Beattie WS, Mosseri M, Jaffe AS Alpert JS. Perioperative myocardial infarction. Circulation. 2009;119(22):2936–44.
7. De Hert S, Imberger G, Carlisle J, Diemunsch P, Fritsch G, Moppett I, et al. Preoperative evaluation of the adult patient undergoing non-cardiac surgery: guidelines from the European Society of Anaesthesiology. Eur J Anaesthesiol. 2011;28(10): 684–722.
8. Mallampati SR, Gatt SP, Gugino LD, Desai SP, Waraksa B, Freiberger D, Liu PL. A clinical sign to predict difficult tracheal intubation; a prospective study. Can Anaesth Soc J. 1985;32(4):429–34.
9. Samsoon GLT, Young JRB. Difficult tracheal intubation: a retrospective study. Anaesthesia. 1987;42(5):487–90.
10. Cros AM, Bourgain JL, Diemunsch P, Francon D, Langeron O. Intubation difficile. Sfar, editor. Conférences d'actualisation. Les Essentiels 2005. 47e Congrès national d'anesthésie et de réanimation; 2005. p.89–401.
11. Cormack RS, Lehane J. Difficult tracheal intubation in obstetrics. Anaesthesia. 1984;39(11):1105–11.
12. Amantea SL, Piva JP, Rodrigues MI, Bruno F, Garcia PCR. Rapid airway access. J Pediatr (Rio J). 2003;79:S127–38.
13. Young T, Palta M, Dempsey J, Skatrud J, Weber S, Badr S. The occurrence of sleep-disordered breathing among middle-aged adults. N Engl J Med. 1993; 328(17):1230–5.
14. Bixler EO, Vgontzas AN, Ten Have T, Tyson K, Kales A. Effects of age on sleep apnea in men: I Prevalence and severity. Am J Respir Crit Care Med. 1998;157(1):144–8.
15. Bixler EO, Vgontzas AN, Lin HM, Ten Have T, Rein J, Vela-Bueno A, Kales A. Prevalence of sleep-disordered breathing in women: effect on gender. Am J Respir Crit Care Med. 2001;163(3 Pt 1):608–13.
16. Frey WC, Pilcher J. Obstructive sleep-related breathing disorders in patients evaluated for bariatric surgery. Obes Surg. 2003;12(5):678–83.
17. Young T, Evans L, Finn L, Palta M. Estimation of the clinically diagnosed proportion of sleep apnea syndrome in middle-aged men and women. Sleep. 1997;20(9):705–6.
18. Seet D, Chung F. Obstructive sleep apnea: preoperative assessment. Anesthesiol Clin. 2010;28:199–215.
19. Chung F, Yegneswaran B, Liao P, Chung SA, Vairavanathan S, Islam S, Khajehdehi A, Shapiro CM. STOP questionnaire: a tool to screen patients for obstructive sleep apnea. Anesthesiology. 2008;108(5):812–21.
20. Akan A, Eryavuz Y, Kamali S, Simsek S, Hot S, Bademci R. A randomized, placebo controlled study: EMLA in minor breast surgery. Minerva Chir. 2012;67(2):181–5.
21. Gan TJ, Ginsberg B, Grant AP, Glass PSA. Double-blind, randomized comparison of ondansetron and intraoperative propofol to prevent postoperative nausea and vomiting. Anesthesiology. 1996;815(5):1036–42.
22. Hohlrieder M, Brimacombe J, von Goedecke A, Keller C. Postoperative nausea, vomiting, airway morbidity and analgesic requirements are lower for the ProSeal laryngeal mask airway than the tracheal tube in females undergoing breast and gynaecological surgery. Br J Anaesth. 2007;99(4):576–80.
23. Schnabel A, Reichl SU, Kranke P, Pogatzki-Zahn EM, Zahn PK. Efficacy and safety of paravertebral blocks in breast surgery: a meta-analysis of randomized controlled trials. Br J Anaesth. 2010;108(6):842–52.

24. Lynch EP, Welch KJ, Carabuena JM, Eberlein TJ. Thoracic epidural anesthesia improves outcome after breast surgery. Ann Surg. 1995;222(5):683–9.
25. Thavaneswaran P, Rubkin GE, Cooter RD, Moyes DC, Perera CL, Maddern GJ. Brief reports: paravertebral block for anesthesia: a systematic review. Anesth Analg. 2010;110(6):1740–4.
26. Moller JF, Nikolajsen L, Rodt SA, Ronning H, Carlsson PS. Thoracic paravertebral block for breast cancer surgery: a randomized double-blind study. Anesth Analg. 2007;105(6):1848–51.
27. Vandepitte C, Pintaric TS, Gautier PE. Sonography of thoracic paravertebral space and considerations for ultrasound-guided thoracic paravertebral block. In: Hadzic A, editor. Hadzic's peripheral nerve blocks and anatomy for ultrasound-guided regional anesthesia. 2nd ed. New York: McGraw Hill; 2012. p. 497–501.
28. Vogt A. Review about ultrasounds in paravertebral blocks. Eur J Pain Suppl. 2011;S2(5):489–94.
29. Hadzic A, Vloka JD. Thoracic paravertebral blocks. In: Hadzic A, Vloka JD, editors. Peripheral nerve blocks: principles and practice. Chicago: McGraw Hill; 2004. p. 194–207.
30. Zielinski J, Jaworski R, Smietanska I, Irga N, Wujtezicz M, Jaskiewicz J. A randomized, double-blind, placebo-controlled trial of preemptive analgesia with bupivacaine in patients undergoing mastectomy for carcinoma of the breast. Med Sci Monit. 2011;17(10):CR589–97.
31. De Oliveira Jr GS, Agarwal D, Benzon HT. Perioperative single dose ketorolac to prevent postoperative pain: a meta-analysis of randomized trials. Anesth Analg. 2012;114(2):424–33.
32. Forget P, Vandenhende J, Berliere M, Machiels JP, Nussbaum B, Legrand C, De Kock M. Do intraoperative analgesics influence breast cancer recurrence after mastectomy? A retrospective analysis. Anesth Analg. 2010;110(6):1630–5.
33. Raghavendra GK, Sreenivasa RH, Ashok K, Chirsabesan P, McLean NR, Youssef M, Piper M, Carr M. Surgically placed wound catheters (SPWC) and local anaesthetic infusion in breast surgery: efficacy and safety analysis. Breast Dis. 2011;33(1):1–8.
34. Huang TT, Parks DH, Lewis SR. Outpatient breast surgery under intercostal block anesthesia. Plast Reconstr Surg. 1979;63(3):299–303.
35. Atanassoff PG, Alon E, Pasch T, Ziegler WH, Gaitschi K. Intercostal nerve block for minor breast surgery. Reg Anesth. 1991;16(1):23–7.
36. Kolawole IK, Adesina MD, Olaoye IO. Intercostal nerve block for mastectomy in two patients with advanced breast malignancy. J Natl Med Assoc. 2006;98(3):450–3.
37. Albi-Feldzer A, Mouret-Fourme E, Hamouda S, Motamed C, Dubois PY, Jouanneau L, Jayr C. A double-blind randomized trial of wound and intercostal space infiltration with ropivacaine during breast cancer surgery: effects on chronic postoperative pain. Anesthesiology. 2013;118(2):318–26.
38. Vilholm OJ, Cold S, Rasmussen L, Sindrup SH. The postmastectomy pain syndrome: an epidemiological study on the prevalence of chronic pain after surgery for breast cancer. Br J Cancer. 2008;99(4):604–10.
39. Macdonald L, Bruce J, Scott NW, Smith WC, Chambers WA. Long-term follow-up of breast cancer survivors with post-mastectomy pain syndrome. Br J Cancer. 2005;92(2):225.
40. Smith WC, Bourne D, Squair J, Phillips DO, Chambers WA. A retrospective cohort study of post mastectomy pain syndrome. Pain. 1999;83(1):91–5.
41. Alves Nogueira Fabro E, Bergmann A, do Amaral Silva E B, Padula Ribeiro AC, De Souza Abrahao K, da Costa Leita Ferriera MG, de Almaida Dias R, Santos Thuler LC. Post-mastectomy pain syndrome: incidence and risks. Breast. 2012;21(3):321–5.
42. Gartner R, Jensen MB, Nielsen J, Ewertz M, Kroman N, Kehlet H. Prevalence of and factors associated with persistent pain following breast cancer surgery. JAMA. 2009;302(18):1985–92.
43. Andreae MH, Andreae DA. Local anaesthetics and regional anaesthesia for preventing chronic pain after surgery. Cochrane Database Syst Rev 2012;(10): CD007105.
44. Juttner T, Werdehausen R, Hermanns H, Monaca E, Danzelsen O, Pannen BH, Janni W, Winterhalter M. The paravertebral lamina technique: a new regional anesthesia approach for breast surgery. J Clin Anesth. 2011;23(6):443–50.
45. Kitowski MJ, Landercasper J, Gundrum JD, De Maiffe BM, Chestnut DH, Bottcher ML, Johnson JM, Johnson RL. Local and paravertebral block anesthesia for outpatient elective breast cancer surgery. Arch Surg. 2010;145(6):592–4.
46. Bakshi SG, Jibhkate B, Sareen R, Badwe R. Nausea and vomiting after breast cancer surgery, and relationship with tumor receptor status. J Anesth. 2012;26(2): 187–95.
47. Gan TJ. Risk factors for postoperative nausea and vomiting. Anesth Analg. 2006;102(6):1884–98.
48. Apfel CC, Heidrich FM, Jukar-Rao S, Jalota L, Hornuss C, Whaelan RP, Zhang K, Cakmakkaya OS. Evidence-based analysis of risk factors for postoperative nausea and vomiting. Br J Anaesth. 2012;109(5):742–53. Epub 2012 Oct 3.
49. Gomez-Hernandez J, Orozco-Alatorre AL, Dominguez-Contreras M, Oceguera-Villanueva A, Gomez-Romo S, Villasenor ASA, Fuentes-Orozco C, Gonzales-Ojeda A. Preoperative dexamethasone reduces postoperative pain, nausea and vomiting following mastectomy for breast cancer. BMC Cancer. 2010;10:692.
50. Singhal AK, Kannan S, Gota VS. 5HT3 antagonists for prophylaxis of postoperative nausea and vomiting in breast surgery: a meta-analysis. J Postgrad Med. 2012;58(1):23–31.
51. Gan TJ, Sinha AC, Kovac AL, Jones RK, Cohen SA, Battikka JP, Deutsch JS, Pergolizzi Jr JV, Glass PS, TDS Study Group. A randomized, double-blind, multicenter trial comparing transdermal scopolamine

plus ondansetron to ondansetron alone for the prevention of postoperative nausea and vomiting in the outpatient setting. Anesth Analg. 2009;105(5): 1498–504.
52. Borgeat A, Wilder-Smith OH, Saiah M, Rifat K. Subhypnotic doses of propofol possess direct antiemetic properties. Anesth Analg. 1992;74(4):539–41.
53. Sadhasivam S, Saxena A, Kathirvel S, Kannan TR, Trikha A, Mohan V. Safety and efficacy of prophylactic ondansetron in patients undergoing radical mastectomy. Anesth Analg. 1999;89(6):1340–5.
54. Exadaktylos AK, Buggy DJ, Moriarty DC, Mascha E, Sessler DI. Can anesthetic technique for primary breast cancer surgery affect recurrence or metastasis? Anesthesiology. 2006;105(4):660–4.
55. Sessler DI. Long-term consequences of anesthetic management. Anesthesiology. 2009;111:1–4.
56. Bar-Yosef S, Melamed R, Page GG, Shakhar G, Shakhar K, Ben-Eliyahu S. Attenuation of the tumor-promoting effect of surgery by spinal blockade in rats. Anesthesiology. 2001;94:1066–73.
57. Snyder GL, Greenberg S. Effect of anaesthetic technique and other perioperative factors on cancer recurrence. Br J Anaesth. 2010;105(2):106–15.
58. Melamed R, Bar-Yosef S, Shakhar G, Shakhar K, Ben-Eliyahu S. Suppression of natural killer cell activity and promotion of tumor metastasis by ketamine, thiopental, and halothane, but not by propofol: Mediating mechanisms and prophylactic measures. Anesth Anal. 2003;97(5):1331–9.
59. Tsuchiya Y, Sawada S, Yoshioka I, Ohashi Y, Matsuo M, Harimaya Y, Tsukada K, Saiki I. Increased surgical stress promotes tumor metastasis. Surgery. 2003;133:547–55.
60. Gottschalk A, Sharma S, Ford J, Durieux ME, Tiouririne M. The role of the perioperative period in recurrence after cancer surgery. Anesth Analg. 2010;110(6):1636–43.
61. Shakhar G, Ben-Eliyahu S. Potential prophylactic measures against postoperative immunosuppression: could they reduce recurrence rates in oncological patients? Ann Surg Oncol. 2003;10:9972–92.
62. Andersen BL, Farrar WB, Golden-Kreutz D, Kutz LA, MacCallum R, Courtney ME, Glaser R. Stress and immune responses after surgical treatment for regional breast cancer. J Natl Cancer Inst. 1998;90(1):30–6.
63. Fried IA. The influence of the anaesthetic on survival rates of breast cancer patients after surgery. Int J Cancer. 1977;20:213–8.
64. Sessler DI, Ben-Eliyahu S, Mascha EJ, Parat MO, Buggy DJ. Can regional analgesia reduce the risk of recurrence after breast cancer? Methodology of a multicenter randomized trial. Contemp Clin Trials. 2008;29(4):5–26.
65. Ben-Eliyahu S, Page GG, Yirmiya R, Shakhar G. Evidence that stress and surgical interventions promote tumor development by suppressing natural killer cell activity. Int J Cancer. 1999;80:880–8.
66. Bovill JG. Surgery for cancer: does anesthesia matter? Anesth Analg. 2010;110(6):1524–6.
67. Kurosawa S, Kato M. Anesthetics, immune cells, and immune responses. J Anesth. 2008;22:263–77.
68. Kundu JK, Surh YJ. Inflammation: gearing the journey to cancer. Mutat Res. 2008;659:15–30.
69. Looney M, Doran P, Buggy DJ. Effect of anesthetic technique on serum vascular endothelial growth factor C and transforming growth factor *b* in women undergoing anesthesia and surgery for breast cancer. Anesthesiology. 2010;113(5):1118–25.
70. Siddiqui RA, Zerouga M, Wu M, Castillo A, Harvey K, Zaloga GP, Stillwell W. Anticancer properties of propofol-docosahexaenoate and propofol-eicosapentaenoate on breast cancer cells. Breast Cancer Res. 2005;7(5):R645–54.
71. Tavare AN, Perry NJS, Benzonana LL, Takata M, Ma D. Cancer recurrence after surgery: direct and indirect effects of anesthetic agents. Int J Cancer. 2012;130(6):1237–50.
72. Gupta K, Kshirsagar S, Chang L, Schwartz R, Law P, Yee D, Hebbel R. Morphine stimulates angiogenesis by activating proangiogenic and survival-promoting signaling and promotes breast tumor growth. Cancer Res. 2002;62:4491–8.
73. Retsky M, Rogers R, Demicheli R, Hrushesky WJM, Gukas I, Vaidya JS, Baum M, Forget P, DeKock M, Pachmann K. NSAID analgesic ketorolac used perioperatively may suppress early breast cancer relapse: particular relevance to triple negative subgroup. Breast Cancer Res Treat. 2012;134(2):881–8.
74. Benish M, Bartal I, Goldfarb Y, Levi B, Avraham R, Raz A, Ben-Eliyahu S. Perioperative use of beta-blockers and COX-2 inhibitors may improve immune competence and reduce the risk of tumor metastasis. Ann Surg Oncol. 2008;15:2042–52.
75. Chaudhry A, Puntis ML, Gikas P, Mokbei K. Does the timing of breast cancer surgery in pre-menopausal women affect clinical outcome?: an update. Int Semin Surg Oncol. 2006;3:37.
76. Wood PA, Bove K, You S, Chambers A, Hrushesky WJM. Cancer growth and spread are saltatory and phase-locked to the reproductive cycle through mediators of angiogenesis. Mol Cancer Ther. 2005;4(7):1065–75.
77. Kucuk AI, Atalay C. The relationship between surgery and phase of the menstrual cycle affects survival in breast cancer. J Breast Cancer. 2012;15(4): 434–40.
78. Oh EY, Wood PA, Yang X, Hrushesky WJM. Discovery of candidate genes and pathways that may help explain fertility cycle stage dependent post-resection breast cancer outcome. Breast Cancer Res Treat. 2009;118:345–59.
79. Yang X, Wood PA, Ansell CM, Quiton DFT, Oh EY, Du-Quiton J, Hrushesky WJM. The circadian clock gene *PER1* suppresses cancer cell proliferation and tumor growth at specific times of day. Chronobiol Int. 2009;26(7):1323–39.
80. Block KI, Hrushesky W, Blask D. In this issue: circadian disruption and cancer. Integr Cancer Ther. 2009;8(4):295–7.

The Multidisciplinary Breast Cancer Program: Patient Navigation

32

Patrice A. Stephens

My initial meeting with Cheryl, a 54-year-old newly diagnosed breast cancer patient, was held in our multidisciplinary oncology breast clinic. After meeting all the team members, her treatment plan was to begin with neoadjuvant chemotherapy. This plan was based on the size and biology of her tumor and her having a "positive" metastatic lymph node at diagnosis. She was single and had great family support, but she initially did express that she was overwhelmed with her treatment plan. Surgery would take place after her chemotherapy was completed, but what exactly that would entail would be discussed later based on her response to chemotherapy.

As her navigator, my first priority was to provide emotional support and discuss her treatment plan while providing education and informational resources. We talked about her fears and concerns, and I assured her that I would be there for her during her treatment. She tolerated her chemotherapy fairly well and completed her treatment without incident. Surgery was then planned and she underwent bilateral mastectomies. Once again, being there for her prior to surgery and after, while providing resources and support, was my major focus in the role as navigator. This concept of patient navigation was founded and pioneered by Dr. Harold Freeman in 1990, for the purpose of eliminating barriers to timely cancer screening, diagnosis, treatment, and supportive care. He established the nation's first navigation program at Harlem Hospital Center in New York City [1].

Patient navigation in cancer care refers to the assistance offered to healthcare consumers (patients, survivors, families, and caregivers) to help them access resources, chart a course through the healthcare system, and overcome barriers that they may encounter during their cancer treatment [2]. The patient navigation concept initially was used to describe a program aimed at reducing the healthcare disparities experienced by people in marginalized communities [3]. There have been several definitions of patient navigation, generally described as a barrier-focused intervention that has the following characteristics:

- Provided to individual patients for a defined episode of cancer-related care (e.g., evaluating an abnormal screening test)
- A definite endpoint when the services are complete (e.g., the patient achieves diagnostic resolution after a screening abnormality), with tracking patients over the course of their cancer care
- Targets a defined set of health services that are required to complete an episode of cancer-related care
- Focus upon the identification of individual patient-level barriers to accessing cancer care
- To reduce delays in accessing the continuum of cancer care services, with an emphasis on

P.A. Stephens, MSN, APN, AOCN-BC
Cancer Institute, 4400 West 95th Street, Outpatient Pavilion, Suite 8326, Oak Lawn, IL 60453, USA
e-mail: patrice.stephens@advocatehealth.com

A.I. Riker (ed.), *Breast Disease: Comprehensive Management*,
DOI 10.1007/978-1-4939-1145-5_32, © Springer Science+Business Media New York 2015

timeliness of diagnosis and treatment, and a reduction in the number of patients lost to follow-up [1, 4–7]

The scope and importance of patient navigation continues to evolve over time, but several core principles remain at the heart of each program. The momentum that patient navigation has received as a community-based intervention (which has expanded and been transformed into a nationally recognized model) stimulated the need to define principles and standards for patient navigation. Dr. Harold Freeman developed and practiced the following principles over the last 20 years:

- A patient-centric healthcare service delivery model.
- Serves to integrate a fragmented healthcare system for the individual patient.
- The elimination of barriers to timely care across all segments of the healthcare system.
- Defined with a clear scope that distinguishes the role and responsibilities of the navigator from those of all other providers.
- Delivery of services should be cost-effective and commensurate with the training and skills necessary to navigate an individual through a particular phase of the care continuum.
- Who should navigate should be determined by the level of the skills required at a given phase of navigation.
- Within a system, there are defined points at which navigation begins and ends.
- There is a need to navigate patients across disconnected systems of care.
- Patient navigation systems require coordination [8].

Each healthcare system brings fragmented pieces of care, whether it is in the physical layout, internal design, political cultures, or other complexities. Patient navigation provides personalized assistance for patients to journey through their care and allows a virtual integration that appears seamless to the traveler [9].

The term patient navigator (PN) has become a healthcare buzzword for many organizations which strive to reduce systematic burdens generated by program inefficiencies. What constitutes a PN? Is it an individual who may periodically assist with the coordination of care, or is it an individual who is educated to provide continuous support to patients along the entire illness trajectory? A review of literature revealed that both definitions are being used to describe the PN role. Characteristics of this role that appeared frequently in the reviewed literature were facilitating access to care, providing information and education, and providing links to resources [3, 10–17].

When a patient is in the treatment phase of the cancer care continuum, they are in a world of staging radiologists, medical oncologists, surgeons, plastic surgeons, radiation oncologists, and genetic consultants—each in their own physical part of a healthcare system. It is important that the navigator is the consistent face and voice throughout the maze of appointments, procedures, tests, and treatments. I find this very true for our specific institution as well. As discussed earlier, our patient Cheryl continued to keep in touch with me throughout her treatment. As concerns or questions arose, we would talk and address these issues. When she was admitted for her surgery, she found my presence prior to and during pre-procedures very supportive. She verbalized that my visit with her post surgery was very important to her.

There remains today the question about the role of the PN, oncology nurse navigators (ONN), or cancer nurse navigator (CNN), depending on whom you are speaking with at the moment. First, we see the title alone varies, depending on what institution you may be working at, and the role varies even to a greater extent. Our institution originally identified and called this role "breast health specialist" back in 1999, as it was a very popular title at that time. We have recently adopted the more common terminology of breast nurse navigator. We have seen the title PN, as identified earlier in this chapter, utilized in other institutions locally as well. Other sources, as you will see later, utilize cancer nurse navigator, or CNN. Whatever the title may be, the function and role of the nurse performing in this capacity vary greatly.

In discussing patient/nurse navigation, it is important to note that there are different models of navigation identified by the AONN (Academy of Oncology Nurse Navigators) [18]. These models may include lay navigators, ACS (American Cancer Society) navigators, social worker navigators, nurse navigators, and APN (advanced practice nurse) navigators. There are strengths and weaknesses with each of these different models. Lay navigators are often in a volunteer capacity and may need supervision as well as training in carrying out their tasks. These tasks may entail connecting patients to educational information resources and community resources or performing clerical functions.

The American Cancer Society (ACS) navigator is trained by their organization and the hospital or breast center where an individual may be working and serves in specific roles. This includes providing some standard information including resources available through the ACS network. The cost of supporting this type of role is usually relatively low as the ACS is providing this individual through a grant. When social workers serve in the navigator role, their background does allow them to assess the patient for barriers and address her psychosocial needs. They are familiar with community resources, but are restricted in their level of medical knowledge. The nurse navigator is seen as the most common model, as the registered nurse can provide patients with medically knowledgeable resources and can perform a nursing assessment. This model is more costly than a social worker or nonclinical navigator, but is a very popular model for many institutions [19].

The model of choice for oncology navigators at our institution at the outset was the APN navigator model, and it still is our model today. We also chose a tumor site-specific model, as it is a more clinically oriented approach. A major strength of this model is that the APN's background tends to bring more credibility to the navigator role from both a physician's and patient's perspective. APNs deliver high-value care to patients and they can effectively support physicians and, therefore, the best interests of the cancer patients. Program development skills are extremely useful and survivorship clinics may be supported by the APN. The success of our program supports the continued use of this model. The collaboration and collegiality among the team members, especially the breast surgeon, radiologist, medical oncologist, and radiation oncologist, have demonstrated support and the need for this model. The team has found the APN navigator model to be successful. The weaknesses may be the additional cost of employing an APN and that most institutions do not bill for their services. This factor has not been a deterrent at our institution. There are recent reports in the literature discussing the value of the nurse navigator model.

One is a first-hand report by a breast cancer nurse navigator at a small community hospital. McDonald explains how the nurse has been an integral part of the navigation team since its inception. The description of the program at her hospital closely resembles our program and the nurse's role. The role of their navigators is primarily a resource role, serving both as providers of care and facilitators of the coordination process, which they refer to as navigation. Initial contact with their patients is similar to our program, as well. Once the plan of care is initiated and developed, the primary focus is support of the patient/family and their decision-making and support in clarification of the information provided by the physician to the patient/family. She summarizes that the nurse navigator makes a significant contribution by providing supportive care to patients facing breast health concerns and facilitating the navigation process. From her perspective, the nurse's hands-on role/care has led to better preparedness and decreased anxiety in their patients [20].

In 2012, the Oncology Nursing Society (ONS) and Oncology Nursing Certification Corporation (ONCC) conducted a role delineation study to understand the function and role of the ONN [21]. The purpose was to examine the job-function activities of the ONN, thus providing a foundation for future ONS-related activities. In an attempt to understand the specific cancer diagnoses of patients with which the nurse navigators worked, respondents were asked which specific cancer sites they provide navigation. Breast-specific navigation was the

Fig. 32.1 The top tasks, knowledge areas, and skills as rated by respondents (Reprinted with permission from Brown et al. [21]. Copyright 2012 by Oncology Nursing Society)

Tasks

- Provide emotional and educational support for patients.
- Practice according to professional and legal standards.
- Advocate on behalf of the patient.
- Demonstrate ethical principles in practice.
- Orient patients to the cancer care system.
- Receive and respond to new patient referrals.
- Pursue continuing education opportunities related to oncology and navigation.
- Collaborate with physicians and other healthcare providers.
- Empower patients to self-advocate.
- Assist patients to make informed decisions.
- Provide education or referrals for coping with the diagnosis.
- Identify patients with a new diagnosis of cancer.

Knowledge Areas

- Confidentiality and informed consent
- Advocacy
- Symptom management
- Ethical principles
- Quality of life
- Goal of treatment
- Therapeutic options
- Evidence-based practice guidelines
- Professional scope of practice
- Legal and professional guidelines

Skills

- Communication
- Problem solving
- Critical thinking
- Multitasking
- Collaboration
- Time management
- Advocacy

most prevalent area reported, followed secondly by navigation for a comprehensive lung cancer program. This is similar at our institution, as we have employed a breast-specific nurse navigator for approximately 8 years, prior to expanding to other cancer programs, specifically lung and eventually gastrointestinal and hepatobiliary malignancies.

As was demonstrated by the ONS (2012), the responsibilities and functions of our disease-specific nurse navigators vary greatly within a single institution. The breast navigator spends the majority of time with her patients in the surgery department. She initially meets most new patients in the multidisciplinary oncology breast clinic. The lung navigator meets most patients in the thoracic surgeon's office, in addition to spending time rounding on lung cancer patients with the physicians as well. We have also seen other smaller hospitals within our own healthcare system utilize an ONN to work with all cancer patients diagnosed at their institutions. Some have nurse navigators working with patients going through the diagnostic phase prior to a cancer diagnosis as well.

Respondents were also asked to indicate which areas of the patient care process that they participated in. Figure 32.1 shows all of the top tasks, knowledge areas, and skills as rated by the respondents. This list is important because it identifies those tasks, knowledge areas, and skills that the respondents most identified with their role as an ONN. The ONS and ONCC Board of Directors are currently exploring the need for additional initiatives to help further define the role and competencies of the ONN [21].

A breast cancer patient navigator fulfills a critical role for many patients who are just learning that they have been diagnosed with breast cancer. It is not unusual for a patient, in retrospect, to say that she felt like her navigator was her "lifeline," her "go-to person," "her support," or "the one with the answers." By navigating a patient, what is usually meant is that someone helps the patient move smoothly through the system, insuring that certain levels and expectations of their care are achieved in an efficient and effective manner [19]. The role of breast nurse navigator is considered crucial at our institution and has been fully supported for over 13 years.

Korber and colleagues [22] completed a study in 2011 examining the effectiveness of navigator programs. They utilized focus groups and a telephone interview with breast cancer patients, finding that all patients identified the critical role of navigators possessing information and education about the entire breast cancer process. We feel this is critical whether it is another specific type of cancer (thoracic, gastrointestinal) or any other cancer nurse navigation program.

This study further showed that the participants discussed the overwhelming nature of the treatment experience, which often made learning difficult. In their study, the navigator was seen as able to repeat, clarify, reinforce, and validate information the patient was receiving from multiple sources. Participants also noted the emotional support provided by the care team, particularly the nurse navigator, and significant others was key to their successful treatment completion.

Having this emotional support, the perception that "just being there" for them was seen as invaluable. In regard to teamwork, the importance of meeting the entire treatment team prior to starting therapy was identified. The multidisciplinary clinic approach was seen as helpful in clarifying roles, reinforcing support of caregivers, and instilling confidence that the collaborative team had a common understanding and acknowledgement of the plan of care. Formal introduction of team members, including a brochure describing each discipline and role, is extremely helpful. For the nurse navigator, a clear list of services, hours of availability, and contact numbers was extremely important to the patient and family members. The navigator was seen as playing a key role in obtaining and coordinating a vast array of medical and social services. Overall, Korber and colleagues felt that as breast navigator programs continue to grow, their impact and effectiveness on clinical outcomes must be examined [22].

One integrative review by Case in 2011 explored the presence of the oncology nurse as navigators on measurable patient outcomes. She identified 18 primary nursing research studies in her exploration, using a combination of keywords. These studies identify nursing-sensitive patient outcomes related to the time to diagnosis and appropriate treatment, effect on mood status, satisfaction, support, continuity of care, and cost outcomes. Of the study patient populations, patients with breast cancer were the predominant populations encountered. In her review, Case discusses how nursing researchers have clearly identified important outcomes that result from the presence of the oncology nurse navigator [23].

One of the studies Case cited was a study that we conducted in 2007, utilizing a telephone interview as part of a follow-up phone call. We identified the many needs and concerns of the newly diagnosed breast cancer patient. Emotional, social, and physical limitations were identified as most important in dealing with a breast cancer diagnosis. Our study indicated that fear of recurrence and anxiety regarding postoperative treatments accounted for more than 65 % of the responses to the question "What concerns you most about your new diagnosis?" These data reinforce the need for early postoperative follow-up and to provide printed materials that patients can use as a resource for their long-term information needs [24].

The provision of both educational materials and emotional support plays a major role at our institution. At the initial meeting among the patient, family members, and the breast nurse navigator, the navigator describes her role and ensures them that she will be with them throughout their cancer journey. The breast nurse navigator works with patients who have been diagnosed with breast cancer and provides up-to-date educational books and many resources to help them understand their diagnosis and treatment plan. The nurse navigator introduces the Multidisciplinary clinic approach for treatment and the importance of all the team members. The nurse navigator's priority is to be accessible and present with the patient and family/caregivers and provide never-ending emotional support.

Navigation has a "ripple effect," or as Webster Dictionary defines it, "a spreading, pervasive, and usually unintentional effect or influence." As patient navigation evolves as a strategy to improve outcomes in cancer patients by removing barriers to diagnosis and treatment, the process and the navigators will have a ripple effect upon patient care. Healthcare systems often bring fragmented pieces of care, whether in physical layout, internal design, political cultures, or other complexities. Gentry reported that the goal of patient navigation is not to compete among healthcare systems but to meet the needs of the patient with personal and accessible healthcare services. Thus, the PN can be the consistent face and voice throughout the maze of appointments, procedures, tests, and treatments. As confidence is gained to access care and patients are empowered to move through the healthcare system, the effects are seen as positive [8, 9, 25].

McDonald and Abella [26] provide an excellent view of the importance of the role of the nurse navigator in their article entitled "The impact of nurse navigation on the patient experience." They recognize and acknowledge that a diagnosis of cancer can be a life-changing event, with the journey from diagnosis to survivorship, and perhaps to end-of-life care, filled with fear, challenges, and uncertainties. They discuss the value of patient navigation provided by a highly experienced, knowledgeable, and compassionate oncology nurse. This may be described best by the patients who share their comments and stories with others members of the healthcare team. They felt fortunate to have been connected with a CNN as their journey began. By being connected to, and supported by, a CNN when newly diagnosed with cancer, this helped the patient and families develop a profound sense of security and safety.

It also helps to decrease fears and anxiety, thus allowing patients to effectively hear and process the tremendous amount of information that is often presented to them about their cancer treatment. Informed and personalized decision-making becomes a much more comfortable process as the CNN begins to outline what patients may experience as well as serve as their guide to support their unique journey. The authors state that having a CNN shepherding a patient's care across the continuum using the clinical expertise embedded in an evidence-based nursing practice is paramount to assure excellence in service and to optimize a patient-centered experience.

They acknowledge that we all know that long after their treatment is completed, patients remember how their nurse navigator treated them, how they made them feel, and how they treated their family and/or loved ones. One can imagine the sense of comfort that patients treasure, knowing that they are personally connected to a CNN who, as their comments illustrate, made their experience so memorable and an experience that will not be forgotten. This experience and connection is often so powerful that one can reasonably assume that patients realized a deeper and more meaningful sense of hope and healing, enabling them to move forward with living beyond cancer, always mindful that the connection with the CNN would continue. The bond they have developed and the assurance that the CNN is readily available and will, at defined intervals, follow-up to address the patients' needs and concerns and provide encouragement to optimize the sense of well-being are powerful.

Thus, a nurse navigation program has the potential to be recognized as the hallmark model for patient-centered care. To ensure this model is consistently provided to every patient regardless of where the navigation begins, the authors feel it is imperative to standardize the role of the CNN. This involves developing a consistent job description, standards, competencies, and educational preparation. The principles of patient-centered care, which were outlined by Gertels and colleagues in 1993 and in 2001 by the Institute of Medicine, are embodied in a nurse navigator program. The intent of standardizing the CNN role is to define an evidence-based model with the most important dimensions of care outlined in the framework to ensure that patients are evaluated consistently for care needs that the evidence has identified as making a difference. Key dimensions of care, including patient education, advocacy, identifying and removing barriers, psychosocial management, and navigating and coordinating care across the continuum, have an impact on patient outcomes [26–28].

It is important to be able to draw on an intimate teamwork between the nurse navigator and the physicians in order to effectively and efficiently coordinate, guide, and navigate patients through the entire duration of treatment and survivorship. I believe this is the most important factor in our institution's success regarding nurse navigation. As the breast nurse navigator, the relationship between our team of physicians and I ensures a consistent high level of patient satisfaction. The respect and camaraderie we have developed over the 12-plus years working together among the team of physicians and myself as the breast nurse navigator has become a hallmark model at our institution. Our goal is to provide that sense of comfort that a patient treasures, knowing that a personal connection with their team will always exist.

As their navigator, I want them to feel there is a personal connection and make the experience memorable, powerful, and one they would not forget, as stated earlier by McDonald and Abella. I also want to help them move forward with living beyond cancer, developing a more meaningful sense of hope and healing, and a bond that will continue between us into the future. Our monthly breast cancer support group is one additional avenue that this connection can be sustained, and all patients are encouraged to come and participate. Survivorship will be discussed next and is extremely important in providing that very important follow-up to address the patients' needs and concerns and provide encouragement to optimize whole-person well-being. It is clear that a diagnosis of cancer can be a time of transformation for a patient and their family. Supporting this challenging transformation, a cancer nurse navigation program will balance the art and science of patient-centered care to ensure a sense of hope, healing, and security regardless of the outcome [26].

References

1. Freeman HP. A model patient navigator program. Oncol Issues. 2004;19(5):44–6.
2. Patient navigation concept. http://crchd.cancer.gov/pnp/concept.html.
3. Freeman HP, Muth BJ, Kerner JF. Expanding access to cancer screening and clinical follow-up among the medically underserved. Cancer Pract. 1995;3(1):19–30.
4. Newman-Horm PA, C-Change. Cancer patient navigation: published information. Washington DC: C-Change; 2005.
5. Cancer Care Nova Scotia. Cancer patient navigation evaluation: final report. Halifax: Cancer Care Nova Scotia; 2004.
6. Fowler T, Steakley C, Garcia AR, Kwok J, Bennett LM. Reducing disparities in the burden of cancer: the role of patient navigators (serial online). PLoS Med. 2006;3:e193.
7. Wells KJ, Battaglia TA, Dudley DJ, Garcia R, Greene A, Calhoun E, et al. Patient navigation: state of the art or is it science. Cancer. 2008;13(8):1999–2010.
8. Gentry S. Navigation principles across the continuum. J Oncol Navig Surviv. 2012;3:30–4.
9. Patient Navigation in Cancer Care Web site. What is patient navigation? http://www.patientnavigation.com. Accessed 26 Dec 2012.
10. NCI. providing information and education, and providing links to resources. 2005. http://www.cancer.gov/cancertopics/cancerlibrary/othersites#top.
11. Battaglia TA, Roloff K, Posner MA, Freund KM. Improving follow-up to abnormal breast cancer screening in an urban population: a patient navigation intervention. Cancer. 2007;109(2 suppl):359–67.
12. BC Cancer Agency. Patient navigation in cancer care: summary report. 2005. http://www.bccancer.bc.ca/WebSummaryNavigation.pdf.

13. Dohan D, Schrag D. Using navigators to improve care of underserved patients: current practices and approaches. Cancer. 2005;104(4):848–55.
14. Ferrante JM, Chen PH, Kim S. The effect of patient navigation on time to diagnosis, anxiety, and satisfaction in urban minority women with abnormal mammograms: a randomized controlled trial. J Urban Health. 2007;85:114–24.
15. Fowler T, Steakley C, Garcia AR, Kwok J, Bennett LM. Reducing disparities in the burden of cancer: the role of patient navigators. PLoS Med. 2006;3:974–6.
16. Freund KM, Battaglia TA, Calhoun E, Dudley DJ, Fiscella K, Paskett E, et al. National Cancer Institute Patient Navigation Research Program: methods, protocol, and measures. Cancer. 2008;113:3391–9.
17. Pedersen A, Hack T. Pilots of oncology health care: a concept analysis of the patient navigator role. Oncol Nurs Forum. 2010;37(1):55–60.
18. Role of the navigator. www.AONNonline.org.
19. Shockney LD. Becoming a breast cancer nurse navigator. Sudbury, MA: Jones and Bartlett; 2011.
20. McDonald C. A first-hand look at the role of the breast cancer nurse navigator. Care Manag. 2011/2012;17(6):11–4.
21. Brown GB, Cantril C, McMullen L, Barkley D, Dietz M, Miller Murphy C, et al. Oncology nurse navigator role delineation study: an oncology nursing society report. Clin J Oncol Nurs. 2010;16:581–5.
22. Korber SF, Padula C, Gray J, Powell M. A breast navigator program: barriers, enhancers, and nursing interventions. Oncol Nurs Forum. 2011;38:44–50.
23. Case MA. Oncology nurse navigator: ensuring safe passage. Clin J Oncol Nurs. 2011;15(1):33–40.
24. Stephens PA, Osowski M, Fidale MS, Spagnoli C. Identifying the educational needs and concerns of the newly diagnosed breast cancer patient after surgery. Clin J Oncol Nurs. 2008;12(2):253–8.
25. Merriam-Webster. www.merriam-webster.com/dictionary/ripple%20effect. Accessed 26 Dec 2012.
26. McDonald J, Abella P. The impact of nurse navigation on the patient experience. J Oncol Navig Surviv. 2012;3(5):10–4.
27. Gertels M, Edgman-Levitah S, Daley J, et al., editors. Through the patient's eyes, understanding and promoting patient-centered care. San Francisco: Jossey-Bass; 1993.
28. Institute of Medicine, Committee on Quality of Health Care in America. Crossing the quality chasm: a new health system for the 21st century. Washington DC: National Academies Press; 2001.

33 Cancer Survivorship

Peggy Kupres

Overview

Survivorship is a very important step in the breast cancer patient's care continuum. The concept of survivorship should be introduced to your patients at diagnosis, so that they are prepared to make the transition into survivorship care when the time comes. The most accepted definition of survivorship from the National Cancer Institute's Office of Cancer Survivorship states: "*An individual is considered a cancer survivor from the time of diagnosis, through the balance of his or her life. Family members, friends, and caregivers are also impacted by the survivorship experience and are, therefore, included in this definition*" [1].

According to McCabe et al., there are over 13 million cancer survivors in the United States today. By the year 2022, this number is expected to increase to over 18 million [2]. Breast cancer survivors make up 25 % of that number [3]. These numbers have increased due to early detection, improvements in treatment, and our aging population. As the population ages, the diagnosis of cancer is also increasing. Due to this fact, cancer survivors will also carry with them the comorbidities of age, which can be exacerbated by the treatment the cancer patient receives. Currently, about 66 % of survivors are living 5 years beyond their original date of their diagnosis. Couple this information with the fact that fewer physicians are specializing in oncology, and we will see the need to change how survivorship is addressed in the future. Oncologists will not be able to provide lifelong care to their cancer patients. It will become increasingly difficult for the oncologist to devote the time needed to his newly diagnosed patients, for those going through treatment and those having completed their treatment. Thus, there is an increasing need to coordinate care between the specialists treating the cancer patient and the primary care physician (PCP). Survivors need surveillance, preventative care, and normal medical care after their cancer diagnosis. Many many of these needs can be addressed and met by adding survivorship to the cancer patient care continuum.

Cancer survivors certainly share many of the same fears at the end of their treatment. They have been carefully monitored and counseled from diagnosis throughout treatment, only to realize that there will now be longer gaps between their visits to their specialists, with limited testing. There is much confusion among the survivors as to who will be there for them if they develop any sort of illness, such as a cold, or something of concern to them. They often will wonder if their cancer has returned and whom should they see in this instance. To address this issue, we have conducted two focus groups comprised of 29 patients who were breast cancer survivors ranging from 7 months to 28 years. The

P. Kupres, BSN, MA
Cancer Institute, Advocate Christ Medical Center, 4440 West 95th Street, Suite 107, Oak Lawn, IL 60453, USA
e-mail: margaret.kupres@advocatehealth.com

A.I. Riker (ed.), *Breast Disease: Comprehensive Management*,
DOI 10.1007/978-1-4939-1145-5_33, © Springer Science+Business Media New York 2015

majority of the patients reported having mixed feelings about the completion of treatment. They were happy that their diagnosis and treatment were behind them, yet apprehensive that it might return. The majority spoke in terms of "what if" it returns, with a few saying, "When it returns." Every one of the patients asked, "What's next? Who watches me now? How will I know if the cancer came back?" In the beginning, patients stated they felt "dropped like a hot potato; abandoned." The emotions patients expressed changed depending on how far out they were from completing treatment. The feelings our patients expressed were no different than those reported by patients in other survivorship programs around the country.

In 1985, Dr. Fitzhugh Mullan identified three "seasons" of survivorship, based on his personal experience as a cancer survivor [4]. *Acute Survivorship*, according to Mullan, deals with diagnosis and treatment. In this phase, emotions and distress are usually very high. Patients regularly are seen by their surgeons, medical oncologists, and radiation oncologists and occasionally their primary care physician (PCP). *Extended Survivorship*, as described by Mullan, extends through the 5-year period after diagnosis. Patients have mixed emotions, they are excited that treatment is finished, yet there is a fear of possible return of the disease. This is the time when patients are trying to find their "new normal." They are no longer being seen weekly or monthly, but have advanced to being followed yearly, creating a feeling of abandonment. Finally, Mullan described *Permanent Survivorship* as a time when the patient can begin to see a future without cancer. Patients begin to feel at ease with their new normal, and many no longer have the feeling of abandonment by their healthcare team. Since this chapter, survivorship itself has begun to emerge as part of the cancer care continuum.

Miller et al. redefined the "seasons of the survival paradigm" for cancer survivorship. In Miller's seasons [5], the A*cute Phase* remains the same, helping the patient through the emotions of a cancer diagnosis. Miller et al. broke the next phase into two phases: Transition and Extended Cancer Survivorship. In *Transition*, the patient is working their way back to normal or finding a "new normal." In this phase patients are dealing with many emotions. They are happy and celebrating their treatment is over, yet they are worried by the perceived lack of observation by their team. *Extended Cancer Survivorship* is described as "a period of watchful waiting and uncertainty about the future." *Chronic Survivorship* addresses the needs of patients living with cancer as a chronic disease as in those with CML or patients living with metastatic disease. *Permanent Survivorship* is broken down into three subgroups: *Cancer Free and Free of Cancer* – these patients are considered cured with minimal treatment and may live for many decades with few or no late or long-term medical or emotional effects. *Cancer Free but Not Free of Cancer* includes patients who are experiencing long-term or late effects of their cancer treatment. The third subgroup consists of patients with *Recurrent Cancers or Secondary Cancers*. The final season is *End of Life*. A patient can enter this season at any time, even during Acute Survivorship if the patient is not responding to treatment. The mixed emotions the patient goes through in Miller's seasons are exactly the same as those described in Mullan's seasons.

In 2004, the Centers for Disease Control (CDC) and over 100 experts in cancer survivorship and public health came together to develop "A National Action for Cancer Survivorship: Advancing Public Health Strategies." The recommendations of this report are as follows [6]:

- *Develop an infrastructure for comprehensive survivorship care.*
- *Develop patient navigation systems to facilitate care.*
- *Establish clinical practice guidelines for each stage of survivorship.*
- *Empower survivors to make informed decisions through education.*
- *Develop quality measures to determine impact of interventions.*
- *Conduct research on preventative interventions.*
- *Educate policy makers on the value of long-term follow-up, economic and insurance barriers, and education for survivors on long-term psychosocial issues.*

- *Educate survivors regarding advocacy.*
- *Educate providers regarding survivorship and the survivor's needs.*
- *Establish timely, high-quality service to survivors.*

In 2005, the National Institute of Medicine (IOM) took the information gained from the above report and recommended that cancer survivors and their PCP receive a comprehensive treatment summary, which is a record of care received, and a care plan for follow-up care. The care plan should include preventive recommendations such as exercise, diet, limited alcohol intake, and smoking cessation, as well as a surveillance schedule. The surveillance recommendations should be specific to include what tests should be ordered, when, and by whom (Hewett et al.), and they should follow evidence-based standards such as those described by the National Comprehensive Cancer Network (NCCN). All recommendations should be evidence based, following the recommendations of organizations like the American Society of Clinical Oncology (ASCO) or the NCCN. This report, called "*From Cancer Patient to Cancer Survivor: Lost in Transition*," also outlines quality care for the cancer survivor and suggestions on how to achieve it [7]. It has become the "bible" and gold standard of survivorship care.

Program Development

To begin the development of a Cancer Survivorship Program, conduct a gap analysis of the programs you have in place for your patients throughout care and at end of treatment. Look for resources in your community to fill the gaps. List what you provide, what you refer out, and what your patients do not have access to. For example, does your program offer physical therapy, financial counseling, psychosocial support, counseling on nutrition, sexuality, etc., or possibly refer your patients elsewhere for these services?.

Create a list of all available resources you provide your patients, both online and in person. This list should include support groups as well as resources on financial aid, legal rights, talking with and caring for your child while in treatment, sources for wigs, exercise, smoking cessation, and weight control to name a few. There are many reputable online resources to help fill in the gaps you may have in your program. Work with marketing to develop a booklet of resources to be given to your physicians, staff, and, of course, your patients. Look to your community for programs that will provide resources to your patients, for instance, American Cancer Society [8], Cancer Support Community [9], LiveSTRONG [10], and Susan G. Komen Foundation [11].

Perhaps there are other departments within your hospital that would be willing to partner with you to develop programs such as rehabilitation services, dietary assistance, and psychosocial support. At our facility, we reached out to our rehabilitation department in order to develop a comprehensive oncology rehabilitation program. After our presentation to their department leadership, they were eager to develop a program with us. They decided to start their program with breast cancer patients. All breast cancer patients that will undergo a sentinel lymph node biopsy and/or mastectomy are preoperatively evaluated in our weekly Multidisciplinary Breast Oncology Clinic (MBOC). A physical therapist performs baseline range of motion and circumferential measurements used as post-op reference for functional limitations or lymphedema. These patients are followed up postoperatively by an occupational therapist in the acute care setting. We shared the cost of an outpatient dietician with our dietary department until they could build the position into their budget. We reached out to our psychiatry department for a counselor for our patients and now share a counselor with our transplant team. These are just a few examples of how to develop your program.

Conducting a focus group or survey for your breast cancer survivors is also very helpful. Ask leading questions to find out how they felt at the end of treatment, what may have been missing for them, and how you can improve their care or emotional wellness. A focus group and survey of your physicians should also be conducted. It may be easier to have the physicians fill out a survey rather than devote time to a focus group. Be sure to send the surveys to all physicians that touch cancer patients. You want to include your surgeons, medical oncologists, radiation oncologists, and primary care physicians as well as specialists such as the plastic/reconstructive surgeons, physiatrists, psychologist, and gynecologists, to name a few. Again, ask leading questions to find out what they feel is missing, what is working well, and what they would like to see added to aid them to better care for their cancer patients. Use this survey to find out if any of your physicians are interested in working on a survivorship advisory committee.

Examine the current available programs in existence, models of care, and statistics on the services that your patients may benefit from. Review the Essential Elements of Survivorship Care Delivery (as described by the LiveSTRONG Foundation) [12], Commission on Cancer Standards on Survivorship [13], and NCCN Guidelines for Survivorship [14]. It is important to present the above information to your senior leadership when requesting personnel, space, or supplies for your survivorship program. Present the information attained from your surveys and focus groups to administration, describing to them what the patients and physicians feel would improve your program. For example, our patients requested loud and clear an educational series that would provide them information that would help them to increase their quality of life. We developed a monthly class that addresses the issues the patients request information on. There are also many helpful statistics to assist with your request for additional personnel and space. This information may help you gain an additional therapist. Our patient's request for more information has allowed us to create a full-time survivorship coordinator position. This person facilitates our lecture series and creates treatment summaries and care plans for our cancer survivors.

It is important to identify a physician champion, which can really be any physician who has an interest in survivorship, such as a medical oncologist, surgical oncologist, radiation oncologist, or PCP. Your physician champion will help with communication of your program to your physicians. It is very important that your medical staff be well educated on issues of survivorship. Many PCPs are unaware of the late and long-term effects of cancer treatment. They need to receive education on survivorship, what the goal of the treatment summary and care plan is, and tests required for surveillance, as well as how to watch for recurrence and secondary cancers. Many programs struggle with this aspect of development. How do you reach your PCPs and specialists? What is the best time and best way to address this education? A physician champion can help to educate your physicians and answer any questions or concerns they may have.

Develop a survivorship advisory committee, which is a team to guide your program and to set and monitor the quality measures and metrics for the survivorship program. This committee should be made up of a representation of those that will be working with your cancer survivors. The committee should have a representative from the specialties: medical oncology, radiation oncology, surgeons, rehabilitation, dietary, PCPs, nursing, psychology, and social work. Be sure to include ad hoc members, such as financial counselors, pharmacy, support organizations in the community, and, of course, cancer survivors. Develop goals within this committee to guide your survivorship program. This committee should set quality measures and those measures should be reported up to this committee yearly. Be sure to make this committee a subgroup of your cancer committee. Your advisory committee should review models of survivorship care and decide what is best for your facility.

Models of Care

You will need to investigate models of care and choose the one that best fits your program. According to Hewitt et al. [6], there are basically three models of survivorship care:

Shared-Care Model – In this model the responsibility of care is shared between individuals; there is a sharing of knowledge between specialists, primary care providers, and the patient. The responsibility can shift back and forth throughout the patient's life, for example, in the instance of recurrence, palliative care, and/or hospice care. In this model, the primary care provider is responsible for meeting all of the patient's physical and emotional needs once treatment is complete. The PCP is responsible for referring the patient to specialists as needed and for caring for the patient's chronic health needs. The specialist's role is to guide the PCP, providing a treatment plan and referring the patient back to the PCP to provide long-term care after treatment and to address other healthcare needs. It is very important to explain to the patient very early on the point at which this transition might occur. The patient may be anxious about returning to their PCP; therefore the specialist must reassure the patient that the PCP is more than competent to attend to their long-term needs.

Nurse-Led Model of Care – In this model, a registered nurse (RN) or an advanced practice nurse (APN) would prepare the treatment summary and care plan for the patient at the end of treatment. The nurse would then meet with the patient to go over the plan in detail. In this model, a nurse acts as the navigator for the patient. The nurse provides the much needed emotional support. At the time of the care plan visit, the nurse stresses routine health screening, lifestyle changes, surveillance for recurrence or secondary cancers, and late and long-term effects of the cancer treatment to the patient. The nurse will go over what tests are needed, how often they should be performed, and who will be ordering them. A copy of the treatment summary and care plan is given to the patient, specialist, and PCP, as well as any other providers the patient requests to receive it. The nurse works with the specialist and PCP to obtain any needed orders or referrals the patient may need. This is usually a one-time visit and the service cannot be billed. It is up to the PCP to see that the patient follows through with the recommendations. Our facility decided to start our program with this model and build up to a Survivorship Follow-Up Program.

Survivorship Follow-up Clinics – This model of care can be led by a nurse practitioner or a physician. The goal of the survivorship clinic is to offer ongoing multidisciplinary care to the patient. Patients are referred to the clinic at the end of treatment. The clinics are usually disease site specific with the needed specialists on hand to see the patient in one visit. The team in the clinic may consist of physical therapist, dietician, pharmacist, social worker, psychologist or counselor, financial services, and other disease site-specific specialists. The information gained is presented to the PCP, who will follow routine health needs of the patient. The team gathers together to create the treatment summary and care plan that is presented to the patient on a subsequent visit. Again, as in all models, the PCP, patient, and any specialists the patient requests receive a copy of the treatment summary and care plan. The patient is eventually transitioned back to the PCP, or in some institutions, the patient is seen in the clinic for life. Although this would be the ideal follow-up care, it is labor and resource intensive and quite costly. It is difficult to start a program at this level, but is certainly one to strive to attain. Some services in this model are billable.

Each model has barriers and advantages. You will need to decide which model best fits what your program is able to provide. Is there clinic space? Is staff available? Choose the model that best fits the design of your program. As the program expands, the model may change to fit your needs. Once you decide on the model you will follow, it is time to decide on the treatment summary and care plan you will use.

Treatment Summary and Care Plans

The treatment summary and care plan are meant to act as a seamless transition from the specialist to the PCP and between healthcare settings. There are many free treatment summary and care plan templates online, for instance, LiveSTRONG [15], JourneyForward [16], National Coalition for Cancer Survivorship [17], or ASCO [18], to name a few. Many programs develop their own care plan utilizing the best of the templates. The Institute of Medicine has clear guidelines of what should be included in the treatment summary and care plans [19]. The CoC will look to see that the following are met in your survivorship treatment summary and care plan.

The Institute of Medicine [19] recommends that the treatment summary include, at a minimum, the following:

- *All diagnostic tests performed and results.*
- *Tumor characteristics – stage, grade, hormone, and marker status.*
- *Summary of all treatment given – surgery, radiation, chemotherapy, and total dose should be included as well as all toxicities patient experienced.*
- *Supportive services provided – such as nutritional, rehab, psychosocial.*
- *Contact information for all providers.*
- *Contact information for coordinator of care.*

The IOM recommends [19] the care plan should include, at a minimum, the following:

- *Course of recovery from treatment.*
- *Ongoing health maintenance.*
- *Necessary cancer screening.*
- *Schedule of testing and examinations and who orders them.*
- *Information on long-term and late effects of treatment.*
- *Information on signs and symptoms of recurrence and second tumors.*
- *If needed, information on effects of treatment on relationships, sexuality, employment, parenting, and potential for future psychosocial support.*
- *If needed, information on legal, insurance, and financial consequences of treatment.*
- *Recommendations for healthy living: diet, exercise, smoking cessation, sunscreen, osteoporosis, and immunizations.*
- *As appropriate, information on genetic counseling. This should include discussing the need for conversations with first-degree relatives when appropriate.*
- *Information on chemoprevention, for example, tamoxifen, and the importance of compliance.*
- *Referrals to specialists as needed.*
- *Information on support groups and online resources and information.*

The American College of Surgeons, Commission on Cancer (ACS-CoC) has added Standard 3.3, Survivorship Care Plan, to be phased in by 2015 [15]. The standard states: "*The cancer committee develops and implements a process to disseminate a comprehensive care summary and follow-up plan to patients with cancer who are completing cancer treatment. The process is monitored, evaluated, and presented annually to the cancer committee and documented in the minutes.*" The CoC recommends the patient receive the treatment summary and care plan at the completion of the first course of treatment. The goal of this standard is to monitor the implementation of survivorship into the patient's continuum of care. The requirements, in addition to assuring the above are covered, necessary to fulfill the standard are as follows [8]:

- *Survivorship care plan is prepared by the provider that coordinated treatment for the patient.*
- *Care plan is given to patient at end of treatment.*
- *The care plan contains a record of the care received, disease characteristics, and a follow-up care plan incorporating recognized evidence-based standards of care.*

The CoC has left the type of care plan and its implementation open-ended to avoid being prescriptive. They understand that there are many different models that require different resources. By leaving the decision on how to implement the treatment summary, care plan, and the discussion of the recommendations with the patient to the discretion of the hospital, even small hospitals with restricted resources will be able to meet the standard. There are minimum requirements as described by the IOM that will need to be met, but the way the hospital meets the standard will be decided by the hospital cancer committee.

In addition to following the IOM recommendations as described above and listed in the resources at the end of this chapter, another guide to developing your survivorship program is the *Essential Elements of Survivorship Care*

Delivery [7]. In 2011, LiveSTRONG held a meeting in Washington, DC, with over 150 leaders in cancer care from across the country. A full list of participants and materials from the meeting can be found at www.LIVESTRONG.org/Essential *Elements*. The team came to the consensus that the following elements are necessary for a survivorship program to meet the needs of the patients that it serves. Survivorship program elements were divided into three tiers [7]:

TIER 1: Consensus Elements (Must Provide)

- *Survivor care plan, psychosocial care plan, and treatment summary*
- *Screening for secondary cancers and surveillance for recurrence*
- *Care coordination between specialists and primary care physicians*
- *Education on healthy living*
- *Symptom management, palliative care, and hospice (when needed)*

TIER 2: High-Need Elements (Should Provide)

- *Education on long-term and late effects*
- *Psychosocial and distress assessment, medical assessment, and care*
- *Nutritional, exercise, rehabilitation, and weight management programs*
- *Transitional visit from cancer to wellness*
- *Support for family and other care givers*
- *Patient navigation throughout continuum of care*
- *Educational series and resources on survivorship issues*

TIER 3: Strive Elements

- *Advocacy training*
- *Counseling*
- *Quality improvement monitoring*
- *Specialty care referrals*
- *Education for physician and staff on survivorship issues*

Each institution should use the above as an outline in developing their program. Even though quality improvement appears in the final tier, it is extremely important to build quality measures into your program at its inception.

Survivorship Education

It is important to educate physicians and staff not only on the program itself, but on late and long-term effects of treatment and surveillance as well. Grand rounds should be held to include the late and long-term effects of cancer such as cardiac issues, rehab needs, and psychosocial needs to name a few. Be sure to educate primary care physicians on acceptable surveillance for the different disease sites. Follow-up care for a breast cancer patient is much different than that for a colon cancer patient. Algorithms are extremely helpful for this. Develop algorithms as a team to help the PCP with follow-up care. Educate your physicians on the treatment summary and care plan, insuring to clarify what it includes, who receives a copy, what they should do with it, and how to use it for guidance. Introduce copies of the care plan and ask for input as to what works well and what could be improved in the document. Although the treatment summary and care plan are important for your patients to receive, it is equally important that you provide your patients with the tools they need to live life to the fullest.

It is extremely important to begin to educate your patient at diagnosis regarding survivorship. At diagnosis, you should define when your patient is considered a survivor as described in the beginning of this chapter. Develop an educational series at your facility that your patient can begin attending at diagnosis. Educate them on issues that many survivors face: How to talk with your doctor, exercise back to health, sexuality after cancer, nutrition, and returning to the work force are just a few examples of topics our patients have requested. Let the patients decide what topics they would like to learn about. Explain the importance of education and provide information on any programs your community has available to help improve your patient's long-term quality of life. Encourage your patients to attend these programs. You should begin discussions about the receipt of a care plan and treatment summary as early as possible. The more your patient hears about survivorship, the more inclined they will be to empower themselves to be able to live life to the fullest.

In conclusion, the goal of a survivorship care plan and treatment summary is coordination of care between the specialist and the primary care physician. The care plan was developed to aid in a seamless transition from cancer care to survivorship. It is a short, yet complete summary of the care the patient received and should include any adverse reactions and the expected late and long-term effects of the patient's treatment. The care plan is an outline for the future. It is designed to help the patients and PCP know what tests the patient should have, when they should have them, and who is responsible for ordering them. As fewer physicians go into oncology as a specialty and more patients are surviving cancer, it becomes more important to integrate survivorship care into your patient's care continuum and to involve PCPs in the long-term care of the patient.

It is essential that in addition to a treatment summary and care plan, your institution include education in your patients' care. We need to provide our patients with the tools and resources they need to live life to the fullest in their "new normal." Education needs to include healthy living: smoking cessation, healthy eating, and importance of exercise, psychosocial distress management, as well as many other topics to empower our patients to survive. It is important the patient know that they are not the only one experiencing fatigue, relationship issues, and weight control, for example.

There is still much research that is needed to enhance what we can offer in terms of survivorship care. We know that participation in survivorship programs increases patient satisfaction, yet we do not know if the changes we suggest and implement are maintained long term. Do survivorship programs make a difference in compliance? Do patients implement suggested changes into their lives? Are we able to hardwire our suggested changes into their lives? Survivorship is a new and important step in the patient care continuum. There are many ways to implement survivorship into your program in a personalized way. Research is needed to improve care and to give us evidence-based benchmarks for survivorship care to strive for in the future.

References

1. National Cancer Institute. About survivorship research: survivorship definitions. 2004. http://dccps.nci.nih.gov/ocs/definitions.html. Accessed 1 Dec 2012.
2. Mullan F. Seasons of survival: reflections of a physician with cancer. N Engl J Med. 1985;313:270–3.
3. Miller K, Ben-Aharon I, Haines L. Seasons of survival: redefining the paradigm for cancer survivorship for 2011. J Oncol Navig Surviv. 2011;2(5):12–5. Accessed Nov 2012.
4. Department of Health and Human Services, CDC, LiveSTRONG Foundation. A national action plan for cancer survivorship: advancing public health strategies. http://www.cdc.gov/cancer/survivorship/pdf/plan.pdf. Accessed 10 Apr 2009.
5. Hewitt M, Greenfield S, Stoval E, editors. From cancer patient to cancer survivor: lost in transition. Washington DC: The National Academies Press; 2006. Institute of Medicine and National Research Council of the National Academies.
6. Institute of Medicine of the National Academies Fact Sheet: Cancer Survivorship Care Planning. 2002. http://www.iom.edu/~/media/files/report%20files/2005/from-cancer-patient-to-cancer-survivor-lost-in-transition/factsheetcareplanning.pdf. Accessed 20 Mar 2011.
7. Institute of Medicine of The National Academies Fact Sheet: Cancer Survivorship Facts and Figures. 2005. http://www.iom.edu/~/media/files/report%20files/2005/from-cancer-patient-to-cancer-survivor-lost-in-transition/factsheetfactsandfigures.pdf. Accessed 20 Mar 2011.
8. Commission on Cancer Standards. 2012. http://www.facs.org/cancer/coc/standards.html. Accessed 12 Dec 2012.
9. LiveSTRONG Foundation. Essential elements of survivorship care: definitions and recommendations. Essential elements of survivorship care meeting summary. Washington DC 9-2011. http://www.livestrong.org/pdfs/3-8/EssentialElementsBrief. Accessed 15 July 2012.
10. Adler N, Page A, editors. Cancer care for the whole patient. Washington DC: The National Academies Press; 2008.
11. American Cancer Society. www.cancer.org.
12. Cancer Support Community. www.cancersupport-community.org.
13. Chubak J, Tuzzio L, Hsu C, Alfano C, Rabin B, Hornbrook M, Spegman A, Von Worley A, Williams A, Nekhlyudov L. Providing care for cancer survivors in integrated healthcare delivery systems: practices, challenges, and research opportunities. J Oncol Pract. 2012;8(3):184–9.
14. Ganz P, Hahn E. Implementing a survivorship care plan for patients with breast cancer. J Clin Oncol. 2008;26:759–67.
15. Greenfield E, et al. Randomized trial of long-term follow-up for early stage breast cancer: a comparison of family physicians versus specialists care. J Clin Oncol. 2006;24(6):848–55.

16. Hewitt M, Ganz P. (rapporteurs) Implementing cancer survivorship care planning – workshop summary. Washington DC: The National Academies Press; 2007.
17. Jackson J, Scheid K, Rolnick S. Development of the cancer survivorship care plan: /what's next? Life after cancer treatment. Clin J Oncol Nurs. 2013;17(3): 280–4.
18. Kendall J, Waddinton C, Bailiff M, Grusenmeyer P. Survivorship care in a community cancer center – a comprehensive multidisciplinary approach. Oncol Issues. 2007:30–34.
19. Ligibel J, Denlinger C. New NCCN guidelines for survivorship care. J Natl Compr Canc Netw. 2013;11: 640–4.
20. LiveSTRONG. http://www.livestrong.org/.
21. McCabe M, Bhatia S, Oeffinger K, Reaman G, Tyne C, Wollins D, Hudson M. American Society of Clinical Oncology Statement: achieving high-quality cancer survivorship care. http://jco.ascopubs.org/cgi/doi/10.1200/JCO.2012.46.6854. Accessed 15 Jan 2013.
22. Mulcahy N. ASCO Blueprint to improve cancer survivorship. http://www.medscape.com/viewarticle/777278_print. Accessed 15 Jan 2013.
23. National Coalition for Cancer Survivorship: Comprehensive Cancer Care Improvement Act. http://www.canceradvocacy.org/cancer-policy/cccia.html. Accessed 10 Dec 2012.
24. Shockney L, Tsangaris T. The Johns Hopkins breast cancer handbook for health care professionals. Sudbury: Jones and Bartlett Publishers; 2008.
25. Shockney L. Breast cancer survivorship care – a resource for nurses. Sudbury: Jones and Bartlett Publishers; 2011.
26. Komen SG. http://ww5.komen.org/.

Benign Breast Pathology

34

Gulbeyaz Omeroglu, Atilla Omeroglu, Yanxia Li, Rasheed Hammadeh, and Çağatay H. Erşahin

Reactive, Inflammatory, and Infectious Lesions

Inflammation of the breast can have different etiologies such as infectious, systemic autoimmune, or unknown, also classified as idiopathic (Tables 34.1 and 34.2) [1]. One important aspect to keep in mind when dealing with an inflamed breast is to be aware of inflammatory breast carcinoma. In the latter, the entire breast may be erythematous and warm to the touch, with areas of skin thickening and the classic "peau d'orange" often associated with inflammatory breast cancer.

Table 34.1 Pathological classification of benign breast diseases

Nonproliferative lesions
Cysts
Mild hyperplasia of the usual type
Epithelial-related calcifications
Fibroadenoma
Papillary apocrine change
Proliferative lesions without atypia
Sclerosing adenosis
Radial and complex sclerosing lesions
Moderate and florid hyperplasia of the usual type
Intraductal papillomas
Atypical proliferative lesions
Atypical ductal hyperplasia
Atypical lobular hyperplasia

Based on Love et al. [1]

Table 34.2 Clinical classification of benign breast diseases

Physiologic swelling and tenderness
Nodularity
Breast pain
Palpable lumps
Nipple discharge
Breast infections and inflammation

Based on Love et al. [1]

Inflammation of the breast can present in a similar fashion [2]. Failure to respond to antibiotic or anti-inflammatory treatment should raise the suspicion for an underlying malignancy, and biopsies should be performed of the skin and subcutaneous tissue

G. Omeroglu, MD (✉) • A. Omeroglu, MD
Department of Pathology, McGill University, 3775 University Street, Montreal, Quebec H3A 2B4, Canada
e-mail: gulbeyaz.omeroglu-altinel@muhc.mcgill.ca; atilla.omeroglu@muhc.mcgill.ca

Y. Li, MD, PhD
Department of Pathology, Loyola University Medical Center, Maywood, IL, USA

Department of Pathology, Adocate Christ Medical Center, 4440 W. 95th Street, Oak Lawn, IL 60514, USA
e-mail: yli@mdpmail.com

R. Hammadeh, MD
Department of Pathology, Advocate Christ Hospital and Medical Center, 4440 W. 95th Street, Oak Lawn, IL 60514, USA
e-mail: rhammadeh@mdpmail.com

Ç.H. Erşahin, MD, PhD
Department of Pathology, Silver Cross Hospital, 1900 Silver Cross Blvd., New Lenox, IL 60451, USA
e-mail: cersahi@hotmail.com

A.I. Riker (ed.), *Breast Disease: Comprehensive Management*,
DOI 10.1007/978-1-4939-1145-5_34, © Springer Science+Business Media New York 2015

(punch biopsy) or possibly a core of any suspicious underlying mass lesion. Similarly, pure squamous cell carcinoma (SCC) of the breast, although a rare entity, can also present with signs and symptoms of mastitis, as it can undergo central cystic changes (in approximately 50 % of cases) that is filled with keratin and necrotic debris eliciting an inflammatory response [3]. In such cases the clinical and radiologic findings might not discriminate benign from malignant lesions; therefore failure to respond to antibiotic therapy and identification of an underlying mass should prompt a core biopsy to clarify the diagnosis.

Most commonly encountered lesions in this segment are (a) lactation-related inflammation (acute mastitis), (b) non-puerperal periareolar inflammatory entities (periductal mastitis, Zuska's disease, and mammary duct ectasia), (c) fat necrosis, (d) sclerosing lymphocytic lobulitis, and (e) granulomatous mastitis. Those entities will be discussed below.

Lactation-Related Inflammation (Acute Mastitis)

Lactation-related inflammation is frequently seen during the first few months of breastfeeding. This is in contrast with inflammatory breast carcinoma, which is usually not associated with pregnancy [2]. The abscess appears as a red mass filled with pus and sometimes can mimic cancer. Biopsy procedures are rarely performed for this disorder, since it is usually managed by nonoperative means [4]. Synonyms are puerperal or acute mastitis, most usually presenting with the classical signs and symptoms of inflammation, such as localized pain, erythema, and associated fevers (Fig. 34.1). This is an inflammation of the breast stroma usually composed of neutrophils and plasma cells, which can lead to abscess formation and septicemia if left untreated [5]. *Staphylococcus aureus* is the most commonly identified infectious agent followed by *Staphylococcus epidermidis* and streptococci. Special stains can sometimes highlight the offending microorganism. It is thought that sleep deprivation, stress, and improper nursing techniques result in milk stasis and cracks of the nipple that lead to inflammation and infection [6]. Early diagnosis and treatment with antibiotics can lower the incidence of abscess formation. One should show due diligence in avoiding the use of antibiotics such as tetracycline that pass into breast milk and have harmful effects on the infant. Once an abscess is formed, aspiration or incision and drainage should be performed. Despite antibiotic therapy and drainage, if there

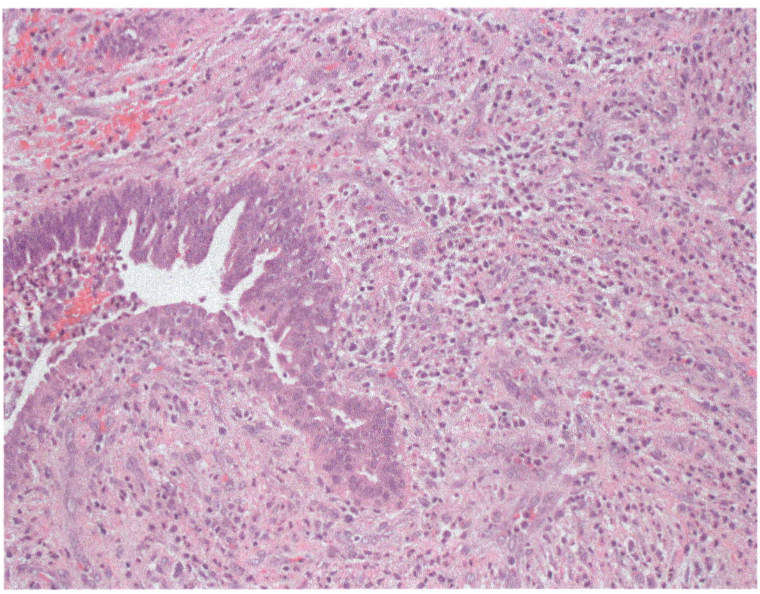

Fig. 34.1 Acute mastitis. Hematoxylin and eosin stain at 200× magnification

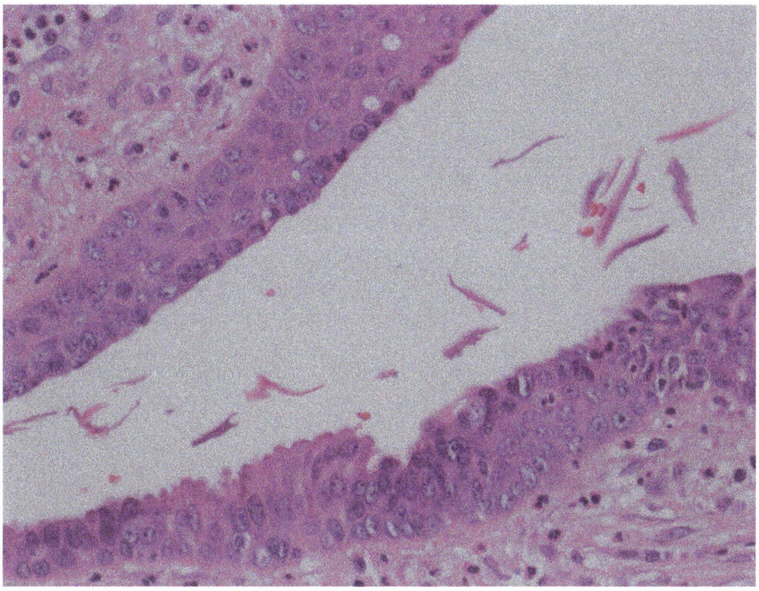

Fig. 34.2 Recurring subareolar abscess: squamous metaplasia. Hematoxylin and eosin stain at 400× magnification

is no response or if solid areas are identified, a tissue biopsy should be obtained to rule out the possibility of carcinoma.

Non-puerperal Periareolar Inflammatory Entities (Periductal Mastitis, Zuska's Disease, and Mammary Duct Ectasia)

The main difference between periductal mastitis and Zuska's disease or recurring subareolar abscess is that the latter occurs due to squamous metaplasia of the lactiferous ducts of the nipple, with secondary keratin plug formation that obstructs the proximal duct causing dilation and infection [5] (Figs. 34.2 and 34.3). This leads to abscess and fistula formation that drains at the margin of the areola [7]. Therefore Zuska's disease is also called SMOLDering (squamous metaplasia of lactiferous ducts) and can present with an inflamed and indurated nipple, nipple retraction, and painful nodules thus potentially mimicking cancer. Abscess drainage and excision of the affected ducts and fistula is the preferred treatment. In one series of 67 cases, half of the patients were successfully managed medically and the other half required surgical intervention [8]. In the same study, it was shown that radial elliptical incision with primary closure gave excellent long-term results. However, another study that looked at 24 women with a subareolar abscess suggests that the abscess together with the plugged duct has to be excised in order to prevent a recurrence [9]. The microbiologic studies performed on the material obtained from the lesions usually identify staphylococcus as the main infectious agent. Recurrent abscesses usually yield a mixed flora.

In a series of 60 patients suffering from recurrent subareolar breast abscess, heavy smoking was found at an unusually high frequency compared to a control group. The authors of the study postulated that cigarette smoking could have either a direct toxic effect on the retroareolar lactiferous ducts or an indirect effect via hormonal stimulation of the breast secretion [10]. Periductal mastitis on the other hand does not show squamous metaplasia, and the ducts are not dilated. It can occur centrally (periareolar) or peripherally. Periductal mastitis affects younger patients and should not be confused with mammary duct ectasia, which is a condition of the perimenopausal and postmenopausal women. Mammary duct ectasia characteristically shows dilation of the major ducts of the nipple with periductal fibrosis and inflammation (Fig. 34.4). The ducts may contain eosinophilic, granular, or inspissated material and sometimes

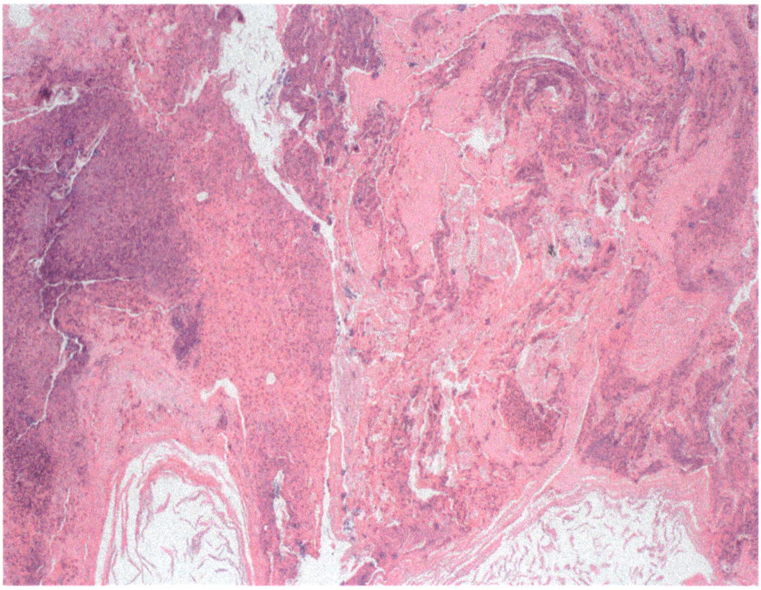

Fig. 34.3 Recurring subareolar abscess: keratin plug with secondary infection. Hematoxylin and eosin stain at 100× magnification

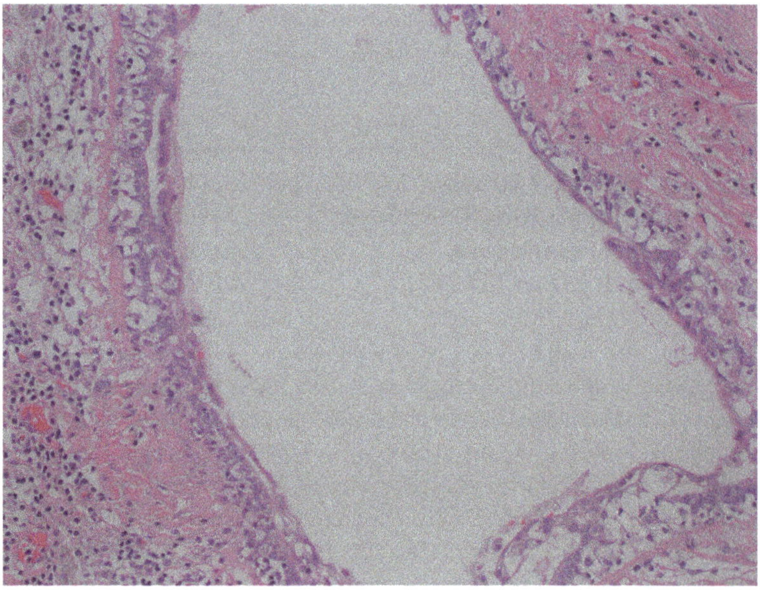

Fig. 34.4 Duct ectasia. Hematoxylin and eosin stain at 200× magnification

may become calcified. On gross examination, the inspissated material may mimic comedo necrosis that is associated with ductal carcinoma in situ. Some suggest that it is also related to smoking [11]. The disease usually affects the middle aged to older women and is usually asymptomatic. Occasionally, patients may present with nipple inversion, retraction, discharge, or a subareolar mass that may mimic a breast cancer [4]. Therefore, some patients with duct ectasia are biopsied to exclude malignancy; otherwise, most can be safely managed with mainly conservative measures [5]. Recurrence is uncommon.

Fat Necrosis

This is another entity that can be clinically confused with cancer, as it may present as an ill-defined, spiculated mass with associated skin retraction. Small areas of fat necrosis are probably not uncommon, but clinically significant

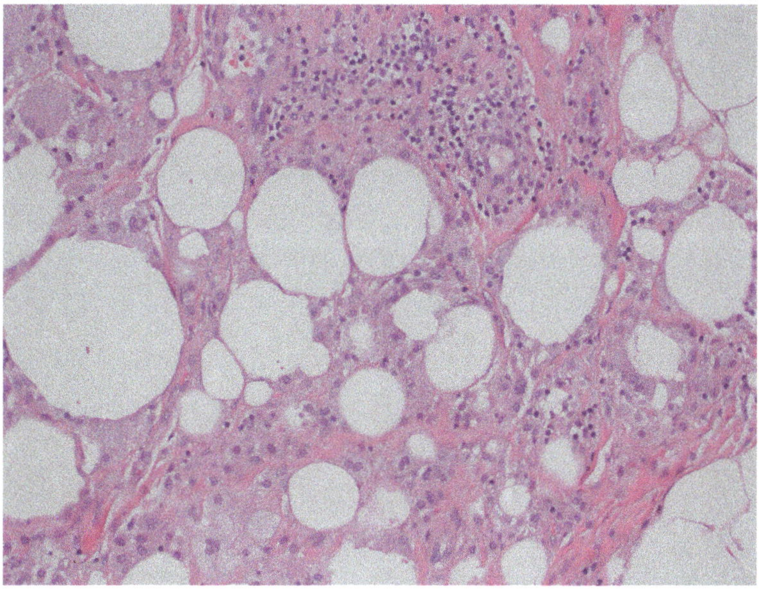

Fig. 34.5 Fat necrosis. Hematoxylin and eosin stain at 200× magnification

lesions are likely due to some sort of trauma, surgical procedure, biopsy, and radiation present in up to 50 % of patients; however the exact etiology is not always identified [12]. The lesion can also be associated with an adjacent malignancy [5]. Grossly, it may appear as a firm, ill-defined mass. Microscopically, the diagnosis is usually straightforward and is characterized by cystic spaces surrounded by lipid-laden histiocytes and foreign body-type giant cells (Fig. 34.5). Hemorrhage, a variable inflammatory infiltrate, and fibrosis can also be identified. When the lesion is fully evolved, it may have the appearance of a cystic cavity with calcified walls sometimes referred to as membranous fat necrosis [13].

Sclerosing Lymphocytic Lobulitis

This is a disorder usually occurring in patients with type 1, insulin-dependent diabetes mellitus. It can also be seen in nondiabetic patients that are affected by other autoimmune disorders such as Hashimoto's thyroiditis [14]. It is characterized by painless, immobile, discrete masses that are clinically suspicious for carcinoma. The lesions are usually bilateral but might also occur as a single mass. Radiologic findings can also be suspicious and usually require a biopsy to rule out a malignant proliferation. The majority of diabetic mastopathy lesions occur in the upper outer quadrant and are irregularly demarcated from the surrounding breast tissue.

Histologically, one usually finds a keloid-like fibrotic stroma; periductal, lobular, or perivascular lymphocytic infiltration by B cells; lobular atrophy; and fibroblasts embedded in fibrous stroma. Some point out that those findings are not specific as they may also be identified in patients with diabetes mellitus type 2 and nondiabetic patients [15]. It is postulated that this represents an immune reaction to hyperglycemia on connective tissue. Others suggest vascular changes as possible factors in the pathogenesis of diabetic mastopathy [16]. Microscopically sclerosing lymphocytic lobulitis shows small lymphocytes extending into epithelial cells, thus potentially mimicking a primary low-grade B cell lymphoma of the breast. Follow-up of patients with diabetic mastopathy is generally recommended.

Granulomatous Mastitis

As in other parts of the body, granulomatous inflammation (Fig. 34.6) of the breast can be infectious, idiopathic, due to foreign material or secondary to a systemic autoimmune disease such as sarcoidosis. The latter rarely involves

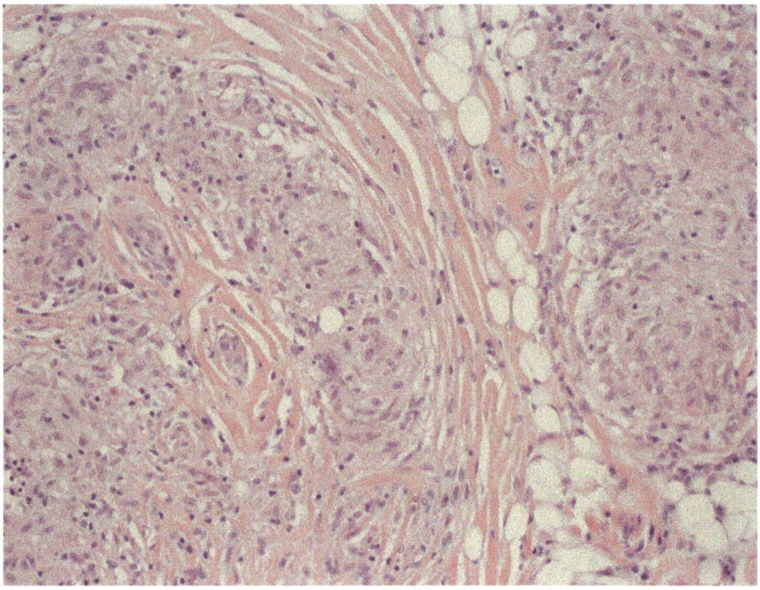

Fig. 34.6 Non-necrotizing granulomatous mastitis. Hematoxylin and eosin stain at 200× magnification

the breast, but it can simulate a neoplasm [17]. It is a diagnosis of exclusion and characterized by non-necrotizing granulomatous inflammation. Idiopathic granulomatous mastitis is an entity without an identifiable cause, thus also a diagnosis of exclusion. It may present as a mass simulating carcinoma, and it usually occurs in young women, often related to a recent pregnancy [18]. The management of this entity requires surgical excision, but sometimes it responds to corticosteroid therapy [4]. Management can be problematic, and despite treatment, recurrence and complications such as abscess and fistula formation are frequent [19]. The treatment sometimes spans over several years. Microscopically there are three neoplastic conditions in the differential diagnosis: histiocytic subtype of lobular carcinoma, carcinoma with osteoclastic giant cells, and granular cell tumor. In cases with abundant histiocytic cells, the inflammation can be confused with a rare variant of invasive lobular carcinoma called histiocytic type, where the neoplastic cells have ample cytoplasm and are disguised as histiocytes. In difficult cases immunohistochemical stains for keratin would confirm the diagnosis of carcinoma. The second tumor is invasive carcinoma with osteoclastic giant cells. In this condition malignant cells are accompanied by numerous reactive giant cells that are CD68 positive pointing to their histiocytic nature. Careful analysis of the surrounding carcinomatous cells should help in arriving at correct diagnosis. Granular cell tumor is another entity that might mimic an inflammatory condition composed of histiocytes. It is a rare neoplasm that usually occurs in other parts of the body, such as the head and neck, oral cavity, and digestive system [20]. It can also involve the breast in approximately 5 % of cases. This is a benign tumor that clinically may show fixation to the pectoral fascia, skin retraction, and ulceration, thus mimicking an invasive carcinoma. It may also occur in the male breast [21]. They are usually small lesions, measuring less than 3 cm, composed of polygonal cells with granular cytoplasm mimicking histiocytes (Fig. 34.7). They express the S100 protein and this is very useful in the confirmation of the diagnosis (Fig. 34.8). The tumor is believed to arise from peripheral nerve sheet cells, i.e., Schwann cells. Rarely, the tumors can be malignant, with the most useful characteristics of malignancy being large size (>5 cm), pleomorphic cells, prominent nucleoli, increased mitotic activity, necrosis, and local recurrence. Both benign and malignant tumors are treated with wide surgical excision. Incomplete excision may result in recurrence. Adjuvant treatment is only reserved for malignant tumors.

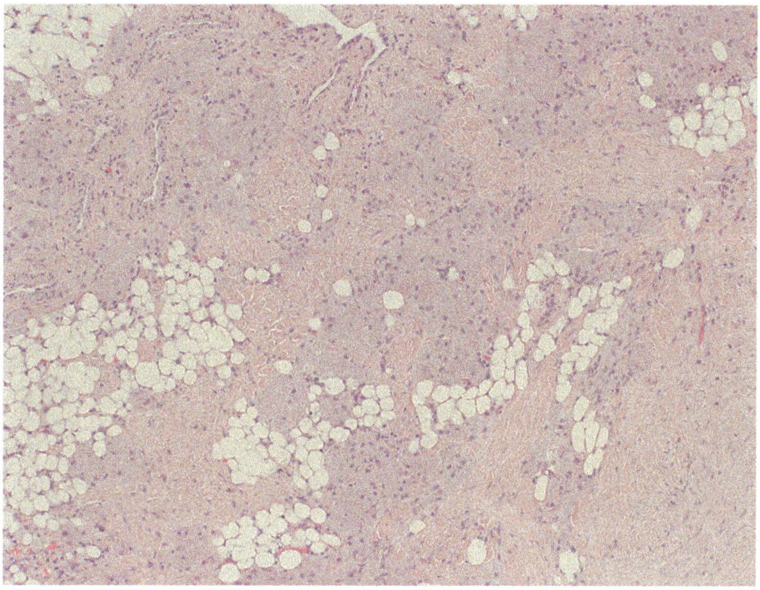

Fig. 34.7 Granular cell tumor. Hematoxylin and eosin stain at 40× magnification

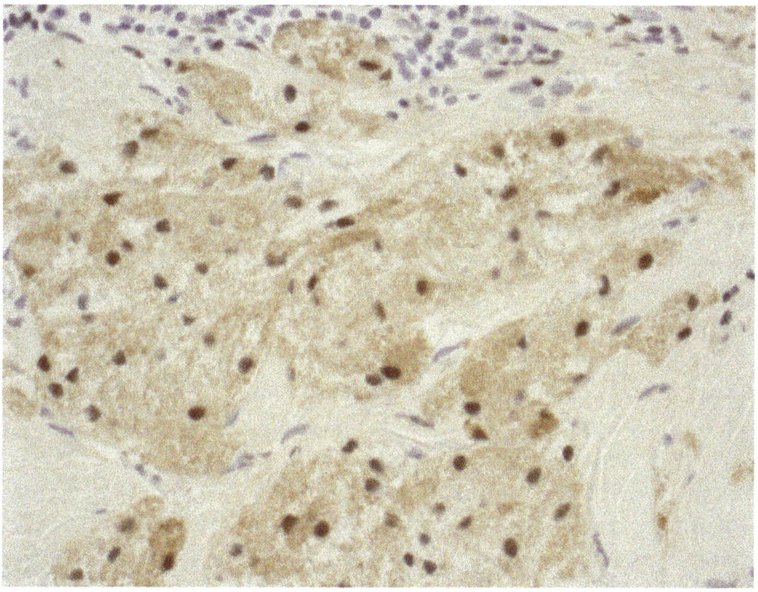

Fig. 34.8 Granular cell tumor: S100 stain at 400× magnification

Fibrocystic Changes (FCC) and Columnar Cell Changes (CCC)

Previously referred to as fibrocystic "disease" of the breast, the term "disease" has been dropped in favor of "changes." This is due to its very high prevalence and because it caused confusion between normal, physiologic changes and pathological ones [22]. Histologically, fibrocystic change can be identified in up to 90 % of all breast tissue examined in women. The most common presenting symptoms are breast pain and palpable nodules or lumps in the breast. It has been noted in a retrospective cohort study that only 6 % of patients between 40 and 70 years of age presenting with breast symptoms had cancer [23]. Cysts are the main component of fibrocystic changes and are characterized by fluid-filled structures that are mostly small and non-palpable, but approximately 20–25 %

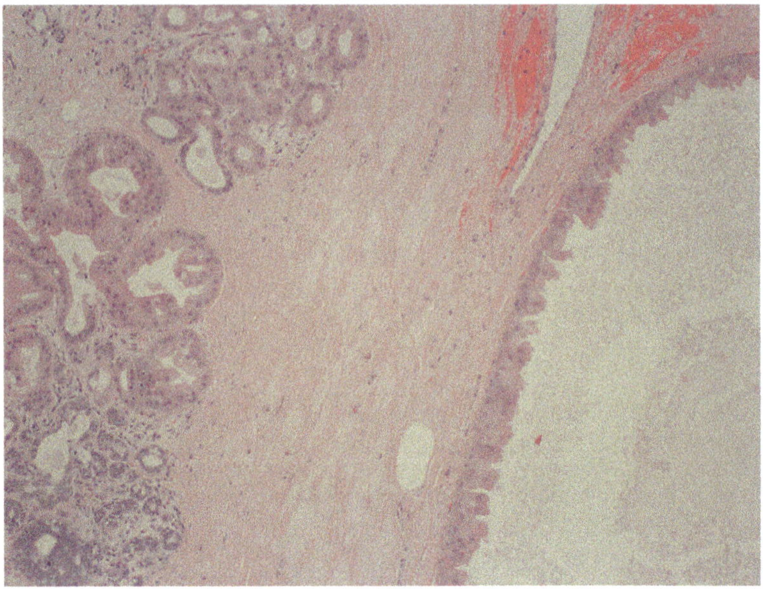

Fig. 34.9 Fibrocystic changes. Hematoxylin and eosin stain at 100× magnification

of them are large enough to present as masses [5, 24]. Mammography and physical examination are not reliable and cannot truly distinguish cysts from solid masses [25]. The utility of ultrasound can help to further define an abnormality identified on mammogram. Simple cysts are usually devoid of a lining or have a flat epithelium that sometimes may show apocrine metaplasia. Complex cysts have internal thin septations, thickened or irregular wall, and absent posterior acoustic enhancement on ultrasound. The malignancy rate in patients with complex cysts is very low, 0.3 % in one study, lower than that of lesions classified as probably benign [26]. If there is concern that the cyst is other than a simple cyst, possibly with internal wall thickening or complex septations, consideration should be given to further evaluation and possible biopsy of these areas in order to exclude a malignancy.

Besides cysts, FCC also comprises other lesions such as apocrine metaplasia (Fig. 34.9), epithelial hyperplasia both atypical and non-atypical, adenosis, radial scar, and papilloma. The most useful way to classify FCC is to divide it into three groups according to their risk of developing breast cancer: nonproliferative lesions (cysts, apocrine metaplasia, mild epithelial hyperplasia, non-sclerosing adenosis), proliferative lesions without atypia (moderate to florid epithelial hyperplasia, sclerosing adenosis, radial scar, papilloma, and papillomatosis), and proliferative lesions with atypia (atypical ductal hyperplasia and atypical lobular hyperplasia) [5] (Table 34.3). Relative to general population, women with nonproliferative lesions have no increased risk for developing breast cancer. On the other hand patients with non-atypical proliferative and atypical proliferative lesions have relative risks ranging from 1.3 to 1.9 and 3.9 to 13, respectively [27–30].

Table 34.3 Classification of fibrocystic changes

Nonproliferative lesions	Proliferative lesions without atypia	Proliferative lesions with atypia
Cysts	Moderate to florid epithelial hyperplasia	Atypical ductal hyperplasia
Apocrine metaplasia	Sclerosing adenosis	Atypical lobular hyperplasia
Mild epithelial hyperplasia	Radial scar	
Non-sclerosing adenosis	Papilloma and papillomatosis	

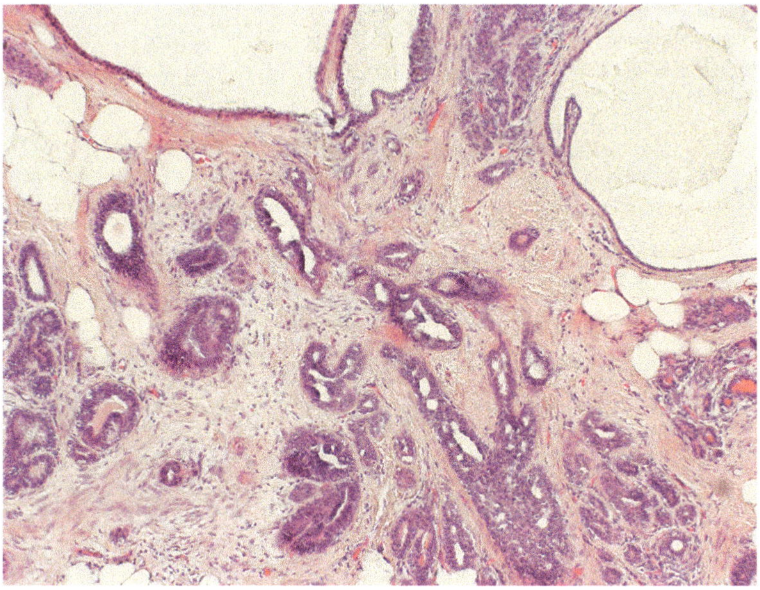

Fig. 34.10 Radial scar. Hematoxylin and eosin stain at 40× magnification

Adenosis and Microglandular Adenosis

Adenosis is defined as a glandular proliferation of the lobular units, with two subtypes that merit mentioning: sclerosing adenosis and microglandular adenosis. Sclerosing adenosis is a disordered proliferation of acini, myoepithelial cells and stromal elements that can be confused for invasive carcinoma both microscopically and grossly [5]. It can present as a mass or a radiologic abnormality such as an asymmetric opacity, cluster of microcalcifications, mass-like lesion, and architectural distortion [31]. In difficult lesions posing a diagnostic challenge, myoepithelial markers can be performed to rule out carcinoma.

On the other hand, microglandular adenosis is characterized by a proliferation of uniform small round glands haphazardly distributed within the breast parenchyma. The most important aspect of this lesion is that it lacks a myoepithelial layer; thus it can be easily confused with carcinoma. The presence of basal lamina encircling glandular structures, which can be confirmed by immunohistochemical stains, and overall round, rather than angulated, morphology of the glands are features that can be used in ruling out a malignant process. There is some evidence that microglandular adenosis can potentially progress to carcinoma, and it can recur if incompletely excised. Occasionally, microglandular adenosis presents as a palpable mass and may be associated with both in situ and invasive carcinoma [32].

Radial Scar and Complex Sclerosing Lesion

Radial scar is characterized by a fibroelastotic core with entrapped glandular structures, radiating ducts that become larger at the periphery of the lesion, and associated epithelial hyperplasia (Fig. 34.10). When larger than 1 cm, some refer to them as a "complex sclerosing lesion," while others require a less organized architecture to classify those as complex sclerosing lesions [4]. Mammographically, they may appear as a spiculated mass mimicking carcinoma [33]. Atypical epithelial proliferations as well as in situ and invasive carcinomas can be associated with radial scars. In general, a radial scar has an increased incidence of malignancy, whereas others found that radial scars are mainly associated with benign breast lesions. Based on its size, radial scars can be either excised or biopsied. Some but

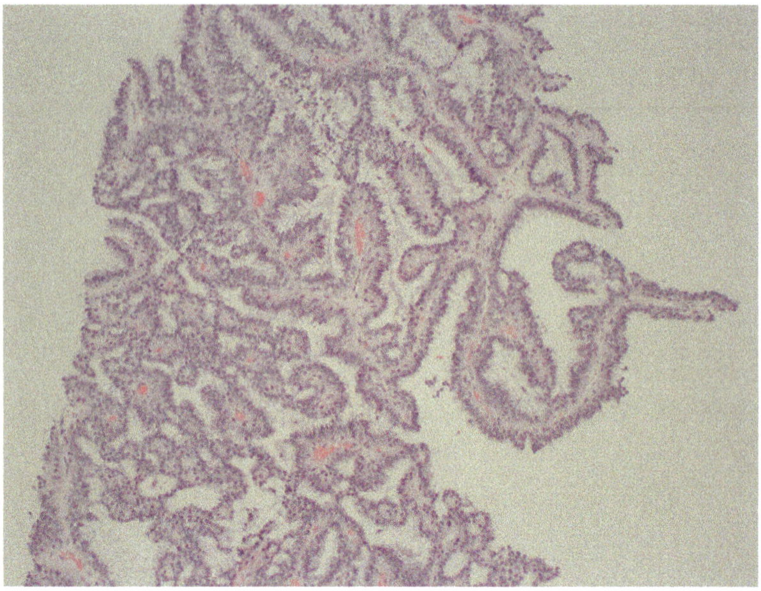

Fig. 34.11 Papilloma. Hematoxylin and eosin stain at 100× magnification

not all believe that radial scars identified on core needle biopsies should be excised due to their association with premalignant and malignant conditions [34]. Radial scars identified on excisional specimens need no further therapy [4].

Papillomas and Papillomatosis

Papillomas are frond-like intraductal proliferations of benign epithelial and myoepithelial cells (Fig. 34.11). They are usually encountered in two types: central and peripheral. Central ones are usually solitary and larger, whereas the peripheral ones tend to be smaller and multiple. Unless associated with atypical epithelial proliferations, central papillomas are not considered premalignant lesions. Certain studies confirm an increased incidence of in situ and invasive carcinoma on excisional specimens in patients with atypical ductal proliferation inside papillomas. On excisional biopsy samples, if the atypical epithelium is confined to the papilloma and the surrounding tissue is non-atypical, then the finding has no prognostic significance. In one study, 29 % of patients diagnosed with intraductal papilloma on core needle biopsy were upstaged to papilloma with atypia on excisional specimens, and 10 % were upstaged to carcinoma [35]. The authors concluded that surgical excision is recommended for benign papillary lesions diagnosed on core needle biopsies (Fig. 34.11).

However, other studies found an upstage rate of only 8.9 % to atypia or malignancy on the excision specimens [36]. Others report that only 3 % of cases diagnosed as benign papilloma on core biopsy are associated with malignancy and recommend follow-up instead of excision [37]. Furthermore, they show a high association with malignancy (67 %) when the diagnosis on biopsy was atypical papilloma and suggest prompt excision for definitive diagnosis. Papillomatosis or multiple papillomas, usually defined as having five or more peripheral papillomas, indicate a slightly elevated risk for subsequent carcinoma. Specimens containing multiple papillomas should be sampled extensively to rule out malignancy. Juvenile papillomatosis is another variant occurring in young patients younger than 30 years old. This is associated with a higher incidence of breast cancer and higher incidence of a family history of breast cancer. Therefore, those patients and their families require long-term follow-up.

Columnar Cell Changes

Columnar cell lesions are encountered with increasing frequency on breast biopsies due to associated microcalcifications detected on

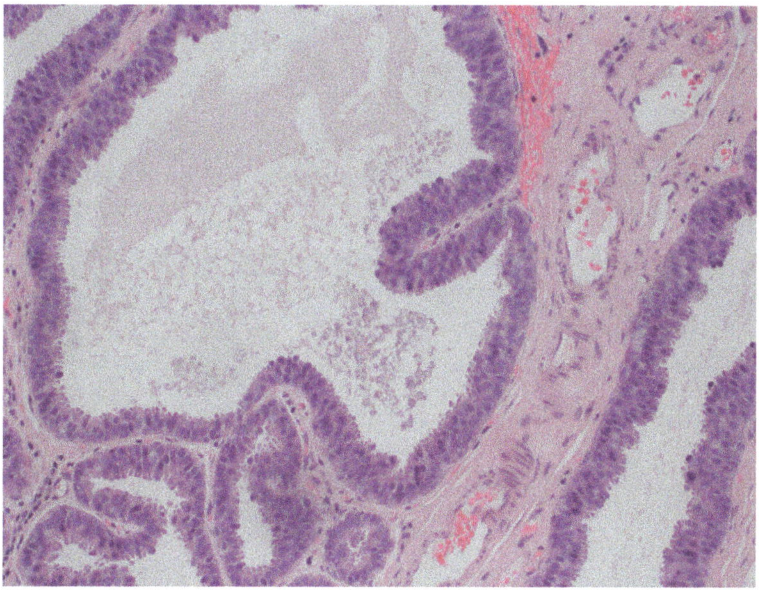

Fig. 34.12 Flat epithelial atypia. Hematoxylin and eosin stain at 200× magnification

screening mammograms [38]. When atypical, it is called "flat epithelial atypia" (FEA) with total excision of the area generally recommended, as there may be a more significant lesion in the surrounding breast tissue [39] (Fig. 34.12). Overall, its progression rate to invasive carcinoma is exceedingly low. However some suggest FEA should just be followed up and not surgically excised. It appears that more studies are needed to determine the significance of atypia in columnar cell alternations.

When flat epithelial atypia is diagnosed on core needle biopsy, the rate in upstaging to carcinoma on subsequent excision is 14 % [40]. The same study shows that the differences in upstaging in subsequent excisions in flat epithelial atypia and atypical ductal hyperplasia group were not statistically different. When FEA microscopically develops architectural changes such as micropapillary and cribriform patterns, the lesion is designated as atypical ductal hyperplasia. Some noted genetic alterations shared with low-grade ductal carcinoma in situ and tubular carcinoma suggesting that flat epithelial atypia might be a precursor of these lesions [41]. One interesting aspect of both atypical and non-atypical columnar cell changes is the diffuse and strong nuclear estrogen and progesterone receptor expression [41]. This is in contrast with normal breast epithelium that is usually only sparsely positive for the same receptors. Nevertheless, when columnar cell changes without atypia are encountered on breast biopsies, patient follow-up is considered sufficient.

Neoplasms

Fibroadenoma and Adenoma

As the most common mass lesion of the breast, fibroadenoma can be identified in up to 25 % of asymptomatic women [42]. This is a hormone-dependent lesion that occurs in young women, during lactational phases of pregnancy, and involutes at menopause. Oral contraceptive use before 20 years of age appears to increase the risk of developing fibroadenoma. It is usually unilateral, but in 20 % of cases, the tumors are multiple and can be bilateral [42]. It develops from the specialized stroma of the lobules. Grossly, the lesions are well-circumscribed, resilient lesions, showing a bulging cut surface and usually measuring less than 3 cm. Tumors reaching more than 10 cm in greatest dimension are often seen in younger patients and are called "giant fibroadenoma." Histologically, fibroadenomas are biphasic tumors that have both stromal and epithelial elements. Some studies suggest that both elements are neoplastic. Based on microscopic

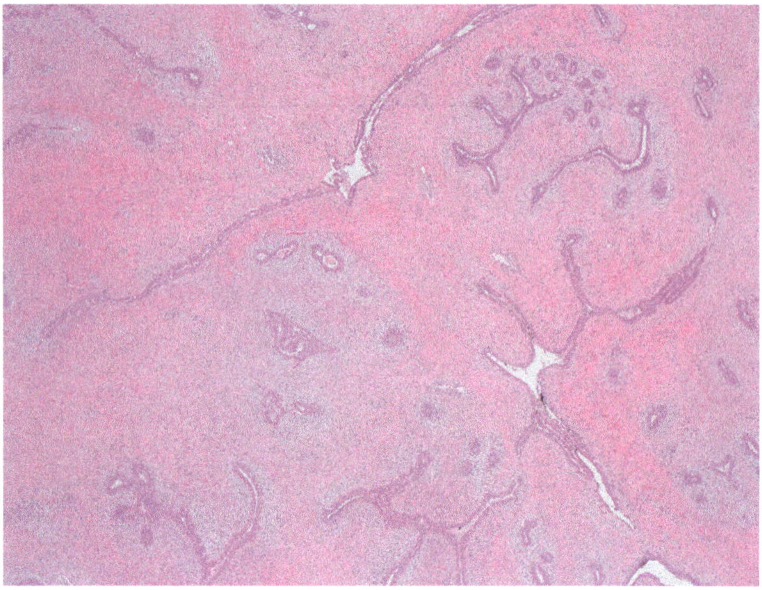

Fig. 34.13 Juvenile fibroadenoma. Hematoxylin and eosin stain at 40× magnification

appearance, the lesions can be divided into pericanalicular and intracanalicular types. The former is characterized by stromal growth around the glandular structures, whereas the latter shows compressed, cleft-like ducts. It is not uncommon that the two patterns occur together in the same tumor.

Histologically the main differential diagnosis for fibroadenomas is the phyllodes tumor, which is also a biphasic tumor. Benign phyllodes tumor can be difficult to distinguish from a fibroadenoma. Features such as stromal atypia, infiltrative margins, increased mitotic activity, and stromal cellularity favor a diagnosis of phyllodes tumor. The importance of distinguishing between the two lesions is that a phyllodes tumor needs to be excised with clear margins. Approximately 50 % of fibroadenomas contain epithelial proliferations such as sclerosing adenosis and epithelial hyperplasia. Those are classified as "complex fibroadenoma." While regular fibroadenoma is not associated with increased risk of developing cancer, patients with complex fibroadenoma have a slightly higher risk of developing breast cancer. Likewise, fibroadenomas in older women or in patients with a family history of breast cancer have a higher incidence of breast cancer.

Management of patients with fibroadenoma varies depending on the treating physicians. Some prefer to excise the tumors, while others will conservatively manage patients without operative removal. One study showed that an expectant management policy of fibroadenomas has not resulted in misdiagnosis of carcinomas. The same study claims that since a significant proportion of fibroadenomas remain static or reduce in size over a 5-year period, many women can avoid excision [43]. In general, there are three reasons to remove a fibroadenoma: persistent pain, rapid growth over a short period of time and cosmetic deformity related to a fibroadenoma just underneath the skin of the breast. A thorough conversation is important in determining the optimal approach to management, discussing both the risks and benefits of operative removal. However, it should be made clear that there is little, if any, risk of malignant degeneration or transformational risk to carcinoma associated with a fibroadenoma.

Some phyllodes tumors show areas compatible with a fibroadenoma on histologic evaluation. In such cases, undersampling of the lesion might result in underestimation of the lesion, i.e., a phyllodes tumor can be misdiagnosed as fibroadenoma on a core needle biopsy. Juvenile fibroadenoma is a rare variant that occurs in patients between the ages of 10 and 18. It is usually a larger mass, with an alarming rapid growth and gross disfigurement, measuring more than 5 cm, and is usually unilateral and painless (Fig. 34.13). Although it is a benign lesion, excision is usually recommended [44].

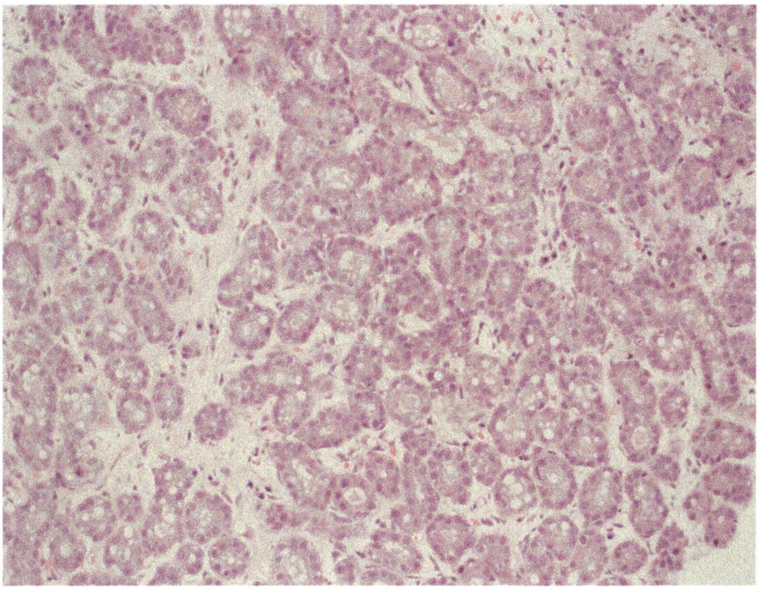

Fig. 34.14 Lactating adenoma. Hematoxylin and eosin stain at 200× magnification

Unlike biphasic fibroadenoma, adenoma is a pure benign epithelial lesion. Several variants exist such as tubular, lactating, apocrine, ductal, and pleomorphic (a lesion similar to a mixed tumor of the salivary glands). Except tubular and lactating adenomas, the remaining lesions are exceedingly rare; therefore, only those two lesions will be discussed. Lactating adenoma is a benign lesion with no malignant potential (Fig. 34.14). It is composed of hyperplastic lobules showing active secretion. It is thought to represent a variant of preexisting tubular adenoma or fibroadenoma [45]. It is usually a small lesion, less than 3 cm in overall diameter, and sometimes involutes post-pregnancy. In certain situations, it is resected due to the mass effect it produces. The lesion does not tend to recur. Tubular adenoma is also characterized by packed tubular and acinar structures with very scant stroma. Clinically and radiographically, such lesions can easily be confused with a fibroadenoma, sometimes showing calcifications. It is a benign lesion usually occurring in patients younger than 35 years old [46].

Nipple Adenoma and Syringomatous Adenoma

Nipple adenoma is an infrequent type of benign breast neoplasm that can show various histologic pictures. Those lesions usually present with nipple discharge and erosion, sometimes mimicking Paget's disease [47]. Histologically, it shows proliferating epithelial structures that might be confused with carcinoma (Fig. 34.15). Identifying a myoepithelial layer usually confirms the diagnosis. The lesions are treated with excision and they may recur if incompletely excised. Nipple adenoma is a benign tumor; however, some describe malignant changes within or adjacent to the lesions [48]. Syringomatous adenoma of the skin can also involve the nipple and is in the differential diagnosis. This is a more infiltrative lesion that requires excision and can recur but does not metastasize. It is characterized by bland infiltrative glands, some showing keratin cyst formation. It resembles the peripherally located low-grade adenosquamous carcinoma of the breast.

Hamartoma

Hamartoma, also known as a fibroadenolipoma, lipofibroadenoma, or adenolipoma, is composed of a mixture of glandular, adipose, and fibrous tissue (Fig. 34.16). Clinically, hamartomas present as a painless mass. It is considered to be a developmental abnormality, rather than a true neoplastic process. Some cases are associated with Cowden's syndrome [49], an autosomal dominant disorder

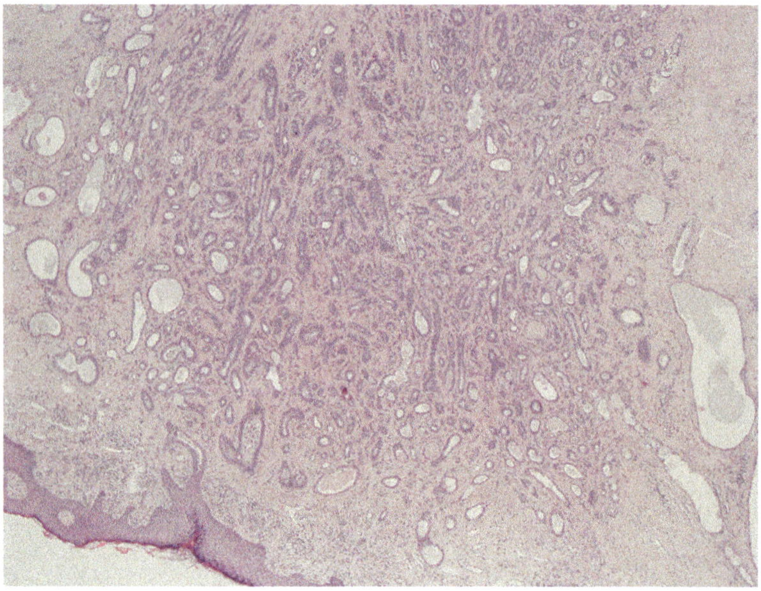

Fig. 34.15 Nipple adenoma. Hematoxylin and eosin stain at 20× magnification

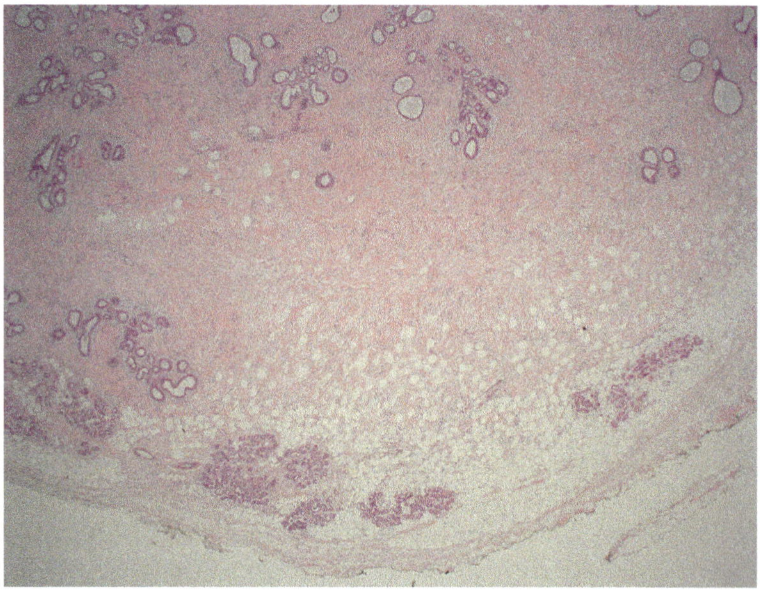

Fig. 34.16 Hamartoma. Hematoxylin and eosin stain at 20× magnification

that is characterized by macrocephaly, hamartomatous intestinal polyps, benign skin tumors, and dysplastic gangliocytoma of the cerebellum. Patients with this syndrome have a predisposition to develop breast, thyroid, and endometrial carcinoma. Macroscopically, those lesions are well-circumscribed tumors. Microscopically one sees normal breast and adipose tissue distributed in a nodular fashion. These lesions may go unrecognized by the pathologists because they show all the constituents of normal breast tissue and maybe reported as "no pathological diagnosis"

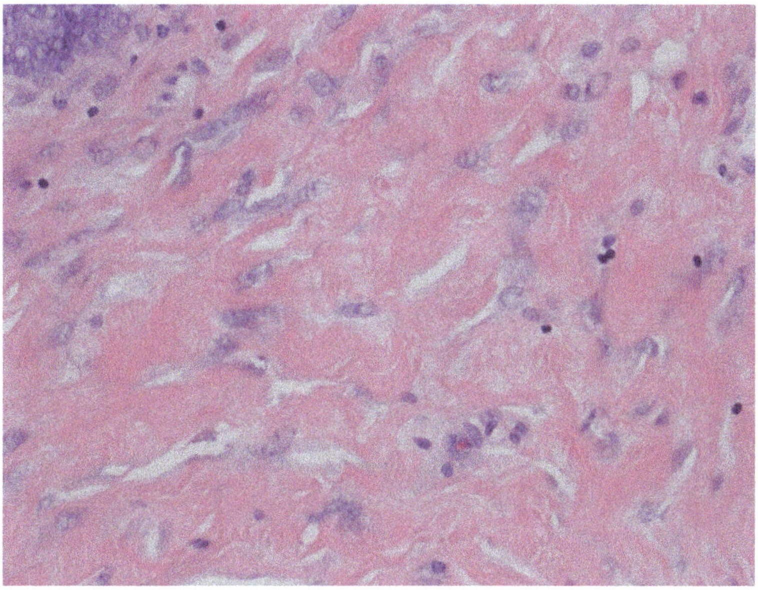

Fig. 34.17 Pseudoangiomatous stromal hyperplasia. Hematoxylin and eosin stain at 400× magnification

or "normal breast tissue" [50]. The treatment of hamartoma is surgical excision.

Pseudoangiomatous Stromal Hyperplasia (PASH) and Myofibroblastoma

Although not considered a true neoplasm, this benign proliferation of myofibroblasts in the breast stroma can present as a clinically palpable mass. It is however mostly an incidental finding on biopsies and excisions performed for other conditions. It may be identified in up to 23 % of breast specimens [51]. Its etiology is unknown; however hormonal stimulation, especially progesterone, is stipulated as a factor for the development of PASH lesions. PASH cells show expression of progesterone receptor and are positive for vimentin and CD34. Smooth muscle actin and desmin are variably expressed [4]. In rare cases where PASH forms a mass, it is usually well circumscribed and mimics a fibroadenoma or a phyllodes tumor. Microscopically, the lesions show anastomosing slit-like spaces within a collagenous stroma (Fig. 34.17). Due to this histologic appearance, one can easily mistake those benign lesions for angiosarcomas (Fig. 34.18). In difficult cases, immunohistochemical stains can be used to confirm the diagnosis. PASH can recur when treated with excision. However, so far malignant transformation has not been described [5].

Myofibroblastoma is a benign tumor that is well circumscribed, slow growing, and mobile. It is frequently mistaken for a fibroadenoma both on physical examination and radiologically [4]. The cells are bland and admixed with a collagenized stroma. Some have abundant stromal collagen and some are more cellular. The cells sometimes appear epithelioid and can form aggregates, thus microscopically mimicking carcinoma. As the lesional cells are also estrogen and progesterone positive, this may further complicate the diagnosis. In difficult cases, a lack of staining with keratin immunohistochemical stains and positivity with CD34 and desmin stains confirm the diagnosis. Some cases of PASH may show areas resembling myofibroblastoma, suggesting that the two entities are related. The treatment of myofibroblastoma is excision, which is considered curative.

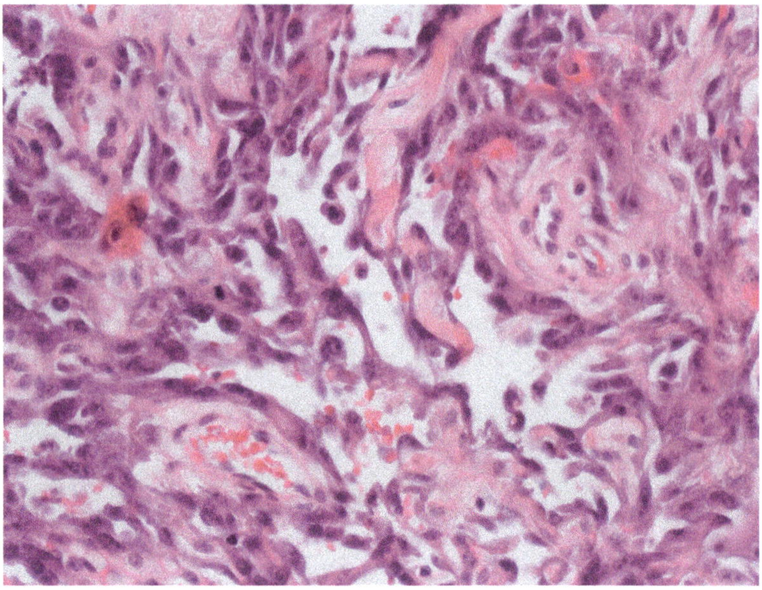

Fig. 34.18 Angiosarcoma. Hematoxylin and eosin stain at 100× magnification

References

1. Love S, Gelman RS, Silen W. Fibrocystic disease of the breast, a nondisease? N Engl J Med. 1982;307:1010–4.
2. Anderson JM. Inflammatory carcinomas of the breast. Ann R Coll Surg Engl. 1980;62(3):195–9.
3. Murialdo R, Bay D, Musizzano Y, et al. Squamous cell carcinoma of the breast: a case report. Case J. 2009;2:7336.
4. Schnitt SJ, Collins LC. Biopsy interpretation of the breast. Philadelphia: Lippincott Williams & Wilkins; 2009.
5. Guray M, Sahin AA. Benign breast diseases: classification, diagnosis, and management. Oncologist. 2006;11:435–49.
6. Foxman B, D'Arcy H, Gillespie B, et al. Lactation mastitis: occurrence and medical management among 946 breast feeding women in the United States. Am J Epidemiol. 2002;155:103–14.
7. Passaro ME, Broughan TA, Sebek BA, et al. Lactiferous fistula. J Am Coll Surg. 1994;178:29–32.
8. Lannin DR. Twenty-two year experience with recurring subareolar abscess and lactiferous duct fistula treated by a single breast surgeon. Am J surg. 2004;188(4):407–10.
9. Meguid MM, Oler A, Numann PJ, Khan S. Pathogenesis based treatment of recurring subareolar abscess. Surgery. 1995;118(4):775–82.
10. Schäfer P, Furrer C, Mermillod B. An association of cigarette smoking with recurrent subareolar breast abscess. Int J Epidemol. 1988;17(4):810–3.
11. Furlong AJ, Al-Nakib L, Knox WF, et al. Periductal inflammation and cigarette smoke. J Am Coll Surg. 1994;179:417–20.
12. Roisman I, Barak V, Manny J, Libson E, Wygoda M, Neuman A, et al. Fat necrosis below musculocutaneous flap mimicking carcinoma of breast. Ann Plast Surg. 1991;26(5):479–82.
13. Coyne JD, Parkinson D, Baildam AD. Membranous fat necrosis of the breast. Histopathology. 1996;28(1):61–4.
14. Dabbs DJ. Breast pathology. Philadelphia: Saunders/Elsevier Inc.; 2012.
15. Ely KA, Tse G, Simpson JF, Clarfeld R, Page DL. Diabetic mastopathy. A clinicopathological review. Am J Clin Pathol. 2000;113:541–5.
16. Dorokhova O, Fineberg S, Koenigsberg T, Wang Y. Diabetic mastopathy, a clinicopathological correlation of 34 cases. Pathol Int. 2012;62:660–4.
17. Gansler TS, Wheeler JE. Mammary sarcoidosis. Two cases and literature review. Arch Pathol Lab Med. 1984;108(8):673–5.
18. Kessler E, Wolloch Y. Granulomatous mastitis: a lesion clinically stimulating carcinoma. Am J Clin Pathol. 1972;58(6):642–6.
19. Azlina AF, Ariza Z, Arni T, et al. Chronic granulomatous mastitis: diagnostic and therapeutic considerations. World J Surg. 2003;27:515–8.
20. Aoyama K, Kamio T, Hirano A, Seshimo A, Kameoka S. Granular cell tumors: a report of six cases. World J Surg Oncol. 2012;10:204.
21. Kim EY, Kang DK, Kim TH, Jung YS, Kim KS, Yim H. Granular cell tumor of the male breast: two case descriptions and brief review of literature. J Ultrasound Med. 2011;30(9):1295–301.
22. Vaidyanathan L, Barnard K, Elnicki DM. Benign breast disease: when to treat, when to reassure, when to refer. Cleve Clin J Med. 2002;69(5):425–32.
23. Barton MB, Elmore JG, Fletcher SW. Breast symptoms among women enrolled in a health maintenance

organization: frequency, evaluation and outcome. Ann Intern Med. 1999;130:651–7.
24. Donegan WL. Common benign conditions of the breast. In: Donegan WL, Spratt JS, editors. Cancer of the breast. 5th ed. St Louis: Saunders; 2002. p. 67–110.
25. Huff JG. The sonographic findings and differing clinical implications of simple complicated, and complex breast cysts. J Natl Compr Canc Netw. 2009;7(101):1101–4.
26. Venta LA, Kim JP, Pelloski CE, Morrow M. Management of complex breast cysts. AJR Am J Roentgenol. 1999;173:1331–6.
27. Dupont WD, Page DL. Risk factors for breast cancer in women with proliferative breast disease. N Engl J Med. 1985;312:146–51.
28. Dupont WD, Parl FF, Hartmann WH, et al. Breast cancer risk associated with proliferative breast disease and atypical hyperplasia. Cancer. 1993;71:1258–65.
29. Palli D, del Turco R, Simoncini R, et al. Benign breast disease and breast cancer: a case control study in a cohort in Italy. Int J Cancer. 1993;71:1258–65.
30. Marshall LM, Hunter DJ, Connolly JL, et al. Risk of breast cancer associated with atypical hyperplasia of lobular and ductal types. Cancer Epidemiol Biomarkers Prev. 1997;6:297–301.
31. Taskin F, Koseoglu K, Unsal A, Erkus M, Ozbas S, et al. Sclerosing adenosis of the breast: radiologic appearance and efficiency of core needle biopsy. Diagn Interv Radiol. 2011;17(40):311–6.
32. Rosen PP. Microglandular adenosis. A benign lesion simulating invasive mammary carcinoma. Am J Surg Pathol. 1983;7(2):137–44.
33. Adler DD, Helvie MA, Oberman HA, et al. Radial sclerosing lesion of the breast: mammographic features. Radiology. 1990;176(3):737–40.
34. Osborn G, Wilton F, Stevens G, Vaughan Williams E, Gower-Thomas K. A review of needle core biopsy diagnosed radial scars in the Welsh breast screening programme. Ann R Coll Surg Engl. 2011;93(2): 123–6.
35. Shouhed D, Amersi FF, Spurrier R, Dang C, Astwatsaturyan K, Bose S, et al. Intraductal papillary lesions of the breast: clinical and pathological correlation. Am Surg. 2012;78(10):1161–5.
36. Richter-Ehrenstein C, Tombokan F, Fallenberg EM, Schneider A, Denkert C. Intraductal papillomas of the breast: diagnosis and management of 151 patients. Breast. 2011;20(6):501–4.
37. Sydnor MK, Wilson JD, Hijaz TA, Massey HD, Shaw de Paredes ES. Underestimation of the presence of breast carcinoma in papillary lesions diagnosed at core needle biopsy. Radiology. 2007;242(1):58–62.
38. Schnitt SJ, Vincent-Salomon A. Columnar cell lesions of the breast. Adv Anat Pathol. 2003;10:113–24.
39. Schnitt SJ. The diagnosis and management of pre-invasive breast disease: flat epithelial atypia – classification, pathological features and clinical significance. Breast Cancer Res. 2003;5:263–8.
40. Mamatha C, Rohit B, George T, David JD. Clinicopathologic implications of "flat epithelial atypia" in core needle biopsy specimens of the breast. Am J Clin Pathol. 2009;131:802–8.
41. Simpson PT, Gale T, Reis-Filho JS, et al. Columnar cell lesions of the breast: the missing link in the breast cancer progression? A morphological and molecular analysis. Am J Surg Pathol. 2005;29(6): 734–46.
42. El-Wakeel H, Umpleby HC. Systematic review of fibroadenoma as a risk factor for breast cancer. Breast. 2003;12:302–7.
43. Carty NJ, Carter C, Rubin C, Ravichandran D, Royle GT, et al. Management of the fibroadenoma of the breast. Ann R Coll Surg Engl. 1995;77(2): 127–30.
44. Abdelhadi MS. Giant juvenile fibroadenoma: experience from a university hospital. J Family Community Med. 2005;12(2):91–5.
45. Choudhury M, Singal MK. Lactating adenoma, cytomorphologic study with review of literature. Indian J Pathol Microbiol. 2001;44(4):445–8.
46. Soo MS, Dash N, Bentley R, Lee LH, Nathan G. Tubular adenomas of the breast: imaging findings with histologic correlation. AJR Am J Roentgenol. 2000;174(3):757–61.
47. Healy CE, Dijkstra B, Walsh M, Hill AD, Murphy J. Nipple adenoma: a differential diagnosis for Paget's disease. Breast J. 2003;9(4):325–6.
48. Vianna LL, Millis RR, Fentiman IS. Adenoma of the nipple: a diagnostic dilemma. Br J Hosp Med. 1994; 50(11):639–42.
49. Sabate JM, Gomez A, Torrubia S, Blancas C, Sanchez G. Evaluation of breast involvement in relation to Cowden syndrome: a radiological and clinicopathological study of patients with PTEN germ-line mutations. Eur Radiol. 2006;16(3): 702–6.
50. Daya D, Trus T, D'Souza TJ, Minuk T, Yemen B. Hamartoma of the breast, an underrecognized breast lesion. A clinicopathological and radiographic study of 25 cases. Am J Clin Pathol. 1995;103(6): 685–9.
51. Ibrahim RE, Sciotto CG, Weidner N. Pseudoangiomatous hyperplasia of the mammary stroma. Some observations regarding its clinicopathologic spectrum. Cancer. 1989;63(6):1154–60.

35 Atypical and Malignant Breast Pathology

Çağatay H. Erşahin, Gülbeyaz Ömeroğlu, Yanxia Li, Rasheed Hammadeh, and Atilla Ömeroğlu

Abbreviations

ADH	Atypical ductal hyperplasia
ALH	Atypical lobular hyperplasia
ASCO/CAP	American Society of Clinical Oncology/College of American Pathologists
CMF	Carcinomas with medullary features
DCIS	Ductal carcinoma in situ
DIALH	Ductal involvement by cells of atypical lobular hyperplasia
ER	Estrogen receptor
FEA	Flat epithelial atypia
HER2	Human epidermal growth factor receptor 2
HPF	High-power field
IHC	Immunohistochemistry
IMPC	Invasive micropapillary carcinoma
MC	Mucinous carcinoma
PD	Paget's disease
PLCIS	Pleomorphic lobular carcinoma in situ
PR	Progesterone receptor
PT	Phyllodes tumor
TC	Tubular carcinoma
TDLU	Terminal duct lobular unit

Ç.H. Erşahin, MD, PhD (✉)
Department of Pathology, Silver Cross Hospital,
1900 Silver Cross Blvd., New Lenox, IL 60451, USA
e-mail: cersahi@hotmail.com

G. Ömeroğlu, MD (✉) • A. Ömeroğlu, MD
Department of Pathology, Duff Medical Building,
3575 University Street, Room A5B,
Montreal, QC H3A 2B4, Canada

Department of Pathology,
McGill University Medical Center,
3575 University Street, Room B18,
Montreal, QC H3A 2B4, Canada
e-mail: gulbeyaz.omeroglu-altinel@muhc.mcgill.ca;
atilla.omeroglu@muhc.mcgill.ca

Y. Li, MD, PhD
Department of Pathology,
Loyola University Medical Center,
2160 South 1st Avenue, Maywood, IL 60153, USA
e-mail: yli6@lumc.edu

R. Hammadeh, MD
Department of Pathology, Advocate Christ Hospital
and Medical Center, Oak Lawn, IL, USA
e-mail: rhammadeh@mdpmail.com

Premalignant Diseases of the Breast

Atypical Ductal Hyperplasia

Atypical ductal hyperplasia (ADH) is a proliferative lesion of the breast, which has only some of the features of ductal carcinoma in situ (DCIS). The major clinical significance with ADH is that it portends a four- to fivefold increased relative risk of developing invasive breast carcinoma compared to the general population [1]. The increased risk is from the time of the diagnosis of ADH, with only 10 % of those with ADH developing invasive breast cancer 10–15 years in the future. The difficulty remains that we still do not have any way to differentiate those that will never develop invasive disease from those that

A.I. Riker (ed.), *Breast Disease: Comprehensive Management*,
DOI 10.1007/978-1-4939-1145-5_35, © Springer Science+Business Media New York 2015

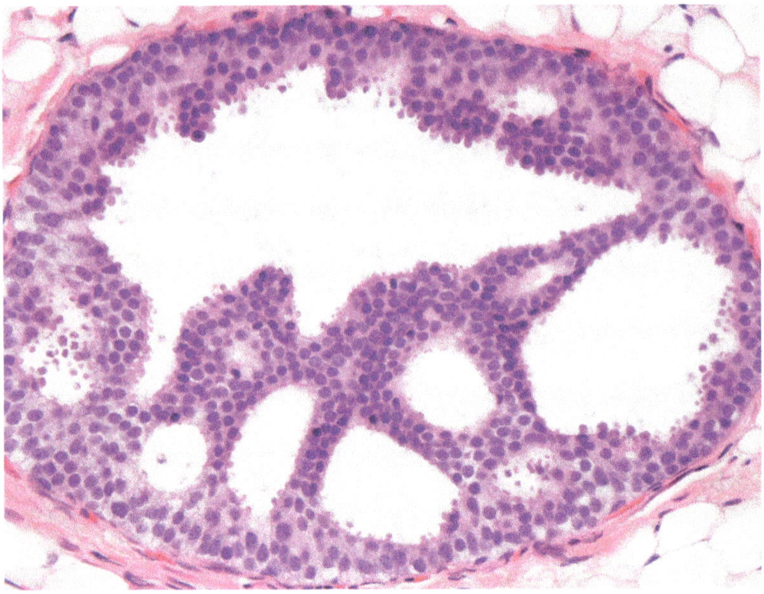

Fig. 35.1 Atypical ductal hyperplasia (*ADH*). The proliferation on the lower side of this lesion has some features of low-grade ductal carcinoma in situ (*DCIS*); however, the upper part of the lesion has features more characteristic of ADH. Overall, a diagnosis of ADH is favored

will. Thus, we must treat all patients with the diagnosis of ADH.

From a pathological perspective, ADH can be considered a lesion with histological characteristics of usual epithelial hyperplasia and those of DCIS. Most areas of ADH are usually smaller than 2 mm in diameter, have a uniform cell population (at least focally), and exhibit architectural features of low-grade DCIS (Fig. 35.1). The quantitative criteria required to diagnose a lesion as ADH or DCIS remain somewhat controversial. Page et al. proposed that low-grade DCIS should be present in at least two separate spaces; therefore, lesions that involve less than two spaces should be considered as ADH [2]. On the other hand, Tavassoli and Norris believe that lesions smaller than 2 mm, with features of low-grade DCIS, should be classified as ADH [1]. Due to such differences in opinion, even the best experts in the field do not always agree on the diagnosis of all proliferative ductal lesions [3].

Molecular studies on ADH have also identified some genetic abnormalities that are similar to low-grade DCIS [4], which supports the view that these lesions are closely related. It is not surprising that immunohistochemical markers, such as cytokeratin 5/6 (CK 5/6), are being used in diagnosing atypical proliferations of the breast. Such markers can be useful in order to differentiate usual non-atypical epithelial hyperplasia from ADH and low-grade DCIS [5]. Most breast pathologists combine qualitative and quantitative criteria for diagnosing atypical proliferations. When in doubt, they favor a diagnosis of ADH over low-grade DCIS and evaluate the lesion further upon complete removal of the area. ADH is frequently present at the periphery of DCIS lesions [6], and due to the reasons mentioned above, biopsy specimens usually underestimate the presence of higher-grade lesions. It has been reported that at least 30–87 % of patients diagnosed with ADH based on a core biopsy will have an occult carcinoma [7–12]. Therefore, complete removal of the lesion with lumpectomy is currently recommended if the core needle biopsy reveals ADH on final pathology [12].

Atypical Lobular Hyperplasia

Atypical lobular hyperplasia (ALH) is always an incidental finding in breast specimens removed for other reasons. It has no grossly identifiable features and usually lacks microcalcifications. ALH is loosely defined as a hyperplasia that has only some features of lobular carcinoma in situ (LCIS); however, this definition is still controversial. Molecularly, ALH can be confirmed with the

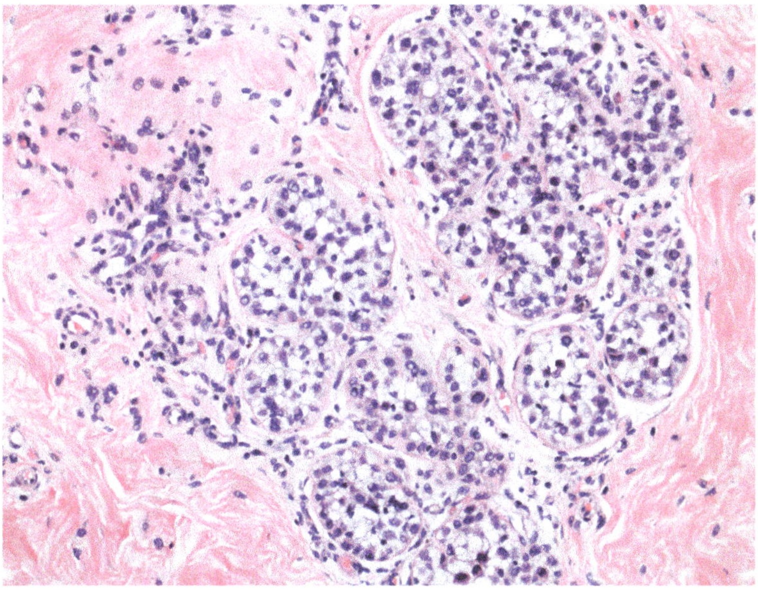

Fig. 35.2 Atypical lobular hyperplasia (*ALH*). ALH shares similar cytologic features with lobular carcinoma in situ and is distinguished by the degree of involvement of lobular structures

absence of E-cadherin expression in tumor cells. Most pathologists use both qualitative and quantitative criteria when making an ALH diagnosis. According to Page et al., less than one half of the spaces in a lobule should be filled with, and distended by, lobular cells in order to make the diagnosis of ALH (Fig. 35.2). Anything more than that should be diagnosed as LCIS [2]. The subsequent risk of developing invasive breast carcinoma once diagnosed with ALH is considered to be four to five times higher than the general population [2]. Previously, lobular neoplasia was considered a risk factor for developing invasive breast cancer in both breasts, which warranted a conservative approach [13]. However, recent studies have shown that invasive carcinoma is more likely to arise in the breast diagnosed with ALH, suggesting that ALH acts more like a premalignant lesion [14]. However, the risk of developing invasive cancer approaches the level of LCIS, with ductal involvement by cells of atypical lobular hyperplasia (DIALH) [15].

The guidelines for the treatment of patients diagnosed with ALH are not clear due to conflicting results in the literature. For instance, the risk of progression to ductal carcinoma in situ and invasive cancer after a core biopsy showing ALH ranges anywhere from 3.1 % to 25 % [16, 17]. The discrepancies in the frequency of worsening diagnoses in different studies may be due to selection criteria in these studies, such as the consideration of various other risk factors within the patient population [17]. The clinical management of ALH is similar to that with ADH, with the current recommendations to completely remove the area with a lumpectomy in most, if not all, cases.

Flat Epithelial Atypia (Columnar Cell Change with Atypia or Columnar Cell Hyperplasia with Atypia)

Flat epithelial atypia (FEA) is characterized by enlarged terminal duct lobular units (TDLU), in which luminal cells are replaced by up to several layers of monomorphic low-grade epithelial cells (Fig. 35.3) [18]. These lesions are *flat* and do not have the same architectural patterns of ADH or DCIS. Cytologically, the epithelial cells are monomorphic, round, and perpendicular to the basement membrane similar to low-grade DCIS [19, 20]. Additionally, columnar cell lesions have been associated with tubular carcinoma and LCIS [21, 22].

Due to its apparent clinical benign nature, FEA was ignored by pathologists for a long time. However, it has gained renewed interest based upon recent observations suggesting that some

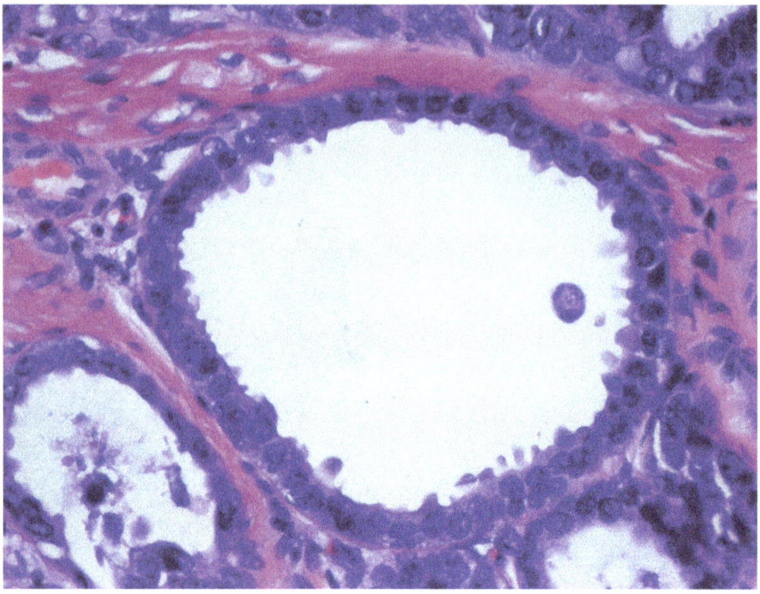

Fig. 35.3 Flat epithelial atypia (*FEA*). A high-power view shows dilated acini with low-grade monomorphic cytologic atypia characteristic of FEA

cases of FEA may progress to invasive breast cancer [23, 24]. For example, one study has shown that there is an approximately twofold increase in breast cancer risk for patients diagnosed with FEA compared to the general population [25]. However, the risk of progression to breast cancer is lower than that of ADH and ALH. Given the limited nature of the data, it is unclear whether the current recommendation for surgical excision following a biopsy diagnosis of FEA is warranted. As a result, radiological-pathological correlation is still recommended in each case [18]. However, many surgeons still recommend complete removal of such areas of FEA, discussing the risks and benefits with each patient.

In Situ Carcinomas

Ductal Carcinoma In Situ

DCIS is a precursor lesion to invasive breast cancer and is defined as a neoplastic proliferation of epithelial cells confined to the ductal lobular unit [18]. Invasive carcinoma, in particular microinvasive carcinoma, ADH, and usual ductal hyperplasia have to be ruled out prior to making the definitive diagnosis of DCIS. Annually, about 14 % of all breast cancers diagnosed in the United States are DCIS, with the risk of death from developing invasive breast cancer after a diagnosis of DCIS very low at about 1–2 % after 10 years [18].

The classification of DCIS can be complex and sometimes problematic [18]. Architecturally, there are five major types of DCIS: cribriform, micropapillary, papillary, solid, and comedo (Fig. 35.4a–c). However, with the newer classification systems, DCIS is divided into only three groups: low grade or grade I (well differentiated or non-high grade without necrosis), intermediate grade or grade II (intermediately differentiated or non-high grade with necrosis), and high grade or grade III (poorly differentiated) [18, 26–28]. Grade I nuclei are defined as large as 1–1.5 red blood cells in diameter with inapparent nucleoli, grade II or intermediate nuclei are 1–2 red blood cells in diameter with coarse chromatin and infrequent nucleoli, and grade III nuclei have >2 red blood cells in diameter with vesicular chromatin and one or two nucleoli [28, 29].

According to the Consensus Conference on the Classification of DCIS, the following features are recommended to be included in the final pathology report: architectural pattern(s), nuclear

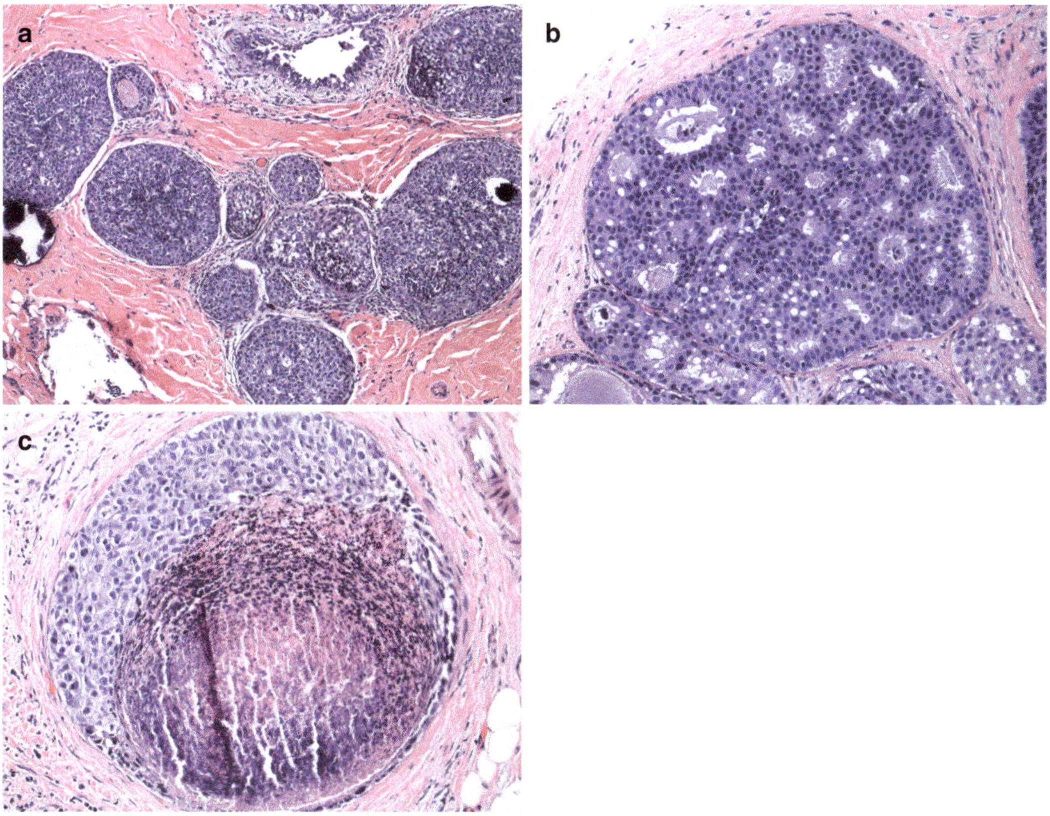

Fig. 35.4 Ductal carcinoma in situ (*DCIS*). DCIS shows different architectural patterns: (**a**) solid type, (**b**) cribriform type, and (**c**) comedo type with necrosis

grade, type of necrosis (punctate or comedo), and cell polarization [30]. Additionally, the size of DCIS, location of calcifications, and margin status should be reported. Reproducibility of DCIS diagnosis is well known; however, using standardized criteria minimizes discrepancies [3]. As mentioned above, in borderline ADH and DCIS cases, ADH diagnosis is usually favored by pathologists based on biopsy specimens. Importantly, 10–15 % of patients with only a DCIS diagnosis have lymph node metastasis, probably due to an unrecognized component of invasive carcinoma. Therefore, analysis of the draining nodal basin with sentinel lymph node biopsy may be considered and discussed with such patients, particularly for patients with extensive high-grade DCIS [31].

Although the clinical validation of biomarkers is not as comprehensive as in invasive breast carcinomas, testing for estrogen receptor (ER) and progesterone receptor (PR) is recommended in DCIS [32, 33]. According to the American Society of Clinical Oncology/College of American Pathologists guideline recommendations, positive result of ER and PR is defined as ≥ 1 % of cells showing nuclear staining by immunohistochemistry [33] (Fig. 35.5).

Ductal Carcinoma In Situ with Microinvasion

Microinvasive carcinoma is described as invasive carcinoma measuring less than or equal to 1 mm, which is most commonly seen in a background of high-grade DCIS (Fig. 35.6). Rarely, it is associated with LCIS, and it can also be present alone [18]. Microinvasive carcinomas are more likely

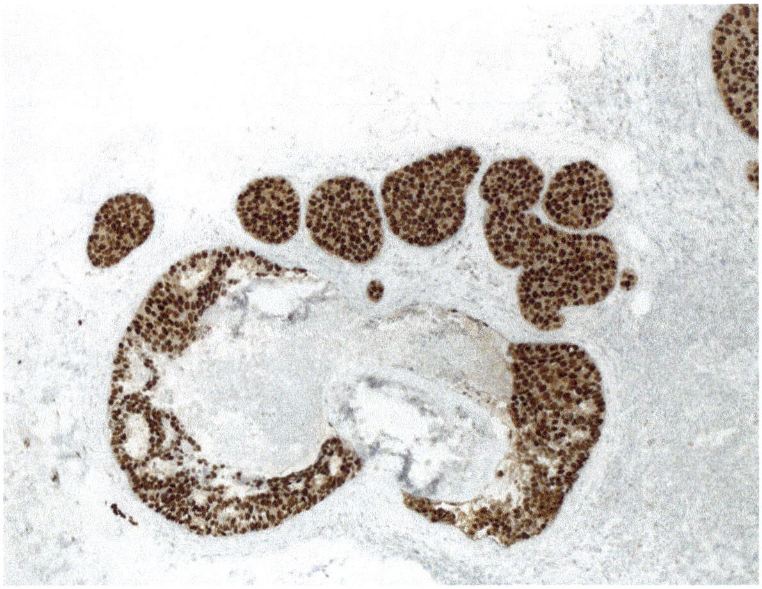

Fig. 35.5 ER (estrogen receptor) staining in ductal carcinoma in situ. Nuclear staining pattern of ER in DCIS

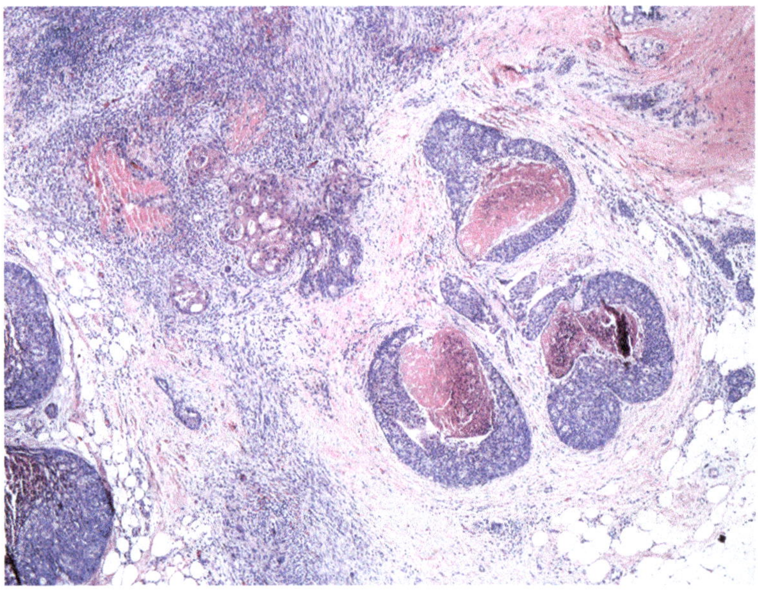

Fig. 35.6 Microinvasive carcinoma. Microinvasive carcinoma is defined by the presence of invasive focus measuring 1 mm or less and is seen next to comedo-type DCIS in the picture

to be multifocal [34]. If there are more than one focus of microinvasive carcinoma, the foci should not be added together to determine the stage of the disease [35]. Microinvasive carcinoma needs to be confirmed by demonstrating the absence of the myoepithelial layer by immunohistochemical staining for p63 and smooth muscle myosin heavy chain, since overdiagnosis is a common problem in classifying these lesions [18].

Biomarkers including ER, PR, and HER2 (ERBB2) can be used for microinvasive carcinomas; however, due to small tumor size, detection of these biomarkers may not be possible for each case. In those instances, biomarkers for DCIS should be reported. If no definitive evidence of invasion is found, a diagnosis of in situ lesion is recommended [18]. Sentinel lymph node biopsy should be performed in patients

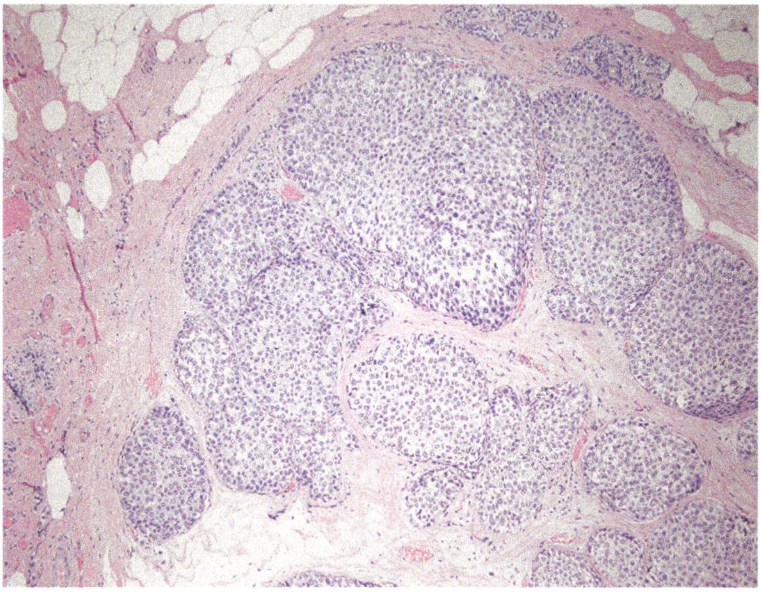

Fig. 35.7 Lobular carcinoma in situ (*LCIS*). The small uniform nuclei fill and distend terminal duct lobular units

with microinvasion, since 10–14 % of these patients exhibit lymph node involvement [18, 36–38]. The prognosis of DCIS with microinvasion is the same with DCIS of equivalent size and grade [18].

Lobular Carcinoma In Situ

Although atypical lobular hyperplasia (ALH) and lobular carcinoma in situ (LCIS) are collectively designated lobular neoplasia [18], the risk of developing invasive breast cancer is nine times higher after LCIS (Fig. 35.7) diagnosis, whereas it is four to five times higher after the diagnosis of ALH [18]. Therefore, we believe that the two entities should remain separate classifications, even though the distinction may be arbitrary as described in Section I.B. The distinction between LCIS and ALH is based on quantitative criteria. According to Page et al., LCIS exhibits that at least half of the acini of a lobular unit are distended by atypical epithelial cells that are E-cadherin negative [2]. According to Rosen, at least 75 % of one lobule should be involved to establish an LCIS diagnosis [18]. Rosen holds that lobular enlargement is not an absolute diagnostic criterion for LCIS, due to lobular atrophy observed in postmenopausal women.

Classic LCIS has monomorphic proliferation of dyscohesive epithelial cells with round nuclei, scant cytoplasm, uniform chromatin, and inconspicuous nucleoli [18]. Particularly, two other variants of LCIS are worthy of mention, as they are being diagnosed more frequently due to screening mammograms, although appropriate management for these LCIS variants is uncertain: (1) classic LCIS with comedo necrosis (Fig. 35.8) and (2) pleomorphic LCIS (Fig. 35.9) with high-grade nuclei, sometimes with apocrine features and comedo necrosis [18]. In fact, there is no consensus regarding the management of patients diagnosed with LCIS via biopsy specimens. In some studies, follow-up surgical excisions revealed infiltrating ductal and/or lobular carcinomas in up to 31 % of cases [16]. The largest retrospective study recently showed that 8.1 % of cases with LCIS diagnosis in biopsy specimens received a higher-stage diagnosis upon follow-up excision [17]. Authors of the latter study stress that excision should be considered on an individual basis, taking into account other parameters including age, previous history of breast carcinoma, and the presence of other high-risk lesions.

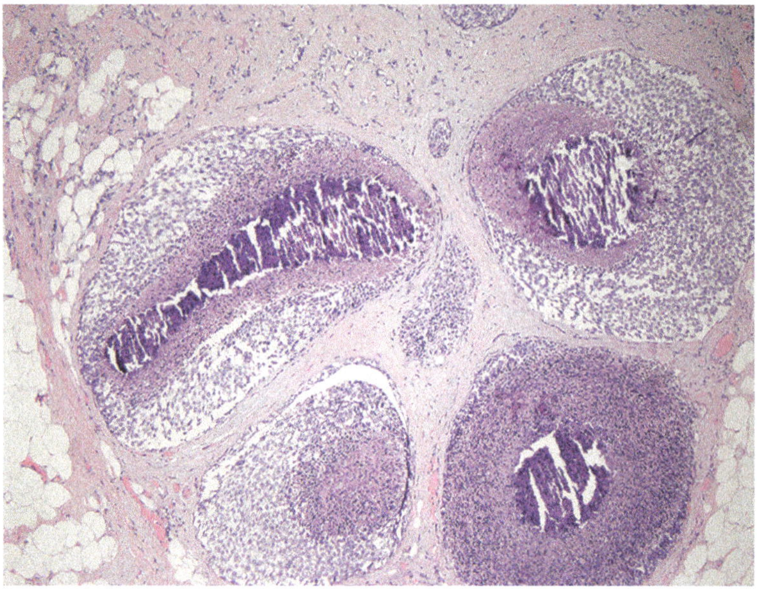

Fig. 35.8 LCIS with comedo-type necrosis mimics ductal carcinoma in situ (DCIS)

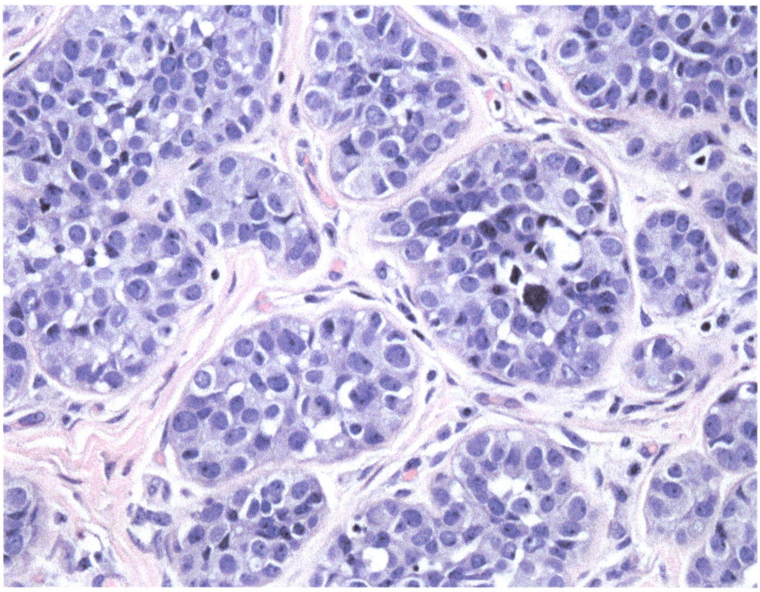

Fig. 35.9 Pleomorphic lobular carcinoma in situ (*PLCIS*). PLCIS is characterized by large cells with marked pleomorphism, abundant cytoplasm, and occasional intracytoplasmic vacuoles. Nuclei are eccentrically located and display conspicuous nucleoli

Histological Classification of Breast Tumors

The WHO classification of the tumors of the breast provides the entire list of breast tumors, including rare types [18]. However, it is beyond the scope of this chapter to cover exceptionally rare types and variants of breast cancer. Instead, we will discuss the most common breast tumors in this chapter. Readers are, therefore, encouraged to refer to classical pathology textbooks for more detailed information about the types of tumors not discussed herein.

Invasive Ductal Carcinoma (Invasive Carcinoma of No Special Type, Ductal Carcinoma NST)

Invasive ductal carcinoma is a default category for the heterogeneous group of tumors that do not show characteristics of a specific histological type,

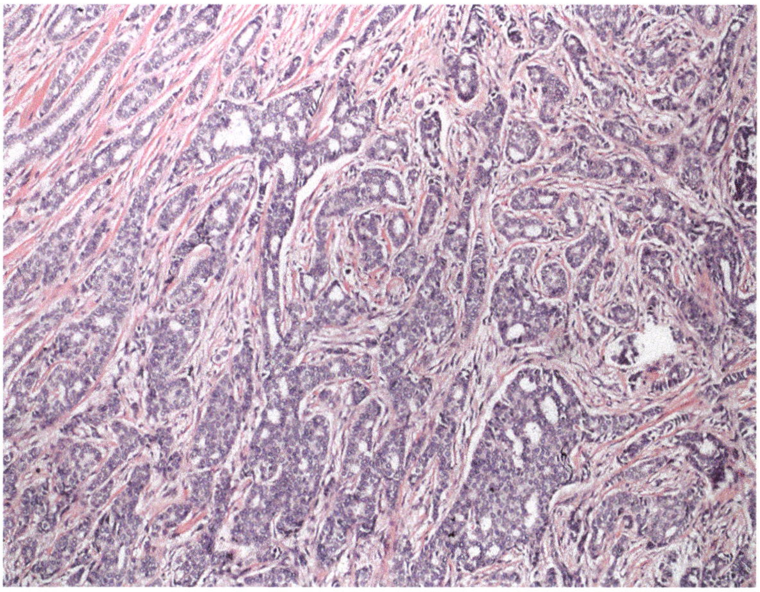

Fig. 35.10 Invasive ductal carcinoma (*IDC*). Low-grade IDC demonstrates tumor cells arranged in trabeculae and cords with diffusely infiltrative pattern

such as mucinous, tubular, or lobular carcinomas [18], and it is the largest group of invasive breast carcinoma (Fig. 35.10), comprising of approximately 40–80 % of all breast tumors [18, 39–41]. Due to tumor cell heterogeneity and differences in grade, microscopic features of invasive ductal carcinomas may vary from case to case. The epithelial component of these tumors may have a glandular architecture, nests, trabecular structures, or solid sheets of tumor tissue in high-grade cancers.

Tissue with clear DCIS features may be entirely separate from the invasive tumor, be incorporated in it, or even dominate it, as up to 80 % of invasive carcinoma cases exhibit a DCIS component [18]. These tumors also can have necrotic foci, minimal to extensive stromal desmoplasia, and lymphoplasmacytic infiltration. Overall, prognosis of invasive carcinoma is influenced by tumor-related factors like histological grade, tumor size, lymph node status, lymphovascular invasion, as well as ER, PR, and HER2 status [18]. Approximately 15–20 % of cases are HER2 positive by gene amplification and/or protein expression [42, 43] and approximately 70–80 % of cases are ER positive [44].

Invasive Lobular Carcinoma

Invasive lobular carcinoma (ILC) represents approximately 5–15 % of all breast cancers (Fig. 35.11) [39, 45–48]. The *classic* variant of invasive lobular carcinoma is a tumor with noncohesive small cells of low nuclear grade in a single-file pattern with less desmoplastic reaction compared to invasive ductal carcinoma [49]. In addition to this classic variant, there are *trabecular*, *alveolar*, and *solid* variants [50, 51]. Another variant mentioned in the WHO classification is tubulolobular carcinoma [18]; however, recent studies suggest that most of these are a variant of ductal/tubular carcinoma [52–54]. Another subtype, pleomorphic lobular carcinoma (PLC; Fig. 35.12), is an aggressive ILC with higher-grade nuclear morphology, mitotic rate, and apocrine differentiation and is associated with pleomorphic lobular carcinoma in situ (PLCIS) in 45 % of cases [55, 56]. The hallmark of ILC is the loss of the cell-cell adhesion molecule and E-cadherin as well as the loss of alpha-, beta-, and gamma-catenin expression [57–59] and the mislocalization of p120 catenin to the cytoplasm [60–62]. A great majority of ILCs are positive for ER and PR and negative for HER2 [18, 63, 64].

Carcinoma of Mixed Type

If more than 50 % of the tumor is a recognized special type, such as lobular, tubular, or mucinous type, and the remainder is a nonspecialized

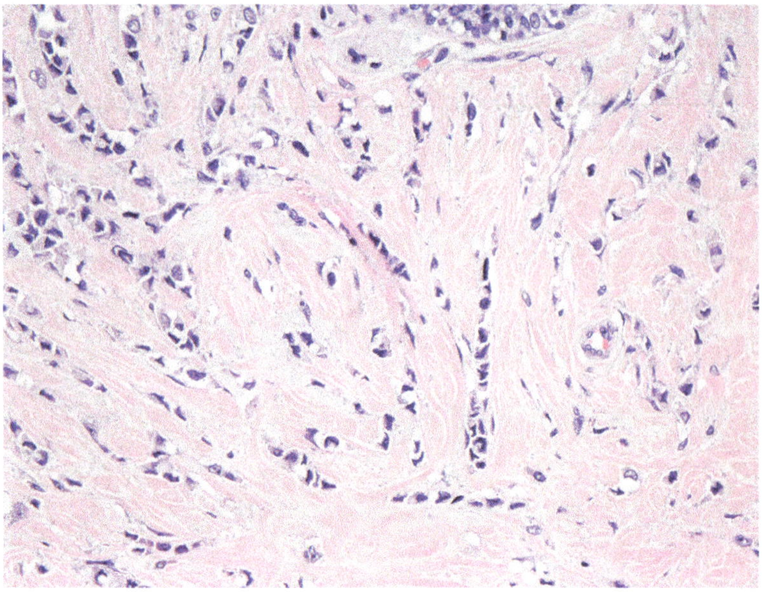

Fig. 35.11 Invasive lobular carcinoma. Tumor cells are small, have relatively uniform nuclei, and invade the stroma in linear strands

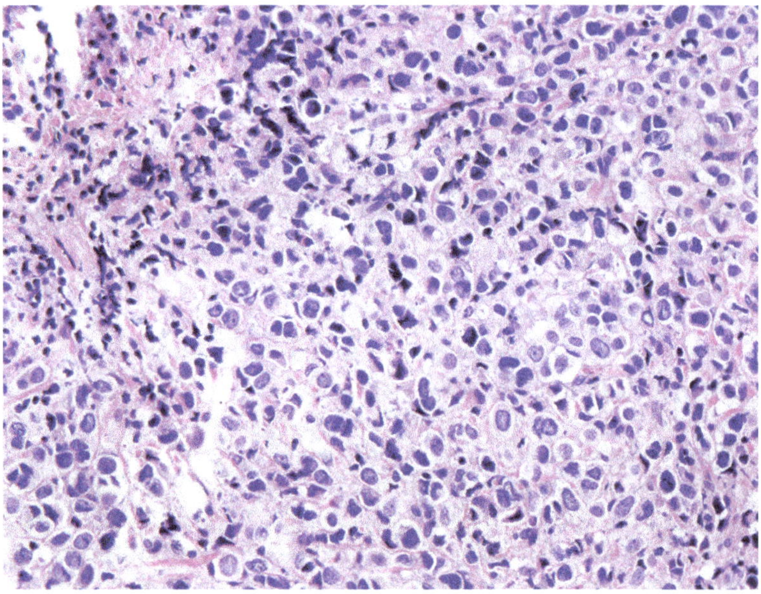

Fig. 35.12 Invasive lobular carcinoma, pleomorphic type with a solid growth pattern

tumor, the tumor is then classified as mixed invasive special type/no special type [18].

Invasive Tubular Carcinoma

Tubular carcinoma (TC) is a special type of invasive breast carcinoma with an excellent prognosis [18, 65]. TC is composed of angulated tubular structures with apical snouts and a cellular desmoplastic stroma (Fig. 35.13). TC may be associated with FEA, low-grade DCIS, and lobular intraepithelial neoplasia [65–67]. TC is almost always positive for ER and PR and negative for HER2 [65, 68].

Mucinous Carcinoma (Colloid Carcinoma)

Mucinous carcinoma (MC) consists of low-grade tumor cells floating in extracellular mucin [18]. Pure MC is associated with a favorable prognosis [69] (Fig. 35.14) and is defined as tumors

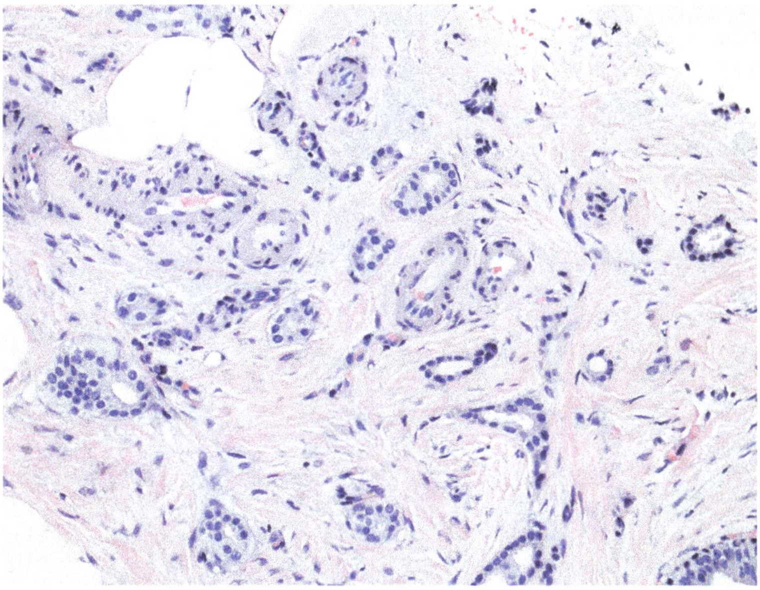

Fig. 35.13 Tubular carcinoma is an extremely well-differentiated carcinoma characterized by well-formed tubules in over 90 % of the lesion

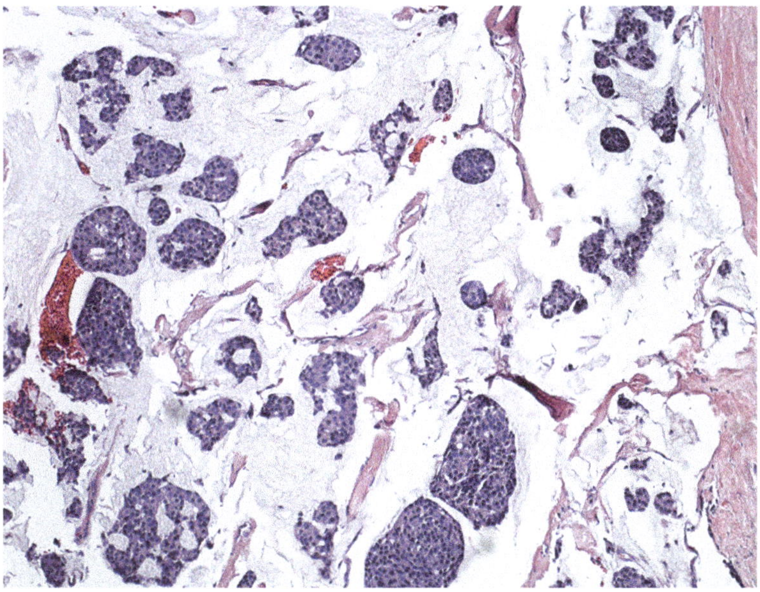

Fig. 35.14 Mucinous carcinoma. Mucinous carcinoma is a well-differentiated carcinoma characterized by the presence of extracellular mucin around the tumor cells in at least 90 % of the tumor

composed of more than 90 % (even close to 100 %, according to some studies) of tumor tissue with characteristic histology [70]. Typically, MCs are positive for ER and PR [69] and negative for HER2 [71].

Carcinomas with Medullary Features

Carcinomas with medullary features (CMF) are a group of breast tumors (Fig. 35.15) including medullary carcinoma, atypical medullary carcinoma, and invasive carcinomas of no special type with similar histological features, such as prominent lymphoid infiltrates pushing borders and high nuclear grade with a syncytial growth pattern [18]. These cancers are grouped together in the latest WHO classification [18] due to poor interobserver reproducibility. The prognosis of medullary carcinoma is unclear, with some studies showing no survival advantage over other types of carcinomas with no special type [39] and others showing favorable long-term prognosis [72]. Similar to basal-like triple-

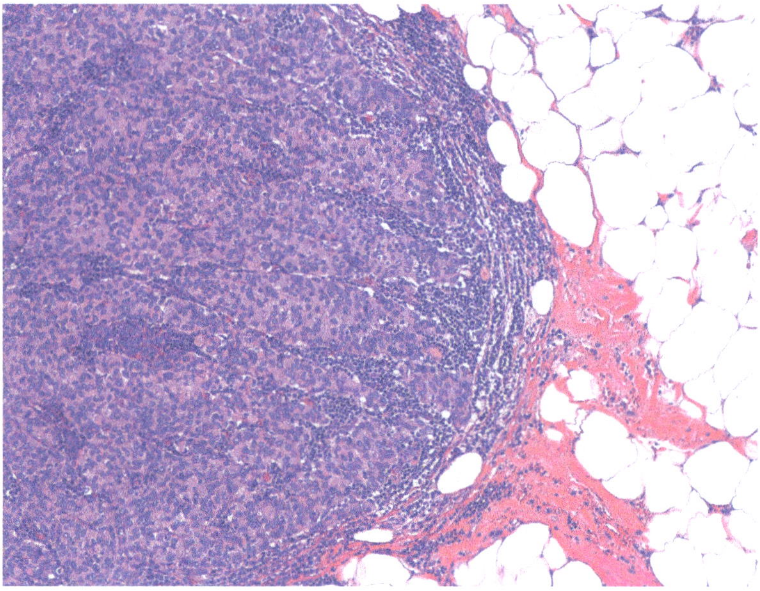

Fig. 35.15 Carcinomas with medullary features are well-circumscribed tumors with high nuclear grade, syncytial growth pattern, and prominent lymphocytic infiltrate

Table 35.1 Characteristics of benign, in situ, and invasive papillary tumors

Tumor type		Myoepithelial cell layer at periphery of involved ducts	Histological characteristics	ER and PR status
Intraductal papilloma	Benign	Present	Benign fibrovascular cores covered by an epithelial and myoepithelial cell layer	Patchy positive
Intraductal papilloma with ADH/DCIS	In situ lesion	Present	Part of the papilloma has features of ADH/DCIS	ADH/DCIS component: diffusely and strongly positive
Intraductal papillary carcinoma	In situ lesion	Present	Papillary DCIS	Diffusely and strongly positive
Encapsulated papillary carcinoma	In situ/ low-grade invasive	Usually not present	Fibrovascular cores covered by neoplastic cells. Absence of myoepithelial cells in the lesion or periphery of the lesion	Diffusely and strongly positive
Solid papillary carcinoma	Invasive	Not present	Expansile, solid growth of tumor with delicate fibrovascular cores and neuroendocrine features	Diffusely and strongly positive for ER/PR and negative for HER2
Invasive papillary carcinoma	Invasive	Not present	Invasive adenocarcinoma with papillary morphology	Not well characterized

negative carcinomas, CMFs are mostly negative for ER, PR, and HER2 (i.e., triple negative) and positive for keratins 5/6 and 14 and EGFR [18].

Intraductal Papillary Lesions and Invasive Papillary Carcinoma

Terminology and accurate diagnosis of papillary lesions of the breast are difficult due to heterogeneous group of lesions. These lesions encompass benign, in situ, and invasive cancers [18] (Table 35.1, Figs. 35.16, 35.17, and 35.18).

Invasive Micropapillary Carcinoma

Invasive micropapillary carcinoma (IMPC) is an aggressive variant of invasive ductal carcinoma (Fig. 35.19) with very frequent lymphovascular

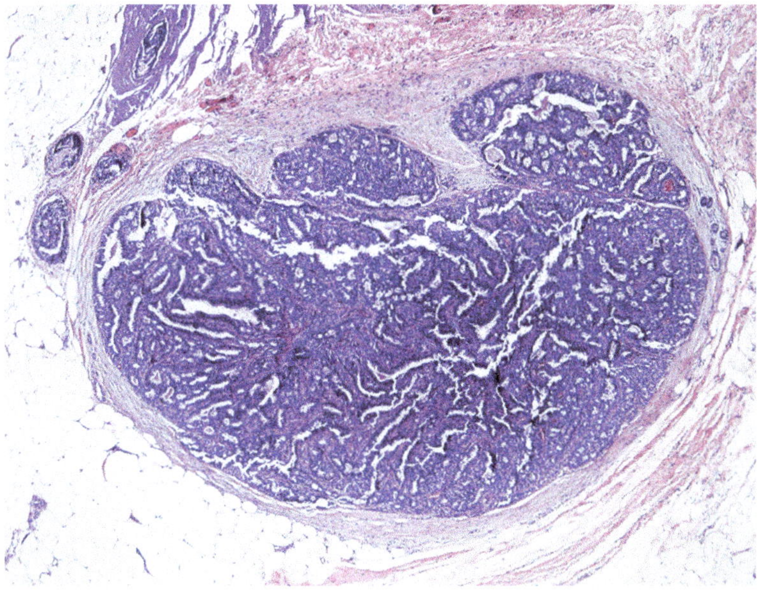

Fig. 35.16 Benign intraductal papilloma. Intraductal papilloma shows well-defined thin fibrovascular cores originating from duct walls lined by myoepithelial and ductal cells. Cytologic atypia is rare

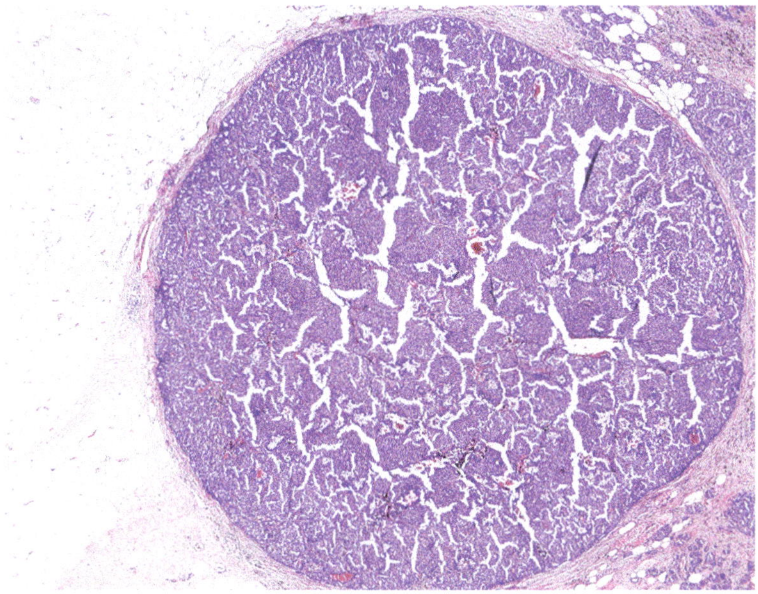

Fig. 35.17 Encapsulated papillary carcinoma. Low-power view shows well-circumscribed lesion with papillary proliferation of uniform neoplastic cells. Myoepithelial cells are absent both in the lesion and periphery of the tumor

invasion and lymph node metastasis [73]. The micropapillary clusters lack fibrovascular cores and have an "inside-out" growth pattern, in which apical cells face the empty stromal spaces rather than the luminal surface [74]. The majority of both pure and mixed micropapillary carcinomas show similar phenotypes, including ER- and PR-positive status and HER2-negative status [75].

Metaplastic Carcinoma

Metaplastic carcinomas (MCs; Fig. 35.20) are a heterogeneous group of tumors with cells differentiated into squamous- and/or mesenchymal-like elements (e.g., spindle, chondroid, osseous, and rhabdomyoid cells) [18, 76–78]. The tumor may be composed of carcinomatous and metaplastic regions or, in some cases, only of

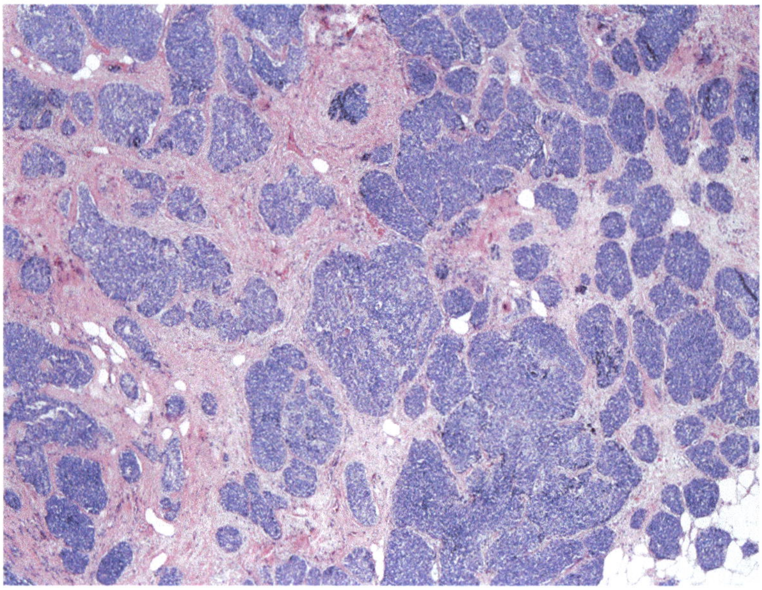

Fig. 35.18 Solid variant of papillary carcinoma. The tumor is composed almost entirely of solid pattern with intermingled fibrovascular network and no apparent papillary structures. The cells are monotonous with a low to intermediate nuclear grade in most of cases

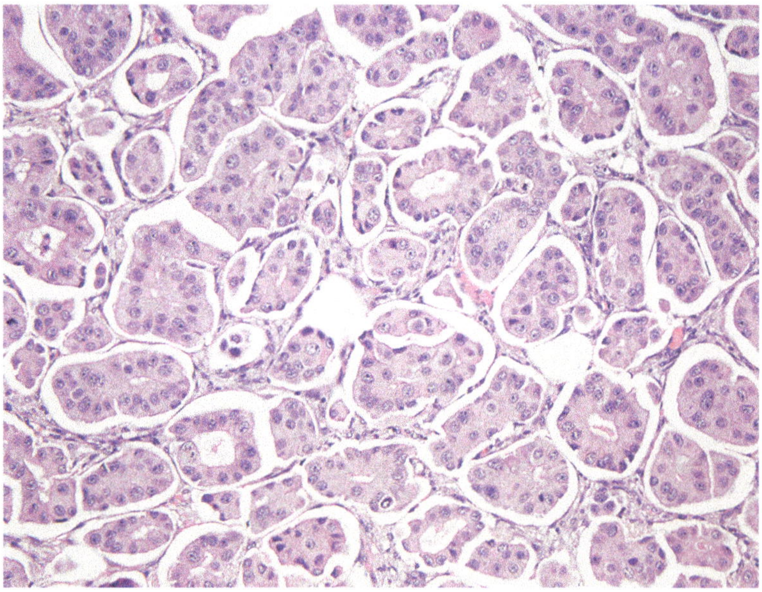

Fig. 35.19 Invasive micropapillary carcinoma. The micropapillary clusters lack fibrovascular cores and apical cells face the empty stromal spaces

metaplastic areas. Variants of this group include low-grade adenosquamous carcinoma, squamous cell carcinoma, spindle cell carcinoma, metaplastic carcinoma with mesenchymal differentiation, and mixed metaplastic carcinomas [18]. Characteristically, metaplastic tumors are ER, PR, and HER2 negative [79]. Overall survival in the metaplastic carcinoma group is worse compared to the poorly differentiated carcinoma group [80].

Phyllodes Tumors

Phyllodes tumors (PT; Fig. 35.21a, b) are included in the general category of fibroepithelial

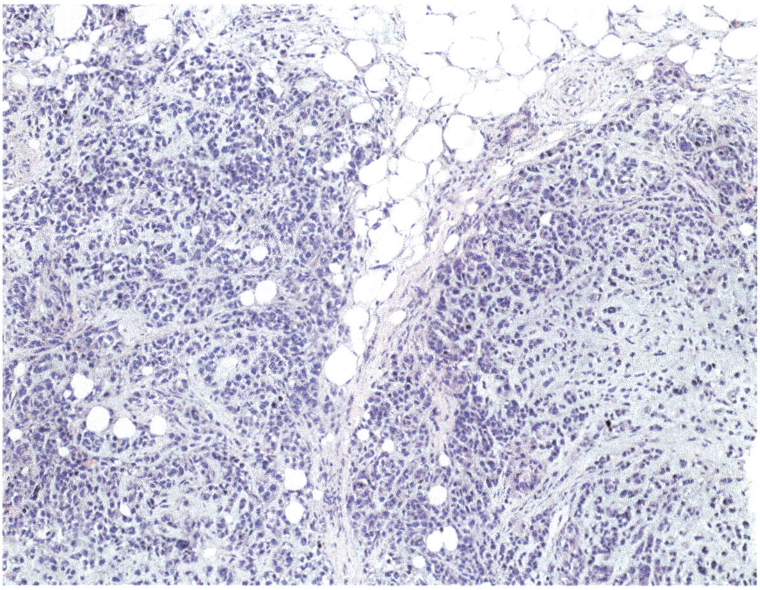

Fig. 35.20 Metaplastic carcinoma. The tumor shows high-grade carcinoma with cartilaginous differentiation

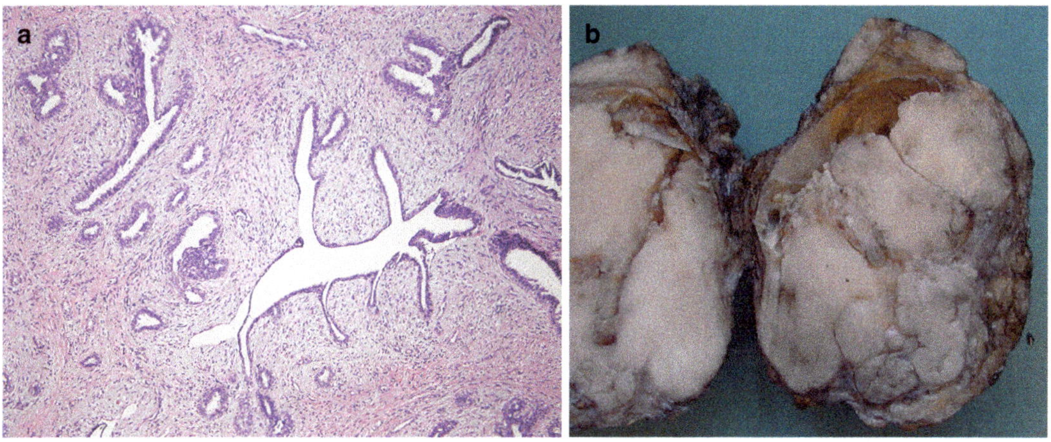

Fig. 35.21 (**a**) Benign phyllodes tumor. This lesion exhibits cleft-like spaces and leaflike projections with a cellular stroma. (**b**) Malignant phyllodes tumor (gross picture)

Table 35.2 WHO classification of phyllodes tumors (PTs)

Histological criteria	Benign PTs	Borderline PTs	Malignant PTs
Tumor borders	Well circumscribed	Generally well circumscribed; may be focally infiltrative	Infiltrative borders
Mitotic activity [81]	<5/10 high-power field (HPF)	5–9/10 HPF	≥10 HPF
Stromal atypia	Not present	Mild to moderate	Severe
Stromal overgrowth	Not present	Focally present	Present

tumors along with fibroadenomas consisting of both epithelial and stromal components [18]. Based on the WHO criteria, PTs are classified into three groups [18] (Table 35.2).

In a recent study, multivariate analysis revealed stromal atypia, stromal overgrowth, and surgical margins to be independently predictive of recurrence [82]. Mitotic activity was also

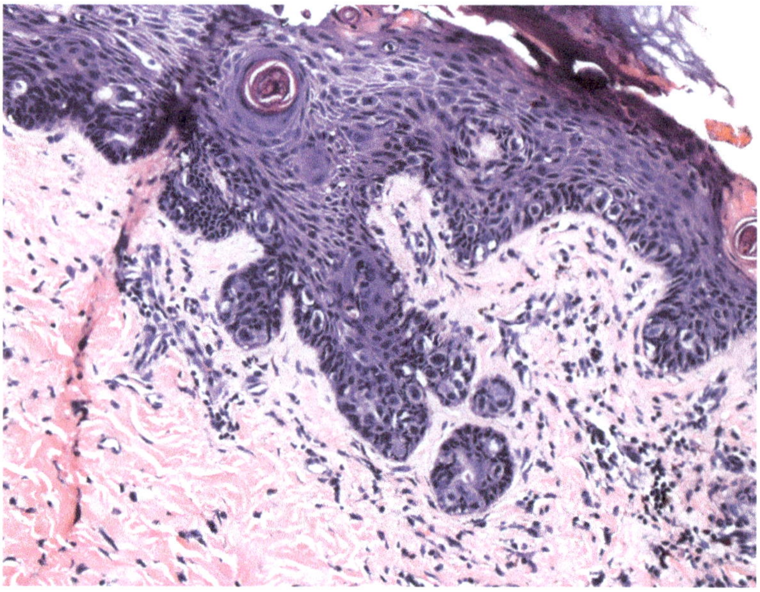

Fig. 35.22 Paget's disease of the nipple. Malignant tumor cells infiltrate epidermis of the nipple in the forms of small nests and single cells

considered important; however, the correlation between recurrence and mitotic activity did not reach statistical significance [82].

Paget's Disease of the Nipple

Paget's disease (PD; Fig. 35.22) is a rare manifestation of breast cancer with Paget cells infiltrating the epidermis of nipple and almost always associated with underlying high-grade invasive ductal carcinoma or ductal carcinoma in situ [18]. Paget cells are malignant cells, which extend from DCIS or invasive cancer into nipple skin. It may be the only manifestation of the disease. Rare cases of PD may not have an underlying invasive or in situ carcinoma [83]. Extensive sampling is recommended to find the underlying disease, since PD prognosis depends on the underlying carcinoma [18].

Mesenchymal Tumors of the Breast

Mesenchymal tumors of the breast are rare and composed of benign, malignant, and tumor-like lesions including nodular fasciitis, benign vascular lesions, pseudoangiomatous stromal hyperplasia, myofibroblastoma, fibromatosis, inflammatory myofibroblastic tumor, lipoma, granular cell tumor and benign peripheral nerve-sheath tumor, angiosarcoma (Fig. 35.23), liposarcoma, rhabdomyosarcoma, osteosarcoma, leiomyoma, and leiomyosarcoma [18].

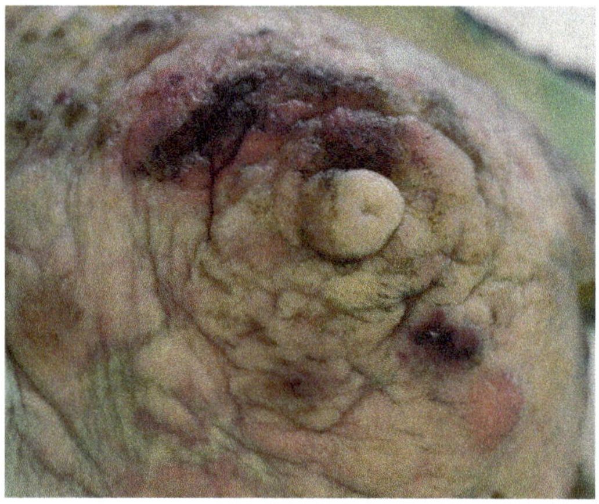

Fig. 35.23 Angiosarcoma, gross appearance. Nipple and surrounding tissue are seen with discoloration reflecting hemorrhage and vascularity of the tumor

Lymphoid and Hematopoietic Tumors of the Breast

Lymphoma may arise in the breast as a primary tumor and include diffuse large B-cell, Burkitt,

Table 35.3 Molecular classification of breast tumors based on immunohistochemistry (IHC)

	Characteristic IHC pattern	Histological grade	Clinical behavior
Luminal A	ER+(strong), HER2−	Often low grade	Overall good prognosis; sensitive to endocrine therapy
Luminal B	ER+(weak/moderate), HER2−	Often higher grade than luminal A	Prognosis poorer than luminal A; tend to respond to endocrine therapy
Basal-like	ER−, PR−, and HER2− (triple negative), CK5+, EGFR+	Often high grade	Poor prognosis; not responsive to endocrine therapy; varying responsiveness to chemotherapy
HER2 positive	ER−, HER2+	Often high grade	Poor prognosis; responsive to anti-HER2 therapy, varying responsiveness to chemotherapy

T-cell, and follicular lymphomas as well as extranodal marginal zone lymphomas of mucosa-associated lymphoid tissue (MALT lymphoma) [18].

Extramammary Malignancies Metastatic to the Breast

Although metastasis to the breast is rare, it must be considered particularly for rare tumor types. Pathologist should be notified regarding the patient's previous cancer history. The most common type of tumor that metastasizes to the breast is melanoma [84]. Some of other types of tumors that spread to the breast include hematological malignancies, lung carcinomas, and ovary, kidney, stomach, and carcinoid tumors, as well as prostate and adrenal cortical carcinomas [84–87]. The prognosis depends on the underlying disease, although it is usually poor [84].

Male Breast Carcinoma

Histological types and prognosis stage by stage of male breast cancers are identical to female breast cancers [18]. Men can present with both in situ and invasive carcinomas.

Molecular Classification of Breast Tumors

Molecular approaches and biomarkers are becoming popular tools to better characterize breast cancers. Perou et al. pioneered the initial molecular taxonomy of breast cancers [88]. Numerous studies have used various molecular techniques, particularly gene expression profiling, to define the molecular classification of breast cancers [89–91]. So far, the molecular subtypes of breast cancers include luminal A, luminal B, HER2-positive, and basal-like types [91]. With the identification of the molecular signature of each individual tumor, researchers hope to shift treatment strategies from a conventional approach to a customized or individualized one, tailored to the specific molecular characteristics of each particular tumor. Immunohistochemistry (IHC) is a reliable surrogate tool for classifying breast cancers according to their gene expression profile classifications (Table 35.3) [92].

Gross Examination of the Breast and Sentinel Lymph Nodes

Gross examination and optimal handling of breast specimens are crucial not only for evaluating tumor size and margins of excision but also for reporting accurate tumor markers such as ER, PR, and HER2 status. According to the American Society of Clinical Oncology/College of American Pathologists (ASCO/CAP) guidelines, specimens should be transported to the pathology laboratory as soon as possible. Specifically, the cold ischemia time (the time from tumor removal to fixation) should be no more than 1 h. In addition, specimens should be fixed in neutral buffered formalin for at least 6 h and no longer than 72 h [93, 94].

In fact, for good practice and optimal results, the entire process should be standardized. The excision specimens must be oriented by the surgeon, using a short suture for the superior margin and a long suture identifying the lateral margin. Lumpectomy specimens are usually inked on six surfaces using six different colors of ink, whereas mastectomy specimens are inked only on their posterior/deep margin. Although there is general agreement to try and achieve negative surgical margins (no tumor at ink), it is not clear what the optimal margin width should be [95, 96]. This definition varies from "tumor not touching the ink" to "1, 2, 5, or even 10 mm of cancer-free margin" [97, 98]. Pathologists may sometimes be consulted on gross evaluation of surgical margins during surgery; however, microscopic evaluation is not encouraged.

Intraoperative evaluation of sentinel lymph nodes has become routine practice. Sentinel lymph node biopsy can be used to detect metastasis via frozen section and/or touch imprint cytology, in which positive results may lead to axillary dissection. The presence of a metastatic tumor and its size should be reported to the surgeon. False-negative rates for frozen section analysis of sentinel lymph nodes for metastatic tumors range from 13 % to 17 % in the literature [95, 96].

Final Surgical Pathology Report

An accurate pathology report is important for patient management. Every pathology report with invasive cancer should include at least the specimen size, cold ischemia time, duration of fixation, tumor size (both invasive and DCIS), histological type and grade, presence of any in situ component, presence or absence of lymphovascular invasion, margin status for any invasive tumor and DCIS, as well as ancillary studies (ER, PR, HER2, and other biomarkers) and cancer staging by the American Joint Committee on Cancer. CAP has published guidelines for reporting common cancers including breast cancer (www.cap.org).

References

1. Tavassoli FA, Norris HJ. A comparison of the results of long-term follow-up for atypical intraductal hyperplasia and intraductal hyperplasia of the breast. Cancer. 1990;65(3):518–29.
2. Page DL, Dupont WD, Rogers LW, Rados MS. Atypical hyperplastic lesions of the female breast. A long-term follow-up study. Cancer. 1985;55(11): 2698–708.
3. Schnitt SJ, Connolly JL, Tavassoli FA, Fechner RE, Kempson RL, Gelman R, et al. Interobserver reproducibility in the diagnosis of ductal proliferative breast lesions using standardized criteria. Am J Surg Pathol. 1992;16(12):1133–43.
4. Simpson PT, Reis-Filho JS, Gale T, Lakhani SR. Molecular evolution of breast cancer. J Pathol. 2005; 205(2):248–54.
5. Otterbach F, Bankfalvi A, Bergner S, Decker T, Krech R, Boecker W. Cytokeratin 5/6 immunohistochemistry assists the differential diagnosis of atypical proliferations of the breast. Histopathology. 2000; 37(3):232–40.
6. Lennington WJ, Jensen RA, Dalton LW, Page DL. Ductal carcinoma in situ of the breast. Heterogeneity of individual lesions. Cancer. 1994; 73(1):118–24.
7. Dahlstrom JE, Sutton S, Jain S. Histological precision of stereotactic core biopsy in diagnosis of malignant and premalignant breast lesions. Histopathology. 1996;28(6):537–41.
8. Jackman RJ, Nowels KW, Rodriguez-Soto J, Marzoni Jr FA, Finkelstein SI, Shepard MJ. Stereotactic, automated, large-core needle biopsy of nonpalpable breast lesions: false-negative and histologic underestimation rates after long-term follow-up. Radiology. 1999;210(3):799–805.
9. Jackman RJ, Nowels KW, Shepard MJ, Finkelstein SI, Marzoni Jr FA. Stereotaxic large-core needle biopsy of 450 nonpalpable breast lesions with surgical correlation in lesions with cancer or atypical hyperplasia. Radiology. 1994;193(1):91–5.
10. Liberman L, Cohen MA, Dershaw DD, Abramson AF, Hann LE, Rosen PP. Atypical ductal hyperplasia diagnosed at stereotaxic core biopsy of breast lesions: an indication for surgical biopsy. AJR Am J Roentgenol. 1995;164(5):1111–3.
11. Moore MM, Hargett 3rd CW, Hanks JB, Fajardo LL, Harvey JA, Frierson Jr HF, et al. Association of breast cancer with the finding of atypical ductal hyperplasia at core breast biopsy. Ann Surg. 1997;225(6):726–31; discussion 31-3.
12. Bassett L, Winchester DP, Caplan RB, Dershaw DD, Dowlatshahi K, Evans 3rd WP, et al. Stereotactic core-needle biopsy of the breast: a report of the Joint Task Force of the American College of Radiology, American College of Surgeons, and College of American Pathologists. CA Cancer J Clin. 1997;47(3): 171–90.

13. Haagensen CD, Lane N, Lattes R, Bodian C. Lobular neoplasia (so-called lobular carcinoma in situ) of the breast. Cancer. 1978;42(2):737–69.
14. Page DL, Schuyler PA, Dupont WD, Jensen RA, Plummer Jr WD, Simpson JF. Atypical lobular hyperplasia as a unilateral predictor of breast cancer risk: a retrospective cohort study. Lancet. 2003; 361(9352):125–9.
15. Page DL, Dupont WD, Rogers LW. Ductal involvement by cells of atypical lobular hyperplasia in the breast: a long-term follow-up study of cancer risk. Hum Pathol. 1988;19(2):201–7.
16. Elsheikh TM, Silverman JF. Follow-up surgical excision is indicated when breast core needle biopsies show atypical lobular hyperplasia or lobular carcinoma in situ: a correlative study of 33 patients with review of the literature. Am J Surg Pathol. 2005;29(4):534–43.
17. Zhao C, Desouki MM, Florea A, Mohammed K, Li X, Dabbs D. Pathologic findings of follow-up surgical excision for lobular neoplasia on breast core biopsy performed for calcification. Am J Clin Pathol. 2012;138(1):72–8.
18. Lakhani SR, Ellis IO, Schnitt SJ, Tan PH, van de Vijver M, editors. Who classification of tumours of the breast. Lyon: IARC Press; 2012.
19. Moinfar F. Flat ductal intraepithelial neoplasia of the breast: evolution of Azzopardi's "clinging" concept. Semin Diagn Pathol. 2010;27(1):37–48.
20. Schnitt SJ. Clinging carcinoma: an American perspective. Semin Diagn Pathol. 2010;27(1):31–6.
21. Abdel-Fatah TM, Powe DG, Hodi Z, Lee AH, Reis-Filho JS, Ellis IO. High frequency of coexistence of columnar cell lesions, lobular neoplasia, and low grade ductal carcinoma in situ with invasive tubular carcinoma and invasive lobular carcinoma. Am J Surg Pathol. 2007;31(3):417–26.
22. Sahoo S, Recant WM. Triad of columnar cell alteration, lobular carcinoma in situ, and tubular carcinoma of the breast. Breast J. 2005;11(2):140–2.
23. Bijker N, Peterse JL, Duchateau L, Julien JP, Fentiman IS, Duval C, et al. Risk factors for recurrence and metastasis after breast-conserving therapy for ductal carcinoma-in-situ: analysis of European Organization for Research and Treatment of Cancer Trial 10853. J Clin Oncol. 2001;19(8):2263–71.
24. Eusebi V, Feudale E, Foschini MP, Micheli A, Conti A, Riva C, et al. Long-term follow-up of in situ carcinoma of the breast. Semin Diagn Pathol. 1994;11(3):223–35.
25. Shaaban AM, Sloane JP, West CR, Moore FR, Jarvis C, Williams EM, et al. Histopathologic types of benign breast lesions and the risk of breast cancer: case-control study. Am J Surg Pathol. 2002;26(4):421–30.
26. Scott MA, Lagios MD, Axelsson K, Rogers LW, Anderson TJ, Page DL. Ductal carcinoma in situ of the breast: reproducibility of histological subtype analysis. Hum Pathol. 1997;28(8):967–73.
27. Holland R, Peterse JL, Millis RR, Eusebi V, Faverly D, van de Vijver MJ, et al. Ductal carcinoma in situ: a proposal for a new classification. Semin Diagn Pathol. 1994;11(3):167–80.
28. Silverstein MJ, Poller DN, Waisman JR, Colburn WJ, Barth A, Gierson ED, et al. Prognostic classification of breast ductal carcinoma-in-situ. Lancet. 1995; 345(8958):1154–7.
29. Lagios MD. Duct carcinoma in situ. Pathology and treatment. Surg Clin North Am. 1990;70(4):853–71.
30. Consensus Conference on the classification of ductal carcinoma in situ. The Consensus Conference Committee. Cancer. 1997;80(9):1798–802.
31. van Deurzen CH, Hobbelink MG, van Hillegersberg R, van Diest PJ. Is there an indication for sentinel node biopsy in patients with ductal carcinoma in situ of the breast? A review. Eur J Cancer. 2007;43(6): 993–1001.
32. Allred DC. Issues and updates: evaluating estrogen receptor-alpha, progesterone receptor, and HER2 in breast cancer. Mod Pathol. 2010;23 Suppl 2:S52–9.
33. Hammond ME, Hayes DF, Dowsett M, Allred DC, Hagerty KL, Badve S, et al. American Society of Clinical Oncology/College of American Pathologists guideline recommendations for immunohistochemical testing of estrogen and progesterone receptors in breast cancer. J Clin Oncol. 2010;28(16):2784–95.
34. Yang M, Moriya T, Oguma M, De La Cruz C, Endoh M, Ishida T, et al. Microinvasive ductal carcinoma (T1mic) of the breast. The clinicopathological profile and immunohistochemical features of 28 cases. Pathol Int. 2003;53(7):422–8.
35. Edge SB, editor. AJCC cancer staging manual. 7th ed. New York: Springer; 2010.
36. Zavotsky J, Hansen N, Brennan MB, Turner RR, Giuliano AE. Lymph node metastasis from ductal carcinoma in situ with microinvasion. Cancer. 1999;85(11):2439–43.
37. Klauber-DeMore N, Tan LK, Liberman L, Kaptain S, Fey J, Borgen P, et al. Sentinel lymph node biopsy: is it indicated in patients with high-risk ductal carcinoma-in-situ and ductal carcinoma-in-situ with microinvasion? Ann Surg Oncol. 2000;7(9): 636–42.
38. Intra M, Zurrida S, Maffini F, Sonzogni A, Trifiro G, Gennari R, et al. Sentinel lymph node metastasis in microinvasive breast cancer. Ann Surg Oncol. 2003;10(10):1160–5.
39. Ellis IO, Galea M, Broughton N, Locker A, Blamey RW, Elston CW. Pathological prognostic factors in breast cancer. II. Histological type. Relationship with survival in a large study with long-term follow-up. Histopathology. 1992;20(6): 479–89.
40. Fisher ER, Gregorio RM, Fisher B, Redmond C, Vellios F, Sommers SC. The pathology of invasive breast cancer. A syllabus derived from findings of the National Surgical Adjuvant Breast Project (protocol no. 4). Cancer. 1975;36(1):1–85.
41. Rosen PP. The pathological classification of human mammary carcinoma: past, present and future. Ann Clin Lab Sci. 1979;9(2):144–56.

42. Yaziji H, Gown AM. Accuracy and precision in HER2/neu testing in breast cancer: are we there yet? Hum Pathol. 2004;35(2):143–6.
43. Owens MA, Horten BC, Da Silva MM. HER2 amplification ratios by fluorescence in situ hybridization and correlation with immunohistochemistry in a cohort of 6556 breast cancer tissues. Clin Breast Cancer. 2004;5(1):63–9.
44. Allred DC, Brown P, Medina D. The origins of estrogen receptor alpha-positive and estrogen receptor alpha-negative human breast cancer. Breast Cancer Res. 2004;6(6):240–5.
45. Li CI, Anderson BO, Daling JR, Moe RE. Trends in incidence rates of invasive lobular and ductal breast carcinoma. JAMA. 2003;289(11):1421–4.
46. Li CI, Uribe DJ, Daling JR. Clinical characteristics of different histologic types of breast cancer. Br J Cancer. 2005;93(9):1046–52.
47. Sastre-Garau X, Jouve M, Asselain B, Vincent-Salomon A, Beuzeboc P, Dorval T, et al. Infiltrating lobular carcinoma of the breast. Clinicopathologic analysis of 975 cases with reference to data on conservative therapy and metastatic patterns. Cancer. 1996;77(1):113–20.
48. Winchester DJ, Chang HR, Graves TA, Menck HR, Bland KI, Winchester DP. A comparative analysis of lobular and ductal carcinoma of the breast: presentation, treatment, and outcomes. J Am Coll Surg. 1998;186(4):416–22.
49. Silverstein MJ, Lewinsky BS, Waisman JR, Gierson ED, Colburn WJ, Senofsky GM, et al. Infiltrating lobular carcinoma. Is it different from infiltrating duct carcinoma? Cancer. 1994;73(6):1673–7.
50. du Toit RS, Locker AP, Ellis IO, Elston CW, Nicholson RI, Blamey RW. Invasive lobular carcinomas of the breast–the prognosis of histopathological subtypes. Br J Cancer. 1989;60(4):605–9.
51. Fechner RE. Histologic variants of infiltrating lobular carcinoma of the breast. Hum Pathol. 1975;6(3): 373–8.
52. Esposito NN, Chivukula M, Dabbs DJ. The ductal phenotypic expression of the E-cadherin/catenin complex in tubulolobular carcinoma of the breast: an immunohistochemical and clinicopathologic study. Mod Pathol. 2007;20(1):130–8.
53. Kuroda H, Tamaru J, Takeuchi I, Ohnisi K, Sakamoto G, Adachi A, et al. Expression of E-cadherin, alpha-catenin, and beta-catenin in tubulolobular carcinoma of the breast. Virchows Arch. 2006;448(4):500–5.
54. Wheeler DT, Tai LH, Bratthauer GL, Waldner DL, Tavassoli FA. Tubulolobular carcinoma of the breast: an analysis of 27 cases of a tumor with a hybrid morphology and immunoprofile. Am J Surg Pathol. 2004;28(12):1587–93.
55. Middleton LP, Palacios DM, Bryant BR, Krebs P, Otis CN, Merino MJ. Pleomorphic lobular carcinoma: morphology, immunohistochemistry, and molecular analysis. Am J Surg Pathol. 2000;24(12):1650–6.
56. Eusebi V, Magalhaes F, Azzopardi JG. Pleomorphic lobular carcinoma of the breast: an aggressive tumor showing apocrine differentiation. Hum Pathol. 1992; 23(6):655–62.
57. De Leeuw WJ, Berx G, Vos CB, Peterse JL, Van de Vijver MJ, Litvinov S, et al. Simultaneous loss of E-cadherin and catenins in invasive lobular breast cancer and lobular carcinoma in situ. J Pathol. 1997;183(4):404–11.
58. Gamallo C, Palacios J, Suarez A, Pizarro A, Navarro P, Quintanilla M, et al. Correlation of E-cadherin expression with differentiation grade and histological type in breast carcinoma. Am J Pathol. 1993;142(4): 987–93.
59. Rasbridge SA, Gillett CE, Sampson SA, Walsh FS, Millis RR. Epithelial (E-) and placental (P-) cadherin cell adhesion molecule expression in breast carcinoma. J Pathol. 1993;169(2):245–50.
60. Dabbs DJ, Bhargava R, Chivukula M. Lobular versus ductal breast neoplasms: the diagnostic utility of p120 catenin. Am J Surg Pathol. 2007;31(3):427–37.
61. Rakha EA, Patel A, Powe DG, Benhasouna A, Green AR, Lambros MB, et al. Clinical and biological significance of E-cadherin protein expression in invasive lobular carcinoma of the breast. Am J Surg Pathol. 2010;34(10):1472–9.
62. Sarrio D, Perez-Mies B, Hardisson D, Moreno-Bueno G, Suarez A, Cano A, et al. Cytoplasmic localization of p120ctn and E-cadherin loss characterize lobular breast carcinoma from preinvasive to metastatic lesions. Oncogene. 2004;23(19):3272–83.
63. Orvieto E, Maiorano E, Bottiglieri L, Maisonneuve P, Rotmensz N, Galimberti V, et al. Clinicopathologic characteristics of invasive lobular carcinoma of the breast: results of an analysis of 530 cases from a single institution. Cancer. 2008;113(7):1511–20.
64. Rakha EA, El-Sayed ME, Menon S, Green AR, Lee AH, Ellis IO. Histologic grading is an independent prognostic factor in invasive lobular carcinoma of the breast. Breast Cancer Res Treat. 2008;111(1):121–7.
65. Rakha EA, Lee AH, Evans AJ, Menon S, Assad NY, Hodi Z, et al. Tubular carcinoma of the breast: further evidence to support its excellent prognosis. J Clin Oncol. 2010;28(1):99–104.
66. Fernandez-Aguilar S, Simon P, Buxant F, Simonart T, Noel JC. Tubular carcinoma of the breast and associated intra-epithelial lesions: a comparative study with invasive low-grade ductal carcinomas. Virchows Arch. 2005;447(4):683–7.
67. Goldstein NS, O'Malley BA. Cancerization of small ectatic ducts of the breast by ductal carcinoma in situ cells with apocrine snouts: a lesion associated with tubular carcinoma. Am J Clin Pathol. 1997;107(5): 561–6.
68. Papadatos G, Rangan AM, Psarianos T, Ung O, Taylor R, Boyages J. Probability of axillary node involvement in patients with tubular carcinoma of the breast. Br J Surg. 2001;88(6):860–4.
69. Barkley CR, Ligibel JA, Wong JS, Lipsitz S, Smith BL, Golshan M. Mucinous breast carcinoma: a large contemporary series. Am J Surg. 2008;196(4): 549–51.

70. Tan PH, Tse GM, Bay BH. Mucinous breast lesions: diagnostic challenges. J Clin Pathol. 2008;61(1): 11–9.
71. Lacroix-Triki M, Suarez PH, MacKay A, Lambros MB, Natrajan R, Savage K, et al. Mucinous carcinoma of the breast is genomically distinct from invasive ductal carcinomas of no special type. J Pathol. 2010;222(3):282–98.
72. Vu-Nishino H, Tavassoli FA, Ahrens WA, Haffty BG. Clinicopathologic features and long-term outcome of patients with medullary breast carcinoma managed with breast-conserving therapy (BCT). Int J Radiat Oncol Biol Phys. 2005;62(4):1040–7.
73. Yu JI, Choi DH, Park W, Huh SJ, Cho EY, Lim YH, et al. Differences in prognostic factors and patterns of failure between invasive micropapillary carcinoma and invasive ductal carcinoma of the breast: matched case-control study. Breast. 2010;19(3):231–7.
74. Luna-More S, Gonzalez B, Acedo C, Rodrigo I, Luna C. Invasive micropapillary carcinoma of the breast. A new special type of invasive mammary carcinoma. Pathol Res Pract. 1994;190(7):668–74.
75. Marchio C, Iravani M, Natrajan R, Lambros MB, Geyer FC, Savage K, et al. Mixed micropapillary-ductal carcinomas of the breast: a genomic and immunohistochemical analysis of morphologically distinct components. J Pathol. 2009;218(3):301–15.
76. Wargotz ES, Deos PH, Norris HJ. Metaplastic carcinomas of the breast. II. Spindle cell carcinoma. Hum Pathol. 1989;20(8):732–40.
77. Wargotz ES, Norris HJ. Metaplastic carcinomas of the breast. III. Carcinosarcoma. Cancer. 1989;64(7):1490–9.
78. Wargotz ES, Norris HJ. Metaplastic carcinomas of the breast. I. Matrix-producing carcinoma. Hum Pathol. 1989;20(7):628–35.
79. Tse GM, Tan PH, Putti TC, Lui PC, Chaiwun B, Law BK. Metaplastic carcinoma of the breast: a clinicopathological review. J Clin Pathol. 2006;59(10): 1079–83.
80. Luini A, Aguilar M, Gatti G, Fasani R, Botteri E, Brito JA, et al. Metaplastic carcinoma of the breast, an unusual disease with worse prognosis: the experience of the European Institute of Oncology and review of the literature. Breast Cancer Res Treat. 2007;101(3):349–53.
81. Tan PH, Jayabaskar T, Chuah KL, Lee HY, Tan Y, Hilmy M, et al. Phyllodes tumors of the breast: the role of pathologic parameters. Am J Clin Pathol. 2005;123(4):529–40.
82. Tan PH, Thike AA, Tan WJ, Thu MM, Busmanis I, Li H, et al. Predicting clinical behaviour of breast phyllodes tumours: a nomogram based on histological criteria and surgical margins. J Clin Pathol. 2012; 65(1):69–76.
83. Caliskan M, Gatti G, Sosnovskikh I, Rotmensz N, Botteri E, Musmeci S, et al. Paget's disease of the breast: the experience of the European Institute of Oncology and review of the literature. Breast Cancer Res Treat. 2008;112(3):513–21.
84. Williams SA, Ehlers 2nd RA, Hunt KK, Yi M, Kuerer HM, Singletary SE, et al. Metastases to the breast from nonbreast solid neoplasms: presentation and determinants of survival. Cancer. 2007;110(4):731–7.
85. Alva S, Shetty-Alva N. An update of tumor metastasis to the breast data. Arch Surg. 1999;134(4):450.
86. Topalovski M, Crisan D, Mattson JC. Lymphoma of the breast. A clinicopathologic study of primary and secondary cases. Arch Pathol Lab Med. 1999;123(12): 1208–18.
87. Gasilionis V, Ersahin C, Gabram S, Bova D, Branch J, Rajan P. Adrenal cortical carcinoma metastatic to the breast. J Clin Pathol. 2006;59(5):546–7.
88. Perou CM, Sorlie T, Eisen MB, van de Rijn M, Jeffrey SS, Rees CA, et al. Molecular portraits of human breast tumours. Nature. 2000;406(6797):747–52.
89. Sorlie T, Perou CM, Tibshirani R, Aas T, Geisler S, Johnsen H, et al. Gene expression patterns of breast carcinomas distinguish tumor subclasses with clinical implications. Proc Natl Acad Sci U S A. 2001;98(19): 10869–74.
90. Sorlie T, Tibshirani R, Parker J, Hastie T, Marron JS, Nobel A, et al. Repeated observation of breast tumor subtypes in independent gene expression data sets. Proc Natl Acad Sci U S A. 2003;100(14):8418–23.
91. Brenton JD, Carey LA, Ahmed AA, Caldas C. Molecular classification and molecular forecasting of breast cancer: ready for clinical application? J Clin Oncol. 2005;23(29):7350–60.
92. Bhargava R, Striebel J, Beriwal S, Flickinger JC, Onisko A, Ahrendt G, et al. Prevalence, morphologic features and proliferation indices of breast carcinoma molecular classes using immunohistochemical surrogate markers. Int J Clin Exp Pathol. 2009;2(5):444–55.
93. Hammond ME, Hayes DF, Dowsett M, Allred DC, Hagerty KL, Badve S, et al. American Society of Clinical Oncology/College of American Pathologists guideline recommendations for immunohistochemical testing of estrogen and progesterone receptors in breast cancer. Arch Pathol Lab Med. 2010;134(6): 907–22.
94. Wolff AC, Hammond ME, Schwartz JN, Hagerty KL, Allred DC, Cote RJ, et al. American Society of Clinical Oncology/College of American Pathologists guideline recommendations for human epidermal growth factor receptor 2 testing in breast cancer. Arch Pathol Lab Med. 2007;131(1):18–43.
95. Schnitt SJ, Morrow M. Should intraoperative frozen section evaluation of breast lumpectomy margins become routine practice? Am J Clin Pathol. 2012;138(5):635–8.
96. Morrow M, Harris JR, Schnitt SJ. Surgical margins in lumpectomy for breast cancer – bigger is not better. N Engl J Med. 2012;367(1):79–82.
97. Hill AD, Tran KN, Akhurst T, Yeung H, Yeh SD, Rosen PP, et al. Lessons learned from 500 cases of lymphatic mapping for breast cancer. Ann Surg. 1999;229(4):528–35.
98. Veronesi U, Paganelli G, Galimberti V, Viale G, Zurrida S, Bedoni M, et al. Sentinel-node biopsy to avoid axillary dissection in breast cancer with clinically negative lymph-nodes. Lancet. 1997;349(9069):1864–7.

Index

A.I. Riker (ed.), *Breast Disease: Comprehensive Management*,
DOI 10.1007/978-1-4939-1145-5, © Springer Science+Business Media New York 2015

B

R

S

CPSIA information can be obtained
at www.ICGtesting.com
Printed in the USA
LVHW06*1853080418
572701LV00004B/485/P

9 781493 911448